Campylobacter

2nd Edition

Campylobacter

2nd Edition

Edited by:

Irving Nachamkin

Department of Pathology and Laboratory Medicine
University of Pennsylvania
Philadelphia, PA 19104-4283

Martin J. Blaser

Division of Infectious Diseases
Vanderbilt University School of Medicine
Nashville, TN 37232-2605

ASM
PRESS

Washington, D.C.

On the cover: Scanning electron micrograph of *Campylobacter jejuni* with eukaryotic cells
(photo courtesy of Michael E. Konkel)

Copyright © 2000   ASM Press
American Society for Microbiology
1752 N Street NW
Washington, DC 20036-2804

Library of Congress Cataloging-in-Publication Data

Campylobacter / edited by Irving Nachamkin, Martin J. Blaser.—2nd ed.
    p. ; cm.
    Rev. ed. of: Campylobacter jejuni. c1992.
    Includes bibliographical references and index.
    ISBN 1-55581-165-5 (alk. paper)
        1. Campylobacter infections.   I. Nachamkin, Irving.   II. Blaser, Martin J.
    [DNLM: 1. Campylobacter—genetics. 2. Campylobacter—pathogenicity. 3.
Campylobacter Infections—Epidemiology. 4. Campylobacter
Infections—physiopathology. 5. Food Contamination—prevention & control. QW 154
C1991 2000]
    QR201.C25 C36 2000
    616′.0145—dc21

                                                                        99-059892

CONTENTS

CONTRIBUTORS

Frank Møller Aarestrup
Danish Veterinary Laboratory, Bülowsvej 27, DK-1790 Copenhagen V, Denmark

Ban Mishu Allos
Department of Medicine, Division of Infectious Diseases, Vanderbilt University School of Medicine, Nashville, TN 37232-2605

Richard Alm
Astra Research Center Boston, 128 Sidney St., Cambridge, MA 02139-4239

Gerald O. Aspinall
Department of Chemistry, York University, North York, Toronto, Ontario M3J 1P3, Canada

Timothy J. Barrett
Foodborne and Diarrheal Diseases Branch, Division of Bacterial and Mycotic Diseases, National Center for Infectious Diseases, Centers for Disease Control and Prevention, 1600 Clifton Road, Mailstop C03, Atlanta, GA 30333

Jeffrey B. Bender
Acute Disease Epidemiology Section, Minnesota Department of Health, 717 Delaware Street SE, Minneapolis, MN 55414

Martin J. Blaser
Division of Infectious Diseases, Vanderbilt University School of Medicine, A3310 MCN, Nashville, TN 37232-2605

Jean-Paul Butzler
WHO Collaborating Center for Enteric Campylobacter, St. Pierre University Hospital, 322 Rue Haute, 1000 Brussels, Belgium

Voon L. Chan
Department of Medical Genetics and Microbiology and Department of Laboratory Medicine and Pathobiology, Medical Sciences Building, University of Toronto, Toronto, Ontario M5S 1A8, Canada

Peter J. Coloe
Department of Applied Biology and Biotechnology, RMIT University, GPO Box 2476V, Melbourne 3001, Australia

B. Duim
Institute for Animal Science and Health (ID-Lelystad), P.O. Box 65, 8200 AB Lelystad, The Netherlands

Jørgen Engberg
Department of Gastrointestinal Infections, Division of Diagnostics, Statens Serum Institute, Artillerivej 5, DK-2300 Copenhagen S, Denmark

James G. Fox
Division of Bioengineering and Environmental Health and Division of Comparative Medicine, Room 16-825, Massachusetts Institute of Technology, Cambridge, MA 02139

C. R. Friedman
Foodborne and Diarrheal Diseases Branch, Centers for Disease Control and Prevention, 1600 Clifton Road, Mailstop A38, Atlanta, GA 30333

J. A. Frost
Campylobacter Reference Unit, Laboratory of Enteric Pathogens, Central Public Health Laboratory, Colindale Avenue, London NW9 5HT, United Kingdom

Benjamin N. Fry
Department of Applied Biology and Biotechnology, RMIT University, GPO Box 2476V, Melbourne 3001, Australia

Patricia Guerry
Enteric Diseases Program, Naval Medical Research Center, National Naval Medical Center, 8901 Wisconsin Ave., Bethesda, MD 20889-5607

Eric Kurt Hani
Department of Microbiology, University of Guelph, Guelph, Ontario N1G 2W1, Canada

Tony W. Ho
Department of Neurology, Johns Hopkins University School of Medicine, Baltimore, MD 21287-7609

Lan Hu
Laboratory of Enteric and Sexually Transmitted Diseases, FDA Center for Biologics Evaluation and Research, Bldg. 29/420, NIH Campus, Bethesda, MD 20892

Wilma Jacobs-Reitsma
ID-Lelystad Institute for Animal Science and Health, P.O. Box 65, 8200 AB Lelystad, The Netherlands

Angela Joe
Department of Microbiology and Immunology, University of Melbourne, Parkville, Victoria 3052, Australia

Lynn A. Joens
Department of Veterinary Science and Department of Microbiology, University of Arizona, Tucson, AZ 85721

Bruce Kaplan
Veterinary Medical Staff Officer, Office of Public Health and Science, Food Safety and Inspection Service, USDA (retired), 4748 Hamlets Grove Drive, Sarasota, FL 34235

Julian M. Ketley
Department of Genetics, University of Leicester, University Road, Leicester LE1 7RH, United Kingdom

Michael E. Konkel
School of Molecular Biosciences, Washington State University, P.O. Box 644233, Pullman, WA 99164-4233

Dennis J. Kopecko
Laboratory of Enteric and Sexually Transmitted Diseases, FDA Center for Biologics Evaluation and Research, Bldg. 29/420, NIH Campus, Bethesda, MD 20892

Victoria Korolik
School of Health Science, Griffith University, Gold Coast, PMB 50, Gold Coast Mail Centre, Queensland, Australia

Albert J. Lastovica
Department of Medical Microbiology, Red Cross Children's Hospital, Rondebosch 7700, and Department of Medical Microbiology, University of Cape Town, Observatory 7925, Cape Town, South Africa

Jennifer Lynett
Department of Laboratory Medicine and Pathobiology, University of Toronto, Toronto, Ontario M5S 1A8, Canada

R. H. Madden
Food Microbiology, DANI/QUB, Agricultural and Food Science Centre, Belfast BT9 5PX, Northern Ireland

Ann Marie McNamara
Sara Lee Foods, Cordova, TN 38108; *formerly* Microbiology Division, Office of Public Health and Science, Food Safety and Inspection Service, USDA, Washington, DC 20250-3700

Richard J. Meinersmann
Poultry Processing and Meat Quality Research Unit, USDA Agricultural Research Service, P.O. Box 5677, Athens, GA 30604

Philip F. Mixter
School of Molecular Biosciences, Washington State University, P.O. Box 644233, Pullman, WA 99164-4233

Anthony P. Moran
Department of Microbiology, National University of Ireland Galway, University Road, Galway, Ireland

Irving Nachamkin
Department of Pathology and Laboratory Medicine, University of Pennsylvania, 3400 Spruce Street, Philadelphia, PA 19104-4283

J. Neimann
Danish Veterinary Laboratory, Danish Zoonosis Centre, Bülowsvej 27, DK-1790 Copenhagen V, Denmark

Diane G. Newell
Veterinary Laboratories Agency (Weybridge), New Haw, Addlestone, Surrey KT15 3NB, United Kingdom

David Ng
Department of Medical Genetics and Microbiology, University of Toronto, Toronto, Ontario M5S 3E2, Canada

Richard A. Oberhelman
Tulane School of Public Health and Tropic Medicine, 1501 Canal Street, New Orleans, LA 70112

Graham M. O'Hanlon
University Department of Neurology, Institute of Neurological Sciences, Southern General Hospital, Glasgow G51 4TF, United Kingdom

Neil J. Oldfield
Department of Genetics, University of Leicester, University Road, Leicester LE1 7RH, United Kingdom

Stephen L. W. On
Danish Veterinary Laboratory, Bülowsvej 27, DK 1790 Copenhagen V, Denmark

Michael T. Osterholm
Acute Disease Epidemiology Section, Minnesota Department of Health, 717 Delaware Street SE, Minneapolis, MN 55414

Simon F. Park
School of Biological Sciences, University of Surrey, Guildford GU2 5XH, United Kingdom

John L. Penner
Department of Medical Genetics and Microbiology, University of Toronto, Toronto, Ontario M5S 1A8, Canada

Carol L. Pickett
Department of Microbiology and Immunology, University of Kentucky, Chandler Medical Center, Lexington, KY 40536

Gerri M. Ransom
Emerging Microbial Issues Branch, Microbiology Division, Office of Public Health and Science, Food Safety and Inspection Service, USDA, Room 3714B Franklin Court Suite, 1400 Independence Avenue, S.W., Washington, DC 20250-3700

David B. Schauer
Division of Bioengineering and Environmental Health and Division of Comparative Medicine, Room 56-787, Massachusetts Institute of Technology, Cambridge, MA 02139

Daniel A. Scott
Enteric Diseases Program, Naval Medical Research Institute, 8901 Wisconsin Avenue, Bethesda, MD 20889-5607

Martin B. Skirrow
Public Health Laboratory, Gloucestershire Royal Hospital, Gloucester GL1 3NN, United Kingdom

Kirk E. Smith
Acute Disease Epidemiology Section, Minnesota Department of Health, 717 Delaware Street SE, Minneapolis, MN 55414

Marina Steele
Department of Pathobiology, University of Guelph, Guelph, Ontario N1G 2W1, Canada

Bala Swaminathan
Foodborne and Diarrheal Diseases Branch, Division of Bacterial and Mycotic Diseases, National Center for Infectious Diseases, Centers for Disease Control and Prevention, 1600 Clifton Road, Mailstop C03, Atlanta, GA 30333

Christine Szymanski
Enteric Diseases Program, Naval Medical Research Center, National Naval Medical Center, 8901 Wisconsin Ave., Bethesda, MD 20889-5607

R. V. Tauxe
Foodborne and Diarrheal Diseases Branch, Centers for Disease Control and Prevention, 1600 Clifton Road, Mailstop A38, Atlanta, GA 30333

David N. Taylor
Department of Enteric Infections, Division of Communicable Diseases and Immunology, Walter Reed Army Institute of Research, Washington, DC 20307-5100

Diane E. Taylor
Departments of Medical Microbiology & Immunology and Biological Sciences, University of Alberta, 128 Medical Sciences Building, Edmonton, Alberta T6G 2H7, Canada

Stuart A. Thompson
Department of Biochemistry and Molecular Biology, Medical College of Georgia, Augusta, GA 30912-2100

David R. Tribble
Enteric Diseases Program, Naval Medical Research Institute, 8901 Wisconsin Avenue, Bethesda, MD 20889-5607

Catharine A. Trieber
Department of Medical Microbiology & Immunology, University of Alberta, 128 Medical Sciences Building, Edmonton, Alberta T6G 2H7, Canada

Trevor J. Trust
Astra Research Center Boston, 128 Sidney St., Cambridge, MA 02139-4239

J. van der Plas
Food Microbiology Department, TNO Nutrition and Food Research Institute, P.O. Box 360, 3700 AJ Zeist, The Netherlands

Peter Vandamme
Laboratorium voor Microbiologie, University of Ghent, Ledeganckstraat 35, B-9000 Ghent, Belgium

I. Kaye Wachsmuth
Office of Public Health and Science, Food Safety and Inspection Service, USDA, Jamie L. Whitten Building, Room 341E, 1400 Independence Avenue, S.W., Washington, DC 20250-3700

Jaap A. Wagenaar
Institute for Animal Science and Health (ID-Lelystad), P.O. Box 65, 8200 AB Lelystad, The Netherlands

Trudy M. Wassenaar
Institute of Medical Microbiology and Hygiene, Johannes Gutenberg University, Hochhaus am Augustusplatz, D-55101 Mainz, Germany

H. C. Wegener
Danish Veterinary Laboratory, Danish Zoonosis Centre, Bülowsvej 27, DK-1790 Copenhagen V, Denmark

Hugh J. Willison
University Department of Neurology, Institute of Neurological Sciences, Southern General Hospital, Glasgow G51 4TF, United Kingdom

Vincent B. Young
Division of Bioengineering and Environmental Health, Room 56-773, Massachusetts Institute of Technology, Cambridge, MA 02139, and Infectious Diseases Unit, Department of Medicine, Massachusetts General Hospital, Boston, MA 02114

PREFACE

In 1991, a symposium on *Campylobacter jejuni,* sponsored by the National Institute of Allergy and Infectious Diseases, was held in Asilomar, California. The purpose of the conference was to bring together the clinicians and scientists most involved in the field to examine the current state of our knowledge and to consider the research needs. From that conference, we, along with Lucy S. Tompkins, edited the predecessor to this book, *Campylobacter jejuni: Current Status and Future Trends.*

We all knew that campylobacters were important pathogens of humans and animals, and since the early 1990s, we have eagerly awaited the public's awareness of these problems. It now is more than eight years since the Asilomar Conference. Research on *Campylobacter* has continued, but the public still has not recognized the medical importance of *Campylobacter.* Clearly, there is a heightened awareness of the need for improved food safety, and the general interest in *Campylobacter* is slowly improving, but not commensurate with the scientific advances.

However, as medical scientists we continued to be fascinated by the campylobacters, both because of their roles in disease and because of their unique biology. Our understanding of the clinical significance of *Campylobacter* infection has increased dramatically with the elucidation of its role as a trigger of the Guillain-Barré syndrome. At the other end of the spectrum, the entire genomic sequence of *Campylobacter jejuni* has been determined, which will permit detailed analysis of the physiology of the organism as well as its interactions with its vertebrate hosts.

In total, we believed that the time was right for a definitive volume that summarizes our current understanding of these organisms. While the major focus remains *C. jejuni,* we have broadened the scope to include related species. We have been fortunate to be joined by our colleagues, leaders in the field, who have contributed their ideas, experiences, and insights. Our goal was to create a state-of-the-art compendium of the knowns and unknowns in the field of "campylobacteriology." It is our hope that this book will aid clinicians, scientists, ecologists, public health workers, and government regulators as they seek solutions to the problems they face. We hope that we will contribute to their providing answers to the important challenges that these organisms pose to society.

Finally, we thank Greg Payne from ASM Press for his foresight and help in making this book a reality, and Ellie Tupper for a superb effort in the production phase of the book. We also thank our families for allowing another love (*Campylobacter*) to intrude on our daily existence.

IRVING NACHAMKIN
MARTIN J. BLASER

FOREWORD

Martin B. Skirrow and Jean-Paul Butzler

So much has happened since campylobacters were identified as a leading cause of acute infective diarrhea that one can hardly believe that it was only 20 years or so ago when the discovery was made. The expansion in our knowledge of these organisms has been phenomenal, although there are many questions still to be answered—hence the reason for this book. We are honored to be asked to write this foreword, with the request that it should include an account of the history of campylobacter infection. In trying to do this we have been selective, concentrating on events that are inherently interesting or instructive. We have always been intrigued by the fact that a bacterial pathogen as common as *Campylobacter jejuni* was overlooked for so long. Indeed, the story has no parallel, but it is an interesting one and it also has a moral.

THE BEGINNINGS

"A discussion of *Vibrio fetus* [*Campylobacter fetus*] can scarcely be limited to the laboratory diagnosis of strains from human infections because to do so would neglect the disease in animals, from which so much can be learned."

So wrote Elizabeth King in 1962 (14). Campylobacters were well known to veterinarians long before they were recognized in human medicine. Indeed, had medical microbiologists paid more attention to the study of comparative pathology, the story might have been very different—and therein lies the moral. Yet there was a point in medical history when campylobacters almost gained a place alongside the classically described enteric bacteria such as *Vibrio cholerae* and shigellae.

At the Third International Campylobacter Workshop held in Ottawa in 1985, Manfred Kist surprised us all with the results of a search of the early German literature (15). He had found a paper, published in 1886, by none other than Theodor Escherich, who described what appear to be typical campylobacters in the colons of infants who had died of what he called "cholera infantum" (Fig. 1) (8). Escherich's attempts to culture these "vibrios" were unsuccessful, and he concluded that their presence was of prognostic rather than causative significance. Other descriptions of spiral bacteria in the gut followed during the ensuing years. Some of these were probably campylobacters, but as all attempts to culture them failed, interest in them waned (15).

THE VETERINARY ERA

How close campylobacters came to being described as enteric pathogens at the end of the 19th century we shall never know. As it turned out, their cultivation and description followed soon afterward but in a very different context. This was the work of a most remarkable man, John McFadyean, who was Principal of the Royal Veterinary College in London and a pioneer veterinary pathologist.

John McFadyean and Stewart Stockman (later to become McFadyean's son-in-law) led

Martin B. Skirrow, Public Health Laboratory, Gloucestershire Royal Hospital, Gloucester GL1 3NN, United Kingdom. *Jean-Paul Butzler,* WHO Collaborating Center for Enteric Campylobacter, St. Pierre University Hospital, 322 Rue Haute, 1000 Brussels, Belgium.

Campylobacter, 2nd Ed., Edited by I. Nachamkin and M. J. Blaser
© 2000 American Society for Microbiology, Washington, D.C.

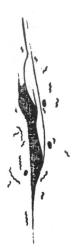

FIGURE 1 Escherich's 1886 drawing of spiral bacteria in the colonic mucus of a child who died of "cholera infantum" (8).

an inquiry set up by the Board of Agriculture and Fisheries to inquire into the causes of epizootic abortion in sheep. This turned out to be a monumental work running for over five lambing seasons and surveying over 250,000 breeding ewes. Much of the work was concerned with *Brucella abortus,* but Part III described abortion due to a "vibrio," first isolated from the uterine mucus of a ewe and the stomach contents of her fetus in February 1906 (18). They went on to describe the microbiology, pathology, and epidemiology of what became known as vibrionic abortion, and from that description it is clear that McFadyean's organism was *Campylobacter fetus*. In 1919, Smith and Taylor, in the United States, described vibrionic abortion in cattle and gave the name *Vibrio fetus* to what was apparently McFadyean's organism (27).

Vibrionic abortion proved to be a major worldwide cause of reproductive loss in cattle and sheep. Later, in 1947, Plastridge et al. in the United States established that there was a cryptic form of the infection transmitted venereally from carrier bulls (21). This infection causes death of the fetus at an early stage and hence apparent infertility in the cow. The work was crucial in that it enabled control to

be effected by excluding carrier bulls from artificial insemination programs. The strains of the "vibrio" causing this infectious infertility were later described by Florent in Belgium in 1959 (9) and accorded subspecies status (now *C. fetus* subsp. *venerealis*).

THE DIARRHEA CONNECTION

The first inkling that campylobacters could cause enteric infection and diarrhea also came from veterinary sources, in the United States. In 1931, Jones et al. isolated a "vibrio" from cattle with "winter dysentery" and from calves with enteritis (10). This work must have entailed singular skill and patience, for they were able to obtain pure cultures, without selective media, by serially diluting material obtained by washing and scraping fragments of jejunal mucosa. The organism they isolated was similar to "*V. fetus*" but antigenically distinct. They named it "*V. jejuni*," and although no cultures survived, the name was retained in current nomenclature as *C. jejuni*. This work was not taken up by others, probably because of technical difficulties and the recognition that much bovine diarrhea is caused by viruses.

A similar circumstance arose in the mid-1940s, when Doyle, also in the United States, isolated another microaerophilic "vibrio" (7), which he thought was the cause of swine dysentery (now know to be caused by *Serpulina hyodysenteriae*). He later called it "*V. coli*," a name likewise retained in modern nomenclature as *C. coli*.

FIRST HUMAN INFECTIONS

Although campylobacters were not generally recognized as fecal pathogens in humans until the late 1970s, occasional isolations of "*V. fetus*" had been obtained from blood or other normally sterile body fluids since 1947, when Vinzent et al. in France isolated the organism from a woman who had suffered septic abortion (30). However, an event that took place in Illinois in May 1938 is now regarded as the first well-documented instance of human campylobacter infection. It was a model investigation of a milk-borne outbreak of diarrhea that affected 355 inmates of two adjacent state institutions (16). Fecal cultures from the 73 victims tested were negative (microscopy was positive in 31), but organisms resembling "*V. jejuni*" were grown in broth cultures of blood samples from 13 victims. Although it was not isolated on solid media, there can be little doubt that the organism was *C. jejuni* (or *C. coli*).

An important milestone was the work of Elizabeth King, whom we quoted earlier. In the late 1950s, she made a systematic study of some 30 bacterial isolates labeled as "*V. fetus*" that had turned up sporadically in blood or other normally sterile body fluids and had been referred to the Center for Disease Control, Atlanta, Ga. (13, 14). She was the first to make the distinction between classical "*V. fetus*" and strains that had the higher optimum growth temperature of 42°C. She recognized the similarity of the latter group to the description by Jones et al. (10) of "*V. jejuni*" and a surviving strain of "*V. coli*" but preferred to give them the provisional name "related vibrio" pending more detailed study. She made three statements about them which perceptively embodied their most medically significant features:

> "The most prominent symptom of this infection in humans is diarrhea."
>
> ". . . chickens . . . are known to have a disease caused by a very similar, if not identical, organism."
>
> ". . . this organism might be more important in childhood diarrhea of unknown etiology than is realized at present. The organism would be exceedingly difficult to isolate from the feces."

Sadly, she died of cancer in 1966, and so she never saw how her "related vibrios" ended up heading the list of enteric pathogens, something that probably far exceeded her expectations.

THE BREAKTHROUGH

That crucial step—the isolation of campylobacters from feces—was accomplished some 10 years later, in 1972, by Dekeyser at the National Institute for Veterinary Research, Brussels, Belgium, in conjunction with Butzler and his team at the St. Pierre University Hospital

(3, 5). It was also accomplished by Slee in Australia at about the same time, but he did not pursue the matter (26).

The initiating event in Butzler's laboratory was the isolation of a "related vibrio" from the blood of a previously healthy young woman with acute febrile hemorrhagic enteritis (5). At that time, fecal samples from patients with diarrhea were routinely preserved by freezing. Thus, after the "vibrio" from her blood had been identified, Butzler had the chance to look for it retrospectively in preserved feces. This is where the help of a veterinary microbiologist proved vital. Butzler turned to Dekeyser, who successfully applied the culture methods (employing selective filtration) used for the isolation of "*V. fetus*" from sheep and cattle with vibrionic abortion (5).

This success led to a more general survey, in which "related vibrios" (*C. jejuni*/*C. coli*) were isolated from 5.3% of 3,000 children with diarrhea but from only 1.6% of 7,200 persons without diarrhea. Evidence that these campylobacters played a causative role was supported by the finding of specific complement-fixing antibodies to the strain of *C. jejuni* isolated from each child with diarrhea and by the excellent clinical response observed in children given erythromycin (2).

Butzler's and Dekeyser's papers (3, 5) inexplicably elicited no response until they were picked up by Skirrow in the United Kingdom several years later (25). Skirrow's first encounter with a campylobacter ("looking impossibly like *Spirillum minus*") was with an organism grown from the blood of a 1-month-old baby with febrile diarrhea. This was an organism that really caught the imagination. A search of the literature turned up Butzler's papers, which were viewed with surprise, and not a little scepticism in view of the absence of any subsequent papers on the subject! However, their potential importance demanded that they be put to the test. Within days, feces were being filtered onto blood agar and isolations were forthcoming from samples from patients with diarrhea.

xx ■ SKIRROW AND BUTZLER

THE OUTCOME

The later development of selective media that obviated the need to filter fecal suspensions brought the isolation of campylobacters into the realm of routine clinical microbiology. From then on, the "balloon went up" in no uncertain manner as the sheer size of the problem of campylobacter diarrhea became apparent. That it was not restricted to the developed world became clear as isolations from Rwanda (6) confirmed an early preliminary report from Zaire by Butzler (1). The year 1979 saw the publication of the first full account of campylobacter enteritis in humans (4).

Those were heady days, exciting but tempered by a lack of basic knowledge. It was truly a daunting experience to be isolating several "related" campylobacters a week without knowing whether *C. jejuni* and *C. coli* were distinct species or, still less, being able to recognize strains or serotypes (very embarrassing when confronted with an outbreak like the Luton one in 1979 [11], although some old-fashioned bacteriology entailing the eyeballing of many plates did achieve something useful on that occasion).

How things have changed! The pioneering studies of John Penner in Toronto (20) and Hermy Lior in Ottawa (17) gave us serotyping schemes of immense value (Canada should be proud). These complimentary schemes, aided by biotyping and phage typing, still form the basis of strain typing, but as this book describes, major advances are being made in genotyping methods. The proliferation of the latter is bewildering, but they will become powerful tools for source tracing and epidemiological studies, provided that standardization can be achieved.

SOURCES OF INFECTION

That there is an urgent need for such tools is clear from the worrying lack of progress in determining the principal sources and modes of transmission of infection and hence strategies for control. Early epidemiological studies at Worcester (25) showed that campylobacter enteritis was a zoonosis and that chickens, both live and dressed, were a prime source of infec-

tion—as King had intimated in 1962 (14). However, a year or two passed before the importance of raw milk and water as vehicles of infection was appreciated. The heralding event, in February 1978, was an outbreak of campylobacter enteritis affecting over 100 people in Somerset, United Kingdom. Power failures caused by a severe blizzard put pasteurizing plants out of action for 2 weeks, so that all distributed milk was raw. This became an all too familiar scenario in the ensuing years (23).

Even more drama attended the first major waterborne outbreak of campylobacter enteritis to be recorded, barely 4 months after the Somerset milk-borne outbreak. The disease struck some 3,000 people in Bennington, Vermont, almost one-fifth of the town's population. This was the first taste of campylobacter enteritis on a grand scale in the United States, and because the disease was not widely known in the country at the time, it took a while to find the cause (31). Faults in municipal water supplies caused similar community outbreaks in Scandinavia.

Despite these spectacular outbreaks, the great majority of campylobacter infections are sporadic single cases or small groups of cases in a single household. The frustrating thing is that we do not know where most of them come from. Chickens are clearly important, but hard data and quantitation on these and other known potential sources are lacking. It is in this area that molecular typing, particularly if used in conjunction with case-control studies, could be so valuable.

NEW CLINICAL PROBLEMS

Once the search for *C. jejuni* and *C. coli* became routine in clinical laboratories, it was not long before other species of *Campylobacter,* such as *C. lari* and *C. upsaliensis,* were discovered. In general, these "other" campylobacter species appear to be of minor clinical significance compared with *C. jejuni* and *C. coli,* although some of them seem to be a significant cause of diarrhea in children in developing countries. This topic is fully discussed in this book.

For a time, campylobacter enteritis due to

C. jejuni and *C. coli* was seen as no more than an unpleasant, temporarily incapacitating illness with fewer serious consequences than those associated with salmonella enteritis. The first hint that there was more to it than this came in 1982 with a report of a patient who developed Guillain-Barré syndrome (GBS) 2 weeks after the onset of campylobacter enteritis (22). The first survey of GBS and campylobacter infection, a retrospective one, was carried out in Australia (12). This study and subsequent prospective studies in the United Kingdom and Japan confirmed the association. It is now clear that campylobacter enteritis is the most frequently identified antecedent event in GBS and that campylobacter-associated GBS patients fare worse than others. Although host factors are undoubtedly important, certain campylobacter strains are particularly associated with this syndrome. Not surprisingly, this has become a topic of intense interest, and it is appropriate that one of the following chapters is devoted to it.

Much work has been done on the pathogenesis of the uncomplicated disease as well as disease complicated by GBS. Over half of this book is given over to molecular biology and the pathogenesis of infection. Perhaps it is a measure of the disparity that exists between the wealth of detail we have on the structure and function of *C. jejuni* and the lack of understanding of how campylobacters actually cause disease.

TAXONOMY

A turning point in the systematic study of this group of bacteria came with the naming of the genus *Campylobacter* by Sebald and Véron in France in 1963 (24). For many years the taxonomic study of campylobacters was fraught with difficulty because we had to rely on phenotypic characters, which are notoriously awkward and difficult to standardize. The advent of molecular and genetic analysis was truly a salvation, and it came in the nick of time to cope with those new and ubiquitous relatives, the helicobacters. The clarity afforded by genetic analysis not only enabled new species to

be neatly categorized but also caused some former campylobacters to be transferred to *Helicobacter* and others to be given a new genus, *Arcobacter* (29). Conversely, *Campylobacter* gained two species from *Wolinella* and one from *Bacteroides*—a fine old shake-up. All are contained in a group called rRNA superfamily VI, which contains the new family *Campylobacteraceae* (28).

SURVEILLANCE

In the United Kingdom, some 6,500 reports of campylobacter isolations were recorded in the first full year of reporting (1978). This has risen steadily to an astonishing 60,000 in 1998. In the early years, the rise was undoubtedly due to increased detection, and this might still be a factor. Even if there is no real increase, the average annual rise of around 10% over the last 5 years is unlikely to represent a decline.

Surveillance in the United States has been more difficult owing to its size and complexity. Passive surveillance figures, for incidence, have remained more or less constant, but active surveillance is needed. We therefore greatly welcome the introduction of FoodNet (Foodborne Diseases Active Surveillance Network), run by the Centers for Disease Control and Prevention, Atlanta, Ga. This active-surveillance scheme should provide a far better picture of campylobacter enteritis in the United States than we have had hitherto.

FINAL REMARKS

As we approach the millennium, the problem of campylobacter enteritis remains undiminished. This is not altogether due to a lack of knowledge of how to control it, although we need to know a lot more. Much of the failure is a lack of will on the part of relevant authorities to take what may sometimes be unpopular action, such as controlling infection in chickens or informing the public on how to handle food correctly. Cost should not be the reason, because the cost of implementing control measures is likely to be far lower than the ultimate cost to society of the unchecked disease (hundreds of millions of dollars per year in the United States alone).

Thus, it was with the aim of increasing the profile of campylobacter infection that a symposium attended by specialist clinicians and scientists was convened in March 1991 in California. The findings were subsequently published by the American Society for Microbiology under the title *Campylobacter jejuni: Current Status and Future Trends* (19). It proved to be one of the most useful publications on the subject of campylobacters ever to appear; many is the time we have cited from it. Thus, we are particularly pleased to be involved with what is, in effect, a progression from that 1992 book. The present book contains accounts of all the aspects of the infection we have mentioned in this foreword and more. We are confident that it will stand as an equally authoritative and valuable source of information as its forerunner.

REFERENCES

1. **Butzler, J.-P.** 1973. Related vibrios in Africa. *Lancet* ii:858. (Letter.)
2. **Butzler, J.-P.** 1974. (Campylobacter, an unrecognized enteropathogen). Ph.D. thesis. Free University of Brussels, Brussels, Belgium. (In Flemish.)
3. **Butzler, J.-P., P. Dekeyser, M. Detrain, and F. Dehaen.** 1973. Related vibrio in stools. *J. Pediatr.* **82**:493–495.
4. **Butzler, J.-P., and M. B. Skirrow.** 1979. Campylobacter enteritis. *Clin. Gastroenterol.* **8**: 737–765.
5. **Dekeyser, P., M. Gossuin-Detrain, J.-P. Butzler, and J. Sternon.** 1972. Acute enteritis due to related vibrio: first positive stool cultures. *J. Infect Dis.* **125**:390–392.
6. **De Mol, P., and E. Bosmans.** 1978. Campylobacter enteritis in central Africa. *Lancet* i:604. (Letter.)
7. **Doyle, L. P.** 1944. A vibrio associated with swine dysentery. *Am. J. Vet. Res.* **5**:3–5.
8. **Escherich, T.** 1886. Articles adding to the knowledge of intestinal bacteria, III. On the existence of vibrios in the intestines and feces of babies. *Münch. Med. Wochenschr.* **33**:815–817. (In German.)
9. **Florent, A.** 1959. Two forms of bovine genital vibriosis: venereal vibriosis due to *V. foetus venerialis,* and vibriosis of intestinal origin due to *V. foetus intestinalis,* p. 953–957. Proceedings of the 16th International Veterinary Congress, Madrid, vol. 2. (In French.)
10. **Jones, F. S., M. Orcutt, and R. B. Little.** 1931. Vibrios (*Vibrio jejuni,* n. sp.) associated with intestinal disorders of cows and calves. *J. Exp. Med.* **53**:853–864.
11. **Jones, P. H., A. T. Willis, D. A. Robinson, M. B. Skirrow, and D. S. Josephs.** 1981. Campylobacter enteritis associated with the consumption of free school milk. *J. Hyg. Camb.* **87**: 155–162.
12. **Kaldor, J., and B. R. Speed.** 1984. Guillain-Barré syndrome and *Campylobacter jejuni:* a serological study. *Br. Med. J.* **288**:1867–1870.
13. **King, E. O.** 1957. Human infections with *Vibrio fetus* and a closely related vibrio. *J. Infect. Dis.* **101**: 119–128.
14. **King, E. O.** 1962. The laboratory recognition of *Vibrio fetus* and a closely related *Vibrio* isolated from cases of human vibriosis. *Ann. N. Y. Acad. Sci.* **98**:700–711.
15. **Kist, M.** 1985. The historical background to campylobacter infection: new aspects, p. 23–27. *In* A. D. Pearson, M. B. Skirrow, H. Lior, and B. Rowe (ed.), *Campylobacter III.* Public Health Laboratory Service, London, United Kingdom.
16. **Levy, A. J.** 1946. A gastro-enteritis outbreak probably due to a bovine strain of vibrio. *Yale J. Biol. Med.* **18**:243–258.
17. **Lior, H., D. L. Woodward, J. A. Edgar, L. J. Roche, and P. Gill.** 1982. Serotyping of *Campylobacter jejuni* by slide agglutination based on heat-labile antigenic factors. *J. Clin. Microbiol.* **15**: 761–768.
18. **McFadyean, J., and S. Stockman.** 1913. *Report of the Departmental Committee appointed by the Board of Agriculture and Fisheries to inquire into Epizootic Abortion. III. Abortion in Sheep.* HMSO, London, United Kingdom.
19. **Nachamkin, I., M. J. Blaser, and L. S. Tompkins (ed.).** 1992. *Campylobacter jejuni: Current Status and Future Trends.* American Society for Microbiology, Washington, D.C.
20. **Penner, J. L., and J. N. Hennessy.** 1980. Passive hemagglutination technique for serotyping *Campylobacter jejuni* subsp. *jejuni* on the basis of heat-stable antigens. *J. Clin. Microbiol.* **12**: 732–737.
21. **Plastridge, W. N., L. F. Williams, and D. Petrie.** 1947. Vibrionic abortion in cattle. *Am. J. Vet. Res.* **8**:178–183.
22. **Rhodes, K. M., and A. E. Tattersfield.** 1982. Guillain-Barré syndrome associated with campylobacter infection. *Br. Med. J.* **285**:173–174.
23. **Robinson, D. A., and D. M. Jones.** 1981. Milk-borne campylobacter infection. *Br. Med. J.* **282**:1374–1376.

24. **Sebald, M., and M. Véron.** 1963. (DNA base content in the classification of vibrios.) *Ann. Inst. Pasteur* **105**:897–910. (In French.)

25. **Skirrow, M. B.** 1977. Campylobacter enteritis: a "new" disease. *Br. Med. J.* **2**:9–11.

26. **Slee, K. J.** 1972. Human vibriosis, an endogenous infection? *Aust. J. Med. Technol.* **3**:7–12.

27. **Smith, T., and M. Taylor.** 1919. Some morphological and biological characters of the spirilla (*Vibrio fetus,* n. sp.) associated with disease of the fetal membranes in cattle. *J. Exp. Med.* **30**:299–311.

28. **Vandamme, P., and J. De Ley.** 1991. Proposal for a new family, *Campylobacteraceae. Int. J. Syst. Bacteriol.* **41**:451–455.

29. **Vandamme, P., E. Falsen, R. Rossau, B. Hoste, P. Segers, R. Tytgat, and J. De Ley.** 1991. Revision of *Campylobacter, Helicobacter,* and *Wolinella* taxonomy: emendation of generic descriptions and proposal of *Arcobacter* gen. nov. *Int. J. Syst. Bacteriol.* **41**:88–103.

30. **Vinzent, R., J. Dumas, and N. Picard.** 1947. (Serious septicemia during pregnancy due to a vibrio, followed by abortion.) *Bull. Acad. Nat. Med.* **131**:90–92. (In French.)

31. **Vogt, R. L., H. E. Sours, T. Barrett, R. A. Feldman, R. J. Dickinson, and L. Witherell.** 1982. Campylobacter enteritis associated with contaminated water. *Ann. Intern. Med.* **96**:292–296.

MICROBIOLOGY OF *CAMPYLOBACTER* INFECTIONS

TAXONOMY OF THE FAMILY
CAMPYLOBACTERACEAE

Peter Vandamme

¦

The taxonomy of *Campylobacter* and related bacteria has undergone drastic changes during the past decade. There are two major reasons for this phenomenon. First, the increased interest in *Campylobacter*-like organisms during the 1980s resulted in the isolation and description of a variety of taxa that could not be assigned unequivocally to one of the existing species. A range of "variants" of established species and a considerable number of novel species had to be inserted in the existing taxonomic framework. Second, like any other science, bacterial taxonomy evolved drastically during this period thanks to the technological progress in molecular biology, biochemistry, and several affiliated disciplines. The general concept of bacterial classification changed too, as a manifold of new data became available.

Whereas previous classification systems were based mainly on morphological and biochemical criteria, present-day classifications are primarily phylogeny based since they are constructed around a backbone derived from similarity studies of highly conserved macromolecules such as rRNA genes. These studies allow us to estimate the divergence between contemporaneous populations of strains, but in the absence of real time units, relationships are expressed in terms of evolutionary changes. The Ad Hoc Committee on Reconciliation of Approaches to Bacterial Systematics (158) stated that taxonomy should be phylogeny based and that the complete genome sequence should therefore be the standard for species delineation. In practice, whole-genome DNA-DNA hybridization studies approach the sequence standard and represent the best applicable procedure at present. A bacterial species was defined as a group of strains (including the type strain) sharing 70% or greater DNA-DNA relatedness with 5°C or less ΔT_m. It was also recommended that phenotypic and chemotaxonomic features should agree with this definition. Preferentially, several simple and straightforward tests should endorse species differentiation based on DNA-DNA hybridization values (137, 158). The integration of all available genotypic, phenotypic, and phylogenetic information into a consensus type of general-purpose classification became the practice of the polyphasic species concept which is now widely accepted (140). The contours of this polyphasic bacterial species are less clear than the ones defined by Wayne et al. (158). Polyphasic classification is empirical, contains elements from both phenetic and phylogenetic classifications, and integrates any significant in-

Peter Vandamme, Laboratorium voor Microbiologie, University of Ghent, Ledeganckstraat 35, B-9000 Ghent, Belgium.

Campylobacter, 2nd Ed., Edited by I. Nachamkin and M. J. Blaser

formation on the organisms. Polyphasic taxonomy is therefore not hindered by conceptual prejudice. Indeed, the more information that can be integrated on a group of organisms, the more likely it is that the outcome will also be a reflection of its biological reality.

It should be underscored that our present view on classification is supposed to reflect the best science of this time. The same was true in the past when only data from morphological and biochemical analyses were available. The technological progress continues and whole-genome sequences of a variety of bacterial organisms, including *Campylobacter jejuni,* are in reach. This is a new "type" of information accessible to microbial taxonomy too. It will be a formidable challenge in the 21st century to use this information to evaluate classifications that have been carefully designed. It is not unlikely that microbial classification will change again when new and better insights are obtained.

TAXONOMIC HISTORY

Discovery and Early History of Campylobacters

In 1886, nonculturable spiral-shaped bacteria were observed and described by Theodor Escherich (31). The reasons why it is very likely that these organisms were campylobacters were summarized by Kist (69): (i) the typical morphology; (ii) the association with enteritis in neonates, infants, and kittins; (iii) the failure to grow on solid medium despite microscopic detection; and (iv) the fact that, to date, no other bacteria with a comparable morphology have been associated with human enteric infections. Bacteria, now known as campylobacters, were probably first successfully isolated at the beginning of this century. In 1913, McFadyean and Stockman isolated *Vibrio*-like bacteria from aborted ovine fetuses (84). Five years later, Smith discovered spiral bacteria in aborted bovine fetuses and concluded that these strains and the vibrios of McFadyean and Stockman belonged to the same species (119), for which he proposed the name *Vibrio fetus* (121). In the

late 1940s, Vinzent and coworkers (153, 154) described *V. fetus* strains isolated from blood cultures from women who aborted. Subsequently, in 1959, Florent (37) showed that two similar vibrios caused fertility problems in cows and ewes. One type of infection affected only cattle and was spread by a symptom-free bull during sexual contact. This condition, in which infected cows failed to become pregnant, was named infectious infertility. A second type of infection caused sporadic abortion but no infertility in cattle and sheep. The organisms causing infectious infertility were named *Vibrio fetus* subsp. *venerealis,* and those causing sporadic abortions were named *Vibrio fetus* subsp. *intestinalis.* The nomenclature of both organisms, nowadays known as *Campylobacter fetus* subsp. *venerealis* and *Campylobacter fetus* subsp. *fetus,* respectively, has been most confusing. A detailed overview of this nomenclatural history was given by Penner (106).

Vibrio jejuni and *Vibrio coli*

In the following decades, several spiral-shaped organisms were detected primarily in veterinary specimens and were gradually classified as *Vibrio* species. In 1927, Smith and Orcutt described another group of *Vibrio*-like bacteria from the feces of cattle with diarrhea (120). Jones and coworkers showed a causal relationship between these microaerophilic vibrios and bovine dysentery and subsequently named the organism *Vibrio jejuni* (62–64). Similar organisms were then detected in blood cultures of humans with gastroenteritis (67, 68, 76) and aborted sheep fetuses (11). In 1944, Doyle isolated yet another vibrio from feces of pigs with diarrhea (25) and classified them as *Vibrio coli* (26).

Vibrio sputorum, Vibrio bubulus, and *Vibrio fecalis*

Bacteria currently classified in one species, *Campylobacter sputorum* (97), were originally described as several different *Vibrio* species. The organism's history starts in 1914, when Tunicliff observed a vibrio, later classified as *Vibrio sputorum* (107), in sputum of a patient with bronchitis (136). Similar bacteria isolated from the bovine vagina and semen were classified *Vibrio bubulus* (36), while strains isolated from normal ovine feces were named *Vibrio fecalis* (35). In 1985, Roop et al. (109) clarified the taxonomic relationships of these bacteria and demonstrated that they all belonged to a single species.

Creation of the Genus *Campylobacter*

Because of their low DNA base composition, their microaerophilic growth requirements, and their nonfermentative metabolism, in 1963 Sebald and Véron (116) transferred *V. fetus* and *V. bubulus* into a new genus, *Campylobacter*. Ten years later, Véron and Chatelain (152) published a more comprehensive study on the taxonomy of the microaerophilic *Vibrio*-like organisms and considered four distinct species in the genus *Campylobacter: Campylobacter fetus* (the type species), *Campylobacter coli, Campylobacter jejuni,* and *Campylobacter sputorum* (the last comprised two subspecies, *C. sputorum* subsp. *sputorum* and *C. sputorum* subsp. *bubulus* to accommodate the organisms described by Prévot [107] and Florent [36], respectively).

Development of Selective Isolation Conditions

A major obstacle to the development of *Campylobacter* research, particularly in human medicine, had been the difficulty encountered in isolating these bacteria. The application of a technique provided by veterinary microbiologists was eventually responsible for a major breakthrough. In the early 1970s, J. P. Butzler and coworkers applied a filtration method, thereby using the small cellular size and the vigorous motily of *Campylobacter* cells to selectively isolate them from stools of humans with diarrhea (12, 20). The main breakthrough, however, was provided a few years later by Skirrow, who described a selective supplement comprising a mixture of vancomycin, polymyxin B, and trimethoprim, that was added to a basal medium (118). This simple isolation procedure thus enabled routine diagnostic mi-

crobiology laboratories to isolate campylobacters and to evaluate their clinical role.

New Campylobacters: the 1980s

The availability of adequate isolation procedures led to a renewed interest in *Campylobacter* research during the early 1980s. As a consequence, manifold *Campylobacter*-like organisms were isolated from a variety of human, animal, and environmental sources, and gradually new species were proposed.

In 1981, novel *Campylobacter* taxa were described for strains isolated from the human oral cavity (*Campylobacter concisus* [131]) and from wounds in the intestines of pigs suffering from intestinal adenomatosis (*C. sputorum* subsp. *mucosalis* [74]).

In 1983, the species *Campylobacter nitrofigilis* was proposed for a group of *Campylobacter*-like organisms isolated from the rhizosphere of *Spartina alterniflora,* a salt marsh plant (82, 83), *Campylobacter hyointestinalis* was proposed for a second group of strains isolated from wounds in the intestines of pigs suffering from intestinal adenomatosis (44), and *Campylobacter laridis* was proposed for thermophilic campylobacters isolated primarily from feces of gulls (*Larus argentus*) (8). The last name was later corrected to *Campylobacter lari* to conform to rules of the International Code for Bacterial Nomenclature (155).

The year 1984 was an important milestone in the history of the genus *Campylobacter* and of human medicine. The name "*Campylobacter pyloridis*" (later corrected to *Campylobacter pylori* [80]) was proposed for a group of human gastric campylobacters (81, 157). The finding that these bacteria were associated with a variety of gastric disorders changed gastroenterology considerably.

Three more names were introduced in 1985 for campylobacters isolated from aborted fetuses of cattle, pigs, and sheep (*Campylobacter cryaerophila* [91]) and for strains isolated from diarrheic stools of homosexual males (*Campylobacter cinaedi* and *Campylobacter fennelliae* [33, 134]). Finally, in 1989, a gastric organism from ferrets, first included in *C. pylori* as a distinct subspecies (41), was elevated to the species level as *Campylobacter mustelae* (42).

CLO Groups

It also became obvious in the early 1980s that the biochemical inertness of these organisms would play a major role in its history. Classical phenotypic tests routinely used for the identification of clinical bacteria often yielded negative or variable results within species. This poor biochemical reactivity and lack of clear-cut differential characters led to the wide application of vernacular names for many groups of *Campylobacter*-like organisms, and the term "*Campylobacter*-like organism" (CLO) became widely used. Some of these CLO groups were later classified as novel species, but several turned out to be biochemical variants of well-known taxa. The terms CLO-1 and CLO-2 campylobacters have rarely been used because they were readily classified as novel species (*C. cinaedi* and *C. fennelliae*, respectively). However, CLO-3 was not formally classified pending the isolation and characterization of additional strains belonging to the same taxon (33, 134) and 15 years later is still known as one of the unnamed *Helicobacter* species. The term "GCLO" was used for gastric *Campylobacter*-like organisms: GCLO-1 strains were classified as *C. pylori*; GCLO-2 and the group of NNC strains (nitrate-negative campylobacters) were shown to represent a distinct subspecies of *C. jejuni*, named *C. jejuni* subsp. *doylei* (128). The name *C. lari* was proposed for the group of NARTC strains (nalidixic acid-resistant thermophilic campylobacters), but later work showed that NASC strains (nalidixic acid-sensitive campylobacters) and UPTC strains (urease-positive thermophilic campylobacters) also belonged to the same species and therefore were to be considered as biochemical variants of *C. lari* (85, 102). Another notorious example is the CNW (catalase negative or weak) campylobacter group. Most CNW strains were shown to represent yet another species, known since the early 1980s (114) but only formally described in 1991: *Campylobacter upsaliensis* (113). These strains were originally isolated from dog and cat feces but were later shown to be important human enteropathogens too. However, some CNW strains represent another biochemical variant of *C. jejuni* subsp. *doylei* (49), and a group of Swiss CNW strains was shown to represent yet another novel species, *Campylobacter helveticus* (125). An overview of these empirical names with their final classification is given in Table 1.

rRNA Homology Studies

In the same period, the study of bacterial phylogeny as imprinted in the degree of rRNA cistron similarity became more popular and was increasingly used to evaluate and revise bacterial classification schemes. Long-standing genera like *Pseudomonas*, *Flavobacterium*, *Bacteroides*, and many others were found to be extremely heterogeneous, and their classification was gradually revised to conform to the new phylogenetic (or "natural") insights. In 1987, Romaniuk et al. and Lau et al. presented the first phylogenetic data on *Campylobacter* species (72, 108). They compared partial 16S rRNA sequences of *C. fetus*, *C. jejuni*, *C. coli*, *C. lari*, *C. sputorum*, and *C. pylori* strains and found that these species formed a previously undescribed bacterial lineage, which was related to other gram-negative bacteria only by very deep branching. *Wolinella succinogenes*, an organism from the bovine rumen (161), belonged to the same phylogenetic lineage, and *C. pylori* was apparently more closely related to *Wolinella* than to the other campylobacters studied. Data on *W. succinogenes* were confirmed by Stackebrandt et al. (123).

One year later, Paster and Dewhirst compared partial 16S rRNA sequences of *C. fetus*, *C. jejuni*, *C. coli*, *C. lari*, *C. concisus*, and *C. pylori* with those of *W. succinogenes*, *Wolinella curva*, *Wolinella recta*, and two oral *Bacteroides* species, *B. gracilis* and *B. ureolyticus* (105). They found a close relationship between *W. curva*, *W. recta*, *B. gracilis*, and *B. ureolyticus* and the so-called "true campylobacters" (i.e., the phylogenetic cluster of *Campylobacter* species containing the type species, *C. fetus*). They also confirmed the close relationship between *W.*

TABLE 1 Overview of *Campylobacter*-like organisms and their present taxonomic designation

Vernacular name	Present affiliation	Reference(s)
CLO-1	*Helicobacter cinaedi*	134
CLO-2	*Helicobacter fennelliae*	134
CLO-3	Unnamed *Helicobacter* sp.	49, 134
CNW	*Campylobacter upsaliensis*	113
	Campylobacter jejuni subsp. *doylei*	49, 128
	Campylobacter helveticus	125
GCLO-1	*Helicobacter pylori*	81
GCLO-2	*Campylobacter jejuni* subsp. *doylei*	128
Ferret GCLO	*Helicobacter mustelae*	38
EF group 22	*Campylobacter concisus*	143
EF group 24	*Helicobacter cinaedi*	144
EF group 25	*Helicobacter cinaedi*	144
NARTC	*Campylobacter lari*	8
NASC	*Campylobacter lari*	102
NNC	*Campylobacter jejuni* subsp. *doylei*	128
UPTC	*Campylobacter lari*	85, 102
Aerotolerant campylobacters	*Arcobacter cryaerophilus* subgroup 1	65, 91, 149
	Arcobacter cryaerophilus subgroup 2	65, 91, 149
	Arcobacter butzleri	65, 91, 149
	Arcobacter skirrowii	91, 149
Free-living *Campylobacter* sp.	*Sulfurospirillum* sp.	70
"*Spirillum* 5175"	*Sulfurospirillum deleyianum*	115, 160

succinogenes and *C. pylori*. The same year, Thompson et al. performed a more comprehensive study of *Campylobacter* taxonomy (133). They compared partial 16S rRNA sequences of 14 *Campylobacter* species and *W. succinogenes*. Their results indicated that *Campylobacter* species belonged to three major phylogenetic clusters: the first cluster contained *C. fetus*, *C. hyointestinalis*, *C. sputorum*, *C. jejuni*, *C. coli*, *C. lari*, *C. upsaliensis*, *C. concisus*, and *C. mucosalis;* the second contained *C. pylori*, *C. fennelliae*, *C. cinaedi*, and *W. succinogenes;* and the third contained *C. nitrofigilis* and *C. cryaerophila*. They concluded that each of these clusters represented a distinct bacterial genus.

Revision of the *Campylobacter* Taxonomy

In 1989, the first step in the revision of *Campylobacter* taxonomy was proposed by Goodwin et al. (47). They summarized genotypic and phenotypic arguments to exclude *C. pylori* from the genera *Campylobacter* and *Wolinella* and proposed a novel genus, *Helicobacter*, to ac-

commodate both *C. pylori* and *C. mustelae*. In 1991, a complete revision of the taxonomy and nomenclature of the genus *Campylobacter* and related bacteria was proposed by Vandamme et al. (145). The results of an extensive DNA-rRNA hybridization study of over 60 strains representing all known *Campylobacter* species, CLO groups, and putative relatives such as *Wolinella*, *Bacteroides* and "*Flexispira*" species corroborated and extended the 16S rRNA sequencing data. *Campylobacter*, together with *Wolinella* and "*Flexispira*" and two generically misnamed *Bacteroides* species, was found to represent a separate, sixth rRNA superfamily sensu De Ley (21) within the group of the gram-negative bacteria. This lineage is now better known as the epsilon subdivision of the *Proteobacteria*. The same although considerably extended three rRNA homology clusters were found. *C. fetus*, *C. hyointestinalis*, *C. concisus*, *C. mucosalis*, *C. sputorum*, *C. jejuni*, *C. coli*, *C. lari*, *C. upsaliensis*, *W. curva*, *W. recta*, *B. gracilis*, and *B. ureolyticus* consitituted the first rRNA homology cluster; *C. nitrofigilis*, *C. cryaerophila*, and several other aerotolerant CLO strains (these strains were later classified as *Arcobacter butzleri* and *Arcobacter skirrowii* [149]) constituted the second rRNA homology cluster, and *H. pylori, H. mustelae, C. cinaedi, C. fennelliae, W. succinogenes,* "*Flexispira rappini,*" and the CLO-3 strain constituted a third rRNA homology cluster. The free-living saprophylic *Campylobacter* strains of Laanbroek et al. (70) and Wolfe and Pfennig (160) (later reclassified as *Sulfurospirillum* species [see below]) belonged to the same phylogenetic lineage but did not belong to one of the three major rRNA homology clusters.

A revised classification, taking into account the phylogenetic results derived from the DNA-rRNA hybridization experiments and published data on the genotype and phenotype of these organisms, was proposed. The genus *Campylobacter* was restricted to species belonging to the rRNA homology cluster containing *C. fetus,* the type species of the genus *Campylobacter.* The generically misnamed *W. curva* and *W. recta* and, in a subsequent study, *B. gracilis* (141) were included in the emended genus *Campylobacter* as *C. curvus, C. rectus,* and *C. gracilis,* respectively. *B. ureolyticus* was obviously a close relative of the emended genus *Campylobacter,* but its taxonomic status was not changed pending further study of this taxon and similar bacteria (141, 145). The name *Arcobacter* (with *A. nitrofigilis* as the type species) was proposed for the organisms belonging to the second rRNA homology cluster. Subsequent studies by Kiehlbauch et al. (65) and Vandamme et al. (149) confirmed the presence of additional taxa in this group of aerotolerant campylobacters, and two additional species were described, *A. butzleri* and *A. skirrowii,* named to honor two pioneers in *Campylobacter* research.

Finally, *C. cinaedi* and *C. fennelliae* were transferred into the genus *Helicobacter* as *H. cinaedi* and *H. fennelliae,* respectively, and an emended genus description was proposed. *Wolinella succinogenes* remained the only species of the genus *Wolinella.*

Proposal of the Family
Campylobacteraceae

The genera *Campylobacter* and *Arcobacter* are phylogenetic neighbors and share several other genotypic and phenotypic features. This close affiliation was reflected in a separate taxonomic and nomenclatural status by the creation of a new bacterial family, the *Campylobacteraceae* (139) (the genera *Helicobacter* and *Wolinella* were recently accommodated in the novel family *Helicobacteraceae* [23]). In addition to the genera *Campylobacter* and *Arcobacter,* the family *Campylobacteraceae* contains the generically misclassified species *Bacteroides ureolyticus* and strains originally described as free-living campylobacters, now known as *Sulfurospirillum* species (115). The phylogenetic tree of the family *Campylobacteraceae* is shown in Fig. 1.

Recent Developments

The cultivation of *H. pylori* from the human gastric mucosa (157) and the demonstration of its relationship to gastritis, peptic ulcer disease, and gastric neoplasia led to renewed interest in the incidence and clinical significance of these microaerophilic bacteria in a variety of hosts. Between 1991 and 1997, a total of 14 novel *Helicobacter* species were added to the 4 species established during the 1980s (*H. pylori, H. cinaedi, H. fennelliae,* and *H. mustelae*): *H. felis* (104), *H. nemestrinae* (10), *H. muridarum* (75), *H. acinonychis* (29), *H. canis* (126), *H. hepaticus* (39), *H. pullorum* (127), *H. pametensis* (24), *H. bilis* (40), *H. bizzozeronii* (52), *H. cholecystus* (43), *H. trogontum* (86), *H. rodentium* (117), and *H. salomonis* (61). A variety of other taxa remain unnamed or have not properly been described, and therefore their names are at present not validated: "*H. westmaedii*" (135), "*H. suncus*" (51), "*F. rappini,*" *Helicobacter* sp. strains bird B and bird C (24), *Helicobacter* sp. strain CLO-3 (134), and *Helicobacter* sp. strain 'Mainz' (59). All of these helicobacters have been isolated from humans and a variety of animal hosts and can be subdivided in a group of gastric species comprising *H. pylori, H. mustelae, H. felis, H. nemestrinae, H. muridarum, H. acino-*

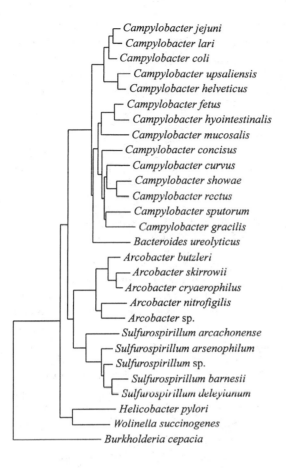

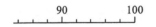

FIGURE 1 Phylogenetic tree of the family *Campylobacteraceae* and its closest phylogenetic neighbors, the genera *Helicobacter* and *Wolinella*, based on the percent 16S rRNA gene sequence similarity. *Burkholderia cepacia* was used as an outgroup organism. The scale represents a 10% sequence dissimilarity. The 16S rRNA gene accession numbers of the strains included are as follows: *C. jejuni*, L04315; *C. lari*, L04316; *C. coli*, L04312; *C. upsaliensis*, L14628; *C. helveticus*, U03022; *C. fetus*, M65012; *C. hyointestinalis*, M65010; *C. mucosalis*, L06978; *C. concisus*, L04322; *C. curvus*, L04313; *C. showae*, L06974; *C. rectus*, L04317; *C. sputorum*, L04319; *C. gracilis*, L04320; *B. ureolyticus*, L04321; *A. butzleri*, L14626; *A. skirrowii*, L14625; *A. cryaerophilus*, L14624; *A. nitrofigilis*, L14627; *Arcobacter* sp., L 42994; *S. arcachonense*, Y11561; *S. arsenophilum*, U85964; *Sulfurospirillum* sp., L 14632; *S. barnesii*, AF038843; *S. deleyianum*, Y13671; *H. pylori*, M88157; *W. succinogenes*, M88159; and *B. cepacia*, M22457.

nychis, *H. bizzozeronii*, and *H. salomonis* and a group of enteric species (all the others). A detailed description of these species is beyond the scope of this present chapter.

GENERAL DESCRIPTION

The Family *Campylobacteraceae*

The genera *Campylobacter*, *Arcobacter*, and *Sulfurospirillum* and the generically misclassified *Bacteroides ureolyticus* form a family of gram-negative, nonsaccharolytic bacteria with microaerobic growth requirements and a low G + C content. This definition is in complete agreement with the original criteria used by Sebald and Véron (116) to separate several *Vibrio* species from the genuine vibrios and to include the former in the new genus *Campylobacter*. Members of the family *Campylobacteraceae* occur primarily as commensals or parasites in humans and domestic animals. The type genus is the genus *Campylobacter* Sebald and Véron 1963.

Members of the family *Campylobacteraceae* have following general characteristics. Cells are curved, S-shaped, or spiral rods that are 0.2 to 0.8 μm wide and 0.5 to 5 μm long. They are gram negative and nonsporeforming. Cells in old cultures may form spherical or coccoid bodies. They are typically motile with a characteristic corkscrew-like motion by means of a single polar unsheathed flagellum at one or both ends of the cell.

Cells grow under microaerobic conditions and have a respiratory and chemoorganotrophic type of metabolism. Some also grow under aerobic or anaerobic conditions. Energy is obtained from amino acids or tricarboxylic acid cycle intermediates, not carbohydrates. Carbohydrates are neither fermented nor oxidized. The optimum growth temperature is 30 to 37°C. Typical biochemical characteristics are reduction of fumarate to succinate; negative methyl red reaction and acetoin and indole production; and for most species, reduction of nitrate, absence of hippurate hydrolysis, and presence of oxidase activity.

Menaquinones are the only respiratory quinones detected, with menaquinone-6 (three different structural types) and menaquinone-5 being the major components (16, 88, 89, 141). rRNA genes (16S as well as 23S) of some strains comprise internal transcribed spacers or intervening sequences. The presence of these internal transcribed spacers is strain specific, not species specific. The DNA base ratio ranges between 27 and 47 mol%.

The Genus *Campylobacter*

GENERAL CHARACTERISTICS

Campylobacter cells are mostly slender, spirally curved rods, 0.2 to 0.8 μm wide and 0.5 to 5 μm long. Cells of some species are predominantly curved or straight rods. Cells in old cultures may form coccoid bodies which are considered degenerative forms rather than a dormant stage of the organism (56). Cells of most species are motile with a characteristic corkscrew-like motion by means of a single polar unsheathed flagellum at one or both ends. Cells of some species are nonmotile (*C. gracilis*) or have multiple flagella (*C. showae*).

In general, biochemical characteristics are as described for the family *Campylobacteraceae*. Several species require anaerobiosis for optimal growth or require fumarate with formate or hydrogen for growth under microaerobic conditions. Gelatin, casein, starch, and tyrosine are not hydrolyzed. Oxidase activity is present in all species except *C. gracilis*. There is no lipase or lecithinase activity. Some species are pathogenic for humans and animals. They are found in the reproductive organs, intestinal tract, and oral cavity of man and animals. The G + C content of the DNA ranges from 29 to 47 mol%. At present, there are 14 validly described *Campylobacter* species, with *Campylobacter fetus* (Smith and Taylor 1919) Sebald and Véron 1963 being the type species.

There is no simple "gold standard" for the routine isolation of all *Campylobacter* species. Simultaneous application of a microaerobic atmosphere containing hydrogen with a filtration method and a selective base is methodologically the optimal solution. However, the predominant species in human infection can be readily grown under a microaerobic atmosphere on selective media without the necessity to use hydrogen. To evaluate the presence of other, less common species, appropriate culture conditions must be applied.

Menaquinone-6 (2-methyl-3-farnesyl-farnesyl-1,4-naphthoquinone) and a methyl-substituted menaquinone-6 (2,[5 or 8]-dimethyl-3-farnesyl-farnesyl-1, 4-naphthoquinone) have been reported as the major respiratory quinones in *Campylobacter* species.

LIST OF THE SPECIES OF THE GENUS *CAMPYLOBACTER*

C. fetus. As described above, *C. fetus* was most probably the first campylobacter isolated. There are two subspecies, *C. fetus* subsp. *fetus* and *C. fetus* subsp. *venerealis,* both of which are considered primary pathogens. *C. fetus* subsp. *fetus* causes abortion in sheep and sporadic abortion in cattle, as well as a sporadic infections in humans. It can be isolated from the placentas and stomach contents of fetuses from aborted sheep and cattle and from the blood, intestinal contents, and bile of infected ewes and cattle. In addition, in humans it is sporadically isolated from blood, spinal fluid, aborted fetuses, and abscesses from most parts of the body. *C. fetus* subsp. *venerealis* causes abortion and infertility in cattle and can be isolated from the vaginal mucus of infected cows, the semen and prepuce of bulls, and the placenta and tissues of aborted bovine fetuses.

Although both subspecies are associated with distinct diseases in animals, their differentiation is not straightforward. Classical biochemical tests useful for the differentiation of these taxa are tolerance to glycine and the ability to produce hydrogen sulfide. Whole-cell protein electrophoresis does not separate the taxa (147). Salama et al. (112) reported the genomes of *C. fetus* subsp. *fetus* strains to be smaller (1.1 Mb) than those of *C. fetus* subsp. *venerealis* strains (1.3 to 1.5 Mb). General differences between the *Sma*I-based macrorestriction profiles of the two subspecies have also been noted (57). A PCR-based assay designed for species and subspecies identification was 98% specific (57).

C. hyointestinalis. *C. hyointestinalis* was originally isolated from pigs with intestinal disorders (44, 45). Subsequent studies identified these organisms in a variety of sources including the intestines of pigs and hamsters, the stomachs of pigs, and cattle, deer, and human feces. There are two subspecies: *C. hyointestinalis* subsp. *hyointestinalis* and *C. hyointestinalis* subsp. *lawsonii.* The former has been isolated from the intestines of pigs and hamsters and from cattle, deer, and human feces; it may be associated with porcine proliferative enteritis and diarrhea in animals and humans, but its pathogenic role is unclear. The latter has been isolated from the stomach of pigs. Its clinical significance is unknown.

When grown on common blood agar bases, only some *C. hyointestinalis* strains grow microaerobically without hydrogen (all strains grow microaerobically in the presence of hydrogen). Whole-cell protein electrophoresis has revealed considerable diversity within this species, and it has been suggested that this offers potential for typing studies (98, 146, 147).

C. sputorum. The taxonomic history of *C. sputorum* is complex and confusing. Strains isolated from the human oral cavity and the genital tract of bulls, initially classified as *Vibrio sputorum* and *Vibrio bubulus,* were later believed to be related at the subspecies level on the basis of their extensive biochemical similarities and named *C. sputorum* subsp. *sputorum* and *C. sputorum* subsp. *bubulus* (152), respectively. In addition, Firehammer described a "fecal-type" vibrio isolated from sheep that differed mainly from *V. bubulus* by the production of large amounts of catalase (35); he proposed the name *Vibrio fecalis.* Subsequent DNA homology studies (109) revealed a high level of DNA-DNA relatedness between *C. sputorum* subsp. *sputorum,* *C. sputorum* subsp. *bubulus,* and *V. fecalis* and also indicated that *C. sputorum* subsp. *mucosalis* (see below) represented a distinct species.

Limited biochemical variation between these taxa had been noted (catalase production and growth on 3.5% NaCl and 1.0% ox-bile media), and therefore Roop et al. (109) proposed that these taxa be referred to as source-specific biovars of *C. sputorum* (*C. sputorum* bv. sputorum, *C. sputorum* bv. bubulus, and *C. sputorum* bv. fecalis). Subsequent studies by On et al. (97, 99) questioned the legitimacy of *C. sputorum* bv. bubulus as a distinct taxon because the results of tests used to distinguish this taxon from other biovars were found to be poorly reproducible. The recent identification of urease-positive variants of *C. sputorum* isolated from cattle feces (3) resulted in the proposal of a new biovar structure, defined by reactions in two simple and reproducible tests: catalase and urease. Strains of *C. sputorum* bv. sputorum produce neither catalase nor urease. They are found in the oral cavity, feces (normal and diarrheic), and abscesses and other skin lesions of humans; the genital tract of bulls; sheep abortions; and the feces of sheep and pigs. Their pathogenicity unknown. Strains of *C. sputorum* bv. faecalis (the biovar epithet was recently corrected to conform to the rules of bacterial nomenclature [142]) produce catalase but not urease. They have been isolated from the feces of sheep and cattle, and their pathogenicity unknown. Finally, strains of *C. sputorum* bv. paraureolyticus produce urease but not catalase. Strains are isolated from the feces of cattle and from humans with diarrhea; their pathogenicity is unknown.

C. mucosalis. The name *C. sputorum* subsp. *mucosalis* was originally proposed for a group of strains thought to be a causal agent of proliferative enteritis in pigs (74). However, subsequent studies have identified *Lawsonia intracellularis* as the principal pathogen in this disease, and DNA-DNA hybridization and 16S rRNA sequence analysis demonstrated that this organism represents a distinct *Campylobacter* species (110, 133).

C. mucosalis strains do not grow microaerobically on common agar bases in an atmosphere without hydrogen. Three distinct serovars, A,

B, and C, which were shown to have strikingly distinct whole-cell protein patterns (17, 147), have been described (74). *C. mucosalis* strains have been isolated from the intestinal mucosa of pigs with porcine intestinal adenamatosis, necrotic enteritis, regional ileitis, and proliferative hemorrhagic enteropathy and from the porcine oral cavity. Their clinical significance is unknown. Human infections supposedly caused by this organism were shown to be misidentified *C. concisus* infections (94).

C. concisus and C. curvus. Tanner et al. (130, 131) described two groups of strains isolated from gingival crevices of persons with gingivitis, periodontitis, and periodontosis, which were named *C. concisus* and *C. curvus* (the latter was originally described as *Wolinella curva* [see above]). Subsequent studies identified these organisms in stool and blood samples of children and adults with and without diarrhea (77, 143, 151). Whole-cell protein electrophoresis and DNA-DNA hybridization experiments (143, 151) revealed that *C. concisus* is a heterogeneous species with many protein electrophoretic and genotypic subgroups; it is also phenotypically diverse, making definitive identification difficult (100). Strains of both species require hydrogen for growth under microaerobic conditions.

C. rectus, C. gracilis, and C. showae. *C. rectus, C. gracilis,* and *C. showae* are hydrogen-requiring campylobacters for which optimal growth is obtained in anaerobic conditions. Their cell morphology is most unusual. *C. rectus* (131) is a rather plump straight rod; its cellular surface is covered with a distinctive array of hexagonal, packed, macromolecular subunits. Strains have been isolated from gingival crevices of humans and from persons with appendicitis and its complications, and the species is considered a putative periodontal pathogen.

C. gracilis cells are straight and nonmotile rods (131). *C. gracilis* is the only oxidase-negative *Campylobacter* species, although the pattern of cytochromes found in *C. gracilis* resembles that reported for other campylobacters. Strains found in humans have been isolated from gingival crevices, from visceral, head, and neck infections; soft tissue abscesses; pneumonia; empyema; and an ischial wound. The association of *C. gracilis* with serious deep tissue infection, coupled with a high frequency of antibiotic resistance, suggests that it is an underestimated pathogen.

C. showae cells are straight rods and have polar bundles of two to five unsheathed flagella (32). Strains have been isolated from human dental plaque and from infected root canals. The pathogenicity is unknown.

C. jejuni and C. coli. *C. jejuni* and *C. coli* are by far the most important human enteropathogens among the campylobacters. *C. jejuni* infection is also a known antecedent of Guillain-Barré syndrome (90). Several other chapters focus on particular characteristics of these species. Within *C. jejuni,* two subspecies are recognized: *C. jejuni* subsp. *jejuni* and *C. jejuni* subsp. *doylei*. Strains of the latter subspecies differ biochemically from the former by the absence of nitrate reduction and, often, catalase activity (a weak reaction may also be observed).

The separation of *C. jejuni* subsp. *jejuni* and *C. coli* remains an important taxonomic problem. The overall phenotype and genotype of both taxa are remarkably similar. The most reliable and commonly used test is the hippurate hydrolysis test (55), in which *C. coli* is negative. However, some strains of *C. jejuni* subsp. *jejuni* also give a negative result. Additional tests that are of use include hydrogen sulfide production in triple-sugar-iron agar, growth on a minimal medium (100), and utilization of propionate (92). The complexity of this taxonomic area has been illustrated by data showing that strains first described as a distinct species, *C. hyoilei,* are in fact *C. coli* (148), despite having a higher 16S rRNA sequence similarity to *C. jejuni* (1). Moreover, the description of strains that closely resemble *C. coli* yet are genotypically more divergent from the type strain (60% DNA-DNA relatedness) (87) than is usual further emphasize the problems associated with the taxonomy of these closely related species.

The pathogenic role of *C. jejuni* subsp. *doylei* is unknown. Strains have been isolated from ulcerated gastric tissue, diarrhea, and blood cultures from humans, notably infants (128).

C. lari. *C. lari* was originally referred to as the group of nalidixic acid–resistant thermophilic campylobacters (the NARTC group). These strains differed from *C. jejuni* and *C. coli* primarily by their resistance to nalidixic acid, their anaerobic growth in the presence of trimethylamine *N*-oxide hydrochloride, and, later, also by the absence of indoxyl acetate hydrolysis. However, nalidixic acid-susceptible strains (NASC strains), urease-producing strains (UPTC strains), and urease-producing nalidixic acid-susceptible strains (30) were also identified as *C. lari* variants by one-dimensional whole-cell protein electrophoresis (102, 146) and semiquantitative DNA-DNA hybridization (85). Endtz et al. (30) described a striking heterogeneity among and within the different groups of *C. lari* variants. The detailed relationships between genuine *C. lari* strains and the various biochemical variants and protein electrophoretic subtypes should be further explored by DNA-DNA hybridization experiments.

C. lari strains have been isolated from intestinal contents of gulls and other animals, river water fish, shellfish, and occasionally human diarrheic feces. Their pathogenicity is unknown.

C. upsaliensis and C. helveticus. Both *C. upsaliensis* and *C. helveticus* are catalase negative or weakly positive campylobacters that have been isolated from the feces of diarrheic and asymptomatic domestic cats and dogs (113, 125). Although *C. upsaliensis* often has been described as a thermophilic species, Goossens et al. (49, 50) demonstrated that only about 80% of the *C. upsaliensis* strains examined grew at 42°C and therefore that it might be more appropriate to refer to these species as thermotolerant. *C. upsaliensis* strains have been isolated from blood specimens from humans and from feces of symptomatic and asymptomatic humans, dogs, and cats; strains associated with a human abortion and a breast abscess have been reported. Evidence to prove that *C. upsaliensis* is a primary human enteropathogen is accumulating in spite of isolation procedures that are generally unfavorable for this organism (9, 49).

At present, *C. helveticus* strains have not been isolated from human sources.

DIFFERENTIATION OF *CAMPYLOBACTER* SPECIES

A variety of different approaches have been used to identify campylobacters to the species level. Some of these are discussed below. The reader is referred to the review papers by On (95) and Vandamme and Goossens (138) for detailed overviews.

Classical Phenotypic Characteristics. Most routine laboratories use basic biochemical tests to identify campylobacters. The lack of application of highly standardized procedures and the well-known biochemical inertness of campylobacters often render biochemical identification of these bacteria difficult, since the discrimination among species or subspecies may rely on one differential character such as the presence of hippuricase or urease activity (95). A computerized scheme of nearly 70 biochemical tests readily differentiated virtually all of the *Campylobacter* strains examined (96, 100). Routine application of such an approach would require a considerably larger number of inexpensive tests to be performed and the availability of a database and experience for handling suitable programs for the numerical analysis and interpretation of the resulting data (95). Biochemical characteristics useful in distinguishing *Campylobacter* species are listed in Table 2.

DNA-DNA Hybridization. In taxonomic studies, the reference method for the delineation of bacterial species is determination of the level of DNA-DNA hybridization (158). A variety of DNA-DNA hybridization studies were performed before the phylogenetic relationships of campylobacters were established

TABLE 2 Differential characteristics between *Campylobacter* and *Arobacter* species and *B. ureolyticus*[a]

Species	Alpha-hemolysis	Catalase	Hippurate hydrolysis	Urease	Nitrate reduction	Selenite reduction	H₂S/TSI (trace amounts)	Indoxyl acetate hydrolysis	Growth: 25°C	42°C	Minimal medium	MacConkey	Glycine (1%)	NaCl (4%)	Resistance to: Cefoperazone (64 mg/lit)	Nalidixic acid	Cephalothin
A. butzleri	−	V	−	−	+	−	−	+	+	V	+	V[b]	−	−	+	V	+
A. cryaerophilus[c]	−	+	−	−	+	−	−	+	+	−	−	V	−	−	+	−	+
A. nitrofigilis	−	+	−	+	+	V	−	+	+	−	−	−	−	+	−	−	−
A. skirrowii	+	+	−	+	+	V	−	+	+	V	−	−	−	+	+	−	+
B. ureolyticus	V	V	−	+	+	−	V	+	−	V	V	V	+	+	−	−	−
C. coli	V	+	−	−	+	+	V	+	−	+	+	V	+	−	+	V	+
C. concisus	V	−	−	−	V	V	V	V	−	+	V[b]	−	V	−	−	V	−
C. curvus	V	−	V	−	+	−	V	V	−	V	V[b]	V[b]	+	−	V[b]	+	−
C. fetus subsp. *fetus*	−	+	−	−	+	V[b]	−	−	+	V[b]	V	V	+	−	+	+	−
C. fetus subsp. *venerealis*	V	V[b]	−	−	+	−	−	−	+	−	V[b]	V	−	−	−	V	−
C. gracilis	−	V	−	−	V[b]	−	−	V	−	V	V	V[b]	+	−	−	V	−
C. helveticus	+	−	−	−	+	−	−	+	−	+	−	−	V	−	V	−	−
C. hyointestinalis subsp. *hyointestinalis*	V	+	−	−	+	+	+	−	V	+	V	V	V	−	V	+	V
C. hyointestinalis subsp. *lawsonii*	−	−	−	−	−	−	−	+	−	−	−	−	V	−	−	−	−
C. jejuni subsp. *doylei*	+	V	+	−	+	V	−	+	−	+	−	−	+	−	+	−	+
C. jejuni subsp. *jejuni*	V	+	−	V	+	V	−	−	−	+	−	V[b]	+	−	+	V	+
C. lari[d]	−	−	−	−	−	−	+	−	−	+	−	−	V	−	V	V[b]	−
C. mucosalis	+	V	−	−	+	−	−	+	−	V	−	−	+	−	−	V[b]	−
C. rectus	+	+	−	−	+	−	V	V	−	V	V	+	V	−	−	V	−
C. showae	+	V	−	V	+	V	+	+	−	V[b]	V	V	+	V	−	V	−
C. sputorum[e]	+	−	−	−	+	+	−	+	−	+	V	−	+	−	V	−	V
C. upsaliensis	+																

[a] Data are taken from On et al. (95, 96). +, characteristic present in over 90% of the strains examined; −, characteristic present in less than 11% of the strains examined; V, strain-dependent reaction.
[b] At least 80% of the strains examined contained this characteristic.
[c] Including subgroup 1 and subgroup 2.
[d] Including NASC and UPTC variants.
[e] Including bv. sputorum, faecalis, and paraureolyticus.

by means of rRNA-directed studies and focused on the species known since the early 1980s (detailed overviews are given by Vandamme and Goossens [138] and On [95]). Significant levels of DNA-DNA hybridization were reported between *C. fetus* and *C. hyointestinalis;* among *C. jejuni, C. coli, C. lari, C. upsaliensis,* and *C. helveticus;* and between *C. rectus* and *C. showae.* DNA-DNA hybridizations among all other *Campylobacter* species have yielded only nonsignificant hybridization values.

Protein Electrophoresis. Although DNA-DNA hybridization is generally considered the reference method, it is not practical to implement this technique in a routine laboratory or to use it to examine large numbers of strains in a reference laboratory. The comparison of whole-cell protein patterns obtained by highly standardized sodium dodecylsulfate–polyacrylamide gel electrophoresis has proven to be extremely reliable for screening and identifying large numbers of strains, since numerous studies revealed a correlation between high similarity in whole-cell protein content and level of DNA-DNA hybridization (140). Polyacrylamide gel electrophoresis of whole-cell proteins has also been a most successful method for the identification of phenotypically aberrant campylobacters (see the reviews by Vandamme and Goossens [138] and On [95]). However, this method is not appropriate for routine identification studies because it is very laborious, time-consuming, and technically demanding to run the patterns in a sufficiently standardized way.

Cellular Fatty Acid Analysis. The total cellular fatty acid methyl ester composition is a stable parameter, provided that highly standardized culture conditions are used. Comparison of fatty acid profiles is of little value if different conditions are used to culture the bacteria or to prepare the extracts. However, fatty acid methyl ester analysis is a simple, cheap, and rapid method that has reached a high degree of automatization. Several authors used cellular fatty acid methyl ester analysis for the differentiation and identification of campylobacters. However, although most species were easily distinguished, "gas–liquid chromatography groups" that consisted of more than one species had to be defined conversely, strains of several species belonged to different gas–liquid chromatography groups (48, 71). Recently, Rosseel et al. (111) used the commercial Microbial Identification System (Microbial ID Inc., Newark, Del.) to develop their own database. Except for *C. jejuni* and *C. coli,* all *Campylobacter* species examined were readily differentiated, suggesting that this approach could serve as an interesting first-line screening method.

rRNA Approach. Sequence analysis of the rRNA genes became the ultimate tool to study bacterial phylogeny during the 1980s, and international databases (22, 93) have been constructed to collect sequences and to present them to the scientific community. Gradually, sequence analysis became more popular and accessible to a wider scientific community. Nowadays, it is not uncommon to identify unknown organisms that are of particular interest by means of total 16S rRNA sequence analysis and comparison with rRNA sequences present in international databases.

Several important points should be addressed here. Although unsurpassed in its capacity to reveal the phylogenetic neighborhood of an unknown bacterium, comparison of the entire 16S rRNA sequence is generally not adequate for the identification of strains to the species level. It has been reported that strains belonging to different species may have identical 16S rRNA sequences and that strains of one species may have 16S rRNA genes that differ up to 3% (124). Recently, Harrington and On (54) demonstrated differences of up to 4.3% of the total 16S rRNA sequence between *C. hyointestinalis* strains. There is definitely a lack of knowledge not only of the strain-to-strain variation within a species but also of the interoperon variation within a single strain, as reported by Clayton et al. (14). Therefore, concluding that an unknown strain belongs to a particular species because it shares a high percentage of its 16S rRNA gene sequence with another strain of that species or concluding that an unknown strain represents a novel species because it shares only 97% of its 16S rRNA gene sequence with its closest neighbor is premature in the absence of other data.

Alternatively, sequence information derived from rRNA cistrons has been used successfully to design and validate many species, group, or genus-specific primers and probes (5 to 7, 18, 28, 46, 57, 73, 78, 79, 92, 103, 148, 150; reviewed in reference 95). Applied in a PCR or a hybridization assay, these primers and probes offer valuable alternatives for the identification of *Campylobacter* taxa.

Finally, broad-spectrum molecular identification schemata based on restriction fragment analysis of PCR amplicons derived from 16S (13) and 23S (58) rRNA genes have also been described.

The Genus *Arcobacter*

GENERAL CHARACTERISTICS

Arcobacter cells are slender, spirally curved rods, 0.2 to 0.9 μm wide and 0.5 to 3 μm long; S-shaped or helical cells are often present. Cells in old cultures may form spherical or coccoid bodies and loose spiral filaments up to 20 μm long. The cells are motile with a characteristic corkscrew-like motion by means of a single polar unsheathed flagellum at one or both ends of the cell.

In general, biochemical characteristics are as described for the family *Campylobacteraceae*. In addition, arcobacters are able to grow under aerobic and anaerobic conditions and at 15°C. Hydrogen is not required. Indoxyl acetate is hydrolyzed, but gelatin, casein, starch, hippurate, and tyrosine are not.

The habitat of this genus is extremely diverse. Some species are pathogenic for humans and animals and are found in the reproductive organs and aborted fetuses of various animals and in the intestinal tract of humans and animals. Arcobacters have been detected in water reservoirs, sewage, oil field communities, and saline environments; one species is a plant-as-sociated nitrogen fixer. The G + C content of the DNA ranges from 27 to 31 mol%. The genus *Arcobacter* presently comprises four species, with *Arcobacter nitrofigilis* Vandamme, Falsen, Rossau, Hoste, Segers, Tytgat, and De Ley 1991 being the type species.

Arcobacters may be isolated by using the selective media or filtration methods described for the isolation of *Campylobacter* species. However, these methods are suboptimal since arcobacters may be overgrown by campylobacters present in the same specimens. Samples should be incubated at 24 to 30°C to enhance the selectivity of the procedure, and an enrichment step is recommended (2, 4). A selective medium developed for the isolation of arcobacters was recently described by de Boer et al. (19) and is based on their swarming capacity in semisolid media.

Menaquinone-6 and a second menaquinone-6, the detailed structure of which has not been determined, have been reported as major respiratory quinones.

Arcobacter is a most unusual genus, unifying species associated with disease or considered pathogenic in humans and animals and a plant-associated nitrogen-fixing bacterium. This combination of plant and animal associated-species within one genus is rarely seen among proteobacteria. Arcobacters were shown to be abundant in particular environmental niches including water reservoirs, sewage, oil field communities, and saline environments. Their role in the environment is not well documented, but some of these organisms are sulfide oxiders (with the production of sulfur), and it has been suggested that they play a role in the sulfur cycle by reoxidizing sulfide formed by microbial sulfate or sulfur reduction (156).

LIST OF THE SPECIES OF THE GENUS *ARCOBACTER*

A. nitrofigilis. *A. nitrofigilis* strains occur in the roots and rhizosphere of salt marsh plants, where they fix nitrogen. They differ from other members of the family *Campylobacteraceae* by their requirement for a high salt concentration (optimum growth is in the presence of 10 to 40 g of NaCl per liter).

A. cryaerophilus. In 1985, Neill et al. (91) performed an extensive phenotypic characterization of aerotolerant *Campylobacter* strains isolated from various animal sources. They concluded that the aerotolerant strains were only distantly related to strains of the other *Campylobacter* species examined and emphasized that they formed a heterogeneous group. Their findings were confirmed by integrated phenotypic, genotypic, and chemotaxonomic studies of, in part, the same isolates (65, 133, 145, 149), which resulted in the description of a novel genus *Arcobacter,* with three separate animal-associated species: *A. cryaerophilus, A. butzleri,* and *A. skirrowii* (65, 145, 149).

Within *A. cryaerophilus,* two subgroups referred to as subgroup 1 or group 1A (65) and subgroup 2 or group 1B (149) have been described. Strains of these subgroups differ in their whole-cell protein and fatty acid patterns and in the restriction fragment length polymorphisms of the rRNA genes. Moderate levels of DNA-DNA hybridization were detected between strains of the different subgroups, suggesting that they could be given a distinct taxonomic rank. However, at present, no formal nomenclatural modifications have been proposed.

A. cryaerophilus strains have been isolated from cases of human bacteremia and diarrhea; from chicken carcasses; from bovine, ovine, and porcine aborted fetuses; from porcine feces; and from cattle with mastitis. Their pathogenicity is unknown.

A. butzleri. *A. butzleri* strains have been isolated from human blood and diarrheic feces; from feces of various animals with diarrhea, including nonhuman primates, pigs, horses, cattle, an ostrich, and a tortoise; from bovine and porcine aborted fetuses; from various food products including ground pork, chicken, and turkey samples; from surface water and drinking-water reservoirs, and from canal waters. This species is associated with enteritis, abdominal cramps, bacteremia, and appendicitis in humans and with enteritis and abortion in animals.

A. skirrowii. *A. skirrowii* strains have been isolated from preputial fluids of bulls; from bovine, ovine, and porcine aborted fetuses; from diarrheic feces of various animals including sheep and cattle; and from chicken carcasses. Their pathogenicity is unknown.

Other Organisms. A number of studies have documented the existence of additional *Arcobacter* taxa in environmental samples including oil field communities (156), cyanobacterial mats (132), and activated sludge of a large municipal wastewater treatment plant (122). Phylogenetic analysis by 16S rRNA gene sequence determination has revealed that these organisms belong to the *Arcobacter* genus, but none has been formally named.

DIFFERENTIATION OF *ARCOBACTER* SPECIES

Basic biochemical tests are also routinely used to identify arcobacters to the species level, and, as with campylobacters, this is hampered by their biochemical inertness. In particular, the separation of *A. cryaerophilus* subgroup 2 and *A. butzleri* is tedious (65, 149). Biochemical characteristics useful to distinguish the various *Arcobacter* species are listed in Table 2.

Whole-cell protein electrophoresis (149) and numerical analysis of 67 phenotypic characters (96, 100) correlated with the percentage of DNA-DNA binding and allowed differentiation of all species. Whole-cell fatty acid analysis did not allow *A. butzleri* to be distinguished from *A. cryaerophilus* subgroup 2, but it differentiated all other *Arcobacter* taxa (149).

The use of 16S rRNA-based DNA probes (159) and PCR assays (53), ribotyping (66), and restriction fragment length polymorphism analysis of a PCR-amplified fragment of the gene coding for 16S rRNA (13) or 23S rRNA (58) differentiated *A. butzleri* from other arcobacters but did not differentiate *A. cryaerophilus* from *A. skirrowii.* Using a variable 23S rRNA region, Bastyns et al. (5) developed genus- and species-specific PCR assays that differentiated *A. butzleri, A. cryaerophilus,* and *A. skirrowii.* Finally, Snaidr et al. (122) described a set of genus-specific PCR primers that enabled the detection of the four named species and an unnamed *A. nitrofigilis*-like taxon.

The Genus *Sulfurospirillum*

The genus *Sulfurospirillum* was created to accommodate various free-living *Campylobacter*-like organisms. Sulfurospirilla are extremely fastidious, and very few strains have been isolated and studied. Species determination is based primarily on differences in 16S rRNA sequence, although there are obvious differences in the metabolism of these organisms too.

S. *deleyianum* was described to accommodate a strain previously known as "*Spirillum* 5175" (160) and isolated from anoxic mud from a forest pond near Heiningen, Germany. S. *arcachonense* was isolated from oxidized surface sediment in an intertidal mud flat near Arcachon (France) (34). S. *arsenophilum* was isolated from arsenic-contaminated watershed sediments in eastern Massachusetts, and S. *barnesii* was isolated from the selenium-contaminated Massie Slough, western Nevada (129).

Cells of all of these species are slender, spiral-shaped curved rods, 0.1 to 0.5 μm wide and 1.0 to 3 μm in length. They may form helical chains of two or more cells. On the basis of available data, their general biochemical profile conforms to that of the family *Campylobacteraceae.* All species produce oxidase activity. Growth occurs between 8 and 36°C. The $G + C$ content of the DNA ranges from 32 to 42 mol%. At present there are four named *Sulfurospirillum* species, with *Sulfurospirillum deleyianum* (Wolfe and Pfenning 1977) Schumacher, Kroneck, and Pfenning 1993 being the type species.

Different isolation procedure have been described, all of which involve enrichment procedures (34, 101, 160).

Menaquinone-6, a methyl-substituted menaquinone-6 (referred to as thermoplasma-quinon-6), and menaquinone-5 have been reported as respiratory quinones in S. *deleyianum.*

Members of this genus are all sulfur reducers but exhibit metabolic versatility. DNA-DNA homology studies confirmed that S. *barnesii,* S. *arsenophilum,* and S. *deleyianum* are separate species, with interspecies DNA-DNA hybridization levels between 31 and 53% (129). Several other presently unnamed organisms also belong to the genus *Sulfurospirillum.* A marine sulfur-reducing bacterium, designated strain SM-5, was isolated by Coleman et al. (15) and implicated as the organism involved in the formation of ferrous nodules. The free-living organism previously known as *Campylobacter* sp. strain "Veldkamp" that was isolated from activated sludge (70) has been reassigned as a strain of S. *deleyianum.* However, phylogenetic analysis of the 16S rRNA sequence of this strain indicates that the strain may represent a separate species.

Bacteroides ureolyticus

B. *ureolyticus* (60) cells are nonmotile rods that grow microaerobically when hydrogen is provided. Representative strains of this species were included in a polyphasic taxonomic study to elucidate its taxonomic status (141). B. *ureolyticus* resembles campylobacters in its respiratory quinone content, its DNA base ratio, and most of its phenotypic characteristics but differs from them in its fatty acid composition and its proteolytic metabolism. Bootstrapping analysis of the 16S rRNA sequence mostly separated B. *ureolyticus* from the *Campylobacter* clade. However, this organism was not formally reclassified pending the isolation and a thorough taxonomic characterization of additional B. *ureolyticus*-like bacteria (27).

Strains have been isolated from superficial ulcers and soft tissue infections, urethritis, and periodontal disease. A pathogenic role is suggested by its predominance in mixed infections and its strong proteolytic activity, which may enable tissue destruction.

ACKNOWLEDGMENTS

P. V. is indebted to the Fund for Scientific Research—Flanders (Belgium) for a position as a postdoctoral fellow.

REFERENCES

1. **Alderton, M. R., V. Korolik, P. Coloe, F. E. Dewhirst, and B. J. Paster.** 1995. *Campylobacter hyoilei* sp. nov., associated with porcine proliferative enteritis. *Int. J. Syst. Bacteriol.* **45:** 61–66.

2. **Atabay, H. I., and J. E. L. Corry.** 1997. The prevalence of campylobacters and arcobacters in broiler chickens. *J. Appl. Microbiol.* **83:**619–626.

3. **Atabay, H. I., J. E. L. Corry, and S. L. W. On.** 1997. Isolation and characterization of a novel catalase-negative, urease-positive *Campylobacter* from cattle faeces. *Lett. Appl. Microbiol.* **24:**59–64.

4. **Atabay, H. I., J. E. L. Corry, and S. L. W. On.** 1998. Diversity and prevalence of *Arcobacter* species in chickens. *J. Appl. Microbiol.* **84:** 1007–1016.

5. **Bastyns, K., D. Cartuyvels, S. Chapelle, P. Vandamme, H. Goossens, and R. De Wachter.** 1995. A variable 23S rDNA region is a useful discriminating target for genus-specific and species-specific amplification of *Arcobacter* species. *Syst. Appl. Microbiol.* **18:**353–356.

6. **Bastyns, K., S. Chapelle, P. Vandamme, H. Goossens, and R. De Wachter.** 1994. Species-specific detection of campylobacters important in veterinary medicine by PCR amplification of 23S rDNA areas. *Syst. Appl. Microbiol.* **17:**563–568.

7. **Bastyns, K., S. Chapelle, P. Vandamme, H. Goossens, and R. De Wachter.** 1995. Specific detection of *Campylobacter concisus* by PCR amplification of 23S rDNA areas. *Mol. Cell. Probes* **9:**247–250.

8. **Benjamin, J., S. Leaper, R. J. Owen, and M. B. Skirrow.** 1983. Description of *Campylobacter laridis*, a new species comprising the nalidixic acid resistant thermophilic *Campylobacter* (NARTC) group. *Curr. Microbiol.* **8:**231–238.

9. **Bourke, B., V. L. Chan, and P. Sherman.** 1998. *Campylobacter upsaliensis:* waiting in the wings. *Clin. Microbiol. Rev.* **11:**440–449.

10. **Bronsdon, M. A., C. S. Goodwin, L. I. Sly, T. Chilvers, and F. D. Schoenknecht.** 1991. *Helicobacter nemestrinae* sp. nov., a spiral bacterium found in the stomach of a pigtailed macaque (*Macaca nemestrina*). *Int. J. Syst. Bacteriol.* **41:** 148–153.

11. **Bryans, J. T., A. G. Smith, and A. G. Baker.** 1960. Ovine vibrionic abortion caused by a new variety of *Vibrio*. *Cornell Vet.* **50:**54–59.

12. **Butzler, J.-P., P. Dekeyser, M. Detrain, and F. Dehaen.** 1973. Related vibrio in stools. *J. Pediatr.* **82:**493–495.

13. **Cardarelli-Leite, P., K. Blom, C. M. Patton,** M. A. Nicholson, A. G. Steigerwalt, S. B. Hunter, D. J. Brenner, T. J. Barrett, and B. Swaminathan. 1996. Rapid identification of *Campylobacter* species by restriction fragment polymorphism analysis of a PCR-amplified fragment of the gene coding for 16S rRNA. *J. Clin. Microbiol.* **34:**62–67.

14. **Clayton, R. A., G. Sutton, P. S. Hinkle, C. Bult, and C. Fields.** 1995. Intraspecific variation in small-subunit rRNA sequences in GenBank: why single sequences may not adequately represent prokaryotic taxa. *Int. J. Syst. Bacteriol.* **45:**595–599.

15. **Coleman, M. L., D. B. Hedrick, D. R. Levley, D. C. White and K. Pye.** 1993. Reduction of Fe(III) in sediments by sulphate-reducing bacteria. *Nature* (London) **361:**436–438.

16. **Collins, M. D., and F. Widdel.** 1986. Respiratory quinones of sulphate-reducing and sulphur reducing bacteria: a systematic investigation. *Syst. Appl. Microbiol.* **8:**8–18.

17. **Costas, M., R. J. Owen, and P. J. H. Jackman.** 1987. Classification of *Campylobacter sputorum* and allied campylobacters based on numerical analysis of electrophoretic protein patterns. *Syst. Appl. Microbiol.* **9:**125–131.

18. **Day, W. A., I. L. Pepper, and L. A. Joens.** 1997. Use of an arbitrarily primed PCR product in the development of a *Campylobacter jejuni*-specific PCR. *Appl. Environ. Microbiol.* **63:** 1019–1023.

19. **de Boer, E., J. J. Tilburg, D. L. Woodward, H. Lior, and W. M. Johnson.** 1996. A selective medium for the isolation of *Arcobacter* from meats. *Lett. Appl. Microbiol.* **23:**64–66.

20. **Dekeyser, P., M. Gossuin-Detrain, J.-P. Butzler, and J. Sternon.** 1972. Acute enteritis due to related vibrio: first positive stools cultures. *J. Infect. Dis.* **125:**390–392.

21. **De Ley, J.** 1978. Modern molecular methods in bacterial taxonomy: evaluation, application, prospects, p. 347–357. *In Proceedings of the 4th International Conference of Plant Pathogenic Bacteria,* vol. 1. Gibert-Clarey, Tours, France.

22. **De Rijk, P., J.-M. Neefs, Y. Van de Peer, and R. De Wachter.** 1992. Compilation of small ribosomal subunit RNA sequences. *Nucleic Acids Res.* **20:**2075–2089.

23. **Dewhirst, F. G.** Personal communication.

24. **Dewhirst, F. E., C. Seymour, G. J. Fraser, B. J. Paster, and J. G. Fox.** 1994. Phylogeny of *Helicobacter* isolates from bird and swine feces and description of *Helicobacter pametensis* sp. nov. *Int. J. Syst. Bacteriol.* **44:**553–560.

25. **Doyle, L. P.** 1944. A vibrio associated with swine dysentery. *Am. J. Vet. Res.* **5:**3–5.

26. **Doyle, L. P.** 1948. The etiology of swine dysentery. *Am. J. Vet. Res.* **9:**50–51.

27. **Duerden, B. I., A. Eley, L. Goodwin, J. T. Magee, J. M. Hindmarch, and K. W. Bennett.** 1989. A comparison of *Bacteroides ureolyticus* isolates from different clinical sources. *J. Med. Microbiol.* **29:**63–73.

28. **Eaglesome, M. D., M. I. Sampath, and M. M. Garcia.** 1995. A detection assay for *Campylobacter fetus* in bovine semen by restriction analysis of PCR amplified DNA. *Vet. Res. Commun.* **19:** 253–263.

29. **Eaton, K. A., F. E. Dewhirst, M. J. Radin, J. G. Fox, B. J. Paster, S. Krakowka, and D. R. Morgan.** 1993. *Helicobacter acinonyx* sp. nov., isolated from cheetahs with gastritis. *Int. J. Syst. Bacteriol.* **43:**99–106.

30. **Endtz, H. P., J. S. Vilegenthart, P. Vandamme, H. W. Weverink, N. P. van den Braak, H. A. Verbrugh, and A. van Belkum.** 1997. Genotypic diversity of *Campylobacter lari* isolated from mussels and oysters in The Netherlands. *Int. J. Food Microbiol.* **34:**79–88.

31. **Escherich, T.** 1886. Beiträge zur Kenntniss der Darmbacterien. III. Über das Vorkommen van Vibrionen im Darmcanal und den Stuhlgängen der Säuglinge. *Münch. Med. Wochenschr.* **33:** 815–817, 833–835.

32. **Etoh, Y., F. E. Dewhirst, B. J. Paster, A. Yamamoto, and N. Goto.** 1993. *Campylobacter showae* sp. nov., isolated from the human oral cavity. *Int. J. Syst. Bacteriol.* **43:**631–639.

33. **Fennell, C. L., P. A. Totten, T. C. Quinn, D. L. Patton, K. K. Holmes, and W. E. Stamm.** 1984. Characterization of *Campylobacter*-like organisms isolated from homosexual men. *J. Infect. Dis.* **149:**58–66.

34. **Finster, K., W. Liesack, and B. J. Tindall.** 1997. *Sulfurospirillum arcachonense* sp. nov., a new microaerophilic sulfur-reducing bacterium. *Int. J. Syst. Bacteriol.* **47:**1212–1217.

35. **Firehammer, B. D.** 1965. The isolation of vibrios from ovine feces. *Cornell Vet.* **55:**482–494.

36. **Florent, A.** 1953. Isolement d'un vibrion saprophyte du sperme du taureau et du vagin de la vache (*Vibrio bubulus*). *C. R. Soc. Biol.* **147:** 2066–2069.

37. **Florent, A.** 1959. Les deux vibrioses génitales: la vibriose due à *Vibrio fetus venerealis* et la vibriose d'origine intestinale due à *V. fetus intestinalis*. *Meded. Veeartsenijsch. Rijksuniv. Gent* **3:**1–60.

38. **Fox, J. G., B. M. Edrise, E. B. Cabot, C. Beaucage, J. C. Murphy, and K. S. Prostak.** 1986. *Campylobacter*-like organisms isolated from the gastric mucosa of ferrets. *Am. J. Vet. Res.* **47:** 236–239.

39. **Fox, J. G., F. E. Dewhirst, J. G. Tully, B. J. Paster, L. Yan, N. S. Taylor, M. J. Collins, P. L. Gorelick, and J. M. Ward.** 1994. *Helicobacter hepaticus* sp. nov., a microaerophilic bacterium isolated from livers and intestinal mucosal scrapings from mice. *J. Clin. Microbiol.* **32:** 1238–1245.

40. **Fox, J. G., L. L. Yan, F. E. Dewhirst, B. J. Paster, B. Shames, J. C. Murphy, A. Hayward, J. C. Belcher, and E. N. Mendes.** 1995. *Helicobacter bilis*, a novel *Helicobacter* species isolated from bile, livers, and intestines of aged, inbred mice. *J. Clin. Microbiol.* **33:**445–454.

41. **Fox, J. G., N. S. Taylor, P. Edmonds, and D. J. Brenner.** 1988. *Campylobacter pylori* subsp. *mustelae* subsp. nov. isolated from the gastric mucosa of ferrets (*Mustela putorius furo*), and an emended description of *Campylobacter pylori*. *Int. J. Syst. Bacteriol.* **38:**367–370.

42. **Fox, J. G., T. Chilvers, C. S. Goodwin, N. S. Taylor, P. Edmonds, L. I. Sly, and D. J. Brenner.** 1989. *Campylobacter mustelae*, a new species resulting from the elevation of *Campylobacter pylori* subsp. *mustelae* to species status. *Int. J. Syst. Bacteriol.* **39:**301–303.

43. **Franklin, C. L., C. S. Beckwith, R. S. Livingston, L. K. Riley, S. V. Gibson, C. L. Besch-Williford, and R. R. Hook.** 1996. Isolation of a novel *Helicobacter* species, *Helicobacter cholecystus* sp. nov., from the gallbladders of Syrian hamsters with cholangiofibrosis and centrilobular pacreatitis. *J. Clin. Microbiol.* **34:** 2952–2958.

44. **Gebhart, C. J., G. E. Ward, K. Chang, and H. J. Kurtz.** 1983. *Campylobacter hyointestinalis* (new species) isolated from swine with lesions of proliferative ileitis. *Am. J. Vet. Res.* **44:**361–367.

45. **Gebhart, C. J., P. Edmonds, G. E. Ward, H. J. Kurtz, and D. J. Brenner.** 1985. "*Campylobacter hyointestinalis*" sp. nov.: a new species of *Campylobacter* found in the intestines of pigs and other animals. *J. Clin. Microbiol.* **21:** 715–720.

46. **Gonzalez, I., K. A. Grant, P. T. Richardson, S. F. Park, and M. D. Collins.** 1997. Specific identification of the enteropathogens *Campylobacter jejuni* and *Campylobacter coli* by using a PCR test based on the *ceuE* gene encoding a putative virulence determinant. *J. Clin. Microbiol.* **35:** 759–763.

47. **Goodwin, C. S., J. A. Armstrong, T. Chilvers, M. Peters, M. D. Collins, L. Sly, W. McConnell, and W. E. S. Harper.** 1989. Transfer of *Campylobacter pylori* and *Campylobacter mustelae* to *Helicobacter* gen. nov. as *Helicobacter pylori* comb. nov. and *Helicobacter mustelae* comb.

nov., respectively. *Int. J. Syst. Bacteriol.* **39:** 397–405.

48. **Goodwin, C. S., W. McConnell, R. K. McCullough, C. McCullough, R. Hill, M. A. Bronsdon, and G. Kasper.** 1989. Cellular fatty acid composition of *Campylobacter pylori* from primates and ferrets compared with those of other campylobacters. *J. Clin. Microbiol.* **27:** 938–943.

49. **Goossens, H., B. Pot, L. Vlaes, C. Van den Borre, R. Van den Abbeele, C. Van Naelten, J. Levy, H. Cogniau, P. Marbehant, J. Verhoef, K. Kersters, J.-P. Butzler, and P. Vandamme.** 1990. Characterization and description of "*Campylobacter upsaliensis*" isolated from human feces. *J. Clin. Microbiol.* **28:** 1039–1046.

50. **Goossens, H., L. Vlaes, M. De Boeck, B. Pot, K. Kersters, J. Levy, P. De Mol, J.-P. Butzler, and P. Vandamme.** 1990b. Is "*Campylobacter upsaliensis*" an unrecognised cause of human diarrhoea? *Lancet* **335:**384–386.

51. **Goto, K., H. Ohashi, S. Ebukuro, K. Itoh, Y. Tohma, A. Takakura, S. Wakana, M. Ito, and T. Itoh.** 1998. Isolation and characterization of *Helicobacter* species from the stomach of the house musk shrew (*Suncus murinus*) with chronic gastritis. *Curr. Microbiol.* **37:**44–51.

52. **Hänninen, M.-L., I. Happonen, S. Saari, and K. Jalava.** 1996. Culture and characteristics of *Helicobacter bizzozeronii*, a new canine gastric *Helicobacter* sp. *Int. J. Syst. Bacteriol.* **46:**160–166.

53. **Harmon, K. M., and I. V. Wesley.** 1997. Multiplex PCR for the identification of *Arcobacter* and differentiation of *Arcobacter butzleri* from other arcobacters. *Vet. Microbiol.* **58:** 215–227.

54. **Harrington, C. S., and S. L. W. On.** 1999. Extensive 16S rRNA gene sequence diversity in *Campylobacter hyointestinalis* strains: taxonomic, and applied implications. *Int. J. Syst. Bacteriol.* **49:** 1171–1175.

55. **Harvey, S. M.** 1980. Hippurate hydrolysis by *Campylobacter fetus. J. Clin. Microbiol.* **11:** 435–437.

56. **Hazeleger, W., C. Arkesteijn, A. Toorop-Bouma, and R. Beumer.** 1994. Detection of the coccoid form of *Campylobacter jejuni* in chicken products with the use of the polymerase chain reaction. *Int. J. Food Microbiol.* **24:** 273–281.

57. **Hum, S., K. Quinn, J. Brunner, and S. L. W. On.** 1997. Evaluation of a PCR assay for identification and differentiation of *Campylobacter fetus* subspecies. *Aust. Vet. J.* **75:**827–831.

58. **Hurtado, A., and R. J. Owen.** 1997. A molecular scheme based on 23S rRNA gene polymorphisms for rapid identification of *Campylobacter* and *Arcobacter* species. *J. Clin. Microbiol.* **35:** 2401–2404.

59. **Husmann, M., C. Gries, P. Jenichen, T. Woelfel, G. Gerken, W. Ludwig, and S. Bhakdi.** 1994. *Helicobacter* sp. strain Mainz isolated from an AIDS patient with septic arthritis: case report and nonradioactive analysis of 16S rRNA sequence. *J. Clin. Microbiol.* **32:** 3037–3039.

60. **Jackson, F. L., and Y. E. Goodman.** 1978. *Bacteroides ureolyticus*, a new species to accommodate strains previously identified as "*Bacteroides corrodens*, anaerobic." *Int. J. Syst. Bacteriol.* **28:** 197–200.

61. **Jalava, K., M. Kaartinen, M. Utriainen, I. Happonen, and M.-L. Hänninen.** 1997. *Helicobacter salomonis* sp. nov., a canine gastric *Helicobacter* sp. related to *Helicobacter felis* and *Helicobacter bizzozeronii. Int. J. Syst. Bacteriol.* **48:** 975–982.

62. **Jones, F. S., and R. B. Little.** 1931. The etiology of infectious diarrhea (winter scours) in cattle. *J. Exp. Med.* **53:**835–844.

63. **Jones, F. S., and R. B. Little.** 1931. Vibrionic enteritis in calves. *J. Exp. Med.* **53:**845–852.

64. **Jones, F. S., M. Orcutt, and R. B. Little.** 1931. Vibrios (*V. jejuni* n. sp.) associated with intestinal disorders in cows and calves. *J. Exp. Med.* **53:**853–863.

65. **Kiehlbauch, J. A., D. J. Brenner, M. A. Nicholson, C. N. Baker, C. M. Patton, A. G. Steigerwalt, and I. K. Wachsmuth.** 1991. *Campylobacter butzleri* sp. nov. isolated from humans and animals with diarrheal illness. *J. Clin. Microbiol.* **29:**376–385.

66. **Kiehlbauch, J. A., B. D. Plikaytis, B. Swaminathan, D. N. Cameron, and I. K. Wachsmuth.** 1991. Restriction fragment length polymorphisms in the ribosomal genes for species identification and subtyping of aerotolerant *Campylobacter* species. *J. Clin. Microbiol.* **29:** 1670–1676.

67. **King, E. O.** 1957. Human infections with *Vibrio fetus* and a closely related *Vibrio. J. Infect. Dis.* **101:**119–128.

68. **King, E. O.** 1962. The laboratory recognition of *Vibrio fetus* and a closely related *Vibrio* isolated from cases of human vibriosis. *Ann. N. Y. Acad. Sci.* **98:**700–701.

69. **Kist, M.** 1986. Who discovered *Campylobacter jejuni/coli*? A historical review. *Zentralbl. Bakteriol. Parasitenkd. Infectionskr. Hyg. I Abt. Orig. A* **261:** 177–186.

70. **Laanbroek, H. J., W. Kingma, and H. Veld-**

kamp. 1977. Isolation of an aspartate-fermenting, free-living *Campylobacter* species. *FEMS Microbiol. Lett.* **1**:99–102.

71. **Lambert, M. A., C. M. Patton, T. J. Barrett, C. W. Moss.** 1987. Differentiation of *Campylobacter* and *Campylobacter*-like organisms by cellular fatty acid composition. *J. Clin. Microbiol.* **25**: 706–713.

72. **Lau, P. P., B. Debrunner-Vossbrinck, B. Dunn, K. Miotto, M. T. Donell, D. M. Rollins, C. J. Pillidge, R. B. Hespell, R. R. Colwell, M. L. Sogin, and G. E. Fox.** 1987. Phylogenetic diversity and position of the genus *Campylobacter*. *Syst. Appl. Microbiol.* **9**:231–238.

73. **Lawson, A. J., D. Linton, J. Stanley, and R. J. Owen.** 1997. Polymerase chain reaction detection and speciation of *Campylobacter upsaliensis* and *C. helveticus* in human faeces and comparison with culture techniques. *J. Appl. Microbiol.* **83**:375–380.

74. **Lawson, G. H. K., J. L. Leaver, G. W. Pettigrew, and A. C. Rowland.** 1981. Some features of *Campylobacter sputorum* subsp. *mucosalis* subsp. nov., nom. rev., and their taxonomic significance. *Int. J. Syst. Bacteriol.* **31**:385–391.

75. **Lee, A., M. W. Philips, J. L. O'Rourke, B. J. Paster, F. E. Dewhirst, G. J. Fraser, J. G. Fox, L. I. Sly, P. J. Romaniuk, T. J. Trust, and S. Kroupach.** 1992. *Helicobacter muridarum* sp. nov., a microaerophilic helical bacterium with a novel ultrastructure isolated from the intestinal mucosa of rodents. *Int. J. Syst. Bacteriol.* **42**:27–36.

76. **Levy, A. J.** 1946. A gastroenteritis outbreak probably due to a bovine strain of vibrio. *Yale J. Biol. Med.* **18**:243.

77. **Lindblom, G.-B., E. Sjögren, J. Hansson-Westerberg, and B. Kaijser.** 1995. *Campylobacter upsaliensis*, *C. sputorum*, and *C. concisus* as common causes of diarrhoea in Swedish children. *Scand. J. Infect. Dis.* **27**:187–188.

78. **Linton, D., A. J. Lawson, R. J. Owen, and J. Stanley.** 1997. PCR detection, identification to species level, and fingerprinting of *Campylobacter jejuni* and *Campylobacter coli* direct from diarrheic samples. *J. Clin. Microbiol.* **35**: 2568–2572.

79. **Linton, D., R. J. Owen and J. Stanley.** 1996. Rapid identification by PCR of the genus *Campylobacter* and of five *Campylobacter* species enteropathogenic for man and animals. *Res. Microbiol.* **147**:707–718.

80. **Marshall, B. J., and C. S. Goodwin.** 1987. Revised nomenclature of *Campylobacter pyloridis*. *Int. J. Syst. Bacteriol.* **37**:68.

81. **Marshall, B. J., H. Royce, D. I. Annear, C.**

S. **Goodwin, J. W. Pearman, J. R. Warren, and J. A. Armstrong.** 1984. Original isolation of *Campylobacter pyloridis* from human gastric mucosa. *Microbios Lett.* **25**:83–88.

82. **McClung, C. R., D. G. Patriquin, and R. E. Davis.** 1983. *Campylobacter nitrofigilis* sp. nov., a nitrogen-fixing bacterium associated with roots of *Spartina alterniflora* Loisel. *Int. J. Syst. Bacteriol.* **33**:605–612.

83. **McClung, C. R., and D. G. Patriquin.** 1980. Isolation of a nitrogen-fixing *Campylobacter* species from the roots of *Spartinal alterniflora* Loisel. *Can. J. Microbiol.* **26**:881–886.

84. **McFadyean, J., and S. Stockman.** 1913. *Report of the Departmental Committee Appointed by the Board of Agriculture and Fisheries To Enquire into Epizootic Abortion*. Appendix to Part II. *Abortion in Sheep*, p. 1–64. His Majesty's Stationery Office, London, United Kingdom.

85. **Mégraud, F., D. Chevrier, N. Desplaces, A. Sedallian, and J. L. Guesdon.** 1988. Urease-positive thermophilic *Campylobacter* (*Campylobacter laridis* variant) isolated from an appendix and from human feces. *J. Clin. Microbiol.* **26**: 1050–1051.

86. **Mendes, E. N., D. M. Queiroz, F. E. Dewhirst, B. J. Paster, S. B. Moura, and J. G. Fox.** 1996. *Helicobacter trogontum* sp. nov., isolated from the rat intestine. *Int. J. Syst. Bacteriol.* **46**:916–921.

87. **Morris, G. K., M. R. El Sheerbeeny, C. M. Patton, H. Kodaka, G. L. Lombard, P. Edmonds, D. G. Hollis, and D. J. Brenner.** 1985. Comparison of four hippurate hydrolysis methods for identification of thermophilic *Campylobacter* spp. *J. Clin. Microbiol.* **22**:714–718.

88. **Moss, C. W., A. Kai, M. A. Lambert, and C. Patton.** 1984. Isoprenoid quinone content and cellular fatty acid composition of *Campylobacter* species. *J. Clin. Microbiol.* **19**:772–776.

89. **Moss, C. W., M. A. Lambert-Fair, M. A. Nicholson, and G. O. Guerrant.** 1990. Isoprenoid quinones of *Campylobacter cryaerophila*, *C. cinaedi*, *C. fennelliae*, *C. hyointestinalis*, *C. pylori*, and "*C. upsaliensis*." *J. Clin. Microbiol.* **28**: 395–397.

90. **Nachamkin, I., B. M. Allos, and T. Ho.** 1998. *Campylobacter* species and Guillain-Barré syndrome. *Clin. Microbiol. Rev.* **11**:555–567.

91. **Neill, S. D., J. N. Campbell, J. J. O'Brien, S. T. C. Weatherup, and W. A. Ellis.** 1985. Taxonomic position of *Campylobacter cryaerophila* sp. nov. *Int. J. Syst. Bacteriol.* **35**:342–356.

92. **Occhialini, A., V. Stonnet, J. Hua, C. Camou, J. L. Guesdon, and F. Mégraud.** 1996. Identification of strains of *Campylobacter*

jejuni and *Campylobacter coli* by PCR and correlation with phenotypic characteristics, p. 217–219. *In* D. G. Newell, J. M. Ketley, and R. A. Feldman (ed.), *Campylobacters, Helicobacters, and Related Organisms.* Plenum Press, New York, N.Y.

93. **Olsen, G. J., G. Larsen, and C. R. Woese.** 1991. The ribosomal RNA database project. *Nucleic Acids Res.* **19**(Suppl.):2017–2021.

94. **On, S. L. W.** 1994. Confirmation of human *Campylobacter concisus* isolates misidentified as *Campylobacter mucosalis* and suggestions for improved differentiation between the two species. *J. Clin. Microbiol.* **32:**2305–2306.

95. **On, S. L. W.** 1996. Identification methods for campylobacters, helicobacters, and related organisms. *Clin. Microbiol. Rev.* **9:**405–422.

96. **On, S. L. W., and B. Holmes.** 1995. Classification and identification of campylobacters, helicobacters and allied taxa by numerical analysis of phenotypic characters. *Syst. Appl. Microbiol.* **18:**374–390.

97. **On, S. L. W., H. I. Atabay, J. E. L. Corry, C. S. Harrington, and P. Vandamme.** 1998. Emended description of *Campylobacter sputorum* and revision of its infrasubspecific (biovar) divisions, including *C. sputorum* bv. paraureolyticus, a urease-producing variant from cattle and humans. *Int. J. Syst. Bacteriol.* **48.**195–206.

98. **On, S. L. W., M. Costas, and B. Holmes.** 1993. Identification and intra-specific heterogeneity of *Campylobacter hyointestinalis* based on numerical analyses of electrophoretic protein profiles. *Syst. Appl. Microbiol.* **16:**37–46.

99. **On, S. L. W., M. Costas, and B. Holmes.** 1994. Classification and identification of *Campylobacter sputorum* using numerical analyses of phenotypic tests and of one-dimensional electrophoretic protein profiles. *Syst. Appl. Microbiol.* **17:**543–553.

100. **On, S. L. W., B. Holmes, and M. Sackin.** 1996. A probability matrix for the identification of campylobacters, helicobacters, and allied taxa. *J. Appl. Bacteriol.* **81:**425–432.

101. **Oremland, R. S., J. Switzer Blum, C. W. Culbertson, P. T. Visscher, G. Miller, P. Dowdle, and F. E. Strohmaier.** 1994. Isolation, growth, and metabolism of an obligately anaerobic, selenate-respiring bacterium, strain SES-3. *Appl. Environ. Microbiol.* **60:**3011–3019.

102. **Owen, R. J., M. Costas, L. L. Sloss, and F. J. Bolton.** 1988. Numerical analysis of electrophoretic protein patterns of *Campylobacter laridis* and allied thermophilic campylobacters from the natural environment. *J. Appl. Bacteriol.* **65:**69–78.

103. **Oyarzabal, O. A., I. V. Wesley, J. M. Barb-**

aree, **L. H. Lauerman, and D. E. Conner.** 1997. Specific detection of *Campylobacter lari* by PCR. *J. Microbiol. Methods* **29:**97–102.

104. **Paster, B. J., A. Lee, J. G. Fox, F. E. Dewhirst, L. A. Tordoff, G. J. Fraser, J. L. O'Rourke, N. S. Taylor, and R. Ferrero.** 1991. Phylogeny of *Helicobacter felis* sp. nov., *Helicobacter mustelae,* and related bacteria. *Int. J. Syst. Bacteriol.* **41:**31–38.

105. **Paster, B. J., and F. E. Dewhirst.** 1988. Phylogeny of campylobacters, wolinellas, *Bacteroides gracilis,* and *Bacteroides ureolyticus* by 16S ribosomal ribonucleic acid sequencing. *Int. J. Syst. Bacteriol.* **38:**56–62.

106. **Penner, J. L.** 1988. The genus *Campylobacter:* a decade of progress. *Clin. Microbiol. Rev.* **1:**157–172.

107. **Prévot, A. R.** 1940. Etudes de systématique bactérienne. V. Essai de classification des vibrions anaérobies. *Ann. Inst. Pasteur* **64:**117–125.

108. **Romaniuk, P. J., B. Zoltowska, T. J. Trust, D. J. Lane, G. J. Olsen, N. R. Pace, and D. A. Stahl.** 1987. *Campylobacter pylori,* the spiral bacterium associated with human gastritis, is not a true *Campylobacter* sp. *J. Bacteriol.* **169:**2137–2141.

109. **Roop, R. M., II, R. M. Smibert, J. L. Johnson, and N. R. Krieg.** 1985. DNA homology studies of the catalase-negative campylobacters and "*Campylobacter fecalis,*" an emended description of *Campylobacter sputorum,* and proposal of the neotype strain of *Campylobacter sputorum. Can. J. Microbiol.* **31:**823–831.

110. **Roop, R. M. II, R. M. Smibert, J. L. Johnson, and N. R. Krieg.** 1985. *Campylobacter mucosalis* (Lawson, Leaver, Pettigrew, and Rowland 1981) comb. nov.: emended description. *Int. J. Syst. Bacteriol.* **35:**189–192.

111. **Rosseel, P., J. Breynaert, P. Vandamme, and S. Lauwers.** 1998. Identification of *Campylobacter* species isolated from human faeces by cellular fatty acid analysis, p. 236–241. *In* A. J. Lastovica, D. J. Newel, and E. Lastovica (ed.), *Proceedings of the IXth International Workshop on Campylobacter, Helicobacter, and Related Organisms,* Cape Town, South Africa. Institute of Child Health, University of Cape Town, Cape Town, South Africa.

112. **Salama, S. M., M. M. Garcia, and D. E. Taylor.** 1992. Differentiation of the subspecies of *Campylobacter fetus* by genome sizing. *Int. J. Syst. Bacteriol.* **42:**446–450.

113. **Sandstedt, K., and J. Ursing.** 1991. Description of *Campylobacter upsaliensis* sp. nov. previously known as the CNW group. *Syst. Appl. Microbiol.* **14:**39–45.

114. **Sandstedt, K., J. Ursing, and M. Walder.**

1983. Thermotolerant *Campylobacter* with no or weak catalase activity isolated from dogs. *Curr. Microbiol.* **8:**209–213.

115. **Schumacher, W., P. M. H. Kroneck, and N. Pfennig.** 1992. Comparative systematic study on "*Spirillum*" 5175, *Campylobacter* and *Wolinella* species. Description of "*Spirillum*" 5175 as *Sulfurospirillum deleyanum* gen. nov., sp. nov. *Arch. Microbiol.* **158:**287–193.

116. **Sebald, M., and M. Véron.** 1963. Teneur en bases de l'ADN et classification des vibrions. *Ann. Inst. Pasteur* **105:**897–910.

117. **Shen, Z., J. G. Fox, F. E. Dewhirst, B. J. Paster, C. J. Foltz, L. Yan, B. Shames, and L. Perry.** 1997. *Helicobacter rodentium* sp. nov., a urease-negative *Helicobacter* species isolated from laboratory mice. *Int. J. Syst. Bacteriol.* **47:**627–634.

118. **Skirrow, M. B.** 1977. *Campylobacter* enteritis: a "new" disease. *Br. Med. J.* **2:**9–11.

119. **Smith, T.** 1918. Spirilla associated with disease of the fetal membranes in cattle (infectious abortion). *J. Exp. Med.* **28:**701–721.

120. **Smith, T., and M. L. Orcutt.** 1927. Vibrios from calves and their serological relation to *Vibrio fetus*. *J. Exp. Med.* **45:**391–397.

121. **Smith, T., and M. S. Taylor.** 1919. Some morphological and biochemical characters of the spirilla (*Vibrio fetus* n. sp.) associated with disease of the fetal membranes in cattle. *J. Exp. Med.* **30:**299–312.

122. **Snaidr, J., R. Amann, I. Huber, W. Ludwig, and K.-H. Schleifer.** 1997. Phylogenetic analysis and in situ identification of bacteria in activated sludge. *Appl. Environ. Microbiol.* **63:**2884–2896.

123. **Stackebrandt, E., V. Fowler, H. Mell, and A. Kröger.** 1987. 16S rRNA analysis and the phylogenetic position of *Wolinella succinogenes*. *FEMS Microbiol. Lett.* **40:**269–272.

124. **Stackebrandt, E., and B. M. Goebel.** 1994. Taxonomic note: a place for DNA-DNA reassociation and 16S rRNA sequence analysis in the present species definition in bacteriology. *Int. J. Syst. Bacteriol.* **44:**846–849.

125. **Stanley, J., A. P. Burnens, D. Linton, S. L. W. On, M. Costas, and R. J. Owen.** 1992. *Campylobacter helveticus* sp. nov., a new thermophilic species from domestic animals: characterization and cloning of a species-specific DNA probe. *J. Gen. Microbiol.* **138:**2293–2303.

126. **Stanley, J., D. Linton, A. P. Burnens, F. E. Dewhirst, R. J. Owen, A. Porter, S. L. W. On, and M. Costas.** 1993. *Helicobacter canis* sp. nov., a new species from dogs: an integrated study of phenotype and genotype. *J. Gen. Microbiol.* **139:**2495–2504.

127. **Stanley, J., D. Linton, A. P. Burnens, F. E. Dewhirst, S. L. W. On, A. Porter, R. J. Owen, and M. Costas.** 1994. *Helicobacter pullorum* sp. nov., genotype and phenotype of a new species isolated from poultry and from human patients with gastroenteritis. *Microbiology* **140:**3441–3449.

128. **Steele, T. W., and R. J. Owen.** 1988. *Campylobacter jejuni* subsp. *doylei* subsp. nov., a subspecies of nitrate-negative campylobacters isolated from human clinical specimens. *Int. J. Syst. Bacteriol.* **38:**316–318.

129. **Stolz, J. F., D. J. Ellis, J. Switzer Blum, D. Ahmann, D. R. Lovley, and R. S. Oremland.** 1999. *Sulfurospirillum barnesii* sp. nov. and *Sulfurospirillum arsenophilus* sp. nov., new members of the *Sulfurospirillum* clade of the Epsilon Proteobacteria. *Int. J. Syst. Bacteriol.,* **49:**1177–1180.

130. **Tanner, A. C. R., M. A. Listgarten, and J. L. Ebersole.** 1984. *Wolinella curva* sp. nov.: "*Vibrio succinogenes*" of human origin. *Int. J. Syst. Bacteriol.* **34:**275–282.

131. **Tanner, A. C. R., S. Badger, C.-H. Lai, M. A. Listgarten, R. A. Visconti, and S. S. Socransky.** 1981. *Wolinella* gen. nov., *Wolinella succinogenes* (*Vibrio succinogenes* Wolin et al.) comb. nov., and description of *Bacteroides gracilis* sp. nov., *Wolinella recta* sp. nov., *Campylobacter concisus* sp. nov., and *Eikenella corrodens* from humans with periodontal disease. *Int. J. Syst. Bacteriol.* **31:**432–445.

132. **Teske, A., P. Sigalevich, Y. Cohen, and G. Muyzer.** 1996. Molecular identification of bacteria from a coculture by denaturing gradient gel electrophoresis of 16S ribosomal DNA fragments as a tool for isolation in pure cultures. *Appl. Environ. Microbiol.* **62:**4210–4215.

133. **Thompson, L. M., R. M. Smibert, J. L. Johnson, and N. R. Krieg.** 1988. Phylogenetic study of the genus *Campylobacter*. *Int. J. Syst. Bacteriol.* **38:**190–200.

134. **Totten, P. A., C. L. Fennell, F. C. Tenover, J. M. Wezenberg, P. L. Perine, W. E. Stamm, and K. K. Holmes.** 1985. *Campylobacter cinaedi* (sp. nov.) and *Campylobacter fennelliae* (sp. nov.): two new *Campylobacter* species associated with enteric disease in homosexual men. *J. Infect. Dis.* **151:**131–139.

135. **Trivett-Moore, N. I., W. D. Rawkuson, M. Yuen, and G. L. Gilbert.** 1997. *Helicobacter westmaedii* sp. nov., a new species isolated from blood cultures of two AIDS patients. *J. Clin. Microbiol.* **35:**1144–1150.

136. **Tunicliff, R.** 1914. An anaerobic vibrio isolated from a case of acute bronchitis. *J. Infect. Dis.* **15:**350–351.

137. **Ursing, J. B., R. A. Rossello-Mora, E. Garcia-Valdes, and J. Lalucat.** 1995. Taxonomic note: a pragmatic approach to the nomenclature of phenotypically similar genomic groups. *Int. J. Syst. Bacteriol.* **45**:604.

138. **Vandamme, P., and H. Goossens.** 1992. Taxonomy of *Campylobacter, Arcobacter,* and *Helicobacter:* a review. *Zentralbl. Bakteriol.* **276**:447–472.

139. **Vandamme, P., and J. De Ley.** 1991. Proposal for a new family, *Campylobacteraceae. Int. J. Syst. Bacteriol.* **41**:451 455.

140. **Vandamme, P., B. Pot, M. Gillis, P. De Vos, K. Kersters, and J. Swings.** 1996. Polyphasic taxonomy, a consensus approach to bacterial classification. *Microbiol. Rev.* **60**:407–438.

141. **Vandamme, P., M. I. Daneshvar, F. E. Dewhirst, B. J. Paster, K. Kersters, H. Goossens, and C. W. Moss.** 1995. Chemotaxonomic analyses of *Bacteroides gracilis* and *Bacteroides ureolyticus* and reclassification of *B. gracilis* as *Campylobacter gracilis* comb. nov. *Int. J. Syst. Bacteriol.* **45**:145–152.

142. **Vandamme, P., F. E. Dewhirst, B. J. Paster, and S. L. W. On.** Genus *Campylobacter* Sebald and Véron 1963, 907. *In* N. R. Krieg, J. Staley, and D. J. Brenner (ed.), *Bergey's Manual of Systematic Bacteriology,* vol. 2, 2nd ed., in press. The Williams & Wilkins Co., Baltimore, Md.

143. **Vandamme, P., E. Falsen, B. Pot, B. Hoste, K. Kersters, and J. De Ley.** 1989. Identification of EF group 22 campylobacters from gastroenteritis cases as *Campylobacter concisus. J. Clin. Microbiol.* **27**:1775–1781.

144. **Vandamme, P., E. Falsen, B. Pot, K. Kersters, and J. De Ley.** 1990. Identification of *Campylobacter cinaedi* isolated from blood and feces of children and adult females. *J. Clin. Microbiol.* **28**:1016–1020.

145. **Vandamme, P., E. Falsen, R. Rossau, B. Hoste, P. Segers, R. Tytgat, and J. De Ley.** 1991. Revision of *Campylobacter, Helicobacter,* and *Wolinella* taxonomy: emendation of generic descriptions and proposal of *Arcobacter* gen. nov. *Int. J. Syst. Bacteriol.* **41**:88–103.

146. **Vandamme, P., B. Pot, and K. Kersters.** 1991. Differentiation of campylobacters and *Campylobacter*-like organisms by numerical analysis of one-dimensional electrophoretic protein patterns. *Syst. Appl. Microbiol.* **14**:57–66.

147. **Vandamme, P., B. Pot, E. Falsen, K. Kersters, and J. De Ley.** 1990. Intra- and interspecific relationships of veterinary campylobacters revealed by numerical analysis of electrophoretic protein profiles and DNA:DNA hybridizations. *Syst. Appl. Microbiol.* **13**:295–303.

148. **Vandamme, P., L.-J. van Doorn, S. T. Al** Rashid, **W. G. V. Quint, J. van der Plas, V. L. Chan, and S. L. W. On.** 1997. *Campylobacter hyoilei* Alderton et al. 1995 and *Campylobacter coli* Véron and Chatelain 1973 are subjective synonyms. *Int. J. Syst. Bacteriol.* **47**:1055–1060.

149. **Vandamme, P., M. Vancanneyt, B. Pot, L. Mels, B. Hoste, D. Dewettinck, L. Vlaes, C. Van Den Borre, R. Higgins, J. Hommez, K. Kersters, J.-P. Butzler, and H. Goossens.** 1992. Polyphasic taxonomic study of the emended genus *Arcobacter* with *Arcobacter butzleri* comb. nov. and *Arcobacter skirrowii* sp. nov., an aerotolerant bacterium isolated from veterinary specimens. *Int. J. Syst. Bacteriol.* **42**:344–356.

150. **van Doorn, L.-J., B. A. J. Giesendorf, R. Bax, B. A. M. van der Zeijst, P. Vandamme, and W. G. V. Quint.** 1997. Molecular discrimination between *Campylobacter jejuni, Campylobacter coli, Campylobacter lari* and *Campylobacter upsaliensis* by polymerase chain reaction based on a novel putative GTPase gene. *Mol. Cell. Probes* **11**:177–185.

151. **Van Etterijck, R., J. Breynaert, H. Revets, T. Devreker, Y. Vandenplas, P. Vandamme, and S. Lauwers.** 1996. Isolation of *Campylobacter concisus* from feces of children with and without diarrhea. *J. Clin. Microbiol.* **34**:2304–2306.

152. **Véron, M., and R. Chatelain.** 1973. Taxonomic study of the genus *Campylobacter* Sebald and Véron and designation of the neotype strain for the type species *Campylobacter fetus* (Smith and Taylor) Sebald and Véron. *Int. J. Syst. Bacteriol.* **23**:122–134.

153. **Vinzent, R.** 1949. Une affection méconnue de la grossesse l'infection placentaire a *Vibrio foetus. Presse Med.* **81**:1230.

154. **Vinzent, R., J. Dumas, and N. Picard.** 1947. Septicemie grave eu cours de la grossesse, due à un vibrion. Avortement consecutif. *C. R. Acad. Med.* **131**:90.

155. **van Graevenitz, A.** 1990. Revised nomenclature of *Campylobacter laridis, Enterobacter intermedium,* and "*Flavobacterium branchiophila*" *Int. J. Syst. Bacteriol.* **40**:211.

156. **Voordouw, G., S. M. Armstrong, M. F. Reimer, B. Foutz, A. J. Telang, Y. Shen, and D. Gevertz.** 1996. Characterization of 16S rRNA genes from oil field microbial communities indicates the presence of a variety of sulfate-reducing, fermentative, and sulfide-oxidizing bacteria. *Appl. Environ. Microbiol.* **5**:1623–1629.

157. **Warren, J. R., and B. Marshall.** 1983. Unidentified curved bacilli on gastric epithelium in active chronic gastritis. *Lancet* **1**:1273–1275.

158. **Wayne, L. G., D. J. Brenner, R. R. Colwell, P. A. D. Grimont, P. Kandler, M. I. Kri-**

chevsky, L. H. Moore, W. E. C. Moore, R. G. E. Murray, E. Stackebrandt, M. P. Starr, and H. G. Trüper. 1987. Report of the ad hoc committee on reconciliation of approaches to bacterial systematics. *Int. J. Syst. Bacteriol.* **37:** 463–464.

159. **Wesley, I. V., L. Schroeder-Tucker, A. L. Baetz, F. E. Dewhirst, and B. J. Paster.** 1995. *Arcobacter*-specific and *Arcobacter butzleri*-specific 16S rRNA-based DNA probes. *J. Clin. Microbiol.* **33:**1691–1698.

160. **Wolfe, R. S., and N. Pfennig.** 1977. Production of sulfur by *Spirillum* 5175 and syntrophism with *Chlorobium*. *Appl. Environ. Microbiol.* **33:** 427–433.

161. **Wolin, M. J., E. A. Wolin, and N. J. Jacobs.** 1961. Cytochrome-producing anaerobic vibrio, *Vibrio succinogenes,* sp. n. *J. Bacteriol.* **81:**911–917.

NEW DEVELOPMENTS IN THE SUBTYPING OF *CAMPYLOBACTER* SPECIES

D. G. Newell, J. A. Frost, B. Duim, J. A. Wagenaar, R. H. Madden, J. van der Plas, and S. L. W. On

2

In England and Wales, where human campylobacter infections have been actively monitored, the incidence of disease has increased annually since the introduction of effective isolation methods and selective media during the 1970s. Although the majority of the 58,000 isolates in 1998 tended to be reported simply as "*Campylobacter*," the available data suggest that the majority (about 90%) are *C. jejuni,* with 10% being *C. coli* and less than 1% being *C. lari* (9, 37).

The subtyping of these *Campylobacter* spp. remains an important requirement for epidemiological studies especially for (i) tracing sources and routes of transmission of human infections, (ii) identifying and monitoring, both temporally and geographically, specific strains with important phenotypic characteris-

tics, and (iii) developing strategies to control organisms within the food chain.

The criteria required for campylobacter subtyping methods have been well defined (58, 79). Given the sheer numbers of campylobacter strains encountered by some reference laboratories speed, cost and ease of use are of prime importance, while discriminatory power is of greater importance for many research purposes. In the former case, the phenotypic methods, such as serotyping and phage typing, are the method of choice (74, 78). In recent years these techniques have been refined and simplified to extend their usefulness for routine purposes in clinical laboratories. However, genetically based methods, with their enhanced sensitivity and discrimination and improving availability, show most promise for research purposes. Genotypic techniques, such as *fla* typing and pulsed-field gel electrophoresis (PFGE), are now being successfully applied to epidemological studies, especially for campylobacters from veterinary sources. Nevertheless, a combination of phenotypic and/or genotypic typing methods may be advisable for some epidemiological studies (78).

A previous review of campylobacter subtyping (79) comprehensively described and evaluated the methods then available. These methods were primarily phenotypic and included

D. G. Newell, Veterinary Laboratories Agency (Weybridge), New Haw, Addlestone, Surrey KT15 3NB, United Kingdom. *J. A. Frost,* Campylobacter Reference Unit, Laboratory of Enteric Pathogens, Central Public Health Laboratory, Colindale Avenue, London NW9 5HT, United Kingdom. *B. Duim and J. A. Wagenaar,* Institute for Animal Science and Health (ID-Lelystad), P.O. Box 65, 8200 AB Lelystad, The Netherlands. *R. H. Madden,* Food Microbiology, DANI/QUB, Agricultural and Food Science Centre, Belfast BT9 5PX, Northern Ireland. *J. van der Plas,* Food Microbiology Department, TNO Nutrition and Food Research Institute, P.O. Box 360, 3700 AJ Zeist, The Netherlands. *S. L. W. On,* Danish Veterinary Laboratory, Bulowsvej 27, DK 1790 Copenhagen V, Denmark.

Campylobacter, 2nd Ed., Edited by I. Nachamkin and M. J. Blaser
© 2000 American Society for Microbiology, Washington, D.C.

serotyping and phage typing. Here we describe both recent modifications to these well-established phenotypic techniques and the recent development and application of genotypic techniques. For a more comprehensive review of *Campylobacter* genotyping techniques and applications, see reference 104. We also speculate about further developments which may enable these techniques to become more readily available and applicable in the near future.

SEROTYPING

Two serotyping schemes for campylobacters were developed in Canada in the 1980s and have been used either separately or together (81). The Penner scheme (82) was based on soluble heat-stable (HS) antigens, while the Lior scheme (51) detected variation in heat-labile (HL) antigens. The Penner scheme has been more extensively applied and was therefore used as the basis for the scheme recently developed in the Laboratory of Enteric Pathogens (LEP), Public Health Laboratory Service, United Kingdom. This new scheme now forms the basis of reference typing in the United Kingdom (19).

The LEP serotyping scheme for *C. jejuni* and *C. coli* has addressed the two principal limitations described for the Penner scheme. Reproducibility problems due to variations in erythrocytes (74) have been eliminated by adopting a direct bacterial agglutination method similar to that used for serogrouping schemes of other enteric pathogens. The nonspecific reactions observed in the original serotyping studies of *Vibrio fetus* (5) have been eliminated by incubating the reaction mixtures at 50°C with gentle shaking and reading the result immediately on removal from the shaker. The Penner method uses passive haemagglutination (PHA); that is, the supernatant from a boiled cell suspension is used to sensitize erythrocytes, which in turn are mixed with antisera to demonstrate agglutination. Although the PHA method is most efficient for soluble antigens, it had been assumed that the *C. jejuni* HS antigens were lipopolysaccharide (LPS) (82). While long-chain LPS has been detected in serotypes of *C. jejuni* in some studies (83), only LPS core

and short-chain polysaccharide have been detected in other studies (52). There is some evidence that the HS antigen may be analogous to the LPS of *Neisseria* and *Haemophilus* (63). It has also been suggested that the antigen detected by PHA and direct agglutination is capsular (11). For a comprehensive review of the nature and function of the HS antigens of the Penner system, see reference 64.

The use of unabsorbed antisera in the Penner scheme resulted in a high proportion of isolates reacting with more than one antiserum (83, 84), and these cross-reactions varied in expression (62). This problem has been addressed by using absorbed antisera. This has resulted in a scheme that currently defines 48 HS serotypes in *C. jejuni* and 17 in *C. coli* (20a).

The LEP method was evaluated by using 2,407 *C. jejuni* and 182 *C. coli* isolates (19). A total of 47 serotypes were identified in *C. jejuni*, of which 20 each accounted for more than 1% of the total and further 16 each accounted for 1 to 5% of the isolates. In *C. coli*, 15 serotypes were identified; 6 of these were represented by a single isolate.

Levels of typeability have always been of concern in serotyping schemes. Certainly, high levels of non-typeability with the Penner serotyping technique have been identified in human isolates (up to 63%) from some countries (3, 68) but in general nontypeability in human and veterinary strains is less than 20% (44, 67). With the LEP serotyping scheme, 19% of human isolates were nontypeable (19.4% *C. jejuni* and 12.1% *C. coli*) (19), however, studies using this scheme indicate that up to 40% of poultry isolates from the United Kingdom are nontypeable (67a).

The high levels of nontypeable strains is not surprising given that the Penner-type strains are representative of campylobacters prevalent in the early 1980s and the majority were isolated in Canada. Antisera raised against recent nontypeable isolates are currently being used to extend the LEP scheme and reduce the proportion of nontypeable isolates in the United Kingdom by defining new types. Prospective new types are identified as clusters of nonserotypeable isolates which are epidemiologically related and have common patterns by one or more other typing or fingerprinting techniques. Three such new types have been defined to date (20a).

PHAGE TYPING

Given the large numbers of isolates belonging to the most prevalent serotypes and the high level of nontypeability observed with the current reagents, further subtyping is usually required for epidemiological studies in which serotyping is the primary method. In some circumstances, phage typing is now being employed as an extension to serotyping.

Campylobacter phage-typing schemes have been described by Grajewski et al. in the United States (30), Salama et al. in the United Kingdom (87), and Khakhria and Lior in Canada (46). All three schemes had some common phages. The original scheme, developed in the United States, used 14 virulent bacteriophages isolated from poultry feces. The scheme developed in the United Kingdom combined 6 phages from the original U.S. collection with 10 virulent phages isolated from various sources in the United Kingdom, including pig and poultry manure and sewage effluent. The U.S. scheme was subsequently extended to form the Canadian scheme by the addition of five phages isolated from chicken litter in Canada.

The U.K. phage-typing scheme is now routinely used as an adjunct to serotyping for the epidemiological typing of strains of *C. jejuni* and *C. coli* in England and Wales (20). To date, a total of 76 defined phage types have been recognized. A phage type is defined as two or more epidemiologically unrelated isolates giving the same phage reaction pattern. The reference phages and propagating strains are available from the National Collection of Type Cultures, London, United Kingdom.

In one study (20), 57 phage types were identified among the 2,407 *C. jejuni* isolates typed. Nearly 60% of the strains were assigned to the 10 most common phage types. The nontypeability rate was about 15%, but a further 7.0% of strains were designated RDNC (React with the phages but Do Not Conform to a designated type). Most strains in this last category had unique phage reaction patterns.

RELATIONSHIP BETWEEN SEROTYPE AND PHAGE TYPE

Serotyping generally classifies strains into broad groups. For example, in the LEP serotyping scheme, the 10 most common serotypes account for 53% of isolates tested (19). However, phage typing enables the subdivision of each of the 20 most common serotypes into 6 to 29 subtypes; the number of types reflects the degree of variation within serotypes (20). Nevertheless, within some serotypes one or two phage types predominate, and these groupings may indicate a closer clonal relationship.

The added value of supplementary subtyping in epidemiological investigations has already been demonstrated in outbreaks (16). This is particularly relevant when dominant serotypes, like HS50, or nonserotypeable strains are observed. Fewer than 3% of *C. jejuni* isolates are nontypeable by both serotyping and phage typing.

Given that there are, to date, 66 serotypes and 76 defined phage types in the two routine typing schemes used in the United Kingdom, a theoretical total of 5,016 different serotype-phage type combinations is possible, assuming that the two characteristics are unrelated. In the only comprehensive study so far, 336 serotype-phage type combinations were identified among a sample of only 2,407 *C. jejuni* isolates (20). This preliminary data suggests that these two phenotypic characteristics are probably related. However, independent expression within a clonal relationship cannot be eliminated.

The adoption of a hierarchical approach to phenotypic subtyping, using serotyping supported by phage typing to give an adequate level of discrimination for epidemiological purposes, is recommended (20).

PULSED-FIELD GEL ELECTROPHORESIS

PFGE is a modification of the more traditional restriction enzyme analysis (REA), which has been used for the subtyping of bacterial strains for several years. Although PFGE and REA both employ restriction site polymorphisms in bacterial DNA, there are several important differences between the methods. For PFGE, bacterial cells are embedded in chromosomal-grade agarose and lysed in situ to prevent DNA shearing. After extensive washing to remove contaminating chemicals (including formaldehyde, used by many workers to deactivate the DNase activity of some thermophilic campylobacter strains), thin slices of the DNA-containing blocks are cut and the restriction enzyme of choice is applied. For PFGE, the aim is to cut the target DNA into a relatively few, comparatively large fragments. Thus, "rare-cut-ting" enzymes are used. *Sma*I, *Sal*I, and *Kpn*I are commonly used for genotyping campylobacters. For this reason, DNA typing by PFGE is often referred to as macrorestriction profiling. The DNA fragments are then separated by a special electrophoretic method. By the coordinated application of pulsed electric fields from different positions in the electrophoresis cell, the DNA fragments are gently oriented and separated, according to size, within the agarose gel matrix. DNA-restriction fragment patterns are visualized by staining in ethidium bromide (Fig. 1).

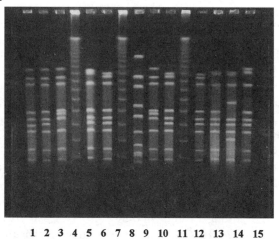

A

1 2 3 4 5 6 7 8 9 10 11 12 13 14 15

B

1 2 3 4 5 6 7 8 9 10 11 12 13 14 15

FIGURE 1 (A) *Sma*I-derived PFGE profiles of Danish isolates of human (lanes 1, 2, 5, 6, 10, 13, and 14: strains DVL 5118, DVL 5146, DVL 5029, DVL 5042b, DVL 5165, and DVL 5057, respectively) and poultry (lanes 3, 9, 12, and 15: strains DVL 992a, DVL 992b, DVL 1123, and DVL 1042, respectively) origin with no known epidemiological relationship. Lanes 4, 7, and 11 contain molecular weight markers (Lambda ladder). (B) *Kpn*I-derived PFGE profiles of *C. jejuni* isolates of human (lanes 9, 10, and 13 to 15: strains DVL 5026, DVL 5061, DVL 5192, DVL 5358, and DVL 5020 respectively), cattle (lanes 4 to 6, 8, 11, and 12; strains DVL 4006, DVL 4010, DVL 4037, DVL 4065, DVL 4111, and DVL 4165, respectively) and poultry (lanes 1 to 3: strains DVL 1203, DVL 1212, and DVL 1256, respectively) origin with no known epidemiological relationship. Lane 7 contains molecular weight markers. Sample preparation and electrophoresis conditions are given in reference 72.

PFGE is generally accepted as one of the most powerful tools currently available for microbial molecular epidemiology. The sensitivity of this technique lies in the fact that whole-genome restriction site polymorphisms are detected and strain differences are far easier to ascertain compared with the highly complex patterns obtained by REA. PFGE was originally used to determine the genome sizes of *C. jejuni, C. coli, C. lari,* and *C. fetus* and to construct a genetic map of a *C. jejuni* strain (10). A subsequent seminal study identified several restriction endonucleases that could be used in conjunction with PFGE to give DNA fragment patterns suitable for epidemiological investigations of *C. jejuni* and *C. coli* (108).

PFGE of *C. jejuni* and *C. coli*

Comparisons of the discriminatory potential of PFGE with other methods of typing *C. jejuni* and *C. coli* consistently show it to be extremely sensitive: only amplified fragment length polymorphism (AFLP) fingerprinting appears to equal its discriminatory capability (50). The contrast in sensitivity is particularly notable between PFGE and phenotypic methods, such as serotyping and phage typing, especially with isolates from nonclinical sources (26, 77, 93). Several studies have shown that *C. jejuni* strains within HS serotypes can be readily differentiated by PFGE, including HS1 (76, 78, 89), HS2 (26), HS4 (76, 77, 89), HS9 (53), HS11 (90), HS38 (53), HS55 (36), and HS63 (53). Interestingly, the levels of discrimination among HS serotypes vary, suggesting that some serotypes are more genetically stable than others. For example, of 90 HS4 isolates examined, 29 distinct *Sma*I-derived PFGE types were identified (76). In contrast, only 6 PFGE types were observed among 29 HS55 strains, of which 9 were outbreak related (36).

PFGE typing is also usually superior, in terms of discriminatory potential, to other molecular typing methods. It appears to be at least twice as discriminatory as ribotyping (26, 39), and two to three times more sensitive than *fla* typing when strains of *C. jejuni* HS1, HS4, HS11, and HS63 are examined (53, 89, 90).

PFGE is also at least as good as, if not marginally better than, a PCR-based fingerprinting method (using a combination of arbitrary and repetitive primer sequences) for the investigation of sporadic and outbreak-related *C. jejuni* strains (42). Similar results indicating the discriminatory power of PFGE have been reported in comparative studies with *C. coli* strains (92).

PFGE has been successfully used to group *C. jejuni* isolates from human outbreaks (14, 26, 42, 76, 97), the same poultry flock (72), and cattle and their drinking-water supply (33), as well as *C. coli* isolates from an outbreak of avian hepatitis (94). Application of the technique to examine sporadically isolated *C. jejuni* strains from Denmark (72), Finland (34), and the United Kingdom (76, 90) has identified groups of strains from human diarrhea and food animals that exhibit common PFGE patterns, suggesting related sources of infection. Similarly, the presence of stable clones of *C. coli* isolates from humans, poultry, cattle, and sheep has been supported by the concordance of *Sma*I-based PFGE profiles, ribotypes, and *flaA* restriction fragment length polymorphism (RFLP) patterns (92). The application of multiple restriction enzymes can be used to dictate especially stringent criteria for strain identity. This approach has been particularly useful to indicate the presence of "genetically identical" strains present among humans, cattle, and poultry (72).

Computer-assisted methods have also been applied to the interpretation of PFGE profiles. A numerical analysis of *Sma*I- and *Kpn*I-based PFGE patterns was used to examine relationships among HS serotype reference *C. jejuni* strains and nonserotypable isolates obtained in the field (27). The analyses presented successfully clustered some reference strains comprising the cross-reacting serotype 4 complex. However, the degree of discordance between clustering results from *Sma*I and *Kpn*I digests (and absence of additional phenotypic or genetic strain data for clarifying the integrity or otherwise of any clusters formed) complicates the evaluation of this approach for determining relationships between *C. jejuni* strains. Numerical analysis of combined *Sma*I and *Sal*I PFGE profiles of six *C. coli* strains maintained under continuous subculture for up to 50 passages did, however, cluster most profiles with the parent strain, even where differences between profiles were observed (70).

PFGE of Other *Campylobacter* Species

C. LARI

There appear to be no published studies evaluating the efficacy of PFGE profiling for epidemiological investigations of *C. lari*. However, PFGE has been used to size the *C. lari* genome (10, 57). Among the restriction enzymes tested, *Apa*I, *Sal*I, and *Sma*I, all appear to be suitable (57). The PFGE fragment profiles obtained by *Sal*I digestion can distinguish multiple profile types (10, 57) which are epidemiologically relevant. Thus, limited data available suggests that *Sal*I−based PFGE profiling may be a sensitive tool for studying the epidemiology of *C. lari*.

C. FETUS

Salama et al. (86) applied PFGE analysis to strains of *C. fetus* subsp. *fetus, C. fetus* subsp. *venerealis,* and *C. fetus* subsp. *venerealis* bv. intermedius (i.e., glycine-tolerant variants of subsp. *venerealis*) and showed that most strains assigned to these taxa could be distinguished by differences in their genome sizes. All subsp. *fetus* strains had a genome size of 1.1 Mb. In contrast, the genome size of most subsp. *venerealis* strains was 1.3 Mb, and subsp. *venerealis* bv. intermedius isolates were characterised by a genome size of 1.5 Mb. However, a few subsp. *venerealis* strains did possess a genome size consistent with subsp. *fetus* strains. The PFGE profiles also distinguish between the two subspecies (22, 39).

Results from published studies indicate that PFGE profiling is an effective means of genotyping *C. fetus,* since most unrelated strains can be readily distinguished. The validity of the method for epidemiological investigations of this species has been proven in outbreaks of human diarrheal illness in a closed community (85), nosocomially acquired meningitis in a neonatal intensive care unit (61), and ovine

abortion (67a). In all investigations, outbreak strains were readily distinguished from unrelated strains. Similarly, PFGE has been used to show that isolates of *C. fetus* subsp. *fetus* from multiple clinical samples (feces, blood, and, in one case, a cellulitis lesion) were identical in the same patient but differed between patients (41).

C. HYOINTESTINALIS

A total of 22 different *Sma*I-derived PFGE profiles were observed from 28 strains representing *C. hyointestinalis* subsp. *hyointestinalis, C. hyointestinalis* subsp. *lawsonii,* and two distinct but unclassified groups of *C. hyointestinalis*-like strains (71). In addition, certain features of the profiles obtained were taxon specific and could thus be used for identification purposes. The choice of restriction enzyme is critical. *Sal*I provided discrimination equal to *Sma*I for PFGE profiling *C. hyointestinalis* subsp. *hyointestinalis* in one study but was significantly less effective for typing the other taxa, since the DNA of most strains resisted digestion (71). Nevertheless, the DNA of the infective strain in an epidemiological investigation of a family outbreak of *C. hyointestinalis* (probably subsp. *hyointestinalis*) was digested only with *Sal*I and not with *Sma*I (88).

C. UPSALIENSIS

A range of restriction enzymes suitable for PFGE profiling of *C. upsaliensis* have been investigated (7). Of the enzymes examined (including *Sal*I, *Sac*II, *Sma*I, *Nru*I, *Nar*I, *Rsr*II, and *Bss*HII), only *Xho*I was able to produce suitable profiles for all strains tested. Although there is considerable genomic heterogeneity among *C. upsaliensis* strains, it appears that strains giving similar profiles are usually members of the same serogroup. However, this putative relationship requires substantiation. In addition, the ability of PFGE to identify outbreak strains of *C. upsaliensis* has apparently not yet been tested.

C. SPUTORUM

PFGE profiling is useful for typing *C. sputorum*. *Sma*I-based profiling demonstrated the long-term (12-month) stability and persistence of *C. sputorum* bv. paraureolyticus genotypes in a single dairy herd (73). Furthermore, most differences between banding patterns could be accounted for by mutational events in restriction sites, suggesting that herd isolates were derived from a single parent strain. Further examinations of unrelated strains with additional restriction enzymes *Sal*I, *Kpn*I, and *Bam*HI indicated that *C. sputorum* bv. sputorum and *C. sputorum* bv. paraureolyticus may represent distinct clonal lines of this species.

Disadvantages of PFGE Profiling

Although the discriminatory potential of PFGE profiling is excellent, a number of disadvantages are recognized. (i) Preparation of the DNA-containing agarose blocks is time-consuming and tedious. Although a rapid method for sample preparation has been described for other bacteria (23), its suitability for *Campylobacter* spp. is unknown. (ii) The DNase of some campylobacter strains must be deactivated to ensure that DNA samples do not degrade before electrophoresis. This generally involves pretreatment of bacterial cells with the toxic chemical formaldehyde (25) (iii) The apparatus used for the electrophoresis is specialized and expensive. (iv) The enzymes commonly used to produce PFGE profiles do not digest the DNA of some strains. (v) Interpretation of the results can be difficult since genetic instability, even during in vitro culture, can lead to minor or major changes in profiles (72, 98, 103; see chapter 18).

fla TYPING

The characteristic motility of *C. jejuni* is due to its possession of a single unsheathed polar flagellum at one end or both ends of the cell. As in many other bacteria, the flagellar filaments are composed of repeats of a flagellin subunit encoded by a gene designated *fla*. However, campylobacters have two flagellin genes (31, 69), designated *flaA* and *flaB*. In *C. jejuni,* these two flagellin genes (of approximately 1.7 kb) are tandemly arranged and separated by an intervening segment of approximately 0.2 kb (18). These genes are highly conserved, with 92% identity between *flaA* and *flaB* genes in individual isolates. However, the *fla* genes vary between isolates, which provides the basis of a typing scheme.

A comparison of *fla* genes from many bacterial species has shown that the N- and C-terminal regions of the encoded proteins are normally conserved and flank a variable domain (107) and that the variable domain can vary in both size and amino acid sequence. Comparison of the published sequences of the *flaA* genes of *C. jejuni* and *C. coli* revealed common regions at the N-terminal (170 amino acids) and C-terminal (100 amino acids) ends of the protein. Such a genetic structure can serve as the basis of a molecular typing method since primers can be synthesized based on the conserved sequences and a product incorporating both the conserved and variable regions can be prepared by PCR. This product can then be digested with appropriate restriction endonucleases to reveal RFLP after the products are separated by gel electrophoresis (Fig. 2).

The suitability of the *fla* genes for PCR-RFLP analysis has been recognized by several

FIGURE 2 *fla*-typing profiles of nine selected human *C. jejuni* strains (A to I) prepared by the method of Ayling et al. (4). Lanes: 2, 4, 6, 8, 10, 12, 14, 16, and 18, *Hin*fI digests of PCR products; 3, 5, 7, 9, 11, 13, 15, 17, and 19, *Dde*I digests of PCR products. Lanes 1 and 20 contain molecular weight markers.

TABLE 1 Regions of flagellin genes targeted in PCR–RFLP analyses and choice of restriction endonucleases

Region amplified	Restriction endonuclease(s)	Reference
Internal regions of *flaA* and *flaB*	*Pst*I + *Eco*RT	1
flaA	*Dde*I	65
flaA	*Hinf*I	75
Intergenic region between *flaA* and *flaB*	*Alu*I + *Dra*I	96
5′ ends of *flaA* and *flaB*	*Dde*I (now extended to include *Hinf*I)	4

groups, and a range of primer sets and restriction endonucleases has been applied (Table 1). The differences between the primers can result in significant variation in the profiles obtained from the same strains. However, there seems to be little variation in the level of discrimination observed. Conversely, the selection of enzymes has a significant effect on discrimination, and the combination of enzymes such as *Dde*I and *Hinf*I has been shown to enhance discrimination substantially in veterinary isolates (4a).

The level of discrimination of *fla* typing is generally reported to be much greater than that of serotyping but lower than that of PFGE, as discussed above. Unlike serotyping, it has a high typeability for human, veterinary, and environmental isolates (4, 55, 66). Both *C. jejuni* and *C. coli* are equally typeable by the method. Failure to *fla* type some isolates can be simply due to problems with DNA extraction. This problem can readily be overcome by alternative extraction methods, unlike the problem in serotyping "rough" strains, which remain nontypeable. Applicability of the technique to other *Campylobacter* spp. will be dependent on conservation of the primer sites, but about 50% of *C. jejuni* subsp. *doylei* strains are also typeable with the primer set of Ayling et al. (4, 50a), and this could be improved by adaptation of the primers.

Because of the presumed association of the HL serotyping scheme with flagellin, there have been several attempts to relate *fla*-type patterns to Lior serotypes. Initial studies indicated that the *flaA* profile was conserved within a given serogroup (1). However, later studies showed that this was an exception and that specific *fla*-types can be found in several serotypes

(8). Conversely, individual Penner serotypes, ribotypes, or PFGE profiles may display more than one *fla* type (89).

fla typing has been successfully applied to campylobacters from broiler flocks (4, 95, 99) in an effort to understand and hence control their manner of infection. Similarly, campylobacters from foodstuffs (55) and from animals and water (49, 53) have been investigated. This method has also been applied as an epidemiological tool to investigate human isolates clustered by Penner serotyping (90) including strains associated with Guillain-Barré syndrome (21).

Disadvantages of *fla* Typing

Application of *fla* typing is relatively simple and quick and involves widely available reagents and equipment. It has been easily adopted by many other laboratories around the world. Typeability is normally very high, but recalcitrant campylobacters may be located in specific geographic areas (56). All these characteristics make *fla* typing a very acceptable subtyping technique. Nevertheless, *fla* typing has a number of disadvantages that limit its applicability.

Comparison of results with those of other groups is currently hampered by the range of techniques used and, where groups used the same method, by the inherent difficulties in comparing electrophoresis profiles. Preliminary attempts at standardization, using software packages to analyze gel patterns and assign *fla* types, have been initiated. Such standardization is essential to address the issue of the difficulties involved in the manual interpretation of the banding patterns arising from PCR–RFLP.

Problems with using gel patterns to examine the variable region of the *fla* genes could be overcome by using relatively simple DNA sequence analysis. A short variable region of approximately 150 bp has been described (59), and sequencing of this region enables fingerprinting of strains. Such a method is now feasible because of the availability of rapid and relatively cheap DNA-sequencing facilities. Such a technique would obviate the need for interpretation of gel patterns and may therefore provide a more definitive *fla* typing scheme. However, the advantages of speed, general availability, and low cost of the PCR-RFLP technique would be lost.

Potentially one of the most significant disadvantages of *fla* typing is related to genetic instability. The ability of *C. jejuni/C. coli* strains to undergo recombinations within the *fla* genes has been previously demonstrated in vitro by using mutants labelled with antibiotic cassettes (2, 102). However, the relevance of this to the natural situation was unclear until Harrington et al. (35), comparing *flaA* sequences from 18 strains of *C. jejuni*, provided strong evidence for intergenomic recombination between *flaA* genes of different strains. Moreover, there was evidence for intragenomic recombination between the *flaA* and *flaB* genes of individual strains. The frequency of such events under natural conditions is currently unknown, but *fla* typing cannot be considered a particularly stable long-term typing method. Given these difficulties, the interpretation of *fla* types should be undertaken with care. For accurate analysis, *fla* typing needs to be supported by alternative phenotypic or genotypic methods.

RANDOM AMPLIFICATION OF POLYMORPHIC DNA

The random amplification of polymorphic DNA (RAPD) method of typing bacteria (105, 106) is based on the use of arbitrary primers which are allowed to bind to target DNA and then amplify sections by normal PCR. The method uses the entire genome of the target organism to generate amplified fragments, and the number and size of fragments are partially controlled by regulating the stringency of the reaction, for example by manipulation of the annealing temperature. Unlike some other PCR-based identification and typing methods, such as *fla* typing, RAPD does not require any prior knowledge of the target DNA sequence; the primers are of arbitrary sequence, and empirical experimentation is used to obtain an acceptable pattern of fragments of variable size.

The band patterns obtained are suitable for comparison of isolates within bacterial species. Moreover, some bands appear to be unique to certain groups of microorganisms (32). In the latter case, the unique bands can subsequently be utilized to detect specific organisms. In this way, species-specific probes have been developed to identify *C. jejuni*, *C. coli*, and *C. lari* from arbitrarily primed PCR products (12, 29). More commonly, the RAPD band patterns are used for subtyping and strain comparison. RAPD can provide a level of discrimination equal to (101) or greater than (6) that of PFGE.

RAPD fingerprinting has been applied to the typing of a range of human, animal, and environmental isolates of *C. jejuni*, *C. coli* and *C. lari* (38, 54). The degree of typeability varies: Hernandez et al. (38) found that 178 out of 208 strains were typeable whereas Madden et al. (54) found that all of 200 *C. coli* porcine isolates and 76 *C. jejuni* clinical isolates were typeable. The technique is highly discriminatory, giving unique profiles in clinical *C. jejuni* isolates except those which are outbreak associated and which give identical RAPD profiles (54). The results indicate a wide genetic diversity in these strains. Similar observations have been made for *C. lari* isolates (15). However, RAPD may be too sensitive for the study of *C. jejuni* isolates under some circumstances, and therefore it is recommended for use only in conjunction with another genotyping method (80).

Disadvantages of RAPD

RAPD is much quicker and cheaper than PFGE and does not require a complex apparatus. It is also less sensitive to genetic instability than *fla* typing. However, significant reproducibility problems have been associated with this method. These problems have largely limited the widespread application of RAPD for campylobacter subtyping. The causes of the lack of reproducibility are multiple. Meunier and Grimont (60) noted that the type of thermocycler used and the source of *Taq* DNA polymerase could significantly affect the patterns obtained and stated that "Unless standardised, the RAPD method does not enable constitution of a data bank of patterns for strain identification." However, recent technical advances in the control of thermocyclers and the commercial availability of preprepared reagents mean that standardized conditions are now more readily obtainable. Nevertheless, the diversity of procedures reported and the complexity of the patterns, with the inherent difficulties in interpretation of weak bands, will probably preclude the widespead acceptance or application of this technique.

AMPLIFIED FRAGMENT LENGTH POLYMORPHISM FINGERPRINTING

AFLP analysis is a new high-resolution genotyping method. It was originally developed for genotyping of plants (45) and has recently been adapted for genotyping bacteria (28, 40, 45, 47, 48, 91, 100). The value of AFLP analysis in the typing of campylobacters has recently been reported (13, 50).

AFLP analysis involves the digestion of chromosomal DNA with two restriction enzymes. Specific oligonucleotide adapters are then ligated to these restriction sites. The oligonucleotides must (i) allow ligation compatible with the restriction enzymes used for digestion, (ii) eliminate the restriction site after ligation, and (iii) create a template sequence for subsequent PCR amplification. By using primers containing one or more selected nucleotides extending beyond the restriction site at the 3′ ends, only a subset of fragments will be amplified under stringent PCR conditions. AFLP is not dependent on prior sequence knowledge, although the choice of restriction enzymes and selective nucleotides extending the primers must be optimized for different organisms to take into account genomic size and G + C content differences.

For the subtyping of campylobacters, two AFLP methods have now been described (13, 50). These methods use either *Hind*III and *Hha*I (13) or *Bgl*II and *Csp*6I (50). Different selective nucleotides, generating either 50 fragments of 50 to 450 bp (13) or 60 fragments of 35 to 500 bp (50) respectively, were also used. In both cases, the fragments generated were detected with fluorescently labelled primers and analyzed on an automated DNA sequencer. Both methods give AFLP banding patterns with excellent discrimination. Unrelated *C. jejuni* and *C. coli* strains show heterogeneous banding patterns (Fig. 3), while analysis of genetically related strains with identical *fla* or PFGE types also shows indistinguishable AFLP banding patterns (13, 50).

A comparison of AFLP with PFGE analysis showed that strains with minor differences in *Sma*I and *Sal*I PFGE profiles but substantive differences with *Bam*HI and *Kpn*I digests contained 17 AFLP fragment differences (50). Thus, AFLP and PFGE appear to provide the same level of discrimination. However, while PFGE involves the use of several restriction enzymes for optimal discrimination, AFLP uses only a single procedure (50).

AFLP has been successfully used to investigate the epidemiology of poultry campylobacters. The variation between AFLP fingerprints was sufficient to differentiate between individual strains (Fig. 3B). Preliminary analysis of AFLP banding patterns suggests that this technique can be used to determine genetic relationships between strains from diverse populations. Dendrograms constructed by using AFLP patterns indicate >95% relatedness between some Dutch human clinical and poultry isolates. Most clinical isolates showed AFLP patterns that grouped with poultry strains in clusters formed at the 60 to 70% similarity level (13). Similar studies in Denmark identified apparent clones of *C. jejuni* in human, poultry, and cattle isolates (50). Perhaps most importantly, AFLP can determine genetic similarity in *C. jejuni* isolates from meat products whereas

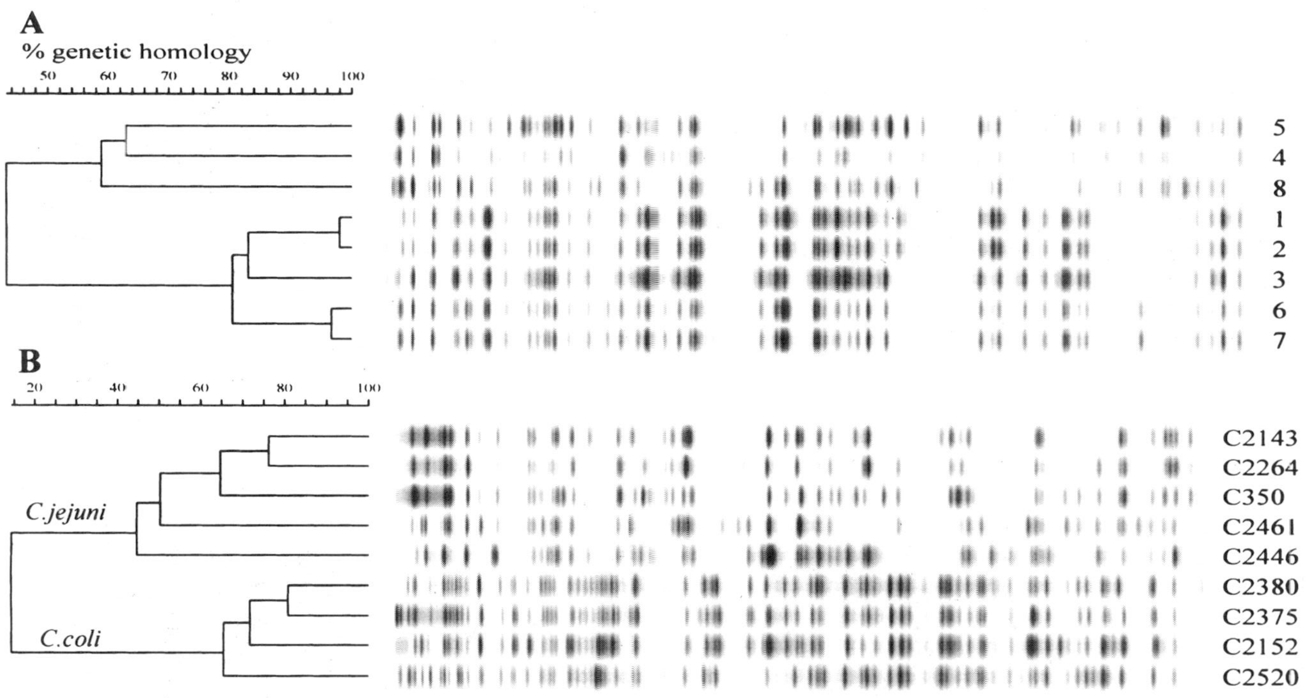

FIGURE 3 AFLP fingerprints generated from *HindIII* and *HhaI* templates by the method of Duim et al. (13). (A) *C. jejuni* strains isolated from poultry meat products as previously described (103). Samples 6 and 7 are *C. jejuni* 302a and 303a, respectively, with identical *SmaI* PFGE and *fla* types. Samples 3 to 5 and 8 are strains 331a, 318a, 307a, and 121a, respectively, which represent distinct PFGE types and *fla* types. Samples 1 and 2 are strain 81116 and its flagellin mutant 81153R, respectively, and are included as genetically related strains. (B) Randomly isolated *C. jejuni* and *C. coli* strains obtained from poultry during a longitudinal study (43). The dendrogram was constructed by the unweighted pair group method with arithmetic mean (UPGMA) with the Pearson product-moment correlation coefficient (GelCompar version 4.1).

PFGE fails to do so due to genetic instability (13).

Numerical analysis of AFLP patterns resulted in separate clusters of *C. jejuni* and *C. coli*. Other *Campylobacter* species (including *C. lari* and *C. fetus*) also show distinctive and species-specific banding patterns (13a).

Disadvantages of AFLP

The possible routine use of AFLP has become feasible because of the increasing availability of automated DNA sequencers. The technique is rapid and easily standardized, but the equipment is expensive. The digitization of AFLP results allows accurate interpretation, ease of data storage, and ready data exchange between laboratories. However, the complex nature of the patterns can make interpretation rather taxing. As with other molecular subtyping techniques, standardized procedures must be established to enable the exchange of AFLP data between laboratories. Although capital equipment costs may restrict the use of this tool to research laboratories, preliminary studies indicate that AFLP is an extremely attractive technique for investigating the molecular epidemiology of *Campylobacter* spp.

AUTOMATED RIBOTYPING

The presence of multiple copies of the rRNA genes (coding for 16S and 23S rRNA) at different positions on the chromosome and the strong conservation of these genes among bacteria make them suitable for typing purposes. The most commonly used technique is Southern blot hybridization of genomic DNA, digested with a six-cutter restriction enzyme and hybridized with a common rRNA probe. Most *Campylobacter* strains have three ribosomal gene copies, which is fewer than many other bacteria. This tends to reduce the discriminatory power of the method, although a 16S ribotyping scheme using a combination of *Hae*III and *Pst*I digestion identified over 80 types within *C. jejuni* (17).

This generally limited discriminatory power, in combination with the tedious nature of the technique, makes ribotyping generally unsuitable for the routine subtyping of campylobacters. However, the RiboPrinter system operates a completely automated and reproducible ribotyping procedure for identification and characterization of bacteria. After normalization to a set of molecular weight markers, the resultant rRNA fingerprint is compared to a dynamic database of RiboPrint patterns for characterization, and also to a fixed identification database. Preliminary experiments have shown that automated ribotyping with *Pst*I as the restriction enzyme could identify 29 different types (ribogroups) in a set of 48 reference strains isolated from geographically unrelated poultry flocks (discriminatory power [D] = 0.97) (99a). On basis of the ribogroups characterized, static patterns can be created and used for automated custom identification. In this way, the interpretation of patterns is more objective and well-defined ribotypes can be catalogued. Thus, automated ribotyping provides a unique opportunity for the interlaboratory exchange of data from a standard typing system. However, the substantial equipment and consumables costs and small sample throughput will certainly restrict the use of this technology.

CONCLUSIONS

Subtyping techniques play an important role in the monitoring of human *Campylobacter* infections, contributing to the identification of foodborne sources and ultimately leading to the development of targeted control strategies. Nevertheless, routine campylobacter subtyping is currently restricted to only a few laboratories. The poor availability of serotyping reagents will continue to restrict its use. However, with the development and refinement of genotyping methods, the routine subtyping of *Campylobacter* strains is feasible. The usefulness of such investigations will depend on the approaches adopted. For other enteric bacterial pathogens, like *Salmonella*, subtyping is used primarily to identify outbreaks. For campylobacters, the identification of outbreaks remains contentious. The majority of human cases are sporadic, and the rare outbreaks observed are usually caused by multiple strains, albeit from single contaminated sources (24). Nevertheless, some veterinary infections are obvious mini-outbreaks. In particular, infections in broiler houses are generally associated with a few strains or even only one strain, indicating single sources. Since the outbreaks are short-term, genetic instability is not generally thought to be a problem. Consequently, subtyping, especially genotyping, techniques are being actively applied to the molecular epidemiology of poultry campylobacters and are enabling the development of strategies to control infection in poultry by targeted biosecurity measures.

With an increasing knowledge of the molecular basis of campylobacter pathogenic mechanisms, it seems likely that virulence factors will be identified in the near future and that it will become feasible to relate the virulence potential of *Campylobacter* strains to phenotypic and genotypic characteristics. The ability to differentiate pathogenic from nonpathogenic strains by using relatively simple typing techniques would greatly improve the accuracy of risk assessment models and more closely define the important sources and route of transmission for human infection.

Finally, increasing interlaboratory collaboration to standardize and harmonize the subtyping techniques already in use and the new technologies under development, combined with rapidly improving numerical analysis software and information technology, will allow the establishment of Internet databases for subtype profiles. Such databases will be invaluable tools in the timely monitoring of worldwide changing trends in *Campylobacter* infections.

ACKNOWLEDGMENTS

All the authors of this chapter are participants in the EC-funded thematic network, CAMPYNET. We acknowledge the financial support of the Ministry of Agriculture, Fisheries and Foods, GB, Department of Health, United Kingdom. We also acknowledge the assistance of Alan Rigter for AFLP analysis and Kirsten Clow for the *fla* typing figure.

REFERENCES

1. **Alm, R. A., P. Guerry, and T. J. Trust.** 1993. Distribution and polymorphism of the flagellin genes from isolates of *Campylobacter coli* and *Campylobacter jejuni. J. Bacteriol.* **175:**3051–3057.
2. **Alm, R. A., P. Guerry, and T. J. Trust.** 1993. Significance of duplicated flagellin genes in *Campylobacter. J. Mol. Biol.* **230:**359–363.
3. **Asrat, D. A., A. Hathaway, E. S. Sjögren, E. Ekwall, and B. Kaijser.** 1997. The serotype distribution of *Campylobacter jejuni* and *Campylobacter coli* isolated from patients with diarrhea and controls in Tikur Anbassa Hospital, Addis Ababa, Ethiopia. *Epidemiol. Infect.* **118:**91–95.
4. **Ayling, R. D., M. J. Woodward, S. Evans, and D. G. Newell.** 1996. Restriction fragment length polymorphism of polymerase chain reaction products applied to the differentiation of poultry campylobacters for epidemiological investigations. *Res. Vet. Sci.* **60:**168–172.
4a. **Ayling, R. D.** Personal communication.
5. **Bokkenheuser, V.** 1972. *Vibrio fetus* infection in man: a serological test. *Infect. Immun.* **5:**222–226.
6. **Bolton, F. J., A. J. Fox, J. Gibson, R. H. Madden, J. E. Moore, L. Moran, P. Murphy, R. J. Owen, T. H. Pennington, T. Stanley, F. Thomson-Carter, D. R. A. Wareing, and T. Wilson.** 1996. A multicentre study of methods for sub-typing *Campylobacter jejuni*, p. 187–189. *In* D. G. Newell, J. M. Ketley, and R. A. Feldman (ed.), *Campylobacters, Helicobacters and Related Organisms.* Plenum Press, London, United Kingdom.
7. **Bourke, B., P. M. Sherman, D. Woodward, H. Lior, and V. L. Chan.** 1996. Pulsed-field gel electrophoresis indicates genotypic heterogeneity among *Campylobacter upsaliensis* strains. *FEMS Microbiol. Lett.* **143:**57–61.
8. **Burnens, A. P., J. Wagner, H. Lion, J. Nicolet, and J. Frey.** 1995. Restriction fragment length polymorphisms and the flagellar genes of the Lior heat-labile serogroup reference strains and field strains of *Campylobacter jejuni* and *Campylobacter coli. Epidemiol. Infect.* **114:**423–431.
9. **CDSC.** 1998. Common gastrointestinal infections, England and Wales. *Commun. Dis. Rep.* **8:**14.
10. **Chang, N., and D. E. Taylor.** 1990. Use of pulsed-field agarose gel electrophoresis to size genomes of *Campylobacter* species and to construct a *Sal*I map of *Campylobacter jejuni* UA580. *J. Bacteriol.* **172:**5211–5217.
11. **Chart, H., J. A. Frost, A. N. Oza, R. T. Thwaites, S. A. Gillanders, and B. Rowe.** 1996. Heat-stable serotyping antigens expressed by strains of *Campylobacter jejuni* are probably capsular and not long-chain lipopolysaccharide. *J. Appl. Bacteriol* **81:**635–640.
12. **Day, W. A., Jr, I. L. Pepper, and L. A. Joens.**

1997. Use of an arbitrarily primed PCR product in the development of *Campylobacter jejuni*-specific PCR. *Appl. Environm. Microbiol.* **63:** 1019–1023.

13. **Duim, B., T. M. Wassenaar, A. Rigter, and J. A. Wagenaar.** 1999. High-resolution genotyping of Campylobacter strains isolated from poultry and humans with AFLP fingerprinting. *Appl. Environ. Microbiol.* **65:**2369–2375.

13a. **Duim, B., and S. L. W. On.** Unpublished data.

14. **Engberg, J., P. Gerner-Smidt, F. Scheutz, E. M. Nielsen, S. L. W. On, and K. Mølbak.** 1998. Waterborne *Campylobacter jejuni* infection in a Danish town—a six-week continuous source outbreak. *Clin. Microbiol. Infect.* **4:** 648–656.

15. **Endtz, H. P., J. S. Vliegenthart, P. Vandamme, H. W. Weverink, N. P. van den Braak, H. A. Verbrugh, and A. van Belkum.** 1997. Genotypic diversity of *Campylobacter lari* isolated from mussels and oysters in The Netherlands. *Int. J. Food Microbiol.* **34:**79–88.

16. **Evans, M. R., W. J. Lane, J. A. Frost, and G. Nylen.** 1998. A campylobacter outbreak associated with stir-fried food. *Epidemiol. Infect.* **121:**275–279.

17. **Fayos, A., R. J. Owen, M. Desai, and J. Hernandez.** 1992. Ribosomal RNA gene restriction fragment diversity amoung Lior biotypes and Penner serotypes of *C. jejuni* and *C. coli.* *FEMS Microbiol. Lett.* **95:**87–94.

18. **Fischer, S. H., and I. Nachamkin.** 1991. Common and variable domains of the flagellin gene, *flaA*, in *Campylobacter jejuni.* *Mol. Microbiol.* **5:**1151–1158.

19. **Frost, J. A., A. N. Oza, R. T. Thwaites, and B. Rowe.** 1998 Serotyping scheme for *Campylobacter jejuni* and *Campylobacter coli* based on direct agglutination of heat stable antigens. *J. Clin. Microbiol.* **36:**335–339.

20. **Frost, J. A., J. M. Kramer, and S. A. Gillanders.** Phage typing of *Campylobacter jejuni* and *Campylobacter coli* and its use as an adjunct to serotyping. *Epidemiol. Infect.* **123:**47–55.

20a. **Frost, J. A.** Unpublished data.

21. **Fujimoto, S., B. M. Allos, N. Misawa, C. M. Patton, and M. J. Blaser.** 1997. Restriction fragment length polymorphism analysis and random amplified polymorphic DNA analysis of *Campylobacter jejuni* strains isolated from patients with Guillain-Barré syndrome. *J. Infect. Dis.* **176:** 1105–1108.

22. **Fujita, M., S. Fujimoto, T. Morooka, and K. Amako.** 1995. Analysis of strains of *Campylobacter fetus* by pulsed-field gel electrophoresis. *J. Clin. Microbiol.* **33:**1676–1678.

23. **Gautom, R. K.** 1997. Rapid pulsed-field gel electrophoresis protocol for typing of *Escherichia coli* O157:H7 and other gram-negative organisms in 1 day. *J. Clin. Microbiol.* **35:**2977–2980.

24. **Gent, R. N., D. R. Telford, and Q, Syed.** 1999. An outbreak of campylobacter food poisoning at a university campus. *Commun. Dis. Public Health* **2:**39–42.

25. **Gibson, J. R., K. Sutherland, and R. J. Owen.** 1994. Inhibition of DNAse activity in PFGE analysis of DNA from *Campylobacter jejuni.* *Lett. Appl. Microbiol.* **19:**357–358.

26. **Gibson, J. R., C. Fitzgerald, and R. J. Owen.** 1995. Comparison of PFGE, ribotyping and phage-typing in the epidemiological analysis of *Campylobacter jejuni* serotype HS2 infections. *Epidemiol. Infect.* **115:**215–225.

27. **Gibson, J., E. Lorenz, and R. J. Owen.** 1997. Lineages within *Campylobacter jejuni* defined by numerical analysis of pulsed-field gel electrophoretic DNA profiles. *J. Med. Microbiol.* **46:** 157–163.

28. **Gibson, J. R., J. R. Slater, J. Xerry, D. S. Tompkins, and R. J. Owen.** 1998. Use of an amplified-fragment length polymorphism technique to fingerprint and differentiate isolates of *Helicobacter pylori.* *J. Clin. Microbiol.* **36:** 2580–2585.

29. **Giesendorf, B. A. J., A. van Belkum, A. Koeken, H. Stegeman, H. H. Henkens, J. van der Plas, H. Goossens, H. G. M. Niesters, and W. G. V. Quint.** 1993. Development of a species specific DNA probes for *Campylobacter jejuni, Campylobacter coli,* and *Campylobacter lari* by PCR fingerprinting. *J. Clin. Microbiol.* **31:** 1541–1546.

30. **Grajewski, B. A., J. W. Kusek, and H. M. Gelfand.** 1985. Development of a bacteriophage typing scheme for *Campylobacter jejuni* and *Campylobacter coli.* *J. Clin. Microbiol.* **22:**13–18.

31. **Guerry, P., R. A. Alm, M. E. Power, S. M. Logan, and T. J. Trust.** 1991. Role of two flagellin genes in *Campylobacter* motility. *J. Bacteriol.* **173:**4757–4764.

32. **Hadrys, H., M. Balick, and B. Schierwater.** 1992. Applications of random amplified polymorphic DNA (RAPD) in molecular ecology. *Mol. Ecol.* **1:**55–63.

33. **Hänninen, M.-L., M. Niskanen, and L. Korhonen.** 1998. Water as a reservoir for *Campylobacter jejuni* infection in cows studied by serotyping and pulsed-field gel electrophoresis (PFGE). *Zentral. Veterinaermed. Reihe C* **45:**37–42.

34. **Hänninen, M.-L., S. Pajarre, M.-L. Klossner, and H. Rautelin.** 1998. Typing of human *Campylobacter jejuni* isolates in Finland by pulsed-field gel electrophoresis. *J. Clin. Microbiol.* **36:** 1787–1789.

35. **Harrington, C. S., F. M. Thomson-Carter, and P. E. Carter.** 1997. Evidence for recombination in the flagellin locus of *Campylobacter jejuni:* implications for the flagellin gene typing scheme. *J. Clin. Microbiol.* **35:**2386–2392.

36. **Harrington, C. S., F. M. Thomson-Carter, and P. E. Carter.** Molecular epidemiological investigation of an outbreak of *Campylobacter jejuni* identifies a dominant clonal line within Scottish serotype HS55 populations. *Epidemiol. Infect.* **122:**367–375.

37. **Healing, T. D., M. H. Greenwood, and A. D. Pearson.** 1992. *Campylobacters* and enteritis. *Rev. Med. Microbiol.* **3:**159–167.

38. **Hernandez, J., A. Fayos, M. A. Ferrus, and R. J. Owen.** 1995. Random amplified polymorphic DNA fingerprinting of *Campylobacter jejuni* and *C. coli* isolated from human faeces, seawater and poultry products. *Res. Microbiol.* **146:**685–696.

39. **Hum, S., K. Quinn, J. Brunner, and S. L. W. On.** 1997. Evaluation of a PCR assay for identification and differentiation of *Campylobacter fetus* subspecies. *Aust. Vet. J.* **75:**827–831.

40. **Huys, G., R. Coopman, P. Janssen, and K. Kersters.** 1996. High-resolution genotypic analysis of the genus Aeromonas by AFLP fingerprinting. *Int. J. Syst. Bacteriol.* **46:**572–580.

41. **Ichiyama, S., S. Hirai, T. Minami, Y. Nishiyama, S. Shimizu, K. Shimokata, and M. Ohta.** 1998. *Campylobacter fetus* subspecies *fetus* cellulitis associated with bacteremia in debilitated hosts. *Clin. Infect. Dis.* **27:**252–255.

42. **Iriarte, M. P., and R. J. Owen.** 1996. Repetitive and arbitary primer DNA sequences in PCR-mediated fingerprinting of outbreak and sporadic isolates of *Campylobacter jejuni*. *FEMS Immunol. Med. Microbiol.* **15:**17–22.

43. **Jacobs-Reitsma, W., N. M. Bolder, and R. W. A. W. Mulder.** 1994. Caecal carriage of *Campylobacter* and *Salmonella* in Dutch broiler flocks at slaughter: a one-year study. *Poult. Sci.* **73:**1260–1266.

44. **Jacobs-Reitsma, W. F., H. M. E. Maas, and W. H. Jansen.** 1995. Penner serotyping of *Campylobacter* isolates from poultry, with absorbed pooled antisera. *J. Appl. Bacteriol.* **79:**286–291.

45. **Janssen, P., R. Coopman, G. Huys, J. Swings, M. Bleeker, P. Vos, M. Zabeau, and K. Kersters.** 1996. Evaluation of the DNA fingerprinting method AFLP as a new tool in bacterial taxonomy. *Microbiology* **142:**1881–1889.

46. **Khakhria, R., and H. Lior.** 1992. Extended phage-typing scheme for *Campylobacter jejuni* and *Campylobacter coli*. *Epidemiol Infect.* **108:**403–414.

47. **Kiem, P., A. Kalif, J. Schupp, K. Hill, S. E. Travis, K. Richmond, D. M. Adair, M. Hugh-Jones, C. R. Kuske, and P. Jackson.** 1997. Molecular evolution and diversity in *Bacillus anthracis* as detected by amplified fragment length polymorphism markers. *J. Bacteriol.* **179:**818–824.

48. **Koeleman, J. G. M., J. Stoof, D. J. Biesmans, P. H. M. Savelkoul, and C. M. J. E. Vandenbroucke-Grauls.** 1998. Comparison of amplified ribosomal DNA restriction analysis random amplified polymorphic DNA analysis, and amplified fragment length polymorphism fingerprinting for identification of *Acinetobacter* genomic species and typing of *Acinetobacter haumannii*. *J. Clin. Microbiol.* **36:**2522–2529.

49. **Koenraad, P. M., R. Ayling, W. C. Hazeleger, F. M. Rombouts, and D. G. Newell.** 1995. The speciation and subtyping of *Campylobacter* isolates from sewage plants and waste water from a connected poultry abattoir using molecular techniques. *Epidemiol. Infect.* **115:**485–494.

50. **Kokotovic, B., and S. L. W. On.** 1999. High-resolution genomic fingerprinting of *Campylobacter jejuni* and *Campylobacter coli* by analysis of amplified fragment length polymorphisms. *FEMS Microbiol. Lett.* **173:**77–84.

50a. **Lustovica, A.** Personal communication.

51. **Lior, H., D. L. Woodward, J. A. Edgar, L. J. Laroche, and P. Gill.** 1982. Serotyping of *Campylobacter jejuni* by slide agglutination based on heat-labile antigenic factors. *J. Clin. Microbiol.* **15:**761–768.

52. **Logan, S. M., and T. J. Trust.** 1984. Structural and antigenic heterogenicity of lipopolysaccharides of *Campylobacter jejuni* and *Campylobacter coli*. *Infect. Immun.* **45:**210–216.

53. **Lorenz, E., A. Lastovica, and R. J. Owen.** 1998. Subtypes of *Campylobacter jejuni* Penner serotypes 9, 38, and 63 from human infections, animals and water by pulsed field gel electrophoresis and flagellin gene analysis. *Lett. Appl. Microbiol.* **26:**179–182.

54. **Madden, R. H., L. Moran, and P. Scates.** 1996. Sub-typing of animal and human *Campylobacter spp.* using RAPD. *Lett. Appl. Microbiol.* **23:**167–170.

55. **Madden, R. H., L. Moran, and P. Scates.** 1998. Genetic typing of *Campylobacter* spp. isolated from retail packs of poultry in Northern Ireland, p. 572–573. *In Proceedings of the 44th International Congress of Meat Science and Technology,* vol. II. IRTA, Barcelona, Spain.

56. **Madden, R. H., L. Moran, and P. Scates.** 1998. Frequency of occurrence of *Campylobacter* spp. in red meats and poultry in Northern Ireland and their subsequent sub-typing using polymer-

ase chain reaction fragment length polymorphism and the random amplified polymorphic DNA method. *J. Appl. Microbiol.* **84:**703–708.

57. **Matsumoto, K., M. Matsuda, and C. Kaneuchi.** 1992. Analysis of chromosome-sized DNA from the bacterial genome of thermophilic *Campylobacter laridis* by pulsed-field gel electrophoresis and physical mapping. *Microbios* **71:** 7–14.

58. **Meinersmann, R. J.** 1998. Criteria for molecular typing methods, p. 582–583. *In* A. J. Lastovica, D. G. Newell, and E. E. Lastovica (ed.), *Campylobacter, Helicobacter and Related Organisms.* Institute of Child Health, University of Cape Town, Cape Town, South Africa.

59. **Meinersmann, R. J., L. O. Helsel, P. I. Fields, and K. L. Heitt.** 1997. Discrimination of *Campylobacter jejuni* isolates by *fla* gene sequences. *J. Clin. Microbiol.* **35:**2810–2814.

60. **Meunier, J.-R., and P. A. D. Grimont.** 1993. Factors affecting reproducibility of random amplified polymorphic DNA fingerprinting. *Res. Microbiol.* **144:**373–379.

61. **Morooka, T., A. Umeda, M. Fujita, H. Matano, S. Fujimoto, K. Yukitake, K. Amako, and T. Oda.** 1996. Epidemiologic application of pulsed-field gel electrophoresis to an outbreak of *Campylobacter fetus* meningitis in a neonatal intensive care unit. *Scand. J. Infect. Dis.* **28:** 269–270.

62. **Mills, S. D., B. Kuznier, B. Shames, B. Kurjanczyk, and J. L. Penner.** 1992. Variation of the O antigen of *Campylobacter jejuni in vivo. J. Med. Microbiol.* **36:**215–219.

63. **Moran, A. P., M. M. Prendergast, and B. J. Appelmelk.** 1996. Molecular mimicry of host structures by bacterial lipopolysaccharides and its contribution to disease. *FEMS Immunol. Med. Microbiol.* **16:**105–115.

64. **Moran, A. P., and J. L. Penner.** 1999. Serotyping of *C. jejuni* based on heat-stable antigens: relevance, molecular basis and implications for pathogenesis. *J. Appl. Microbiol.* **86:**361–377.

65. **Nachamkin, I., K. Bohachick, and C. M. Patton.** 1993. Flagellin gene typing of *Campylobacter jejuni* by restriction fragment length polymorphism analysis. *J. Clin. Microbiol.* **31:** 1531–1536.

66. **Nachamkin, I., H. Ung, and C. M. Patton.** 1996. Analysis of HL and O serotypes of *Campylobacter* strains by the flagellin gene typing system. *J. Clin. Microbiol.* **34:**277–281.

67. **Neilsen, E. M., J. Engberg, and M. Mogens.** 1997. Distribution of serotypes of *Campylobacter jejuni* and *C. coli* from Danish patients, poultry, cattle and swine. *FEMS Immunol. Med. Microbiol.* **19:**47–56.

67a. **Newall, D. G.** Unpublished data.

68. **Nishimura, M., M. Nukina, J. M. Yuan, B. Q. Shen, J. J. Ma, M. Ohta, T. Saida, and T. Uchiyama.** 1996. PCR-based restriction fragment length polymorphism (RFLP) analysis and serotyping of *Campylobacter jejuni* isolates from diarrhoeic patients in China and Japan. *FEMS Microbiol. Lett.* **142:**133–138.

69. **Nultjen, P. M. J., A. J. A. M. VanAsten, W. Gaastra, and B. A. M. van der Zeijst.** 1990. Structural and functional analysis of two *Campylobacter jejuni* flagellin genes. *J. Biol. Chem.* **265:** 17798–17804.

70. **On, S. L. W.** 1998. In vitro genotypic variation of *Campylobacter coli* documented by pulsed-field gel electrophoretic DNA profiling: implications for epidemiological studies. *FEMS Microbiol. Lett.* **165:**341–346.

71. **On, S. L. W., and P. Vandamme.** 1997. Identification and epidemiological typing of *Campylobacter hyointestinalis* subspecies by phenotypic and genotypic methods and description of novel subgroups. *Syst. Appl. Microbiol.* **20:**238–247.

72. **On, S. L. W., E. M. Nielsen, J. Engberg, and M. Madsen.** 1998. Validity of *Sma*I-defined genotypes of *Campylobacter jejuni* examined by *Sal*I, *Kpn*I, and *Bam*HI polymorphisms: evidence of identical clones infecting humans, poultry, and cattle. *Epidemiol. Infect.* **120:**231–237.

73. **On, S. L. W., H. I. Atabay, and J. E. L. Corry.** 1999. Clonality of *Campylobacter sputorum* bv. paraureolyticus determined by macrorestriction profiling and biotyping, and evidence for long-term persistence in cattle. *Epidemiol. Infect.* **122:**175–182.

74. **Owen, R. J., and J. R. Gibson.** 1995. Update on epidemiological typing of *Campylobacter. PHLS Microbiol. Digest* **12:**2–6.

75. **Owen, R. J., C. Fitzgerald, K. Sutherland, and P. Borman.** 1994. Flagellin gene polymorphism analysis of *Campylobacter jejuni* infecting man and other hosts and comparison with biotyping and somatic antigen serotyping. *Epidemiol. Infect.* **113:**221–234.

76. **Owen, R. J., K. Sutherland, C. Fitzgerald, J. Gibson, P. Borman, and J. Stanley.** 1995. Molecular subtyping scheme for serotypes HS1 and HS4 of *Campylobacter jejuni. J. Clin. Microbiol.* **33:**872–877.

77. **Owen, R. J., E. Slater, D. Telford, T. Donovan, and M. Barnham.** 1997. Subtypes of *Campylobacter jejuni* from sporadic cases of diarrhoeal disease at different locations in England are highly diverse. *Eur. J. Epidemiol.* **13:**837–840.

78. **Patton, C. M. I., K. Wachsmuth, G. M. Evins, J. A. Keihlbauch, B. D. Plikaytis, N. Troup, L. Tompkins, and H. Lior.** 1991.

Evaluation of 10 methods to distinguish epidemic-associated *Campylobacter* strains. *J. Clin. Microbiol.* **29**:680–688.

79. **Patton, C. M., and I. K. Wachsmuth.** 1993. Typing schemes: are current methods useful? p. 110–128. *In* I. Nachamkin, M. J. Blaser, and L. S. Tompkins (ed.), *Campylobacter jejuni: Current Status and Future Trends.* ASM Press, Washington, D.C.

80. **Payne, R. E., M. D. Lee, D. W. Dreesen, and H. M. Barnhart.** 1999. Molecular epidemiology of *Campylobacter jejuni* in broiler flocks using randomly amplified polymorphic DNA-PCR and 23S rRNA PCR and role of litter in its transmission. *Appl. Environ. Microbiol.* **65**:260–263.

81. **Penner, J. L.** 1988. The genus *Campylobacter:* a decade of progress. *Clin. Microbiol. Rev.* **1**:157–172.

82. **Penner, J. L., and J. N. Hennessey.** 1980. Passive haemagglutination technique for serotyping *Campylobacter fetus* subsp. *jejuni* on the basis of soluble heat stable antigens. *J. Clin. Microbiol.* **12**:732–737.

83. **Preston, M. A., and J. L. Penner.** 1987. Structural and antigenic properties of lipopolysaccharides from serotype reference strains of *Campylobacter jejuni. Infect. Immun.* **55**:1806–1812.

84. **Preston, M. A., and J. L. Penner.** 1989. Characterization of cross- reacting serotypes of *Campylobacter jejuni. Can. J. Microbiol.* **35**:265–273.

85. **Rennie, R. P., D. Strong, D. E. Taylor, S. M. Salama, C. Davidson, and H. Tabor.** 1994. *Campylobacter fetus* diarrhea in a hutterite colony: epidemiological observations and typing of the causative organism. *J. Clin. Microbiol.* **32**:721–724.

86. **Salama, S. M., M. M. Garcia, and D. E. Taylor.** 1992. Differentiation of the subspecies of *Campylobacter fetus* by genomic sizing. *Int. J. Syst. Bacteriol.* **42**:446–450.

87. **Salama, S. M., F. J. Bolton, and D. N. Hutchinson.** 1990. Application of a new phage-typing scheme to campylobacters isolated during outbreaks. *Epidemiol. Infect.* **104**:405–411.

88. **Salama, S. M., H. Tabor, M. Richter, and D. E. Taylor.** 1992. Pulsed-field gel electrophoresis for epidemiologic studies of *Campylobacter hyointestinalis* isolates. *J. Clin. Microbiol.* **30**:1982–1984.

89. **Santesteban, E., J. Gibson, and R. J. Owen.** 1996. Flagellin gene profiling of *Campylobacter jejuni* heat-stable serotype 1 and 4 complex. *Res. Microbiol.* **147**:641–649.

90. **Slater, E., and R. J. Owen.** 1998. Subtyping of *Campylobacter jejuni* Penner heat-stable (HS) serotype 11 isolates from human infections. *J. Med. Microbiol.* **47**:353–357.

91. **Sloos, J. H., P. Janssen, C. P. A. van Boven, and L. Dijkshoorn.** 1998. AFLP typing of *Stapylococcus epidermidis* in multiple sequential blood cultures. *Res. Microbiol.* **149**:221–228.

92. **Stanley, J., D. Linton, K. Sutherland, C. Jones, and R. J. Owen.** 1995. High-resolution genotyping of *Campylobacter coli* identifies clones of epidemiologic and evolutionary significance. *J. Infect. Dis.* **172**:1130–1134.

93. **Steele, M., B. McNab, L. Fruhner, S. DeGrandis, D. Woodward, and J. A. Odumeru.** 1998. Epidemiological typing of *Campylobacter* isolates from meat processing plants by pulsed-field gel electrophoresis, fatty acid profile typing, serotyping, and biotyping. *Appl. Environ. Microbiol.* **64**:2346–2349.

94. **Stephens, C. P., S. L. W. On, and J. A. Gibson.** 1998. An outbreak of infectious hepatitis in commercially reared ostriches associated with *Campylobacter coli* and *Campylobacter jejuni. Vet. Microbiol.* **61**:183–190.

95. **Stern, N. J., M. A. Myszewski, H. M. Barnhart, and D. W. Dreesen.** 1997. Flagellin A gene restriction polymorphism patterns of *Campylobacter* spp. isolates from broiler production sources. *Avian Dis.* **14**:899–905.

96. **Studer, E., M. Domke, B. Wegmüller, J. Lüthy, S. Schmid, and U. Candrian.** 1998. RFLP and sequence analysis of *Campylobacter jejuni* and *Campylobacter coli* PCR products amplified directly from environmental samples. *Lebensm. Wiss. Technol.* **31**:537–545.

97. **Suzuki, Y., M. Ishihara, M. Saito, N. Ishikawa, and T. Yokochi.** 1994. Discrimination by means of pulsed-field gel electrophoresis between strains of *Campylobacter jejuni* Lior type 4 derived from sporadic cases and from outbreaks of infection. *J. Infect.* **29**:183–187.

98. **Tenover, F. C., R. C. Arbeit, R. V. Goering, P. A. Mickelsen, B. E. Murray, D. H. Persing, and B. Swaminathan.** 1995 Interpreting chromosomal DNA restriction patterns produced by pulsed-field gel electrophoresis: criteria for bacterial strain typing. *J. Clin. Microbiol.* **33**:2233–2239

99. **Thomas, L. M., K. A. Long, R. T. Good, M. Panaccio, and P. R. Widders.** 1997. Genotypic diversity among *Campylobacter jejuni* isolates in a commercial broiler flock. *Appl. Environm. Microbiol.* **63**:1874–1877.

99a. **van der Plas, J.** Unpublished data.

100. **Vos, P., R. Hogers, M. Bleeker, M. Reijans, T. van der Lee, M. Hames, A. Frijters, J. Pot, J. Peleman, J. Kuiper, et al.** 1996. AFLP:

a new technique for DNA fingerprinting. *Nucleic Acids Res.* **23**:4407–4414.

101. **Vu-Thien, H., C. Dulot, D. Moissenet, B. Fauroux, and A. Garbarg-Chenon.** 1999. Comparison of randomly amplified polymorphic DNA analysis and pulsed-field gel electrophoresis for typing of *Moraxella catarrhalis* strains. *J. Clin. Microbiol.* **37**:450–452.

102. **Wassenaar, T. M., B. N. Fry, and B. A. M. van der Zeijst.** 1995. Variation of the flagellin gene locus of *Campylobacter jejuni* by recombination and horizontal gene transfer. *Microbiology* **141**:95–101.

103. **Wassenaar, T. M., B. Geilhausen, and D. G. Newell.** 1998. Evidence of genomic instability in *Campylobacter jejuni* isolated from poultry meat. *Appl. Environ. Microbiol.* **64**:1816–1821.

104. **Wassenaar, T. M., and D. G. Newell.** 2000.

Genotyping of *Campylobacter* spp. *Appl. Environ. Microbiol.* **66**:1–9.

105. **Welsh, J., and M. McClelland.** 1990. Fingerprinting genomes using PCR with arbitrary primers. *Nucleic Acids Res.* **18**:7213–7218.

106. **Williams, J. G. K., A. R. Kubelik, K. L. Livak, J. A. Rafalski, and S. V. Tingey.** 1990. DNA polymorphisms amplified by arbitrary primers are useful as genetic markers. *Nucleic Acids Res.* **18**:6531–6535.

107. **Winstanley, C., and J. A. W. Morgan.** 1997. The bacterial flagellin gene as a biomarker for detection, population genetics and epidemiological analysis. *Microbiology* **143**:3071–3084.

108. **Yan, W., N. Chang, and D. E. Taylor.** 1991. Pulsed-field gel electrophoresis of *Campylobacter jejuni* and *Campylobacter coli* genomic DNA and its epidemiologic application. *J. Infect. Dis.* **163**:1068–1072.

DIAGNOSIS AND ANTIMICROBIAL SUSCEPTIBILITY OF *CAMPYLOBACTER* SPECIES

Irving Nachamkin, Jørgen Engberg, and Frank Møller Aarestrup

3

Campylobacter jejuni subsp. *jejuni* (referred to as *C. jejuni* throughout this chapter) and *C. coli* have been recognized since the late 1970s as important agents of gastrointestinal infections. Within the genus *Campylobacter, C. jejuni* and *C. coli* are the most common species associated with diarrheal illness in humans and cause clinically similar illnesses (153). Although most laboratories do not routinely distinguish these organisms, 80 to 90% of *Campylobacter* infections in industrialized countries are probably due to *C. jejuni* and 5 to 10% are due to *C. coli,* when the diagnosis is performed solely on the basis of culture on selective media. The distribution of species may be different in other parts of the world and when a nonselective isolation technique, such as the filter technique, is applied in conjunction with a selective medium (7, 97, 168).

C. jejuni and *C. coli* cause a spectrum of illnesses in humans. Fever, abdominal cramping, and diarrhea (with or without blood or fecal leukocytes) are prominent features of uncomplicated illness and may last for as little as a few days to more than 1 week. *Campylobacter* infections are generally self-limited, with a relapse rate of 5 to 10% in untreated patients (17). Patients with *Campylobacter* infection may present with signs and symptoms of acute appendicitis, resulting in unnecessary surgery. Bacteremia, endocarditis, meningitis, urinary tract infection, and other extraintestinal diseases may result from *Campylobacter* infection (17). Bacteremia occurs at an estimated rate of 1.5 per 1,000 intestinal infections, with the highest rate occurring in the elderly (160). Patients with immunodeficiencies such as those with human immunodeficiency virus infection may develop persistent diarrheal illness and bacteremia (130). *C. jejuni* is now the most widely recognized antecedent cause of Guillain-Barré syndrome, an acute paralytic disease of the peripheral nervous system, which is reviewed in chapter 8. Death following *C. jejuni* infection is rare but does occur (46, 167).

CLASSIFICATION

Campylobacter and *Arcobacter* are included in the family *Campylobacteraceae* (179–181). The family *Campylobacteraceae* includes, at present, 18 species and subspecies in the genus *Campylobacter* and 4 species in the genus *Arcobacter* (see Chapter 1, Table 2). *C. hyoilei,* associated with

Irving Nachamkin, Department of Pathology and Laboratory Medicine, University of Pennsylvania, 3400 Spruce Street, Philadelphia, PA 19104-4283. *Jørgen Engberg,* Department of Gastrointestinal Infections, Division of Diagnostics, Statens Serum Institut, Artillerivej 5, DK-2300 Copenhagen S, Denmark. *Frank Møller Aarestrup,* Danish Veterinary Laboratory, Bülowsvej 27, DK-1790 Copenhagen V, Denmark.

porcine proliferative enteritis and previously thought to be a distinct species (6), is now considered to be identical to *C. coli* (182). *Bacteroides gracilis* was reclassified as *C. gracilis* (178), and *Bacteroides ureolyticus* is thought to be closely related to the genus *Campylobacter;* however, this classification is still uncertain. Some phenotypically unusual isolates of *C. gracilis* were recently reclassified into a new genus and species, *Sutterella wadsworthensis* (193). The classification of *C. sputorum* has been amended recently to include three biovars (123). Lawson et al. recently detected 16S rRNA sequences representing a new putative noncultivatable *Campylobacter* sp. isolated from stool samples of healthly individuals (94). The authors termed this uncultivated species "*Candidatus Campylobacter hominis.*" Daneshvar et al. recently described a group of aerobic, oxidase-positive, slightly curved gram-negative rods termed CDC group O-3, that grows well on Campylobacter CVA selective agar and may be misidentified as *Campylobacter* species (32). An extensive review on the taxonomy of *Campylobacter* is given in chapter 1.

SPECIMEN CONSIDERATIONS

Fecal samples from patients with diarrheal illness should routinely be submitted to the laboratory for isolation of *Campylobacter* species. Although not ideal, rectal swabs are also acceptable for culture. Like the other common enteric pathogens (*Salmonella, Yersinia enterocolitica,* and *Shigella*), *Campylobacter* infections are usually community acquired, and therefore, routine cultures for *Campylobacter* should not be performed on hospitalized patients with diarrhea according to the "3-day" rule (68). Two fecal samples may be required to rule out infection (177). Transport medium, such as Cary-Blair medium, is suitable for common enteric pathogens including *Campylobacter* and may be beneficial when transporting fecal specimens to the laboratory if a delay of more than 2 h is anticipated and when transporting rectal swabs (190). Specimens received in Cary-Blair medium should be stored at 4°C if processing is not performed immediately.

Blood cultures may yield *Campylobacter* species, primarily *C. fetus, C. jejuni,* and *C. upsaliensis.* The optimal conditions for isolating *Campylobacter* from blood culture systems are not known. Both the Bactec system (aerobic bottles) and the Septi-Chek system appear to support the growth of the common *Campylobacter* species (83, 93, 189), but their isolation in blood cultures may be difficult in the laboratory. If curved gram-negative rods are observed by Gram stain, broth media should be subcultured to a nonselective blood agar medium and incubated at 37°C under microaerobic conditions. If the Isolator system is used to obtain blood cultures, primary plating should be performed on nonselective media. Acridine orange may also be useful for detecting campylobacters in blood culture bottles if the Gram stain is negative.

DIRECT DETECTION IN STOOL SAMPLES

The Gram stain procedure has been used successfully to detect *Campylobacter* directly in stool samples. The procedure should be modified, however, to include carbol fuchsin or basic fuchsin, rather than safranin, as a counterstain to visualize the characteristic spirals (126, 150). For samples from patients with acute *Campylobacter* enteritis, the sensitivity of direct microscopic examination has been reported to range from 66 to 94% and the specificity is very high (126, 150).

The presence of fecal leukocytes in patients with *Campylobacter* infection has been found in as few as 25% to as many as 80% of culture-proven cases (42, 56). Although the likelihood of isolating *Campylobacter* or other enteroinvasive pathogens may be higher in the presence of fecal leukocytes, their absence does not rule out disease (177). Thus, submitting stool samples to the laboratory for fecal leukocyte analysis is not recommended as a test for predicting bacterial infection or for selective culturing for *Campylobacter* or other stool pathogens (42).

CULTURE AND ISOLATION

Enrichment broth cultures have been used to enhance the recovery of *Campylobacter* from stool samples. Several media, such as Preston enrichment broth (19), Campythio (18), Campylobacter enrichment broth (104), and other formulations (5, 27, 86, 156), have been used regularly. The use of enrichment broth in the workup of patients with acute *Campylobacter* diarrhea has been controversial, but enrichment cultures may be beneficial in instances where small numbers of organisms may be expected due to delayed transport to the laboratory or after the acute stage of disease, when the concentration of organisms may be low (113, 170).

A number of approaches to isolating *C. jejuni, C. coli,* and other species on primary selective media and by filtration methods have been described. Selective media include blood-free media such as charcoal cefoperazone deoxycholate agar (CCDA) (76), charcoal-based selective medium (CSM) (82), and semisolid blood-free motility medium (SSM) (61), and blood-containing media such as Campy-CVA medium (145) and Skirrow medium (158). A charcoal-based medium containing cefoperazone, amphotericin, and teichoplanin (CAT medium) has been described for the primary isolation of *C. upsaliensis* (13).

Some antimicrobial agents present in selective media may be inhibitory to *Campylobacter* species. Cephalothin, colistin, and polymyxin B, which are present in some selective-medium formulations, may be inhibitory to some strains of *C. jejuni* and *C. coli* (58, 118) and are inhibitory to *C. fetus* subsp. *fetus, C. jejuni* subsp *doylei, C. upsaliensis,* and *A. butzleri.* For this reason, the incidence of infection by different *Campylobacter* spp. may be understated. When choosing selective media for primary isolation of *Campylobacter* from fecal samples, laboratories should use cefoperazone-containing media and discontinue the use of cephalothin-containing formulations.

Since some species of *Campylobacter* and *Arcobacter* may be susceptible to various antibiotics present in selective media, a filtration method has been used to isolate these organisms from fecal samples (58, 60, 85, 191). In contrast to selective media, filtration with nonselective media is not as sensitive as primary culture with selective media (60). Thus, filtration should be used to complement selective plating media and not as a replacement. A combination of a selective medium and the filtration technique may improve the sensitivity of detecting *Campylobacter* in stool samples, even though this is rather inconvenient and expensive for the average routine diagnostic laboratory with a high flow of samples (39, 63).

Because of the expense of including several types of media and filtration in the initial workup for *Campylobacter,* one reasonable approach would be to include one or two selective plates (a blood-free formulation and blood-containing formulation) incubated at 42°C. If cultures are negative and no other organism is identified, additional samples should be plated on selective media, processed by the filtration method, and incubated at 37°C under microaerobic conditions.

Most *Campylobacter* species require a microaerobic atmosphere containing approximately 5% O_2, 10% CO_2, and 85% N_2 for optimal recovery (109, 175). Candle jars have been used to isolate *Campylobacter* species; however, the concentration of oxygen generated in candle jars is suboptimal and is not recommended for routine use (103). An atmosphere containing an increased concentration of hydrogen may be required to isolate some species of *Campylobacter,* such as *C. sputorum, C. concisus, C. mucosalis, C. curvus, C. rectus,* and *C. hyointestinalis.* A hydrogen-enriched atmosphere is not necessary for the isolation of *C. jejuni* and *C. coli,* but hydrogen also strongly supports the growth of these species. A gas mixture of 6% O_2, 6% CO_2, 3% H_2, and 85% N_2 is sufficient for isolating hydrogen-requiring species (112).

Campylobacter and *Arcobacter* species have different optimal temperatures for growth, and the choice of temperature for routine laboratory use will determine the spectrum of species that will be isolated. Many laboratories use 42°C as the primary incubation temperature which will allow growth of *C. jejuni* and *C. coli* on selective media. Although *C. upsaliensis* grows well at 42°C, it is usually not recovered on selective media. However, an increased isolation rate of *C. jejuni* and *C. coli* is obtained if the plates are incubated at 37 rather than 42°C (19a). In addition, *C. fetus* may be overlooked in stool samples plated on media incubated at 42°C. Nonthermophilic bacteria such as *Arcobacter* spp. will generally not be recovered at 42°C.

Most *Campylobacter* and *Arcobacter* species grow well at 37°C. However, several of the selective media, such as Skirrow medium and SSM, were devised for use at 42°C and have poor selective properties at 37°C, whereas CCDA and CSM show good selective properties at 37°C (39). At either 42 or 37°C, plates should be incubated for 72 h before being reported as negative.

Arcobacter spp. were first isolated on semisolid media designed to isolate *Leptospira* spp. (181, 192). *Arcobacter* species are aerotolerant and have been recovered on Campy-CVA (9) incubated under microaerobic conditions at 37°C and on nonselective media used in the filtration method. *Arcobacter* species have been recovered on several other media but have not been studied in clinical settings (9, 20, 33, 181). Additional information about the microbiology of non-*C. jejuni* species can be found in chapter 5.

IDENTIFICATION

Culture-Based Methods

Depending on the medium used, *Campylobacter* colonies may have different appearances. *Campylobacter* spp. generally produce grey, flat, irregular, and spreading colonies, particularly on freshly prepared media. As the moisture content decreases, colonies may form round, convex, and glistening colonies with little spreading observed. Hemolysis on blood agar is usually not observed. *Arcobacter* spp. are morphologically similar to *Campylobacter* spp. (181).

For initial analysis, a Gram stain or saline wet mount phase-contrast examination of the colony should be performed, along with an oxidase test. Oxidase-positive colonies exhibiting a characteristic Gram stain appearance (e.g., curved, S-shaped, or spiral rods that are 0.2 to

0.9 μm wide and 0.5 to 5 μm long) when isolated from selective media incubated under microaerobic conditions can be reliably reported as *Campylobacter* spp. until other biochemical tests are performed. Upon prolonged exposure to air or in old cultures, cells become spherical or coccoid and may be difficult to identify. *Arcobacter* are slightly curved, curved, S-shaped, or helical gram-negative, non-spore-forming rods that are 0.2 to 0.9 μm wide and 1 to 3 μm long (180). The appearance of *Arcobacter* may differ from that of typical *Campylobacter* colonies. *A. butzleri* is only slightly curved, and *A. cryaerophilus* tends to be much more helical.

Many of the common *Campylobacter* species can be identified by phenotypic assays. Molecular methods may be necessary for identifying certain species, however, because of phenotypic similarity between them. *C. jejuni* is relatively easy to identify phenotypically; however, hippurate-negative strains are sometimes encountered. *C. coli* are biochemically similar to *C. jejuni* except for hippuricase activity, and molecular methods are needed to definitively identify *C. coli*. PCR analysis of the hippuricase gene, *hipO,* may be used to confirm an isolate as *C. jejuni* (64, 161). *C. jejuni* and *C. coli* have been reported to be reliably differentiated based on polymorphism in the *ceuE* gene (55), the GTPase gene (184), the 16S rDNA gene (26, 100), the 23S rDNA gene (74), and other sequences (117, 148, 194) by using PCR, PCR-restriction fragment length polymorphism, and/or reverse transcription-PCR analysis.

Several phenotypic tests for identifying *Campylobacter* spp. have been described. The most routinely useful tests for initial identification include growth temperature studies (e.g., growth at 25, 37, and 42°C), catalase, hippurate hydrolysis, indoxyl acetate hydrolysis, nitrate reduction, production of H_2S, and antibiotic sensitivity by the disk method (15). The methods used for the routinely useful tests have been previously published (15, 78, 109, 112, 122).

The use of antibiotic disk identification with cephalothin and nalidixic acid is becoming more problematic in the laboratory due to the increasing frequency of fluoroquinolone resistance in *Campylobacter*. Nalidixic acid-resistant *C. jejuni*/*C. coli* strains have been noted by a number of investigators, and an increasing resistance to fluoroquinolones has also been registered (38, 141). Thus, the finding of nalidixic acid resistance does not exclude the identification of *C. jejuni* or *C. coli*. Hippurate-positive strains should be reported as *C. jejuni* regardless of the nalidixic acid disk results. Detection of a nalidixic acid-resistant strain of *C. jejuni* should also alert the laboratory and suggest to the physician that the strain may be resistant to fluoroquinolones; further susceptibility testing may be warranted if antimicrobial therapy with this class of drugs is used.

Unfortunately, *Campylobacter* species are difficult to differentiate from *Arcobacter* species based on phenotypic tests. However, an aerotolerant isolate (i.e., growth under aerobic conditions) that grows on MacConkey agar (under microaerobic conditions) could be presumptively identified as *Arcobacter*. Failure to grow on MacConkey agar, however, does not rule out the presence of *Arcobacter* species. PCR-based assays may ultimately be the most useful approach for accurately identifying *Arcobacter* species and have recently been described (16, 66, 74).

Nonculture Methods

Several commercial assays to aid in identifying *Campylobacter* spp. at the genus level are available. Two immunologic assays (ID Campy [Integrated Diagnostics, Baltimore, Md.] and Campyslide [BBL Microbiology Systems, Cockeysville, Md.]) (70, 114) can detect *C. jejuni* and *C. coli* but cannot differentiate between them. The ID Campy assay may not reliably identify *C. lari* (114). A commercial probe assay directed against *Campylobacter* RNA (Accuprobe [Gen-Probe Inc., San Diego, Calif.]) detects *C. jejuni* subsp. *jejuni*, *C. jejuni* subsp. *doylei*, *C. coli*, and *C. lari* and is highly sensitive (138, 174); however, cross-hybridization with *C. hyointestinalis* has been noted for some isolates (138).

Several investigators have evaluated PCR as a method of directly detecting *Campylobacter* in stool samples (95, 100, 124, 125, 166, 188). A commercial enzyme-linked immunosorbent assay for detecting *Campylobacter* antigen directly in stool samples was recently introduced (Alexon-Trend, Minneapolis, Minn.), and published evaluations should be forthcoming.

EPIDEMIOLOGIC TYPING SYSTEMS

Several typing systems have been developed to study the epidemiology of *Campylobacter* infections, and they vary in their complexity and ability to discriminate between strains. These methods include phenotypic and genotypic approaches, and each has advantages and disadvantages. Serotyping based on O antigens (i.e., lipopolysaccharide) (the Penner scheme [127, 128]) and serotyping based on heat-labile antigens (the Lior scheme [8, 10]) are the two most common serotyping systems used for typing *C. jejuni* and *C. coli*. Serotyping is performed in only a few reference laboratories because of the time and expense needed to maintain high-quality serotyping antisera. Commercially available HL serotyping reagents are generally of very poor quality (119). Other methods used by various investigators include biotyping, bacteriocin sensitivity, detection of preformed enzymes, auxotyping, lectin binding, phage typing, and molecular methods such as pulsed-field gel electrophoresis, multilocus enzyme electrophoresis, ribotyping, and PCR (127). A combination of serotyping and molecular methods should be used for surveillance and outbreak investigations of *Campylobacter* infections. A detailed discussion of subtyping systems is given in chapter 2.

SEROLOGY

Serologic assays may be used to study the epidemiology of *Campylobacter* infections, but the role of serology in the diagnosis of *Campylobacter* enteritis is limited. However, it can be an aid to determine the antecedent cause of the Guillain-Barré syndrome as well as the role of *Campylobacter* in cases of reactive arthritis. Immunoglobulin G (IgG) IgM, and IgA levels in serum rise in response to infection, but IgA levels in serum and feces increase during the first few weeks of infection and then fall rapidly (17). Serum antibody assays vary in both sensitivity and specificity for detecting *Campylobacter* infection, and test performance appears to be population dependent. Patients with *Campylobacter* infection may give false-positive *Legionella* antibody tests (21).

TREATMENT

Campylobacter enteritis is given supportive and symptomatic treatment, as for any other case of acute diarrhea, including the use of oral rehydration therapy. Patients with severe illness may be hospitalized for observation, rehydration, and antimicrobial treatment. Additional information about the treatment of *C. jejuni* infections can be found in chapter 4.

IN VITRO SUSCEPTIBILITY PROFILES

Species identification of campylobacters in relation to susceptibility testing is important for surveillance and epidemiological purposes but less important in the routine clinical laboratory, where timely susceptibility testing and reporting is more important to facilitate and ensure appropriate treatment.

Interpretation of susceptibility results when testing *Campylobacter* is difficult due to the lack of standards for testing methods and accepted breakpoints for determining resistance. In general, however, *C. jejuni* and *C. coli* are almost universally resistant to penicillins, cephalosporins (except a few broad-spectrum cephalosporins), trimethoprim, sulfamethoxazole, rifampin, and vancomycin. They were originally described as highly susceptible to erythromycin, fluoroquinolones, tetracyclines, aminoglycosides, and clindamycin and moderately susceptible to chloramphenicol, cefotaxime, ceftazidime, and cefpirone (106, 159); unfortunately, this is not universally the case any more.

Macrolides and Clindamycin

Since the recognition of *Campylobacter* enteritis in the 1970s, erythromycin has been commonly used to treat patients with uncomplicated enteritis (36, 81, 120, 185). Erythromycin resistance rates in *C. jejuni* range from 0 to 11%; they are generally higher in *C. coli*, ranging from 0 to 68.4% (Table 1). Trends over time for erythromycin resistance show stable and low rates in Japan, Canada, Finland, and Denmark, whereas recent data from Thailand

TABLE 1 Erythromycin and azithromycin resistance rates among *C. jejuni, C. coli* and *C. jejuni/C. coli* combined, isolated from human sources around the world since 1989

Country	Resistance rate (%) among:			Reference(s)
	C. jejuni	*C. coli*	*C. jejuni/C. coli*	
Austria	0.7	5.5	<1	44
Canada	0			52
Denmark	0	14.0	0–2.0	3, 10
Finland			<1–3	65, 140, 141
Hungary			0	186
Italy	1.2	68.4	7.8–9.8	43, 135
Japan	0.8			79
New Zealand			1.5	34
Singapore			51	99
Spain	0–11.0	0–35.0	3.2–7.3	116, 144, 146, 149
Sweden	6.4[a]	11.1[a]	6.1[b]/25.5[b]	155, 157
Taiwan	10.0	50.0	18.3	98
Thailand			0–31.0	71
United Kingdom	1	13		48
United States	0–7.8			11, 111

[a] 90% of the isolates were acquired abroad.
[b] Isolates acquired domestically.
[c] Isolates acquired abroad.

and Sweden document the development of resistance (67, 157). It is unclear whether erythromycin resistance develops during therapy, although posttreatment resistant isolates have been described (49, 137, 163).

The activity of clindamycin against *C. jejuni* is equivalent to that of erythromycin, and the drug may be a useful alternative for the treatment of serious infections in children. However, reported resistance rates are variable (11, 98, 144, 169).

In conclusion, macrolides are the treatment of choice for most cases of complicated *C. jejuni-C. coli* enteritis. The data stress the need for additional studies of antimicrobial use in the human and animal populations and that empiric antimicrobial therapy of *Campylobacter* enteritis should be based on locally assessed susceptibility profiles.

Quinolones

The fluoroquinolones are active against most major pathogens causing bacterial enteritis, and the introduction in the 1980s of this class of antibiotic offered a new approach to antibiotic intervention. Fluoroquinolones had good in vitro activity against all *Campylobacter* species as well as against members of the family *Enterobacteriaceae*. Due to an advantageous pharmacokinetic profile with few serious adverse effects, it looked as though there was finally a class of agents that could be used as the drug of choice for acute bacterial diarrhea including *Campylobacter* enteritis. Early clinical trials of both community-acquired acute diarrhea and traveler's diarrhea demonstrated good clinical response (132, 195). Unfortunately, it soon became apparent that resistance in *Campylobacter* spp. can arise in vivo, sometimes even after just one or two administrations of fluoroquinolones (4). Additionally, an increasing number of reports claimed that fluoroquinolone-resistant strains were isolated from patients who had not received any medical treatment for their illness, suggesting that strains were fluoroquinolone resistant prior to causing the infection (28, 53, 98, 132, 144, 149).

The 1990s have been notable for a striking emergence of resistance to nalidixic acid and fluoroquinolones among campylobacters and other enteric pathogens (Tables 2 and 3). Before 1990, quinolone resistance among campylobacters was rarely reported. With the introduction of enrofloxacin (a derivative of ciprofloxacin) in veterinary medicine and, less important, fluoroquinolones in human medicine in mainland Europe, a rapid emergence of quinolone resistance in *Campylobacter* isolates from patients were registered (4, 28, 141, 142). Surveillance data on resistance rates in human isolates from Asia soon indicated an equal and worrisome increase (87, 172). Recent data from Taiwan, Thailand, and Spain show rates of fluoroquinolone resistance in *C. jejuni* or *C. jejuni/C. coli* of 56.9, 84, and 88%, respectively (50, 71, 98). With the approval of quinolones for veterinary use in the United Kingdom and the United States in late 1993 and 1995, respectively, recent reports from these countries show increasing quinolone resistance profiles (11, 48, 111). Antimicrobial resistance in animals and its relevance to human infections are discussed in more detail in chapter 25.

Induction of fluoroquinolone resistance during treatment is well recognized and frequently reported (4, 37, 152, 171). It has been predicted that in 10 to 20% of patients treated with a fluoroquinolone for *Campylobacter* enteritis, the *Campylobacter* strains will develop quinolone resistance (133, 195). However, in a recent study by Ellis et al. (37), the organism in between 18 and 28% of the patients in their prospective trial developed fluoroquinolone resistance. Development of resistance has been registered in short-term treatments, but prolonged therapy, i.e., in immunosuppressed patients, is a risk factor and has been associated with both clinical and bacteriological failures (4, 108, 152, 171, 172).

In conclusion, the available information on fluoroquinolone resistance, frequent and rapid in vivo development of high-grade resistance, and lack of clear clinical efficacy on community-acquired diarrhea suggests that fluoroquinolones may now be of limited use, if any at all, in the treatment of *Campylobacter* infections

TABLE 2 Nalidixic acid and fluoroquinolone resistance among *C. jejuni* and *C. coli* from human sources around the world

Organism and country	Resistance (%)[a] in:										Reference(s)
	Pre-1989	1989	1990	1991	1992	1993	1994	1995	1996	1997 & later	
C. jejuni											
Austria	(0)								(27.4)		44, 69
Canada	0–0.6 (0)				4.7–13.6 (3.5–11.5)			13.9 (12.7)			51, 67, 81, 91
Denmark								12 (3)			3
Italy		1.7									187
Japan	0 (0)			10.7 (7)							79, 147
Spain	0–2.3 (0–2.3)	3.4–18.2 (3.4–9)	15–19 (7.5–13)	31.8–60 (30.5–51.6)	36.7–63.5 (32.9–63.5)	44.7–73 (48.8–73)	88 (88)		88 (88)		50, 143, 144, 146, 149
Sweden	(0.9–1.8)	(0.9–1.8)									155
Thailand			0								131
United Kingdom	(0) (0)									(11)	48, 134
United States	0			0	1.3					23.9 (10.8–13.4)	11, 14, 111, 162
C. coli											
Austria	(0)								47.3		44, 69
Canada						29 (24.6)					51, 67
Denmark								0 (29)			3
Italy		26.3									187
Japan	10 (0)										147
Spain	0 (0)		0 (0)	29.6 (25.9)	33.3 (33.3–43)						147, 149
Sweden	(0)	(0)									155
Thailand			0								131
United Kingdom										22	134
United States	(0)			0	(0)						11, 14

[a] Numbers without parentheses refer to nalidixic acid; numbers in parentheses indicate percentage of isolates resistant to a fluoroquinolone.

TABLE 3 Nalidixic acid and fluoroquinolone resistance rates in percentage among *C. coli*/*C. jejuni* combined from human sources around the world

Country	Resistance (%) in:										Reference(s)
	Before 1989	1989	1990	1991	1992	1993	1994	1995	1996	1997	
Austria	2.3 (0)	1.8	1.3	3	21.1 (15.9)	23.3 (22.1)			25.9 (25.2)	34.9 (34.1)	44, 45, 69
Canada						16.4 (13.2)					67
Denmark								11–14 (4.9–13)		14 (12)	1, 11
Finland	(0–4)		(9–11)				(17)	(20)	(32)	(35–37)	65, 140, 141
Italy		4.2		(8.5)		(25.9)					135, 187
Japan	0.8 (0)										147
Spain	1.4 (0–2.3)	5.8 (3.4–4.2)	6.8–16.3 (10.4–13)	29–43.4 (29.8–37.4)	42.5–45 (46.3)	50.3					116, 129, 142, 143, 146, 149
Sweden	(1–5)	(1.5)				6.1[b]/25.5[c]					155, 157
Thailand	0		0			(40–50)	(69–79)	(84)			71, 87, 110
United Kingdom		(0)	(0)	(1.9–3)	(4.9)			(7.8)	(8.8)	15.8 (8.8–11.7)	23, 24, 48, 105, 134
The Netherlands	(0–12)						(11)	(22)	(26)	(29)	164
United States	(0)		(0)		1.3					23.9 (10.8–13.4)	11, 14, 111, 162

[a] Numbers without parentheses indicate percent resistant to nalidixic acid; numbers in parentheses indicate percent resistant to a fluoroquinolone.
[b] Isolates acquired domestically.
[c] Isolates acquired abroad.

in many regions (37, 67, 71, 87, 98, 110, 136, 141, 146, 157).

β-Lactam Agents

With the exception of imipenem, the majority of *C. jejuni*/*C. coli* strains are resistant to β-lactam agents, principally penicillins and cephalosporins. However, they are moderately susceptible to cefotaxime, ceftazidime, and cefpirone (183). β-Lactamase-producing strains of *C. jejuni*/*C. coli* are frequently identified. The β-lactamase of *C. jejuni*/*C. coli* seems to play a role only in resistance to amoxicillin, ampicillin, and ticarcillin. With penicillin G, piperacillin, and cephalosporins, the mechanism of resistance in *C. jejuni*/*C. coli* is primarily considered dependent on their limited ability to bind to penicillin-binding proteins and their permeability (89, 90, 165). Ampicillin is not recommended for the treatment of *C. jejuni* infections (52). The rate of resistance to amoxicillin-clavulanic acid has been reported fairly low, but data on the efficacy for treatment of *Campylobacter* bacteremia are sparse (136). Imipenem may be useful for serious systemic infections in patients with renal damage, where the use of aminoglycosides may be problematic (159).

Tetracycline

Although tetracyclines have been suggested as an alternative choice in the treatment of *C. jejuni* and *C. coli* enteritis, large geographical differences in the susceptibility of these species to tetracycline have been reported. The rate of resistance in Denmark ranges from 0 to 11% (3, 10), in Spain it is 25% (54), in the United States it is 48% (11, 111), in Israel it is 70% (151), in Singapore it is 79% (99), and in Taiwan it is 85 to 95% (98). In a recent Canadian study, Gaudreau and Gilbert (52) noticed a significant increase in the resistance of *C. jejuni* to tetracycline from 19.1% in 1985–1986 to 55.7% in 1995–1997. Tetracyclines are ecologically disadvantageous drugs, with a broad antibacterial spectrum, and their use is contraindicated in children. General use of tetracycline is not recommended, but it can be used

in areas of low resistance or, better, after susceptibility testing of the clinical isolate in situations when other agents are contraindicated because of strain resistance or idiosyncratic responses in patients.

Multidrug Resistance

Multidrug resistance in *Campylobacter* species appears to be occurring more frequently and poses the risk that an effective antimicrobial regimen to treat infection may be lacking. Hoge et al. (71), in a study in Thailand, found 100% coresistance to azithromycin and ciprofloxacin in the latest 2 years of investigation. In addition, the level of tetracycline and ampicillin resistance in this area is now so high that these agents can play no role in the treatment of *Campylobacter* or noncholera diarrhea in general. Li et al. (98) reported that concomitant resistance rates among their nalidixic acid-resistant *C. jejuni* isolates from patients (exclusively children) in Taiwan were as follows: gentamicin, 2%; erythromycin, 12%; clindamycin, 12%; tetracyline, 97%; and ciprofloxacin, 66%. All of their human erythromycin-resistant *C. jejuni* isolates and 90% of their *C. coli* isolates were concomitantly resistant to clindamycin.

C. lari

Until the 1990s, *C. lari* could easily be distinguished from other thermophilic species based on resistance to nalidixic acid (115). However, since then resistance to nalidixic acid and fluoroquinolones has emerged among *C. jejuni* and *C. coli* isolates, and nalidixic acid-sensitive biovars of *C. lari* have been described (107). Thus, more reliable tests are required to identify this species. The indication for treatment with antimicrobial agents is similar to that of *C. jejuni*/*C. coli,* with the same classes of drugs, e.g., macrolides, aminoglycosides, imipenem, clindamycin, tetracycline, and fluoroquinolones according to susceptibility testing results (25, 29, 41, 154). As with the other thermophilic *Campylobacter* spp., fluoroquinolone resistance has also been described for this species (41).

C. upsaliensis

No controlled trials of antibiotic treatment of *C. upsaliensis* enteritis have been performed, and experience with antimicrobial treatment is limited. The organism is typically sensitive to aminoglycosides, cephalosporins, tetracycline, and nalidixic acid and resistant to vancomycin, methicillin, piperacillin, and chloramphenicol (22, 139). *C. upsaliensis* is usually sensitive to erythromycin, but up to 10% resistance has been observed (59). In a recent study, Jenkin and Tee (80) reported resistance to fluoroquinolones in three isolates from two human immunodeficiency virus seropositive patients, suggesting that routine susceptibility testing for this species, as for any other species in this genus, is advised.

C. fetus subsp. fetus

Reported *C. fetus* infections most often involve bloodstream and extraintestinal infections, which are often prolonged and relapsing. The prognosis depends largely on the severity of the underlying illnesses. Immunocompetent patients with uncomplicated enteritis may not require antibiotics. Systemic infections require parenteral therapy, but erythromycin is not always effective and is no longer a recommended treatment for systemic *C. fetus* infections (7, 47, 88, 176). Appropriate antimicrobial therapy for serious infections due to *C. fetus* has not been fully assessed for two reasons. Firstly, *C. fetus* infection is rare, and second, many patients die, despite intensive therapy, as a result of associated predisposing factors (57). However, patients with endovascular infections due to *C. fetus* require at least 4 weeks of treatment, and gentamicin plus ampicillin seems to be the combination of choice (17, 57). Imipenem may be a useful alternative (35, 176). Recently, an abdominal aortic aneurism infected by *C. fetus* was successfully treated with surgery and ciprofloxacin (92).

Most studies have used agar dilutions to assess the susceptibility of *C. fetus*. However, Tremblay and Gaudreau (176), compared MIC, disk diffusion, and E-test results on 59 *C. fetus* subsp. *fetus* isolates and found relatively good agreement among the three methods for most antimicrobial agents; however, the results for cefotaxime and erythromycin varied from 0 to 90% and 39 to 100% susceptible, respectively. In general, *C. fetus* isolates were found to be susceptible to most antimicrobials, except tetracycline, with 27% resistant isolates.

A. butzleri and A. cryaerophila

Kiehlbauch et al. (84) studied 78 human and animal isolates of *A. butzleri* and *A. cryaerophila* for susceptibility to 22 antimicrobial agents. Most isolates were resistant to macrolides including erythromycin, cephalosporins except cefotaxime, ampicillin, ampicillin-sulbactam, clindamycin, chloramphenicol, and trimethoprim-sulfamethoxazole, whereas the fluoroquinolones, aminoglycosides, and one tetracycline (minocycline) demonstrated the most activity. Fluoroquinolone resistance has also been reported (96).

C. concisus

Taxonomically, *C. concisus* is not a homogeneous species, and it is difficult to identify. Very little information is available on its antimicrobial susceptibility. Greig et al. from South Africa (62) have tested the MIC for eight isolates and found that ciprofloxacin was the most active agent. All strains were also sensitive to tetracycline, ampicillin, and gentamicin. In contrast, all but one of the strains were resistant to erythromycin. The activity of cephalosporins was variable.

SUSCEPTIBILITY TESTING OF CAMPYLOBACTER

Antimicrobial susceptibility testing can be performed by either dilution or diffusion methods. The choice of method depends on several factors, including preference, ease of performance, and availability of methods in individual laboratories. Susceptibility tests for *Campylobacter* are not standardized, and consequently the literature contains some variability in susceptibility data reported. Recommendations for the agar dilution method include using Mueller-Hinton agar supplemented with 5%

horse or sheep blood, incubated for 16 to 18 h under microaerobic conditions (173). For *Campylobacter,* a number of different diffusion methods (disks, tablets, and E-test strips) have been used and in some cases compared to results obtained by MIC determinations assessed by dilution methods (14, 40, 51, 73, 77). The E-test (PDM Epsilometer [AB Biodisk, Solna, Sweden]) with Mueller-Hinton agar with 5% sheep blood has been found to compare favorably with agar dilution methods for most drugs except clindamycin (14, 40, 72).

For interpretation of the results, breakpoints recommended by the National Committee for Clinical Laboratory Standards for bacterial isolates grown aerobically have been chosen in most cases. However, national breakpoints or breakpoints established through population distribution have also been used. The interpretation of MIC in relation to clinical outcome of infections has not been established, and until this has been done, the classification of MIC results into groups of susceptibilities has to be empirically based.

With the lack of internationally accepted performance standards, the procedures for susceptibility testing must be managed locally. We recommend that isolates be routinely tested for susceptibility to a macrolide and a quinolone. Disk diffusion methods with either disks, tablets, or E-test strips will probably give reliable results in most cases.

In the future, the direct determination of the actual resistance genes by using molecular methods may become important as a supplement to the conventional phenotypic tests (30, 31). Simple and rapid determinations of the genetic mechanism determining resistance to the drugs of choice may have great potential in the future clinical microbiology laboratory. Husmann and colleagues (75) used sequence analysis of a 30-bp fragment of the quinolone resistance–determining region of campylobacters to determine both the species and possible development of quinolone resistance. Since quinolones in several countries are the drugs of choice for undiagnosed gastrointestinal infections, this could have potential value for future

diagnostics. However, the major drawback of these methods is that they will not detect resistance if a new, unexpected resistance mechanism is present.

SURVEILLANCE FOR RESISTANCE

Antimicrobial treatment is often initiated before the results of susceptibility testing are available. Thus, a general knowledge of the expected susceptibility of *Campylobacter* species causing infections in a given geographic region is a prerequisite to initiate treatment with the most appropriate antimicrobial treatment. Infections with *Campylobacter* are most commonly treated with macrolides or fluoroquinoles, but with the recent emergence of resistance to these compounds in several regions around the world, these antimicrobials cannot always be used. Thus, surveillance of the general occurrence of antimicrobial resistance in a given region can help the clinician to choose the most appropriate antimicrobial for treatment.

Most knowledge about the occurrence of antimicrobial resistance is based on experience at individual institutions and often on single surveys in different countries. In addition, in most cases only information from a single sample from one reservoir at a single point in time is available. These uncertain factors makes it difficult to compare studies conducted in different countries or different reservoirs or at different points in time and are in most cases only of limited value in assisting the clinician in the choice of antimicrobial treatment.

Surveillance of antimicrobial resistance in *Campylobacter* is a requirement to measure and monitor the occurrence of antimicrobial resistance. When establishing a surveillance program, several factors have to be taken into consideration before a meaningful program can be established (102, 121). These include decisions on the criteria for identification, sampling strategies, susceptibility testing methods, data recording, computing, and reporting.

Monitoring of the occurrence of resistance among *Campylobacter* species is included in only a very few surveillance systems (11, 12), and systems combining surveillance of antimicrobial resistance among isolates from food animals, food, and humans have so far only been described in the Danish DANMAP surveillance system (12). The DANMAP surveillance system is the first of its kind in the world and includes studies on the occurrence of resistance to antimicrobial agents used both for therapy and for growth promotion in a variety of bacterial pathogens and indicator organisms (1, 2). In this surveillance system, *Campylobacter* isolates are collected randomly among clinical isolates from humans and among isolates from randomly chosen healthy broilers, pigs, and cattle at slaughter. Food animals are collected as a systematic random sample covering the entire country.

It is not feasible to perform a surveillance such as DANMAP in all geographic regions. In relation to *Campylobacter* species of human origin, it is possible only to collect data on resistance in isolates received at laboratories for susceptibility testing. Results obtained from such isolates may be biased, since requisition varies among different medical practitioners and since fecal samples from severe infections are more likely to be sent for culture and susceptibility testing. Data obtained from such collections must be reported with caution, and it will be necessary to consider the value of each individual sample based on epidemiological considerations. Data can be collected from different regional laboratories and compiled centrally. Differences in susceptibility testing methods might include testing biases. However, careful standardization and calibration between laboratories can improve the value of such programs significantly (40).

Data recording, computing, and reporting are essential for an appropriate surveillance system. Thus, the database must include information on the sample population and patient origin (ideally including travel history, history of antimicrobial treatment, suspected source of infection, time of bacterial isolation, bacterial species identification, and testing procedure). Furthermore, to enable later studies on the emergence of resistance, it would be advisable if all or some isolates were stored centrally. The establishment of such relatively simple surveillance programs may be of great assistance to doctors and may improve the implementation of correct treatment.

REFERENCES

1. **Aarestrup, F. M., F. Bager, N. E. Jensen, M. Madsen, A. Meyling, and H. C. Wegener.** 1998. Resistance to antimicrobial agents used for animal therapy in pathogenic-, zoonotic- and indicator bacteria isolated from different food animals in Denmark: a baseline study for the Danish Integrated Antimicrobial Resistance Monitoring Programme (DANMAP). *APMIS* **106:**745–770.

2. **Aarestrup, F. M., F. Bager, N. E. Jensen, M. Madsen, A. Meyling, and H. C. Wegener.** 1998. Surveillance of antimicrobial resistance in bacteria isolated from food animals to antimicrobial growth promoters and related therapeutic agents in Denmark. *APMIS* **106:** 606–622.

3. **Aarestrup, F. M., E. M. Nielsen, M. Madsen, and J. Engberg.** 1997. Antimicrobial susceptibility patterns of thermophilic *Campylobacter* spp. from humans, pigs, cattle, and broilers in Denmark. *Antimicrob. Agents Chemother.* **41:** 2244–2250.

4. **Adler, M., H. Luthy, L. Martinetti, A. Burnens, and M. Altwegg.** 1991. Development of resistance to quinolones in five patients with campylobacteriosis treated with norfloxacin or ciprofloxacin. *Eur. J. Clin. Microbiol. Infect. Dis.* **10:**953–957.

5. **Agulla, A., F. J. Merino, P. A. Villasante, J. V. Saz, A. Diaz, and A. C. Velasco.** 1987. Evaluation of four enrichment media for isolation of *Campylobacter jejuni*. *J. Clin. Microbiol.* **25:** 174–175.

6. **Alderton, M. R., V. Korolik, P. J. Coloe, F. E. Dewhirst, and B. J. Paster.** 1995. *Campylobacter hyoilei* sp. nov., associated with porcine proliferative enteritis. *Int. J. Syst. Bacteriol.* **45:** 61–66.

7. **Allos, B. M., A. J. Lastovica and M. J. Blaser.** 1995. Atypical campylobacters and related organisms, p. 849–865. *In* M. J. Blaser, P. D. Smith, J. I. Ravdin, H. B. Greenberg, and R. L. Guerrant (ed.), *Infections of the Gastrointestinal Tract.* Raven Press, New York, N.Y.

8. **Alm, R. A., P. Guerry, M. E. Power, H. Lior, and T. J. Trust.** 1991. Analysis of the role of flagella in the heat-labile Lior serotyping scheme of thermophilic campylobacters by mutant allele exchange. *J. Clin. Microbiol.* **29:** 2438–2445.

9. **Anderson, K. F., J. A. Kiehlbauch, D. C. Anderson, H. M. McClure, and I. K. Wachsmuth.** 1993. *Arcobacter (Campylobacter) butzleri* associated diarrheal illness in a nonhuman primate. *Infect. Immun.* **61**:2220–2223.

10. **Anonymous.** 1998. *Danmap 97—Consumption of Antimicrobial Agents and Occurrence of Antimicrobial Resistance in Bacteria from Food Animals, Food and Humans in Denmark,* p. 3–59. Danish Zoonosis Centre, Copenhagen, Denmark.

11. **Anonymous.** 1998. *National Antimicrobial Resistance Monitoring System (NARMS)—1997 Annual Report Revised.* Centers for Disease Control and Prevention, Atlanta, Ga.

12. **Anonymous.** 1998. The Danish integrated antimicrobial resistance monitoring and research programme (DANMAP). *APMIS* **106**:605–605.

13. **Aspinall, S. T., D. R. A. Wareing, P. G. Hayward, and D. N. Hutchinson.** 1996. A comparison of a new campylobacter selective medium (CAT) with membrane filtration for the isolation of thermophilic campylobacters including *Campylobacter upsaliensis. J. Appl. Bacteriol.* **80**:645–650.

14. **Baker, C. N.** 1992. The E-test and *Campylobacter jejuni. Diagn. Microbiol. Infect. Dis.* **15**:469–472.

15. **Barrett, T. J., C. M. Patton, and G. K. Morris.** 1988. Differentiation of *Campylobacter* species using phenotypic characterization. *Lab. Med.* **19**:96–102.

16. **Bastyns, K., D. Cartuyvels, S. Chapelle, P. Vandamme, H. Goossens, and R. De Wachter.** 1995. A variable 23S rDNA region is a useful discriminating target for genus-specific and species-specific PCR amplification in *Arcobacter* species. *Syst. Appl. Microbiol.* **18**:353–356.

17. **Blaser, M. J.** 1995. *Campylobacter* and related species, p. 1948–1956. *In* G. L. Mandell, J. E. Bennett, and R. Dolin (ed.), *Principles and Practice of Infectious Diseases.* Churchill Livingstone, Inc., New York, N.Y.

18. **Blaser, M. J., I. D. Berkowitz, F. M. LaForce, J. Craven, L. B. Reller, and W. L. Wang.** 1979. Campylobacter enteritis: clinical and epidemiologic features. *Ann. Intern. Med.* **91**:179–185.

19. **Bolton, F. J., and L. Robertson.** 1982. A selective medium for isolating *Campylobacter jejuni/coli. J. Clin. Pathol.* **35**:462–467.

19a. **Bolton, F. J., D. N. Hutchinson, and G. Parker.** 1988. Reassessment of selective agars and filtration techniques for isolation of campylobacter species from feces. *Eur. J. Clin. Microbiol. Infect. Dis.* **7**:155–160.

20. **Borczyk, A., S. D. Rosa, and H. Lior.** 1991. Enhanced recognition of *Campylobacter cryaerophila* in clinical and environmental specimens, abstr. C-267, p. 386. *In Abstract of the 91st Annual Meeting of the American Society for Microbiology* 1991. American Society for Microbiology, Washington, D.C.

21. **Boswell, T. C. J., and G. Kudesia.** 1992. Serological cross-reactions between *Legionella pneumophila* and *Campylobacter* in the indirect fluorescent antibody test. *Epidemiol. Infect.* **109**:291–295.

22. **Bourke, B., V. L. Chan, and P. Sherman.** 1998. *Campylobacter upsaliensis:* waiting in the wings. *Clin. Microbiol. Rev.* **11**:440–449.

23. **Bowler, I., and D. Day.** 1992. Emerging quinolone resistance in campylobacters. *Lancet* **340**:245–245. (Letter.)

24. **Bowler, I. C. J. W., M. Connor, M. P. A. Lessing, and D. Day.** 1996. Quinolone resistance and *Campylobacter* species. *J. Antimicrob. Chemother.* **38**:315.

25. **Bruneau, B., L. Burc, C. Bizet, Z. Lambert, and C. Branger.** 1998. Purulent pleurisy caused by *Campylobacter lari. Eur. J. Clin. Microbiol. Infect. Dis.* **17**:185–188.

26. **Cardarelli-Leite, P., K. Blom, C. M. Patton, M. A. Nicholson, A. G. Steigerwalt, S. B. Hunter, D. J. Brenner, T. J. Barrett, and B. Swaminathan.** 1996. Rapid identification of *Campylobacter* species by restriction fragment length polymorphis analysis of a PCR amplified fragment of the gene coding for 16S rRNA. *J. Clin. Microbiol.* **34**:62–67.

27. **Chan, F. T. H., and A. M. R. Mackenzie.** 1984. Advantage of using enrichment-culture techniques to isolate *Campylobacter jejuni* from stools. *J. Infect. Dis.* **149**:481–482.

28. **Chatzipanagiotou, S., E. Papavasiliou, and L. Malamou.** 1993. Isolation of *Campylobacter jejuni* strains resistant to nalidixic acid and fluoroquinolones from children with diarrhea in Athens, Greece. *Eur. J. Clin. Microbiol. Infect. Dis.* **12**:566–568. (Letter.)

29. **Chiu, C. H., C. Y. Kuo, and J. T. Ou.** 1995. Chronic diarrhea and bacteremia caused by *Campylobacter lari* in a neonate. *Clin. Infect. Dis.* **21**:700–701. (Letter.)

30. **Cockerill, F. R., III.** 1999. Genetic methods for assessing antimicrobial resistance. *Antimicrob. Agents Chemother.* **43**:199–212.

31. **Courvalin, P.** 1996. Interpretive reading of in vitro antibiotic susceptibility tests (the antibiogramme). *Clin. Microbiol. Infect.* **2**:26–34.

32. **Daneshvar, M. I., B. Hill, D. G. Hollis, C. W. Moss, J. G. Jordan, J. P. Macgregor, F. C. Tenover, and R. S. Weyant.** 1998. CDC group O-3: phenotypic characteristics, fatty acid composition, isoprenoid quinone content, and in

vitro antimicrobic susceptibilities of an unusual gram-negative bacterium isolated from clinical specimens. *J. Clin. Microbiol.* **36:**1674–1678.

33. **de Boer, E., J. J. H. C. Tilburg, D. L. Woodward, H. Lior, and W. M. Johnson.** 1996. A selective medium for the isolation of *Arcobacter* from meats. *Lett. Appl. Microbiol.* **23:**64–66.

34. **Dowling, J., D. MacCulloch, and A. J. Morris.** 1998. Antimicrobial susceptibility of *Campylobacter* and *Yersinia enterocolitica* isolates. *N. Z. Med. J.* **111:**281–281. (Letter.)

35. **Dronda, F., I. Garcia-Arata, E. Navas, and L. de Rafael.** 1998. Meningitis in adults due to *Campylobacter fetus* subspecies *fetus*. *Clin. Infect. Dis.* **27:**906–907.

36. **Elharrif, Z., F. Megraud, and A. M. Marchand.** 1985. Susceptibility of *Campylobacter jejuni* and *Campylobacter coli* to macrolides and related compounds. *Antimicrob. Agents Chemother.* **28:**695–697.

37. **Ellis, P., L. K. Hyman, R. J. Ingram, and M. McCarthy.** 1995. A placebo controlled evaluation of lomefloxacin in the treatment of bacterial diarrhoea in the community. *J. Antimicrob. Chemother.* **36:**259–263.

38. **Endtz, H. P., G. J. Ruijs, B. van Klingeren, W. H. Jansen, T. van der Reyden, and R. P. Mouton.** 1991. Quinolone resistance in campylobacter isolated from man and poultry following the introduction of fluoroquinolones in veterinary medicine. *J. Antimicrob. Chemother.* **27:**199–208.

39. **Endtz, H. P., G. J. Ruijs, A. H. Zwinderman, T. van der Reijden, M. Biever, and R. P. Mouton.** 1991. Comparison of six media, including a semisolid agar, for the isolation of various *Campylobacter* species from stool specimens. *J. Clin. Microbiol.* **29:**1007–1010.

40. **Engberg, J., S. Andersen, R. Skov, F. M. Aarestrup, and P. Gerner-Smidt.** Comparison of two agar dilution methods and three agar diffusion methods including the E-test for antibiotic susceptibility testing of thermophilic *Campylobacter* species. Submitted for publication.

41. **Evans, T. G., and D. Riley.** 1992. *Campylobacter laridis* colitis in a human immunodeficiency virus-positive patient treated with a quinolone. *Clin. Infect. Dis.* **15:**172–173. (Letter.)

42. **Fan, K., A. J. Morris, and L. B. Reller.** 1993. Application of rejection criteria for stool cultures for bacterial enteric pathogens. *J. Clin. Microbiol.* **31:**2233–2235.

43. **Farthing, M., R. Feldman, R. Finch, R. Fox, C. Leen, B. Mandal, P. Moss, D. Nathwant, F. Nye, A. Percival, R. Read, L. Ritchie, W. T. Todd, and M. Wood.** 1996. The management of infective gastroenteritis in adults.

A consensus statement by an expert panel convened by the British Society for the Study of Infection. *J. Infect.* **33:**143–152.

44. **Feierl, G., C. Berghold, T. Furpass, and E. Marth.** 1999. Further increase in ciprofloxacin-resistant *Campylobacter jejuni/coli* in Styria, Austria. *Clin. Microbiol. Infect.* **5:**59–60.

45. **Feierl, G., A. Pschaid, B. Sixl, and E. Marth.** 1994. Increase of ciprofloxacin resistance in *Campylobacter* species in Styria, Austria. *Int. J. Med. Microbiol. Virol. Parasitol. Infect. Dis.* **281:**471–474.

46. **Font, C., A. Cruceta, A. Moreno, O. Miro, B. Coll-Vinent, M. Almela, and J. Mensa.** 1997. Estudio de 30 pacientes con bacteriemia por *Campylobacter* spp. *Med. Clin.* (Barcelona) **108:**336–340.

47. **Francioli, P., J. Herzstein, J. Grob, J. J. Valloton, G. Mombelli, and M. P. Glauser.** 1985. *Campylobacter fetus* subspecies *fetus* bacteremia. *Arch. Intern. Med.* **145:**289–292.

48. **Frost, J. A., and R. T. Thwaites.** 1998. *Drug Resistance in C. jejuni, C. coli and C. lari Isolated from Humans in Wales and North West England during 1997.* Working paper 20.10b. World Health Organization, Geneva, Switzerland.

49. **Funke, G., R. Baumann, J. L. Penner, and M. Altwegg.** 1994. Development of resistance to macrolide antibiotics in an AIDS patient treated with clarithromycin for *Campylobacter jejuni* diarrhea. *Eur. J. Clin. Microbiol. Infect. Dis.* **13:**612–615.

50. **Gallardo, F., J. Gascon, J. Ruiz, M. Corachan, M. T. de Anta, and J. Vila.** 1998. *Campylobacter jejuni* as a cause of traveler's diarrhea: clinical features and antimicrobial susceptibility. *J. Travel Med.* **5:**23–26.

51. **Gaudreau, C., and H. Gilbert.** 1997. Comparison of disc diffusion and agar dilution methods for antibiotic susceptibility testing of *Campylobacter jejuni* subsp. *jejuni* and *Campylobacter coli*. *J. Antimicrob. Chemother.* **39:**707–712.

52. **Gaudreau, C., and H. Gilbert.** 1998. Antimicrobial resistance of clinical strains of *Campylobacter jejuni* subsp. *jejuni* isolated from 1985 to 1997 in Quebec, Canada. *Antimicrob. Agents Chemother.* **42:**2106–2108.

53. **Gaunt, P. N., and L. J. Piddock.** 1996. Ciprofloxacin resistant *Campylobacter* spp. in humans: an epidemiological and laboratory study. *J. Antimicrob. Chemother.* **37:**747–757.

54. **Gomez, G., R. Cogollos, and J. L. Alos.** 1995. Susceptibilities of fluoroquinolone-resistant strains of *Campylobacter jejuni* to 11 oral antimicrobial agents. *Antimicrob. Agents Chemother.* **39:**542–544.

55. **Gonzalez, I., K. A. Grant, P. T. Richardson,**

S. F. Park, and M. D. Collins. 1997. Specific identification of the enteropathogens *Campylobacter jejuni* and *Campylobacter coli* by using a PCR test based on the *ceuE* gene encoding a putative virulence determinant. *J. Clin Microbiol.* **35:** 759–763.

56. Goodman, L. J., G. M. Trenholme, R. L. Kaplan, J. Segreti, D. Hines, R. Petrak, J. A. Nelson, K. W. Mayer, W. Landau, and G. W. Parkhurst. 1990. Empiric antimicrobial therapy of domestically acquired acute diarrhea in urban adults. *Arch. Intern. Med.* **150:**541–546.

57. Goossens, H., H. Coignau, L. Vlaes, and J. P. Butzler. 1989. In-vitro evaluation of antibiotic combinations against *Campylobacter fetus*. *J. Antimicrob. Chemother.* **24:**195–201.

58. Goossens, H., M. De Boeck, H. Coignau, L. Vlaes, C. Van den Borre, and J.-P. Butzler. 1986. Modified selective medium for isolation of *Campylobacter* spp. from feces: comparison with Preston medium, a blood-free medium, and a filtration system. *J. Clin. Microbiol.* **24:**840–843.

59. Goossens, H., B. Pot, L. Vlaes, C. Van den Borre, R. Van den Abbeele, C. Van Naelten, H. Cogniau, P. Marbehant, and J. Verhoef. 1990. Characterization and description of "*Campylobacter upsaliensis*" isolated from human feces. *J. Clin. Microbiol.* **28:**1039–1046.

60. Goossens, H., L. Vlaes, M. De Boeck, B. Pot, K. Kersters, J. Levy, P. de Mol, J. P. Butzler, and P. Vandamme. 1990. Is "*Campylobacter upsaliensis*" an unrecognised cause of human diarrhoea? *Lancet* **335:**584–586.

61. Goossens, H., L. Vlaes, I. Galand, C. Van den Borre, and J. P. Butzler. 1989. Semisolid blood-free selective-motility medium for the isolation of campylobacters from stool specimens. *J. Clin. Microbiol.* **27:**1077–1080.

62. Greig, A., D. Hanslo, E. Le Roux, and A. Lastovica. 1993. In-vitro activity of eight antimicrobial agents against paediatric isolates of *C. concisus* and *C. mucosalis*. *Acta Gastro-Enterol. Belg.* **56:**12–12.

63. Gun-Monro, J., R. P. Rennie, J. H. Thornley, H. L. Richardson, D. Hodge, and J. Lynch. 1987. Laboratory and clinical evaluation of isolation media for *Campylobacter jejuni*. *J. Clin. Microbiol.* **25:**2274–2277.

64. Hani, E., and V. L. Chan. 1995. Expression and characterization of *Campylobacter jejuni* benzoylglycine amidohydrolase (hippuricase) gene in *Escherichia coli*. *J. Bacteriol.* **177:**2396–2402.

65. Hanninen, M. L., S. Pajarre, M. L. Klossner, and H. Rautelin. 1998. Typing of human *Campylobacter jejuni* isolates in Finland by pulsed-field gel electrophoresis. *J. Clin. Microbiol.* **36:** 1787–1789.

66. Harmon, K. M., and I. V. Wesley. 1996. Identification of *Arcobacter* isolates by PCR. *Lett. Appl. Microbiol.* **23:**241–244.

67. Harnett, N., S. Mcleod, Y. A. Yong, C. Hewitt, M. Vearncombe, and C. Krishnan. 1995. Quinolone resistance in clinical strains of *Campylobacter jejuni* and *Campylobacter coli*. *J. Antimicrob. Chemother.* **36:**269–270. (Letter.)

68. Hines, J., and I. Nachamkin. 1996. Effective use of the clinical microbiology laboratory for diagnosing diarrheal diseases. *Clin. Infect. Dis.* **23:** 1292–1301.

69. Hirschl, A. M., D. Wolf, J. Berger, and M. L. Rotter. 1990. In vitro susceptibility of *Campylobacter jejuni* and *Campylobacter coli* isolated in Austria to erythromycin and ciprofloxacin. *Zentbl. Bakteriol.* **272:**443–447.

70. Hodinka, R. L., and P. H. Gilligan. 1988. Evaluation of the Campyslide agglutination test for confirmatory identification of selected *Campylobacter* species. *J. Clin. Microbiol.* **26:** 47–49.

71. Hoge, C. W., J. M. Gambel, A. Srijan, C. Pitarangsi, and P. Echeverria. 1998. Trends in antibiotic resistance among diarrheal pathogens isolated in Thailand over 15 years. *Clin. Infect. Dis.* **26:**341–345.

72. Huang, M. B., C. N. Baker, S. Banerjee, and F. C. Tenover. 1992. Accuracy of the E test for determining antimicrobial susceptibilities of staphylococci, enterococci, *Campylobacter jejuni,* and gram-negative bacteria resistant to antimicrobial agents. *J. Clin. Microbiol.* **30:** 3243–3248.

73. Huang, M. B., C. N. Baker, S. Banerjee, and F. C. Tenover. 1992. Accuracy of the E test for determining antimicrobial susceptibilities of staphylococci, enterococci, *Campylobacter jejuni,* and gram-negative bacteria resistant to antimicrobial agents. *J. Clin. Microbiol.* **30:** 3243–3248.

74. Hurtado, A., and R. J. Owen. 1997. A molecular scheme based on 23S rRNA gene polymorphisms for rapid identification of *Campylobacter* and *Arcobacter* species. *J. Clin. Microbiol.* **35:** 2401–2404.

75. Husmann, M., A. Feddersen, A. Steitz, C. Freytag, and S. Bhakdi. 1997. Simultaneous identification of campylobacters and prediction of quinolone resistance by comparative sequence analysis. *J. Clin. Microbiol.* **35:**2398–2400.

76. Hutchinson, D. N., and F. J. Bolton. 1984. Improved blood free selective medium for the isolation of *Campylobacter jejuni* from faecal specimens. *J. Clin. Pathol.* **37:**956–957.

77. Huysmans, M. B., and J. D. Turnidge. 1997.

Disc susceptibility testing for thermomphilic campylobacters. *Pathology* **29**:209–216.

78. **Isenberg, H.** 1992. *Clinical Microbiology Procedures Handbook.* American Society for Microbiology, Washington, D.C.

79. **Itoh, T., K. Tadano, H. Obata, M. Shingaki, A. Kal, K. Saito, M. Takahashi, Y. Yanagawa, K. Ohta, and Y. Kudoh.** 1995. Emergence of quinolones-resistance in clinical isolates of Campylobacter jejuni in Japan, p. 83–83. *In* D. G. Newell, J. Ketley, and R. A. Feldman (ed.), *8th International Workshop on Campylobacters, Helicobacters and Related Organisms.* Abstracts from the meeting held at Winchester, United Kingdom, 10 to 13 July 1995. Central Veterinary Laboratory, New Haw, United Kingdom.

80. **Jenkin, G. A., and W. Tee.** 1998. Campylobacter upsaliensis-associated diarrhea in human immunodeficiency virus-infected patients. *Clin. Infect. Dis.* **27**:816–821.

81. **Karmali, M. A., S. De Grandis, and P. C. Fleming.** 1981. Antimicrobial susceptibility of Campylobacter jejuni with special reference to resistance patterns of Canadian isolates. *Antimicrob. Agents Chemother.* **19**:593–597.

82. **Karmali, M. A., A. E. Simor, M. Roscoe, P. C. Flemming, S. S. Smith, and J. Lane.** 1986. Evaluation of a blood-free, charcoal based, selective medium for the isolation of Campylobacter organisms from feces. *J. Clin. Microbiol.* **23**:456–459.

83. **Kasten, M. J., F. Allerberger, and J. P. Anhalt.** 1991. Campylobacter bacteremia: clinical experience with three different blood culture systems at Mayo Clinic 1984–1990. *Infection* **19**:88–90.

84. **Kiehlbauch, J. A., C. N. Baker, and I. K. Wachsmuth.** 1992. In vitro susceptibilities of aerotolerant Campylobacter isolates to 22 antimicrobial agents. *Antimicrob. Agents Chemother.* **36**:717–722.

85. **Kiehlbauch, J. A., D. J. Brenner, M. A. Nicholson, C. N. Baker, C. M. Patton, A. G. Steigerwalt, and I. K. Wachsmuth.** 1991. Campylobacter butzleri sp. nov. isolated from humans and animals with diarrheal illness. *J. Clin. Microbiol.* **29**:376–385.

86. **Korhonen, L. K., and P. J. Martikainen.** 1990. Comparison of some enrichment broths and growth media for the isolation of thermophilic campylobacters from surface water samples. *J. Appl. Bacteriol.* **68**:593–599.

87. **Kuschner, R. A., A. F. Trofa, R. J. Thomas, C. W. Hoge, C. Pitarangsi, S. Amato, R. P. Olafson, P. Echeverria, J. C. Sadoff, and D. N. Taylor.** 1995. Use of azithromycin for the treatment of Campylobacter enteritis in travelers to Thailand, an area where ciprofloxacin resistance is prevalent. *Clin. Infect. Dis.* **21**:536–541.

88. **Kwon, S. Y., D. H. Cho, S. Y. Lee, K. Lee, and Y. Chong.** 1994. Antimicrobial susceptibility of Campylobacter fetus subsp. fetus isolated from blood and synovial fluid. *Yonsei Med. J.* **35**:314–319.

89. **Lachance, N., C. Gaudreau, F. Lamothe, and L. A. Lariviere.** 1991. Role of the beta-lactamase of Campylobacter jejuni in resistance to beta-lactam agents. *Antimicrob. Agents Chemother.* **35**:813–818.

90. **Lachance, N., C. Gaudreau, F. Lamothe, and F. Turgeon.** 1993. Susceptibilities of beta-lactamase-positive and -negative strains of Campylobacter coli to beta-lactam agents. *Antimicrob. Agents Chemother.* **37**:1174–1176.

91. **Lariviere, L. A., C. L. Gaudreau, and F. F. Turgeon.** 1986. Susceptibility of clinical isolates of Campylobacter jejuni to twenty-five antimicrobial agents. *J. Antimicrob. Chemother.* **18**:681–685.

92. **La Scola, B., S. Chambourller, C. Mercier, and J. P. Casalta.** 1998. Abdominal aortic aneurysm infected by Campylobacter fetus subsp. fetus. *Clin. Microbiol. Infect.* **4**:527–529.

93. **Lastovica, A. J., E. Le Roux, and J. L. Penner.** 1989. "Campylobacter upsaliensis" isolated from blood cultures of pediatric patients. *J. Clin. Microbiol.* **27**:657–659.

94. **Lawson, A. J., D. Linton, and J. Stanley.** 1998. 16S rRNA gene sequences of "Candidatus Campylobacter hominis," a novel uncultivated species, are found in the gastrointestinal tract of healthy humans. *Microbiology* **144**:2063–2071.

95. **Lawson, A. J., D. Linton, J. Stanley, and R. J. Owen.** 1997. Polymerase chain reaction and speciation of Campylobacter upsaliensis and C. helveticus in human faeces and comparison with culture techniques. *J. Appl. Microbiol.* **83**:375–380.

96. **Lerner, J., V. Brumberger, and M. Preac.** 1994. Severe diarrhea associated with Arcobacter butzleri. *Eur. J. Clin. Microbiol. Infect. Dis.* **13**:660–662.

97. **Le Roux, E., and A. J. Lastovica.** 1998. The Cape Town protocol: how to isolate the most campylobacters for your dollar, pound, franc, yen, etc. p. 30–33. *In* A. L. Lastovica, D. G. Newell, and E. E. Lastovica (ed.), *Campylobacter, Helicobacter and Related Organisms.* Institute of Child Health, Cape Town, South Africa.

98. **Li, C. C., C. H. Chiu, J. L. Wu, Y. C. Huang, and T. Y. Lin.** 1998. Antimicrobial susceptibilities of Campylobacter jejuni and coli by

using E-test in Taiwan. *Scand. J. Infect. Dis.* **30:** 39–42.

99. **Lim, Y. S., and L. Tay.** 1992. A one-year study of enteric *Campylobacter* infections in Singapore. *J. Trop. Med. Hyg.* **95:**119–123.

100. **Linton, D., A. J. Lawson, R. J. Owen, and J. Stanley.** 1997. PCR detection, identification to species level, and fingerprinting of *Campylobacter jejuni* and *Campylobacter coli* direct from diarrheic samples. *J. Clin. Microbiol.* **35:** 2568–2572.

101. **Lior, H., D. L. Woodward, J. A. Edgar, L. J. Laroche, and P. Gill.** 1982. Serotyping of *Campylobacter jejuni* by slide agglutination based on heat-labile antigenic factors. *J. Clin. Microbiol.* **15:**761–768.

102. **Livermore, D. M., A. P. Macgowan, and M. C. Wale.** 1998. Surveillance of antimicrobial resistance. Centralised surveys to validate routine data offer a practical approach. *Br. Med. J.* **317:** 614–615. (Editorial.)

103. **Luechtefeld, N. W., L. B. Reller, M. J. Blaser, and W. -L. L. Wang.** 1982. Comparison of atmospheres of incubation for primary isolation of *Campylobacter fetus* subsp. *jejuni* from animal specimens: 5% oxygen versus candle jar. *J. Clin. Microbiol.* **15:**53–57.

104. **Martin, W. T., C. M. Patton, G. K. Morris, M. E. Potter, and N. D. Puhr.** 1983. Selective enrichment broth for isolation of *Campylobacter jejuni. J. Clin. Microbiol.* **17:**853–855.

105. **McIntyre, M., and M. Lyons.** 1993. Resistance to ciprofloxacin in *Campylobacter* spp. *Lancet* **341:**188–188. (Letter.)

106. **McNulty, C. A.** 1987. The treatment of campylobacter infections in man. *J. Antimicrob. Chemother.* **19:**281–284.

107. **Megraud, F., D. Chevrier, N. Desplaces, A. Sedallian, and J. L. Guesdon.** 1988. Urease-positive thermophilic *Campylobacter* (*Campylobacter laridis* variant) isolated from an appendix and from human feces. *J. Clin. Microbiol.* **26:** 1050–1051.

108. **Molina, J., I. Casin, P. Hausfater, E. Giretti, Y. Welker, J. Decazes, V. Garrait, P. Lagrange, and J. Modai.** 1995. *Campylobacter* infections in HIV-infected patients: clinical and bacteriological features. *AIDS* **9:**881–885.

109. **Morris, G. K., and C. M. Patton.** 1985. *Campylobacter,* p. 302–308. *In* E. Lennette, A. Balows, W. J. Hausler, Jr., and H. J. Shadomy (ed.), *Manual of Clinical Microbiology,* 4th ed. American Society for Microbiology, Washington, D.C.

110. **Murphy, G. S., Jr., P. Echeverria, L. R. Jackson, M. K. Arness, C. LeBron, and C. Pitarangsi.** 1996. Ciprofloxacin- and azithro-mycin-resistant *Campylobacter* causing traveler's diarrhea in U.S. troops deployed to Thailand in 1994. *Clin. Infect. Dis.* **22:**868–869.

111. **Nachamkin, I.** 1994. Antimicrobial susceptibility of *Campylobacter jejuni* and *Campylobacter coli* to ciprofloxacin, erythromycin and tetracycline from 1982 to 1992. *Med. Microbiol. Lett.* **3:** 300–305.

112. **Nachamkin, I.** 1995. *Campylobacter* and *Arcobacter,* p. 483–491. *In* P. R. Murray, E. J. Baron, M. A. Pfaller, F. C. Tenover, and R. H. Yolken, (ed.), *Manual of Clinical Microbiology,* 6th ed. ASM Press, Washington, D.C.

113. **Nachamkin, I.** 1997. Microbiologic approaches for studying *Campylobacter* in patients with Guillain-Barré syndrome. *J. Infect. Dis.* **176**(Suppl 2): S106–S114.

114. **Nachamkin, I., and S. Barbagallo.** 1990. Culture confirmation of *Campylobacter* spp. by latex agglutination. *J. Clin. Microbiol.* **28:** 817–818.

115. **Nachamkin, I., C. Stowell, D. Skalina, A. M. Jones, R. M. Roop, and R. M. Smibert.** 1984. *Campylobacter laridis* causing bacteremia in an immunosuppressed patient. *Ann. Intern. Med.* **101:**55–57.

116. **Navarro, F., E. Miro, B. Mirelis, and G. Prats.** 1993. *Campylobacter* spp. antibiotic susceptibility. *J. Antimicrob. Chemother.* **32:** 906–907. (Letter.)

117. **Ng, L.-K., C. I. B. Kingombe, W. Yan, D. E. Taylor, K. Hiratsuka, N. Malik, and M. M. Garcia.** 1997. Specific detection and confirmation of *Campylobacter jejuni* by DNA hybridization and PCR. *Appl. Environ. Microbiol.* **63:** 4558–4563.

118. **Ng, L. -K., D. E. Taylor, and M. E. Stiles.** 1988. Characterization of freshly isolated *Campylobacter coli* strains and suitability of selective media for their growth. *J. Clin. Microbiol.* **26:** 518–523.

119. **Nicholson, M. A., and C. M. Patton.** 1993. Evaluation of commercial antisera for serotyping heat-labile antigens of *Campylobacter jejuni* and *Campylobacter coli. J. Clin. Microbiol.* **31:**900–903.

120. **Nolan, C. M., K. E. Johnson, M. B. Coyle, and K. Faler.** 1983. *Campylobacter jejuni* enteritis: efficacy of antimicrobial and antimotility drugs. *Am. J. Gastroenterol.* **78:**621–626.

121. **O'Brien, T. F.** 1997. The global epidemic nature of antimicrobial resistance and the need to monitor and manage it locally. *Clin. Infect. Dis.* **24**(Suppl. 1):S2–S8.

122. **On, S. L.** 1996. Identification methods for campylobacters, helicobacters, and related organisms. *Clin. Microbiol. Rev.* **9:**405–422.

123. **On, S. L. W., H. I. Atabay, J. E. L. Corry,**

C. S. Harrington, and P. Vandamme. 1998. Emended description of *Campylobacter sputorum* and revision of its infrasubspecific (biovar) divisions, including *C. sputorum* biovar paraureolyticus, a urease-producing variant from cattle and humans. *Int. J. Syst. Bacteriol.* **48**:195–206.

124. Oyofo, B. A., Z. S. Mohran, S. El-Etr, M. O. Wasfy, and L. F. Peruski. 1996. Detection of enterotoxigenic *Escherichia coli*, *Shigella*, and *Campylobacter* spp. by multiplex PCR assay. *J Diarrheal Dis Res.* **14**:207–210.

125. Oyofo, B. A., S. A. Thornton, D. H. Burr, T. J. Trust, O. R. Pavlovskis, and P. Guerry. 1992. Specific detection of *Campylobacter jejuni* and *Campylobacter coli* by using polymerase chain reaction. *J. Clin. Microbiol.* **30**:2613–2619.

126. Park, C. H., D. L. Hixon, A. S. Polhemus, C. B. Ferguson, S. L. Hall, C. C. Risheim, and C. B. Cook. 1983. A rapid diagnosis of campylobacter enteritis by direct smear examination. *Am. J. Clin. Pathol.* **80**:388–390.

127. Patton, C. M., and I. K. Wachsmuth. 1992. Typing schemes: are current methods useful? p. 110–128. *In* I. Nachamkin, M. J. Blaser, and L. S. Tompkins (ed.), *Campylobacter jejuni: Current Status and Future Trends.* American Society for Microbiology, Washington, D.C.

128. Penner, J. L., and J. N. Hennessy. 1980. Passive hemagglutination technique for serotyping *Campylobacter fetus* subsp. *jejuni* on the basis of soluble heat-stable antigens. *J. Clin. Microbiol.* **12**:732–737.

129. Perez, T., M. Urbieta, C. L. Lopategui, C. Zigorraga, and I. Ayestaran. 1993. Antibiotics in veterinary medicine and public health. *Lancet* **342**:1371–1372. (Letter.)

130. Perlman, D. M., N. M. Ampel, R. B. Schifman, D. L. Cohn, C. M. Patton, M. L. Aguirre, W.-L. L. Wang, and M. J. Blaser. 1988. Persistent *Campylobacter jejuni* infections in patients infected with human immunodeficiency virus (HIV). *Ann. Intern. Med.* **108**:540–546.

131. Petruccelli, B. P., G. S. Murphy, J. L. Sanchez, S. Walz, R. DeFraites, J. Gelnett, R. L. Haberberger, P. Echeverria, and D. N. Taylor. 1992. Treatment of traveler's diarrhea with ciprofloxacin and loperamide. *J. Infect. Dis.* **165**:557–560.

132. Piddock, L. J. 1995. Quinolone resistance and *Campylobacter* spp. *J. Antimicrob. Chemother.* **36**:891–898.

133. Piddock, L. J. 1997. Quinolone resistance and *Campylobacter*, p. 191–199. *In The Medical Impact of the Use of Antimicrobial Use in Food Animals.* Report and Proceedings of a WHO meeting, Berlin, Germany, 13 to 17 October 1997. Division of Emerging and Other Communicable Diseases Surveillance and Control, World Health Organization, Geneva, Switzerland.

134. Piddock, L. J. 1998. *Quinolone Resistant Campylobacter in the United Kingdom*, p. 1–9. Working paper 20.09. World Health Organization, Geneva, Switzerland.

135. Piersimoni, C., D. Crotti, D. Nista, G. Bornigia, and G. De Sio. 1995. Evolution of resistance to erythromycin, norfloxacin and tetracycline in thermophilic campylobacters, p. 88–88. *In* D. G. Newell, J. Ketley, and R. A. Feldman (ed.), *8th International Workshop on Campylobacters, Helicobacters and Related Organisms.* Abstracts from the meeting held at Winchester, United Kingdom, 10 to 13 July 1995. Central Veterinary Laboratory, New Haw, United Kingdom.

136. Pigrau, C., R. Bartolome, B. Almirante, A. M. Planes, J. Gavalda, and A. Pahissa. 1997. Bacteremia due to *Campylobacter* species: clinical findings and antimicrobial susceptibility patterns. *Clin. Infect. Dis.* **25**:1414–1420.

137. Pitkanen, T., T. Pettersson, A. Pomka, and T. U. Kosunen. 1982. Effect of erythromycin on the fecal excretion of *Campylobacter fetus* subspecies *jejuni*. *J. Infect. Dis.* **145**:128–128.

138. Popovic-Uroic, T., C. M. Patton, I. K. Wachsmuth, and P. Roeder. 1991. Evaluation of an oligonucleotide probe for identification of *Campylobacter* species. *Lab. Med.* **22**:533–539.

139. Preston, M. A., A. E. Simor, S. L. Walmsley, S. A. Fuller, A. J. Lastovica, K. Sandstedt, and J. L. Penner. 1990. In vitro susceptibility of "*Campylobacter upsaliensis*" to twenty-four antimicrobial agents. *Eur. J. Clin. Microbiol. Infect. Dis.* **9**:822–824.

140. Rautelin, H. 1999. Personal communication.

141. Rautelin, H., O. V. Renkonen, and T. U. Kosunen. 1991. Emergence of fluoroquinolone resistance in *Campylobacter jejuni* and *Campylobacter coli* in subjects from Finland. *Antimicrob. Agents Chemother.* **35**:2065–2069.

142. Reina, J., N. Borrell, and A. Serra. 1992. Emergence of resistance to erythromycin and fluoroquinolones in thermotolerant *Campylobacter* strains isolated from feces 1987–1991. *Eur. J. Clin. Microbiol. Infect. Dis.* **11**:1163–1166.

143. Reina, J., M. J. Ros, and B. Fernandez. 1995. Resistance to erythromycin in fluoroquinolone-resistant *Campylobacter jejuni* strains isolated from human faeces. *J. Antimicrob. Chemother.* **35**:351–352. (Letter.)

144. Reina, J., M. J. Ros, and A. Serra. 1994. Susceptibilities to 10 antimicrobial agents of 1,220 *Campylobacter* strains isolated from 1987 to 1993

from feces of pediatric patients. *Antimicrob. Agents Chemother.* **38:**2917–2920.

145. **Reller, L. B., S. Mirrett, and L. G. Reimer.** 1983. Controlled evaluation of an improved selective medium for isolation of *Campylobacter jejuni,* abstr. C-274, p. 357. *In Abstracts of the 83rd Annual Meeting of the American Society for Microbiology 1983.* American Society for Microbiology, Washington, D.C.

146. **Ruiz, J., P. Goni, F. Marco, F. Gallardo, B. Mirelis, D. A. Jimenez, and J. Vila.** 1998. Increased resistance to quinolones in *Campylobacter jejuni:* a genetic analysis of *gyrA* gene mutations in quinolone-resistant clinical isolates. *Microbiol. Immunol.* **42:**223–226.

147. **Sagara, H., A. Mochizuki, N. Okamura, and R. Nakaya.** 1987. Antimicrobial resistance of *Campylobacter jejuni* and *Campylobacter coli* with special reference to plasmid profiles of Japanese clinical isolates. *Antimicrob. Agents Chemother.* **31:**713–719.

148. **Sails, A. D., F. J. Bolton, A. J. Fox, D. R. Wareing, and D. L. A. Greenway.** 1998. A reverse transcriptase polymerase chain reaction assay for the detection of thermophilic *Campylobacter* spp. *Mol. Cell. Probes* **12:**317–322.

149. **Sanchez, R., B. Fernandez, M. D. Diaz, P. Munoz, C. Rodriguez, and E. Bouza.** 1994. Evolution of susceptibilities of *Campylobacter* spp. to quinolones and macrolides. *Antimicrob. Agents Chemother.* **38:**1879–1882.

150. **Sazie, E. S. M., and A. E. Titus.** 1982. Rapid diagnosis of *Campylobacter* enteritis. *Ann. Intern. Med.* **96:**62–63.

151. **Schwartz, D., H. Goossens, J. Levy, J. P. Butzler, and J. Goldhar.** 1993. Plasmid profiles and antimicrobial susceptibility of *Campylobacter jejuni* isolated from Israeli children with diarrhea. *Int. J. Med. Microbiol. Virol. Parasitol. Infect. Dis.* **279:**368–376.

152. **Segreti, J., T. D. Gootz, L. J. Goodman, G. W. Parkhurst, J. P. Quinn, B. A. Martin, and G. M. Trenholme.** 1992. High-level quinolone resistance in clinical isolates of *Campylobacter jejuni. J. Infect. Dis.* **165:**667–670.

153. **Shallow, S., P. Daily, G. Rothrock, A. Reingold, D. Vugia, S. Waterman, T. Florentino, R. Marcus, R. Ryder, P. Mshar, J. L. Hadler, W. Vaughman, J. Koehler, P. Blake, K. E. Toomey, J. Hogan, V. Deneen, C. Hedberg, M. T. Osterholm, M. Cassidy, J. Townes, B. Shiferaw, P. Cieslak, K. Hedberg, and D. Fleming.** 1997. Foodborne diseases active surveillance network, 1996. *Morbid. Mortal. Weekly Rep.* **46:**258–261.

154. **Simor, A. E., and L. Wilcox.** 1987. Enteritis associated with *Campylobacter laridis. J. Clin. Microbiol.* **25:**10–12.

155. **Sjogren, E., B. Kaijser, and M. Werner.** 1992. Antimicrobial susceptibilities of *Campylobacter jejuni* and *Campylobacter coli* isolated in Sweden: a 10-year follow-up report. *Antimicrob. Agents Chemother.* **36:**2847–2849.

156. **Sjogren, E., G. B. Lindblom, and B. Kaijser.** 1987. Comparison of different procedures, transport media, and enrichment media for isolation of *Campylobacter* species from healthy laying hens and humans with diarrhea. *J. Clin. Microbiol.* **25:**1966–1968.

157. **Sjogren, E., G. B. Lindblom, and B. Kaijser.** 1997. Norfloxacin resistance in *Campylobacter jejuni* and *Campylobacter coli* isolates from Swedish patients. *J. Antimicrob. Chemother.* **40:**257–261.

158. **Skirrow, M. B.** 1977. Campylobacter enteritis: a "new" disease. *Br. Med. J.* **2:**9–11.

159. **Skirrow, M. B., and M. J. Blaser.** 1995. *Campylobacter jejuni,* p. 825–848. *In* M. J. Blaser, P. D. Smith, J. I. Ravdin, H. B. Greenberg, and R. L. Guerrant (ed.), *Infections of the Gastrointestinal Tract.* Raven Press, New York, N.Y.

160. **Skirrow, M. B., D. M. Jones, E. Sutcliffe, and J. Benjamin.** 1993. *Campylobacter* bacteremia in England and Wales, 1981–1991. *Epidemiol. Infect.* **110:**567–573.

161. **Slater, E. R., and R. J. Owen.** 1997. Restriction fragment length polymorphism analysis shows that the hippuricase gene of *Campylobacter jejuni* is highly conserved. *Lett. Appl. Microbiol.* **25:**274–278.

162. **Smith, K. E., J. M. Besser, C. W. Hedberg, F. T. Leano, J. B. Bender, J. H. Wicklund, B. P. Johnson, K. A. Moore, and M. T. Osterholm.** 1999. Quinolone-resistant *Campylobacter jejuni* infections in Minnesota, 1992–1998. *N. Engl. J. Med.* **340:**1525–1532.

163. **Snijders, F., E. J. Kuijper, B. de Wever, L. van der Hoek, S. A. Danner, and J. Dankert.** 1997. Prevalence of *Campylobacter*-associated diarrhea among patients infected with human immunodeficiency virus. *Clin. Infect. Dis.* **24:**1107–1113.

164. **Stobberingh, E., A. van den Bogaard, D. Mevius, and H. Endtz.** 1998. *Examples of In-Vitro Quinolone Resistance Prevalence Trends in Humans and Animal Isolates of Food-Borne Salmonella and Campylobacter.* Working paper 20.09. World Health Organization, Geneva, Switzerland.

165. **Tajada, P., G. Gomez, J. I. Alos, D. Balas, and R. Cogollos.** 1996. Antimicrobial susceptibilities of *Campylobacter jejuni* and *Campylobacter coli* to 12 beta-lactam agents and combinations with beta-lactamase inhibitors. *Antimicrob. Agents Chemother.* **40:**1924–1925.

166. **Takeshi, K., T. Ikeda, A. Kubo, Y. Fuji-naga, S. Makino, K. Oguma, E. Isogai, S. Yoshida, H. Sunagawa, T. Ohyama, and H. Kimura.** 1997. Direct detection by PCR of *Escherichia coli* O157 and enteropathogens in patients with bloody diarrhea. *Microbiol. Immunol* **41:**819–822.

167. **Tauxe, R. V.** 1992. Epidemiology of *Campylobacter jejuni* infections in the United States and other industrialized nations, p. 9–19. *In* I. Nachamkin, M. J. Blaser, and L. S. Tompkins (ed.), *Campylobacter jejuni: Current Status and Future Trends.* American Society for Microbiology, Washington, D.C.

168. **Taylor, D. N.** 1992. *Campylobacter* infections in developing countries, p. 20–30. *In* I. Nachamkin, M. J. Blaser, and L. S. Tompkins (ed), *Campylobacter jejuni: Current Status and Future Trends.* American Society for Microbiology, Washington, D.C.

169. **Taylor, D. N., M. J. Blaser, P. Echeverria, C. Pitarangsi, L. Bodhidatta, and W. L. Wang.** 1987. Erythromycin-resistant *Campylobacter* infections in Thailand. *Antimicrob. Agents Chemother.* **31:**438–442.

170. **Taylor, D. N., P. Echeverria, C. Pitarangsi, J. Seriwatana, L. Bodhidatta, and M. J. Blaser.** 1988. Influence of strain characteristics and immunity on the epidemiology of *Campylobacter* infections in Thailand. *J. Clin. Microbiol.* **26:**863–868.

171. **Tee, W., and A. Mijch.** 1998. *Campylobacter jejuni* bacteremia in human immunodeficiency virus (HIV)-infected and non-HIV-infected patients: comparison of clinical features and review. *Clin. Infect. Dis.* **26:**91–96.

172. **Tee, W., A. Mijch, E. Wright, and A. Yung.** 1995. Emergence of multidrug resistance in *Campylobacter jejuni* isolates from three patients infected with human immunodeficiency virus. *Clin. Infect. Dis.* **21:**634–638.

173. **Tenover, F. C., C. N. Baker, C. L. Fennell and C. A. Ryan.** 1992. Antimicrobial resistance in *Campylobacter* species, p. 66–73. *In* I. Nachamkin, M. J. Blaser, and L. S. Tompkins (ed.), *Campylobacter jejuni: Current Status and Future Trends.* American Society for Microbiology, Washington, D.C.

174. **Tenover, F. C., L. Carlson, S. Barbagallo, and I. Nachamkin.** 1990. DNA probe culture confirmation assay for identification of thermophilic *Campylobacter* species. *J. Clin. Microbiol.* **28:**1284–1287.

175. **Thompson, J. S., D. S. Hodge, D. E. Smith, and Y. A. Yong.** 1990. Use of tri-gas incubator for routine culture of *Campylobacter* species from fecal specimens. *J. Clin. Microbiol.* **28:**2802–2803.

176. **Tremblay, C., and C. Gaudreau.** 1998. Antimicrobial susceptibility testing of 59 strains of *Campylobacter fetus* subsp. *fetus. Antimicrob. Agents Chemother.* **42:**1847–1849.

177. **Valenstein, P., M. Pfaller, and M. Yungbluth.** 1996. The use and abuse of routine stool microbiology: a college of american pathologists Q-probes study of 601 institutions. *Arch. Pathol. Lab. Med.* **120:**206–211.

178. **Vandamme, P., M. I. Daneshvar, F. E. Dewhirst, B. J. Paster, K. Kersters, H. Goossens, and C. W. Moss.** 1995. Chemotaxonomic analyses of *Bacteroides gracilis* and *Bacteroides ureolyticus* and reclassification of *B. gracilis* as *Campylobacter gracilis* comb. nov. *Int. J. Syst. Bacteriol.* **45:**145–152.

179. **Vandamme, P., and J. De Ley.** 1991. Proposal for a new family, *Campylobacteraceae. Int. J. Syst. Bacteriol.* **41:**451–455.

180. **Vandamme, P., E. Falsen, R. Rossau, B. Hoste, P. Segers, R. Tytgat, and J. De Ley.** 1991. Revision of *Campylobacter, Helicobacter,* and *Wolinella* taxonomy: emendation of generic descriptions and proposal of *Arcobacter* gen. nov. *Int. J. Syst. Bacteriol.* **41:**81–103.

181. **Vandamme, P., M. Vancanneyt, B. Pot, L. Mels, B. Hoste, D. Dewettinck, L. Vlaes, C. Van den Borre, R. Higgins, and J. Hommez.** 1992. Polyphasic taxonomic study of the emended genus *Arcobacter* with *Arcobacter butzleri* comb. nov. and *Arcobacter skirrowii* sp. nov., an aerotolerant bacterium isolated from veterinary specimens. *Int. J. Syst. Bacteriol.* **42:**344–356.

182. **Vandamme, P., L. J. VanDoorn, S. T. Alrashid, W. G. V. Quint, J. VanderPlas, V. L. Chan, and S. L. W. On.** 1997. *Campylobacter hyoilei* Alderton et al. 1995 and *Campylobacter coli* Veron and Chatelain 1973 are subjective synonyms. *Int. J. Syst. Bacteriol* **47:**1055–1060.

183. **Van der Auwera, P., and B. Scorneaux.** 1985. In vitro susceptibility of *Campylobacter jejuni* to 27 antimicrobial agents and various combinations of beta-lactams with clavulanic acid or sulbactam. *Antimicrob. Agents Chemother.* **28:**37–40.

184. **VanDoorn, L. J., B. A. J. Glesendorf, R. Bax, B. A. M. Van Der Zeijst, P. Vandamme, and W. G. V. Quint.** 1997. Molecular discrimination between *Campylobacter jejuni, Campylobacter coli, Campylobacter lari* and *Campylobacter upsaliensis* by polymerase chain reaction based on a novel putative GTPase gene. *Mol. Cell. Probes* **11:**175–185.

185. **Vanhoof, R., M. P. Vanderlinden, R. Dierickx, S. Lauwers, E. Yourassowsky, and J.**

P. Butzler. 1978. Susceptibility of *Campylobacter fetus* subsp. *jejuni* to twenty-nine antimicrobial agents. *Antimicrob. Agents Chemother.* **14:** 553–556.

186. **Varga, J., and L. Fodor.** 1998. Biochemical characteristics, serogroup distribution, antibiotic susceptibility and age-related significance of *Campylobacter* strains causing diarrhoea in humans in Hungary. *Zentbl. Bakteriol.* **288:**67–73.

187. **Varoli, O., M. Gatti, M. T. Montella, and M. La Placa, Jr.** 1991. Observations made on strains of *Campylobacter* spp. isolated in 1989 in northern Italy. *Microbiologica* **14:**31–35.

188. **Waegel, A. and I. Nachamkin.** 1996. Detection and molecular typing of *Campylobacter jejuni* in fecal samples by polymerase chain reaction. *Mol. Cell. Probes* **10:**75–80.

189. **Wang, W.-L. L., and M. J. Blaser.** 1986. Detection of pathogenic *Campylobacter* species in blood culture systems. *J. Clin. Microbiol.* **23:** 709–714.

190. **Wang, W.-L. L., L. B. Reller, B. Smallwood, N. W. Luechtefeld, and M. J. Blaser.** 1983. Evaluation of transport media for *Campylobacter jejuni* in human fecal specimens. *J. Clin. Microbiol.* **18:**803–807.

191. **Wells, J. G., N. D. Puhr, C. M. Patton, M. A. Nicholson, M. A. Lambert, and R. C. Jerris.** 1989. Comparison of selective media and filtration for the isolation of *Campylobacter* from feces, abstr. C-231, p. 432. *In Abstracts of the 89th Annual Meeting of the American Society for Microbiology 1989.* American Society for Microbiology, Washington, D.C.

192. **Wesley, I. V.** 1994. *Arcobacter* infections, p. 181–190. *In* G. W. Beran. (ed.), *CRC Handbook of Zoonosis.* CRC Press, Inc., Boca Raton, Fla.

193. **Wexler, H. M., D. Reeves, P. H. Summanen, E. Molitoris, M. McTeague, J. Duncan, K. H. Wilson, and S. M. Finegold.** 1996. *Sutterella wadsworthensis* gen. nov., sp. nov., bile-resistant microaerophilic *Campylobacter gracilis*-like clinical isolates. *Int. J. Syst. Bacteriol* **46:** 252–258.

194. **Winters, D. K., A. E. O'Leary, and M. F. Slavik.** 1997. Rapid PCR with nested primers for direct detection of *Campylobacter jejuni* in chicken washes. *Mol. Cell. Probes* **11:**267–271.

195. **Wistrom, J., and S. R. Norrby.** 1995. Fluoroquinolones and bacterial enteritis, when and for whom? *J. Antimicrob. Chemother.* **36:**23–39.

CLINICAL AND EPIDEMIOLOGICAL ASPECTS OF *CAMPYLOBACTER* INFECTIONS

CLINICAL ASPECTS OF *CAMPYLOBACTER* INFECTION

Martin B. Skirrow and Martin J. Blaser

4

In this chapter we describe the clinical aspects of infection with *Campylobacter jejuni* subsp. *jejuni* and *C. coli*, which are the main cause of *Campylobacter* enteritis in humans. Our account includes extraintestinal infections that may arise either as a complication of enteritis or as an apparently spontaneous event, but it does not include infections due to species other than *C. jejuni* and *C. coli*, which are described in chapter 5 (which includes infection due to *C. jejuni* subsp. *doylei*). *Campylobacter*-associated Guillain-Barré syndrome has taken on such importance that it also merits its own chapter (see chapter 8).

DESCRIPTION OF DISEASE

Campylobacter enteritis is an acute diarrheal disease with clinical manifestations like those of other acute bacterial gut infections of the intestinal tract, such as salmonellosis or shigellosis. Clinically it cannot be distinguished from these infections, although the presence of a prodromal period of fever without diarrhea, intense abdominal pain, or prostration would favor a diagnosis of *Campylobacter* enteritis. A definitive

diagnosis can be made only by detecting campylobacters in the feces. There does not seem to be any clear difference between infections caused by *C. jejuni* and *C. coli*. In one study *C. coli* was found to cause milder disease (137), whereas in another the opposite was reported (54).

Clinical Pathology

The essential lesion in *Campylobacter* enteritis is an acute inflammatory enteritis, which commonly extends down the intestine to affect the colon and rectum. Terminal ileitis and cecitis, with mesenteric adenitis, are prominent features. Since autopsy or surgical material is rare, nearly all our knowledge of the histological changes in the gut are derived from biopsy specimens obtained at proctosigmoidoscopy. These are described below in the section on *Campylobacter* colitis.

For infection to become established, campylobacters must first survive the acidic conditions in the stomach and then colonize the jejunum and ileum. Thus, lowering of gastric acidity facilitates infection, which is well established in relation to salmonella infections. A case-control study indicated that omeprazole therapy roughly doubles the risk of acquiring campylobacter enteritis; interestingly, this ef-

Martin B. Skirrow, Public Health Laboratory, Gloucestershire Royal Hospital, Gloucester GL1 3NN, United Kingdom. *Martin J. Blaser*, Division of Infectious Diseases, Vanderbilt University School of Medicine, A3310 MCN, Nashville, TN 37232-2605.

Campylobacter, 2nd Ed., Edited by I. Nachamkin and M. J. Blaser
© 2000 American Society for Microbiology, Washington, D.C.

fect was not seen with H_2 receptor antagonists (120).

Colonization of the gut mucosa depends on unimpaired bacterial motility and the ability to attach to the surface of mucosal cells. The rapid motility and spiral shape of campylobacters enables them to move easily through viscous mucus overlying the mucosa. These and other aspects of pathogenesis are discussed in chapters 9 to 16.

Immune Response

Antibodies to *Campylobacter* antigens appear in the serum from about day 5 of illness, peak within 2 to 4 weeks, and then decline over several months (10, 13). Intestinal antibodies are also produced (11). Volunteer studies show that *Campylobacter* infection confers short-term immunity to the homologous strain (10, 11), but it is not known how long it lasts or how broad is the immunity from a single infection. Sequential infections arising 6 to 18 months apart have been recorded, invariably with a strain that is different from the original one (80, 161). However, under natural conditions, immunity is gained from relatively few infections, despite the heterogeneity of *C. jejuni* strains.

In developing countries, where repeated infection is common in early childhood, infection rates decline with age, fewer infections are associated with diarrhea, and the duration and magnitude of convalescent-phase excretion of campylobacters are reduced. This is paralleled by a progressive rise in specific immunoglobulin A (IgA) antibody levels in serum (19). In developing countries, *Campylobacter* enteritis is virtually absent in older children and adults, but it is not clear whether sustaining this immunity depends on repeated reexposure to the organism.

Relative resistance to infection has also been observed in groups of people who habitually drink raw milk, a high-risk food (18, 74). The importance of the humoral response is indicated by the problems experienced by subjects with hypogammaglobulinemia, who are likely to develop prolonged and sometimes severe infections (see p. 74). *Campylobacter*-specific IgA antibody is secreted in the breast milk of immune mothers and confers some protection against infection in their infants (117). Considerations of the immune response are clinically relevant in that illness becomes increasingly mild with age among children in developing countries.

Infective Dose

There are many influencing factors, but in general the infective dose of *C. jejuni* often is low. Infection has been induced with doses as low as 500 bacteria in experimental human infection (10, 147). This low dose is consistent with the large size of milk-borne and waterborne outbreaks of *Campylobacter* enteritis, which may further lower the infective dose by exerting a buffering action or enabling rapid wash through of stomach contents.

Incubation Period

The mean incubation period of *Campylobacter* enteritis calculated from 17 point-source outbreaks is 3.2 days, with a range of 18 h to 8 days. The extremes of the range are somewhat suspect, since the outliers might not represent infection from the defined source. A working range of 1 to 7 days is a reasonable compromise. We emphasize that the mean incubation period of 3 days is longer than that of most other intestinal infections, a point of significance when questioning patients with suspected foodborne infection.

Onset and Prodrome

The clinical consequences depend in part on the virulence of the infecting strain, the challenge dose, and the susceptibility of the patient. As described above, people who have had previous *Campylobacter* infection, such as those who habitually drink raw milk, or children brought up in developing countries, will probably experience no symptoms. Others are likely to become ill. The disease described below is that experienced by patients sufficiently ill to seek medical attention, but unrecorded milder illness is undoubtedly common.

The onset is often abrupt, with cramping

pains in the abdomen quickly followed by diarrhea, but about 30% of patients suffer a nonspecific influenza-like prodrome with one or more symptoms of fever, headache, dizziness, and myalgia. Rigors have been recorded in up to 22% of patients, and fever may be sufficiently high to cause convulsions in children (75) or delirium in adults. Meningismus also has been observed. The prodrome can be highly misleading in the absence of abdominal symptoms, which may not appear for 2 or even 3 days. Patients with prodromal symptoms tend to have more severe illness than those whose illness starts with diarrhea.

Diarrheal Stage

The onset of diarrhea betrays the intestinal nature of the infection. It is commonly profuse, watery, bile stained, and sometimes prostrating. Surveys have shown that at least 50% of patients attending emergency rooms have 10 or more bowel actions per day. After 1 or 2 days of diarrhea, frank blood appears in the stools in about 15% of patients (30% of hospital patients), indicating a progression of infection into the colon and rectum (see the section on colitis, below). In two studies, gross or occult blood in the stools was shown to be more frequent than in *Salmonella* or *Shigella* enteritis (20, 142). Nausea is a frequent symptom, but only about 15% of patients vomit.

A particular feature of *Campylobacter* enteritis is abdominal pain, which may become continuous and sufficiently intense to mimic acute appendicitis; this is the most frequent reason for admission of *Campylobacter* enteritis patients to the hospital. Although the pain usually is central, it can radiate to the right iliac fossa and make the diagnosis difficult (see below). Outbreaks of *Campylobacter* enteritis in schools in which 30% of children had abdominal pain without diarrhea have been reported (93, 183). The acute-stage clinical features are shown in Table 1.

Recovery Stage

After a variable period, usually about 3 to 4 days into the illness, the diarrhea begins to ease

TABLE 1 Clinical features of *Campylobacter* enteritis derived from surveys of community outbreaks in which 50 or more people were affected and analyzed[a]

Symptom[b]	Frequency (%)	
	Mean/median	Range
Fever (25)	50/52	6–75
Diarrhea (26)	84/85	52–100
Headache (21)	41/47	6–69
Abdominal pain (26)	79/80	56–99
Myalgia (5)	42/37	28–59
Vomiting (20[c])	15/11	1–42
Blood in feces (7)	15/13	0.5–32

[a] Compiled from references 52, 68, 71, 75, 93, 98, 102, 105, 138, 139, 148, 149, 152, 166, 167, 172, 175, and 180.
[b] Numbers in parentheses are the number of outbreaks from which data were obtained.
[c] Excluding waterborne outbreaks, since the exceptionally high frequency of vomiting in several waterborne outbreaks suggested the additional presence of Norwalk-like viruses.

and the patient's condition improves, although the abdominal pain may persist for several more days. The mistake many patients make at this stage is to eat too much too soon, which invites a prompt return of symptoms, especially abdominal pain. Minor relapses have been reported in 15 to 25% of patients who present to physicians (12, 43, 134). Weight loss of up to 5 kg is a common outcome.

Patients continue to excrete campylobacters in their feces for several weeks after they have clinically recovered, unless the infection has been treated with antibiotics. Estimation of the excretion period depends heavily on the sensitivity of the detection methods. With direct-plating methods, 50% of patients are culture negative after 3 weeks, but in a study involving more sensitive methods, a mean excretion period of 37.6 days (maximum, 69 days) was found (76). Long-term carriage has been observed only in patients with immune deficiency, notably hypogammaglobulinemia and AIDS (see below). The question of *Campylobacter* excretion is somewhat academic, since it has never been proved that such patients have ever transmitted infection. The typical course of *Campylobacter* enteritis is shown diagrammatically in Fig. 1.

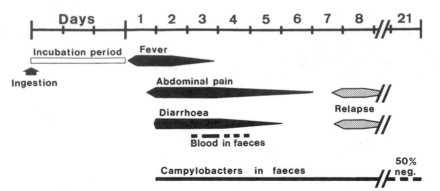

FIGURE 1 Diagram illustrating the typical course of *Campylobacter* enteritis. Reprinted from D. Greenwood, R. Slack, and J. Peutherer (ed.), *Medical Microbiology*, 15th ed., 1997, Churchill Livingstone, Edinburgh, United Kingdom, with permission.

Morbidity

The average duration of illness is difficult to measure, because there are so many variables, such as the immune status of the host, the virulence of the infecting strain, and the criteria used to define illness. The average figure covering nine outbreaks affecting about 1,500 people was 4.6 days, but in one of the outbreaks one-third of the patients were ill for more than 7 days (110). A survey of sporadic cases in Norway recorded mean durations of 3.8 days lost from work or school and 14.6 days for the presence of symptoms (76). There is a remarkable case of a young man who allegedly had campylobacter enteritis for 17 years, which was ultimately cured by a course of erythromycin (126). The proportion of patients admitted to the hospital shows even greater variation between surveys (0.5 to 32%). Most surveys indicate the range of 5 to 10%. A fatal outcome is rare and is usually confined to elderly patients or those already suffering from another serious disease (163, 164).

SPECIAL ASPECTS OF INFECTION

Appendicitis

Abdominal pain in *Campylobacter* enteritis may be highly intense and continuous and radiate to the right iliac fossa. In most patients the appendix is not affected ("pseudo-appendicitis")

and the pain is caused by terminal ileitis and mesenteric adenitis. However, occasionally there is genuine appendicitis, and campylobacters can be isolated from the inflamed appendices (28, 101, 112, 127). True guarding and rebound tenderness demand surgical attention whether or not *Campylobacter* infection is thought to be present.

Although seemingly rare, appendicitis associated with *Campylobacter* enteritis is probably overlooked, since surgically removed appendices are not routinely cultured. A survey of 251 children admitted to a surgical unit with suspected appendicitis showed that 6 (2.4%) had *Campylobacter* infection, 3 of whom (1.2%) had genuine appendicitis and 3 had mesenteric adenitis with normal appendices (127). In a larger survey of 533 older children and adults, the *Campylobacter* infection rate was almost the same (2.8%), but only 1 patient showed minor histological evidence of acute appendicitis (141). The other infected patients were shown by graded-compression ultrasonography to have a characteristic picture of mural thickening of the terminal ileum and cecum with enlarged mesenteric lymph nodes but no image of the appendix. As a result of these sonographic tests, 26 planned appendectomies were cancelled (141).

The proportion of *Campylobacter* enteritis patients referred for suspected appendicitis is small. In a large milk-borne outbreak in the United Kingdom (75), the fraction was 0.1%, and among sporadic infections reported the Communicable Disease Surveillance Centre, London, the figure was 0.27% (unpublished data).

Colitis

Sigmoidoscopy and rectal biopsy shows that an element of colitis and proctitis is present in most patients with *Campylobacter* enteritis sufficiently severe to have these tests done (17, 30, 86, 96, 140). In some patients, colitis is a dominant feature, and then the problem is to distinguish the condition from acute nonspecific inflammatory bowel disease (IBD). Stool cultures should be performed as soon as possible, and it is worth finding whether the local laboratory can undertake rapid diagnosis by direct microscopic examination of feces for campylobacters. Cultures involving filtration techniques to identify other *Campylobacter* and related species also should be done.

There are conflicting views on how reliably the distinction between *Campylobacter* infection and IBD can be made by sigmoidoscopy and rectal biopsy, with some workers finding little difficulty (100, 140) but others encountering problems in some patients (86, 96). The first point to make is that the changes seen in *Campylobacter* enteritis are indistinguishable from those of other acute bacterial infections of the gut, such as salmonella and shigella infection. Endoscopic appearances range from mildly hyperemic intact epithelium to mucosal edema, granularity, friability, spontaneous bleeding, and patchy aphthous-type ulceration (30, 86, 96, 100). Active colitis may extend at least as far as the splenic flexure, and one patient has been described as having ulcers measuring up to 3 by 5 cm and a "cobblestone" mucosa, but with "skip areas" of normal mucosa (90).

Histology shows acute inflammation of the mucosa with edema, infiltration by polymorphonuclear leukocytes, and crypt abscess formation (30, 86, 96, 140, 179). In one study, the degree of histological abnormality was graded and found to correlate with a history of blood in the stools but not with fever, abdominal pain, or diarrhea (30). In contrast to IBD, the lesions are focal and there is little or no distortion of the crypts or mucosa, nor is there a striking depletion of mucus cells. However, the appearances overlap, especially in *Campylobacter* enteritis patients who have had the infection for more than 1 week, in whom chronic inflammatory cells may be numerous (96). The main distinguishing histological features are shown in Table 2.

It is important to remember that an apparent flare-up of IBD may be due to an intercurrent intestinal infection, such as *Campylobacter* enteritis (60, 121). It is mandatory to look for pathogens in such patients, so that appropriate antimicrobial treatment can be started at the earliest opportunity. It is unlikely that *Campylobacter* infection plays any part in the cause of IBD, since no excess of patients with antibodies

TABLE 2 Comparison of histological features that help to differentiate *Campylobacter* and other infective causes of proctocolitis from acute IBD[a]

Feature	Infective colitis	IBD
Distribution of lesions	Focal and segmental	Diffuse and general
Crypt architecture	Preserved	Distored, atrophic
Mucus cell depletion	Absent or mild	Pronounced
Inflammatory cells	Mainly polymorphs in focal collections; crypt abscess formation	Chronic inflammatory cells (especially plasma cells)
Distribution of cells	Mainly mucosal	Submucosa may be involved
Epitheliod granulomata	Absent	Often present
Basal lymphoid aggregates	Absent	Present
Isolated giant cells	In upper part of glandular epithelium	Basally located

[a] Based on data from reference 169.

to campylobacter antigens were found in serological surveys of patients with IBD (14, 15, 103).

Toxic Megacolon

Toxic megacolon complicating *Campylobacter* enteritis has been reported in three patients, all adult women (62, 97, 168). Unless perforation of the bowel is suspected, it is best to avoid surgical treatment in such patients and to rely on vigorous antimicrobial treatment.

CAMPYLOBACTER ENTERITIS IN CHILDREN

The pattern of infection in children, especially newborns, differs sufficiently from the above description to warrant special consideration. Fortunately, illness is seldom severe. Fever is often absent, but vomiting and the passage of blood in the stools is more frequent. In a hospital-based study, 92% of infected children under 1 year of age had frank blood in their stools (77). In the newborn, the passage of blood, often without obvious diarrhea, can mimic intussusception, with the risk of an unnecessary laparotomy being performed. In cases in which the infant shows more severe illness, the picture can resemble necrotizing enterocolitis (176).

The high frequency of blood in the stools of infected children reflects the frequency of colitis, although few have performed sigmoidoscopic examinations in the young (63). Chronic colitis also has been described (66). Pancolitis was recorded in a 14-year-old boy (86) and a 4-year-old girl who apparently died of *Campylobacter* infection superimposed on Crohn's disease (29). In another case, a 7-year-old boy with suspected bowel obstruction was found on radiography to have colonic distension, fluid levels, and aphthous ulcers of his colon, all apparently due to *Campylobacter* infection (9).

Neonatal Infection

Neonatal infection usually is acquired from infected mothers at birth. The mother may not be having diarrhea at the time, nor is there always a history of diarrhea (2, 78). At least five outbreaks in neonatal nurseries in which there has been nosocomial spread of infection from some communally used items, such as inadequately disinfected thermometers or baby baths, have been reported (61, 65, 150, 174, 178). In one such case, *C. jejuni* was isolated from a rubber bath plug in the affected nursery (178). In another outbreak, 11 infants developed *C. jejuni* meningitis (61). There is a single report of a 3½-week-old boy with hemolytic anemia associated with *C. jejuni* gastroenteritis (31).

RASHES

Urticaria appearing late in *Campylobacter* enteritis has been described on several occasions (22, 24, 68, 89). Most remarkable was when 12 boys presented with urticaria near the end of an outbreak of campylobacter enteritis in a British boarding school, in which some 400 boys had symptoms; not all of the 12 boys with urticaria had had diarrheal symptoms (68).

Erythema nodosum appearing 1 to 2 weeks after campylobacter enteritis has been found in four patients, all women (6, 47, 50, 85). A patient whose forearms and elbows, as well as her shins, were affected had terminal ileitis (85). Immune complex vasculitis has been found in association with campylobacter enteritis, but the patients had underlying diseases that could have contributed to the skin pathology (7, 118, 157).

INFECTION IN IMMUNODEFICIENT PATIENTS

Hypogammaglobulinemia and AIDS are the conditions most often associated with more severe *Campylobacter* infection. Chronic carriage of campylobacters with recurrent enteritis, often with bacteremia, is a typical problem.

A study of *Campylobacter* infection in human immunodeficiency virus-infected patients, 76% of whom had AIDS, showed that 10% had bacteremia (111). Another study showed that bacteremia in human immunodeficiency virus-infected patients was often a severe, debilitating, febrile illness requiring multiple and prolonged courses of antimicrobial therapy (173).

The incidence of campylobacter infection in patients with AIDS has been calculated to be 40-fold higher than in immunocompetent patients (165).

In a survey of 41 hypogammaglobulinemic patients, 5 had experienced at least one episode of *C. jejuni* septicemia, 3 with an erysipelas-like cellulitis (81). Repeated courses of antimicrobial treatment are often needed in these patients, and this carries the risk that the infecting strain will become resistant, thus leading to an intractable problem. Limited experience suggests that the best approach is to combine an antimicrobial agent with an immunoglobulin preparation. A commercial IgM-containing preparation (Pentaglobin) has been used successfully with antibiotics to cure two hypogammaglobulinemic patients of *C. jejuni* infection (21), and the bactericidal properties of the preparation have been demonstrated in vitro against several serotypes of *C. jejuni* (8). The anti–campylobacter IgM antibodies present in this preparation appear essential, since eight other immunoglobulins containing only IgG lacked a bactericidal effect (8). Another report describes the successful combination of maternal plasma with ciprofloxacin on an intractable 2-year-long *C. jejuni* infection in a 7-year-old boy with X-linked agammaglobulinemia (7).

OTHER INTESTINAL COMPLICATIONS

Intestinal Hemorrhage
Severe intestinal hemorrhage has been reported once. The patient was a previously healthy 24-year-old nurse who had to undergo emergency hemicolectomy for a massively bleeding ulcer in the terminal ileum (109).

Ileostomy Stoma Ulceration
Patients with an ileostomy may experience partial strangulation of their stoma with *Campylobacter* enteritis, presumably through congestion and edema. In two women with long-established ileostomies after total colectomy for IBD, the stoma became extensively ulcerated but eventually healed without lasting damage (107, 162).

Perirectal Abscess
A perirectal abscess in a 64-year-old woman yielded *C. jejuni* and *Citrobacter freundii* on culture 3 weeks after she had suffered diarrhea presumed to have been caused by the *C. jejuni* strain (84).

EXTRAINTESTINAL INFECTION

Bacteremia
Bacteremia in *Campylobacter* enteritis is seldom reported, but it probably occurs commonly as a transient event in the early stages of infection, especially in patients with rigors and high fever. There are three reasons why *C. jejuni* bacteremia is not detected more frequently: (i) blood cultures are rarely performed early in the disease; (ii) *C. jejuni* generally is sensitive to the bactericidal properties of normal serum, unlike *C. fetus,* which is serum resistant; and (iii) not all methods to detect bacteremia are equally sensitive for *Campylobacter* species (181).

A survey of laboratory reports made to the Communicable Disease Surveillance Centre, London, showed an average bacteremia rate of 1.5 per 1,000 intestinal infections, but there was wide variation with age (163). The highest rate (5.9 per 1,000) was in patients aged 65 years or more, and the lowest (0.3 per 1,000) was in children aged 1 to 4 years (Fig. 2). The rates were nearly twice as high in males than in females. Although some patients had immunodeficiency or some underlying disease, 71% were apparently normal (in sharp contrast to patients with *C. fetus* infection, most of whom had some predisposing disorder). *C. jejuni* strains belonging to Penner serogroups O4 and O18 were more frequent among blood than fecal isolates, but subsequent genotypic analysis cf these and additional strains did not suggest that blood isolates were especially invasive or serum resistant (72). In another study, systemic isolates were found to be less susceptible to normal human serum than intestinal isolates, but the ranges showed considerable overlap (16). In a more recent study in Denmark, the bacteremia rate was found to be 8 per 1,000 intestinal infections (157).

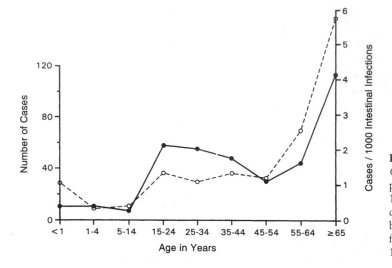

FIGURE 2 Distribution of *Campylobacter* bacteremia cases with patient age in England and Wales 1981 to 1991. Solid line, number of cases (*n* = 374); dashed line, number of cases per 1,000 intestinal infections. Reprinted from reference 163 with permission.

C. jejuni can cause serious septicemic infection in patients whose immune system is severely compromised (see above). A fatal outcome was reported in two patients who had undergone splenectomy for thalassemia, both of whom had iron overload (73, 108).

Infection of the Hepatobiliary System

HEPATITIS

A mild degree of hepatitis may be a regular feature of *Campylobacter* enteritis. Several reports have shown slightly raised transaminase levels in serum in hospital patients with campylobacter enteritis (43, 96, 134). Some strains of *C. jejuni* produce hepatotoxic factors in mice (82), and the liver and gallbladder were found to be the most consistently colonized organs after the intestines in experimentally infected rhesus monkeys (55).

Obvious clinical hepatitis is rare. Two young men were found to have enlarged livers and raised liver enzyme levels 1 week after the onset of *Campylobacter* enteritis (70). In three other patients with clinical hepatitis, liver biopsy showed evidence of hepatitis: a 52-year-old man had mild mononuclear cell infiltration in portal areas, with variation in hepatocyte and nuclear size (144); a 48-year-old alcoholic man had cholestatic hepatitis with lymphohistiocytic infiltration of portal tracts and *C. jejuni*

bacteremia (119); and a previously healthy 50-year-old woman, also with bacteremia (with *C. coli*), had neutrophil infiltration of the portal tracts with adjacent areas of necrosis (1). More recently, an 82-year-old woman admitted to the hospital with rigors, fever, and watery diarrhea due to *C. jejuni* was found to have acute hepatitis (83). Significantly, the hepatitis resolved in all six of these patients after treatment directed against the infecting campylobacter strain.

CHOLECYSTITIS

C. jejuni is a bile-tolerant organism, and so it is not surprising that it is sometimes found in the gallbladder in association with acute cholecystitis or acute-complicating-chronic cholecystitis (32, 38, 44, 106, 177). Patients may or may not give a history of recent diarrhea. Prospective searches for campylobacters in bile from several hundred cholecystectomy samples yielded none; therefore, biliary infection appears to be uncommon (32).

PANCREATITIS

Acute pancreatitis has been reported in a few patients, all adults, during the acute stages of *Campylobacter* enteritis. Abdominal pain was a dominant symptom in each (26, 34, 46, 58, 135). An 88-year-old woman had acute pancreatitis and *C. jejuni* bacteremia without diarrhea (51). The pancreatitis resolved satisfactorily in all of these patients after they had received appropriate antimicrobial treatment. The mechanism by which campylobacters cause pancreatitis is unknown.

The possibility that a mild degree of pancreatitis is a regular feature of the disease was suggested by a Finnish study of 188 hospitalized patients with *Campylobacter* enteritis. In that study, 22% of patients were considered to have pancreatitis based on elevated amylase or lipase levels in serum (134). However, in a study of 22 other patients, none was found to have raised enzyme levels (115).

Abortion and Perinatal Infection

C. fetus has been traditionally regarded as the cause of epizootic abortion of sheep, but it was only after the advent of *C. jejuni* and *C. coli* in human medicine that the role of these organisms in veterinary medicine became apparent. A survey in the United Kingdom showed that *C. jejuni* and *C. coli* account for about 40 and 20% of ovine abortion cases respectively, only 40% are caused by *C. fetus*. This predilection of campylobacters for uterine and fetal tissues in ruminants is fortunately low in humans. Nevertheless, there have been nearly 30 reports of septic abortion or stillbirth due to campylobacter infection. About half were caused by *C. fetus,* one was caused by *C. hyointestinalis* (see chapter 5), and the remaining half were caused by *C. jejuni* or *C. coli*. The average stage of gestation for women infected with *C. fetus* or with *C. jejuni* is 28 and 19 weeks, respectively. However, five infants infected in utero with *C. fetus* were born sufficiently late in gestation to survive premature birth, whereas none of the *C. jejuni*-infected infants survived; indeed, only two were born late enough to have a chance of survival.

The pathology resembles that of campylobacter abortion in sheep, namely, an acute placentitis that is severe enough to cause fetal death as a result of placental insufficiency, although infection eventually reaches the fetus via amniotic fluid. The bacteria probably reach the placenta by hematogenous spread from the intestinal tract, although this is unproven. There is no evidence that infection ascends from the genital tract. Most infected mothers have fever and about half have diarrhea shortly before or at the time of abortion. However, maternal illness is seldom pronounced and there may be little to indicate the nature of the problem.

Twenty patients with *Campylobacter* abortion have been described by Simor et al. (160), and several more patients have been described since then (37, 114, 159). There is a report of a 28-year-old woman with acquired agammaglobulinemia who had recurrent abortions after a persistent attack of *C. jejuni* diarrhea (133). The factors that allow campylobacters to infect the human placenta are unknown. In a study in the United Kingdom, *C. jejuni*/*C. coli* was isolated from 0.2% of women in labour (rectal swabs), most of whom had no symptoms relating to the organism (185). Thus, many thousands of pregnant women must develop the infection without any untoward effect. Some infections are almost certainly overlooked, but even allowing for this, campylobacter abortion remains a rare event.

Renal and Urinary Tract Disease

HEMOLYTIC-UREMIC SYNDROME

There are reports of eight patients, including five children younger than 5 years, who developed hemolytic-uremic syndrome within a few days of developing campylobacter enterocolitis (27, 36, 40, 95, 158). An exception was the case of an adult patient, in whom the interval was 1 month (35). Most of the patients had blood in their stools, and all recovered except one, a 4-month-old Bangladeshi infant who died (64). A further report describes a 72-year-old woman who developed the closely related syndrome of thrombotic thrombocytopenic purpura 5 days after the onset of nonbloody *C. jejuni* diarrhea (113). Since only one of these reports states that enterohemorrhagic *Escherichia coli* (EHEC) was not isolated, it is possible that the isolation of campylobacters was coincidental to undiscovered EHEC infection. Several of the incidents arose before the role of EHEC in hemolytic-uremic syndrome was known or routine measures for their isolation were implemented.

NEPHRITIS

Rare instances of nephritis, mainly glomerulonephritis, complicating *Campylobacter* enteritis have been reported. An 18-year-old man developed mild acute glomerulonephritis during an attack of *C. jejuni* enteritis (104). A 33-year-old man had moderately severe diffuse proliferative endocapillary glomerulonephritis on renal biopsy a few days into an attack of *C. jejuni* diarrhea; he required hemodialysis but recovered completely (91). A 5-year-old girl developed glomerulonephritis with pulmonary hemorrhage and anemia (Goodpasture's syndrome) 3 to 4 weeks after the onset of *C. jejuni* diarrhea. Renal biopsy showed immune complex-mediated crescentic glomerulonephritis, and *C. jejuni* antigen was identified in the glomeruli. The patient developed progressive renal failure (4). Mesangial IgA glomerulonephritis has been observed in two males 15 and 26 years old, both of whom had hematuria within 2 days of the onset of diarrhea (25, 161). There is a single report of self-limited tubulointerstitial nephritis diagnosed in a 20-year-old man 8 days after the onset of *C. jejuni* enteritis (143).

PROSTATITIS AND URINARY TRACT INFECTION

The urinary tract seems an unlikely place to find campylobacters, since they do not easily tolerate acidic conditions, but there are two reports of apparent *C. jejuni* urinary tract infection. In the first, the main site of infection was thought to be the prostate (33), but the other appeared to involve cystitis in a 6-year-old girl (53). The authors of that report saw campylobacter-like organisms in the urine and performed appropriate cultures for them. As they indicate, infections will be missed unless cultures specific for campylobacters are set up when morphologically suspect bacteria are seen in urine samples.

Miscellaneous Extraintestinal Infections

FOCAL INFECTION

Focal infection with *C. jejuni* or *C. coli* is rare. Most such infections are in subjects with immunodeficiency or other predisposing conditions such as cirrhosis, and presumably they arise from bacteremia. Reports of focal infection, other than infection of the female reproductive tract (see above), are listed in Table 3.

PERITONITIS

There are four reports of spontaneous peritonitis, two due to *C. jejuni,* one to *C. coli,* and one in which the differentiation was not made. Three patients had long-standing alcoholic cirrhosis, and the other had cirrhosis secondary to congestive heart failure (42, 67, 99, 156).

TABLE 3 Focal infections due to *C. jejuni* and *C. coli*

Focus of infection (reference)	Age (yr)/sex of patient	Predisposing condition	Organism
Chest wall abscess (116)	72F	Mastectomy scar, postirradiation	*C. jejuni*
Osteitis of foot (128)	57M	Site of previously removed histiocytoma	*C. jejuni*
Prosthetic hip sepsis (130)	60M	AIDS	*C. jejuni*
Septic arthritis of knee (125)	51F	Rheumatoid arthritis	*C. jejuni*
Septic arthritis of shoulder (unpublished)[a]	90M	Not known	*Campylobacter* sp.
Acute bursitis (155)	81M	Chronic bursitis	*C. jejuni*
Meningitis, non-neonatal (123)	34M	Long-standing ventricular shunt	*C. jejuni*
Subdural sepsis (145)	2.5F	Previous hemispherectomy	*C. jejuni*
Empyema (unpublished)[a]	70M	Not known	*C. jejuni*
Empyema (unpublished)[a]	52M	Not known	*C. coli*

[a] Public Health Laboratory Service, London, United Kingdom.

Less rare is *Campylobacter* peritonitis complicating continuous ambulatory peritoneal dialysis, which usually arises during an attack of *Campylobacter* enteritis. Whether the bacteria seed the peritoneal cavity from the bloodstream by transluminal migration from the intestine or by contamination of the catheter fittings is unknown. A report of eight patients and a review of other case reports are given by Wood et al. (184), and there has been one other subsequent report (182).

MYOCARDITIS

Myocarditis within 1 week of *C. jejuni* enteritis in two young men has been reported. The cardinal feature in both patients was severe chest pain radiating to the right arm. The first patient, aged 27 years, was believed to have perimyocarditis (136). The second patient, aged 23 years, had more convincing evidence of cardiac damage in that his cardiac enzyme levels were greatly elevated (56). Electrocardiographic changes were observed in both cases: T-wave inversion, slight elevation of the S-T segment, and lengthening of the PR interval on serial tracings. No signs of lasting damage was found in either patient 2 months after the episode. There is a brief report of transient atrial fibrillation associated with *C. jejuni* enteritis in three patients, all older than 50 years (79).

SPLENIC RUPTURE

Spontaneous rupture of the spleen was reported in a 71-year-old man 1 week after the onset of explosive diarrhea due to *C. jejuni* enteritis (57). Recovery was uneventful after partial splenectomy. There was no other factor to account for the rupture, but the authors indicated that spontaneous splenic rupture has been associated with other enteric pathogens, including *Salmonella dublin*.

LATE-ONSET COMPLICATIONS

Reactive Arthritis and Reiter's Syndrome

The reactive arthritis that sometimes follows *Campylobacter* enteritis is no different from that associated with *Salmonella* or other intestinal

bacterial infections. In a review of 29 patients, the mean interval between the onset of bowel symptoms and the appearance of pain and swelling of the joints was 14 days, with a range of 3 days to 6 weeks (131). The ankles, knees, wrists, and the small joints of the hands and feet are most commonly affected, often in migratory fashion (131, 154). The duration of arthritis ranges from several weeks to several months or occasionally a year. Although the arthritis can be incapacitating, full recovery is the rule. Acute erosions of the hamate bone of the wrist and distal ends of the clavicles were found in a 46-year-old man (49). The full Reiter's syndrome has been observed in some patients with *Campylobacter*-associated arthritis (87, 131, 151, 154), and uveitis in the absence of arthritis has been found in two middle-aged women, one of whom had hypogammaglobulinemia (88) and one of whom had conjunctivitis several weeks before the onset of uveitis (69).

Possession of the HLA B27 tissue antigen carries a strong predisposition to reactive arthritis, and patients with this antigen have, on average, higher erythrocyte sedimentation rates than do B27-negative patients (84.6 and 44.6 mm/h, respectively) (131). At least 60% (and probably closer to 80%) of reactive arthritis victims possess the antigen. It is difficult to generalize about the frequency of reactive arthritis in *Campylobacter* enteritis patients, since much depends on the prevalence of HLA B27 in the population. Estimates ranging from 0 to 1.7% have been given in community outbreaks of the disease (48, 75, 102, 105, 110). A calculated frequency of 5% in hospital patients has been reported in Scandinavia, where 14% of the population are HLA B27 positive (134). A long-term followup of 66 patients affected in a food-borne outbreak of *C. jejuni* enteritis in Sweden suggested that nonspecific rheumatic disorders are a common sequel of infection (23). Four patients suffered chronic or relapsing rheumatic symptoms beginning 3 to 8 months after infection and persisting for 5 years, but the significance of this finding is questionable in the absence of a control group.

Guillain-Barré Syndrome

The association of *Campylobacter* enteritis with Guillain-Barré syndrome, which emerged during the mid-1980s, greatly increased our concept of the morbidity of the disease. In view of the importance of Guillain-Barré syndrome and the complexity of its pathogenesis, it is given special consideration in chapter 8.

DIAGNOSIS AND CLINICAL INVESTIGATIONS

Bacteriology

As mentioned above, a definitive diagnosis of *Campylobacter* enteritis can be made only bacteriologically. Since the laboratory diagnosis of the infection is described in chapter 3, all that is necessary here is to stress the importance of delivering fecal samples to the laboratory with the minimum delay. Samples should be refrigerated while awaiting transport. If delays of more than 1 day are likely, transport medium, such as a standard Cary-Blair-type medium, should be used. Rectal swabs should be used as a substitute for feces only as a last resort, in which case the use of transport medium is essential.

RAPID DIAGNOSIS

Rapid diagnosis may be helpful in patients with suspected appendicitis or with acute colitis masquerading as acute IBD, or for definitive early anti-bacterial therapy. The microscopic examination of wet feces or fecal smears for campylobacters can provide a rapid diagnosis, but the sensitivity of microscopy is variable (36 to 90%), and it may not be available in all laboratories. The detection of campylobacters in feces by latex agglutination, DNA probes, or PCR is under development (see chapter 3).

SERODIAGNOSIS

Serological tests are occasionally useful for the retrospective diagnosis of *Campylobacter* enteritis in patients with late complications in whom cultures were not performed. Such tests are available only in reference or research laboratories.

Hematology and Biochemistry

Hematological and biochemical analyses are likely to be needed only in patients with complications, but it is useful to be aware of the changes found in patients with *Campylobacter* enteritis. These values relate mainly to series of patients treated in hospital. Leukocyte counts are usually normal or only slightly raised (134). Mean leukocyte counts in three series of patients were 7.9×10^9/liter (170), 8.9×10^9/liter (129), and 10.0×10^9/liter (39). In the last series, a particular feature of *Campylobacter* enteritis not seen in other forms of acute diarrhea, except shigellosis, was a high percentage of band forms (mean 15.1%), especially in the presence of only a moderate total leukocyte count (39). The erythrocyte sedimentation rate is usually raised; mean values of 25 to 30 mm/h were found in surveys of hospital patients. Elevated C-reactive protein levels were recorded in all acutely ill patients in one series (134).

Biochemical values in *Campylobacter* enteritis are usually normal, although metabolic acidosis was detected in 32% of hospital patients in one study (134). Mildly raised transaminase levels in serum have been reported in 14 to 25% of patients (43, 96, 134), and slightly raised alkaline phosphatase levels have been found in 10% (43).

Endoscopy and Radiography

The place of endoscopy and rectal biopsy in the management of patients has been described in the section on *Campylobacter* colitis. Only patients with severe or complicated infection are likely to require radiographic investigation. Dilated loops of intestine with fluid levels on plain abdominal radiographs were observed in 5 of 20 patients in one study of hospital patients (22) but not in 14 patients in another study (129). Contrast radiography has shown the presence of pancolitis (17, 86), nodular thickening of the terminal ileum (85), right-sided colonic ulceration and dilation (97), and multiple aphthous–type ulceration, which in one patient mimicked Crohn's disease (9). Barium enema examination strongly suggested colonic carcinoma in two patients, so much so that one patient was subjected to hemicolectomy for what turned out to be nothing more than inflammatory edema, congestion, and lymphoid hyperplasia (41, 122). The increasing availability and usage of abdominal computed tomography should facilitate the differentiation between appendicitis and mesenteric adenitis.

TREATMENT

No specific treatment is required for the great majority of patients with *Campylobacter* enteritis, other than the oral replacement of fluid and electrolytes lost through diarrhea and vomiting. Antimicrobial therapy plays only a limited role, because the patient is likely to be showing signs of improvement by the time a bacteriological diagnosis has been made. This is not necessarily a reflection of a slow laboratory service, since it has repeatedly been shown that patients seek medical advice only after they have been ill for 4 to 6 days on average (3, 92, 124).

This late presentation of patients invalidated early trials of antibiotic therapy, but anecdotal evidence suggested that antimicrobial agents were effective when given early in the disease. This prompted trials of erythromycin and fluoroquinolones given empirically when patients first presented with diarrhea. Such studies confirmed that the illness was shortened and that campylobacters disappeared from the feces, provided that the infecting strain was susceptible to the antimicrobial used (45, 59, 94, 132, 153). Trials in developing countries showed less effect, but the results were confounded by the simultaneous presence of other pathogens (146) or the high frequency of antibiotic-resistant strains (171). Clear instances of improvement after antimicrobial therapy have been observed in patients with severe or chronic infection, often in cases where other measures have failed (9, 17, 121, 122).

Erythromycin

Erythromycin was the first antimicrobial agent to be used, and in general it remains the agent of choice. Erythromycin resistance has remained below 5% in most regions, although there are some exceptions, such as Thailand, where up to 50% of strains are resistant. Erythromycin resistance is much more frequent in *C. coli* than *C. jejuni*. Unfortunately there is cross-resistance between erythromycin and other macrolides.

The choice of preparation probably matters little, except that enteric-coated forms of the antibiotic should not be used in patients with diarrhea, since they are likely to be passed intact without releasing their contents. Erythromycin stearate has the theoretical advantage that some remains unabsorbed in the gut, where it can have a contact effect on campylobacters; a suitable dosage is 500 mg twice daily for 5 days. For children the recommended preparation is erythromycin ethyl succinate (40 mg/kg/day) in divided doses for 5 days.

Fluoroquinolones and Other Antimicrobials

Ciprofloxacin and other fluoroquinolones were hailed with great enthusiasm when they first appeared, but their use has been severely compromised by increasing resistance rates in some countries. Fortunately, most quinolone-resistant campylobacters remain susceptible to erythromycin. Tetracyclines and chloramphenicol are alternative antibiotics when resistance or some other reason excludes the former drugs, but up to 60% of strains may be resistant to tetracyclines. Serious systemic infection should be treated with an aminoglycoside, such as gentamicin, or imipenem. Erythromycin may still be needed to clear infection from the gut.

Indications for Antimicrobial Therapy

The categories of patients likely to benefit from antimicrobial therapy are those who (i) remain acutely ill and show no signs of improvement at the time a bacteriological diagnosis is made; (ii) have unusually severe or complicated infection; (iii) have systemic infection; (iv) are immunosuppressed or suffering from other predisposition to infection; and/or (v) live in an institution or closed group where the risks of spread are high. In this last case, treatment is given to eliminate the organism from the stools of infected patients. Erythromycin was used successfully in this way to control a persistent outbreak of *Campylobacter* infection in a day care nursery in Israel (5).

REFERENCES

1. **Ampelas, M., C. Perez, J. Jourdan, B. Nalet, A. Raynaud, J. M. Emberger, and H. Michel.** 1982. Hépatite à *Campylobacter coli*. *Nouv. Presse Med.* **11:**593–595.
2. **Anders, B. J., B. A. Lauer, and J. W. Paisley.** 1981. *Campylobacter* gastroenteritis in neonates. *Am. J. Dis. Child.* **135:**900–902.
3. **Anders, B. J., B. A. Lauer, J. W. Paisley, and L. W. Reller.** 1982. Double-blind placebo controlled trial of erythromycin for treatment of *Campylobacter* enteritis. *Lancet* **i:**131–132.
4. **Andrews, P. I., G. Kainer, L. C. J. Yong, V. H. Tobias, and A. R. Rosenberg.** 1989. Glomerulonephritis, pulmonary hemorrhage and anemia associated with *C. jejuni* infection. *Aust. N. Z. J. Med.* **19:**721–723.
5. **Ashkenazi, S., Y. Danziger, Y. Varsano, J. Peilan, and M. Mimouni.** 1987. Treatment of *Campylobacter* gastroenteritis. *Arch. Dis. Child.* **62:**84–85.
6. **Ashworth, J., and J. S. C. English.** 1984. Recurrent erythema nodosum and prolonged *Campylobacter jejuni* excretion. *Br. Med. J.* **288:**830.
7. **Autenrieth, I. B., V. Schuster, J. Ewald, D. Harmsen, and H. W. Kreth.** 1996. An unusual case of refractory *Campylobacter jejuni* infection in a patient with X-linked agammaglobulinemia: successful combined therapy with maternal plasma and ciprofloxacin. *Clin. Infect. Dis.* **23:**526–531.
8. **Autenrieth, I. B., A. Schwarzkopf, J. H. Evald, H. Karch, and R. Lissner.** 1995. Bactericidal properties of *Campylobacter jejuni*-specific immunoglobulin M antibodies in commercial immunoglobulin preparations. *Antimicrob. Agents Chemother.* **39:**1965–1969.
9. **Bentley, D., J. Lynn, and J. W. Laws.** 1985. *Campylobacter* colitis with intestinal aphthous ulceration mimicking obstruction. *Br. Med. J.* **291:**634.
10. **Black, R. E., M. M. Levine, M. L. Clements, T. P. Hughes, and M. J. Blaser.** 1988. Experimental *Campylobacter jejuni* infection in humans. *J. Infect. Dis.* **157:**472–479.
11. **Black, R. E., D. Perlman, M. L. Clements, M. M. Levine, and M. J. Blaser.** 1992. Human volunteer studies with *Campylobacter jejuni*, p. 207–215. *In* I. Nachamkin, M. J. Blaser, and L. S. Tompkins (ed.), *Campylobacter jejuni: Current Status and Future Trends*. American Society for Microbiology, Washington, D.C.
12. **Blaser, M. J., I. D. Berkowitz, F. M. LaForce, J. Cravens, L. B. Reller, and W.-L. L. Wang.** 1979. *Campylobacter* enteritis: clinical and epidemiologic features. *Ann. Intern. Med.* **91:**179–185.
13. **Blaser, M. J., and D. Duncan.** 1984. Human serum antibody response to *Campylobacter jejuni* infection as measured in an enzyme-linked immunosorbent assay. *Infect. Immun.* **44:**292–298.
14. **Blaser, M. J., D. Hoverson, I. G. Ely, D. J. Duncan, W. L. L. Wang, and W. R. Brown.** 1984. Studies of *Campylobacter jejuni* on patients with inflammatory bowel disease. *Gastroenterology* **86:**33–38.
15. **Blaser, M. J., R. A. Miller, J. Lacher, and J. W. Singleton.** 1984. Patients with active Crohn's disease have elevated serum antibodies to antigens of seven enteric bacterial pathogens. *Gastroenterology* **87:**888–894.
16. **Blaser, M. J., G. Pérez-Pérez, P. F. Smith, C. Patton, F. C. Tenover, A. J. Lastovica, and W. L. L. Wang.** 1986. Extraintestinal *Campylobacter jejuni* and *Campylobacter coli* infections: host factors and strain characteristics. *J. Infect. Dis.* **153:**552–559.
17. **Blaser, M. J., R. B. Parsons, and W. L. L. Wang.** 1980. Acute colitis caused by *Campylobacter fetus ss. jejuni*. *Gastroenterology* **78:**448–453.
18. **Blaser, M. J., E. Sazie, and P. Williams.** 1987. The influence of immunity on raw milk-associated *Campylobacter* infection. *JAMA* **257:**43–46.
19. **Blaser, M. J., D. N. Taylor, and P. Echeverria.** 1986. Immune response to *Campylobacter jejuni* in a rural community in Thailand. *J. Infect. Dis.* **153:**249–254.
20. **Blaser, M. J., J. G. Wells, R. A. Feldman, R. A. Pollard, and J. R. Allen.** 1983. *Campylobacter* enteritis in the United States. A multicenter study. *Ann. Intern. Med.* **98:**360–365.
21. **Borleffs, J. C. C., J. F. Schellekens, E. Brouwer, and M. Rozenberg-Arska.** 1993. Use of an immunoglobulin M-containing preparation for treatment of two hypogammaglobulinemic patients with persistent *Campylobacter jejuni* infection. *Eur. J. Clin. Microbiol. Infect. Dis.* **12:**772–775.
22. **Bradshaw, M. J., R. Brown, J. H. Swallow, and J. A. Rycroft.** 1980. *Campylobacter* enteritis in Chelmsford. *Postgrad. Med. J.* **56:**80–84.
23. **Bremell, T., A. Bjelle, and Å. Svedhem.** 1991. Rheumatic symptoms following an outbreak of *Campylobacter* enteritis: a five year follow up. *Ann. Rheum. Dis.* **50:**934–938.

24. **Bretag, A. H., R. S. Archer, H. M. Atkinson, and W. H. Woods.** 1984. Circadian urticaria: another *Campylobacter* association. *Lancet* **i:** 954.

25. **Carter, J. E., and N. Cimolai.** 1991. IgA nephropathy associated with *Campylobacter jejuni* enteritis. *Nephron* **58:**101–102.

26. **Castilla, L., M. Castro, and P. Guerrero.** 1989. Acute pancreatitis associated with *Campylobacter* enteritis. *Dig. Dis. Sci.* **34:**961–962.

27. **Chamovitz, B. N., A. I. Hartstein, S. R. Alexander, A. B. Terry, P. Short, and R. Katon.** 1983. *Campylobacter jejuni*-associated hemolytic-uremic syndrome in a mother and daughter. *Pediatrics* **71:**253–256.

28. **Chan, F. T. H., G. Stringel, and A. M. R. Mackenzie.** 1983. Isolation of *Campylobacter jejuni* from an appendix. *J. Clin. Microbiol.* **18:** 422–424.

29. **Coffin, C. M., P. L'Heureaux, and L. P. Dehner.** 1982. *Campylobacter*-associated colitis in childhood: report of a fatal case. *Am. J. Clin. Pathol.* **78:**117–123.

30. **Colgan, T., J. R. Lambert, A. Newman, and S. C. Luk.** 1980. *Campylobacter jejuni* enterocolitis. *Arch. Pathol. Lab. Med.* **104:**571–574.

31. **Damani, N. N., C. A. Humphrey, and B. Dell.** 1993. Haemolytic anaemia in *Campylobacter* enteritis. *J. Infect.* **26:**109–110.

32. **Darling, W. M., R. N. Peel, M. B. Skirrow, and A. E. J. L. Mulira.** 1979. *Campylobacter* cholecystitis. *Lancet* **i:**1302.

33. **Davies, J. S., and J. B. Penfold.** 1979. *Campylobacter* urinary infection. *Lancet* **i:**1091.

34. **De Bois, M. H. W., M. C. Shoemaker, S. D. J. vander Werf, and J. B. C. M. Pulyeart.** 1989. Pancreatitis associated with *Campylobacter jejuni* infection: diagnosis by ultrasonography. *Br. Med. J.* **298:**1004.

35. **Delans, R. J., J. D. Biuso, S. R. Saba, and G. Ramirez.** 1984. Hemolytic-uremic syndrome after *Campylobacter*-induced diarrhea in an adult. *Arch. Intern. Med.* **144:**1074–1076.

36. **Denneberg, T., M. Freidberg, L. Holmberg, C. Mathiasen, K. O. Nilsson, R. Takolander, and M. Walder.** 1982. Combined plasmapheresis and hemodialysis treatment for severe hemolytic-uremic syndrome following *Campylobacter* colitis. *Acta Pediatr. Scand.* **71:** 243–245.

37. **Denton, K. J., and T. Clarke.** 1992. Role of *Campylobacter jejuni* as a placental pathogen. *J. Clin. Pathol.* **45:**171–172.

38. **De Sa Pereira, M., S. D. Lipton, and J. K. Kim.** 1981. Acute cholecystitis and *Campylobacter fetus*. *Ann. Intern. Med.* **94:**821.

39. **De Witt, T. G., K. F. Humphrey, and G. V. Doern.** 1985. White blood cell counts in patients with *Campylobacter*-induced diarrhea and controls. *J. Infect. Dis.* **152:**427–428.

40. **Dickgiesser, A.** 1983. Campylobakterfektion und hämolytischurämisches Syndrom. *Immun. Infeckt.* **11:**71–74.

41. **Doberneck, R. C.** 1983. *Campylobacter* colitis mimicking colonic cancer during barium enema examination. *Surgery* **93:**508–509.

42. **Domingo, P., B. Mirelis, A. Gimeno, and R. Cabezas.** 1985. Peritonitis espontánea por *Campylobacter jejuni* en un paciento cirrótico. *Med. Clin.* **84:**416.

43. **Drake, A. A., M. J. R. Gilchrist, J. A. Washington, K. A. Huizenga, and R. E. Van Scoy.** 1981. Diarrhea due to *Campylobacter fetus* subspecies *jejuni*. *Mayo Clin. Proc.* **56:**414–423.

44. **Drion, S., C. Wahlen, and P. Taziaux.** 1988. Isolation of *Campylobacter jejuni* from the bile of a cholecystic patient. *J. Clin. Microbiol.* **26:** 2193–2194.

45. **Dryden, M. S., R. J. E. Gab, and S. K. Wright.** 1996. Empirical treatment of severe acute community-acquired gastroenteritis with ciprofloxacin. *Clin. Infect. Dis.* **22:**1019–1025.

46. **Dutronc, Y., M. Duong, M. Buisson, P. Chavanet, and H. Porter.** 1995. Pancréatite aiguë et infection à *Campylobacter jejuni*. *Med. Mal. Infect.* **25:**1168–1169.

47. **Eastmond, C. J., and T. M. S. Reid.** 1982. *Campylobacter* enteritis and erythema nodosum. *Br. Med. J.* **285:**1421–1422.

48. **Eastmond, C. J., J. A. N. Rennie, and T. M. S. Reid.** 1983. An outbreak of *Campylobacter* enteritis: a rheumatological follow-up survey. *J. Rheumatol.* **10:**107–108.

49. **Ebright, J. R., and L. M. Ryan.** 1984. Acute erosive reactive arthritis associated with *Campylobacter jejuni*-induced colitis. *Am. J. Med.* **76:** 321–323.

50. **Ellis, M. E., J. Pope, A. Mokashi, and E. Dunbar.** 1982. *Campylobacter* colitis associated with erythema nodosum. *Br. Med. J.* **285:**937.

51. **Ezpeleta, C., P. Rojo de Ursua, F. Obregon, F. Goñi, and R. Cisterna.** 1992. Acute pancreatitis associated with *Campylobacter jejuni* bacteremia. *Clin. Infect. Dis.* **15:**1050.

52. **Fahey, T., D. Morgan, C. Gunnenburg, G. K. Adak, F. Mauid, and E. Kaczmarski.** 1995. An outbreak of *Campylobacter jejuni* enteritis associated with failed milk pasteurisation. *J. Infect.* **31:**137–143.

53. **Feder, H. M., M. Rasoulpour, and A. J. Rodriguez.** 1986. *Campylobacter* urinary tract infection: value of the urine Gram's stain. *JAMA* **256:**2389.

54. **Figura, N., and P. Guglielmetti.** 1988. Clini-

cal characteristics of *Campylobacter jejuni* and *C. coli* enteritis. *Lancet* **i:**942–943.

55. **Fitzgeorge, R. B., A. Baskerville, and K. P. Lander.** 1981. Experimental infection of Rhesus monkeys with a human strain of *Campylobacter jejuni. J. Hyg.* **86:**343–351.

56. **Florkowski, C. M., R. B. Ikram, I. M. Crozier, H. Ikram, and M. E. Berry.** 1984. *Campylobacter jejuni* myocarditis. *Clin. Cardiol.* **7:**558–560.

57. **Frizelle, F. A., and J. A. Rietveld.** 1993. Spontaneous splenic rupture associated with *Campylobacter jejuni* infection. *Br. J. Surg.* **81:**716–718.

58. **Gallagher, P., P. Chadwick, D. M. Jones, and L. Turner.** 1981. Acute pancreatitis associated with campylobacter infection. *Br. J. Surg.* **68:**383.

59. **Goodman, L. J., G. N. Trenholme, R. L. Kaplan, J. Segreti, D. Hines, R. Petrak, G. A. Nelson, K. W. Mayer, W. Landau, G. W. Parkhurst, and S. Levin.** 1990. Empiric antimicrobial therapy of domestically acquired acute diarrhea in urban adults. *Arch. Intern. Med.* **150:**541–546.

60. **Goodman, M. J., K. W. Pearson, D. McGhie, S. Dutt, and S. G. Deodhar.** 1980. Campylobacter and *Giardia lamblia* causing exacerbation of inflammatory bowel disease. *Lancet* **ii:**1247.

61. **Goossens, H., G. Henocque, L. Kremp, J. Rocque, R. Boury, G. Alanio, L. Vlaes, W. Hemelhof, C. Van den Borre, M. Macart, and J. P. Butzler.** 1986. Nosocomial outbreak of *Campylobacter jejuni* meningitis in newborn infants. *Lancet* **ii:**146–149.

62. **Gould, S. R.** 1985. Toxic megacolon complicating *Campylobacter* colitis. *Br. Med. J.* **291:**1580.

63. **Guandalini, S., S. Cucchiara, G. de Ritis, G. Capano, A. Caprioli, V. Falbo, V. Giraldi, A. Guarino, P. Vairano, and A. Rubino.** 1983. *Campylobacter* colitis in infants. *J. Pediatr.* **102:**72–74.

64. **Haq, J. A., K. M. Rahman, and M. S. Akbar.** 1985. Haemolytic-uraemic syndrome and campylobacter. *Med. J. Aust.* **142:**662–663.

65. **Hershkowici, S., M. Barak, A. Cohen, and J. Montag.** 1987. An outbreak of *Campylobacter jejuni* infection in a neonatal intensive care unit. *J. Hosp. Infect.* **9:**54–59.

66. **Heyman, M. B., V. I. Paterno, and M. E. Ament.** 1982. *Campylobacter* colitis: a cause of chronic diarrhea in children. *West. J. Med.* **137:**243–245.

67. **Ho, H., M. J. Zuckerman, and S. M. Polly.** 1987. Spontaneous bacterial peritonitis due to

Campylobacter coli. Gastroenterology **92:**2024–2025.

68. **Hoskins, T., and J. W. Davies.** 1983. Clinical features of a large outbreak of milk-borne *Campylobacter* enteritis in a boys' boarding school, p. 14. *In* A. D. Pearson, M. B. Skirrow, B. Rowe, J. R. Davies, and D. M. Jones (ed.), *Campylobacter II. Proceedings of the Second International Workshop on Campylobacter Infections.* Public Health Laboratory Service, London, United Kingdom. (Abstract.)

69. **Howard, R. S., N. J. C. Sarkies, and M. D. Sanders.** 1987. Anterior uveitis associated with *Campylobacter jejuni* infection. *J. Infect.* **14:**186–187.

70. **Humphrey, K. S.** 1993. Campylobacter infection and hepatocellular injury. *Lancet* **341:**49.

71. **Itoh, T., K. Saito, Y. Yanagawa, A. Kai, M. Takahashi, M. Inaba, I. Takano, S. Sakai, and M. Ohashi.** 1983. Epidemiological and bacteriological studies on fifteen outbreaks of *Campylobacter* enteritis in Tokyo. *J. Jpn. Assoc. Infect. Dis.* **57:**576–586. (In Japanese.)

72. **Jackson, C. J., A. J. Fox, D. R. A. Wareing, E. M. Sutclliffe, and D. M. Jones.** 1997. Genotype analysis of human blood isolates of *Campylobacter jejuni* in England and Wales. *Epidemiol. Infect.* **118:**81–89.

73. **Jackson, N., M. Zaki, A. R. Rahman, M. Nazim, M. N. Win, and S. Osman.** 1997. Fatal *Campylobacter jejuni* infection in a patient splenectomised for thalassaemia. *J. Clin. Pathol.* **50:**436–437.

74. **Jones, D. M., D. A. Robinson, and J. Eldridge.** 1981. Serological studies in two outbreaks of *Campylobacter jejuni* infection. *J. Hyg.* **87:**163–170.

75. **Jones, P. H., A. T. Willis, D. A. Robinson, M. B. Skirrow, and D. S. Josephs.** 1981. *Campylobacter* enteritis associated with the consumption of free school milk. *J. Hyg.* **87:**155–162.

76. **Kapperud, G., J. Lassen, S. M. Ostroff, and S. Aasen.** 1992. Clinical features of sporadic campylobacter infections in Norway. *Scand. J. Infect. Dis.* **24:**741–749.

77. **Karmali, M. A., and P. C. Fleming.** 1979. *Campylobacter* enteritis in children. *J. Pediatr.* **94:**527–533.

78. **Karmali, M. A., B. Norrish, H. Lior, B. Heyes, and A. Montgomery.** 1984. *Campylobacter* enterocolitis in a neonatal nursery. *J. Infect. Dis.* **149:**874–877.

79. **Kell, R. J. A., and M. E. Ellis.** 1985. Transient atrial fibrillation in *Campylobacter jejuni* infection. *Br. Med. J.* **291:**1542.

80. **Kendall, E. J. C., and E. I. Tanner.** 1982.

Campylobacter enteritis in general practice. *J. Hyg.* **88**:155–163.

81. **Kerstens, P. J. S. M., H. P. Endtz, J. F. G. M. Meis, W. J. G. Oyen, R. J. I. Koopman, P. J. van den Broek, and J. W. M. van der Meer.** 1992. Erysipelas-like skin lesions associated with *Campylobacter jejuni* septicemia in patients with hypogammaglobulinemia. *Eur. J. Clin. Microbiol. Infect. Dis.* **11**:842–847.

82. **Kita, E., F. Nishikawa, N. Kamikaidou, A. Nakano, N. Katsui, and S. Kashiba.** 1992. Mononuclear cell response in the liver of mice infected with hepatotoxigenic *Campylobacter jejuni. J. Med. Microbiol.* **37**:326–331.

83. **Korman, T. M., C. C. Varley, and D. W. Spelman.** 1997. Acute hepatitis associated with *Campylobacter jejuni* bacteraemia. *Eur. J. Clin. Microbiol. Infect. Dis.* **16**:678–681.

84. **Krajden, S., C. J. Burul, and M. Fuska.** 1986. *Campylobacter jejuni* associated with a perirectal abscess. *Can J Surg.* **29**:228.

85. **Lambert, M., E. Marion, E. Coche, and J.-P. Butzler.** 1982. *Campylobacter* enteritis and erythema nodosum. *Lancet* **i**:1409.

86. **Lambert, M. E., P. F. Schofield, A. G. Ironside, and B. K. Mandal.** 1979. *Campylobacter* colitis. *Br. Med. J.* **1**:857–859.

87. **Leung, F. Y.-K., G. O. Littlejohn, and C. Bombardier.** 1980. Reiter's syndrome after *Campylobacter jejuni* enteritis. *Arthritis Rheum.* **23**:948–950.

88. **Lever, A. M. L., J. M. Dolby, A. D. B. Webster, and A. B. Price.** 1984. Chronic *Campylobacter* colitis and uveitis in patient with hypogammaglobulinaemia. *Br. Med. J.* **288**:531.

89. **Lopez-Brea, M., P. M. Fontelas, M. Baquero, and L. Aragon.** 1984. Urticaria associated with *Campylobacter* enteritis. *Lancet* **i**:1354.

90. **Loss, R. W., J. C. Mangla, and M. Pereira.** 1980. *Campylobacter* colitis presenting as inflammatory bowel disease with segmental colonic ulcerations. *Gastroenterology* **79**:138–140.

91. **Maidment, C. G. H., D. B. Evans, R. A. Coulden, and S. Thiru.** 1985. *Campylobacter jejuni* enteritis complicated by glomerulonephritis. *J. Infect.* **10**:177–178.

92. **Mandal, B. K., M. E. Ellis, E. M. Dunbar, and K. Whale.** 1984. Double-blind placebo-controlled trial of erythromycin in the treatment of clinical campylobacter infection. *J. Antimicrob. Chemother.* **13**:619–623.

93. **Matsusaki, S., and A. Katayama.** 1984. Studies on outbreaks of food poisoning due to *Campylobacter jejuni* between 1980 and 1982 in Yamaguchi prefecture, Japan. *Yamaguchi J. Vet. Med.* **11**:53–56.

94. **Mattila, L., H. Peltola, A. Siitonen, H. Kyrönseppä, I. Simula, and M. Kataja.** 1993. Short-term treatment of traveler's diarrhea with norfloxacin: a double-blind, placebo-controlled study during two seasons. *Clin. Infect. Dis.* **17**:779–782.

95. **May, T., A. Gerard, P. Voiriot, J. L. Schmit, C. Lion, and Ph. Canton.** 1986. Entérite à *Campylobacter jejuni* associée à un syndrome hémolytique et urémique. *Presse Med.* **15**:803–804.

96. **McKendrick, M. W., A. M. Geddes, and J. Gearty.** 1982. *Campylobacter* enteritis: a study of clinical features and rectal mucosal changes. *Scand. J. Infect. Dis.* **14**:35–38.

97. **McKinley, M. J., M. Taylor, and M. H. Sangree.** 1980. Toxic megacolon with *Campylobacter* colitis. *Conn. Med.* **44**:496–497.

98. **McNaughton, R. D., R. Leyland, and L. Mueller.** 1982. Outbreak of *Campylobacter* enteritis due to consumption of raw milk. *Can. Med. Assoc. J.* **126**:657–658.

99. **McNeil, N. I., S. Buttoo, and G. L. Ridgway.** 1984. Spontaneous bacterial peritonitis due to *Campylobacter jejuni. Postgrad. Med. J.* **60**:487–488.

100. **Mee, A. S., M. Shield, and M. Burke.** 1985. *Campylobacter* colitis: differentiation from inflammatory bowel disease. *J. R. Soc. Med.* **78**:217–223.

101. **Megraud, F., C. Tachoire, J. Latrille, and J. M. Bondonny.** 1982. Appendicitis due to *Campylobacter jejuni. Br. Med. J.* **285**:1165–1166.

102. **Melby, K., O. P. Dahl, L. Crisp, and J. L. Penner.** 1990. Clinical and serological manifestations in patients during a waterborne epidemic due to *Campylobacter jejuni. J. Infect.* **21**:309–316.

103. **Melby, K., and S. Kildebo.** 1988. Antibodies against *Campylobacter jejuni/coli* in patients suffering from campylobacteriosis or inflammatory bowel disease. *NIPH Ann.* **11**:47–52.

104. **Menck, H.** 1981. *Campylobacter jejuni* enteritis kompliceret med glomerulonephritis. *Ugeskr. Laeg.* **143**:1020–1021.

105. **Mentzing, L. O.** 1981. Waterborne outbreaks of *Campylobacter* enteritis in central Sweden. *Lancet* **ii**:352–354.

106. **Mertens, A., and M. De Smet.** 1979. *Campylobacter* cholecystitis. *Lancet* **i**:1092.

107. **Meuwissen, S. G. M., P. J. M. Bakkar, and P. J. G. M. Rietra.** 1981. Acute ulceration of ileal stoma due to *Campylobacter fetus* subspecies *jejuni. Br. Med. J.* **282**:1362.

108. **Meyrieux, V., G. Monnaret, A. Lepape, M. Chomorat, and V. Banssillon.** 1996. Fatal shock with multiple organ failure due to *Campylobacter jejuni. Clin. Infect. Dis.* **22**:183–184.

109. **Michalak, D. M., J. Perrault, M. J. Gilchrist,**

R. R. Dozois, J. A. Carney, and P. F. Sheedy. 1980. *Campylobacter fetus* ss. *jejuni:* a cause of massive lower gastrointestinal hemorrhage. *Gastroenterology* **79:**742–745.

110. Millson, M., M. Bokhout, J. Carlson, L. Spielberg, R. Idis, A. Borczyk, and H. Lior. 1991. An outbreak of *Campylobacter jejuni* gastroenteritis linked to meltwater contamination of a municipal well. *Can. J. Public Health* **82:**27–31.

111. Molina, J.-M., I. Casin, P. Hausfater, E. Giretti, Y. Welker, J.-M. Decazes, V. Garrait, P. Lagrange, and J. Modai. 1995. *Campylobacter* infections in HIV-infected patients: clinical and bacteriological features. *AIDS* **9:**881–885.

112. Morlet, N., and R. Glancy. 1986. *Campylobacter jejuni* appendicitis. *Med. J. Aust.* **145:**56–57.

113. Morton, A. R., R. Yu, S. Waldek, A. M. Holmes, A. Craig, and K. Mundy. 1985. *Campylobacter*-induced thrombocytopenic purpura. *Lancet* **ii:**1133–1134.

114. Moscuna, M., Z. Gross, R. Korenblum, M. Volfson, and M. Oettinger. 1989. Septic abortion due to *Campylobacter jejuni. Eur. J. Clin. Microbiol. Infect. Dis.* **8:**800–801.

115. Murphy, S., N. J. Beeching, S. J. Rogerson, and A. D. Harries. 1991. Pancreatitis associated with *Salmonella* enteritis. *Lancet* **338:**571.

116. Muytjens, H. L., and J. Hoogenhout. 1982. *Campylobacter jejuni* isolated from a chest wall abscess. *Clin. Microbiol. Newsl.* **4:**166.

117. Nachamkin, I., S. H. Fischer, X.-H. Yang, O. Benitez, and A. Cravioto. 1994. Immunoglobulin A antibodies directed against *Campylobacter jejuni* flagellin present in breast milk. *Epidemiol. Infect.* **112:**359–365.

118. Nagaratnam, N., T. K. Goh, and D. Ghoughassian. 1990. *Campylobacter jejuni*-induced vasculitis. *Br. J. Clin. Pract.* **44:**636–637.

119. Nahum, H. D., E. Kaloustian, P. Baumer, A. Felten Papiconomou, and J. Lubetski. 1982. Syndrome de rétention biliaire au cours d'une septicémie à *Campylobacter jejuni. Nouv. Presse Med.* **11:**1805–1806.

120. Neal, K. R., H. M. Scott, R. C. B. Slack, and R. F. A. Logan. 1996. Omeprazole as a risk factor for *Campylobacter* gastroenteritis: case-control study. *Br. Med. J.* **312:**414–415.

121. Newman, A., and J. R. Lambert. 1980. *Campylobacter jejuni* causing flare-up in inflammatory bowel disease. *Lancet* **ii:**919.

122. Noble, C. J., D. J. Hibbert, and G. J. Patel. 1982. *Campylobacter* colitis: a case with unusual radiological features. *J. Infect.* **5:**199–200.

123. Norrby, R., R. V. McCloskey, G. Zackrisson, and E. Falsen. 1980. Meningitis caused by *Campylobacter fetus* ssp. *jejuni. Br. Med. J.* **280:**1164.

124. Pai, C. H., F. Gillis, E. Tuomanen, and M. I. Marks. 1983. Erythromycin in treatment of *Campylobacter* enteritis in children. *Am. J. Dis. Child.* **137:**286–288.

125. Pasticci, B., E. Baratta, A. Del Favero, A. Gillio, F. Baldelli, and S. Pauluzzi. 1992. *Campylobacter jejuni:* an unusual cause of infectious arthritis. *Postgrad. Med. J.* **68:**150–152.

126. Paulet, P., and M. Coffernils. 1990. Very long term diarrhoea due to *Campylobacter jejuni. Postgrad. Med. J.* **66:**410–411.

127. Pearson, A. D., D. P. Drake, D. Brookfield, S. O'Connel, W. G. Suckling, M. J. Knill, E. Ware, and J. R. Knott. 1982. Campylobacter infections in patients presenting with diarrhoea, mesenteric adenitis and appendicitis, p. 147–151. *In* D. G. Newell (ed.), *Campylobacter: Epidemiology, Pathogenesis and Biochemistry.* MTP Press, Lancaster, United Kingdom.

128. Pedler, S. J., and A. J. Bint. 1984. Osteitis of the foot due to *Campylobacter jejuni. J. Infect.* **8:**84–85.

129. Pentland, B. 1979. *Campylobacter* enteritis: an in-patient study. *Scott. Med. J.* **24:**299–301.

130. Peterson, M. C., R. W. Farr, and M. Castiglia. 1993. Prosthetic hip infection and bacteremia due to *Campylobacter jejuni* in a patient with AIDS. *Clin. Infect. Dis.* **16:**439–440.

131. Peterson, M. C. 1994. Rheumatic manifestations of *Campylobacter jejuni* and *C. fetus* infections in adults. *Scand. J. Rheumatol.* **23:**167–170.

132. Pichler, H. E. T., G. Diridl, K. Stickler, and D. Wolf. 1987. Clinical efficacy of ciprofloxacin compared with placebo in bacterial diarrhea. *Am. J. Med.* **82**(Suppl. 4A):329–332.

133. Pines, A., E. Golhammer, J. Bregman, N. Kaplinski, and O. Frankl. 1983. *Campylobacter* enteritis associated with recurrent abortions in agammaglobulineamia. *Acta Obstet. Gynecol. Scand.* **62:**279–280.

134. Pitkänen, T., A. Pönkä, T. Pettersson, and T. U. Kosunen. 1983. *Campylobacter* enteritis in 188 hospitalized patients. *Arch. Intern. Med.* **143:**215–219.

135. Pönkä, A., and T. U. Kosunen. 1981. Pancreas infection associated with enteritis due to *Campylobacter fetus* ssp. *jejuni. Acta Med. Scand.* **209:**239–240.

136. Pönkä, A., T. Pitkänen, T. Pettersson, S. Aittoniemi, and T. U. Kosunen. 1980. Carditis and arthritis with *Campylobacter jejuni* infection. *Acta Med. Scand.* **208:**495–496.

137. Popovic-Uroic, T., B. Gmajnicki, S. Kalenic, and I. Vodopija. 1988. Clinical compar-

ison of *Campylobacter jejuni* and *C. coli* diarrhoea. *Lancet* **i:**176–177.

138. **Porter, I. A., and T. M. S. Reid.** 1980. A milk-borne outbreak of campylobacter infection. *J. Hyg.* **84:**415–419.

139. **Potter, M. E., M. J. Blaser, R. K. Sykes, A. F. Kaufmann, and J. G. Wells.** 1983. Human campylobacter infection associated with certified raw milk. *Am. J. Epidemiol.* **117:**475–483.

140. **Price, A. B., J. Jewkes, and P. J. Sanderson.** 1979. Acute diarrhoea: *Campylobacter* colitis and the role of rectal biopsy. *J. Clin. Pathol.* **32:**990–997.

141. **Puylaert, J. B. C. M., R. J. Vermeiden, S. D. J. van der Werf, L. Doornbos, and R. K. J. Koumans.** 1989. Incidence and sonographic diagnosis of bacterial ileocaecitis masquerading as appendicitis. *Lancet* **ii:**84–86.

142. **Rao, G. G., and M. Fuller.** 1992. A review of hospitalized patients with bacterial gastroenteritis. *J. Hosp. Infect.* **20:**105–111.

143. **Rautelin, H. I., A. V. Outinen, and T. U. Kosunen.** 1987. Tubulointerstitial nephritis as a complication of *Campylobacter jejuni* enteritis. *Scand. J. Urol. Nephrol.* **21:**151–152.

144. **Reddy, K. R., and E. Thomas.** 1982. *Campylobacter jejuni* enterocolitis and hepatitis. *Gastroenterology* **82:**1156. (Abstract.)

145. **Ritchie, P. M. A., J. C. Forbes, and P. Steinbok.** 1987. Subdural space campylobacter infection in a child. *Can. Med. Assoc. J.* **137:**45–46.

146. **Robbins-Browne, R. M., H. M. Coovadia, M. N. Bodasing, and M. K. R. Mackenjee.** 1983. Treatment of acute nonspecific gastroenteritis of infants and young children with erythromycin. *Am. J. Trop. Med. Hyg.* **32:**886–890.

147. **Robinson, D. A.** 1981. Infective dose of *Campylobacter jejuni* in milk. *Br. Med. J.* **282:**1584.

148. **Robinson, D. A.** 1981. Unpublished observations.

149. **Rogol, M., I. Sechter, H. Falk, Y. Shtark, S. Alfi, Z. Greenberg, and R. Mirachi.** 1983. Waterborne outbreak of *Campylobacter* enteritis. *Eur. J. Clin. Microbiol.* **2:**588–590.

150. **Rusu, V., and S. Lucinescu.** 1988. The value of *Campylobacter jejuni/coli* serotyping for the evaluation of an enteritis outbreak in newborn infants, p. 138–139. *In* B. Kaijser and E. Falsen (ed.), *Campylobacter IV: Proceedings of the Fourth International Workshop on Campylobacter Infections.* University of Göteborg, Göteborg, Sweden.

151. **Saari, K. M., and O. Kauranen.** 1980. Ocular inflammation in Reiter's syndrome associated with *Campylobacter jejuni* enteritis. *Am. J. Ophthalmol.* **90:**572–573.

152. **Sacks, J. J., S. Lieb, L. M. Baldy, S. Berta, C. M. Patton, M. C. White, W. J. Bigler, and J. J. Witte.** 1986. Epidemic campylobacteriosis associated with a community water supply. *Am. J. Public Health* **76:**424–429.

153. **Salazar-Lindo, E., R. B. Sack, E. Chea-Woo, B. A. Kay, Z. A. Piscoya, R. Leon-Barua, and Y. August.** 1986. Early treatment with erythromycin of *Campylobacter jejuni*-associated dysentery in children. *J. Pediatr.* **109:**355–360.

154. **Schaad, U. B.** 1982. Reactive arthritis associated with *Campylobacter* enteritis. *Pediatr. Infect. Dis.* **1:**328–332.

155. **Schieven, B. C., D. Baird, C. L. Leatherdale, and Z. Hussain.** 1991. *Campylobacter jejuni* infected bursitis. *Diagn. Microbiol. Infect. Dis.* **14:**507–508.

156. **Schmidt, U., H. Chmel, Z. Kaminsky, and P. Sen.** 1980. The clinical spectrum of *Campylobacter fetus* infections: report of five cases and review of the literature. *Q. J. Med. New Ser.* **49:**431–442.

157. **Schonheyder, H. C., P. Sogaard, and W. Frederiksen.** 1995. A survey of bacteremia in three Danish counties, 1989 to 1994. *Scand. J. Infect. Dis.* **27:**145–148.

158. **Shulman, S. R., and D. Moel.** 1983. *Campylobacter* infection. *Pediatrics* **72:**437. (Letter.)

159. **Simor, A. E., and S. Ferro.** 1990. *Campylobacter jejuni* infection occurring during pregnancy. *Eur. J. Clin. Microbiol. Infect. Dis.* **9:**141–144.

160. **Simor, A. E., M. A. Karmali, T. Jadavji, and M. Roscoe.** 1986. Abortion and perinatal sepsis associated with campylobacter infection. *Rev. Infect. Dis.* **8:**397–402.

161. **Skirrow, M. B.** Unpublished data.

162. **Skirrow, M. B.** 1981. Acute ulceration of ileal stoma due to *Campylobacter fetus* subspecies *jejuni*. *Br. Med. J.* **282:**1978.

163. **Skirrow, M. B., D. M. Jones, J. Sutcliffe, and J. Benjamin.** 1993. *Campylobacter* bacteraemia in England and Wales, 1981–91. *Epidemiol. Infect.* **110:**567–573.

164. **Smith, G. S., and M. J. Blaser.** 1985. Fatalities associated with *Campylobacter jejuni* infections. *JAMA* **253:**2873–2875.

165. **Sorvillo, F. J., L. E. Lieb, and S. H. Waterman.** 1991. Incidence of campylobacteriosis among patients with AIDS in Los Angeles County. *J. Acquired Immun. Defic. Syndr.* **4:**598–602.

166. **Stalder, H., R. Isler, W. Stutz, M. Salfinger, S. Lauwers, and W. Vischer.** 1983. Outbreak of *Campylobacter* enteritis involving over 500 participants in a jogging rally, p. 143. *In* A. D. Pear-

son, M. B. Skirrow, B. Rowe, J. R. Davies, and D. M. Jones (ed.), *Campylobacter II. Proceedings of the Second International Workshop on Campylobacter Infections.* Public Health Laboratory Service, London, United Kingdom. (Abstract.)

167. **Stehr-Green, J., P. Mitchell, C. Nicholls, S. McEwan, and A. Payne.** 1991. *Campylobacter* enteritis—New Zealand, 1990. *Morbid. Mortal. Weekly Rep.* **40:**116–117, 123.

168. **Stephenson, T. J., and D. W. K. Cotton.** 1985. Toxic megacolon complicating *Campylobacter* colitis. *Br. Med. J.* **291:**1242.

169. **Surawicz, C. A., and L. Belic.** 1984. Rectal biopsy helps to distinguish acute self-limited colitis from idiopathic inflammatory bowel disease. *Gastroenterology* **86:**104–113.

170. **Svedhem, Å., and B. Kaijser** 1980. *Campylobacter fetus* subspecies *jejuni:* a common cause of diarrhea in Sweden. *J. Infect. Dis.* **142:**353–359.

171. **Taylor, D. N., M. J. Blaser, P. Echeverria, C. Pitarangsi, L. Bodhidatta, and W.-L. L. Wang.** 1987. Erythromycin-resistant campylobacter infections in Thailand. *Antimicrob. Agents Chemother.* **31:**438–442.

172. **Taylor, D. N., B. W. Porter, C. A. Williams, H. G. Miller, C. A. Bopp and P. A. Blake.** 1982. *Campylobacter* enteritis: a large outbreak traced to commercial raw milk. *West. J. Med.* **137:**365–369.

173. **Tee, W., and A. Mijch.** 1998. *Campylobacter jejuni* bacteremia in human immunodeficiency virus (HIV)-infected and non-HIV-infected patients: comparison of clinical features and review. *Clin. Infect. Dis.* **26:**90–96.

174. **Terrier, A., M. Altwegg, P. Bader, and A. von Graevenitz.** 1985. Hospital epidemic of neonatal *Campylobacter jejuni* infection. *Lancet* **ii:**1182.

175. **Tettmar, R. E., and E. J. Thornton.** 1981. An outbreak of *Campylobacter* enteritis affecting an operational Royal Air Force unit. *Public Health* **95:**69–73.

176. **Torphy, D. E., and W. W. Bond.** 1979. *Campylobacter fetus* infections in children. *Pediatrics* **64:**898–903.

177. **Van der Hoop, A. G., and E. M. Veringa.** 1993. Cholecystitis caused by *Campylobacter jejuni. Clin. Infect. Dis.* **17:**133.

178. **Van Dijk, W. C., and P. J. C. van der Straaten.** 1988. An outbreak of *Campylobacter jejuni* infection in neonatal intensive care unit. *J. Hosp. Infect.* **11:**91–92.

179. **Van Spreeuwel, J. P., G. C. Duursma, C. J. L. M. Meijer, R. Bax, P. C. M. Rosekrans, and J. Lindeman.** 1985. *Campylobacter* colitis: histological immunohistochemical and ultrastructural findings. *Gut* **26:**945–951.

180. **Vogt, R. L., H. E. Sours, T. Barrett, R. A. Feldman, R. J. Dickinson, and L. Witherell.** 1982. *Campylobacter* enteritis associated with contaminated water. *Ann. Intern. Med.* **96:**292–296.

181. **Wang W. L. L., and M. J. Blaser** 1986. Detection of pathogenic *Campylobacter* species in blood culture systems. *J. Clin. Microbiol.* **23:**709–714.

182. **Webster, P. B., and D. J. Farrell.** 1993. *Campylobacter* peritonitis as a complication of continuous ambulatory peritoneal dialysis. *Aust. J. Med. Sci.* **14:**68–70.

183. **Wilson, P. G., J. R. Davies, T. W. Hoskins, K. P. Lander, H. Lior, D. M. Jones, and A. D. Pearson.** 1983. Epidemiology of an outbreak of milk-borne enteritis in a residential school, p. 143. *In* A. D. Pearson, M. B. Skirrow, B. Rowe, J. R. Davies, and D. M. Jones (ed.), *Campylobacter II. Proceedings of the Second International Workshop on Campylobacter Infections.* Public Health Laboratory Service, London, United Kingdom. (Abstract.)

184. **Wood, C. J., V. Fleming, J. Turnidge, N. Thomson, and R. C. Atkins.** 1992. *Campylobacter* peritonitis in continuous ambulatory peritoneal dialysis: report of eight cases and a review of the literature. *Am. J. Kidney Dis.* **19:**257–263.

185. **Youngs, E. R., and C. Roberts.** 1985. Campylobacter carriage and pregnancy. *Br. J. Obstet. Gynaecol.* **92:**541–542.

CLINICAL SIGNIFICANCE OF *CAMPYLOBACTER* AND RELATED SPECIES OTHER THAN *CAMPYLOBACTER JEJUNI* AND *C. COLI*

Albert J. Lastovica and Martin B. Skirrow

5

Campylobacter is the most frequently identified bacterial causative agent of diarrhea in humans, particularly in very young children, in both developed and developing countries. ·*Campylobacter* has also been associated with other clinical conditions such as bacteremia, Guillain-Barré syndrome, hemolytic-uremic syndrome, pancreatitis, and reactive arthritis. The genus *Campylobacter* currently comprises 14 species, of which 12 have been isolated from humans. Historically, more than 95% of *Campylobacter* strains isolated and identified in cases of human disease have been *C. jejuni* subsp. *jejuni* or *C. coli.* However, the isolation techniques currently used in many diagnostic laboratories may not support the growth of other, potentially pathogenic non-*jejuni*/*coli Campylobacter* species. These organisms may be fastidious, requiring special atmospheric and temperature conditions or prolonged incubation, or may be unable to tolerate the antibiotics commonly included in selective-medium plates. The disease potential of·these non-*jejuni*/*coli Campylobacter* species is beginning to be appreciated, particu-

larly in areas where they have been looked for. This chapter describes the microbiology, epidemiology, and clinical features of infection with *Campylobacter* species other than *C. jejuni* subsp. *jejuni* and *C. coli* that are associated with human disease. Details of the distribution, sources, characteristics, and clinical features of these organisms are also given.

CAMPYLOBACTER FETUS

Early this century McFadyean and Stockman (120) first recognized campylobacters as causative agents of fetal infection and abortion in sheep. In 1919, these organisms, then called *Vibrio fetus,* were reported to cause abortion in cattle (171). Evidence indicates that these strains were *C. fetus* subsp. *fetus,* which is now recognized as a major cause of septic abortion in domestic animals (56). Since 1947, *C. fetus* has also been implicated as a causative agent of a range of human intestinal and extraintestinal illnesses.

C. fetus is the type species of the genus *Campylobacter* (214) and it is separated into two subspecies, *C. fetus* subsp. *fetus* and *C. fetus* subsp. *venerealis.* This division stems from the realization that two distinct disease entities could be attributed to two varieties of strains (50), which were subsequently accorded subspecies status. DNA-DNA hybridization stud-

Albert J. Lastovica, Department of Medical Microbiology, Red Cross Children's Hospital, Rondebosch 7700, and Department of Medical Microbiology, University of Cape Town, Observatory 7925, Cape Town, South Africa. *Martin B. Skirrow,* Public Health Laboratory, Gloucestershire Royal Hospital, Gloucester GL1 3NN, United Kingdom.

Campylobacter, 2nd Ed., Edited by I. Nachamkin and M. J. Blaser
© 2000 American Society for Microbiology, Washington, D.C.

TABLE 1 Distribution of *Campylobacter* and related species isolated from the diarrhetic stools of pediatric patients at the Red Cross Children's Hospital, Cape Town, South Africa, from 1 October 1990 to 30 April 1999[a]

Species or subspecies	No. (%)
C. jejuni subsp. *jejuni*, biotype 1[b]	1,107 (28.55)
C. concisus	911 (23.49)
C. upsaliensis	882 (22.28)
C. jejuni subsp. *doylei*	358 (9.23)
H. fennelliae	253 (6.52)
C. jejuni subsp. *jejuni*, biotype 2[b]	113 (2.91)
C. coli	109 (2.81)
C. hyointestinalis	51 (1.31)
H. cinaedi	37 (0.95)
CLO/HLO[c]	23 (0.59)
A. butzleri	15 (0.37)
C. fetus subsp. *fetus*	6 (0.15)
"*H. rappini*"	4 (0.10)
C. lari	2 (0.05)
C. curvus	2 (0.05)
C. rectus	2 (0.05)
C. sputorum biovar sputorum	2 (0.05)
Total	3,877 (100.00)

[a] Data from reference 111 and unpublished results.
[b] Biotype of Skirrow and Benjamin (168).
[c] CLO/HLO, *Campylobacter* or *Helicobacter* organisms that could not be fully characterized.

ies showed that these subspecies are intimately related (76). *C. fetus* subsp. *fetus* colonizes the intestine and causes sporadic abortion in sheep and cattle, usually late in gestation. *C. fetus* subsp. *venerealis* is adapted to the bovine genital tract and causes infertility by destroying the embryo early in gestation. This disease, known as bovine vibriosis or infectious infertility, is of major concern to the cattle industry (56). The principal habitat of *C. fetus* subsp. *venerealis* is the prepuce of asymptomatic bulls, which form a reservoir of infection for cows.

The status of *C. fetus* subsp. *venerealis* as a human pathogen is apparently minimal, but owing to the difficulty of separating subsp. *venerealis* from subsp. *fetus* by phenotypic methods (mainly growth in the presence of 1% glycine), uncertainty remains. Hum et al. (80) have developed a PCR assay for the identification and differentiation of the two subspecies, which, when compared with traditional phe-

notyping, indicates that they are often misidentified in diagnostic microbiology laboratories. Nevertheless, strains confirmed as subsp. *venerealis* by genotyping methods have been isolated from the vagina of a woman with bacterial vaginosis in Sweden and from two homosexual men in Australia (78, 160). The sexual transmission of *C. fetus* in humans has not been demonstrated. Additional research is required to define the role of *C. fetus* subsp. *venerealis* in human disease. Thus, our main concern in this section is with *C. fetus* subsp. *fetus,* which we refer to hereafter simply as *C. fetus.*

Microbiology

C. fetus, like other campylobacters, grows in a microaerobic atmosphere (6 to 12% CO_2). These organisms do not ferment carbohydrates, and they are catalase, oxidase, and nitrate reductase positive (Table 3). *C. fetus* strains grow well at 25 and 37°C, but unlike *C. jejuni,* they usually do not grow at 42°C (39). *C. fetus* is resistant to nalidixic acid and susceptible to cephalothin and lacks pyrazimidase activity (24), characteristics which are useful in distinguishing it from *C. jejuni.*

Although early investigators (26) reported that the isolation of *C. fetus* from stools was rare, its natural habitat is the intestine. The susceptibility of *C. fetus* to cephalothin and the fact that most strains do not grow at 42°C may explain why the organism is not isolated from stools more frequently. Most clinical laboratories incubate samples at 42°C and may use a medium that contains cephalothin (77), and many laboratories incubate blood cultures for only 7 days. *C. fetus* grows slowly, and primary isolation from blood culture can take several weeks (55, 219). Radiometric aerobic bottles are reportedly superior to anaerobic bottles for the isolation of *C. fetus* from blood cultures (218). Since other members of the enteric flora grow more rapidly than campylobacteria, antibiotic-containing media traditionally have been used for the isolation of campylobacters from stool specimens. However, isolation of *C. fetus* and other non-*jejuni Campylobacter* species from stools may be unsuccessful due to the use of cephalothin-containing media, on which

TABLE 2 Sources and disease associations of non *jejuni/coli Campylobacter* and related bacteria[a]

Species or subspecies	Recognized sources	Human disease association	Animal disease association
C. fetus subsp fetus	Cattle, sheep	Septicemia, enteritis, abortion, meningitis	Bovine and ovine spontaneous abortion
C. fetus subsp. venerealis	Cattle	Septicemia (rarely)	Bovine infectious infertility
C. upsaliensis	Cats, dogs, ducks, monkeys	Enteritis, septicemia	Canine and feline gastroenteritis
C. hyointestinalis subsp. hyointestinalis	Pigs, cattle, hamsters	Enteritis, septicemia[b]	Porcine and bovine enteritis
C. hyointestinalis subsp. lawsonii	Pigs, birds (including poultry)	None	?[c]
C. lari	Cats, dogs, chickens, monkeys, seals, mussels, oysters, river water, seawater	Enteritis, septicemia	?
C. concisus[d]	Humans	Periodontal disease, enteritis, septicemia[b]	?
C. mucosalis	Pigs	None	Porcine necrotic enteritis
C. sputorum bv. sputorum	Humans, cattle, pigs, sheep	Abscesses	?
C. jejuni subsp doylei	Humans	Enteritis, septicemia[b]	?
H. cinaedi	Humans, hamsters	Enteritis, septicemia,[b] proctocolitis	Hamster enteritis
H. fennelliae	Humans	Enteritis, septicemia,[b] proctocolitis	?
H. pullorum	Poultry	Enteritis	Avian hepatitis
A. butzleri	Pigs, bulls, horses, cattle, chickens, primates, ostriches, ducks, water, sewage	Enteritis, septicemia	Porcine, bovine, primate gastroenteritis, porcine abortion
A. cryaerophilus	Pigs, bulls, poultry, sheep, sewage, horses	Enteritis, septicemia	Bovine, porcine, ovine, equine abortion
A. skirrowii	Sheep, bulls, pigs, chickens, ducks	None	Porcine equine abortion; ovine and bovine gastroenteritis
H. rappini	Humans, mice, sheep	Enteritis, septicemia[b]	Ovine abortion

[a] Data from references 11, 54, 56, 59, 62, 77, 93, 111, 140, 154, 176, and 198.
[b] Children and HIV patients.
[c] Unknown.
[d] Includes *C. curvus* and *C. rectus*.

TABLE 3 Phenotypic and biochemical characteristics of *Campylobacter*, *Arcobacter*, and intestinal *Helicobacter* species of clinical significance[a]

Species or subspecies	Catalase	Nitrate reduction	Arylsulfatase	Pyrazin-amidase	Hippurate hydrolysis	Nalidixic acid[b]	Cephalothin[b]	H2S production			Growth at:		Indoxyl acetate	H2 required	Urease
								Rapid[c]	Lead acetate	TSI	25°C	42°C			
C. jejuni subsp. jejuni biotype 1[d]	+	+	−	+	+	(S)	R	−	++	−	−	+	+	−	−
C. jejuni subsp. jejuni biotype 2[d]	+	+	+	+	+	(S)	R	+	++	−	−	+	+	−	−
C. jejuni subsp. doylei[d]	+	−	−	+	(+)	S	(S)	−	−	−	−	(+)	+	−[e]	−
C. coli	+	+	−	+	−	S	R	−	++	−	−	+	+	−	−
C. fetus subsp. fetus	+	+	−	−	−	R	S	−	+	−	+	(−)	−	−	−
C. upsaliensis	(+)	+	−	+	−	S	S	−	(+)	−	−	(+)	+	−[e]	−
C. lari	+	+	−	+	−	R	R	+	+	−	(−)	+	−	−[e]	(−)[f]
C. hyointestinalis	+	+	−	+	−	R	S	−	5+	3+	(+)	+	−	−[e]	−
C. sputorum	−	+	+	(+)	−	R	S	+	5+	3+	−	+	−	−	(−)[g]
C. concisus	−	+	+	+	−	(R)	(S)	−	3+	(+)	(−)	(−)	(−)	+	−
C. mucosalis	−	+	−	−	−	R	S	−	5+	+	−	(−)	−	+	−
C. curvus[h]	−	+	+	+	−	R	S	−	5+	+	−	+	+	+	−
C. rectus[h]	−	+	+	+	−	(R)	S	−	3+	+	−	+	+	+	−
C. showae	+	+	+	ND	−	R	S	ND	ND	+	ND	ND	+	+	−
C. gracilis[h,i]	−	+	ND	ND	−	S	R	ND	ND	+	ND	ND	ND	+	−
A. butzleri[j]	(+)	+	−	−	−	S	(R)	−	−	−	+	(+)	+	−	−
A. cryaerophilus[j]	(+)	+	−	−	−	S	(R)	−	−	−	+	−	+	−	−
H. cinaedi[k]	+	+	−	−	−	S	(S)	−	(+)	−	−	−	−	+	−
H. fennelliae[k,l]	+	−	+	−	−	S	(S)	−	+	+	−	−	+	−	−
H. pullorum	(+)	+	ND	ND	−	S	R	ND	ND	+	ND	ND	ND	+	−

[a] +, positive; (+), most strains positive; −, negative; (−), most strains negative; ND, not determined; R, resistant; (R), most strains resistant; S, susceptible; (S), most strains susceptible.
[b] 30-µg disk.
[c] Method of Skirrow and Benjamin (168).
[d] Biotypes 1 and 2 of Skirrow's scheme (168).
[e] Some strains grow better under H2-enhanced microaerophilic conditions.
[f] UPTC variant positive.
[g] Biovar paraureolyticus positive.
[h] Pitting colonies on blood agar.
[i] Nonmotile and oxidase negative.
[j] Aerobic growth at 30°C.
[k] Spreading, noncolonial growth.
[l] Hypochlorite odor.

TABLE 4 Clinical features of infection with non-*jejuni/coli Campylobacter* species and related organisms obtained from children in Cape Town, South Africa, 1990 to 1999

Organisms	No. of patients	% of patients with:					
		Diarrhea	Vomiting	Fever	Coexisting enteric pathogen:		Preexisting conditions
					Bacterial	Parasitic	
C. concisus	911	80	3	9	3	6	18
C. upsaliensis	882	88	9	6	3	7	13
C. jejuni subsp. *doylei*	358	78	6	4	4	8	10
H. fennelliae	253	79	8	5	5	10	31
C. hyointestinalis	51	75	12	4	6	12	39
H. cinaedi	37	79	9	9	9	9	27
A. butzleri	15	100	60	20	20	0	40
C. fetus subsp. *fetus*	6	100	17	17	17	0	100

these organisms will not grow. Filtration of stools through 0.45- or 0.65-μm-pore-size filters onto the surface of antibiotic-free blood agar plates allows for the isolation of the smaller *C. fetus* bacteria from larger contaminating microorganisms (Fig. 1) (177).

A PCR assay based on 16S rRNA DNA has proved useful for the identification of *C. fetus* (146).

Epidemiology

During the period from 1987 to 1989, 122 *C. fetus* isolates were reported to the Centers for Disease Control and Prevention surveillance systems (201). For the 66 isolates for which the site of infection was known, 18 were from blood, 41 were from stool, and 7 were from other sites. In the northern hemisphere, the incidence of *C. fetus* infection peaks in late summer and early fall.

The source of many *C. fetus* infections in humans is probably zoonotic. The major habitat of *C. fetus* is the intestine, and it is commonly isolated from healthy sheep and cattle (Table 2). The organism is found in abundance in the genital tracts of aborting sheep and cattle and their products of conception (56). It has also been found in poultry, swine, and reptiles (170). Feces from infected animals may contaminate soil, fresh water, and carcasses during abattoir processing (9), and human infection most probably results from consumption of contaminated food or water. Several such incidents have been documented. The only exposure common to 10 Californian patients with cancer or other serious disease, who developed *C. fetus* sepsis, was "nutritional therapy" entailing consumption of raw calf liver during the week before they became ill (29). Exposure to raw meat (raw beef, raw beef liver, or improperly cooked pork) shortly before illness has been reported in several patients with *C. fetus* bacteremia (82, 155). Klein et al. reported an outbreak of *C. jejuni* and *C. fetus* infection caused by drinking raw milk in Wisconsin (96).

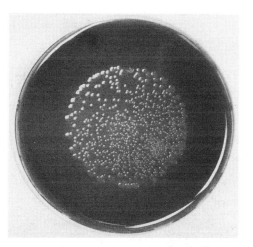

FIGURE 1 A 4–day-old pure growth of *C. fetus* after filtration of a stool specimen onto an antibiotic-free blood-agar plate.

The presence of *C. fetus* was detected solely because the *C. fetus* strains grew (atypically) at 42°C, the standard temperature for isolating *C. jejuni*. In another outbreak of *C. fetus* diarrhea affecting 18 of 90 members of a Hutterite colony in Alberta, Canada, persons who worked in the colony's abattoir were 2.03 times more likely to have diarrhea than others, although this difference did not reach statistical significance (156). The mode of transmission of *C. fetus* infection in humans is not well understood, despite the evidence which indicates zoonotic transmission. More than two-thirds of patients with *C. fetus* bacteremia lived in an urban environment with no known exposure to farm animals (10). There is a single report of the nosocomial spread of infection in a neonatal intensive care unit, in which four infants developed meningitis (130).

Clinical Features

The clinical features of diarrheal disease due to *C. fetus* infection in healthy individuals is similar to infection by *C. jejuni* (156). Sequelae are uncommon, and most patients do not require antibiotic treatment. *C. fetus* infection usually occurs in immunocompromised patients, more than 75% of whom are men who suffer from serious medical conditions such as diabetes mellitus, atherosclerosis, liver cirrhosis, chronic alcoholism, or AIDS or who are undergoing treatment with immunosuppressive agents (10, 36, 55, 71). Intestinal infections are associated with serious complications such as toxic megacolon (89). *C. fetus* accounts for more bacteremia in adults than any other *Campylobacter* species except *C. jejuni* and *C. coli* (104, 169). Infections due to *C. fetus* were previously considered primarily to cause bacteremia in elderly men with chronic underlying illness, but AIDS patients may now represent the most typical population with *C. fetus* infection (155). *C. fetus* may cause a prolonged, relapsing illness characterized by chills, fever, and myalgia but without an identified focus of infection (10, 71). Secondary seeding to an organ may occur, which can lead to complications and an occasional fatal outcome (31). *C. fetus* is rarely iso-lated from pediatric patients, since one laboratory, using filtration onto antibiotic-free media and incubation in an H_2-enriched microaerophilic atmosphere, isolated only 6 *C. fetus* strains (0.15%) out of a total of 3,877 campylobacters (Table 1). Clinical details of these isolates are given in Table 4. This laboratory, in a study of 221 pediatric *Campylobacter* blood culture strains, isolated 8 (3.6%) *C. fetus* strains (104).

Bacteremia due to *C. fetus* can be primary, presumably arising from the gastrointestinal tract, or secondary, arising from infection of another site. *C. fetus* infection can occur as a direct result of invasion of the bloodstream via venipuncture or by an intravenous line (71). Although the organism is rarely isolated from feces, diarrhea precedes or accompanies bacteremia in nearly half the cases (55, 71, 104). High fevers frequently occur but usually are well tolerated, and the mortality is approximately 20% (37, 155).

C. fetus exhibits a distinct affinity for vascular tissue, and infections have been associated with thrombophlebitis, cellulitis, and mycotic aneurysms (27, 82, 125, 128, 131). Recent reviews describe 26 cases of *C. fetus*-associated endocarditis (5, 44); all of the patients had some kind of predisposing disorder such as liver or hepatic cirrhosis, rheumatic or ischemic heart disease, or alcoholism. Rahman described a woman with diffuse lymphoma who died of *C. fetus* pericarditis (153).

Earlier this century, *C. fetus* was recognized as a causative agent of septic abortions in animals, and it is now known to cause perinatal sepsis and fetal loss in humans. In pregnant animals, ingestion of *C. fetus* leads to intestinal infection followed by bacteremia, and since the organism has a high affinity for placental tissues (116), there is a risk of infection of the placenta and fetus (126). A similar mechanism, gastrointestinal colonization with or without enteritis, followed by hematogenous spread and then a placental infection, probably occurs in the rare cases of infection in women. *C. fetus* infection in pregnant women is usually recognized during the third trimester, although abortions at

9.5 and 14 weeks have been reported (57, 182). The illness is usually mild in the mothers, but outcome is often poor in the infants. Neonates may be infected transplacentally or during delivery. Even with appropriate antimicrobial therapy, the average mortality of fetuses and neonates is about 70% (57, 164, 182). The possibility of miscarriage when women are infected with *C. fetus* early in their pregnancy has not been established. Fetal infection and abortion may become apparent only several weeks after infection in the mother. Salpingitis and tubo-ovarian abscess due to *C. fetus* has been described in nonpregnant women (20, 112, 121).

The central nervous system may be infected by *C. fetus,* with meningoencephalitis being the most common presentation in adults (38, 70, 72). Subarachnoid hemorrhages, brain abscesses (98, 117), cerebral infarctions, and subdural abscesses (124) have been reported; although two-thirds of the patients survive, neurological sequelae are frequent. In neonates the prognosis is usually, but not invariably, worse (99). The cerebrospinal fluid typically shows polymorphonuclear pleocytosis. Subdural effusion may also be present (72).

C. fetus can remain latent after bacteremic seeding in a bony focus of an immunocompromised host, only to be reactivated years later (133). Eradication of such an infection probably requires surgical excision of the infected area. Postoperative prosthetic hip joint infections due to *C. fetus* have been reported (6,224), and so has chronic osteomyelitis of the ankle (17). *C. fetus* may be an unobtrusive inhabitant of the gut, but with decreased host immunity, it may invade the mucosa and cause generalized infection. Other forms of *C. fetus* infection are vertebral osteomyelitis, septic arthritis (48), lung abscess (109), empyema (189), gluteal abscess (35a), salpingitis, and cholecystitis (184). Infection of the peritoneum by *C. fetus* in peritoneal dialysis patients has been reported; it was postulated that direct contamination of the catheter had occurred (220). Spontaneous *C. fetus* peritonitis has occurred in alcoholic cirrhosis patients (188), possibly as a result of impaired reticuloendothelial clearance of portal bacteremia.

The pathogenesis of *C. fetus* infection is covered in detail in chapter 16.

Treatment

C. fetus infections are often prolonged and relapsing, but most patients recover if appropriate antibiotic treatment and medical procedures are instituted. The prognosis depends on the severity of the underlying illness and the rapidity of application of antibiotic treatment. Infection by *C. fetus* is lethal in some debilitated persons and could hasten the demise of others. Healthy patients usually have self-limited bacteremia with no sequelae. Immunocompetent patients with uncomplicated intestinal infections usually do not need antibiotics. However, patients with systemic *C. fetus* infection usually require parenteral therapy. Erythromycin may not be sufficient to treat infections due to *C. fetus* (55). Patients with *C. fetus* endocarditis may require up to a month of antibiotic therapy. Ampicillin or cephalosporins are usually effective against established *C. fetus* infections (133). Patients with central nervous system or other serious infections due to *C. fetus* have been treated successfully with aminoglycosides, ampicillin, or chloramphenicol. Patients with hypogammaglobulinemia and persistent *C. fetus* bacteremia may require lifelong antibiotic therapy. Intravenous immunoglobulins are not effective in treating immunodeficient persons with *C. fetus* infection, since the serum from normal persons usually does not contain opsonizing antibodies to *C. fetus* (133).

CAMPYLOBACTER UPSALIENSIS

C. upsaliensis is a recognized human pathogen in both healthy and immunocompromised patients, in whom it causes acute as well as chronic, recurrent diarrhea. This organism, originally described as a catalase-negative or weak campylobacter, can cause bacteremia in debilitated and immunocompromised patients. It has been associated with hemolytic-uremic syndrome (28), Guillain-Barré syndrome (105), and spontaneous human abortion (73). *C.*

upsaliensis was first isolated from the stools of healthy and diarrhetic dogs in 1983. DNA-DNA hybridization studies indicated that this was a new species (162), and the name "*upsaliensis*" was proposed in honor of Uppsala in Sweden, where the organism was first isolated (83). *C. helveticus* is a closely related species found in dogs and cats, but to date it has not been isolated from humans (174). A recent review by Bourke et al. (16) has summarized the available data on *C. upsaliensis*.

Microbiology

C. upsaliensis is a thermotolerant *Campylobacter* species that usually grows well at 42°C but not at 25°C. However, some strains grow better in an H_2-enhanced microaerophilic atmosphere (Table 3). This organism is catalase negative or only weakly positive (163), hippurate and aryl sulfatase negative, but nitrate reductase and indoxyl acetate positive. A striking and distinguishing characteristic of *C. upsaliensis* is its intense susceptibility to both nalidixic acid and cephalothin, with inhibitory zones of up to 80 mm for cephalothin (100). Since cephalothin is frequently used in media for the isolation of *Campylobacter,* cephalothin-sensitive campylobacters such as *C. upsaliensis* are not isolated, which may account for suboptimal isolation of the organism in some laboratories (64).

Detection and the Cape Town Protocol

Wareing et al. (219) examined 950 stool samples both by passive filtration through 0.45- and 0.65-μm-pore-size membrane filters and with a *Campylobacter* selective agar medium, CAT agar (cefoperazone, amphotericin, and teicoplanin). The results indicated that CAT agar is as sensitive as membrane filtration. However, in this study, some of the cultures were overgrown when membrane filters were used (219). In an Australian study of 676 hospitalized gastroenteritis patients, 75 *Campylobacter* strains were isolated on blood-free medium with a selective supplement but concurrent isolation onto antibiotic-free blood agar overlaid with a membrane filter yielded 213 *Campylo-*

bacter strains. Some of these could be isolated only by the membrane filter technique (2). Some studies have recommended both membrane filtration and selective media for the optimal isolation of *Campylobacter* (2). However, an optimal protocol, the "Cape Town protocol," for the isolation of *C. upsaliensis* and other campylobacters from stool specimens without the use of selective media has been developed. The method involves filtration of stools through a membrane filter onto antibiotic-free blood agar plates (Fig. 1) and subsequent incubation in an H_2-enhanced microaerobic atmosphere (111).

With the use of this protocol since 1990, stool cultures positive for *Campylobacter* or related microorganisms rose to 21.8% from the 7.1% obtained with antibiotic-containing selective plates and conventional microaerobic incubation used previously (111). The above diagnostic microbiology laboratory could begin to isolate *C. upsaliensis* from stool specimens only when the isolation protocol was changed from antibiotic-containing media to the Cape Town protocol (111). The use of membrane filtration in this protocol has the added advantage of permitting the isolation of antibiotic-susceptible campylobacters other than *C. upsaliensis*. Based on the difference in colony morphology on primary isolation and subsequent biochemical and serological confirmation, 16.2% of the stools of South African children suffering gastroenteritis had multiple isolates of two to five species or of several different serotypes of *C. jejuni* or *C. coli* (111). In this study, *C. upsaliensis* was frequently coisolated with other campylobacters such as *C. jejuni* subsp. *jejuni, C. jejuni* subsp. *doylei,* and, particularly, *Helicobacter fennelliae* (111). If infection by more than one species is suspected, considerable care must be taken to separate the domed colonies of *C. upsaliensis* from the spreading, noncolonial growth of *H. fennelliae* or *H. cinaedi* before positive identification can be undertaken (Fig. 2).

Antibiotic-containing media have a limited shelf life, and a selection of different media, each with a different antibiotic formulation,

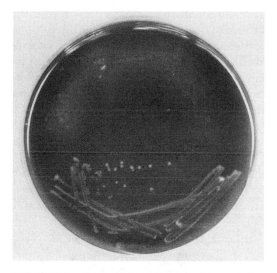

FIGURE 2 Culture plate showing the spreading, noncolonial growth of *H. fennelliae* (top) contrasted with the domed colonies of *C. upsaliensis* (bottom).

may be required to isolate the whole spectrum of clinically relevant *Campylobacter*, *Helicobacter*, and *Arcobacter* species. Membrane filtration onto antibiotic-free media and incubation in an H_2-enhanced microaerophilic atmosphere is a simple, efficient, and cost-effective alternative to the use of antibiotic-containing selective media (111).

Epidemiology

Sandstedt et al. (162) originally identified *C. upsaliensis* in the stools of dogs, and they found that *C. upsaliensis* comprised 63 (64%) of the 98 *Campylobacter* strains isolated from dogs over a 2-year period. *C. upsaliensis* was also isolated from a dog with chronic diarrhea (34). The organism has been isolated from healthy puppies and kittens (74), asymptomatic cats (54), and asymptomatic vervet monkeys (101). While the exact source of *C. upsaliensis* infection in humans in unknown, zoonotic transmission is a distinct possibility. Evidence to support the transmission of *C. upsaliensis* infection from animals to humans comes from several sources. Four of seven patients with *C. upsaliensis* infection in one study reported animal contact (148). Stool isolates of *C. upsaliensis*

that appeared to be the same strain were isolated from a 53-year-old man with bloody diarrhea and his healthy 3-year-old dog (65). In another study, identical plasmid profiles were detected in human and dog isolates (145). Gurgan and Diker (73) documented the isolation of *C. upsaliensis* in blood and fetoplacental specimens of a woman suffering a spontaneous abortion at 18 weeks gestation. A *C. upsaliensis* strain was isolated from her asymptomatic cat, and protein profile analysis confirmed a strong similarity between the human and feline isolates (73). While these observations are suggestive, animal-to-human transmission of *C. upsaliensis* still remains to be unequivocally proved.

Indirect evidence suggests that person-to-person transmission of *C. upsaliensis* is possible. Goossens et al. (66) documented *C. upsaliensis* infection in 34 children in four day-care centers in Brussels, Belgium. Based on multiple typing methods, it was demonstrated that the outbreaks of *C. upsaliensis* infection in three of the four centers were due to the same strain. Also, the *C. upsaliensis* isolates implicated in these outbreaks were closely related to the strain isolated from an outbreak in the fourth day care center.

C. upsaliensis infection occurs in all seasons, but two separate studies of patients at pediatric hospitals in Toronto and in Cape Town indicated that the majority of isolates were obtained in the respective autumns of the northern and southern hemispheres (111,217). The proportion of all campylobacters that are *C. upsaliensis* is relatively high when fecal samples are prospectively cultured for *C. upsaliensis*. From 1990 to 1999, at a pediatric hospital in South Africa, 882 strains of *C. upsaliensis* were isolated, which accounted for 22.3% of all the campylobacters isolated and identified (Table 1). This high isolation rate of *C. upsaliensis* is attributed to membrane filtration of liquefied stools onto antibiotic-free blood agar plates and subsequent incubation in an H_2-enriched microaerophilic atmosphere (111). In a Belgian study of 15,185 fecal samples, 802 yielded *Campylobacter* strains, and of these, 99 (12%) were identified as *C. upsaliensis* (64). However, only a single *C. upsaliensis* strain was obtained in a study of 631 stools from Thai children (194). A Canadian study of 915 *Campylobacter* stool isolates indicated that only 7 (0.1%) were *C. upsaliensis* (192). In a survey of 394 *Campylobacter* blood culture strains isolated from patients in England and Wales, 2 (0.8%) were *C. upsaliensis* (169). By contrast, a South African study of 221 *Campylobacter* strains obtained from the blood cultures of pediatric patients indicated that 39 (18%) were *C. upsaliensis* (104). Differences in the isolation and culture protocol used in various laboratories could account for part of the wide variation in *C. upsaliensis* prevalence. Alternatively, data from South Africa compared with other studies may reflect differences in prevalence and exposure to *C. upsaliensis* or, possibly, differences in colonization and the nature of *C. upsaliensis* infection in different geographical areas.

Characterization of Isolates

C. upsaliensis has a plasmid carriage rate of about 90%, much higher than other species of *Campylobacter* (33, 64, 145). Digestion of *C. upsaliensis* chromosomal DNA with *Hae*III has indicated that fewer than 20% of the strains examined were related (145), but the epidemiology remains to be clarified. While serotyping of *C. upsaliensis* strains has been of limited value (100), sodium dodecyl sulfate-polyacrylamide gel electrophoresis (SDS-PAGE) protein profile analysis (144) has proved useful for the differentiation of individual isolates of *C. upsaliensis*. Pulsed-field gel electrophoresis has indicated molecular heterogeneity in a study of 20 *C. upsaliensis* strains (15).

C. upsaliensis can be identified by PCR techniques based on the 16S rRNA gene (114) or the GTPase gene (209). Based on restriction fragment length polymorphism and PCR assays, the strains obtained from the 44 children at day care centers in Brussels (66) could be divided into two strongly related clonal variants. One variant was isolated only from children in one center, and the second was isolated only from children in the other three centers (66).

Clinical Features

The usual symptoms associated with *C. upsaliensis* infection are gastrointestinal and include watery diarrhea, abdominal cramps, vomiting, and low-grade fever (122, 149, 193). While most patients recover quickly, some are ill for several weeks (122, 148, 192, 217). In a study of 99 patients with *C. upsaliensis* in their stools, in whom the onset of the symptoms was abrupt, 92% had diarrhea, 14% had vomiting, and only 6% had fever (64). The symptoms persisted for more than 1 week in 16% of these patients, 25% had blood in their stools, and 10% had fecal leukocytes. In a study of 882 *C. upsaliensis*-infected pediatric patients (Table 4), the average age was 19.4 months (range, 1 month to 10 years). Loose stools were present in 89%, watery stools were present in 10%, and formed stools were present in <1% of the children. Gastroenteritis symptoms were present in 88%, vomiting was present in 9%, and fever (>38°C) was present in 6% of these patients. Less than 4% were coinfected with *Salmonella* or *Shigella;* however, 7% of these patients had *Ascaris, Trichuris, Cryptosporidium,* or *Giardia* detected in their stools. Underlying illnesses such as kwashiorkor, marasmus, convulsions, protein-losing enteropathy, hepatitis, anemia, or tuberculosis were present in 13% of these children (100).

Two of eight patients with *C. upsaliensis* bacteremia had recent abdominal surgery (148), and 8 of 16 children with *C. upsaliensis* bacteremia had gastrointestinal symptoms. These observations suggest that the bacteremias may have been secondary to intestinal infections (100). Most patients with *C. upsaliensis* bacteremia have other serious underlying medical conditions (30, 100, 148). *C. upsaliensis* has also been isolated from the breast abscess of a patient who reported no animal contact or gastrointestinal symptoms (58), and it has been linked to hemolytic-uremic syndrome (28), and Guillain-Barré syndrome (105).

Pathogenesis

The mechanisms of pathogenicity of *C. upsaliensis* have not been fully characterized. Sylvester et al. (183) demonstrated that *C. upsaliensis* is capable of binding to CHO and HEp-2 cells in tissue culture. These authors also detected surface proteins in the range 50 to 90 kDa on *C. upsaliensis* isolates that are capable of binding to phosphatidylethanolamine, a putative cell membrane receptor. Biotin-labeled *C. upsaliensis* strains also bound in a concentration-dependent fashion to human small-intestine mucin, implying that *C. upsaliensis* express an adhesin(s) capable of recognizing a specific mucin epitope(s) (183). The binding of mucins may influence bacterial access to cell membrane receptors and thus may influence host resistance to infection. The occurrence of *C. upsaliensis* sepsis in a boy with hypogammaglobulinemia (30) suggests that antibody-mediated killing of *C. upsaliensis* is important. Pickett et al. (149) confirmed the presence of a cytolethal distending toxin homologue on *C. upsaliensis*. However, the appropriate *cdt* gene(s) has yet to be cloned. Although these observations, particularly the association of *C. upsaliensis* with outbreaks of disease (66), are suggestive, proof of its role as a human enteropathogen will require controlled studies such as comparison of isolation rates in asymptomatic and symptomatic subjects and animal challenge experiments.

Treatment

The most active antimicrobial agents available for treatment of *C. upsaliensis* infection are fluoroquinolones (151). Erythromycin was once considered the preferred antibiotic for *Campylobacter* infections, but 4 to 18% of *C. upsaliensis* isolates are resistant to erythromycin (33, 64, 148). Infections with *C. upsaliensis* have been treated successfully with augmentin, cefotaxime, and doxycycline (30, 65, 148).

CAMPYLOBACTER HYOINTESTINALIS

In 1983, *C. hyointestinalis* was identified and suggested as a possible cause of proliferative enteritis in pigs (Table 2) (59). This organism has subsequently been isolated from human stools and may be a cause of diarrhea, particularly a watery, nonbloody diarrhea in children. The name *hyointestinalis* is derived from the Latin *hyo,* meaning hog, and *intestinalis,* meaning pertaining to the intestine. Based on phenotypic and genomic methods, On et al. (138) described *C. hyointestinalis* subsp. *lawsonii* subsp. nov. and *C. hyointestinalis* subsp. *hyointestinalis* subsp. nov. The pathogenic role of *C. hyointestinalis* subsp. *lawsonii* in animals and humans is unknown (140).

Microbiology and Diagnosis

C. hyointestinalis is closely related to *C. fetus* and, like *C. fetus*, is catalase and nitrate reductase positive, indoxyl acetate negative, susceptible to cephalothin, and resistant to nalidixic acid. *C. hyointestinalis* differs from *C. fetus* in its copious production of H_2S in triple sugar iron agar in the presence of H_2. Lead acetate strips are often entirely blackened (Table 3). *C. hyointestinalis* grows under microaerophilic conditions, but some strains require additional hydrogen (40, 111). These isolates can be differentiated from other H_2-requiring isolates by the catalase and other tests (Table 3) (205). All strains of *C. hyointestinalis* will grow at 37°C, but some strains will also grow at 42°C. Lack of aryl sulfatase activity and intolerance to 3.5% NaCl are useful phenotypic tests for the diagnosis of *C. hyointestinalis* (24).

Since cephalothin is a constituent of many *Campylobacter* selective media, *C. hyointestinalis,* similar to other cephalothin-sensitive campylobacters, is underdetected. Filtration onto antibiotic-free blood agar media and incubation under microaerobic conditions or in an H_2-enhanced microaerobic atmosphere at 37°C has proved to be extremely efficient for the isolation of *C. hyointestinalis* (111).

Pulsed-field gel electrophoresis and SDS-PAGE have been used to differentiate strains of *C. hyointestinalis* from each other as well as from other *Campylobacter* species (32, 161, 203). DNA probes have been useful for the detection of *C. hyointestinalis* in swine with proliferative enteritis (62). Oligodeoxynucleotide probes have been constructed for both *C. hyointestinalis* and *C. fetus* based on 16S rRNA sequence data (221). A PCR assay based on the

16S rRNA gene has been developed for the detection of *C. hyointestinalis* (114).

Epidemiology

C. hyointestinalis has been consistently isolated from the intestines of pigs with proliferative enteritis but not from asymptomatic pigs or pigs with other enteric diseases (60). Its role in this disease still remains uncertain. *C. hyointestinalis* has been isolated from hamsters, cattle, and nonhuman primates (Table 2) (159, 216). Ohya and Nakazawa (135) reported that 21 (77%) of 29 *C. hyointestinalis* strains from swine with proliferative enteropathy can produce a cytotoxin, although at present the role of this cytotoxin in human disease is uncertain.

Clinical Features and Treatment

In 1986 the first episode of human illness was reported with the isolation of a *C. hyointestinalis* strain from the stool of a homosexual man with proctitis; no other pathogens were recognized. The patient's symptoms resolved and the organism disappeared after appropriate antibiotic treatment (46). Since then, *C. hyointestinalis* strains have been isolated from stool specimens from four patients, all of whom had nonbloody, watery diarrhea (40). An 8-month-old girl, the youngest patient, had drunk unpasteurized milk, and the oldest, a 78-year-old woman, experienced fever and vomiting. There were no leukocytes present in their stools, and both patients recovered with appropriate antibiotic therapy. The other two patients, both homosexual men, had abdominal cramps, and one was febrile. One patient recovered after treatment with trimethoprim-sulfamethoxazole. No antibiotic treatment was administered to the other patient, who continued to have intermittent diarrhea and cramps for several months (40).

An additional case of *C. hyointestinalis*-associated diarrhea was reported in a 52-year-old woman who was immunodeficient because of an evolutive chronic myeloid leukemia (127). This patient was febrile and had a nonbloody, watery diarrhea. In another study, five strains of *C. hyointestinalis* were isolated from five members of the same family who had previously drunk unpasteurized milk (161). In this family outbreak, only in the index case, a 5-month-old female, was diarrhea present, and this infant was also infected with *C. jejuni*. Genomic DNA of these five *C. hyointestinalis* strains, after digestion with *Sal*I, was examined by pulsed-field gel electrophoresis. Three of the strains had identical genome patterns, while the other two had completely different patterns and appeared to be unrelated (161).

In a recent review of patients infected with *C. hyointestinalis*, Breynaert et al. (19) examined the clinical features of nine patients. Seven of the patients (four males and three females with a mean age of 63 years) were adults, while two were young children. Six of the patients experienced diarrhea, and five had abdominal pain. The youngest asymptomatic patient was a 1-year-old girl with constipation, and the oldest was an 89-year-old woman with a myocardial infarction. None of these patients was seriously immunocompromised, but most of the adult patients had a history of neurological or vascular disease (19).

Fifty-one strains of *C. hyointestinalis* (1.3%) were recognized in a study of 3,877 South African pediatric *Campylobacter* stool isolates examined over a 103-month period (Table 1). The average age of the patients infected with *C. hyointestinalis* was 16 months (range, 1 month to 7 years). Stools from these children were loose in 77% of the cases, watery in 21%, and formed in <2%. Blood was present in 13% of the stools, and fecal leukocytes were present in 18%. Thirty-nine percent of these patients suffered underlying illness such as anemia, hepatitis, tuberculosis, convulsions, kwashiorkor, and marasmus. Other clinical features are indicated in Table 4. The only known extraintestinal isolations of *C. hyointestinalis* were from the blood cultures of a 22-year-old man after a bone marrow transplant (104) and subsequently, in March 1999, from a 7-month-old girl with chronic diarrhea.

CAMPYLOBACTER LARI

C. lari is a nalidixic-acid resistant, thermophilic *Campylobacter* which was first identified in 1980 by Skirrow and Benjamin (168). Initially, most strains were isolated from gulls (genus *Larus*), and the name *C. laridis* was proposed; it was changed to *C. lari* in 1990 (215). Although the first human isolate was from an asymptomatic 6-year-old boy, *C. lari* can produce acute diarrheal illness in immunocompetent hosts and can cause bacteremia in immunocompromised patients. A subgroup of *C. lari* has the unusual capability (for a *Campylobacter* species) of hydrolyzing urea; strains are usually sensitive to nalidixic acid. Known by the acronym UPTC (urease-positive thermophilic *Campylobacter*), they are plentiful in natural water and shellfish.

C. lari strains are microaerophilic (some isolates may require H$_2$-enhanced microaerobic growth conditions) campylobacters which grow at 42°C but not usually at 25°C. They are resistant to nalidixic acid, cephalosporins, vancomycin, and trimethoprim. Most are oxidase and nitrate reductase positive and do not hydrolyze hippurate (Table 3) (191).

Epidemiology

C. lari has been isolated from a variety of environmental and animal sources (Table 2). Of 312 riverine samples collected in a study in the United Kingdom, 134 yielded campylobacters; and 7 (5%) of these were *C. lari* (11). In another survey of surface waters in Norway, 2 (2%) of 96 *Campylobacter* samples cultured were *C. lari* (18). These isolations may be significant, since water is an established vehicle for the transmission of campylobacters to humans (193). *C. lari* isolation rates were 25% from gulls (215), 8% from herring gulls, (29%) from kittiwakes (63), and 5 to 7% from crows (119). In a study of the prevalence of *Campylobacter* spp. in oysters and mussels in the Netherlands, Van Doorn et al. (210) found that of 44 *Campylobacter* isolates, 38 were *C. lari*. When 1,564 samples of fresh vegetables were examined in a Canadian study, 3% yielded campylobacters, and *C. lari* comprised 8% of them (147). *C. lari* was isolated from 8 (17%) of 47 pigs in Sweden (113), from poultry in Peru (199) and Tanzania (91), and occasionally from dogs (7, 88). *C. lari* is a potential pathogen that is infrequently isolated from human stools, since in a South African study of 3,877 campylobacters isolated from pediatric diarrhetic stools, *C. lari* was isolated only twice (Table 1).

Diagnosis

Since the spectrum of clinical disease described in association with *C. lari* is similar to that seen with other campylobacters, the diagnosis of *C. lari* depends on the isolation and identification of the organisms from cultured specimens. *C. lari* differs from *C. jejuni* in several ways, most notably in its resistance to nalidixic acid, to which most *C. jejuni* strains are sensitive. Correct identification of *C. lari* may not be made since many clinical microbiology laboratories may not routinely test isolates for nalidixic acid resistance. Nalidixic acid-susceptible isolates of *C. lari* have been reported (11, 123), as well as nalidixic acid-resistant *C. jejuni* strains (217), but *C. lari* is negative in the hippurate hydrolysis test while *C. jejuni* is positive (Table 3), and *C. jejuni* strains hydrolyze indoxylacetate while *C. lari* does not (150).

Based on the nucleotide sequence of the 16S rRNA gene, Linton et al. (114) have developed a PCR assay specific for *C. lari*. Van Doorn and associates (209) have developed a PCR assay that is based on a novel putative GTPase gene and uses species-specific probes for *C. jejuni*, *C. coli*, *C. lari*, and *C. upsaliensis*. This PCR hybridization assay offers rapid and specific identification of thermophilic *Campylobacter* spp. In a study of 38 *C. lari* strains isolated from mussels and oysters, Van Doorn et al. (210) found that the *C. lari* isolates were a more heterogeneous group, when compared to *C. jejuni*, *C. coli*, and *C. upsaliensis*, than was previously thought. Based on sequence information, a novel PCR reverse hybridization line probe assay was developed by these researchers to permit the specific and rapid detection of different *C. lari* variants (210).

Clinical Features

C. lari is an enteric pathogen for both immunocompetent and immunocompromised hosts. While the first human isolates of *C. lari* were found in asymptomatic persons (7, 167), the pathogenicity of *C. lari* was realized only in 1984, with the description of a fatal case of *C. lari* bacteremia in a severely immunocompromised patient (132). The finding of other bloodstream isolates has confirmed its pathogenic potential. Another human immunodeficiency virus (HIV)-infected patient with *C. lari* bacteremia had persistently positive blood cultures in spite of aminoglycoside treatment (213). Bacteremia was associated with a purulent pleurisy in an 80-year-old debilitated patient (21). *C. lari* accounted for 2 (0.8%) of 394 *Campylobacter* strains isolated from blood cultures of patients in England and Wales (169).

C. lari is also associated with diarrheal disease. *C. lari* induced colitis in a 32-year-old HIV-positive woman, who required extensive antimicrobial therapy before her symptoms improved (43). *C. lari* was isolated from the diarrhetic stools of five immunocompetent persons, two of whom were hospitalized. The illness lasted from 1 week to 4 months (median, 2 weeks), and all the patients recovered completely (191). None of these patients was febrile, but four had abdominal cramps, four reported contact with pets, and four had eaten chicken in the week before symptoms became apparent. Simor and Wilcox (166) reported a patient with *C. lari* enteritis for whom they were able to demonstrate specific serum antibodies to the isolated *C. lari* strain, indicating an association between enteritis and infection by *C. lari*. A common-source waterborne outbreak of *C. lari* infection occurred in Ontario in 1985 (12). Gastroenteritis occurred among construction workers who drank water that had become contaminated with surface water from Lake Ontario, which has a large population of gulls. Of 162 ill persons, 87% had diarrhea, 70% had abdominal pain, and 20% had fever; vomiting, nausea, malaise, and headaches were also noted (12). Only one patient reported bloody stools, and the mean duration of illness was 4 days (range, 1 to 10 days). Of the 125 stool samples cultured, 7 yielded *C. lari*, which is probably an underestimate, since collection was delayed and specimens were transported in dry containers, reducing bacterial viability.

Urease-positive, nalidixic-acid susceptible variants of *C. lari* (UPTC) were isolated in France from the stools of two compromised adult patients (an ovarian cancer patient and an alcoholic person) with diarrhea, from the inflamed appendix of an immunocompetent 10-year-old boy (123), and from the blood of a 79-year-old woman with leukemia (165). A urinary tract infection due to a UPTC variant was reported in an alcoholic man with cirrhosis (8). There is a single report of a young man with *C. lari*-associated reactive arthritis (67). *C. lari* strains are capable of producing both cytotoxic and cytotonic factors (87); however, the role of these factors in the disease process is still unknown.

Treatment

C. lari infections involving uncomplicated diarrhea are usually self-limiting and generally do not require antibiotic therapy. When there are severe symptoms such as fever, aminoglycosides, erythromycin, clindamycin, and chloramphenicol have been successfully used (43, 132, 166). *C. lari* is resistant to broad-spectrum cephalosporins, vancomycin, penicillin, and trimethoprim-sulfamethoxazole (43, 166). Fluoroquinolone-resistant strains have been isolated from HIV-infected persons (43).

CAMPYLOBACTER JEJUNI SUBSP. DOYLEI

Based on DNA hybridization studies, *C. jejuni* has been divided into two subspecies: *C. jejuni* subsp. *jejuni* and *C. jejuni* subsp. *doylei* (178). *C. jejuni* subsp. *doylei* was named after L. P. Doyle, who isolated vibrios from pig intestines (179). The pathogenic potential of *C. jejuni* subsp. *doylei* is just beginning to be appreciated. Clinical and other aspects of *C. jejuni* subsp. *jejuni* are covered in detail in chapter 4.

Microbiology and Diagnosis

The inability to reduce nitrate to nitrite (179) is the determining phenotypic characteristic which distinguishes *C. jejuni* subsp. *doylei* from

C. jejuni subsp. *jejuni* and all other campylobacters (Table 3). While *H. fennelliae* is also nitrate reductase negative, it has a spreading colony morphology on blood agar plates and a strong hypochlorite smell (45) and is resistant to polymyxin B (24). These characteristics readily differentiate *C. jejuni* subsp. *doylei* from *H. fennelliae*. *C. jejuni* subsp. *doylei* grows poorly at 42°C and is usually hippuricase and catalase positive (Table 3). These organisms are sensitive to nalidixic acid but, unlike *C. jejuni* subsp. *jejuni*, are also susceptible to cephalothin (Table 3). Filtration of stools onto antibiotic-free blood agar plates is a simple and efficient method of obtaining these microorganisms (Fig. 1). Differences in colony morphology on primary isolation and subsequent characterization by biochemical and serological tests indicates that *C. jejuni* subsp. *doylei* can be coisolated with *C. jejuni* subsp. *jejuni*, *C. upsaliensis*, and *H. fennelliae* (100, 102, 111). Care must taken to separate the discrete, domed colonies of *C. jejuni* subsp. *doylei* from the noncolonial spreading growth of *H. fennelliae* in suspected cases of mixed infection, as indicated in Fig. 2.

Epidemiology and Clinical Features

C. jejuni subsp. *doylei* can be present in the upper gastrointestinal tract (90, 143). Urease-negative, gastric *Campylobacter*-like organisms, which were originally called GCLO2 isolates and then *C. jejuni* subsp. *doylei*, were identified in gastric antral biopsy specimens from six patients (90, 143). Almost identical microorganisms were found in the feces of young Australian children hospitalized with gastritis (178, 180). Other studies have shown that this microorganism may be associated with pediatric diarrhea (47, 102, 129). In a study of 631 Thai children with diarrhea, 93 (15%) had campylobacters isolated from their stool and 1 (1.1%) of these was a *C. jejuni* subsp. *doylei* strain (194). In a Belgian investigation of 15,185 stools, 802 *Campylobacter* isolates were cultured and *C. jejuni* subsp. *doylei* accounted for 4 (0.5%) of them (65).

In a South African study of 3,877 *Campylobacter*/*Helicobacter* isolates obtained from the diarrheal stools of children over a 103-month period, 358 (9.2%) of the strains were *C. jejuni* subsp. *doylei* (Table 1). These 358 isolates were obtained from gastroenteritis patients whose average age was 20 months (range, 1 month to 11 years). Of these children 82% had loose stools, and 18% had watery stools; 15% of the patients had blood in their stools, and 24% had fecal leukocytes. Other clinical features are indicated in Table 4. In a separate study of *Campylobacter* blood cultures from South African children 53 of 221 isolates (24.0%) were *C. jejuni* subsp. *doylei* (104). The average age of these children was 12 months (range, 2 to 30 months) Of the 53 children 26 had diarrhea, often chronic, suggesting that intestinal infection preceded systemic infection. Of these 53 patients, 30 were suffering from severe protein deficiency diseases, such as marasmus and kwashiorkor. *C. jejuni* subsp. *doylei* made up less than 10% of the campylobacters found in stool (Table 1) but accounted for 24% of the *Campylobacter* blood cultures seen at the same pediatric hospital (104). Similar findings were reported by Morey (129) in disadvantaged aboriginal children in central Australia, where *C. jejuni* subsp. *doylei* accounted for a staggering 85% of *Campylobacter* bacteremias. These observations suggest a pathogenic and invasive role for *C. jejuni* subsp. *doylei*.

⁺H₂-REQUIRING CAMPYLOBACTERS

There are six *Campylobacter* species that have an essential growth requirement for hydrogen or formate. Five of them are found in the gingival flora of the human mouth, notably in periodontal pockets of diseased gums. *C. rectus* (Latin: *rectus* meaning straight) and *C. curvus* (Latin: *curvus* meaning curved) were originally described as *Wolinella* species (186, 187). *C. concisus* (Latin: *concisus* meaning concise) and *C. showae* (Latin: *showae* referring to Showa University, where the organism was first isolated) are biochemically similar organisms (42, 185). *C. gracilis* was formerly regarded as a *Bacteroides* species but was reclassified in 1995 (208). A similar organism, also wrongly classified as a

Bacteroides sp., "*B. ureolyticus,*" is now considered to belong to the family *Campylobacteraceae* and is awaiting a suitable generic assignment (208). *C. mucosalis* is an H_2-requiring species that has been associated with proliferative enteritis in pigs (110) but not so far with human disease (Table 2).

Microbiology

Apart from the H_2 or formate requirement of these species, the other feature they have in common is that they are all, except for *C. showae,* catalase negative. Many, but not all, isolates are susceptible to cephalothin and nalidixic acid (30-μg disks), often with inhibitory zones up to 50 mm in diameter (103, 204). *C. curvus* may be difficult to differentiate from *C. concisus* since the indoxyl acetate assay is not always infallible (108), and serological (186) or other methods may be required. Two suspected cases of *C. mucosalis* enteritis in Italian schoolchildren have been reported (49). However, these isolates were characterized only by variable phenotypic criteria, such as colony color. A subsequent investigation of these presumptive *C. mucosalis* strains by another researcher using DNA-DNA hybridization techniques indicated that these strains were misidentified *C. concisus* strains (103). Occasionally, some isolates of *C. hyointestinalis, C. jejuni* subsp. *doylei, C. upsaliensis,* or *C. lari* require an H_2-enriched microaerophilic atmosphere for growth. However, these strains can easily be differentiated from the above four hydrogen-requiring species by differences in the available phenotypic tests (Table 3). *C. rectus, C. curvus, C. gracilis,* and "*B. ureolyticus*" can produce agar-corroding (pitting) colonies. *C. gracilis* is unique (for a *Campylobacter* species) since it is nonmotile (aflagellate) and oxidase negative. *C. rectus* and *C. curvus* may appear oxidase negative in traditional tests, but they are positive in the modified test of Tarrand and Gröschel (190).

Epidemiology and Clinical Features

C. rectus was isolated from 80% of 1,654 adults and children with periodontitis in a 2-year study (154). *C. rectus* has also been isolated from periodontitis patients with inflammatory bowel disease (211). Two isolates of *C. rectus* have been identified in the diarrheal stools of South African children (Table 1). Reports of additional *C. rectus* isolates associated with gastroenteritis have not been published, possibly because less than optimal conditions were used for the isolation of this fastidious microorganism. *C. curvus* has been recovered from patients with periodontal disease or septicemia (187). It has also been isolated from diarrheal stools of children in Belgium (108) and South Africa (Table 1).

The association of *C. concisus* with human periodontal disease is well known (185, 187), but a direct causal role has not been established. *C. concisus* may have been responsible for osteomyelitis of the sacrum in a patient with diabetes and a sacral decubitus ulcer (86). Evidence that *C. concisus* is an enteric pathogen is equivocal. Among 14 isolates of *C. concisus* studied in Belgium, 7 were from patients with diarrhea and 1 was from the blood of a man with carcinoma of the bronchus (202). However, in a subsequent study, the same Belgian team found no significant difference in *C. concisus* isolation rates between patients with diarrhea and controls (212). Zhi et al. (226) found that concentrations in serum of an antibody to a *C. concisus* antigen preparation were higher in infected patients than in control groups, but the differences were not large; some infected patients had low or undetectable antibody levels. The average antibody titers in healthy adults were higher than in infected children.

In a South African study of 1,519 *Campylobacter* isolates, 187 (12.3%) required hydrogen for growth (103); 184 isolates were from pediatric diarrheal stools, 1 was from an adult diarrheal stool, 1 was from the blood culture of an 18-day-old infant, and 1 was from a duodenal biopsy specimen from an adult. All 187 H_2-requiring *Campylobacter* isolates were characterized as *C. concisus* on the basis of phenotypic testing. In addition, 92 of the isolates were chosen for further testing, and all 92 were confirmed as *C. concisus* by DNA-DNA hybridization studies (103). The mean age of the *C. concisus* gastroenteritis patients was 24 months (range, 4 days to 11 years). In these patients, 21% of the stools were watery, and the remainder were loose. Blood was present in 14% of the stools, and fecal leukocytes were detected in 27%. Preexisting clinical conditions in 18% of the patients included anemia, metabolic disturbances, tuberculosis, and kwashiorkor. Additional data are provided in Table 4. Thirty of the *C. concisus* isolates from pediatric stools were tested against eight antimicrobial agents (69). Ciprofloxacin was the most effective agent examined. All strains were susceptible to tetracycline, ampicillin, and gentamicin. All but one of the strains was resistant to erythromycin (MIC, >1 mg/ml). The activity of the cephalosporins was variable.

C. gracilis and "*B. ureolyticus*" are both associated with periodontal disease, but they have also been isolated from other sites. *C. gracilis* has been found in deep-seated abscesses, particularly in the head and neck region, and "*B. ureolyticus*" has been isolated from more superficial lesions such as ulcers, soft tissue infections, and urethritis (85, 208). Strains from the urethra are distinguishable from those from soft tissue infections (1).

C. mucosalis can be recovered at high concentrations (up to 10^8 CFU/g) from the diseased intestinal mucosa in cases of porcine intestinal adenomatosis, but experimental infection does not always cause the disease (110). At present, there is no known association of *C. mucosalis* and human disease.

CAMPYLOBACTER SPUTORUM

Although not strictly hydrogen requiring, *C. sputorum* has many of the features of the foregoing species, notably in being catalase negative, and it also forms part of the human gingival flora. Until recently, *C. sputorum* was considered to have three biovars: biovar sputorum, living in the mouth and intestinal tract; biovar bubulus, living in the healthy genital tracts of cattle and sheep; and biovar fecalis, found mainly in the feces of sheep and cattle. It has now been shown that the biochemical differences between biovar bubulus and biovar sputorum are unreliable and that absolute validity of the source-specific biovars is questionable. Thus, biovar bubulus is no longer recognized (141). On the other hand, a group of catalase-negative, urease-positive *Campylobacter* strains isolated from cattle feces were found to belong to *C. sputorum,* and they now form a new biovar, paraureolyticus. This biovar has been isolated from a patient with enteritis in Canada (141).

C. sputorum biovar sputorum has been isolated from the human lung and abscesses of the groin and axillary areas (13, 137) and from the blood of a patient with a knee abscess (197). It has also been isolated from patients with gastroenteritis, but it can be found in about 2% of normal stools; however, this could be coincidental.

ARCOBACTER BUTZLERI AND ARCOBACTER CRYAEROPHILUS

The genus *Arcobacter* now comprises four species which were previously included in the genus *Campylobacter: A. nitrofigilis, A. cryaerophilus* group 1A and group 1B, *A. butzleri,* and *A. skirrowii* (203). These organisms, following DNA-rDNA and DNA-DNA hybridization studies, were moved from the genus *Campylobacter* to the genus *Arcobacter* (204, 207).

Arcobacters are morphologically similar to campylobacters, but they differ sharply in that they are able to grow in air. The type species, *A. nitrofigilis,* originally isolated from plant roots and associated sediment, has not been isolated from humans or animals. *A. skirrowii* has been isolated from aborted cattle, sheep, and pig fetuses but not from humans. The clinical significance of these organisms is limited, and the majority of human isolates described to date belong to the species *A. butzleri.*

A. butzleri was first described by Kiehlbauch et al., who recognized two distinct genetic groups among 78 isolates of aerotolerant "campylobacters" referred to the Centers for Disease Control and Prevention (93). Group 1 contained the type strain of *C. cryaerophila* (now *A. cryaerophilus*). Group 2 was named *C. butz-*

leri (now *A. butzleri*) in honor of Jean–Paul Butzler, a Belgian microbiologist and pioneer of campylobacter research. Differences in the biochemical features of these two species are outlined in Table 3. *A. cryaerophilus* and *A. butzleri* grow poorly or not at all at 42°C on blood agar plates, but they grow on McConkey plates and are generally resistant to cephalothin (Table 3).

Epidemiology

A total of 100 strains of *A. butzleri* and 41 strains of *A. butzleri*-like or *Arcobacter* spp. were isolated recently from six drinking-water plants in Germany (84). Two strains of *A. butzleri* were isolated from a contaminated well in Idaho (157). Survival studies, conducted at 5°C, a temperature typical of groundwater, indicated that *A. butzleri* can remain viable for up to 16 days in groundwater (157). *A. cryaerophilus* was first isolated from porcine, equine, and bovine feces and aborted porcine and bovine fetuses (14, 41). An Australian traveler with gastroenteritis was thought to be the first human infected with *A. cryaerophilus,* but this organism was later correctly identified as *A. butzleri* (195). *A. cryaerophilus* has been found in urban sewage (173). In a study of 15 broiler chickens obtained from a poultry abattoir and 10 broiler chickens from a supermarket, all 25 carcasses yielded *A. butzleri*. Three supermarket and 10 abattoir carcasses also carried *A. cryaerophilus,* while 2 of the abattoir carcasses carried *A. skirrowii* (4). A Canadian study (97) indicated that poultry appears to be a major reservoir for *A. butzleri,* since 121 of 125 broiler chicken carcasses examined were positive for *A. butzleri* after primary abattoir processing. *A. butzleri* was also recovered from whole chicken and ground chicken and turkey samples from retail stores (97). In a study of 130 raw–meat samples, one strain of *A. butzleri* was identified in a pork sample (225).

Characterization of Isolates

A serotyping scheme based on heat-labile antigens can discriminate 65 serotypes of *A. butzleri* (115). A multiplex PCR assay has been devel-oped to identify *Arcobacter* isolates and to distinguish *A. butzleri* from other arcobacters (75). Based on 23S rRNA gene polymorphisms, Hurtado and Owen (81) have proposed a PCR scheme for the rapid identification of *Campylobacter* and *Arcobacter* spp. Digestion of the PCR amplicons with four restriction endonucleases (*Hae*III, *Cfo*I, *Hpa*II, and *Hinf*I) enabled species differentiation of *Campylobacter* and *Arcobacter* at the genomic level. With this scheme, *A. butzleri* and *A. nitrofigilis* gave unique profiles. However, *A. cryaerophilus* and *A. skirrowii* produced profiles that were identical to each other but different from those of *A. butzleri* and *A. nitrofigilis* (81). Ribotyping and restriction fragment polymorphisms are able to distinguish between *A. cryaerophilus* and *A. butzleri* (94).

Clinical Features

A. butzleri can cause diarrhea and associated gastrointestinal symptoms in humans. In the collection studied by Kiehlbauch et al., mentioned above (93), there were 64 *A. butzleri* isolates. Of these, 43 had been isolated from patients with diarrhea, 3 from the abdominal contents or peritoneal fluid of patients with acute appendicitis, and 3 from blood cultures. Some of these isolates were from children in Thailand, where *A. butzleri* was isolated from the feces of 2.4% of children (16.1% of all *Campylobacter/Arcobacter* isolates) (194). *A. butzleri* was isolated less frequently from children in South Africa, where they accounted for 0.4% of isolates (Table 1). Underlying illness such as anemia, tuberculosis, and pneumonia were present in 40% of these children, whose average age was 19 months (102). Additional clinical details are given in Table 4.

In a 15-month survey of routine fecal samples in Belgium, Dediste et al. (35) found that *A. butzleri* made up 7.4% of *Campylobacter/Arcobacter* isolations. The absence of fever (<38°C) was noted in most patients, but watery diarrhea occurred in 13 of the 16 patients and vomiting and abdominal pain occurred in about half of them. Neither blood nor inflammatory exudate was detected on microscopy of stools. Half the patients were treated with amoxicillin and clavulanate, and they rapidly recovered. The remaining patients improved spontaneously with conservative management. Only one patient, who had chronic diarrhea, had an underlying pathology, namely, HIV infection.

Of particular interest is an outbreak of *A. butzleri* infection affecting 10 Italian children, aged 2 to 5 years, none of whom had diarrhea or fever but all of whom had episodes of recurrent abdominal cramps. Each episode lasted up to 2 h and occurred several times a day for up to 10 days (206). These children felt well between attacks, and the illness was self-limiting. All isolates belonged to a single serogroup and had identical protein profiles. Most of the children seroconverted to this strain. The sequential timing of these infections suggested person-to-person spread.

A. butzleri was isolated from the blood of a preterm neonate, which was probably infected in utero (139). Treatment with penicillin and cefotaxime was successful in resolving the infection.

A. butzleri appears to be pathogenic for nonhuman primates. It was found in 14 (6%) of 222 nonhuman primates with diarrhea. It was isolated from colonic specimens obtained at necroscopy from 3 (4%) of 76 macques. All three animals had active colitis (3). The stools of 7 (39%) of 18 infant *Macaca nemestrina* monkeys (apparently asymptomatic) when cultured weekly from birth to 1 year of age also yielded *A. butzleri* (159).

A. cryaerophilus is infrequently isolated from humans. Only two isolations were made in the Belgian study of routine fecal samples mentioned above (35). *A. cryaerophilus* was the sole potential pathogen in one patient, who had watery diarrhea, fever, and abdominal pain, while the other patient had no symptoms. There were three isolates of *A. cryaerophilus* of human origin in the collection studied by Kiehlbauch et al. (93), two from blood and one from stool. An *A. cryaerophilus* group 1B strain was isolated from the blood of a 72-year-old uremic woman with hematogenous pneumonia secondary to an infected atrioventricular

fistula (79). She had suffered a period of diarrhea 2 months before this episode. She was successfully treated with ceftizoxime and tobramycin.

Pathogenicity

Neonatal piglets have been used as models to determine relative pathogenicities, based on fecal shedding and tissue colonization of *Arcobacter* (222). One-day-old cesarean-derived colostrum-deprived piglets were infected, per os, with three field strains and type strains of *A. butzleri, A. cryaerophilus,* and *A. skirrowii.* *Arcobacter* spp. were detected at least once in rectal swab samples from all but one of the experimentally infected piglets. At necroscopy, *Arcobacter* spp. were cultured from the liver, kidney, ileum, or brain tissue in two of four *A. butzleri*-infected piglets. However, no severe gross pathology was noted. These data suggest that *Arcobacter* spp., particularly *A. butzleri,* can colonize neonatal pigs (222).

HELICOBACTER CINAEDI AND *HELICOBACTER FENNELLIAE*

Initially, *H. cinaedi* and *H. fennelliae* were called CLOs (*Campylobacter*-like organisms) and were divided into three phenotypic groups, CLO1, CLO2, and CLO3. Subsequently, CLO1 was found to comprise two genetically distinct groups, CLO1A and CLO1B, that could not be separated solely on the basis of phenotypic criteria (198). Both CLO1A and CLO1B were initially called *Campylobacter cinaedi,* from the Latin word *cinaedi* meaning "of a homosexual." CLO2 isolates were initially called *C. fennelliae* after Cynthia Fennell, the microbiologist who first isolated these organisms from the rectal swabs of homosexual men. The names of these organisms were subsequently amended to *Helicobacter cinaedi* and *Helicobacter fennelliae* (205).

Microbiology

H. cinaedi and *H. fennelliae* grow under microaerobic conditions, but some strains require H_2-enhanced microaerobic conditions for optimum growth. These bacteria grow at 37°C but grow poorly or not at all at 42°C (Table 3). *H. fennelliae* may be differentiated from *H.*

cinaedi by SDS-PAGE profiles (136), serology (52), and differences in aryl sulfatase activity (24) (Table 3). A useful diagnostic test is the odor of a mature growth of *H. fennelliae,* which is similar to hypochlorite (bleach) and which is absent in *H. cinaedi* and campylobacters (45). While *Campylobacter* and *Arcobacter* species form domed colonies on agar plates, both *H. cinaedi* and *H. fennelliae* produce, on freshly prepared agar plates, a flat spreading growth without discrete colonies (45). This growth may be missed on primary isolation plates, particularly if the domed colonies of a *Campylobacter* species are present as well. *H. fennelliae* is often coisolated with *C. jejuni* subsp. *jejuni, C. jejuni* subsp. *doylei,* or *C. upsaliensis* (2, 102, 111). In cases of suspected mixed infection, extreme care must be taken the separate the noncolonial spreading growth of *H. fennelliae* or *H. cinaedi* from the domed colonies of other campylobacters (Fig. 2).

Strain Characterization

Thirty-four human and animal strains of *H. cinaedi* and two animal and two human strains of *H. fennelliae* have been characterized by phenotypic and molecular tests (95). The results indicated that most isolates of *H. cinaedi* formed a single group, both phenotypically and by DNA-DNA hybridization studies. Subgroups were distinguishable by ribotyping. The two human *H. fennelliae* strains had similar but different ribotyping patterns from those of the type strains and from each other and had no bands in common with either of the animal *H. fennelliae* strains.

Epidemiology and Clinical Features

CLOs were first recognized as human pathogens when they were isolated from the stools of 26 of 158 homosexual men with diarrhea or proctitis examined at a sexually transmitted disease clinic (152). These organisms were also isolated from 6 of 75 asymptomatic homosexual men but were not isolated from 150 heterosexual men and women (152). In a study of the diarrheal stools of homosexual or bisexual men in Baltimore and Washington, D.C., 9 (27%)

of 33 patients had *Campylobacter* or *Helicobacter* in their stools, while 2 had an *H. cinaedi* strain and one had a CLO3 strain (107). Two CLO3 strains have been isolated from the stools of homosexual men with proctitis (51, 198). CLOs have been isolated from up to 8% of the stools of homosexual men with diarrhea or proctitis (106). In another investigation based in California, CLOs were not identified in the stools or colonic brushings of 27 homosexual men with diarrhea (223). In the initial descriptions of patients with gastroenteritis symptoms attributed to CLO infections, the clinical features, which included diarrhea, abdominal cramps, and hematochezia, were similar to those in *C. jejuni*-infected patients (152). CLO infections were also noted as causing fever, anal discharge, and pain (152). Sigmoidoscopic examinations of infected patients indicated mucosal bleeding and ulcers. Fecal leukocytes were present in most patients, and histological examination revealed crypt abscesses and polymorphonuclear leukocytes scattered through the lamina propria. A subsequent report has described HIV-infected patients with *H. cinaedi* in their stools who experienced chronic but mild symptoms lasting several weeks (68) but without blood or polymorphonuclear leukocyte cells in the stools. Diarrhea consisted of three to four loose stools per day and was not associated with fever or other indications of systemic illness.

In addition to gastroenteritis, *H. cinaedi* and *H. fennelliae* are capable of causing bacteremia, particularly in HIV-positive patients (22). Chills, low-grade fever, lethargy, and malaise are usually present in patients with *H. cinaedi* bacteremia, but not all have preceding gastrointestinal symptoms. A homosexual man with AIDS developed recurrent *H. cinaedi* bacteremia during 2 months of intermittent diarrhea and fecal incontinence. His blood cultures yielded a second organism, which was identified as *H. fennelliae,* and cultures were consistently positive, despite treatment with ciprofloxacin and trimethoprim-sulfamethoxazole. The patient died 4 months later, although the role of the *H. cinaedi* and *H. fennelliae* isolates was not clearly defined (134). Another AIDS patient developed bacteremia due to *H. fennelliae* (92). In a survey of 394 blood culture *Campylobacter* isolates from patients in England and Wales, 2 isolates (0.50%) were *H. fennelliae* and 1 (0.25%) was *H. cinaedi* (169).

A study of 221 pediatric blood culture isolates in a pediatric hospital in South Africa indicated that 7 strains (3.2%) were *H. fennelliae* and 5 (2.3%) were *H. cinaedi* (104). At the same hospital, 3,877 *Campylobacter* or *Helicobacter* isolates were obtained from 17,386 diarrheal stools (Table 1). There were 253 strains of *H. fennelliae* (6.5%) and 37 strains of *H. cinaedi* (0.95%) detected in this study (Table 1). The average age of the infected children was 18 months (range, 2 weeks to 11 years). Of the stools, 73% contained blood and 8% had fecal leukocytes. More than 25% of these patients had underlying illnesses such as anemia, pneumonia, metabolic disturbances, and nutritional problems. Additional-clinical details are shown in Table 4.

These reports suggest that *H. cinaedi* and *H. fennelliae* infections may occur more frequently than previously thought in the immunocompetent and heterosexual populations. Gastroenteritis due to *H. cinaedi* or *H. fennelliae* has been found in heterosexual men, women, and children in various studies (25, 68, 223).

The source of human infection by these organisms is not known, although apparent transmission from animals has been recorded. *H. cinaedi* was isolated from the cerebrospinal fluid and blood of a 5-day-old neonate whose mother had a mild diarrheal illness during the third trimester of her pregnancy. The mother had cared for pet hamsters during the first two trimesters of her pregnancy (142). *H. cinaedi* has been isolated from 72% of commercially available hamsters (61) and from the stools of diarrhetic dogs (23).

Pathogenesis

Evidence for the pathogenicity of *H. cinaedi* and *H. fennelliae* comes from several sources. The association of these organisms with homosexual men who had proctitis and enteritis, but not with asymptomatic men, suggests a causal relationship. Bacteremia in immunocompromised patients, as well as the presence of fecal leukocytes, indicates that these organisms play a pathogenic role. Flores et al. (53) studied the effects of experimental *H. cinaedi* and *H. fennelliae* infection in infant macaque monkeys. Four monkeys were challenged with *H. cinaedi,* two animals subsequently developed diarrhea, and *H. cinaedi* was isolated from the stools and blood cultures of all four monkeys. When challenged with *H. fennelliae,* all three monkeys became bacteremic and two developed diarrhea. *H. fennelliae* was isolated from their stools, and prolonged rectal colonization was observed in all the animals examined (53).

Treatment

Although *H. cinaedi* and *H. fennelliae* infections have not resulted in deaths to date, some patients have displayed a slow clinical response to antimicrobial therapy. Antimicrobial agents that have demonstrated in vitro activity against *H. cinaedi* and *H. fennelliae* include ampicillin, tetracycline, rifampin, nalidixic acid, chloramphenicol, and gentamicin (51). However, 28% of strains were resistant to erythromycin and clindamycin and 17% were resistant to sulfamethoxazole (51). Like campylobacters, these organisms are resistant to trimethoprim and most are resistance to metronidazole. In South Africa, 13% of *H. cinaedi* and *H. fennelliae* stool and blood culture isolates from pediatric patients were resistant to erythromycin (102). Oral fluoroquinolones may be the best treatment for severe or persistent *H. cinaedi* and *H. fennelliae* infection. Two patients with persistent *H. cinaedi* bacteremia were successfully treated with oral ciprofloxacin (22).

OTHER *HELICOBACTER* SPECIES AND *CAMPYLOBACTER*-LIKE ORGANISMS

H. canis is a species that resembles *H. fennelliae*. It was originally found in dogs (with and without diarrhea), but it has also been isolated from a 5.5-year old boy with diarrhea (175). Stanley and colleagues described *H. pullorum,* a species isolated from poultry liver, duodenum and cecum, and from humans with diarrhea (176, 181). *H. westmeadii* is another newly recognized species isolated from the blood of two AIDS patients with febrile diarrhea in Australia (200). *H. rappini* (formerly called *Flexispira rappini*) is a fusiform bacterium with spiral periplasmic fibrils and bipolar tufts of sheathed flagella. These organisms were first isolated from aborted lambs. Subsequently they have been isolated from patients with diarrhea (158), from the blood cultures of a 7-year-old girl with pneumonia (196), and from a 65-year-old febrile man undergoing hemodialysis (172).

Anaerobiospirillum succiniciproducens does not belong in this group of organisms, but on several occasions when it has been isolated from blood and feces of human patients, it has been mistaken for a campylobacter (118).

CONCLUSION

New species of *Campylobacter* and related genera are being identified on a regular basis. Many of these "atypical" campylobacters may play a greater role in causing human and animal disease than previously recognized. Since methods originally formulated for the isolation of *C. jejuni* often fail to support the growth of non-*jejuni/coli Campylobacter* species, these fastidious organisms are most probably underdetected in clinical specimens. Appreciation and application of a correct protocol is essential for the isolation of non-*jejuni/coli Campylobacter* species for surveillance, epidemiological, and other studies. Reservoirs of newly described non-*jejuni/coli Campylobacter* species have been found in animals such as pigs, cattle, dogs, foxes, and rodents. Moreover, nonmammalian species such as birds and shellfish recently have been implicated as reservoirs of these organisms, and surface water and ground water are known to harbor non-*jejuni/coli Campylobacter* species and related organisms. At present, the role that these newly described *Campylobacter* species play in the disease process is not fully understood. Additional research is required to

better define the prevalence and scope of potential illness associated with these organisms.

REFERENCES

1. **Akhtar, N., and A. Eley.** 1992. Restriction endonuclease analysis and ribotyping differentiate genital and nongenital strains of *Bacteroides ureolyticus. J. Clin. Microbiol.* **30:**2408–2414.

2. **Albert, M. J., W. Tee, A. Leach, V. Asche, and J. L. Penner.** 1992. Comparison of a blood free medium and a filtration technique for the isolation of a *Campylobacter* spp. from diarrhoeal stools of hospitalized patients in central Australia. *J. Med. Microbiol.* **37:**176–179.

3. **Anderson, K. F., J. A. Kiehlbauch, D. C. Anderson, H. M. McClure and I. K. Wachmuth.** 1993. *Arcobacter (Campylobacter) butzleri*-associated diarrheal illness in a non-human primate population. *Infect. Immun.* **61:**2220–2223.

4. **Atabay, H. I., J. E. Corry, and S. L. On.** 1998. Diversity and prevalence of *Arcobacter* spp. in broiler chickens. *J. Appl. Microbiol.* **84:** 1007–1016.

5. **Bär, W., G. Márquez de Bär, H.-M. Nitschke, A. Schiessler, G. Mauff, A. Goldmann, B. Steinbrueckner, G. Härter, and M. Kist.** 1998. Endocarditis associated with *Campylobacter fetus,* p. 162–165. *In* A. J. Lastovica, D. G. Newell, and E. E. Lastovica (ed.), *Campylobacter, Helicobacter and Related Organisms.* Institute of Child Health, Cape Town, South Africa.

6. **Bates, C. J., T. C. Clarke, and R. C. Spencer.** 1994. Prosthetic hip joint infection due to *Campylobacter fetus. J. Clin. Microbiol.* **32:**2037. (Letter.)

7. **Benjamin, J., S. Leaper, R. J. Owen, and M. B. Skirrow.** 1983. Description of *Campylobacter laridis,* a new species comprising the nalidixic acid resistant thermophilic *Campylobacter* (NARTC) group. *Curr. Microbiol.* **8:**231–238.

8. **Bézian, M. C., G. Ribou, C. Barberis-Giletti, and F. Mégraud.** 1990. Isolation of a urease positive thermophilic variant of *Campylobacter lari* from a patient with urinary tract infection. *Eur. J. Clin. Microbiol. Infect. Dis.* **9:**895–897.

9. **Blaser, M. J., D. N. Taylor, and R. A. Feldman.** 1983. Epidemiology of *Campylobacter jejuni* infections. *Epidemiol. Rev.* **5:**157–176.

10. **Bokkenheuser, V.** 1970. *Vibrio fetus* infection in man. Ten new cases and some epidemiological observations. *Am. J. Epidemiol.* **91:**400–409.

11. **Bolton, F. J., D. Coates, D. N. Hutchinson, and A. F. Godfree.** 1987. A study of thermophilic *Campylobacter* in a river system. *J. Appl. Bacteriol.* **62:**167–176.

12. **Borczyk, A., S. Thompson, D. Smith, and**

H. Lior. 1987. Water-borne outbreak of *Campylobacter laridis*-associated gastroenteritis. *Lancet* **1:**164–165.

13. **Borczyk, A., H. Lior, A. McKeown, and H. Svendsen.** 1987. Isolations of *Campylobacter sputorum* associated with human infection, p. 166–167. *In* B. Kaijser, and E. Falsen (ed.), *Campylobacter IV.* University of Göteborg, Göteborg, Sweden.

14. **Boudreau, M., R. Higgins, and K. R. Mittal.** 1991. Biochemical and serological characterization of *Campylobacter cryaerophila. J. Clin. Microbiol.* **29:**54–58.

15. **Bourke, B., P. M., Sherman, D. Woodward, H. Lior, and V. L. Chan.** 1996. Pulsed-field gel electrophoresis indicates genotypic heterogeneity among *Campylobacter upsaliensis* strains. *FEMS Microbiol. Lett.* **143:**57–61.

16. **Bourke, B., V. L. Chan, and P. Sherman.** 1998. *Campylobacter upsaliensis:* waiting in the wings. *Clin. Microbiol. Rev.* **11:**440–449.

17. **Bracikowski, J. P., I. E. Hess, and M. F. Rein.** 1984. *Campylobacter* osteomyelitis. *South. Med. J.* **77:**1611–1613.

18. **Brennhoud, O., G. Kapperud, and G. Langeland.** 1992. Survey of thermotolerant *Campylobacter* spp. and *Yersinia* spp. in three surface water sources in Norway. *Int. J. Food Microbiol.* **15:**327–328.

19. **Breynaert, J., P. Vandamme, and S. Lauwers.** 1998. Review of 9 cases of human infection with *Campylobacter hyointestinalis*, p. 428–431. *In* A. J. Lastovica, D. G. Newell, and E. E. Lastovica (ed.), *Campylobacter, Helicobacter and Related Organisms.* Institute of Child Health, Cape Town, South Africa.

20. **Brown, W. J., and R. Sautter.** 1997. *Campylobacter fetus* septicemia with concurrent salpingitis. *J. Clin. Microbiol.* **6:**72–75.

21. **Bruneau, B., L. Burc, C. Bizet, N. Lambert-Zechovsky, and C. Branger.** 1998. Purulent pleurisy caused by *Campylobacter lari. Eur. J. Clin. Microbiol. Infect. Dis.* **17:**185–188.

22. **Burman, W. J., D. L. Cohn, R. R. Reeves, and M. L. Wilson.** 1995. Multifocal cellulitis and monoarticular arthritis as manifestations of *Helicobacter cinaedi* bacteremia. *Clin. Infect. Dis.* **20:**564–570.

23. **Burnens, A. P., B. Angeloy-Wick and J. Nicolet.** 1992. Comparison of *Campylobacter* carriage rates in diarrheic and healthy pet animals. *J. Vet. Med. Ser. B* **39:**175–180.

24. **Burnens, A. P., and J. Nicolet.** 1993. Three supplementary diagnostic tests for *Campylobacter* species and related organisms. *J. Clin. Microbiol.* **31:**708–710.

25. **Burnens, A. P., J. Stanley, V. B. Schaad, and J. Nicolet.** 1993. Novel *Campylobacter*-like organism resembling *Helicobacter fennelliae* isolated from a boy with gastroenteritis and from dogs. *J. Clin. Microbiol.* **31:**1916–1917.

26. **Butzler, J. P., and M. B. Skirrow.** 1979. *Campylobacter* enteritis. *Clin. Gastroenterology* **8:**737–765.

27. **Carbone, K. M., M. C. Heinrich, and T. C. Quinn.** 1985. Thrombophlebitis and cellulitis due to *Campylobacter fetus* ssp. *fetus, Medicine* **64:**244–250.

28. **Carter, J. E., and N. Cimolai.** 1996. Hemolytic-uremic syndrome associated with acute *Campylobacter upsaliensis* gastroenteritis. *Nephron* **74:**489. (Letter.)

29. **Centers for Disease Control.** 1981. *Campylobacter* sepsis associated with 'nutritional therapy'—California. *Morbid. Mortal. Weekly Rep.* **30:**294–295.

30. **Chusid, M. J., D. W. Wortmann, and W. M. Dunne.** 1990. "*Campylobacter upsaliensis*" sepsis in a boy with acquired hypogamaglobulinemia. *Diagn. Microbiol. Infect. Dis.* **13:**367–369.

31. **Collins, H. S., A. Blevins, and E. Baxter.** 1964. Protracted bacteremia and meningitis due to *Vibrio fetus. Arch. Intern. Med.* **113:**361–364.

32. **Costas, M., R. J. Owen, and P. H. J. Jackman.** 1987. Classification of *Campylobacter sputorum* and allied campylobacters based on numerical analysis of electrophoretic patterns. *Syst. Appl. Microbiol.* **9:**125–131.

33. **Da Silva Tatley, F., A. J. Lastovica, and L. M. Steyn.** 1992. Plasmid profiles of "*Campylobacter upsaliensis*" isolated from blood cultures and stools of paediatric patients. *J. Med. Microbiol.* **37:**8–14.

34. **Davies, A. P., C. J. Beghart, and S. A. Meric.** 1984. *Campylobacter* associated chronic diarrhea in a dog. *Am. J. Vet. Med.* **184:**469–471.

35. **Dediste, A., A. Aeby, A. Ebraert, L. Vlaes, R. Tridiani, O. Vandenberg, J.-M. Devaster, P. Vandamme, and J.-P. Butzler.** 1998. *Arcobacter* in stools: clinical features, diagnosis and antibiotic susceptibility, p. 436–439. *In* A. J. Lastovica, D. G. Newell, and E. E. Lastovica (ed.), *Campylobacter, Helicobacter and Related Organisms.* Institute of Child Health, Cape Town, South Africa.

35a.**de Otero, J. C. Pigrau, M. Buti, and R. Bartolomé.** 1994. Isolation of *Campylobacter fetus* subspecies *fetus* from a gluteal abscess. *Clin. Infect. Dis.* **19:**557–558.

36. **Devlin, H. R., and L. McIntyre.** 1983. *Campylobacter fetus* subsp. *fetus* in homosexual males. *J. Clin. Microbiol.* **18:**999–1000.

37. **Dickgiesser, N., G. Kasper, and W. Kihm.**

1983. *Campylobacter fetus* ssp. *fetus* bacteraemia: a patient with liver cirrhosis. *Infection* **11**:288.

38. **Dronda, F., I. Garcia-Arata, E. Navas, L. de Rafael.** 1998. Meningitis in adults due to *Campylobacter fetus* subspecies *fetus*. *Clin. Infect. Dis.* **27**:906–907.

39. **Edmonds, P., C. M. Patton, T. J. Barrett, G. K. Morris, A. G. Steigerwalt, and D. J. Brenner.** 1985. Biochemical and genetic characteristics of atypical *Campylobacter fetus* subsp. *fetus* strains isolated from humans in the United States. *J. Clin. Microbiol.* **21**:936–940.

40. **Edmonds, P., C. M. Patton, P. M. Griffin, T. J. Barett, G. P. Schmid, C. N. Baker, M. A. Lambert, and D. J. Brenner.** 1987. *Campylobacter hyointestinalis* associated with human gastrointestinal disease in the United States. *J. Clin. Microbiol.* **25**:685–691.

41. **Ellis, W. A., S. D. Neill, J. J. O'Brien, H. W. Ferguson, and J. Hanna.** 1977. Isolation of spirillium/vibrio-like organisms from bovine fetuses. *Vet. Rec.* **100**:451–452.

42. **Etoh, Y., F. E. Dewhirst, B. J. Paster, A. Yamamoto, and N. Goto.** 1993. *Campylobacter showae* sp. nov., isolated from the human oral cavity. *Int. J. Syst. Bacteriol.* **43**:631–639.

43. **Evans, T. G., and D. Riley.** 1992. *Campylobacter laridis* colitis in a human immunodeficiency virus-positive patient treated with a quinolone. *Clin. Infect. Dis.* **15**:172–173.

44. **Farrugia, D. C., S. J. Eykyn, and E. G. Smyth.** 1994. *Campylobacter fetus* endocarditis: two case reports and review. *Clin. Infect. Dis.* **18**:443–446.

45. **Fennell, C. J., P. A. Totten, T. C. Quinn, C. L. Patton, K. K. Holmes, and W. E. Stamm.** 1984. Characterization of *Campylobacter*-like organisms isolated from homosexual men. *J. Infect. Dis.* **149**:58–66.

46. **Fennell, C. L., A. M. Rompalo, P. A. Totten, K. L. Bruch, B. M. Flores, and W. E. Stamm.** 1986. Isolation of "*Campylobacter hyointestinalis*" from a human. *J. Clin. Microbiol.* **24**:146–148.

47. **Férnandez, H., U. Fagundes, S. Ogatha, U. F. Neto, and U. S. Ogatha.** 1997. Acute diarrhoea associated with *Campylobacter jejuni* subsp. *doylei* in Sao Paulo, Brazil. *Infect. Dis. J.* **16**:1098–1099. (Letter.)

48. **Fick, R. B., R. Isturiz, and E. C. Cadman.** 1979. *Campylobacter fetus* septic arthritis: report of a case. *Yale J. Biol. Med.* **52**:339–344.

49. **Figura, N., P. Gugliemetti, A. Zanchi, N. Partini, D. Armellini, P. F. Bayeli, M. Bugnoli, and S. Verdiani.** 1993. Two cases of *Campylobacter mucosalis* enteritis in children. *J. Clin. Microbiol.* **31**:727–728.

50. **Florent, A.** 1959. Les deux vibriosis génitales: la vibriose due à *V. foetus venerialis* et la vibriose d'origine intestinale due à *V. foetus intestinalis*. *Meded. Veeartsenijsch. Rijksuniv. Gent.* **3**:1–60.

51. **Flores, B. M., C. L. Fennell, K. K. Holmes, and W. E. Stamm.** 1985. In vitro susceptibility of *Campylobacter*-like organisms to twenty antimicrobial agents. *Antimicrob. Agents Chemother.* **28**:188–191.

52. **Flores, B. M., C. L. Fennell, and W. E. Stamm.** 1989. Characterization of *Campylobacter cinaedi* and *Campylobacter fennelliae* antigens and analysis of human immune response. *J. Infect. Dis.* **159**:635–640.

53. **Flores, B. M., C. L. Fennell, L. Kuller, M. A. Brondson, W. R. Morton, and W. Stamm.** 1990. Experimental infection of pig-tailed macaques (*Macaca nemestrina*) with *Campylobacter cinaedi* and *Campylobacter fennelliae*. *Infect. Immun.* **58**:3947–3953.

54. **Fox, J. O., K. O. Maxwell, N. S. Taylor, C. D. Runsick, P. Edmonds, and D. J. Brenner.** 1989. "*Campylobacter upsaliensis*" isolated from cats as identified by DNA relatedness and biochemical features. *J. Clin. Microbiol.* **27**:2376–2378.

55. **Francioli, P., J. Herzstein, J.-P. Grob, J.-J. Vallotton, G. Mombelli, and M. P. Glauser.** 1985. *Campylobacter fetus* subspecies *fetus* bacteremia. *Arch. Intern. Med.* **145**:289–292.

56. **Garcia, M. M., M. D. Eaglesome, and C. Rigby.** 1983. Campylobacters important in veterinary medicine. *Vet. Bull.* **53**:793–818.

57. **Garcier, F., G. Aubert, B. Coppéré, and A. Claudy.** 1983. Hypodermite nodulaire et infection a *Campylobacter fetus*. *Ann. Dermatol. Venereol.* **110**:449–453.

58. **Gaudreau, C., and F. Lamonthe.** 1992. *Campylobacter upsaliensis* isolated from a breast abscess. *J. Clin. Microbiol.* **30**:1354–1356.

59. **Gebhart, C. J., G. E. Ward, K. Chang, and H. J. Kurtz.** 1983. *Campylobacter hyointestinalis* (new species) isolated from swine with lesions of proliferative ileitis. *Am. J. Vet. Res.* **44**:361–367.

60. **Gebhart, C. J., P. Edmonds, G. E. Ward, H. J. Kurtz, and D. J. Brenner.** 1985. "*Campylobacter hyointestinalis*" sp. nov.: a new species of *Campylobacter* found in the intestines of pigs and other animals. *J. Clin. Microbiol.* **21**:715–720.

61. **Gebhart, C. J., C. L. Fennell, M. P. Murtaugh, and W. E. Stamm.** 1989. *Campylobacter cinaedi* is the normal intestinal flora in hamsters. *J. Clin. Microbiol.* **27**:1692–1694.

62. **Gebhart, C. J., M. P. Murtaugh, G. F. Lin, and G. E. Ward.** 1990. Species-specific DNA probes for *Campylobacter* species isolated from

pigs with proliferative enteritis. *Vet. Microbiol.* **24:**367–379.

63. **Glunder, G., and S. Petermann.** 1989. The occurrence and characterization of *Campylobacter* spp. in silver gulls (*Larus argentatus*), three toed gulls (*Rissa tridactyla*), and house sparrows (*Passer domesticus*). *Zentbl. Veterinaemed. Reihe B* **36:** 123–130.

64. **Goossens, H., B. Pot, L. Vlaes, C. Van den Borre, R. Van den Abbeele, C. Van Naelten, J. Levy, H. Gogniau, P. Marbehant, J. Verhoef, K. Kersters, J. P. Butzler, and P. Vandamme.** 1990. Characterization and description of "*Campylobacter upsaliensis*" isolated from human feces. *J. Clin. Microbiol.* **28:** 1039–1046.

65. **Goossens, H., L. Vlaes, and J. P. Butzler, A. Adnet, P. Hanicq, S. N'Jufom, D. Massart, G. DeSchrijver, and W. Blomme.** 1991. *Campylobacter upsaliensis* associated with canine infections. *Lancet* **337:**1486–1487.

66. **Goossens, H., B. A. J. Giesendorf, P. Vandamme, L. Vlaes, C. Van den Borre, A. Koeken, W. G. V. Quint, W. Blomme, P. Hanicq, D. S. Koster, H. Hofstra, J.-P. Butzler, and J. Van der Plas.** 1995. Investigation of an outbreak of *Campylobacter upsaliensis* in day care centers in Brussels: analysis of relationships among isolates by phenotypic and genotypic typing methods. *J. Infect. Dis.* **172:**1298–1305.

67. **Goudswaard, J., L. Sabbe, and W. te Winkel.** 1995. Reactive arthritis as a complication of *Campylobacter lari* enteritis. *J. Infect.* **31:**171. (Letter.)

68. **Grayson, M. L., W. Tee, and B. Dwyer.** 1989. Gastroenteritis associated with *Campylobacter cinaedi. Med. J. Aust.* **150:**214.

69. **Greig, A., D. Hanslo, E. Le Roux, and A. Lastovica.** 1993. In-vitro activity of eight antimicrobial agents against pediatric isolates of *C. concisus* and *C. mucosalis. Acta Gasteroenterol. Belg.* **56**(Suppl.)**:12.**

70. **Gubina, M., J. Zajc-Satler, J. Mehle, B. Drinovec, P. Pikelj, A. Radsel-Medvescek, and M. Suhac.** 1976. Septicaemia and meningitis with *Campylobacter fetus* subspecies *intestinalis. Infection* **4:**115–118.

71. **Guerrant, R. L., R. G. Lahita, W. C. Winn Jr., and R. B. Roberts.** 1976. Campylobacteriosis in man: pathogenic mechanisms and review of 91 bloodstream infections. *Am. J. Med.* **65:** 584–592.

72. **Gunderson, C. H., and G. E. Sack.** 1971. Neurology of *Vibrio fetus. Neurology* **21:**307.

73. **Gurgan, T., and K. S. Diker.** 1994. Abortion associated with *Campylobacter upsaliensis. J. Clin. Microbiol.* **32:**93–94.

74. **Hald, B., and M. Madsen.** 1997. Healthy puppies and kittens as carriers of *Campylobacter* spp., with special reference to *Campylobacter upsaliensis. J. Clin. Microbiol.* **35:**3351–3352.

75. **Harmon, K. M., and I. V. Wesley.** 1997. Multiplex PCR for the identification of *Arcobacter* and differentiation of *Arcobacter butzleri* from other arcobacters. *Vet. Microbiol.* **58:** 215–278.

76. **Harvey, S. M., and J. R. Greenwood.** 1983. Relationships among catalase-positive campylobacters determined by deoxyribonucleic acid–deoxyribonucleic acid hybridization. *Int. J. Syst. Bacteriol.* **33:**275–284.

77. **Harvey, S. M., and J. R. Greenwood.** 1983. Probable *Campylobacter fetus* subsp. *fetus* gastroenteritis. *J. Clin. Microbiol.* **18:**1278–1279.

78. **Holst, E., C. Schalén, and P.-A. Mårdh.** 1987. Isolation of *Campylobacter* spp. from the vagina, p. 167–168. *In* B. Kaijser and E. Falsen (ed.), *Campylobacter IV.* University of Göteborg, Göteborg, Sweden.

79. **Hsueh, P.-R., L.-J. Teng, P.-C. Yang, S.-K. Wang, S.-C. Chang, S.-W. Ho. W.-C. Hsieh, and K.-T. Luh.** 1997. Bacteraemia caused by *Arcobacter cryaerophilus* 1B. *J. Clin. Microbiol.* **35:**489–491.

80. **Hum, S., K. Quinn, J. Brunne, and S. L. On.** 1997. Evaluation of a PCR assay for the identification and differentiation of *Campylobacter fetus* subspecies. *Aust. Vet. J.* **75:**827–831.

81. **Hurtado, A., and R. J. Owen.** 1997. A molecular scheme based on 23S rRNA gene polymorphisms for rapid identification of *Campylobacter* and *Arcobacter* species. *J. Clin. Microbiol.* **35:** 2401–2404.

82. **Ichiyama, S., S. Hirai, T. Minami, Y. Nishiyama, S. Shimizu, K. Shimokata, and M. Ohta.** 1998. *Campylobacter fetus* subspecies *fetus* cellulitis associated with bacteremia in debilitated hosts. *Clin. Infect. Dis.* **27:**252–255.

83. **International Union of Microbiological Societies.** 1991. Validation of the publication of new names and new combinations previously published outside the IJSB. *Int. J. Syst. Bacteriol.* **41:**331.

84. **Jacob, J., D. Woodward, I. Feuerpfeil, and W. M. Johnson.** 1998. Isolation of *Arcobacter butzleri* in raw water and drinking water treatment plants in Germany. *Zentbl. Hyg. Umweltmed.* **201:** 189–198.

85. **Johnson, C. C., J. F. Reinhardt, M. A. C. Edelstein, M. E. Mulligan, W. L. George, and S. M. Finegold.** 1985. *Bacteroides gracilis,* an important anaerobic bacterial pathogen. *J. Clin. Microbiol.* **22:**799–802.

86. **Johnson, C. C., and S. M. Finegold.** 1987.

Uncommonly encountered motile, anaerobic gram-negative bacilli associated with infection. *Rev. Infect. Dis.* **9:**1150–1162.

87. **Johnson, W. M., and H. Lior.** 1986. Cytotoxic and cytotonic factors produced by *Campylobacter jejuni, Campylobacter coli* and *Campylobacter laridis. J. Clin. Microbiol.* **24:**275–281.

88. **Kakkar, M., and S. C. Dogra.** 1990. Prevalence of *Campylobacter* infections in animals and children in Haryana, India. *J. Diarrhocal Dis. Res.* **8:**34–36.

89. **Kalkay, M. N., Z. S. Ayanian, E. A. Lehaf, and A. Baldi.** 1983. Campylobacter-induced toxic megacolon. *Am. J. Gastroenterol.* **78:** 557–559.

90. **Kaspar, G., and N. Dickgiesser.** 1985. Isolation from the gastric epithelium of *Campylobacter*-like bacteria that are distinct from *Campylobacter pyloridis. Lancet* **i:**111–112.

91. **Kazawala, R. R., S. F. H. Jiwa, and A. E. Nkya.** 1993. The role of management systems in the epidemiology of thermophilic campylobacters among poultry in the eastern zone of Tanzania. *Epidemiol. Infect.* **110:**273–278.

92. **Kemper, C. A., P. Mickelson, A. Morton, B. Walton, and S. C. Deresinski.** 1993. *Helicobacter (Campylobacter) fennelliae*-like organisms as an important but occult phase of bacteraemia in a patient with AIDS. *J. Infect.* **26:**97–101.

93. **Kiehlbauch, J. A., D. J. Brenner, M. A. Nicholson, C. N. Baker, C. M. Patton, A. G. Steigerwalt, and I. K. Wachsmuth.** 1991. *Campylobacter butzleri* sp. nov. isolated from humans and animals with diarrheal illness. *J. Clin. Microbiol.* **29:**376–385.

94. **Kiehlbauch, J. A., B. D. Plikaytis, B. Swaminathan, C. N. Cameron, and I. K. Wachsmuth.** 1991. Restriction fragment length polymorphisms in the ribosomal genes for specific identification and subtyping of aerotolerant *Campylobacter* species. *J. Clin. Microbiol.* **29:** 1670–1676.

95. **Kiehlbauch, J. A., D. J. Brenner, D. N. Cameron, A. G. Steigerwalt, J. M. Markowski, C. N. Baker, C. M. Patton, and I. K. Wachsmuth.** 1995. Genotypic and phenotypic characterization of *Helicobacter cinaedi* and *Helicobacter fennelliae* strains isolated from humans and animals. *J. Clin. Microbiol.* **33:**2940–2947.

96. **Klein, B. S, J. M. Vergeront, M. J. Blaser, P. Edmonds, D. J. Brenner, D. Janssen, and J. P. Davis.** 1986. *Campylobacter* infection associated with raw milk: an outbreak of gastroenteritis due to *Campylobacter jejuni* and thermotolerant *Campylobacter fetus* subsp. *fetus. JAMA* **255:** 361–364.

97. **Lammerding, A. M., J. E. Harris, H. Lior,** D. E. Woodward, L. Cole, and C. A. Muckle. 1996. Isolation method for recovery of *Arcobacter butzleri* from fresh poultry and poultry products, p. 329–323. *In* D. G. Newell, J. M. Ketley, and R. A. Feldman (ed.), *Campylobacters, Helicobacters and Related Organisms.* Plenum Press, New York, N.Y.

98. **La Scola, B., S. Chambourlier, and P. Bouillot.** 1998. *Campylobacter fetus* ssp. *fetus* brain abscess. *J. Infect.* **37:**309–310. (Letter.)

99. **La Scolea, L. J.** 1985. *Campylobacter fetus* subsp. *fetus* meningitis in a neonate. *Clin. Microbiol. Newsl.* **7:**125–126.

100. **Lastovica, A. J., E. Le Roux, and J. L. Penner.** 1989. "*Campylobacter upsaliensis*" isolated from the blood cultures of pediatric patients. *J. Clin. Microbiol.* **27:**657–659.

101. **Lastovica, A. J., E. Le Roux and M. Jooste.** 1991. "*Campylobacter upsaliensis*" isolated from vervet monkeys. *Microb. Ecol. Health Dis.* **4**(Suppl.):S87.

102. **Lastovica, A. J., and E. Le Roux.** 1993. Prevalence and distribution of *Campylobacter* spp. in the diarrhoeic stools and blood cultures of paediatric patients. *Acta Gastroenterol. Belg.* **56**(Suppl.): 34.

103. **Lastovica, A. J., E. Le Roux, R. Warren, and H. Klump.** 1993. Clinical isolates of *Campylobacter mucosalis. J. Clin. Microbiol.* **31:** 2835–2836.

104. **Lastovica, A. J.** 1996. *Campylobacter/Helicobacter* bacteraemia in Cape Town, South Africa, 1977–1995, p. 475–479. *In* D. G. Newell, J. M. Ketley, and R. A. Feldman (ed.), *Campylobacters, Helicobacters and Related Organisms.* Plenum Press, New York, N.Y.

105. **Lastovica, A. J., E. A. Goddard, and A. C. Argent.** 1997. Guillain-Barré syndrome in South Africa associated with *Campylobacter jejuni* O:41 strains. *J. Infect. Dis.* **176**(Suppl.): S139–S143.

106. **Laughton, B. E., A. A. Vernon, D. A. Druckman, R. Fox, T. C. Quinn, B. F. Polk, and J. G. Bartlett.** 1988. Recovery of *Campylobacter* species from homosexual men. *J. Infect. Dis.* **158:**464–467.

107. **Laughton, B. E., D. A. Druckman, A. Vernon, T. C. Quinn, B. F. Polk, J. F. Modlin, R. H. Yolken, and J. G. Bartlett.** 1988. Prevalence of enteric pathogens in homosexual men with and without acquired immunodeficiency syndrome. *Gastroenterology* **94:**984–993.

108. **Lauwers, S., T. Devreker, R. Van Etterijck, J. Breynaert, A. Van Zeebroeck, L. Smekens, K. Kersters, and P. Vandamme.** 1991. Isolation of *Campylobacter concisus* from human faeces. *Microb. Ecol. Health Dis.* **4**(Suppl.):S91.

109. **Lawrence, R., A. F. Nibbe, and S. Lewis.** 1971. Lung abscess secondary to *Vibrio fetus* malabsorption syndrome and acquired agammaglobulinemia. *Chest* **60:**191–194.

110. **Lawson, G. H. K., and A. C. Rowland.** 1984. *Campylobacter sputorum* subsp. *mucosalis,* p. 207–225. In J.-P. Butzler (ed.), *Campylobacter Infection in Man and Animals.* CRC Press, Inc., Boca Raton, Fla.

111. **Le Roux, E., and A. J. Lastovica.** 1998. The Cape Town protocol: how to isolate the most campylobacters for your dollar, pound, franc, yen, etc., p. 30–33. In A. J. Lastovica, D. G. Newell, and E. E. Lastovica (ed.), *Campylobacter, Helicobacter and Related Organisms.* Institute of Child Health, Cape Town, South Africa.

112. **Lichtenberger, C. J., and C. A. Perlino.** 1982. Campylobacter and pelvic inflammatory disease. *Ann. Intern. Med.* **97:**147–148. (Letter.)

113. **Lindblom, G. B., M. Johny, K. Khalil, K. Mazhar, G. M. Ruiz-Palacios, and B. Kaijser.** 1990. Enterotoxigenicity and frequency of *Campylobacter jejuni, C. coli* and *C. laridis* in human and animal isolates from different countries. *FEMS Microbiol. Lett.* **54:**163–167.

114. **Linton, D., R. J. Owen, and J. Stanley.** 1996. Rapid identification by PCR of the genus *Campylobacter* and five *Campylobacter* species enteropathogenic for man and animals. *Res. Microbiol.* **147:**707–718.

115. **Lior, H., and D. L. Woodward.** 1993. *Arcobacter butzleri:* a serotyping scheme. *Acta Gastroenterol. Belg.* **56**(Suppl.)**:**29.

116. **Lowrie, D. B., and J. H. Pearce.** 1970. The placental localisation of *Vibrio fetus. J. Med. Microbiol.* **3:**607–614.

117. **Lucht, F., P. Fournel, G. Aubert, G. Clavreul, G. Dorche, J. Brunon, and H. Rousset.** 1983. Abcès cérébral à *Campylobacter fétus* subsp. *fétus* chez un adulte. *Med. Mal. Infect.* **13:**565–567.

118. **Malnick, H., K. Williams, J. Phil-Ebosie, and A. S. Levy.** 1990. Description of a medium for isolating *Anaerobiospirillum* spp., a possible cause of zoonotic disease, from diarrheal feces and blood of humans and use of the medium in a survey of human, canine, and feline feces. *J. Clin. Microbiol.* **28:**1380–1384.

119. **Maruyama, M., T. Tanaka, Y. Katsube, H. Nakanishi, and M. Nukina.** 1990. Prevalence of thermophilic campylobacters in crows (*Corvus lavaillantii, Corvus corone*) and serogroups of the isolates. *Jpn. J. Vet. Sci.* **52:**1237–1244.

120. **McFadyean, J., and S. Stockman.** 1913. *Report of the Departmental Committee Appointed by the Board of Agriculture and Fisheries to Inquire into Epizootic Abortion.* Appendix to part III. *Abortion in Sheep,* p. 1–29. His Majesty's Stationery Office, London, United Kingdom.

121. **McGechie, D. B., T. B. Teoh, and V. W. Bamford.** 1982. Campylobacter enteritis in Hong Kong and Western Australia, p. 19–21. In D. G. Newell (ed.), *Campylobacter: Epidemiology, Pathogenesis and Biochemistry.* MTP Press, Lancaster, United Kingdom.

122. **Mégraud, F., and F. Bonnet.** 1986. Unusual *Campylobacters* in human feces. *J. Infect.* **12:**275–276.

123. **Mégraud, F., D. Chevrier, N. Desplaces, A. Sedallian, and J. L. Guesdon.** 1988. Urease-positive thermophilic *Campylobacter* (*Campylobacter laridis* variant) isolated from an appendix and from human feces. *J. Clin. Microbiol.* **26:**1050–1051.

124. **Mendelson, M. H., P. Nicholas, M. Malowany, and S. Lewin.** 1986. Subdural empyema caused by *Campylobacter fetus* ssp. *fetus. J. Infect Dis.* **153:**1183–1184. (Letter.)

125. **Mii, S., K. Tanaka, K. Furugaki, H. Sakata, H. Katoh, and A. Mori.** 1998. Infected abdominal aortic aneurysm caused by *Campylobacter fetus* subspecies *fetus:* report of a case. *Surg. Today* **28:**661–664.

126. **Miller, V. A., R. Jenson, and J. J. Gilroy.** 1959. Bacteremia in pregnant sheep following oral administration of *Vibrio fetus. Am. J. Vet. Res.* **20:**677–679.

127. **Minet, J., B. Grosbois, and F. Mégraud.** 1988. *Campylobacter hyointestinalis:* an opportunistic enteropathogen? *J. Clin. Microbiol.* **26:**2659–2660.

128. **Montero, A., X. Corbella, J. A. López, M. Santín, and I.-H. Ballón.** 1997. *Campylobacter fetus*-associated aneurysms: report of a case involving the popliteal artery and review of the literature. *Clin. Infect. Dis.* **24:**1019–1021.

129. **Morey, F.** 1996. Five years of *Campylobacter* bacteraemia in Central Australia, p. 491–494. In D. G. Newell, J. M. Ketley, and R. A. Feldman (ed.), *Campylobacters, Helicobacters and Related Organisms.* Plenum Press, New York, N.Y.

130. **Morooka, T., A. Umeda, M. Fujita, H. Matano, S. Fujimoto, K. Yukitake, Z. Amako, and T. Oda.** 1996. Epidemiologic application of pulsed-field gel electrophoresis to an outbreak of *Campylobacter fetus* meningitis in a neonatal intensive care unit. *Scand. J. Infect. Dis.* **28:**269–270.

131. **Morrison, V. A., B. K. Lloyd, J. K. S. Chia, and C. U. Tuazon.** 1990. Cardiovascular and bacteremic manifestations of *Campylobacter fetus* infection: case report and review. *Rev. Infect. Dis.* **12:**387–392.

132. **Nachamkin, I., C. Stowell, D. Skalina, A.**

M. Jones, R. M. Roop, and R. M. Smibert. 1984. *Campylobacter laridis* causing bacteraemia in an immunosuppressed patient. *Ann. Intern. Med.* **101**:55–57.

133. **Neuzil, K., E. Wang, D. Haas, and M. J. Blaser.** 1994. Persistence of *Campylobacter fetus* bacteraemia associated with absence of opsonizing antibodies. *J. Clin. Microbiol.* **32**:1718–1720.

134. **Ng, V. L., W. K. Hadley, C. L. Fennell, B. M. Flores, and W. E. Stamm.** 1987. Successive bacteremias with "*Campylobacter cinaedi*" and "*Campylobacter fennelliae*" in a bisexual male. *J. Clin. Microbiol.* **25**:2008–2009.

135. **Ohya, T., and M. Nakazawa.** 1992. Production and some properties of cytotoxins produced by *Campylobacter* species isolated from proliferative enteropathy in swine. *J. Vet. Med. Sci.* **54**:1031–1033.

136. **On, S. L. W., R. J. Owen, A. J. Lastovica, M. Costas, and B. Lopez-Urquijo.** 1991. Taxonomic study of *Helicobacter* (*Campylobacter*) *fennelliae* from clinical material by numerical analysis of one-dimensional electrophoretic protein patterns. *Microb. Ecol. Health Dis.* **4**(Suppl.): S103.

137. **On, S. L., F. Ridgewell, B. Cryan, and B. S. Azadian.** 1992. Isolation of *Campylobacter sputorum* biovar sputorum from an axillary abscess. *J. Infect.* **24**:175–179.

138. **On, S. L., B. Bloch, B. Holmes, B. Hoste, and P. Vandamme.** 1995. *Campylobacter hyointestinalis* subsp. *lawsonii* subsp. nov., isolated from the porcine stomach, and an emended description of *Campylobacter hyointestinalis*. *Int. J. Syst. Bacteriol.* **45**:767–774.

139. **On, S. L. W., A. Stacey, and J. Smyth.** 1995. Isolation of *Arcobacter butzleri* from a neonate with bacteraemia. *J. Infect.* **31**:225–227.

140. **On, S. L. W.** 1996. Identification methods for campylobacters, helicobacters and arcobacters. *Clin. Microbiol. Rev.* **9**:405–422.

141. **On, S. L. W., H. I. Atabay, J. E. L. Corry, C. S. Harrington, and P. Vandamme.** 1998. Emended description of *Campylobacter sputorum* and revision of its infrasubspecific (biovar) divisions, including *C. sputorum* biovar paraureolyticus, a urease-producing variant from cattle and humans. *Int. J. Syst. Bacteriol.* **48**:195–206.

142. **Orlicek, S. L., D. F., Welch and T. L. Kuhls.** 1993. Septicemia and meningitis caused by *Helicobacter cinaedi* in a neonate. *J. Clin. Microbiol.* **31**: 569–571.

143. **Owen, R. J., A. Beck, and P. Borman.** 1985. Restriction endonuclease digest patterns of chromosomal DNA from nitrate-negative *Campylobacter jejuni*-like organisms. *Eur. J. Epidemiol.* **1**: 281–287.

144. **Owen, R. J., D. D. Morgan, M. Costas, and A. J. Lastovica.** 1989. Identification of "*Campylobacter upsaliensis*" and other catalase-negative *Campylobacters* from pediatric blood cultures by numerical analysis of electrophoretic protein patterns. *FEMS Microbiol. Lett.* **58**: 145–150.

145. **Owen, R. J., and J. Hernandez.** 1990. Occurrence of plasmids in "*Campylobacter upsaliensis*" (catalase negative or weak group) from geographically diverse patients with gastroenteritis or bacteremia. *Eur. J. Epidemiol.* **6**:111–117.

146. **Oyarzabal, O. A., I. V. Wesley, K. M. Harmon, L. Schroeder-Tucker, J. M. Barbaree, L. H. Lauerman, S. Backert, and D. E. Conner.** 1997. Specific identification of *Campylobacter fetus* by PCR targeting variable regions of the 16S rRNA. *Vet. Microbiol.* **58**:61–71.

147. **Park, C. E., and G. W. Sanders.** 1992. Occurrence of thermotolerant campylobacters in fresh vegetables sold at farmer's outdoor markets and supermarkets. *Can. J. Microbiol.* **38**:313–316.

148. **Patton, C. M., N. Shaffer, P. Edmonds, T. J. Barrett, M. A. Lambert, C. Baker, D. M. Perlman, and D. J. Brenner.** 1989. Human disease associated with "*Campylobacter upsaliensis*" (catalase-negative or weakly positive *Campylobacter* species) in the United States. *J. Clin. Microbiol.* **27**:66–73.

149. **Pickett, C. L., E. C. Pecsi, D. L. Cottle, G. Russell, A. N. Erdem, and H. Zeytin.** 1996. Prevalence of cytolethal distending toxin production in *Campylobacter jejuni* and relatedness of *Campylobacter* sp. *cdtB* genes. *Infect. Immun.* **64**: 2070–2078.

150. **Popovic-Uroic, T., C. M. Patton, M. A. Nicholson, and J. A. Kiehlbauch.** 1990. Evaluation of indoxylacetate hydrolysis test for rapid differentiation of *Campylobacter, Helicobacter,* and *Wolinella* species. *J. Clin. Microbiol.* **28**: 2335–2339.

151. **Preston, M. A., A. E. Simor, S. L. Walmsley, S. A. Fuller, A. J. Lastovica, K. Sandstedt, and J. L. Penner.** 1990. In vitro susceptibility of "*Campylobacter upsaliensis*" to twenty-four antimicrobial agents. *Eur. J. Clin. Microbiol. Infect. Dis.* **9**:822–824.

152. **Quinn, T. C., S. E., Goodell and C. L. Fennell, S. P. Wang, M. D. Schufler, K. K. Holmes, and E. W. Stamm.** 1984. Infections with *Campylobacter jejuni* and *Campylobacter*-like organisms in homosexual men. *Ann. Intern. Med.* **101**:187–192.

153. **Rahman, M.** 1979. Bacteraemia and pericarditis from *Campylobacter* infection. *Br. J. Clin. Pract.* **33**:331–334.

154. **Rams, T. E., D. Feik, and J. Slots.** 1993.

Campylobacter rectus in human periodontitis. *Oral Microbiol. Immunol.* **8:**230–235.

155. **Rao, G. G., Q. N. Karim, A. Maddocks, R. J. Hillman, J. R. W. Harris, and A. J. Pinching.** 1990. *Campylobacter fetus* infections in two patients with AIDS. *J. Infect.* **20:**170–172.

156. **Rennie, R. P., D. Strong, D. E. Taylor, S. M. Salama, C. Davidson, and H. Tabor.** 1994. *Campylobacter fetus* diarrhea in a Hutterite colony: epidemiological observations and typing of the causative organism. *J. Clin. Microbiol.* **32:**721–724.

157. **Rice, E. W., M. R. Rodgers, I. V. Wesley, C. H. Johnson, and S. A. Tanner.** 1999. Isolation of *Arcobacter butzleri* from ground water. *Lett. Appl. Microbiol.* **28:**31–35.

158. **Romero, S., J. R. Archer, M. E. Hamacher, S. M. Bologna, and R. F. Schell.** 1988. Case report of an unclassified microaerophilic bacterium associated with gastroenteritis. *J. Clin. Microbiol.* **26:**142–143.

159. **Russell, R. G., J. A. Kiehlbauch, C. J. Gebhart, and L. J. De Tolla.** 1992. Uncommon *Campylobacter* species in infant *Macaca nemestrina* monkeys housed in a nursery. *J. Clin. Microbiol.* **30:**3024–3027.

160. **Salama, S. M., M. M. Garcia, and D. E. Taylor.** 1992. Differentiation of the sub-species of *Campylobacter fetus* by genomic sizing. *Int. J. Syst. Bacteriol.* **42:**446–450.

161. **Salama, S. M., H. Tabor, M. Richter, and D. E. Taylor.** 1992. Pulsed-field gel electrophoresis for epidemiological studies of *Campylobacter hyointestinalis* isolates. *J. Clin. Microbiol.* **30:**1982–1984.

162. **Sandstedt, K., J. Ursing, and M. Walder.** 1983. Thermotolerant campylobacter with no or weak catalase activity isolated from dogs. *Curr. Microbiol.* **8:**209–213.

163. **Sandstedt, K., and J. Ursing.** 1991. Description of *Campylobacter upsaliensis* sp. nov. previously known as the CNW group. *Syst. Appl. Microbiol.* **14:**39–48.

164. **Sauerwein, R. W., J. Bisseling, A. M. Horrevorts.** 1993. Septic abortion associated with *Campylobacter fetus* subsp. *fetus* infection: case report and review of the literature. *Infection* **21:**331–333.

165. **Schrader, J. A., R. A. Venezia, and J. Tillotson.** 1991. Urease-positive thermophilic *Campylobacter* isolated from human blood. *Clin. Microbiol. Newsl.* **13:**158–160.

166. **Simor, A. E., and L. Wilcox.** 1987. Enteritis associated with *Campylobacter laridis*. *J. Clin. Microbiol.* **25:**10–12.

167. **Skirrow, M. B., and J. Benjamin.** 1980. "1001" campylobacters from man and animals. *J. Hyg.* **85:**427–442.

168. **Skirrow, M. B., and J. Benjamin.** 1980. Differentiation of enteropathogenic campylobacter. *J. Clin. Pathol.* **33:**1122.

169. **Skirrow, M. B., D. M. Jones, E. Sutcliffe, and J. Benjamin.** 1993. *Campylobacter* bacteraemia in England and Wales, 1981–91. *Epidemiol. Infect.* **110:**567–573.

170. **Smibert, R. M.** 1984. Genus *Campylobacter*, p. 111–118. *In* N. R. Kreig and H. G. Holt (ed.), *Bergey's Manual of Systematic Bacteriology*, vol. 1. The Williams & Wilkins Co., Baltimore, Md.

171. **Smith, T.** 1919. The etiological relation of spirilla (*Vibrio fetus*) to bovine abortion. *J. Exp. Med.* **30:**313–322.

172. **Sorlin, P., P. Vandamme, J. Nortier, B. Hoste, C. Rossi, S. Pavlof, and M. J. Struelens.** 1999. Recurrent "*Flexispira rappini*" bacteremia in an adult patient undergoing hemodialysis: case report. *J. Clin. Microbiol.* **37:**1319–1323.

173. **Stamp, S., O. Varoli, F. Zanetti, and G. De Luca.** 1993. *Arcobacter cryaerophilus* and thermophilic campylobacters in a sewage treatment plant in Italy: two secondary treatments compared. *Epidemiol. Infect.* **110:**633–639.

174. **Stanley, J., A. P. Burnens, D. Linton, S. L. W. On, M. Costas, and R. J. Owen.** 1992. *Campylobacter helveticus* sp. nov., a new thermophilic species from domestic animals: characterization, and cloning of a species-specific DNA probe. *J. Gen. Microbiol.* **138:**2293–2303.

175. **Stanley, J., D. Linton, A. P. Burnens, F. E. Dewhirst, R. J. Owen, A. Porter, S. L. W. On, and M. Costas.** 1993. *Helicobacter canis* sp. nov., a new species from dogs: an integrated study of phenotype and genotype. *J. Gen. Microbiol.* **139:**2495–2504.

176. **Stanley, J., D. Linton, A. P. Burnens, F. E. Dewhirst, S. L. W. On, A. Porter, R. J. Owen and M. Costas.** 1994. *Helicobacter pullorum* sp. nov.—genotype and phenotype of a new species isolated from poultry and human patients with gastroenteritis. *Microbiology* **140:**3441–3449.

177. **Steele, T. W., and J. N. McDermott.** 1984. Technical note: the use of membrane filters applied directly to the surface of agar plates for the isolation of *Campylobacter jejuni* from feces. *Pathology* **16:**263–265.

178. **Steele, T. W., N. Sangster, and J. A. Lanser.** 1985. DNA relatedness and biochemical features of *Campylobacter* spp. isolated in central and south Australia. *J. Clin. Microbiol.* **22:**71–74.

179. **Steele, T. W., and R. J. Owen.** 1988. *Campylobacter jejuni* subspecies *doylei* (subsp. nov.), is a

subspecies of nitrate-negative campylobacters isolated from clinical specimens. *Int. J. Syst. Bacteriol.* **38:**316–318.

180. **Steele, T. W., J. A. Lanser, and N. Sangster.** 1985. Nitrate-negative *Campylobacter*-like organisms. *Lancet* **i:**294.

181. **Steinbrueckner, B., G. Haerter, K. Pelz, S. Weiner, J.-A. Rump, W. Deissler, S. Bereswill, and M. Kist.** 1997. Isolation of *Helicobacter pullorum* from patients with enteritis. *Scand. J. Infect. Dis.* **29:**315–318.

182. **Steinkraus, G. E., and B. D. Wright.** 1994. Septic abortion with intact fetal membranes caused by *Campylobacter fetus* subsp. *fetus. J. Clin. Microbiol.* **32:**1608–1609.

183. **Sylvester, F. A., D. Philpott, B. Gold, A. Lastovica, and J. F. Forstner.** 1996. Adherence to lipids and intestinal mucin by a recently recognized human pathogen, *Campylobacter upsaliensis. Infect. Immun.* **64:**4060–4066.

184. **Takatsu, M., S. Ichiyama, T. Nada, Y. Iinuma, H. Toyoda, Y. Fukuda, and N. Nakashima.** 1997. *Campylobacter fetus* subsp. *fetus* cholecystitis in a patient with advanced hepatocellular carcinoma. *Scand. J. Infect. Dis.* **29:**197–198.

185. **Tanner, A. C. R., S. Badger, C. H. Lai, M. A. Listgarten, R. A. Visconti, and S. S. Socransky.** 1981. *Wolinella* gen. nov., *Wolinella succinogenes* (*Vibrio succinogenes* Wolin et al.) comb. nov., and description of *Bacteroides gracilis* sp. nov., *Wolinella recta* sp. nov., *Campylobacter concisus* sp. nov., and *Eikenella corrodens* from humans with periodontal disease. *Int. J. Syst. Bacteriol.* **31:**432–435.

186. **Tanner, A. C. R., M. A. Listgarten, and J. L. Ebersole.** 1984. *Wolinella curva* sp. nov.: "*Vibrio succinogenes*" of human origin. *Int. J. Syst. Bacteriol.* **34:**275–282.

187. **Tanner, A. C. R., J. L. Dzink, J. L. Ebersole, and S. S. Socransky.** 1987. *Wolinella recta, Campylobacter concisus, Bacteroides gracilis,* and *Eikenella corrodens* from periodontal lesions. *J. Periodontal Res.* **22:**327–330.

188. **Targan, S. R., A. W. Chow, and L. B. Guze.** 1976. Spontaneous peritonitis of cirrhosis due to *Campylobacter fetus. Gastroenterology* **71:**311–313.

189. **Targan, S. R., A. W. Chow, and L. B. Guze.** 1977. *Campylobacter fetus* associated with pulmonary abscess and empyema. *Chest* **71:**105–108.

190. **Tarrand, J. J., and D. H. M. Gröschel.** 1982. Rapid, modified oxidase test for oxidase-variable bacterial isolates. *J. Clin. Microbiol.* **16:**772–774.

191. **Tauxe, R. V., C. M. Patton, P. Edmonds, T. J. Barrett, D. J. Brenner, and P. A. Blake.** 1985. Illness associated with *Campylobacter laridis,*

a newly recognized *Campylobacter* species. *J. Clin. Microiol.* **21:**222–225.

192. **Taylor, D. E., K. Hiratsuka, and L Mueller.** 1989. Isolation and characterization of catalase-negative and catalase-weak strains of *Campylobacter* species, including "*Campylobacter upsaliensis,*" from humans with gastroenteritis. *J. Clin. Microbiol.* **27:**2042–2045.

193. **Taylor, D. N., K. T. McDermott, J. R. Little, J. G. Wells, and M. J. Blaser.** 1983. *Campylobacter* enteritis from untreated water in the Rocky Mountains. *Ann. Intern. Med.* **99:**38–40.

194. **Taylor, D. N., J. A. Kiehlbauch, W. Tee, C. Pitarangsi, and P. Echeverria.** 1991. Isolation of group 2 aerotolerant *Campylobacter* species from Thai children with diarrhea. *J. Infect. Dis.* **163:**1062–1067.

195. **Tee, W., R. Baird, M. Dyall-Smith, and B. Dwyer.** 1988. *Campylobacter cryaerophila* isolated from a human. *J. Clin. Microbiol.* **26:**2469–2473.

196. **Tee, W., K. Leder, E. Karroum, and M. Dyall-Smith.** 1998. '*Flexispira rappini*' bacteraemia in a child with pneumonia. *J. Clin. Microbiol.* **36:**1679–1682.

197. **Tee, W., M. Luppino, and S. Rambaldo.** 1998. Bacteremia due to *Campylobacter sputorum* biovar sputorum. *Clin. Infect. Dis.* **27:**1544–1545.

198. **Totten, P. A., C. L. Fennell, F. C. Tenover, J. M. Wezenberg, P. L. Perine, W. E. Stamm, and K. K. Holmes.** 1985. *Campylobacter cinaedi* (sp. nov.) and *Campylobacter fennelliae* (sp. nov.): two new *Campylobacter* species associated with enteric disease in homosexual men. *J. Infect. Dis.* **151:**131–139.

199. **Tresierra-Ayala, A., M. E. Bendayan, A. Bermuy, G. Pereyra, and H. Fernandez.** 1994. Chicken as potential contamination source of *Campylobacter lari* in Iquitos, Peru. *Rev. Inst. Med. Trop. Sao Paulo* **36:**497–499.

200. **Trivett-Moore, N. L., W. D. Rawlinson, M. Yuen, and G. L. Gilbert.** 1997. *Helicobacter westmeadii* sp. nov., a new species isolated from blood cultures in two AIDS patients. *J. Clin. Microbiol.* **35:**1144–1150.

201. **U.S. Department of Health and Human Services, Public Health Service: Centers for Disease Control.** 1990. *Campylobacter* annual tabulation, 1987–89, p. 5–10. U.S. Dept. of Health and Human Services, Washington, D.C.

202. **Vandamme, P., E. Falsen, B. Pot, B. Holste, K. Kersters, and J. De Ley.** 1989. Identification of EF group 22 campylobacters from gastroenteritis cases as *Campylobacter concisus. J. Clin. Microbiol.* **27:**1775–1782.

203. **Vandamme, P., B. Pot, E. Falsen, K. Kers-**

ters, and J. De Ley. 1990. Intra- and interspecific relationships of veterinary campylobacters revealed by numerical analysis of electrophoretic protein profiles and DNA:DNA hybridizations. *Syst. Appl. Microbiol.* **13**:295–303.

204. **Vandamme, P., and J. De Ley.** 1991. Proposals for a new family, *Campylobacteraceae. Int. J. Syst. Bacteriol.* **41**:451–455.

205. **Vandamme, P., E. Falsen, R. Rossau, B. Hoste, R. Tygat, and J. De Ley.** 1991. Revision of *Campylobacter, Helicobacter* and *Wolinella* taxonomy: emendation of generic descriptions and proposal of *Arcobacter* gen. nov. *Int. J. Syst. Bacteriol.* **41**:88–103.

206. **Vandamme, P., P. Pugina, G. Benzi, R. Van Etterijck, L. Vlaes, K. Kersters, J.-P. Butzler, H. Lior, and S. Lauwers.** 1992. Outbreak of recurrent abdominal cramps associated with *Arcobacter butzleri* in an Italian school. *J. Clin. Microbiol.* **30**:2335–2337.

207. **Vandamme, P., M. Vancanneyt, B. Pot, L. Mels, B. Holste, D. Dewettinck, L. Vlaes, C. Van den Borre, R. Higgins, J. Hommez, K. Kersters, J.-P. Butzler, and H. Goossens.** 1992. Polyphasic taxonomic study of the emended genus *Arcobacter* with *Arcobacter butzleri* comb. nov. and *Arcobacter skirrowii* sp. nov., an aerotolerant bacterium isolated from veterinary specimens. *Int. J. Syst. Bacteriol.* **42**:344–356.

208. **Vandamme, P., M. I. Daneshvar, F. E. Dewhirst, B. J. Paster, K. Kersters, H. Goossens, and C. W. Moss.** 1995. Chemotaxonomic analyses of *Bacteroides gracilis* and *Bacteroides ureolyticus* and reclassification of *B. gracilis* as *Campylobacter gracilis* comb. nov. *Int. J. Syst. Bacteriol.* **45**:145–152.

209. **Van Doorn, L. J., B. A. Giesendorf, R. Bax, B. A. Van der Zeijst, P. Vandamme, and W. G. Quint.** 1997. Molecular discrimination between *Campylobacter jejuni, Campylobacter coli, Campylobacter lari* and *Campylobacter upsaliensis* by polymerase chain reaction based on a novel putative GTPase gene. *Mol. Cell. Probes* **11**:177–185.

210. **Van Doorn, L. J., W. G. Verschuuren-Van Haperen, A. Van Belkum, H. P. Endtz, J. S. Vliegenthart, P. Vandamme, and W. G. Quint.** 1998. Rapid identification of diverse *Campylobacter lari* strains isolated from mussels and oysters using a reverse hybridization line probe assay. *J. Appl. Microbiol.* **84**:545–550.

211. **Van Dyke, T. E., V. R. Dowell, S. Offenbacher, S. Synder and W. Hersh.** 1986. Potential role of microorganisms isolated from periodontal lesions in the pathogenesis of inflammatory bowel disease. *Infect. Immun.* **53**:671–677.

212. **Van Etterijck, R., J. Breynaert, H. Revets, T. Devreker, Y. Vandenplas, P. Vandamme, and S. Lauwers.** 1996. Isolation of *Campylobacter concisus* from feces of children with and without diarrhea. *J. Clin. Microbiol.* **34**:2304–2306.

213. **Vargas, J., J. E. Corzo, M. J. Perez, F. Lozano, and E. Martin.** 1992. Bacteriemia por *Campylobacter* e infeccion por VIH. Enfern. *Infecc. Microbiol. Clin.* **10**:155–157.

214. **Véron, M., and R. Chatelain.** 1973. Taxonomic study of the genus *Campylobacter* Sebald and Véron and designation of the neotype strain for the type species, *Campylobacter fetus* (Smith and Taylor) Sebald and Véron. *Int. J. Syst. Bacteriol.* **23**:122–134.

215. **Von Graevenitz, A.** 1990. Revised nomenclature of *Campylobacter laridis, Enterobacter intermedium,* and "*Flavobacterium brachophilia.*" *Int. J. Syst. Bacteriol.* **40**:211.

216. **Walder, M., K. Sandstedt, and J. Ursing.** 1983. Phenotypic characteristics of thermotolerant *Campylobacter* from human and animal sources. *Curr. Microbiol.* **9**:291–296.

217. **Walmsley, S. L., and M. A. Karmali.** 1989. Direct isolation of thermophilic *Campylobacter* species from human feces on selective agar medium. *J. Clin. Microbiol.* **27**:688–670.

218. **Wang, W. L., and M. J. Blaser.** 1986. Detection of pathogenic *Campylobacter* species in blood culture systems. *J. Clin. Microbiol.* **23**:709–714.

219. **Wareing, D. R. A., S. T. Aspinall, P. G. Hayward, and D. N. Hutchinson.** 1998. Improved selective medium (CAT) for thermophilic campylobacters including *Campylobacter upsaliensis*, p. 46–49. *In* A. J. Lastovica, D. G. Newell, and E. E. Lastovica (ed.), *Campylobacter, Helicobacter and Related Organisms.* Institute of Child Health, Cape Town, South Africa.

220. **Wens, R., M. Dratwa, C. Potvliege, C. Hansen, C. Tielemans, and F. Collart.** 1985. *Campylobacter fetus* peritonitis followed by septicaemia in a patient on continuous ambulatory dialysis. *J. Infect.* **10**:249–251.

221. **Wesley, I. V., R. D. Wesley, M. Cardella, F. E., Dewhirst, and B. J. Paster.** 1991. Oligodeoxynucleotide probes for *Campylobacter fetus* and *Campylobacter hyointestinalis* based on 16S rRNA sequences. *J. Clin. Microbiol.* **29**:1812–1817.

222. **Wesley, I. V., A. L. Baetz, and D. J. Larson.** 1996. Infection of cesarean-derived colostrum-deprived 1 day-old piglets with *Arcobacter butzleri, Arcobacter cryaerophilus* and *Arcobacter skirrowii. Infect. Immun.* **64**:2295–2299.

223. **Wilcox, C. M., B. A. Byford, C. E. Forsmark, W. K. Hadley, J. P. Cello, and M. A.**

Jacobson. 1990. *Campylobacter*-like organisms are uncommon pathogens in patients infected with the human immunodeficiency virus. *J. Clin. Microbiol.* **28:**2370–2371.

224. Yao, J. D. C., H. M. C. Ng, and I. Campbell. 1993. Prosthetic hip joint infection due to *Campylobacter fetus*. *J. Clin. Microbiol.* **31:** 3323–3324.

225. Zanetti, F., O. Varoli, S. Stampi, and G. De Luca. 1996. Prevalence of thermophilic *Campylobacter* and *Arcobacter butzleri* in food of animal origin. *Int. J. Food Microbiol.* **33:**315–321.

226. Zhi, N., H. Revets, A. Van Zeebroek, and S. Lauwers. 1996. Serological response to *Campylobacter concisus* infection, p. 673–678. *In* D. G. Newell, J. M. Ketley, and R. A. Feldman (ed.), *Campylobacters, Helicobacters, and Related Organisms*. Plenum Press, New York, N.Y.

EPIDEMIOLOGY OF *CAMPYLOBACTER JEJUNI* INFECTIONS IN THE UNITED STATES AND OTHER INDUSTRIALIZED NATIONS

C. R. Friedman, J. Neimann, H. C. Wegener, and R. V. Tauxe

6

Campylobacter organisms have long been recognized as a cause of diarrhea in cattle and of septic abortion in both cattle and sheep, but they have been recognized as an important cause of human illness for only the last 25 years. *Campylobacter* organisms may have been what Escherich observed in the stools of infants with diarrhea in Germany in 1880 (30). However, *Campylobacter* appeared to be a rare and perhaps opportunistic human pathogen when it was isolated from cultures of blood isolated from humans in the 1950s (53). The most commonly identified species, *Campylobacter jejuni,* was first isolated from human diarrheal stools in 1972 by a filtration technique developed for veterinary diagnosis (25). The subsequent development of selective *Campylobacter* stool culture media led to the recognition that *C. jejuni* was a common cause of human diarrheal illness in many countries.

NATIONAL *CAMPYLOBACTER* SURVEILLANCE IN THE UNITED STATES

Passive Surveillance
The Centers for Disease Control and Preven-

tion (CDC) began national *Campylobacter* surveillance through the Public Health Laboratory Information System in 1982 (31, 79, 97, 98). Reports of isolates were mailed weekly to CDC by state health departments in the same format as that used for *Salmonella* and *Shigella* surveillance data in the United States. The reported data included the *Campylobacter* species isolated, the date of reporting to CDC, the age and sex of the person from whom the isolate came, the county of residence of the person, and the clinical source of the culture. No other clinical information was included, and deaths were not reported.

During the first year of *Campylobacter* reporting, the number of reported isolations increased from 4,027 in 1982 to over 8,630 in 1983. This was related to a dramatic rise in the number of states reporting *Campylobacter* isolates. Since 1983, the number of states reporting has remained relatively constant each year; however, since 1990, the number of isolations reported and the isolation rate per 100,000 have decreased, and the rate reached a low of 2.5 per 100,000 in 1995. This decrease does not represent a decrease in *Campylobacter* incidence but, rather, decreased reporting in this passive-surveillance system.

Passive surveillance relies on clinical laboratories to report or refer isolates to local or state

C. R. Friedman and R. V. Tauxe, Foodborne and Diarrheal Diseases Branch, Centers for Disease Control and Prevention, 1600 Clifton Road, Mailstop A38, Atlanta, GA 30333. *J. Neimann and H. C. Wegener,* Danish Veterinary Laboratory, Danish Zoonosis Centre, Bülowsvej 27, DK-1790 Copenhagen V, Denmark.

Campylobacter, 2nd Ed., Edited by I. Nachamkin and M. J. Blaser
© 2000 American Society for Microbiology, Washington, D.C.

health departments, which then report them to CDC. Participating states vary widely in their internal reporting requirements for *Campylobacter* species. Unlike *Salmonella* species, *Campylobacter* isolates are not routinely referred for serotyping or confirmation except in the outbreak setting or for an unusual isolate; therefore, we are largely dependent on species identification by the local laboratory. Many clinical laboratories may not routinely culture for non-*jejuni Campylobacter* species, and others may not use optimal culture methods.

Several studies and data from active surveillance provide evidence that *Campylobacter* is the most commonly isolated enteric bacterial pathogen (10, 17, 90). However, the reported incidence rate of *Salmonella* via passive surveillance (13 per 100,000 in 1997) is five times greater than that of Campylobacter. It is estimated that only 5% of *Campylobacter* isolates are reported to the CDC through passive surveillance.

In 1995, the species was reported for 83% of *Campylobacter* isolates received through passive surveillance; *C. jejuni* represented 99% of the reported species. Reported isolations of *Campylobacter* organisms show a consistent seasonal distribution (Fig. 1). The number of *Campylobacter* isolates is small in the first 4 months of the year, and then there is a marked surge beginning in May and June, a peak in

July and August, and a sustained plateau for the rest of the year.

Active Surveillance

In 1995, CDC, the U.S. Department of Agriculture, and the Food and Drug Administration developed the Foodborne Diseases Active Surveillance Network (FoodNet) to better determine the frequency and severity of food-borne disease (5). FoodNet is an active population-based surveillance system, which began conducting surveillance in 1996 in five sites, Minnesota, Oregon, and selected counties in California, Connecticut, and Georgia. In 1998, there were seven FoodNet sites, which represented 7.8% of the U.S. population (17). Public health officials from each site regularly contact microbiology laboratories to collect information on all culture-confirmed cases of food-borne diseases. Data are collected from over 300 clinical microbiology laboratories that test stool samples in participating sites; therefore, the total number of culture-confirmed cases that occur in these populations can be determined. Information is collected on culture-confirmed cases of *Campylobacter, Salmonella, Shigella, Escherichia coli* O157:H7, *Listeria,* and *Yersinia* infection. The information is then transmitted electronically to CDC.

All clinical laboratories in the FoodNet catchment routinely culture diarrheal stool

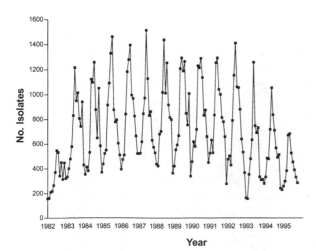

FIGURE 1 Reported *Campylobacter* isolates by month in the United States, 1982 to 1995.

TABLE 1 Number of *Campylobacter* isolates and isolation rate from five original FoodNet sites

Year	No. of isolates	No. of cases per 100,000
1996	3,359	23.5
1997	3,642	25.2
1998	3,132	21.7

TABLE 2 Isolation rate of specific bacterial food-borne pathogens for the five original FoodNet sites, 1998

Pathogen	No. of cases per 100,000
Campylobacter	21.7
Salmonella	12.4
Shigella	8.5
E. coli O157:H7	2.8
Yersinia	1.0
Listeria	0.5
Vibrio	0.3
Total	47.2

specimens for *Campylobacter* (5). Thus, Food-Net provides a timely database of *Campylobacter* infections in a well-defined population. Comparative data on the *Campylobacter* isolation rate per 100,000 in 1996 to 1998 from the original five FoodNet sites are listed in Table 1. The isolation rate per 100,000 decreased from 23.5 in 1996 to 21.7 in 1998 (18). *Campylobacter* has the highest incidence rates of all pathogens under surveillance in FoodNet (Table 2).

In 1992, a CDC study was conducted at 10 U.S. hospitals whose microbiology laboratories cultured all stool specimens for *E. coli* O157, *Campylobacter*, *Salmonella*, and *Shigella* species routinely from diarrheal stool specimens (89, 90). The percentage of stool cultures that yielded *Campylobacter*, *Salmonella*, *Shigella*, and *E. coli* O157:H7 species varied with the ages of the patients (Table 3). Overall, *Campylobacter* species were isolated 1.5 times more often than *Salmonella* species, 1.7 times more often than *Shigella* species, and 5.8 times more often than

E. coli O157:H7. In 1980, CDC conducted a similar study to determine the frequency of diagnosed infection with *C. jejuni* compared with other enteric pathogens in eight U.S. hospitals. For all age groups combined, *Campylobacter* species were isolated twice as often as *Salmonella* species and 4.5 times as often as *Shigella* species (10). Since the proportion of stools yielding *Salmonella* and *Shigella* did not change substantially between 1980 and 1992, it is possible that these findings offer additional evidence that the rates of *Campylobacter* have decreased.

Epidemiologic Characteristics

The age- and sex-specific incidence of *Campylobacter* isolates shows a unique pattern. In 1998,

TABLE 3 Isolation proportion from fecal specimens of enteric bacterial pathogens in stool cultures of diarrheal patients by age group at 10 hospitals in the United States, 1990 to 1992[a]

Age (yr)	% of cultures with:				Ratio of *Campylobacter* spp. to:		
	Campylobacter spp.	*Salmonella* spp.	*Shigella* spp.	*E. coli* O157:H7	*Salmonella* spp.	*Shigella* spp.	*E. coli* O157:H7
<1	1.1	3.6	0.2	0.1	0.3	4.6	18.7
1–4	2.7	3.9	3.7	0.7	0.7	0.7	4.1
5–9	2.8	1.8	7.0	0.9	1.6	0.4	3.1
10–19	5.1	2.5	1.8	0.7	2.1	2.9	7.4
20–29	5.0	1.8	1.1	0.5	2.7	4.5	10.5
30–39	3.4	1.7	0.4	0.3	2.0	7.7	9.9
40–49	1.7	0.5	0.5	0.4	3.5	3.3	4.3
50–59	2.6	1.3	0.3	0.9	2.0	7.9	2.9
60+	1.3	0.8	0.2	0.2	1.6	5.8	5.6
Total	2.9	2.0	1.7	0.5	1.5	1.7	5.8

[a] Data from reference 90. A total of 30,463 fecal specimens were examined.

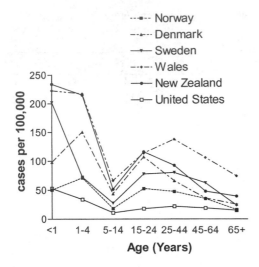

····■··· Norway
···▲··· Denmark
──▲── Sweden
···◆··· Wales
──●── New Zealand
──□── United States

FIGURE 2 Incidence of *Campylobacter* infections by age group in developed countries.

for children younger than 1 year, the rate of *Campylobacter* infection was 53 per 100,000, substantially higher than for other age groups (Fig. 2). A second, lesser peak occurred in young adults aged 15 to 44 years. This may reflect specific exposures in that age group. Rates of *Campylobacter* infection were 30% higher in males than females. The incidence rate was higher for males in all age groups. It is difficult to explain this difference entirely by a sex-specific behavior difference, such as a greater willingness on the part of males to eat undercooked chicken.

The infectious dose of *C. jejuni* for humans appears to be low. Robinson reported his own experience following ingestion of 500 organisms (81). Human volunteer studies at the University of Maryland have shown that *Campylobacter* organisms can produce infection at a variety of doses ranging from 800 organisms, the lowest tested, to 10^6 organisms (9). The attack rates did not vary significantly with the dose, being in the neighborhood of 10%. Therefore, it is difficult to determine the minimum dose required to make 50% of exposed persons ill. However, these data clearly demonstrate that relatively low doses of 500 to 800 organisms are sufficient to cause illness.

In 1998, the rate of hospitalization for patients with *Campylobacter* infection was 11% in FoodNet sites. *Campylobacter* has a relatively low case fatality rate compared to other bacterial enteric pathogens; in 1998, it was 0.05%. During 1998, the vast majority of *Campylobacter* isolates came from stool specimens; less than 1% of *Campylobacter* isolations were from normally sterile sites. This is in contrast to *Salmonella* isolates, of which 7% came from normally sterile sites (18).

Persons with AIDS are also at increased risk of acquiring *Campylobacter* infections, but it is not known if this risk is increased during early human immunodeficiency virus infection (4). The reported incidence of laboratory-confirmed campylobacteriosis in persons with AIDS in Los Angeles County between 1983 and 1987 was 519 per 100,000, much higher than the reported rate in the general population (93). Host factors play a role in the risk of development of *C. jejuni* bacteremia. However, it is not known whether patients with AIDS are at increased risk for invasive disease from *Campylobacter*. In the same study in Los Angeles County, patients with AIDS were more likely to develop bacteremia from *Campylobacter* infection than were controls, who were patients without AIDS who had *Campylobacter* infection and were matched by age, sex, race, and year of onset of *Campylobacter* infection (93). No association with invasive disease was seen in a study of 30 human immunodeficiency virus-infected patients in a study at a London hospital between 1986 and 1991 (65). In addition, in FoodNet sites between 1996 and 1998, the number of *Campylobacter* isolates that were from a body site considered to be invasive remained constant at 0.2% (13, 14).

Burden of Disease

The true annual incidence *Campylobacter* infections in the United States is much greater than the 2.5 per 100,000 reported in 1995 through passive surveillance; it is even higher than the 21.7 per 100,000 reported through active FoodNet surveillance in 1998. This is because many infections go undiagnosed, and in passive

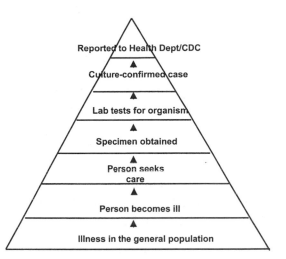

FIGURE 3 Estimation of the burden of food-borne diseases (from reference 14).

surveillance, most diagnosed infections are not reported.

To estimate the true incidence of *Campylobacter* infections, we must take additional factors into account. To calculate the true incidence of *Salmonella* infections Voetsch and colleagues (20) used a multiplier of 37.7. This multiplier takes into account the loss of cases at each step of the reporting chain (Fig. 3). By assuming that the population in FoodNet sites is representative of the total U.S. population, we can estimate the actual number of *Campylobacter* isolations in the United States. Using the 1996 to 1998 FoodNet average incidence rate of 23.5 per 100,000, and the U.S. Census Bureau 1997 U.S. population size of 267,636,061 million, we can estimate that there are 62,886 isolations of *Campylobacter* in the United States each year. Applying the *Salmonella* multiplier of 37.7 to *Campylobacter*, we estimate that there are 2.4 million *Campylobacter* infections in the United States each year.

The mortality associated with *Campylobacter* can also be estimated. The case fatality rate from FoodNet data for 1996 to 1998 was 0.08%, or 8 per 10,000 culture-confirmed cases. Smith and Blaser reported two *Campylobacter* deaths among 600 culture-confirmed cases in Colorado, giving a case fatality rate of 24 per 10,000 culture-confirmed cases (91). Applying these case fatality rates to the 62,886

isolations of *Campylobacter* in the United States, we can estimate that there are between 50 and 151 deaths per year due to *Campylobacter* infections.

SURVEILLANCE AND ESTIMATES OF INCIDENCE IN THE REST OF THE DEVELOPED WORLD

Campylobacter is one of the most frequently reported causes of acute bacterial gastroenteritis in many developed countries around the world. Variations in incidence rates have been observed between countries and even among regions within countries (11, 22, 70). These differences in incidence rates may be due to differences in infection rates in food animals, differences in food production systems, or different patterns of food consumption. Variations in incidence rates can also occur because of differences in diagnosis, reporting systems, or case definitions used in each country's surveillance systems (11). For example, in France, *Campylobacter* isolates are received at the national reference center but are collected mainly from patients who have been diagnosed in hospitals (58). In Latvia, diarrheal stool specimens are not routinely cultured for *Campylobacter* and there is no national *Campylobacter* surveillance system (74), and a number of other Central and Eastern European countries do not have national *Campylobacter* surveillance (21, 22, 58).

Surveillance and Reporting of Human Campylobacteriosis

There are large differences in *Campylobacter* incidence rates in countries with laboratory-based surveillance. In countries that have free health care and good laboratory support, such as those in Northern Europe, reported incidence rates range from 60 to 90 cases per 100,000. Even these incidence rates, which rely on laboratory reporting, represent a fraction of the true number of infections. From studies in the Netherlands and the United Kingdom, the true rate of *Campylobacter* is estimated to be 10 to 100 times higher than that reported, corresponding to an incidence of 1,100 to 2,300 per 100,000 (49, 68, 88).

Trends

Many developed countries have experienced an increase in the number of reported cases during the last 20 years (Fig. 4). In some countries there has been a steady increase during the entire period, whereas in other countries the increase has occurred primarily in the 1990s. New Zealand had a nearly nine-fold increase in incidence (per 100,000 population), from 14 to 120 cases, between 1981 and 1990, and another three-fold increase, from 128 to 363 cases, from 1991 to 1998 (11). Denmark reported no increase between 1980 and 1990 but had a nearly threefold increase between 1990 and 1998 (24).

Part of this increase in *Campylobacter* incidence is probably due to increased physician awareness about this pathogen, increased culturing by laboratories, improved laboratory methods for detection, and improved reporting (11, 23, 50, 86, 88). This may explain the increase in reported isolations during the 1980s. However, the increase observed during the last 10 years, when culturing for *Campylobacter* has become routine in many laboratories (50), more probably reflects a true increase in infections. It is unclear why these changes are occurring and whether they reflect shifts in the underlying ecology of the organism.

Age and Sex Distribution

The age distribution of patients in the developed world in general is similar to that in the United States (Fig. 2). *Campylobacter* affects all age groups but has a bimodal age distribution, with one peak in children younger than 4 years and a second peak in young adults between 15 and 44 years. It has been postulated that the higher incidence rates seen in children may be due to oversampling in this age group, because parents may be more likely to seek medical care for their children (50, 94). It has also been postulated that the peak in incidence in young adults may be related to increased foreign travel in this age group compared to other age groups (50, 94). The sex distribution of *Campylobacter* infection in developed countries in other parts

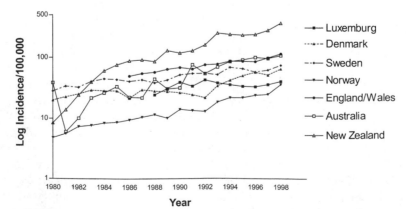

FIGURE 4 Incidence of human *Campylobacter* infections in selected countries, 1980 to 1998.

of the world is also similar to the distribution in the United States. The incidence is 1.2 to 1.5 times higher in males than in females. This difference is more pronounced in persons younger than 30 to 40 years (50, 87).

Seasonal Distribution

Countries in Europe, especially in temperate zones, observe a seasonal distribution, with a well-defined summer peak (50, 69, 87, 88). When comparing surveillance data from five countries in Europe, Nylen et al. found a more pronounced seasonal variation with increasing latitude (69). A study conducted in Norway found a similar south-to-north gradient within that country (50). A distinct seasonality is also observed in New Zealand, with a peak incidence in the warmer months of the year (11), whereas in Australia the seasonal trend seems to vary from year to year with only a slightly higher incidence during warmer months (94). The trends in seasonality observed suggest that the incidence of *Campylobacter* infections peaks worldwide when climatic conditions are similar to the Northern Hemisphere's summer (85). However, there have been anecdotal reports from Israel and Hong Kong of a larger number of infections during winter and spring (40, 57, 85). This phenomenon remains unexplained.

COMMON-SOURCE OUTBREAKS IN THE UNITED STATES

In the United States, CDC receives reports of food-borne and waterborne disease outbreaks, including those caused by *Campylobacter* species, as part of the national food- and water-borne disease outbreak surveillance systems (6, 56). The first outbreak was also the largest and occurred in Burlington, Vt., when a contaminated community water supply affected an estimated 3,000 persons (102). Between 1978 and 1996, 111 outbreaks of *Campylobacter* infections were reported, affecting a total of 9,913 persons (Table 4). Of these, all but three were caused by *C. jejuni*. Three were caused by *C. fetus* subsp. *fetus,* including one mixed-species outbreak of gastroenteritis, caused by both *C. jejuni* and *C. fetus* infections, and two bacteremia

TABLE 4 Food-borne and waterborne outbreaks of *Campylobacter* infections reported in the United States, by vehicle, 1978 to 1996

Origin	No. of outbreaks	No. of outbreak associated cases
Food-borne		
Milk	30	1,212
Chicken	2	16
Turkey	1	11
Beef	1	24
Other meat	2	30
Eggs	1	26
Fruits	4	227
Other foods	4	251
Multiple foods	10	411
Unknown food	42	2,775
Waterborne		
Community water supply	8	5,068
Other water supply	4	104
Total	111	10,155

outbreaks, one affecting cancer patients consuming raw liver, and one affecting nursing home patients (16, 20, 55).

Even though *Campylobacter* is the most common bacterial cause of sporadic diarrheal illness, outbreaks are relatively rare. They represent approximately 1% of reported food-borne and reported waterborne outbreaks in the period between 1980 and 1996. This is not an artifact of limited surveillance. In 1998, the seven FoodNet sites, with a combined population of 20.5 million, reported a total of 77 food-borne outbreaks affecting at least 10 persons (17). Of these, only one was caused by *Campylobacter*.

Over the last two decades, the sources of outbreaks has changed. Between 1978 and 1987, water and unpasteurized milk accounted for 56% of outbreaks, while between 1988 and 1996, other foods accounted for 83% of all outbreaks (Fig. 5). Large waterborne outbreaks have occurred in municipal water systems as a result of a break in chlorination or when a nonchlorinated groundwater supply becomes contaminated. *Campylobacter* is quite susceptible to chlorination. A recent regulatory shift by the Environmental Protection Agency to

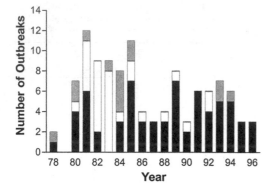

FIGURE 5 Food-borne and waterborne outbreaks of *Campylobacter* infections by year in the United States, 1978 to 1996. Gray bars, waterborne; white bars, milk borne; black bars, other food.

require disinfection of groundwater and surface water before distributing it in community systems may have decreased outbreaks in recent years (Fig. 5). Among food-borne outbreaks, milk, usually raw, unpasteurized milk, has historically been the most common single food source. Milk-associated outbreaks account for 55% of the food-borne outbreaks with known identified food sources (Table 4). The most typical scenario for these outbreaks is a school field trip to a dairy farm where a drink of raw milk is part of the experience (103). This was particularly common in the early 1980s. Public health warnings following such events may have decreased their frequency since such outbreaks have been rare in recent years. Milk that is of high quality, or even "certified," offers little protection unless it is also pasteurized (76). Milk can become contaminated by cattle feces or as a result of asymptomatic *Campylobacter* mastitis, which has been found in dairy cattle (45, 47). Routine pasteurization of all milk can easily prevent such outbreaks.

The broad variety of other foods implicated in outbreaks is consistent with cross-contamination events in the kitchen from raw meat, poultry in particular, to a variety of other foods. Transmission from ill food handlers occurs occasionally but is not common. Unlike *Salmonella, Campylobacter* does not tend to multiply on foods left out for many hours; indeed, it

does not tolerate exposure to atmospheric oxygen or to drying. This would explain the rarity of large outbreaks related to solid foods (33). Typical scenarios involve simple cross-contamination between raw poultry and other foods in the kitchen. However, more complex events can occur. In one curious recent outbreak affecting at least 30 patrons of one restaurant, garlic butter used on multiple sandwiches in a restaurant was implicated, suggesting that butter contaminated in the kitchen was a likely vehicle (7). *Campylobacter* was shown to survive in butter for many days and can also survive the process of melting butter onto garlic bread (27). Presumably the oil content protected it from atmospheric oxygen. In another unusual outbreak, an atypical *C. fetus* subsp. *fetus* strain caused an outbreak of bacteremia in nursing-home residents who ate commercial cottage cheese (20). The implicated lot of cheese was noted to have a high coliform count and could have been contaminated from raw milk at the dairy, suggesting that at least some campylobacters might survive well in this product.

Outbreaks exhibit a curious seasonal distribution. Milk-borne and waterborne outbreaks are most likely to occur in the spring and fall but are rare in the summer, when sporadic cases are at their height (Fig. 6). It is possible that surface-water sources become contaminated during spring and fall bird migrations, leading

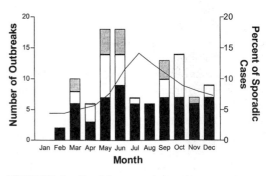

FIGURE 6 Food-borne and waterborne outbreaks of *Campylobacter* infections, 1978 to 1996, and distribution of sporadic cases by month, 1982 to 1995, in the United States. Gray bars, waterborne; white bars, milk borne; black bars, other food.

to seasonal waterborne outbreaks, and that cattle also acquire the infections at that time from drinking water from streams or shallow wells. Sporadic infections have a very different seasonality, with a summer peak, which suggests that a different ecology is at work. Sporadic cases may peak in summer because of the seasonal acquisition and carriage of *Campylobacter* by broiler flocks. Food-borne outbreaks from other sources begin to occur in early spring and continue steadily through December, without a summer peak, and may reflect cross-contamination events from raw poultry or other sources in the kitchen.

COMMON-SOURCE OUTBREAKS IN OTHER DEVELOPED NATIONS

Outbreaks reported from other developed nations are also less common than those caused by other bacterial food-borne pathogens and are predominantly caused by contaminated water, milk and poultry. Combining three recent series, from the United Kingdom, Sweden, and Germany, 21 (37%) of 56 general outbreaks of campylobacteriosis were waterborne (22, 73, 96). Waterborne outbreaks have been traced to both surface and ground drinking-water sources (3, 15, 29, 61, 73). In a Norwegian outbreak that occurred in 1990, a small unfenced reservoir may have been contaminated by runoff from a nearby sheep pasture following heavy rain (59). In another Norwegian outbreak, surface water contamination by sheep, cattle, or wild animals was presumed to have occurred (60). Similar episodes may have contaminated spring water in two outbreaks in Christchurch, New Zealand, that were attributed to water (12, 15). During investigation of an outbreak in England in 1993, a dead lamb was found in the water supply of a university dormitory (73). Contamination of a municipal groundwater supply with sewage led to a prolonged 6-week outbreak in a Danish town, associated with an attack rate of 87.5% (29). *Campylobacter* species are rapidly inactivated by chlorine, and failures in disinfection or poor water system maintenance are frequent con-

tributing causes (12, 60, 73). As in the United States, most of these outbreaks occur in the springtime, perhaps reflecting a seasonality in the contamination of water.

Milk, including raw and inadequately pasteurized milk, is the most common food associated with outbreaks. Such outbreaks occur regularly in Sweden and in the United Kingdom (73, 96). In a survey of retail raw milk in southwestern England, 5.9% of samples yielded *Campylobacter* (46). Undercooked poultry is also identified as a source of outbreaks; six of seven outbreaks reported in Denmark between 1993 and 1997 were associated with poultry (101). Cross-contamination in the kitchen may explain a prolonged Australian outbreak traced to cucumber served at a salad bar (54) and an outbreak in England in 1993 that was associated with a melon and prawn appetizer (73).

SOURCES OF SPORADIC INFECTIONS

The vast majority of *Campylobacter* infections are not related to outbreaks but occur as sporadic individual infections. As noted above, the sources of sporadic infections may be quite different from those of outbreaks. While it is difficult to determine the sources of an individual case, epidemiologic investigations by the case-control method can identify the exposures that are most likely to be associated with *C. jejuni* infection, from which the sources can be inferred. Several such studies have been done in the United States, and a large nationwide case-control study is currently under way. At least eight similar investigations have been conducted in other developed nations (1, 28, 51, 62, 64, 74, 83, 100). Although these case-control studies differ in the technique used and in the array of hypotheses tested, they consistently indicate several dominant sources: contact with and consumption of poultry, transmission from pets and other animals, and contaminated drinking water (Fig. 7). *Campylobacter* is also a cause of traveler's diarrhea, probably through similar exposures occurring during travel.

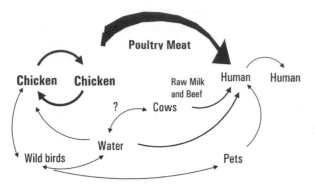

FIGURE 7 *C. jejuni* transmission—the 1999 model.

Case-Control Studies in the United States

A large case-control study conducted at a Health Maintenance Organization in Seattle, Wash., in 1981 showed that eating poultry, including chicken, turkey, and Cornish game hen, accounted for over 50% of all the cases (39). Five percent of the cases were attributed to raw milk, including both cow and goat milk; 6% of the cases were attributed to contact with pets; 8% were attributed to drinking contaminated surface water; and 9% were attributed to exposure during overseas travel (38). In a second study, conducted among students at a Georgia university, 70% of cases were attributed to eating chicken and 30% were attributed to contact with cats (26). In a case-control study of sporadic cases in Colorado, the identified risk factors were drinking untreated water or raw milk, having contact with cats, and eating undercooked chicken (43). In a second Colorado study, handling raw chicken, as opposed to eating it, emerged as a risk factor (44). In some rural parts of the United States, where drinking raw milk remains popular, raw milk can be an important source of sporadic cases as well as of outbreaks. In a study of sporadic cases in Dubuque, Iowa, an etiologic fraction of 47% can be calculated for drinking raw milk, which was the only risk factor identified (82).

Case-Control Studies in Other Developed Nations

Of eight studies conducted in Europe and New Zealand, consumption of poultry was identified as a risk factor in seven, accounting for a variable percentage of cases ranging from slightly less than 10% of cases in Denmark to approximately 50% of cases in New Zealand. Drinking untreated water was identified as a risk factor in five of the studies (1, 28, 51, 64, 100), and drinking raw milk was identified in the New Zealand study, where 5% of the cases reported this exposure (28). Two studies identified occupational contact with raw meat as risk factors for infection (1, 28), four identified contact with pets or farm animals as a risk factor (1, 28, 62, 63), and four identified foreign travel as a risk factor (28, 62, 64, 83).

Sporadic Infections and Poultry

The above studies shed some epidemiologic light on how poultry can cause so much infection. The U.S. and European studies often identified chicken prepared in the home as a risk factor, but one British study and the New Zealand study identified chicken eaten outside of the home as risk factors, while eating chicken in the home was protective (1, 28). How the chicken is cooked can be a risk modifier; usually eating chicken that is perceived to be undercooked is a clear risk factor. In studies in the Netherlands and New Zealand, barbecuing or frying chicken was associated with higher risk (28, 71).

Seasonal changes in contamination of poultry with *Campylobacter* have rarely been described but may be common. In a survey conducted in Denmark and Sweden, the overall seasonal pattern of contamination of local

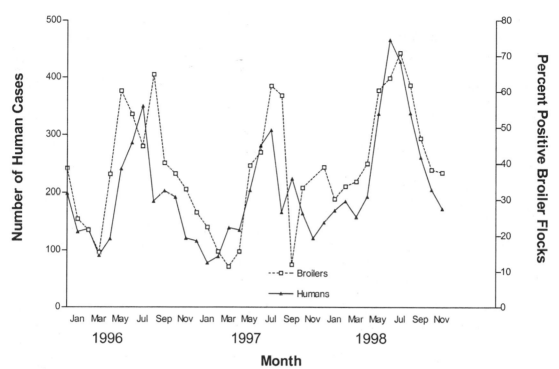

FIGURE 8 Number of human *Campylobacter* infections and prevalence of *Campylobacter* infection in broiler flocks at slaughter by month, 1996 to 1998, Denmark.

broilers and of human cases is similar (Fig. 8) (8, 36). By itself, this may indicate that humans acquire *Campylobacter* from eating fresh broilers or that humans and broilers are becoming infected from the same source. Similar evidence is provided by serotyping, which has been applied systematically in a Danish study of isolates from cattle, chicken, and humans (66). The finding of substantial overlap in serotype distribution indicates that these cases are linked to those animal reservoirs.

The case-control study in Seattle also identified a separate association between infection and not washing the kitchen cutting board with soap, a marker for cross-contamination. In the second Colorado case-control study, it was the food preparer rather than the food consumer who became ill, perhaps because of direct exposure to raw poultry during the preparation of meals. In studies among students at the University of Georgia, we identified three pathways by which contaminated poultry could easily cause *C. jejuni* infections. The first was tasting raw chicken, which some respondents reported doing. The second was eating it undercooked, defined operationally as still bloody and pink near the bone. This seems to be a relatively common exposure among male college students. The third was using a knife and cutting board first to prepare raw chicken and then to prepare other food without washing it in between.

These relatively simple errors in food handling are consistent with the low infectious dose. The quantity of *Campylobacter* organisms on the surface of a fresh chicken carcass has been estimated to be 10^3 to 10^6 per chicken in one study in the United Kingdom (42). Ingestion of a drop of raw chicken juice could easily provide the infectious dose of 500 organisms. This means that reducing the proportion of carcasses that are contaminated could have a greater impact on the public health than reducing the number of organisms on each carcass.

Until other control strategies emerge that greatly reduce contamination, the most effective strategy would appear to be cold pasteurization of poultry carcasses by irradiation or similar technologies.

Several important questions about transmission from poultry meat remain unanswered. First, because bacteria on the surface of poultry would be destroyed by limited cooking, the recurrent association of illness with undercooked poultry suggests either that the poultry is regularly recontaminated after cooking or that *Campylobacter* is somehow present deep in the tissues of a single poultry carcass, where it survives limited cooking. Is *Campylobacter* introduced into deep tissue via the cooking fork, or is it there already in the slaughtered carcass, perhaps via the avian intramuscular respiratory tree? Second, *Campylobacter* is likely to colonize the liver and biliary tree of the live hen, but an association with handling or eating liver or other organ meats has been demonstrated only infrequently. The role of bile in carcass contamination needs exploration. Third, it has been well documented that freezing can diminish counts of viable *Campylobacter* (95). However, a protective effect of freezing chicken carcasses has yet to be demonstrated epidemiologically. Finally, the source of infection among chickens and the means by which this can be prevented remain unclear. Although some poultry flocks remain unaffected, the organisms can rapidly spread horizontally in chickens, presumably through a common water source or fecal contact (84). The observation that chlorinating the drinking water of poultry is associated with lower infection rates in flocks in Norway and in the United Kingdom suggests that environmental interventions at the flock level may be useful (52, 72).

Sporadic Infections and Other Foods

Raw milk has been implicated as a source of sporadic cases in the largest studies, where there is sufficient power, such as the Seattle or New Zealand studies (28, 39), or in areas where raw-milk consumption may be very high, such as Dubuque, Iowa (82). Regular raw-milk consumption may ultimately immunize a population against prevalent Campylobacters, so that little risk is observed in some areas, such as rural Scandinavia, where raw-milk consumption is reported by 10% of cases and controls alike. Other foods have also been implicated, including consumption of sausages at a barbecue in Norway (51) or consumption of barbecued red meat in general in Denmark (64).

Sporadic Infections and Water

The contribution of drinking water to the burden of sporadic cases varies around the world but may be substantial in many parts of the developed and developing world. Even pristine mountain streams can be a sources of infection, presumably as a result of contamination by the feces of wild birds (99). In Denmark, drinking water from a private well that had a bad taste or smell was associated with infection (64). In New Zealand, drinking rainwater collected from a roof where birds might roost was associated with infection (28). Small unprotected rural water supplies may be a particular source in many parts of the world. Routine disinfection of drinking water can prevent these infections at extremely low cost (77). If poultry ultimately acquire and spread infection through water, and if cattle are also infected in the springtime by drinking contaminated surface water, the waterborne route may be the common underlying pathway linking waterborne, milkborne, and poultry-associated campylobacteriosis in humans to an underlying cycle involving birds and the water they drink (Fig. 7).

Sporadic Infections and Contact with Animals, and Secondary Transmission

Contact with live animals continues to be a small but important challenge. Contact with pets has been demonstrated repeatedly as a risk factor, and contact with other animals has occasionally been shown to be a risk factor for *Campylobacter* infections in humans. In addition to established reservoirs in domesticated poultry, cattle, and pigs, wild birds (such as oystercatchers, gulls, lapwings, and geese) have been shown to be carriers of *Campylobacter* (24, 32, 37). Wild birds may contribute to contamination of water supplies, but direct linkage to human illness is difficult to establish epidemiologically. In the United Kingdom, illness has been associated with drinking pasteurized milk from bottles that have been pecked at by jackdaws (80). These birds have learned to pierce the foil tops of bottles delivered to the front door and may have contaminated the milk directly. The nature of the contact with an infected dog or cat that actually transmits the illness remains to be defined, as does the means by which the pets become contaminated in the first place. Anecdotally, contact can be quite casual, the animal need not be sick, and there need not be direct contact with animal feces.

Another unexplained observation concerning the transmission of this organism is that despite the low infectious dose in experimental challenge trials with humans and despite the fact that vast numbers of motile organisms are present in the feces of ill persons, sustained transmission between humans does not occur. Secondary infections in households are distinctly unusual. Outbreaks in settings such as day care centers or mental institutions, where person-to-person transmission has been common for other enteric pathogens such as *Shigella* or *Giardia,* are unheard of in the United States. Although infection rates in homosexual men have been reported to be high (78), they do not appear to be higher than infection rates in heterosexual men of the same age, and transmission through sexual contact has not been conclusively demonstrated. It is as though the infectiousness of the organism depends on the immediate growth conditions; passage through the human gut may render it largely noninfectious for humans, while passage in the bird or cow and the subsequent cold-processing steps of slaughter may enhance its infectiousness for humans.

Sporadic Infections and Foreign Travel

Travel in other countries is a complex exposure, including foods that may be unusual and water of unknown quality. In both the Swiss and Danish studies, cases had more frequently traveled to the developing world and Southern Europe (63, 83). In addition, many countries identify foreign travel-associated cases as part of routine surveillance. Such exposure is reported in 10 to 15% of cases in Britain and Denmark (23, 50) and in 50 to 65% of cases in Sweden and Norway (2, 49, 67). Identifying travel as a risk factor does not by itself identify the actual sources of infection. A case-control study comparing the specific exposures of those who are ill with other travelers to similar destinations who remain well remains to be done. It is likely that both food and water play a role. Since, travel to warm climates is more likely in winter and summer holidays, the impact of travel on the overall seasonality is worthy of examination.

SURVEILLANCE FOR EMERGING ANTIMICROBIAL RESISTANCE

Fluoroquinolones, such as ciprofloxacin, are commonly used for the treatment of infections caused by *Campylobacter*. Fluoroquinolone-resistant *Campylobacter* infections in humans have been reported from Europe and Asia since the end of the last decade (35, 41, 75). This was not the case in the United States. In a survey conducted between 1989 and 1990 in 19 U.S. counties, no *C. jejuni* or *C. coli* strains were resistant to fluoroquinolones (20). In 1997, 217 *Campylobacter* isolates from five states were tested for antimicrobial susceptibility as part of the National Antimicrobial Resistance Monitoring System (NARMS). Of these isolates, 186 (86%) were resistant to one or more antimicrobials and 108 (50%) were resistant to two or more agents. Overall, 81 (37%) strains were resistant to two quinolone antibiotics tested, 53 (24%) were resistant to nalidixic acid, and 28 (13%) were resistant to ciprofloxacin (Fig. 9) (19).

A retrospective survey was conducted in four FoodNet sites to determine risk factors for ciprofloxacin-resistant *Campylobacter* infections that occurred in 1997. Although foreign travel was identified as a risk factor, the majority of patients surveyed acquired their ciprofloxacin-

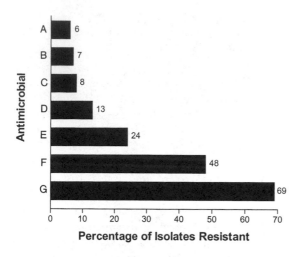

FIGURE 9 Resistance among *C. jejuni* isolates at five FoodNet Sites, 1997. Antimicrobial agent: A, chloramphenicol; B, clindamycin; C, erythromycin; D, ciprofloxacin; E, nalidixic acid; F, tetracycline; G, trimethoprim-sulfamethoxazole.

resistant *Campylobacter* infections in the United States, and these infections were not associated with previous fluoroquinolone use (34). Thus, neither foreign travel nor the use of fluoroquinolones by humans can easily explain the emergence of ciprofloxacin-resistant *Campylobacter* in the United States. Reports from Europe suggest that the rise in fluoroquinolone-resistant *Campylobacter* isolations in humans is associated with fluoroquinolone use in poultry, which has led to fluoroquinolone-resistant *Campylobacter* strains in poultry which have spread to humans via the food chain (35, 75). Veterinary use of fluoroquinolones in poultry in the United States, approved since 1995, may explain the rise in domestically acquired ciprofloxacin-resistant *Campylobacter* infections in humans in recent years. A 1997 study conducted in Minnesota showed that 14% of 91 *C. jejuni* isolates obtained from raw chicken bought at grocery stores were ciprofloxacin resistant. In that same year, domestically acquired cases of ciprofloxacin-resistant *Campylobacter* infections in Minnesota doubled (92). In contrast, in Australia, where the use of fluoroquinolone antibiotics in poultry is still prohibited, a recent study revealed that none of 98 *C. jejuni* or *C. coli* human isolates were resistant to fluoroquinolones (48).

CONCLUSIONS

Campylobacter is the most common bacterial enteric pathogen in the United States and many developed countries throughout the world. Although the organism is usually not invasive, infection is occasionally fatal. In the last 20 years, *Campylobacter* infection rates have risen in many developed countries. Part of this increase may be due to improvements in detection and reporting, but part may reflect a true increase in infections. The vast majority of *Campylobacter* infections occur as sporadic individual infections. Consumption of untreated water, raw milk, or milk products and contact with pets are important sources of infection; however, most of the sporadic cases appear to be due to consumption of or contact with raw or undercooked poultry in most developed countries. Outbreaks of *Campylobacter* in developed countries are caused predominantly by contaminated water, milk, and poultry. In the United States, outbreaks due to raw milk and water have become less common in the last decade; this may be because of recent requirements for the disinfection of groundwater and surface water before distribution and public health warnings about the hazards of raw milk consumption. Veterinary use of fluoroquinolones in poultry may explain the recent rise in ciprofloxacin-resistant *Campylobacter* infections in humans.

REFERENCES

1. **Adak, G. K., J. M. Cowden, S. Nicholas, and H. S. Evans.** 1995. The Public Health Lab-

oratory Service national case-control study of primary indigenous sporadic cases of *Campylobacter* infection. *Epidemiol. Infect.* **115**:15–22.

2. **Andersson, Y.** Personal communication.

3. **Andersson, Y., B. Jong, and A. Studahl.** 1997. Waterborne *Campylobacter* in Sweden: the cost of an outbreak. *Water Sci. Technol.* **35**:11–14.

4. **Angulo, F. J., and D. L. Swerdlow.** 1995. Bacterial enteric infections in persons infected with human immunodeficiency virus. *Clin. Infect. Dis.* **21**:S84–S93.

5. **Angulo, F. J., A. C. Voetsch, D. Vugia, J. L. Hadler, M. Farley, C. Hedberg, P. Cieslak, D. Morse, D. Dwyer, and D. L. Swerdlow.** 1998. Determining the burden of human illness from food borne diseases. CDC's emerging infectious disease program Food Borne Diseases Active Surveillance Network (FoodNet). *Vet. Clin. North Am. Food Anim. Pract.* **14**:165–172.

6. **Bean, N. H., J. S. Goulding, C. Lao, and F. J. Angulo.** 1996. Surveillance for foodborne disease outbreaks—United States, 1988–1992. *Morbid. Mortal. Weekly Rep. CDC Surveill. Summ.* **45**:1–66.

7. **Berg, D. E., T. Farley, L. McFarland, and T. Zhao.** 1996. Program and Abstracts of the 36th Interscience Conference on Antimicrobial Agents and Chemotherapy. American Society for Microbiology, Washington, DC.

8. **Berndtson, E.** 1996. Campylobacter in broiler chickens. Thesis. Swedish University of Agricultural Sciences, Uppsala, Sweden.

9. **Black, R. E., M. M. Levine, M. L. Clements, T. P. Hughes, and M. J. Blaser.** 1988. Experimental *Campylobacter jejuni* infection in humans. *J. Infect. Dis.* **157**:472–479.

10. **Blaser, M. J., J. G. Wells, R. A. Feldman, R. A. Pollard, and J. R. Allen.** 1983. *Campylobacter* enteritis in the United States. A multicenter study. *Ann. Intern. Med.* **98**:360–365.

11. **Brieseman, M. A.** 1990. A further study of the epidemiology of *Campylobacter jejuni* infections. *N. Z. Med. J.* **103**:207–209.

12. **Brieseman, M. A.** 1987. Town water supply as the cause of an outbreak of *Campylobacter* infection. *N. Z. Med. J.* **100**:212–213.

13. **Centers for Disease Control and Prevention.** 1996. *1996 Final FoodNet Surveillance Report.* Centers for Disease Control and Prevention, Atlanta, Ga.

14. **Centers for Disease Control and Prevention.** 1997. *1997 Final FoodNet Surveillance Report.* Centers for Disease Control and Prevention, Atlanta, Ga.

15. **Centers for Disease Control and Preven-**

tion. 1991. *Campylobacter* enteritis—New Zealand, 1990. *Morbid. Mortal. Weekly Rep.* **40**:116–117, 123.

16. **Centers for Disease Control and Prevention.** 1981. *Campylobacter* sepsis associated with "nutritional therapy"—California. *Morbid. Mortal. Weekly Rep.* **30**:294–295.

17. **Centers for Disease Control and Prevention.** 1999. *FoodNet 1998 Surveillance Results—Preliminary Report.* Centers for Disease Control and Prevention, Atlanta, Ga.

18. **Centers for Disease Control and Prevention.** 1999. Incidence of foodborne illnesses: preliminary data from the Foodborne Diseases Active Surveillance Network (FoodNet) United States, 1998. *Morbid. Mortal. Weekly Rep.* **48**:189–194.

19. **Centers for Disease Control and Prevention.** 1997. *National Antimicrobial Resistance Monitoring System.* 1997 annual report. Centers for Disease Control and Prevention, Atlanta, Ga.

20. **Centers for Disease Control and Prevention.** Unpublished data.

21. **Cherkasskiy, B. L.** 1998. Foodborne infections in Russia, p. 317–318. *In Proceedings of the 4th World Congress on Foodborne Infections and Intoxications.* June 5, 1998, Berlin, Germany.

22. **Community Reference Laboratory on the Epidemiology of Zoonoses.** 1997. *Reporting on Trends and Sources of Zoonotic Agents in Animals, Feeding Stuff, Food and Man in the European Union in 1997.* Community Reference Laboratory on the Epidemiology of Zoonoses, Berlin, Germany.

23. **Cowden, J.** 1992. *Campylobacter:* epidemiological paradoxes. *Br. Med. J.* **305**:132–133. (Editorial.)

24. **Danish Zoonosis Centre.** 1998. *Annual Report on Zoonoses in Denmark, 1997.* Danish Zoonosis Centre, Veterinary Laboratory, Copenhagen, Denmark.

25. **Dekeyser, P., M. Gossuin-Detrain, J. P. Butzler, and J. Sternon.** 1972. Acute enteritis due to related vibrio: first positive stool cultures. *J. Infect. Dis.* **125**:390–392.

26. **Deming, M. S., R. V. Tauxe, P. A. Blake, S. E. Dixon, B. S. Fowler, T. S. Jones, E. A. Lockamy, C. M. Patton, and R. O. Sikes.** 1987. *Campylobacter* enteritis at a university: transmission from eating chicken and from cats. *Am. J. Epidemiol.* **126**:526–534. (Erratum, 126:1220.)

27. **Doyle, M.** Personal communication.

28. **Eberhart-Phillips, J., N. Walker, N. Garrett, D. Bell, D. Sinclair, W. Rainger, and M. Bates.** 1997. *Campylobacter*iosis in New Zealand:

results of a case-control study. *J. Epidemiol. Community Health* **51**:686–691.

29. **Engberg, J., P. Gerner-Smidt, F. Scheutz, E. M. Nielsen, S. L. W. On, and K. Moelbak.** 1998. Waterborne *Campylobacter jejuni* infection in Danish town—a 6 week continuous source outbreak. *Clin. Microbiol. Infect.* **4**:648–656.

30. **Escherich, T.** 1881. Beitraege zur Kenntniss der Darmbacterien. III. Ueber das Vorkommen von Vibrionen in Darmcanal und den Stuhlgaengen der Saeuglinge. *Muench. Med. Wochenschr.* **33**:815–817.

31. **Finch, M. J., and L. W. Riley.** 1984. *Campylobacter* infections in the United States. Results of an 11-state surveillance. *Arch. Intern. Med.* **144**:1610–1612.

32. **Fitzgerald, C., K. Jones, S. Anderton, and S. Andrew.** 1997. Campylobacters in wild birds: identification and molecular characterization, p. 80. *In Proceedings of the 9th International Workshop on Campylobacter, Helicobacter and Related Organisms,* Cape Town, South Africa, 15–19 September 1997.

33. **Franco, D. A.** 1988. *Campylobacter* species: considerations for controlling a food-borne pathogen. *J. Food Prot.* **51**:145–153.

34. **Friedman, C. R., S. Yang, J. Rocourt, K. Stamey, D. Vugia, R. Marcus, S. Segler, B. Shiferaw, and F. J. Angulo.** 1998. *In Proceedings of the Infectious Diseases Society of America 36th Annual Meeting.*

35. **Gaunt, P. N., and L. J. Piddock.** 1996. Ciprofloxacin resistant *Campylobacter* spp. in humans: an epidemiological and laboratory study. *J. Antimicrob. Chemother.* **37**:747–757.

36. **Hald, T.** 1999. Zoonoseudviklingen. *ZoonoseNyt.* **6**:4, 2–5. (In Danish.).

37. **Hänninen, M. L., and H. Rautelin.** 1997. *In Proceedings of the 9th International Workshop on Campylobacter, Helicobacter, and Related Organisms.*

38. **Harris, N. V.** 1984. *Surveillance of the Flow of Salmonella and Campylobacter in a Community.* Communicable Disease Control Section, Seattle-King County Health Department, Seattle, Wash.

39. **Harris, N. V., N. S. Weiss, and C. M. Nolan.** 1986. The role of poultry and meats in the etiology of *Campylobacter jejuni/coli* enteritis. *Am. J. Public Health* **76**:407–411.

40. **Ho, B. S., and W. T. Wong.** 1985. A one-year survey of *Campylobacter* enteritis and other forms of bacterial diarrhoea in Hong Kong. *J. Hyg.* **94**:55–60.

41. **Hoge, C. W., J. M. Gambel, A. Srijan, C. Pitarangsi, and P. Echeverria.** 1998. Trends in antibiotic resistance among diarrheal pathogens isolated in Thailand over 15 years. *Clin. Infect. Dis.* **26**:341–345.

42. **Hood, A. M., A. D. Pearson, and M. Shahamat.** 1988. The extent of surface contamination of retailed chickens with *Campylobacter jejuni* serogroups. *Epidemiol. Infect.* **100**:17–25.

43. **Hopkins, R. S., R. Olmsted, and G. R. Istre.** 1984. Endemic *Campylobacter jejuni* infection in Colorado: identified risk factors. *Am. J. Public Health* **74**:249–250.

44. **Hopkins, R. S., and A. S. Scott.** 1983. Handling raw chicken as a source for sporadic *Campylobacter jejuni* infections. *J. Infect. Dis.* **148**:770. (Letter.)

45. **Hudson, P. J., R. L. Vogt, J. Brondum, and C. M. Patton.** 1984. Isolation of *Campylobacter jejuni* from milk during an outbreak of campylobacteriosis. *J. Infect. Dis.* **150**:789. (Letter.)

46. **Humphrey, T. J., and R. J. Hart.** 1988. *Campylobacter* and *Salmonella* contamination of unpasteurized cows' milk on sale to the public. *J. Appl. Bacteriol.* **65**:463–467.

47. **Hutchinson, D. N., F. J. Bolton, P. M. Hinchliffe, H. C. Dawkins, S. D. Horsley, E. G. Jessop, P. A. Robertshaw, and D. E. Counter.** 1985. Evidence of udder excretion of *Campylobacter jejuni* as the cause of milk-borne *Campylobacter* outbreak. *J. Hyg.* **94**:205–215.

48. **Huysmans, M. B., and J. D. Turnidge.** 1997. Disc susceptibility testing for thermomphilic *Campylobacters. Pathology* **29**:209–216.

49. **Kapperud, G.** 1994. *Campylobacter* infection. Epidemiology, risk factors and preventive measures. *Tidsskr. Nor. Laegeforen.* **114**:795–799.

50. **Kapperud, G., and S. Aasen.** 1992. Descriptive epidemiology of infections due to thermotolerant *Campylobacter* spp. in Norway, 1979–1988. *APMIS* **100**:883–890.

51. **Kapperud, G., E. Skjerve, N. H. Bean, S. M. Ostroff, and J. Lassen.** 1992. Risk factors for sporadic *Campylobacter* infections: results of a case-control study in southeastern Norway. *J. Clin. Microbiol.* **30**:3117–3121.

52. **Kapperud, G., E. Skjerve, L. Vik, K. Hauge, A. Lysaker, I. Aalmen, S. M. Ostroff, and M. Potter.** 1993. Epidemiological investigation of risk factors for *Campylobacter* colonization in Norwegian broiler flocks. *Epidemiol. Infect.* **111**:245–255.

53. **King, E. O.** 1962. The laboratory recognition of *Vibrio fetus* and closely related *Vibrio* species isolated from cases of human vibriosis. *Ann. N. Y. Acad. Sci.* **98**:700–711.

54. **Kirk, M., R. Waddell, C. Dalton, A. Creaser, and N. Rose.** 1997. A prolonged outbreak of *Campylobacter* infection at a training facility. *Commun. Dis. Intell.* **21**:57–61.

55. **Klein, B. S., J. M. Vergeront, M. J. Blaser, P. Edmonds, D. J. Brenner, D. Janssen, and J. P. Davis.** 1986. *Campylobacter* infection associated with raw milk. An outbreak of gastroenteritis due to *Campylobacter jejuni* and thermotolerant *Campylobacter fetus* subsp *fetus. JAMA* **255:** 361–364.

56. **Levy, D. A., M. S. Bens, G. F. Craun, R. L. Calderon, and B. L. Herwaldt.** 1998. Surveillance for waterborne-disease outbreaks—United States, 1995–1996. *Morbid. Mortal. Weekly Rep. CDC Surveill. Summ.* **47:**1–34.

57. **McGechie, D. B., T. B. Teoh, and V. W. Bamford.** 1982. *Campylobacter* enteritis in Hong Kong and Western Australia, p. 19–21. *In* D. G. Newell (ed.), *Campylobacter: Epidemiology, Pathogenesis and Biochemistry. Proceedings of the International Workshop on Campylobacter Infection.* MTP Press Ltd., Lancaster, United Kingdom.

58. **Mégraud, F.** 1999. Les infections à *Campylobacter* en France: bilan du Centre National de Référence. *Bulletin Epidémiologique Annual 1997.* Réseau National de Santé Publique, in press.

59. **Melby, K., O. P. Dahl, L. Crisp, and J. L. Penner.** 1990. Clinical and serological manifestations in patients during a waterborne epidemic due to *Campylobacter jejuni. J. Infect.* **21:**309–316.

60. **Melby, K., L. A. Holmen, J. G. Svendby, T. Eggebø, and B. M. Andersen.** 1991. Epidemisk udbrudd av *Campylobacter* infeksjon. *Tidsskr. Nor. Laegeforen.* **12:**111.

61. **Mentzing, L. O.** 1981. Waterborne outbreaks of *Campylobacter* enteritis in central Sweden. *Lancet* **ii:**352–354.

62. **Neal, K. R., and R. C. Slack.** 1997. Diabetes mellitus, anti-secretory drugs and other risk factors for *Campylobacter* gastroenteritis in adults: a case-control study. *Epidemiol. Infect.* **119:** 307–311.

63. **Neimann, J.** Personal communication.

64. **Neimann, J., J. Engberg, K. Moelbak, and H. C. Wegener.** 1998. Foodborne risk factors associated with sporadic campylobacteriosis in Denmark. *Dansk Veterinaertidsskrift.* **81:**702–705.

65. **Nelson, M. R., D. C. Shanson, D. A. Hawkins, and B. G. Gazzard.** 1992. *Salmonella, Campylobacter* and *Shigella* in HIV-seropositive patients. *AIDS* **6:**1495–1498.

66. **Nielsen, E. M., J. Engberg, and M. Madsen.** 1997. Distribution of serotypes of *Campylobacter jejuni* and *C. coli* from Danish patients, poultry, cattle and swine. *FEMS Immunol. Med. Microbiol.* **19:**47–56.

67. **Norkrans, G., and A. Svedhem.** 1982. Epidemiological aspects of *Campylobacter jejuni* enteritis. *J. Hyg.* **89:**163–170.

68. **Notermans, S.** 1994. Epidemiology and surveillance of *Campylobacter* infections. *Bull. W. H. O.* **94:**135.

69. **Nylen, G., S. R. Palmer, F. Bager, G. Feierl, K. Molbak, P. Ruutu, and L. P. Sanchez Serrano.** 1998. Campylobacter seasonality in Europe, p. 293–297. *In Proceedings of the 4th World Congress on Foodborne Infections and Intoxications.* 7–12 June 1998, Berlin, Germany.

70. **O'Brien, E., R. D'Souza, N. Gilroy, M. Burgess, S. Lister, P. McIntyre, S. Torvaldsen, K. Moser, and A. Milton.** 1999. Australia's notifiable diseases status, 1997. *Commun. Dis. Intell.* **23:**1–27.

71. **Oosterom, J., C. H. den Uyl, J. R. Banffer, and J. Huisman.** 1984. Epidemiological investigations on *Campylobacter jejuni* in households with a primary infection. *J. Hyg.* **93:**325–332.

72. **Pearson, A. D., M. Greenwood, T. D. Healing, D. Rollins, M. Shahamat, J. Donaldson, and R. R. Colwell.** 1993. Colonization of broiler chickens by waterborne *Campylobacter jejuni. Appl. Environ. Microbiol.* **59:** 987–996.

73. **Pebody, R. G., M. J. Ryan, and P. G. Wall.** 1997. Outbreaks of *Campylobacter* infection: rare events for a common pathogen. *Commun. Dis. Rep. CDR Rev.* **7:**R33–R37.

74. **Perevoscikovs, J.** Personal communication.

75. **Piddock, L. J.** 1995. Quinolone resistance and Campylobacter spp. *J. Antimicrob. Chemother.* **36:** 891–898.

76. **Potter, M. E., M. J. Blaser, R. K. Sikes, A. F. Kaufmann, and J. G. Wells.** 1983. Human *Campylobacter* infection associated with certified raw milk. *Am. J. Epidemiol.* **117:**475–483.

77. **Quick, R. E., L. V. Venczel, E. D. Mintz, L. Soleto, J. Aparicio, M. Gironaz, L. Hutwagner, K. Greene, C. Bopp, K. Maloney, D. Chavez, M. Sobsey, and R. V. Tauxe.** 1999. Diarrhea prevention in Bolivia through point-of-use water treatment and safe water storage: a promising new strategy. *Epidemiol. Infect.* **122:**83–90.

78. **Quinn, T. C.** 1997. Diversity of *Campylobacter* species and its impact on patients infected with human immunodeficiency virus *Clin. Infect. Dis.* **24:**1114–1117. (Editorial.)

79. **Riley, L. W., and M. J. Finch.** 1985. Results of the first year of national surveillance of *Campylobacter* infections in the United States. *J. Infect. Dis.* **151:**956–959.

80. **Riordan, T., T. J. Humphrey, and A. Fowles.** 1993. A point source outbreak of *Campylobacter* infection related to bird-pecked milk. *Epidemiol. Infect.* **110:**261–265.

81. **Robinson, D. A.** 1981. Infective dose of

Campylobacter jejuni in milk. *Br. Med. J. Clin. Res. Ed.* **282:**1584.

82. **Schmid, G. P., R. E. Schaefer, B. D. Plikaytis, J. R. Schaefer, J. H. Bryner, L. A. Wintermeyer, and A. F. Kaufmann.** 1987. A one-year study of endemic campylobacteriosis in a midwestern city: association with consumption of raw milk. *J. Infect. Dis.* **156:**218–222.

83. **Schorr, D., H. Schmid, H. L. Rieder, A. Baumgartner, H. Vorkauf, and A. Bumens.** 1994. Risk factors for *Campylobacter* enteritis in Switzerland. *Zentbl. Hyg Umweltmed.* **196:** 327–337.

84. **Shane, S. M.** 1991. Environmental factors associated with *Campylobacter jejuni* colonization of poultry, p. 29–46. *In* L. C. Blankenship and S. M. Shane (ed.), *Colonization Control of Human Bacterial Enteropathogens in Poultry.* Academic Press, Inc., San Diego, Calif.

85. **Shmilovitz, M., B. Kretzer, and N. Rotman.** 1982. *Campylobacter jejuni* as an etiological agent of diarrheal diseases in Israel. *Isr. J. Med. Sci.* **18:**935–940.

86. **Skirrow, M. B.** 1989. *Campylobacter* perspectives. *Public Health Lab. Serv. Microbiol. Digest.* **6:** 113–117.

87. **Skirrow, M. B.** 1987. A demographic survey of *Campylobacter, Salmonella* and *Shigella* infections in England. A Public Health Laboratory Service Survey. *Epidemiol. Infect.* **99:**647–657.

88. **Skirrow, M. B.** 1991. Epidemiology of *Campylobacter* enteritis. *Int. J. Food Microbiol.* **12:**9–16.

89. **Slutsker, L., J. Guarner, and P. Griffin.** 1998. *Escherichia coli* O157:H7, p. 259–82. *In* A. M. Nelson and C. R. Horsburgh Jr. (ed.), *Pathology of Emerging Infections.* ASM Press, Washington, D.C.

90. **Slutsker, L., A. A. Ries, K. D. Greene, J. G. Wells, L. Hutwagner, and P. M. Griffin.** 1997. *Escherichia coli* O157:H7 diarrhea in the United States: clinical and epidemiologic features. *Ann. Intern. Medicine.* **126:**505–513.

91. **Smith, G. S., and M. J. Blaser.** 1985. Fatalities associated with *Campylobacter jejuni* infections. *JAMA* **253:**2873–2875.

92. **Smith, K. E., J. M. Besser, C. W. Hedberg, F. T. Leano, J. B. Bender, J. H. Wicklund, B. P. Johnson, K. A. Moore, and M. T. Osterholm.** 1999. Quinolone-resistant *Campylobacter jejuni* infections in Minnesota, 1992–1998. *N. Engl. J. Med.* **340:**1525–1582.

93. **Sorvillo, F. J., L. E. Lieb, and S. H. Waterman.** 1991. Incidence of campylobacteriosis among patients with AIDS in Los Angeles County. *J. Acquired Immune Defic. Syndr.* **4:** 598–602.

94. **Stafford, R., T. Tenkate, and B. McCall.** 1996. A five year review of *Campylobacter* infection in Queensland. *Commun. Dis. Intell.* **20:** 478–482.

95. **Stern, N. J., S. S. Green, N. Thaker, D. Krout, and J. Chiu.** 1984. Recovery of *Campylobacter jejuni* from fresh and frozen meat and poultry collected at slaughter. *J. Food Prot.* **47:** 372–374.

96. **Swedish Institute of Infectious Disease Control.** 1997. *Reported Foodborne and Waterborne Outbreaks in Sweden.* Swedish Institute of Infectious Disease Control, Stockholm, Sweden.

97. **Tauxe, R. V., N. Hargrett-Bean, C. M. Patton, and I. K. Wachsmuth.** 1988. *Campylobacter* isolates in the United States, 1982–1986. *Morbid. Mortal. Weekly Rep. CDC Surveill. Summ.* **37:**1–13.

98. **Tauxe, R. V., D. A. Pegues, and N. Hargrett-Bean.** 1987. *Campylobacter* infections: the emerging national pattern. *Am. J. Public Health* **77:**1219–1221.

99. **Taylor, D. N., K. T. McDermott, J. R. Little, J. G. Wells, and M. J. Blaser.** 1983. *Campylobacter* enteritis from untreated water in the Rocky Mountains. *Ann. Intern. Med.* **99:** 38–40.

100. **Thurm, V., and E. Dinger.** 1998. Subtyping of outbreak-related strains as a useful method in the surveillance of *Campylobacter* infections. *In Proceedings of the 4th World Congress on Foodborne Infections and Intoxications.* 7–12 June 1998, Berlin, Germany.

101. **VFD.** 1997. *Annual Survey of Foodborne Diseases in Denmark.* Ministry of Food Agriculture and Fisheries, Copenhagen, Denmark.

102. **Vogt, R. L., H. E. Sours, T. Barrett, R. A. Feldman, R. J. Dickinson, and L. Witherell.** 1982. *Campylobacter* enteritis associated with contaminated water. *Ann. Intern. Med.* **96:** 292–296.

103. **Wood, R. C., K. L. MacDonald, and M. T. Osterholm.** 1992. *Campylobacter* enteritis outbreaks associated with drinking raw milk during youth activities. A 10-year review of outbreaks in the United States. *JAMA* **268:**3228–3230.

CAMPYLOBACTER INFECTIONS IN DEVELOPING COUNTRIES

Richard A. Oberhelman and David N. Taylor

7

Campylobacter species occur in the animal food chain of humans from the most to the least economically developed cultures. Although *Campylobacter* species are recognized as among the most common causes of diarrhea worldwide, the epidemiology of *Campylobacter* infections in the developing world differs markedly from that in the developed world. Given the differences in climate, population density, and ethnic background of the inhabitants of the developing world from those in the developed world, it is not surprising that there are geographic differences in the disease patterns. However, there are also great geographic and cultural diversities among the developing countries of Asia, Africa, and Latin America, yet a definite developing world pattern of disease has emerged. The epidemiological differences in developed and developing countries described in this chapter are best explained by increased exposure and high infection rates early in life in developing-world populations, which in turn induce high levels of immunity early in life. This situation is somewhat analogous to the development of partial immunity to malaria during childhood in areas of endemic infection, where repeated infections may result in milder symptomatic disease or chronic asymptomatic carriage with reinfection.

EPIDEMIOLOGIC FEATURES

Magnitude of Infection in Indigenous Populations

Most, if not all, of the many differences in the epidemiology of *Campylobacter* infection can be traced to the concept that the incidence of disease in developing countries is higher by several orders of magnitude than in developed countries. In England and the United States, *Campylobacter* species are isolated from about 5% of patients with diarrhea and the annual incidence of *Campylobacter* enteritis is approximately 50/100,000 population for all persons and about 300/100,000 for children 1 to 4 years old (42, 64). The isolation rates are considerably higher than for *Salmonella* species, which are isolated from 2 to 3% of patients, and *Shigella* species, which are isolated from 1% of patients (12, 64). In the former Yugoslavia, a region intermediate in its economic development, the annual incidence of disease in all persons is about 90/100,000 and increases to 2,500/100,000 in children 1 to 4 years old (52). The

Richard A. Oberhelman, Tulane School of Public Health and Tropic Medicine, 1501 Canal Street, New Orleans, LA 70112. David N. Taylor, Department of Enteric Infections, Division of Communicable Diseases and Immunology, Walter Reed Army Institute of Research, Washington, DC 20307-5100.

Campylobacter, 2nd Ed., Edited by I. Nachamkin and M. J. Blaser
© 2000 American Society for Microbiology, Washington, D.C.

incidence of *Campylobacter* enteritis in developing countries is much higher, i.e., 0.4 episode per child per year, or 40,000/100,000 for children younger than 5 years old, based on studies from Thailand and Mexico in 1988 (14, 72) and on a more recent (1997) survey of pediatric diarrhea in a periurban shantytown in Peru (51). Although these rates seem extraordinarily high, they are substantiated by *Campylobacter* diarrhea rates in travelers to these countries of 2 to 3% per month (or 27,000 to 38,000/ 100,000 per year) (21, 71, 77). Although the diarrhea rates in young children in the developing world are over 100 times greater than those seen in England, the rates of symptomatic illness in school-age children and adults in developing countries are lower than in England. Thus, the incidence of *Campylobacter* enteritis for all age groups in the developing world may not be much higher than in Yugoslavia.

Most studies report cross-sectional prevalence of *Campylobacter* among persons with diarrhea, rather than longitudinal incidence. In developing parts of Asia, Africa, and Latin America, *Campylobacter* isolation rates have ranged from 5 to 20% in surveys of children with diarrhea (36, 61, 67). *Campylobacter* species are commonly isolated as often as or more often than rotavirus and enterotoxigenic *Escherichia coli* and are frequently more commonly isolated than nontyphoidal *Salmonella* and *Shigella* species (19, 72, 73). In studies from Latin America and Africa, *Campylobacter* is the most commonly isolated bacterial pathogen from children with diarrhea (36, 51, 61). Recovery of *Campylobacter* among children with diarrhea declines with age (14, 76); for example, in Thailand *Campylobacter* species were associated with 18.8% of cases among children younger than 12 months, 12.3% of cases among those aged 12 to 23 months, and 10.3% of cases among those aged 24 to 59 months. While *Campylobacter* enteritis is most common in the first year of life in Thailand and Peru, the number of *Shigella* infections increases steadily with age and peaks between 2 and 4 years. Data from other cross-sectional prevalence studies (3, 36,

59) suggest that this demographic pattern is common in many developing countries.

In the developed world, infections with multiple enteric pathogens are infrequent, while in developing areas, recovery of more than one pathogen from a patient with diarrhea is relatively common. *Campylobacter* species were isolated from 18% of Thai children with diarrhea (72), and another enteric pathogen was isolated from half of the patients in whom *Campylobacter* was isolated. This is typical of studies throughout the developing world, and the proportion of mixed infections may be more dependent on the number of pathogens looked for than on any true differences in proportion.

C. jejuni as a Cause of Traveler's Diarrhea

Studies on diarrhea in travelers to the developing world have shown that *Campylobacter* is an important cause of traveler's diarrhea (Table 1), although isolation rates vary by geographical location and tend to be lower in studies where laboratory studies were performed in the home country than in studies where the laboratory studies were performed in the field. The lower recovery rate in some studies of returning travelers is likely to be related to the inclusion of specimens sent by mail, which may not be cultured for several days after collection and may not be transported under optimal conditions. *Campylobacter* species are associated with a disproportionately larger number of cases of diarrhea among travelers than among indigenous persons of similar age, probably because of lack of immunity provided by prior infection. In a 1995 study of traveler's diarrhea in Nepal (32), *Campylobacter* was associated with 28% of diarrhea cases among travelers but only 17% of cases among expatriate residents of Nepal. A 1998 study from Austria found that *C. jejuni* was the leading bacterial cause of diarrhea among 322 travelers returning from destinations in Asia, Africa, and Latin America (54). During the last 10 years, *Campylobacter* has consistently been the leading cause of traveler's diarrhea among U.S. troops participating in

TABLE 1 Isolation rates of *Campylobacter* spp. and other enteric pathogens from travelers in the developing world[a]

Origin	Travel location	% Isolation of:		
		Campylobacter spp.	ETEC[b]	*Salmonella* spp.
Finland	Morocco	29	5	10
United States	Egypt	0	57	2
Switzerland	The Gambia	1	42	4
United States	Thailand	39	6	18
Japan	Asia	5	34	11
Japan	Far East	5	33	15
Japan	India	11	39	6
Western world	Bangladesh	15	ND[c]	0
Western world	Nepal	14	27	3
United States	Mexico	3	20	1
United States	Mexico	1	24	1
Western world[d]	Thailand	10	17	8
Western world[d]	Nepal	28	28	3
Austria[d]	Various	3	2	2

[a] Data from references 7, 10, 24, 32, 44, 54, 65, 70, 71, 74, and 78.
[b] ETEC, enterotoxigenic *E. coli*.
[c] ND, not determined.
[d] Based on data collected in 1992 or later.

military exercises in Thailand, with isolation rates as high as 39%, while it accounts for only 10 to 15% of cases among indigenous residents, who experience diarrhea associated with *Shigella* and enterotoxigenic *E. coli* just as frequently (31, 77). The rates in Thailand may have been increased because the soldiers received doxycycline (tetracycline) daily for malaria prophylaxis. However, doxycycline was shown to have decreased the number of cases of diarrhea due to enterotoxigenic *E. coli* rather than to have increased the number of cases due to *C. jejuni*.

Campylobacter infections in returning travelers may contribute significantly to reports of this organism in more developed countries. In Sweden, over 70% of cases of *Campylobacter* enteritis were acquired outside the country (66). Thus, some studies in developed countries may reflect the symptoms associated with *C. jejuni* strains acquired in the developing world. Studies in Morocco and in South and Southeast Asia usually describe very high rates of *Campylobacter* diarrhea in travelers, suggesting that these are high-risk areas for *Campylobacter* infections. When a group of 380 Finnish tourists went

to Morocco in January and February 1989, *C. jejuni* was isolated from 29% of 80 persons with diarrhea (60). Among Japanese travelers, *C. jejuni* enteritis was more common in travelers to the Indian subcontinent than in travelers to other countries in the Far East (70). The Japanese studies, as well as studies of travelers to Bangladesh and Nepal, have consistently indicated that over 10% of diarrhea in travelers to South Asia is caused by *C. jejuni* (65, 70, 74).

Sources and Modes of Transmission

In developed countries, outbreaks of *Campylobacter* enteritis are most frequently transmitted by food such as contaminated milk and water (10). Eating undercooked chicken appears to be the most common cause of sporadic cases of *Campylobacter* enteritis (16). In general, the transmission is similar to that of *Salmonella* infection.

In the developing world, *Campylobacter* species are frequently isolated in populations at every stage of economic development. In Bangkok, Thailand, *Campylobacter* and *Salmonella* species are now well established in the food chain (53). *Campylobacter* was isolated from 40% of chicken samples from Bangkok markets, and the serotypes of the organisms were similar to those of organisms isolated from humans. This is in contrast to *Salmonella* infections, which are very rare in less developed countries such as India and African countries, except in institutional settings such as orphanages. *Salmonella* species are not common in the least developed areas of the world, where livestock are not mass produced and where institutional and nosocomial outbreaks are uncommon. It appears that food-associated pathogens can be acquired very early in life from the foods themselves, from other humans who are excreting the organisms, or from environmental contamination. This may explain why there is little seasonality associated with infections due to these organisms. In contrast, *Shigella* species and rotavirus were not detected in foods, were not associated with a high rate of asymptomatic infections, and showed seasonality. Since *Campylobacter* organisms do not multiply at ambient temperatures and oxygen concentrations, recontamination of cooked foods, theoretically, should not occur.

Close direct contact with animals was reported to be an important risk factor in both rural and periurban areas of developing countries (5, 17, 29). In Lima, Peru, and in Cameroon, exposure to living chickens in the household was a significant risk factor for *Campylobacter* infection (5, 29, 36). Recent studies of free-roaming chickens in households of periurban shantytowns in Lima, Peru, demonstrated that 37% of chickens had *Campylobacter* in the stool. Identical strains of *Campylobacter,* based on random–primer and restriction fragment length polymorphism (RFLP) analyses, were isolated from chickens and humans from 11 of 18 households with both human and avian *Campylobacter* isolates, suggesting that intrahousehold transmission in these communities is common (50a).

Seasonality

In the developed world, *Campylobacter* isolations typically increase during the summer and fall months (22, 64), and although most cases appear to be sporadic, epidemics do occur (10).

In the developing world, there is less seasonal variation (3, 69) and epidemics are not reported, although in some studies from Peru and Thailand, infections tend to increase in the hot, dry season (66a). One study of Finnish travelers to Morocco (44) suggested that *Campylobacter* was associated with more traveler's diarrhea in the winter (isolated from 28% of persons with diarrhea in January and February; mean temperatures, 13.8 to 15.0°C) than in the fall (isolated from 7% of persons with diarrhea in October and November; mean temperatures, 20.5 to 18.1°C). However, the higher attack rate of traveler's diarrhea in the fall than in the winter (31 versus 15%, respectively) suggests that part of this observation is based on more pronounced seasonality of other pathogens, such as enterotoxigenic *E. coli* and *Salmonella,* while rates of *Campylobacter* enteritis remained relatively stable despite seasonal changes.

The lack of seasonality might be explained by the lack of extreme temperature variations in tropical climates, and the apparent lack of epidemics might be explained by poor surveillance. However, the combination of milder illness, the high rates of asymptomatic illness, and the high rates of infections with multiple pathogens suggest a different epidemiological process. Transmission of *Campylobacter* in developing countries appears to be related to sources with little seasonal variation, such as infected chicken meat and feces of infected chickens, rather than to human contamination of previously uninfected food sources, which are accentuated at higher ambient temperature.

Asymptomatic Infections

Campylobacter species are rarely isolated from healthy persons in developed countries (10, 67). However, from the first studies in the developing world, it was recognized that *Campylobacter* species could be isolated from children who were well as often as from children who had diarrhea. In 1979, Bokkenheuser et al. (13) found that after the age of 9 months, there was no difference in the isolation rate of *Campylobacter* species between children with diarrhea and well children in South Africa. When cultures were made from samples isolated from South African schoolchildren over a 16-month period, 6 of 73 children apparently excreted the organism for several months without showing signs of illness (55). A high rate of asymptomatic carriage was also found in Bangladesh (28) and the Central African Republic (27), and the rate of asymptomatic infection is three to four times the rate of symptomatic infections in children in Mexico and Thailand (14, 72). Immunity to infection appears to affect both symptomatic and asymptomatic infection, since both rates decline steadily in Mexican and Peruvian children between 1 and 5 years of age (14, 66a). In Mexico, children were repeatedly infected with new serotypes when follow-up cultures were taken, and multiple *Campylobacter* serotypes were isolated from 42% of 62 patients (63). There was no difference between the serotypes isolated from persons with symptomatic and asymptomatic infection (63).

Not all enteropathogens were isolated so frequently from healthy children in the developing world. In surveys done in Thailand, rotavirus and *Shigella* species were infrequently found in asymptomatic controls whereas *Campylobacter* and *Salmonella* species were isolated nearly as often in children without diarrhea as in those with diarrhea (19, 73). Although frequent isolation from asymptomatic persons is a typical feature of *Campylobacter* infection throughout the developing world, some studies did find a difference in isolation rates of *Campylobacter* species in children with and without diarrhea who were younger than 6 months (17, 19, 41). However, a number of studies have found no difference in rates in any age group (25, 27, 28, 80).

The dynamics of symptomatic and asymptomatic *Campylobacter* infection were studied by Calva et al. (14) in 1985 to 1988 in a cohort of 179 children younger than 5 years in San Pedro Martir, a low-income area on the outskirts of Mexico City. For 1 year, these children were visited twice a week, and samples were obtained and cultured for *Campylobacter* species. Typical of many developing countries, there were 2.7 episodes of diarrhea per child-

year but only 0.4 of these episodes was associated with *Campylobacter* species. Over the year, 66% of the cohort had a *Campylobacter* infection and 30% had an illness associated with *Campylobacter* infection. *Campylobacter* infections occurred at an early age; they peaked at 12 to 17 months of age and declined steadily thereafter, presumably due to the development of partial immunity. The illness-to-infection ratio was highest in the first 6 months of age (0.46) and declined steadily to values between 0.14 and 0.17 for children ages 24 to 71 months. Data from other populations demonstrating the highest incidence of symptomatic *Campylobacter* infection in children younger than 12 months (51) suggest that this is a common epidemiological pattern. This observation is consistent with a changing clinical disease pattern among children younger and older than 12 months, with younger patients experiencing higher rates of bloody diarrhea (i.e., severe invasive disease), while older children with prior immunologic exposure had relative protection against invasive disease.

Excretion of Organisms in Infected Individuals

In the developed world, the mean duration of convalescent-phase excretion of *Campylobacter* organisms after an acute infection is 2 to 3 weeks (33, 66). In Thailand, the average duration of convalescent-phase excretion of *Campylobacter* organisms was 14 days for children younger than 1 year and 8 days for children 1 to 5 years old, a significant difference ($P < 0.02$) (72). In a subsequent study, both the duration of excretion and the quantity of organisms excreted were inversely proportional to age among Thai children with *Campylobacter*-associated diarrhea (76). Children shed 1 to 8 log units of campylobacters, and quantitative fecal excretion of *C. coli* and group 2 aeotolerant *Campylobacter* was generally lower than that of *C. jejuni*. Fecal *Campylobacter* loads tended to be higher in children with fecal leukocytes, suggesting that inflammatory reactions may be associated with a higher infectious inoculum.

In Mexico, the median duration of excretion in patients with *Campylobacter* diarrhea was 3 days (range, 1 to 29 days) (14), and when infections were asymptomatic, the duration of excretion was 7 days. Studies in Thailand and Mexico, which have examined serotype-specific excretion rates, have demonstrated that frequent isolation of *Campylobacter* species from healthy persons in the developing world is not a function of prolonged carriage, as was postulated previously (55), but of constant reinfection. The average length of excretion for Thai and Mexican children is actually shorter than that for children in developed countries, probably because the children in developing countries are partially immune.

CLINICAL ILLNESS

In the developed world, *Campylobacter* enteritis can be quite severe. The most prominent features among patients presenting to medical attention are diarrhea, abdominal pain, and fever (7, 12, 33, 66). Grossly bloody stools are common and are often the reason for seeking medical attention. Abdominal pain is the most characteristic manifestation of illness. In hospital surveys, bloody diarrhea occurs in about half of the patients.

In developing countries, *C. jejuni* infection is milder than in patients in developed countries (25, 28, 72). In Thailand, about one-third of symptomatic infections were associated with

TABLE 3 Clinical symptoms of patients with diarrhea associated with *C. jejuni*, *Shigella* spp., and enterotoxigenic *E. coli* in Bangladesh, 1980[a]

Symptom	No. of patients with symptom due to:		
	C. jejuni (*n* = 164)	*Shigella* spp. (*n* = 413)	ETEC[b] (*n* = 624)
Watery diarrhea	66	30	78
Abdominal pain	45	69	54
Bloody stool	17	55	10
Mucoid stool	61	86	46
Vomiting	66	37	67
Fever	50	52	42
Dehydration	20	13	26

[a] Adapted from reference 28.
[b] ETEC, enterotoxigenic *E. coli*.

bloody diarrhea, one-third with watery diarrhea, and one-third with mucoid diarrhea (Table 2). In the developing world, bloody diarrhea is seen with *Shigella* infections at a considerably higher frequency than with *Campylobacter* infections (Table 3). In Thailand, *Shigella* organisms were associated with grossly bloody diarrhea in 37% of cases in which only one pathogen was detected whereas *Campylobacter* and *Salmonella* organisms were associated with bloody stools in 14 and 26%, respectively. More than 10 fecal leukocytes per high-power microscopic field, an indicator of invasive diarrheal disease, were present in 67% of patients infected with *Shigella* species and in 24 to 36%

TABLE 2 Clinical features of diarrheal disease in children infected with a single enteric pathogen in Bangkok, Thailand[a]

Organism	Total no. of patients (%)[b]	No. with single pathogen	No. with fever (>38°C)	No. with bloody stools	No. with >10 leukocytes	No. given i.v. fluid[c]	No. hospitalized
Shigella spp.	155 (13)	94	42	37	67	3	2
EIEC[d]	19 (2)	11	45	18	36	9	0
Salmonella spp.	151 (12)	81	27	26	27	3	4
Campylobacter spp.	163 (13)	80	28	14	24	4	0
Rotavirus	220 (20)	141	28	5	6	19	4
ETEC[d]	112 (9)	48	17	4	6	6	2

[a] Adapted from reference 19.
[b] expressed as percentage of single-pathogen infection.
[c] i.v., intravenous.
[d] EIEC, enteroinvasive *E. coli*; ETEC, enterotoxigenic *E. coli*.

TABLE 4 Symptoms associated with *Campylobacter* infections among U.S. military personnel during an outbreak in Fort Knox, Ky., and a field maneuver in Thailand

Symptom	% of persons with symptoms in:	
	Kentucky ($n = 34$)	Thailand ($n = 43$)
Diarrhea	88	100
Cramps	76	75
Fever	68	—[a]
Headache	65	70
Vomiting	59	51
Bloody diarrhea	26	30

[a] Data not collected.

of patients infected with enteroinvasive *E. coli*, *Salmonella* species, or *Campylobacter* species (Table 2). The incidence of bloody diarrhea and the duration of illness decrease with increasing age among children from most developing countries (see "Systemic Immunity" below).

Most *Campylobacter* infections in travelers cause symptoms, although frank dysentery is rare. Asymptomatic infections were found in only 2% of 313 Finnish tourists who went to Morocco (60). The symptoms associated with *C. jejuni* infections acquired by travelers in the developing world were similar to the symptoms associated with domestically acquired infections (Table 4), although symptoms in travelers were generally more severe than those in children from the developing world with *Campylobacter* infections. In a recent study of Spanish travelers with *Campylobacter* enteritis acquired in developing countries (23), 23 of 24 patients (96%) had watery diarrhea and only 1 of 24 had dysentery. Abdominal cramps were present in 83% of patients, fever in 46%, nausea and vomiting in 42%, and gross blood in only 3%. *Campylobacter* diarrhea persisted for at least 14 days in 79% of patients in this study, which is longer than in most previous reports, although most of these patients experienced a fluctuating course of disease, with remissions and recrudescence.

C. jejuni has been associated with sporadic cases of Guillain-Barré syndrome (GBS) in several parts of the developing world (9, 38, 42, 47, 50, 58). To our knowledge, *Campylobacter*-associated GBS is rarely if ever reported from countries in the lowest per capita income group in Asia, Africa, and Latin America, even though many of these countries have high rates of *Campylobacter* infection. It is not clear if this is due to inadequate reporting, inadequate recognition of the disease, or a relative paucity of *Campylobacter*-associated GBS cases. One possible explanation is that in areas of the world where polio is endemic, cases of postinfectious GBS may be misdiagnosed as paralytic polio. If this is the case, further progress in polio eradication may unmask *Campylobacter*-associated GBS in other parts of the developing world.

STRAIN DIFFERENCES

Strain differences have been cited as one possible explanation for the epidemiological differences in developed and developing countries. These differences could include differences in serotype, in virulence factors or in *Campylobacter* species. *Campylobacter* strains isolated in developing countries are biochemically and serotypically similar to strains isolated in developed countries (1, 40, 72). Most *Campylobacter* strains isolated in the developing world can be typed by using typing antisera from the developed world; for example, 0 of 31 strains isolated from patients in Mexico and only 3 of 104 strains from patients in Thailand were nontypeable by the Lior system (63, 72). There is little evidence that serotype differences can account for these markedly different clinical and epidemiological patterns (63). Furthermore, as described above, the spectrum of illness in travelers is similar to the illness observed in the developed world.

However, with newer strain typing tools such as RFLP patterns for flagellar genes, several new observations of strain differences have emerged. In a study of 59 clinical isolates of *C. jejuni* from Egypt (46), more extensive heterogeneity of RFLP patterns was observed than in North American isolates, with the addition of five new polymorphism groups, even though the Egyptian isolates corresponded to common

TABLE 5 Relative isolation rates of *C. jejuni* by geographic location[a]

Location (yr)	Proportion of infection due to:	
	C. jejuni	*C. coli*
Algeria (1990)	85	15
Central African Republic (1986)	56	44
Chile (1990)	56	44
Ethiopia (1992)	82	18
France (1987)	78	22
Mexico (1985)	90	10
Taiwan (1994–1996)	78	22
Tanzania (1990)	80	20
Thailand (1985)	87	13
Thailand (1987)	67	15
Thailand (1988)	87	7
Yugoslavia (1987)	64	35
Zimbabwe (1996)	73	27

[a] Adapted from references 1, 14, 26, 30, 39, 45, 45a, 52, 61, 72, and 73.

Lior serotypes. One RFLP group of the nine found in the Egyptian isolates, group 5, was uniquely associated with febrile diarrhea.

Although *C. jejuni* is the species most commonly associated with diarrhea, other species associated with diarrhea include *C. coli, C. lari, C. hyointestinalis, C. fetus* subsp. *fetus, C. cinaedi, C. fennelliae,* and *C. upsaliensis* (20, 35, 62). The proportion of infections due to *C. coli* or other hippurate-negative strains can be much higher in developing than developed countries (Table 5). *C. coli* was isolated from 12% of children with *Campylobacter* infections in Thailand but accounted for 41 and 39% of isolates in Hong Kong and the Central African Republic, respectively (26, 30). In Europe and the United States, *C. coli* infections account for less than 5% of all *Campylobacter* infections. By using the membrane filter technique, *C. jejuni* was isolated from 10%, *C. coli* was isolated from 2%, and atypical campylobacters were isolated from 3% of 631 Thai children with diarrhea (75). In this study, 15 of 17 atypical strains were aerotolerant strains, designated group 2 aerotolerant *Campylobacter* species or *Arcobacter butzleri* (34). The inability of group 2 aerotolerant strains to grow at 42°C suggests that poultry or another

avian reservoir is unlikely, and other environmental sources such as contaminated waters may be implicated. Atypical campylobacters were also isolated in Australia from persons returning from India or Indonesia, suggesting that atypical strains may be more common in developing countries in general and possibly also more common in Asian countries (79).

C. coli was as often isolated from cases as from controls and was not associated with bloody diarrhea in Thailand, whereas *C. jejuni* was associated with bloody diarrhea in about one-third of cases. Thus, the spectrum of *Campylobacter* infections appears to be milder in areas where *C. coli* is frequently isolated. The clinical illness associated with group 2 aerotolerant hippurate-negative *Campylobacter* infections in Thailand was also milder than that associated with *C. jejuni* infections in children of the same age (75). These findings support our conclusions, and those of others who found that *C. coli* infections tended to be milder than *C. jejuni* infections (72). Determination of the importance of these organisms in developed countries awaits large-scale studies involving nonselective isolation methods.

IMMUNOLOGIC FEATURES

Systemic Immunity

The hyperendemnicity of *Campylobacter* species appears to be the most important factor in defining the epidemiological pattern of infection in the developing world. Healthy children in Bangladesh, Thailand, and the Central African Republic develop serum antibodies to *Campylobacter* species very early in life and have much higher levels of *Campylobacter*-specific antibodies than do children in the United States (8, 11, 43). In Thai children there is an early rise in the level of antibodies to *Campylobacter* species that parallels the peak in isolation rate (72). In the Central African Republic the rise in the level of antiflagellar antibody inversely correlated with rates of *Campylobacter* enteritis (43). The development of immunity to these or other antigens appears to play an important role in the age-related decreases in the case-to-infection ratio and the duration of convalescent-phase excretion (72, 76). Further exposure to *Campylobacter* species probably continues to stimulate gut immunity and prevent tissue involvement and subsequent symptomatic infection but has less effect on asymptomatic infections.

In Thailand, *Campylobacter* infection was most often associated with bloody diarrhea in the first year of life, most probably as a result of a primary infection (72). These observations suggest that immunity may prevent bloody diarrhea from developing and eventually prevents any disease from occurring. This is supported by volunteer studies, which have found that rechallenge with the same organism led to infection but not to disease (4), and by observations of Mexican children, of whom those with symptom-producing infections during the first 6 months of life were less likely to develop subsequent *Campylobacter* infection (symptomatic or asymptomatic) than were those with diarrhea-free infection (14).

In a subsequent study, the effect of age, symptoms, excretion pattern, and coinfection with other enteric pathogens on the immune response to *Campylobacter* infection and on the quantitative excretion of the organism in Thai children was examined (76). In theory, nonpathogenic organisms might not cause a serum immune response and might be excreted for shorter periods or in smaller numbers. For 6 months, stool samples from children younger than 5 years who came to the Bangkok Children's Hospital with diarrhea were cultured. Any patient whose stool culture was positive for *Campylobacter* species or *Shigella* species was seen at 2 and 4 weeks after the initial visit. Serum samples were collected at the initial presentation and at the time of the two home visits. In 37 of 416 children with diarrhea, *Campylobacter* species were the only pathogens found, and in 24 there was a mixed infection. Compared with the United States, where bloody diarrhea was seen in 50% of patients with *Campylobacter* infection, in Thailand only 25% of patients had bloody diarrhea, and most of these children were younger than 2 years.

There were no differences between the illnesses in children with *Campylobacter* species as the sole pathogens and those in children with mixed infection.

This study demonstrated several important features of immunity to *Campylobacter*. (i) *Campylobacter* antibody production is age dependent. As the age increases, baseline levels of antibody also increase. During the first 6 months of life, immunoglobulin A (IgA), IgM, and, to a lesser extent, IgG levels in serum did not appear to rise in response to infection. After that age, rises were seen in all Ig subclasses in response to infection. A poor seroresponse in the first 6 months of life may occur because it is a primary response to *Campylobacter* species and/or because maternal antibodies are present from placental transfer or breast feeding. Previous studies in the same population have shown that 38% of children younger than 1 year receive breast milk. (ii) The antibody response is not dependent on symptoms or the presence of coinfections. (iii) Better antibody responses in older children correlate with excretion of few organisms and with the presence of milder, nonbloody diarrhea, findings consistent with the development of immunity. The presence of asymptomatic *Campylobacter* infections suggested that *Campylobacter* species were nonpathogenic in an immune host. These immunologic features parallel responses to other hyperendemic infections among children in developing countries, such as malaria, demonstrating progressive acquisition of partial immunity that offers some protection against severe disease while providing lesser protection against reinfection with strains causing milder or no apparent disease. This is in contrast to the epidemiology of *Campylobacter* in the developed world, where most cases are primary infections in a wider age group, with more severe clinical symptoms (Table 6). These observations are also consistent with results of studies in Swedish abattoirs (15), where new and presumably immunologically naïve workers suffered many more episodes of *Campylobacter* diarrhea than did persons who had been employed for many years, who had significantly

TABLE 6 Comparison of the features of *C. jejuni* infections in developed with those in developing countries[a]

Feature	Developed countries	Developing countries
Isolation rate among persons with diarrhea (%)	5	15–40
Isolation rate among well persons (%)	<1	15–40
Average no. of infections/lifetime	0–1	>5
Widespread immunity among adults	Absent	Present
Affected age groups (yr)	<5, 20–30	<2
Principal manifestation of illness	Inflammatory diarrhea	Simple diarrhea
Illness severity	Severe	Mild
Bloody diarrhea (%)	50	15
Epidemics reported	Yes	No
Seasonal increase in incidence	Yes	No
Duration of excretion (days)	16	8

[a] Adapted from reference 6.

higher titers of antibody to *Campylobacter*. These Swedish workers with intense exposure over time, like children in developing countries, still experienced regular asymptomatic *Campylobacter* colonization which was not completely prevented by systemic immunity.

Mucosal Immunity from Breast-Feeding

In Mexico, where 98 infants were monitored from birth to 2 years of age, breast-feeding decreased the number of episodes and the duration of diarrhea (56). The diarrhea rate caused by *C. jejuni* was significantly greater for non-breast-fed infants than for breast-fed infants. Secretory IgA antibody titers to *Campylobacter* surface antigens were highest in colostrum but persisted throughout lactation. Human milk consumed by children with *Campylobacter* diarrhea did not contain secretory *Campylobacter* antibodies. The author's conclusion that *Campylobacter* antibodies in human milk prevented *Campylobacter* diarrhea was supported by another cohort study in Mexico, in which anti-*Campylobacter* flagellin antibody titers were measured in breast milk. In this study, infants receiving breast milk with IgA antibodies against flagellin proteins had significantly fewer *Campylobacter* infections than did non-breast-fed children, while infants receiving milk that was anti-flagellin negative also had fewer infec-

tions than did non-breast-fed infants but at a level that did not reach statistical significance.

In Algeria, *Campylobacter* species were isolated from 58 infants younger than 6 months (45); 35 had diarrhea, and 23 did not. The difference in isolation rate was not significant. Only 4 children with diarrhea (15%) were exclusively breast-fed, whereas 10 children without diarrhea (40%) were exclusively breast-fed. This study suggested that exclusively breast-fed infants had fewer symptomatic *Campylobacter* infections than did infants who were both breast- and bottle-fed.

A cohort of 127 African infants were monitored from birth until 6 months of age (27). None of 11 *Campylobacter* infections in the first month of life was associated with symptoms, compared with 13 (20%) of 71 infections in children 2 to 6 months old. The presence of maternal antibody was suggested as one reason for the lack of symptoms in children younger than 1 month. However, in contrast to the Algerian study, infants in this study who were exclusively breast-fed were actually more likely to have a symptomatic *Campylobacter* infection than were infants who were both breast- and bottle-fed.

ANTIBIOTIC RESISTANCE

Antimicrobial resistance among *Campylobacter* isolates is an increasing problem in the developing world. Because stool culture is not generally available for travelers with diarrhea or children with diarrhea in developing countries, antimicrobial therapy is usually empirical and selected to cover a broad range of pathogens. Trimethoprim-sulfamethoxazole was initially the drug of choice for traveler's diarrhea, even though *C. jejuni* is intrinsically resistant to trimethoprim, leading to many treatment failures in cases of *Campylobacter* enteritis. Erythromycin has traditionally been the drug of choice for *Campylobacter,* where it remains active against 80 to 90% of isolates in Taiwan (39), but use of this drug is limited because it is inadequate to treat the other major causes of traveler's diarrhea, such as *E. coli, Salmonella,* or *Shigella,* and in some areas resistance among *Campylobacter* isolates is also increasing (57, 68). Doxycycline, used extensively for malaria prophylaxis among American troops stationed in Thailand, is no longer effective against 95% of *Campylobacter* isolates from Taiwan and Thailand (2, 39).

Currently, the fluoroquinolone antibiotics, principally ciprofloxacin, are the most widely used drugs for empirical treatment of traveler's diarrhea because of their broad spectrum of activity against a wide variety of pathogens, but resistance to these agents has also been reported in increasing proportions of strains from the developing world, especially in Southeast Asia. In Taiwan, 57% of *Campylobacter* isolates from children with diarrhea and 91% of isolates from chicken products were resistant to ciprofloxacin (39). This high rate of ciprofloxacin resistance in isolates from humans is even more remarkable because all the patients studied were children, who generally do not receive fluoroquinolone drug therapy in Taiwan. In most areas of the developing world with high rates of ciprofloxacin resistance among *Campylobacter* isolates, this phenomenon is probably attributed to the extensive use of ciprofloxacin in poultry feed to promote the growth of chickens (18, 39). Ciprofloxacin resistance is unlikely to be due to use in travelers, who comprise a relatively small proportion of the total number of cases, or to use in the indigenous population, where high cost limits the use of fluoroquinolone antibiotics in most developing countries. In recent studies in Thailand, ciprofloxacin resistance among *Campylobacter* strains from U.S. troops with diarrhea has increased rapidly, with resistance rates increasing from 0% in 1987 and 1990 to 69–79% in 1994 (48) and 84% in 1995 (31). Ciprofloxacin resistance in *Campylobacter* can occur rapidly and exists in several continents, and so this drug, like other fluoroquinolones, cannot reliably treat *Campylobacter* infections in the developing world.

With the problem of fluoroquinolone resistance, azithromycin has become increasingly popular as an alternative drug for empirical therapy in traveler's diarrhea. Unlike erythromycin, this newer macrolide antibiotic is active against most common bacterial enteric pathogens. In a randomized study of azithromycin versus ciprofloxacin for treatment of traveler's diarrhea in U.S. troops in Thailand in 1993 (37), azithromycin recipients had a shorter duration of diarrhea and more rapid eradication of *Campylobacter* from the stool, although patients not infected with *Campylobacter* recovered faster if they received ciprofloxacin. Of 44 *Campylobacter* isolates in this study, 22 (50%) were ciprofloxacin resistant, while none were azithromycin resistant. However, azithromycin resistance has been reported in Thailand as well (15% of Campylobacter strains in 1994 and 7% of strains in 1995), paralleling the development of azithromycin resistance among *E. coli* and *Salmonella* isolates from the same region (Fig. 1) (31), so that the clinical management of *Campylobacter* infections remains an ever-changing challenge.

CONCLUSIONS

Both strain and host factors play important roles in the divergent clinical and epidemiological features of *Campylobacter* infections in the developed and developing world. In the developing world, where *Campylobacter* infections are endemic, the peak isolation rate occurs in children younger than 2 years old and is associated with a humoral response to *C. jejuni* antigens.

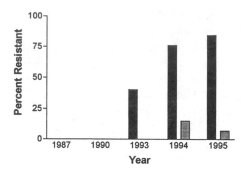

FIGURE 1 Percentage of *C. jejuni* strains resistant to ciprofloxacin (solid bars) and azithromycin (shaded bars), 1987 to 1995. Strains were recovered from U.S. military troops and travelers with diarrhea in Thailand, and 50 to 60 strains were examined each year.

The development of immunity to these antigens plays an important role in decreasing the case-to-infection ratio and the duration of convalescent-stage excretion. Further *Campylobacter* exposure continues to stimulate gut immunity and prevent tissue involvement and subsequent symptomatic infection but does not prevent asymptomatic infection. The most well-defined strain difference is the increase in the proportion of hippurate-negative strains in some parts of the developing world. These strains appear to be less pathogenic than *C. jejuni*. The role of other virulence factors in the clinical illness is unclear.

REFERENCES

1. **Asrat, D. A., A. Hathaway, E. Sjogren, E. Ekwall, and B. Kaijser.** 1997. The serotype distribution of *Campylobacter jejuni* and *C. coli* isolated from patients with diarrhea and controls at Tukur Anbassa Hospital, Addis Ababa, Ethiopia. *Epidemiol. Infect.* **118:**91–95.

2. **Beecham, J. H., III, C. I. Lebron, and P. Echeverria.** 1997. Short report. Impact of traveler's diarrhea on United States troops deployed to Thailand. *Am. J. Trop. Med. Hyg.* **57:**699–701.

3. **Biswas, R., D. J. Lyon, A. S. Nelson, D. Lau, and P. J. Lewindon.** 1996. Aetiology of acute diarrhoea in in hospitalized children in Hong Kong. *Trop. Med. Int. Health* **1:**679–683.

4. **Black, R. E., M. M. Levine, M. L. Clements, T. P. Hughes, and M. J. Blaser.** 1988. Experimental *Campylobacter jejuni* infection in humans. *J. Infect. Dis.* **157:**472–479.

5. **Black, R. E, G. Lopez de Romana, K. H. Brown, N. Bravo, O. G. Bazalar, and H. C. Kanashiro.** 1989. Incidence and etiology of infantile diarrhea and major routes of transmission in Huascar, Peru. *Am. J. Epidemiol.* **129:**785–799.

6. **Blaser, M. J.** 1997. Epidemiologic and clinical features of *Campylobacter jejuni* infections. *J. Infect. Dis.* **176**(Suppl. 2)**:**S103–S105.

7. **Blaser, M. J., L. D. Berkowitz, F. M. LaForce, F. M. Cravens, L. B. Reller, and W. L. L. Wang.** 1979. *Campylobacter* enteritis: clinical and epidemiologic features. *Ann. Intern. Med.* **91:**179–185.

8. **Blaser, M. J., R. E. Black, D. J. Duncan, and J. Amer.** 1985. *Campylobacter jejuni*-specific serum antibodies are elevated in healthy Bangladeshi children. *J. Clin. Microbiol.* **21:**164–167.

9. **Blaser, M. J., A. Olivares, D. N. Taylor, D. R. Cornblath, and G. M. McKhann.** 1991. Campylobacter serology in patients with Chinese paralytic syndrome. *Lancet* **338:**308.

10. **Blaser, M. J., and L. B. Reller.** 1981. *Campylobacter* enteritis. *N. Engl. J. Med.* **305:**1444–1452.

11. **Blaser, M. J., D. N. Taylor, and P. Echeverria.** 1986. Immune response to *Campylobacter jejuni* in a rural community in Thailand. *J. Infect. Dis.* **153:**249–254.

12. **Blaser, M. J., J. G. Wells, R. A. Feldman, R. A. Pollard, J. R. Allen, and the Collaborative Diarrheal Disease Study Group.** 1983. *Campylobacter* enteritis in the United States: a multicenter study. *Ann. Intern. Med.* **98:**360–365.

13. **Bokkenheuser, V. D., N. J. Richardson, J. H. Bryner, D. J. Roux, A. B. Schutte, H. J. Koornhof, I. Freiman, and E. Hartman.** 1979. Detection of enteric campylobacteriosis in children. *J. Clin. Microbiol.* **9:**227–232.

14. **Calva, J. J., G. M. Ruiz-Palacios, A. B. Lopez-Vidal, A. Ramos, and R. Bojalil.** 1988. Cohort study of intestinal infection with *Campylobacter* in Mexican children. *Lancet* **i:**503–506.

15. **Christenson, B., A. Ringner, C. Blucher, H. Billaudelle, K. N. Gundtoft, G. Eriksson, and M. Bottinger.** 1983. An outbreak of *Campylobacter* enteritis among the staff of a poultry abattoir in Sweden. *Scand. J. Infect. Dis.* **15:**167–172.

16. **Deming, M. S., R. V. Tauxe, P. A. Blake, S. E. Dixon, B. S. Fowler, T. S. Jones, E. A. Lockamy, C. M. Patton, and R. O. Sikes.** 1987. *Campylobacter* enteritis at a university: transmission from eating chicken and from cats. *Am. J. Epidemiol.* **126:**526–534.

17. **De Mol, P., D. Brasseur, W. Hemelhof, T. Kalala, J. P. Butzler, and H. L. Vis.** 1983. Enteropathogenic agents in children with diarrhoea in rural Zaire. *Lancet* **i:**516–518.

18. **Du Pont, H. L.** 1995. Editorial response. Antimi-

crobial-resistant *Campylobacter* species—a new threat to travelers to Thailand. *Clin. Infect. Dis.* **21**:542–543.

19. **Echeverria, P., D. N. Taylor, U. Lexsomboon, M. Bhaibulaya, N. R. Blacklow, and R. Sakazaki.** 1989. Case-control study of endemic diarrheal disease in Thai children under 5 years old. *J. Infect. Dis.* **159**:543–548.

20. **Edmonds, P. C., M. Patton, P. M. Griffin, T. J. Barrett, G. P. Schmid, C. N. Baker, M. A. Lambert, and D. J. Brenner.** 1987. *Campylobacter hyointestinalis* associated with human gastrointestinal disease in the United States. *J. Clin. Microbiol.* **25**:685–691.

21. **Ericsson, C. D., H. L. DuPont, J. J. Mathewson, M. S. West, P. C. Johnson, and J. M. Bitsura.** 1990. Treatment of traveler's diarrhea with sulfamethoxazole and trimethoprim and loperamide. *JAMA* **263**:257–261.

22. **Finch, M. J., and L. W. Riley.** 1984. *Campylobacter* infections in the United States: results of an 11-state surveillance. *Arch. Intern. Med.* **144**:1610–1612.

23. **Gallardo, F., J. Gascon, J. Ruiz, M. Corachan, M. Jimenez de Anta, and J. Vila.** 1998. *Campylobacter jejuni* as a cause of traveler's diarrhea: clinical features and antimicrobial susceptibility. *J. Travel Med.* **5**:23 26.

24. **Gaudio, P. A., P. Echeverria, C. W. Hoge, C. Pitarangsi, and P. Goff.** 1996. Diarrhea among expatriate residents in Thailand: correlation between reduced *Campylobacter* prevalence and longer duration of stay. *J. Travel Med.* **3**:77–79.

25. **Georges, M. C., I. K. Wachsmuth, D. M. V. Meunier, N. Nebout, F. Didier, M. R. Siopathis, and A. J. Georges.** 1984. Parasitic, bacterial, and viral enteric pathogens associated with diarrhea in the Central African Republic. *J. Clin. Microbiol.* **19**:571–575.

26. **Georges-Courbot, M. C., C. Baya, A. M. Beraud, D. M. Y. Meunier, and A. J. Georges.** 1986. Distribution and serotypes of *Campylobacter jejuni* and *Campylobacter coli* in enteric *Campylobacter* strains isolated from children in the Central African Republic. *J. Clin. Microbiol.* **23**:592–594.

27. **Georges-Courbot, M. C., A. M. Beraud-Cassel, I. Gouandjika, and A. J. Georges.** 1987. Prospective study of enteric *Campylobacter* infections in children from birth to 6 months in the Central African Republic. *J. Clin. Microbiol.* **25**:836–839.

28. **Glass, R. I., B. J. Stoll, M. I. Huq, M. J. Struelens, M. J. Blaser, and A. K. G. Kibriya.** 1983. Epidemiology and clinical features of endemic *Campylobacter jejuni* infection in Bangladesh. *J. Infect. Dis.* **148**:292–296.

29. **Grados, O., N. Bravo, R. E. Black, and J.-P.**

Butzler. 1988. Pediatric *Campylobacter* diarrhoea from household exposure to live chickens in Lima, Peru. *Bull. W. H. O.* **66**:369–374.

30. **Ho, D. D., and W. T. Wong.** 1985. A one-year survey of *Campylobacter* enteritis and other forms of bacterial diarrhoea in Hong Kong. *J. Hyg.* (Cambridge) **94**:55–60.

31. **Hoge, C. W., J. M. Gambel, A. Srijan, C. Pitarangsi, and P. Echeverria.** 1998. Trends in antibiotic resistance among diarrheal pathogens isolated in Thailand over 15 years. *Clin. Infect. Dis.* **26**:341–345.

32. **Hoge, C. W., D. R. Shlim, P. Echeverria, R. Rajah, J. E. Herrmann, and J. H. Cross.** 1996. Epidemiology of diarrhea among expatriate residents living in a highly endemic environment. *JAMA* **275**:533–538.

33. **Karmali, M. A., and P. C. Fleming.** 1979. *Campylobacter* enteritis in children. *J. Pediatr.* **94**:527–533.

34. **Kiehlbauch, J. A., D. J. Brenner, M. A. Nicholson, C. N. Baker, C. M. Patton, A. G. Steigerwalt, and I. K. Wachsmuth.** 1991. *Campylobacter butzleri* sp. nov. isolated from humans and animals with diarrheal illness. *J. Clin. Microbiol.* **29**:376–385.

35. **Klein, B. S., J. M. Vergeront, M. J. Blaser, P. Edmonds, D. J. Brenner, D. Janssen, and J. P. Davis.** 1986. *Campylobacter* infection associated with raw milk: an outbreak of gastroenteritis due to *Campylobacter jejuni* and thermotolerant *Campylobacter fetus* subsp. *fetus*. *JAMA* **255**:361–364.

36. **Koulla-Shiro, S., C. Loe, and T. Ekoe.** 1995. Prevalence of *Campylobacter* enteritis in children from Yaounde (Cameroon). *Centr. Afr. J. Med.* **41**:91–94.

37. **Kuschner, R. A., A. F. Trofa, R. J. Thomas, C. W. Hoge, C. Pitarangsi, S. Amato, R. P. Olafson, P. Echeverria, J. C. Sadoff, and D. N. Taylor.** 1995. Use of azithromycin for the treatment of *Campylobacter* enteritis in travelers to Thailand, an area where ciprofloxacin resistance is prevalent. *Clin. Infect. Dis.* **21**:536–541.

38. **Lastovica, A. J., E. A. Goddard, and A. C. Argent.** 1997. Guillan-Barré syndrome in South Africa associated with *Campylobacter jejuni* O:41 strains. *J. Infect. Dis.* **176**(Suppl. 2):S139–S143.

39. **Li, C. C., C. H. Chiu, J. L. Wu, Y. C. Huang, and T. Y. Lin.** 1998. Antimicrobial susceptibility of *Campylobacter jejuni* and *coli* by using E-test in Taiwan. *Scand. J. Infect. Dis.* **30**:39–42.

40. **Lior, H., D. L. Woodward, J. A. Edgar, L. J. Laroche, and P. Gill.** 1982. Serotyping of *Campylobacter jejuni* by slide agglutination based on heat-labile antigenic factors. *J. Clin. Microbiol.* **15**:761–768.

41. Luo, N. P., K. S. Baboo, D. Mwenya, A. Diab, C. U. Perera, C. Cummings, H. L. DuPont, J. R. Murphy, and A. Zumla. 1996. Isolation of *Campylobacter* species from Zambian patients with acute diarrhoea. *East Afr. Med. J.* **73:** 395–396.

42. MacDonald, K. L., M. J. O'Leary, M. L. Cohen, P. Norris, J. G. Wells, E. Noll, J. M. Kobayashi, and P. A. Blake. 1988. *Escherichia coli* O157:H7: an emerging gastrointestinal pathogen: results of a one-year, prospective, population-based study. *JAMA* **259:**3567–3570.

43. Martin, P. M. V., J. Mathiot, J. Ipero, M. Kirimat, A. J. Georges, and M. C. Georges-Courbot. 1989. Immune response to *Campylobacter jejuni* and *Campylobacter coli* in a cohort of children from birth to 2 years of age. *J. Clin. Microbiol.* **57:**2542–2546.

44. Mattila, L., A. Siitonen, H. Kyronseppa, I. Simula, P. Oksanen, M. Stenvik, P. Salo, H. Peltola, and the Finnish-Moroccan Study Group. 1992. Seasonal variation in etiology of traveler's diarrhea. *J. Infect. Dis.* **165:**385–388.

45. Megraud, F., G. Boudraa, K. Bessaoud, S. Bensid, F. Dabis, R. Soltana, and M. Touhami. 1990. Incidence of *Campylobacter* infection in infants in western Algeria and the possible protective role of breast feeding. *Epidemiol. Infect.* **106:** 73–78.

45a. Megraud, F., A. M. Gavinet, and J. Camou-Junca. 1987. Serogroups and biotypes of human strains of *Campylobacter jejuni* and *Campylobacter coli* isolated in France. *Eur. J. Clin. Microbiol.* **6:** 641–645.

46. Mohran, Z. S., P. Guerry, H. Lior, J. R. Murphy, A. El-Gendy, M. M. Mikhail, and B. A. Oyofo. 1996. Restriction fragment length polymorphisms of flagellin genes of *Campylobacter jejuni* and/or *C. coli* isolates from Egypt. *J. Clin. Microbiol.* **34:**1216–1219.

47. Monos, D. S., M. Papaioakim, T. W. Ho, C. Y. Li, and G. M. McKhann. 1997. Differential distribution of HLA alleles in two forms of Guillan-Barré syndrome. *J. Infect. Dis.* **176**(Suppl. 2): S180–S182.

48. Murphy, G. S., P. Echeverria, L. R. Jackson, M. K. Arness, C. LeBron, and C. Pitarangsi. 1995. Ciprofloxacin and azithromycin-resistant *Campylobacter* causing traveler's diarrhea in U.S. troops deployed to Thailand in 1994. *Clin. Infect. Dis.* **22:**868–869.

49. Nachamkin, I., S. H. Fischer, X.-H. Yang, O. Benitez, and A. Cravioto. 1994. Immunoglobulin A antibodies directed against *Campylobacter jejuni* flagellin present in breast milk. *Epidemiol. Infect.* **112:**359–365.

50. Nishimura, M., M. Nukina, J. M. Yuan, B.

Q. Shen, J. J. Ma, M. Ohta, T. Saida, and T. Uchiyama. 1996. PCR-based restriction fragment length polymorphisms (RFLP) analysis and serotyping of *Campylobacter jejuni* isolates from diarrheic patients in China and Japan. *FEMS Microbiol. Lett.* **142:**133–138.

50a. Oberhelman, R. A. Unpublished data.

51. Oberhelman, R. A., R. H. Gilman, D. N. Taylor, R. E. Black, P. Sheen, L. Cabrera, G. Madico, and A. G. Lescano. 1999. A placebo-controlled trial of *Lactobacillus* GG to prevent diarrhea in Peruvian children. *J. Pediatr.* **134:**15–20.

52. Popovic-Uroic, T. 1989. *Campylobacter jejuni* and *Campylobacter coli* diarrhoea in rural and urban populations in Yugoslavia. *Epidemiol. Infect.* **102:** 59–67.

53. Rasrinaul, L., O. Suthienkul, P. D. Echeverria, D. N. Taylor, J. Seriwatana, and A. Bangtrakulnonth. 1988. Foods as a source of antibiotic resistant enteropathogens causing childhood diarrhea in Thailand. *Am. J. Trop. Med. Hyg.* **39:** 97–102.

54. Reinthaler, F. F., G. Feierl, D. Stunzner, and E. Marth. 1998. Diarrhea in returning Austrian tourists: epidemiology, etiology, and cost-analyses. *J. Travel Med.* **5:**65–72.

55. Richardson, N. J., H. J. Koornhoff, and V. D. Bokkenheuser. 1981. Long-term infections with *Campylobacter fetus* subsp. *jejuni*. *J. Clin. Microbiol.* **13:**846–849.

56. Ruiz-Palacios, G. M., J. J. Calva, L. K. Pickering, Y. Lopez-Vidal, P. Volkow, H. Pezzarossi, and M. S. West. 1990. Protection of breast-fed infants against *Campylobacter* diarrhea by antibodies in human milk. *J. Pediatr.* **116:** 707–713.

57. Sack, R. B., M. Rahman, M. Yunus, and E. H. Khan. 1997. Antimicrobial resistance in organisms causing diarrheal disease. *Clin. Infect. Dis.* **24**(Suppl. 1):S102–S105.

58. Saida, T., S. Kuroki, Q. Hao, M. Nishimura, M. Nukina, and H. Obayashi. 1997. *Campylobacter jejuni* isolates from Japanese patients with Guillan-Barré syndrome. *J. Infect. Dis.* **176**(Suppl. 2):S129–S134.

59. Saidi, S., Y. Iijima, W. Sang, A. K. Mwangudza, J. O. Oundo, K. Taga, M. Aihara, K. Nagyama, H. Yamamoto, P. G. Waiyaki, and T. Honda. 1997. Epidemiological study of infectious diarrheal diseases in children in a coastal rural area of Kenya. *Microbiol. Immunol.* **41:** 773–778.

60. Siitonen, A., L. Kotola, H. Kyrönseppä, P. Oksanen, B. Naouri, A. Mechbal, and H. Peltola. 1989. *Campylobacter* spp. is the leading cause of travelers' diarrhea among Finnish tourists to Morocco, abstr. 44. *In Program and Abstracts of*

the *29th Interscience Conference on Antimicrobial Agents and Chemotherapy*. American Society for Microbiology, Washington, D.C.

61. **Simango, C., and M. Nyahanana.** 1997. *Campylobacter* enteritis in children in an urban community. *Centr. Afr. Med. J.* **43:**172–175.

62. **Simor, A. E., and L. Wilcox.** 1987. Enteritis associated with *Campylobacter laridis. J. Clin. Microbiol.* **25:**10–12.

63. **Sjögren, E., G. Ruiz-Palacios, and B. Kaijser.** 1989. *Campylobacter jejuni* isolations from Mexican and Swedish patients, with repeated symptomatic and/or asymptomatic diarrhoea episodes. *Epidemiol. Infect.* **102:**47–57.

64. **Skirrow, M. B.** 1987. A demographic survey of *Campylobacter, Salmonella,* and *Shigella* infections in England. *Epidemiol. Infect.* **99:**647–657.

65. **Speelman, P., M. J. Struelens, and R. I. Glass.** 1983. Detection of *Campylobacter jejuni* and other potential pathogens in travellers' diarrhea in Bangladesh. *Scand. J. Gastroenterol.* **18**(Suppl. 84)**:**1923.

66. **Svedhem, A., and B. Kaijser.** 1980. *Campylobacter fetus* subspecies *jejuni:* a common cause of diarrhea in Sweden. *J. Infect. Dis.* **142:**353–359.

66a. **Taylor, D. N.** Unpublished data.

67. **Taylor, D. N., and M. J. Blaser.** 1991. *Campylobacter* infections, p. 151–172. *In* A. S. Evans and P. S. Brachman (ed.), *Bacterial Infections of Humans. Epidemiology and Control.* Plenum Publishing Corp., New York, N.Y.

68. **Taylor, D. N., M. J. Blaser, P. Echeverria, C. Pitarangsi, L. Bodhidatta, and W. L. L. Wang.** 1987. Erythromycin-resistant *Campylobacter* infections in Thailand. *Antimicrob. Agents Chemother.* **31:**438–442.

69. **Taylor, D. N., L. Bodhidatta, and P. Echeverria.** 1991. Epidemiologic aspects of shigellosis and other causes of dysentery in Thailand. *Rev. Infect. Dis.* **13**(Suppl. 4)**:**S226–S230.

70. **Taylor, D. N., and P. Echeverria.** 1986. The etiology and epidemiology of travelers' diarrhea in Asia. *Rev. Infect. Dis.* **8**(Suppl. 2)**:**S136–S141.

71. **Taylor, D. N., P. Echeverria, M. Blaser, C. Pitarangsi, N. R. Blacklow, J. H. Cross, and B. Weniger.** 1985. The polymicrobial etiology of travelers' diarrhea. *Lancet* **i:**381–383.

72. **Taylor, D. N., P. Echeverria, C. Pitarangsi, J. Seriwatana, L. Bodhidatta, and M. Blaser.**
1988. Influence of strain characteristics and immunity on the epidemiology of *Campylobacter* infections in Thailand. *J. Clin. Microbiol.* **26:**863–868.

73. **Taylor, D. N., P. Echeverria, O. Sethabutr, C. Pitarangsi, U. Leksomboon, N. R. Blacklow, B. Rowe, R. Gross, and J. Cross.** 1988. Clinical and microbiologic features of *Shigella* and enteroinvasive *Escherichia coli* infections detected by DNA hybridization. *J. Clin. Microbiol.* **26:**1362–1366.

74. **Taylor, D. N., R. Houston, D. R. Shlim, P. Echeverria, M. Bhaibulaya, and B. L. P. Ungar.** 1988. Etiology of diarrheal disease among travelers and foreign residents in Nepal. *JAMA* **260:**1245–1248.

75. **Taylor, D. N., J. A. Kiehlbauch, W. Tee, C. Pitarangsi, and P. Echeverria.** 1991. Isolation of group 2 aerotolerant *Campylobacter* species from Thai children with diarrhea. *J. Infect. Dis.* **163:**1062–1067.

76. **Taylor, D. N., D. M. Perlman, P. D. Echeverria, U. Lexomboon, and M. J. Blaser.** 1993. Campylobacter immunity and quantitative excretion rates in Thai children. *J. Infect. Dis.* **168:**754–758.

77. **Taylor, D. N., C. Pitarangsi, P. Echeverria, and B. M. Diniega.** 1988. *Campylobacter* enteritis during doxycycline prophylaxis for malaria in Thailand. *Lancet* **ii:**578–579. (Letter.)

78. **Taylor, D. N., J. L. Sanchez, W. Candler, S. Thornton, C. McQueen, and P. Echeverria.** 1991. Treatment of travelers' diarrhea: ciprofloxacin plus loperamide compared with ciprofloxacin alone: a placebo-controlled, randomized trial. *Ann. Intern. Med.* **114:**731–734.

79. **Tee, W., B. N. Anderson, B. C. Ross, and B. Dwyer.** 1987. Atypical campylobacters associated with gastroenteritis. *J. Clin. Microbiol.* **25:**1248–1252.

80. **Zaki, A. M., H. L. DuPont, M. A. El Alamy, R. R. Arafat, K. Amin, M. M. Awad, L. Bassiouni, I. Z. Imam, G. S. El Malih, A. El Marsafie, M. S. Mohieldin, T. Naguib, M. A. Rakha, M. Sidaros, N. Wasef, C. E. Wright, and R. G. Wyatt.** 1986. The detection of enteropathogens in acute diarrhea in a family cohort population in rural Egypt. *Am. J. Trop. Med. Hyg.* **35:**1013–1022.

CAMPYLOBACTER JEJUNI INFECTION AND THE ASSOCIATION WITH GUILLAIN-BARRÉ SYNDROME

Irving Nachamkin, Ban Mishu Allos, and Tony W. Ho

8

Campylobacter jejuni is well documented as the most common cause of bacterial gastroenteritis in the United States and other developed countries, but only during the past decade has there been increasing evidence that *C. jejuni* is an important factor in the development of Guillain-Barré syndrome (GBS). Since the early 1980s, numerous case reports and series have been published supporting the role of *C. jejuni* as a cause of GBS. Further insights into the mechanisms by which *C. jejuni* might cause GBS have come to light in the past few years as well. This chapter summarizes our current understanding of the clinical, epidemiologic, and pathogenesis aspects of *Campylobacter* and GBS.

GUILLAIN-BARRÉ SYNDROME

In 1916, Guillain, Barré, and Strohl described a syndrome defined clinically by flaccid paralysis, areflexia, and albuminocytological dissociation in the spinal fluid (52). This syndrome, GBS, is an autoimmune-mediated disorder of the peripheral nervous system. With the virtual elimination of poliomyelitis, the most common cause of acute flaccid paralysis is now GBS. Affected persons rapidly develop weakness of the limbs and of the respiratory muscles and areflexia. Cerebrospinal fluid examination reveals an elevation of protein levels without an increase in the number of cells. The disease is self-limited, with muscle strength usually reaching a nadir within 2 to 3 weeks, followed by partial or complete recovery over weeks to months (2).

Although most people have an uneventful recovery, a significant proportion of patients may require mechanical ventilation (83, 131, 173) and 15 to 20% may have severe neurologic deficits (7, 20, 28, 53, 134, 138, 172). Mortality rates of GBS have been reduced to 2 to 3% in the developed world but remain higher elsewhere in the world (31, 173). GBS remains a major public health burden, despite two beneficial treatments: plasmapheresis and intravenous immunoglobulin (40, 53, 124, 167).

The hallmark study by Asbury and colleagues nearly 30 years ago identified lymphocytic infiltration and macrophage-mediated demyelination as characteristic features of the early pathology (7, 60, 127, 128). Thus, the clinical term "GBS" has often been used inter-

Irving Nachamkin, Department of Pathology and Laboratory Medicine, University of Pennsylvania School of Medicine, Philadelphia, PA 19104-4283. *Ban Mishu Allos,* Department of Medicine, Division of Infectious Diseases, Vanderbilt University School of Medicine, Nashville, TN 37232-2605. *Tony W. Ho,* Department of Neurology, Johns Hopkins University School of Medicine, Baltimore, MD 21287-7609.

Campylobacter, 2nd Ed., Edited by I. Nachamkin and M. J. Blaser
© 2000 American Society for Microbiology, Washington, D.C.

changeably with the pathologic term "acute inflammatory demyelinating polyneuropathy" (AIDP). In severe cases, axonal degeneration may accompany the demyelination (7, 60). However, recent studies have shown that GBS is a diverse disorder that can be divided into several patterns (65, 89, 101, 102, 133, 152, 163). The most frequent pattern of GBS in Europe and North America continues to be AIDP. However, axonal patterns, in which axons appear to be the target of immune system attack, are common in China (65, 101, 102, 175), Japan (89, 152), Mexico (54, 130), and other regions of the world, even though they are not frequently encountered in North America and Europe.

Two patterns of predominantly axonal involvement can be distinguished. The first pattern resembles the "axonal GBS" cases initially described by Feasby et al. and more recently termed acute motor-sensory axonal neuropathy (AMSAN) (35–38). The second pattern has a nearly pure motor axonal involvement, a pattern termed acute motor axonal neuropathy (AMAN) (65, 101, 102). A final related disorder, Fisher's syndrome, is characterized by acute onset of ataxia (unsteadiness of gait), areflexia (loss of reflexes), and ophthalmoplegia (an inability to move the eyes) and is usually associated with nonreactive pupils (39). A suggested physiological and pathological classification of GBS by Griffin et al. (48) is shown in Fig. 1. The different clinical, electrophysiological, and serological manifestations of these GBS subtypes suggest that there are different targets of immune system attacks.

EPIDEMIOLOGY OF GBS

GBS, as clinically defined, ranges in incidence from 0.4 to 4.0 cases per 100,000 population (median, 1.3/100,000) (16, 68). Seasonal variation of GBS is not usually observed in developed countries; however, summertime peaks do occur in China and perhaps in Mexico, Spain, and Korea (65, 101, 102, 130, 164, 165). Summertime peaks in northern China are largely attributed to the AMAN form of GBS (65, 101). GBS is, with rare exceptions, a sporadic illness, but outbreaks have been reported (19, 79). In an outbreak of gastroenteritis affecting over 5,000 individuals, 16 people developed GBS (80, 151).

GBS occurs more commonly in males than in females, and in the United States it may be slightly more common in whites than in blacks (67, 69). GBS occurs in patients of all ages, and the incidence appears to increase with age. Some studies have shown an early peak among

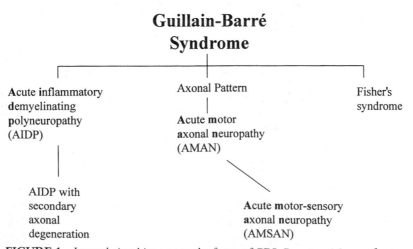

FIGURE 1 Interrelationships among the forms of GBS. Reprinted from reference 64 with permission.

persons 15 to 30 years old, and suggesting a possible bimodal distribution of cases (33, 148). In developed countries, AIDP appears to affect an older population whereas in northern China, AMAN affect primarily children and young adults (101).

C. jejuni Infection and the Link to GBS

The occurrence of an infectious illness preceding GBS, primary viral respiratory disease, has been known for a century (32, 43, 68, 120, 145, 162, 164). Diarrheal illness preceding GBS in up to 20% of patients was recognized several decades ago (23). Rhodes and Tattersfield reported the first case of *Campylobacter* infection preceding GBS in 1982 (136). Following this case report, numerous reports described patients who developed GBS following infection with *C. jejuni* (29, 107, 129, 153, 174). A number of important observations were apparent from these initial reports. It appeared that male GBS patients outnumbered females by 3 to 1 (104). GBS following *Campylobacter* infection appeared to be more severe and more likely to involve axonal injury (29, 107, 136, 138, 184).

Serologic studies of patients with GBS for evidence of *Campylobacter* infection have played an important role in understanding the pathogenesis of GBS. Isolation of *Campylobacter* from stool samples of patients with GBS is difficult, since the median period of excretion of *Campylobacter* in stools of infected persons is only 16 days (157). Thus, GBS patients frequently have negative stool cultures because of the 1- to 3-week lag time between infection and the onset of GBS. Because of the limitations of culture techniques, serologic studies in combination with cultures and clinical histories are useful in identifying patients likely to have had a previous *Campylobacter* infection (104).

Numerous antibody assays for detecting isotype-specific antibodies have been developed, but there are no standards for serologic testing, with regard to either the antigens used or the end points for positivity (17, 61, 77, 90, 99, 115, 176). Enzyme-linked immunosorbent assay appears to be the most commonly used method to measure antibody levels in serum (17, 61, 105, 114). Protein extracts containing surface proteins with cross-reactive epitopes of *Campylobacter* are commonly used in antibody assays and are not serotype specific. In general, a high prevalence of serum antibodies against *Campylobacter* can be found in patients with GBS (14, 51, 65, 74, 78, 82, 87, 139, 154, 172).

Gruenwald et al. found that 3 (18%) of 17 patients in an uncontrolled population with GBS had elevated antibody titers in two or more immunoglobulin classes (51). Winer et al. found that 14% of 99 patients with GBS had positive *C. jejuni* serologic tests, compared to only 2% of controls (172). In a nonblinded study of 56 GBS patients and 57 controls, Kaldor and Speed found that 38% of the patients and none of the controls met their criteria for positive serologic responses (78). In a blinded case-control study by Mishu et al., 36% of GBS patients were seropositive for *Campylobacter* and GBS patients were more than five times as likely to have serologic evidence of recent *Campylobacter* infection than were the controls (105). In a study of GBS patients in Japan, 36% of patients were seropositive (87). Ho et al. showed that *Campylobacter* infections were common in both AMAN and AIDP patients in a prospective study conducted in northern China (65). Depending on the definition of seropositivity, the number of patients with positive results ranged from 24 to 76% for AMAN patients.

Despite the difficulties in isolating *Campylobacter* from GBS patients, several investigators have succeeded in isolating *C. jejuni* from the stools of patients with GBS at the onset of their neurologic symptoms (Table 1). Determining the isolation rate of *Campylobacter* from GBS patients is difficult because there are few prospective studies. In a study by Kuroki et al. (87), 30% of GBS patients had positive stool cultures, but in a prospective study in England, only 8% of patients had positive cultures (133). An uncontrolled study by Ropper recovered *Campylobacter* organisms from 4 (44.4%) of 9 patients with diarrhea preceding GBS (139).

TABLE 1 Isolation of *C. jejuni* from patients with GBS

Study	Country	Yr	No. of patients	% with positive cultures
Speed et al. (154)	Australia	1987	4	25
Ropper (139)	United States	1988	9	44
Gruenwald et al. (51)	United States	1991	4	50
Kuroki et al. (87)	Japan	1993	46	30
Enders et al. (34)	Germany	1994	26	15
Rees et al. (133)	England	1995	100	8
Hariharan et al. (57)	India	1996	8	38
Goddard et al. (44)	South Africa	1997	14	64
Gregson et al. (47)	England	1997	103	6
Sheikh et al. (149)	China	1998	90	6
Ohtsuka et al. (118)	Japan	1998	4[a]	100
Hao et al. (56)	Japan	1998	76	17

[a] Four consecutive cases of Fisher syndrome.

It appears that 8 to 50% of GBS patients had *Campylobacter* cultured from their stools very soon after the onset of neurologic symptoms, based on various reports (51, 87, 133, 139, 153). Culture and serologic data showed that approximately 30 to 40% of patients with GBS have evidence of preceding *Campylobacter* infection, but this may be an underestimate.

C. jejuni appears to be the most common species identified from patients with GBS. *C. upsaliensis* was recently recovered from a U.S. patient with AMAN (62), suggesting that other *Campylobacter* species may be involved in GBS.

CAMPYLOBACTER SEROTYPES AND GBS

The epidemiology of *Campylobacter*-associated GBS could not have been determined without the use of typing systems. O serotyping (123) has been especially important in linking particular types with GBS. The Penner O serotyping scheme (123) detects 60 types of *C. jejuni* and *C. colt* (121) and is based on detection of lipopolysaccharide (LPS) antigens.

Using O serotyping, Kuroki et al. solidified the association of *Campylobacter* and GBS in a prospective study of 46 GBS patients (87). In that study conducted in Japan, *C. jejuni* was isolated from 14 (30.4%) of 46 GBS patients compared with only 6 (1.2%) of 503 persons in a healthy control population. Of 12 GBS-associated strains characterized by O serotyping, 10 (83%) were serotype O:19. When 1,150 enteritis-associated isolates of *C. jejuni* were serotyped, only 1.7% were of this serotype. Yuki et al. also found that serotype O:19 strains were overrepresented in GBS patients, accounting for 52% of 31 GBS-associated strains but only in 5% of 215 control isolates (180). Another serotype, O:2, was also found to be overrepresented in patients with Miller-Fisher syndrome (it was found in 71% patients versus 38% of controls), although only seven patients were studied (180). More recently, O:19 was found to be an important serotype in patients with AMAN in northern China (149) and in Mexico City (115a).

Although O:19 is an important serotype involved in GBS, other O serotypes have been isolated from these patients. Of particular note is the isolation of O:41 strains from GBS patients in South Africa (44, 92). Of 14 children admitted to a Cape Town hospital with GBS, 9 had positive stool cultures for *C. jejuni* and 6 of the 9 isolates were serotype O:41 (biotype 2) (44). This particular serotype had been identified in only 0.1% of enteritis strains isolated over a 19-year period.

Serotypes that occur frequently as a cause of diarrheal disease also have been isolated from GBS patients and include O:1, O:2, O:4, O:4 complex, O:5, O:10, O:16, O:23, O:37, O:44, and O:64 (8, 73, 87, 133, 144, 149, 180, 182, 183).

O:19 serotypes do cause uncomplicated diarrheal illness in approximately 1 to 6% of patients (3, 42, 76, 103). Laboratory animals including dogs, cats, and primates have also harbored this serotype (160). Outbreaks of *Campylobacter* infection where O:19 serotypes have been implicated have been reported (76, 122); however, only one patient whose case was associated with O:19 developed GBS (143).

Risk of Developing GBS after *C. jejuni* Infection

C. jejuni infections are quite common in the general population, but the risk of developing GBS following infection is low. The incidence of *C. jejuni* infection is approximately 1,000 per 100,000 population per year (158). In 1995, the National Center for Health Statistics Hospital Discharge data documented 7,874 GBS cases in the United States. Assuming that the U.S. population is 250 million and that 30% of GBS cases are preceded by *C. jejuni*, approximately 1 case of GBS occurs per 1,058 cases of *C. jejuni* infection.

The risk of developing GBS following infection with *C. jejuni* O:19 is difficult to establish but may be higher. Over 80% of *C. jejuni* organisms isolated from GBS patients in Japan were O:19, but this serotype accounted for only 2% of isolates from patients with enteritis (87). In northern China, serotype O:19 accounted for three of seven isolates from GBS patients (149). Two of seven GBS-associated *Campylobacter* isolates were serotype O:19 in a U.S. study (106). None of four isolates from GBS patients in a British study were O:19 (133). If 20% of GBS-associated *C. jejuni* isolates are serotype O:19, it is estimated that one case of GBS will occur for every 158 infections with serotype O:19.

Severity of GBS after *Campylobacter* Infection

GBS following *Campylobacter* infection may be more severe than GBS following other inciting events. Thirty percent of patients with evidence of prior *Campylobacter* infection, compared with no patients without evidence of prior *Campylobacter* infection, had severe disease in a study by Vriesendorp et al. (170). "Severe" was defined as fulminating disease with quadriplegia and ventilatory dependence within 24 to 48 h of onset. Rees et al. found that 23% of patients with evidence of *Campylobacter* infection were unable to walk unassisted one year after the onset of symptoms (133). In GBS patients without prior *Campylobacter* infection, only 9% were unable to walk unassisted after 1 year. Over half of GBS patients in a Dutch study (14 of 24 patients) treated with plasmapheresis were unable to walk unassisted 6 months after developing GBS, compared with 12% of patients without evidence of *Campylobacter* infection infection (75). Thus, these studies suggest that *Campylobacter* infection induces more severe disease in GBS patients than do other putative causes. Larger prospective studies that define GBS according to clinical and electrophysiological criteria are needed to clarify this issue.

PATHOGENESIS OF GBS

Peripheral nerves are composed of motor and sensory nerve fibers. The motor fibers originate from motor neurons in the ventral horns of the spinal cord and carry nerve impulses to the muscles. The sensory fibers carry nerve impulses from the specialized sensory receptors in the periphery to the spinal cord. Their cell bodies reside in the dorsal root ganglia next to the spinal cord. To speed the conduction of the nerve impulses, insulating layers of myelin formed by Schwann cells are wrapped around some of these fibers. Between two adjacent myelin sheaths is the node of Ranvier, a gap where sodium channels are concentrated and nerve impulses are regenerated. The myelin sheaths prevent impulses from leaking away and allow impulses to jump from one node to the next up to 75 m/s.

Access to the peripheral nervous system by the immune system requires penetration of the blood-nerve barrier. Specialized endothelial cells line the endoneurium blood vessels. The lumens of these vessels are heavily glycosylated with negatively charged, sialic acid–containing glycoconjugates (94, 125). They form the first part of the blood-nerve barrier and repel negatively charged molecules (94, 125). The tight junctions between endothelial cells from the next part of the blood-nerve barrier. The entry of molecules around the nerve is further limited by the perineurium, which consists of layers of specialized fibroblasts bounded by a basal lamina in each layer with tight junctions between adjacent perineurial cells. However, the blood-nerve barrier is not as "tight" as the blood-brain barrier; consequently, small amounts of circulating proteins such as albumin, immunoglobulin G (IgG), and exogenously administered horseradish peroxidase (100), none of which can enter the central nervous system, can gain entrance to the endoneurial space (6). This relative leakiness may render the PNS more vulnerable than the CNS to antibody-mediated disorders. The blood-nerve barrier is particularly leaky within the dorsal root ganglia and is altogether absent at nerve terminals in the periphery (for example, at the neuromuscular junction), making these areas especially vulnerable to immune system-mediated attacks.

AIDP

Patients with AIDP present with flaccid paralysis, areflexia, and usually some sensory loss. Electrophysiologic testing suggests that demyelination has occurred in both motor and sensory nerves (41, 62, 175). Pathologically, macrophage-mediated demyelination and lymphocytic infiltrates are evident (7, 49). AIDP has long been presumed to be a T-cell-mediated disorder, based on the lymphocytic inflammation found in many patients (7) and on the analogy to experimental allergic neuritis (EAN) (for reviews, see references 5, 58, and 59). Many markers of T-cell activation can be detected in the serum of AIDP patients, including soluble interleukin-2 receptor and gamma interferon (13). However, several lines of evidence have suggested the importance of anti-body-mediated nerve fiber damage in AIDP; these include the response to plasmapheresis (40, 161), the presence of anti-myelin antibodies by complement activation assays (85, 86), the frequent presence of anti-glycoconjugate antibodies, and the demonstration of demyelinating immunoglobulins in sera by either intraneural injection (156) or incubation with nerve or Schwann cells in vitro (15, 85, 146, 147).

The immunopathology of early AIDP showed lymphocytic inflammation and complete demyelination (49, 55) (Fig. 2). Complement activation products (C3d and the membrane attack complex C5b-9) can be seen diffusely on the outermost surface of the Schwann cell (Fig. 2A). This suggests that the target of attack is on the Schwann cell surface (55). Electron microscopy showed that most of these fibers had early vesicular changes in the myelin sheaths, usually beginning in the outer lamellae of the sheath (Fig. 2B). A model for the pathogenesis of AIDP is that an antibody directed against antigens on the outermost surface of the Schwann cell (the abaxonal Schwann cell plasmalemma) binds complement which results in sublytic complement activation and the development of transmembrane pores formed by complement. The resulting entry of calcium might be sufficient to activate calcium-sensitive enzymes, potentially including phospholipase A_2 and proteases capable of degrading myelin proteins. Macrophages then participate in the removal of damaged myelin (Fig. 2C and D) (127).

The nature of the antigen on the abaxonal Schwann cell plasmalemma that may be involved in AIDP is uncertain, but it is likely to be a glycolipid (70, 71). Recent studies by Kusunoki et al. (88) suggest that galactocerebroside could be such an antigen in at least some cases. It is likely that other immune system mechanisms operate in others. In Chinese patients, the chief role of T cells may be to breach the blood-nerve barrier (126), but in some cases demyelination may be more directly T-cell mediated and comparable to that in EAN.

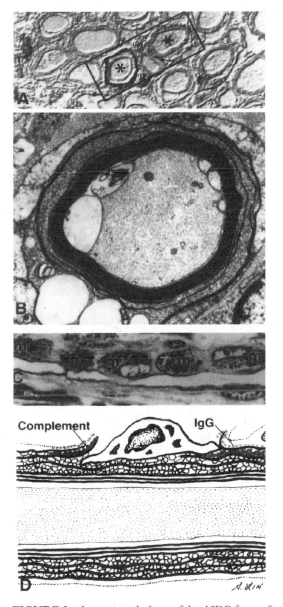

FIGURE 2 Immunopathology of the AIDP form of GBS. (A) Nerve fiber stained with markers of complement activation C3d on the outermost surface of the Schwann cell. (B) Electron micrograph showing early vesicular changes in the myelin sheath. (C) Macrophages participate in the removal of damaged myelin. (D) Cartoon of the overall process. Reprinted from reference 64 with permission.

AMAN

More recently, another pattern of GBS, purely motor by clinical and electrodiagnostic findings and termed AMAN, has been identified (49, 50, 65, 101) and can usually be distinguished from other forms of GBS (65). AMAN is characterized by weakness or paralysis without sensory loss. Electrodiagnostic data suggest that motor fibers can be lost selectively while sensory nerve fibers are preserved, and features of demyelination are absent (65, 101).

The clinical features of the AMAN pattern have largely been established by studies in northern China. Every summer, hundreds of children and young adults with GBS inundate the hospitals of northern China. Over 70% of GBS patients studied at one hospital, the Second Teaching Hospital in Shijiazhuang, showed the clinical and electrodiagnostic picture of AMAN (65, 101). It is now clear that the AMAN pattern of GBS occurs frequently in other parts of Asia (27) but less often in North America (63, 72) and Europe. The AMAN pattern is closely associated with antecedent *Campylobacter* infection (65, 132, 133, 184) and the presence of IgG anti-GD1a antibody (66).

In these axonal patterns, lymphocytic infiltration is usually absent or scanty (36, 38, 49, 101). The earliest identifiable change is found in the nodes of Ranvier of motor fibers (50, 54). The nodal gap lengthens at a time when the fibers appear otherwise normal. Immunopathologically, this change correlates with the binding of IgG and the activation of complement, as reflected by the presence of the complement activation marker C3d on those nodes of Ranvier (Fig. 3A) (54). Also, in these early cases, macrophages are recruited to the nodes of Ranvier (Fig. 3B) (50, 54), perhaps as a result of the elaboration of C5a and other chemoattractants. These macrophages insert processes into the nodal gap, penetrate the overlying basal lamina of the Schwann cell (50), and then encircle the node. They frequently dissect beneath the myelin sheath attachment sites of the paranode and enter the periaxonal space of the internode (Fig. 3C and D).

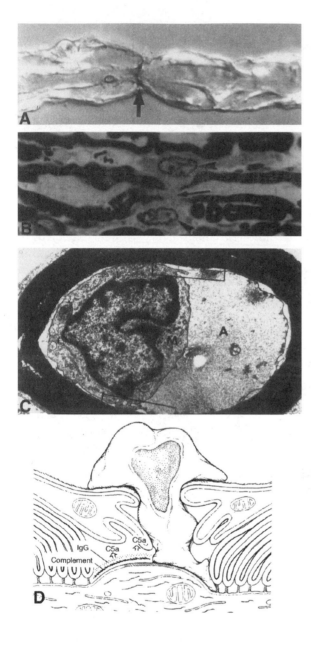

FIGURE 3 Immunopathology of the AMAN form of GBS. (A) Immunostaining of a nerve fiber, showing the presence of C3d on the node of Ranvier. (B) Macrophage recruitment to the node and insertion into the nodal gap. (C) Electron micrograph showing a macrophage surrounding the axon in the periaxonal space without damage to the myelin. (D) Cartoon depicting the entire process. Reprinted from reference 64 with permission.

Many fibers express complement activation markers in the periaxonal space—that is, the 11-nm space between the axolemma and the Schwann cell. Normally, this periaxonal space is extremely regular in its spacing, and it is sealed from both ions and macromolecules of the endoneurial fluid by junctional complexes between the myelin terminal loops and the axolemma. The intrusion of the macrophage probably opens the periaxonal space to endoneurial constituents and allows the antibody and complement to enter the internodal region. Immunocytochemical studies have demonstrated that the antigen to which IgG binds is on the axolemma (as it is in the node of Ranvier). As the macrophages invade the periaxonal space, the axon collapses away from the Schwann cell, resulting in a marked dilatation of the periaxonal space (50). However, most of the axon evidently survives for some period, even though it is surrounded by macrophages. The end stage of this process occurs when motor axons interrupt and degenerate, extending as far up as the ventral root exit zone (49, 101).

Fisher Syndrome

Fisher syndrome, characterized by ataxia, ophthalmoparesis, and areflexia, is usually accompanied by serum antibodies that recognize the ganglioside GQ1b (26, 171, 179). Recent studies have shown that these anti-GQ1b antibodies can alter synaptic release at motor nerve terminals (21, 137). This result at first seems anomalous, since weakness is not a feature of Fisher syndrome; however, this finding suggests that a small amount of antigen is present even in motor nerve terminals of somatic musculature and that the anti-ganglioside antibody can block normal quantal release. The population of motor fibers most heavily enriched in GQ1b-reactive antigens is the oculomotor fibers, i.e., the fibers whose function is affected in Fisher syndrome (25). Whether the ataxia is due to sensory abnormalities with loss of proprioception (sensory ataxia) or to cerebellar disease (cerebellar ataxia) remains controversial, but anti-GQ1b antibodies are known to stain both sensory neurons in the dorsal root ganglia and a population of cerebellar neurons (179).

GLYCOCONJUGATES AND GBS

Gangliosides are negatively charged glycoconjugates of the plasma membrane, whose oligosaccharides are oriented toward the extracellular space. Gangliosides are the major surface molecules in both the PNS and CNS (109). They are synthesized in neuronal somata and are actively transported to specific sites of enrichment, such as the synapses and the nodes of Ranvier. Many anti-glycoconjugate antibodies have been described in GBS patients. A detailed discussion on antiganglioside antibodies in GBS can be found in chapter 13.

The strongest association is between Fisher syndrome and IgG anti-GQ1b (26, 171, 179).

However, in AIDP and AMAN, the association with anti-glycoconjugate antibodies has varied from report to report (132). Tissue-bound GM1 was proposed as a possible target in GBS, especially in the axonal form (84), but Enders et al. and Vriesendorp et al. found no correlation between anti-GM1 antibodies and GBS subtypes as determined electrophysiologically (34, 170). Rees and colleagues detected IgG anti-GM1 antibodies in 25% of their AIDP cases versus 57% of their AMAN and AMSAN cases ($p = 0.07$) (34, 46, 84, 132, 168, 170, 184). One reason for the confusion is that most of these studies have involved GBS populations composed mostly, if not exclusively, of AIDP patients.

Recently, a prospective study by Ho et al. of GBS patients consisting of both AMAN and AIDP patients showed that IgG anti-GD1a was a specific marker for AMAN, being present in 60% of AMAN patients but in only 4% of AIDP patients (66). Although anti-GM1 antibodies are more common in GBS patients than non-GBS controls, there was no significant difference between AMAN and AIDP patients (57 and 35%). The study suggests that the IgG anti-GD1a antibody may be important in the pathogenesis of AMAN and that anti-GM1 antibodies are only modestly correlated with different subtypes of GBS.

An important issue in evaluating the possible role of anti-glycoconjugate antibodies in GBS is whether appropriate antigens are at the sites of known antibody bindings in nerve fibers. Localization of different gangliosides can be determined by using toxins and lectins that have high specificity toward different oligosaccharides epitopes. Cholera toxin, which has a high affinity to the GM1 epitope, binds to the nodes of Ranvier and paranodes, including the paranodal Schwann cell (30, 149). Peanut agglutinin, which has high affinity to asialo-GM1, binds only to the nodes of Ranvier (4, 149). Tetanus toxin, which binds to the B-series gangliosides (disialosyl gangliosides, e.g., GT1b and GD1b), shows binding to both nodal and internodal axons (149). With regard to the predominantly motor involvement in AMAN cases, it is noteworthy that Ogawa-Goto and Nagashima et al. found that motor nerve myelin contained abundant GM1 (15% of total gangliosides) whereas sensory nerve myelin contained only trace amounts (117). GT1b and possibly GD1a also appear to be concentrated on the axolemma and may act as ligands for the myelin-associated glycoprotein. Myelin-associated glycoprotein is concentrated on the Schwann cell adaxonal surface (177) and has been postulated to bind to axonal GT1b or GD1a in the periaxonal space.

MOLECULAR MIMICRY AND GBS

Certain O serotypes of *C. jejuni* contain LPS outer core structures that are identical to a number of different glycoshingolipids of the ganglioside group (see chapter 12 by Moran and colleagues for detailed structures). Studies by several groups showed that serotype O:19, in particular, had structural similarity to ganglioside GM1 (181) as well as to GD1a, GT1a, and GD3 (10). The repeating O-antigenic region from serotype O:19 and O:19 strains from two patients with GBS has been deduced as well and contains a disaccharide repeating unit similar to that in hyaluronic acid (9). Other O serotypes such as O:1, O:23, and O:36 show structural similarity to GM2, and serotype O:4 shows similarity to that of GD1a (12). The type strain of O:2 does not show similarity to any known glycolipid (11). Similarly, the type strain of O:3 does not show ganglioside mimicry (110). Ganglioside-like epitopes have also been found in isolates of *C. jejuni* by using toxin binding and immunochemical analysis (8, 73, 113, 119, 178–180, 182, 183). The molecular basis for these ganglioside-like epitopes is only now beginning to be studied. For a detailed summary of the molecular analysis of LPS genes in *C. jejuni,* see chapter 19.

Several lines of evidence support the hypothesis that *Campylobacter* is involved in the pathogenesis of GBS. Certain O serotypes of *C. jejuni* contain ganglioside-like epitopes in the LPS outer core moiety, such as GM1, GD1a, and GQ1b. Some patients with GBS produce antibodies against gangliosides, and relevant gangliosides are present on peripheral nerve fibers.

Specific anti-ganglioside antibodies have been associated with different forms of GBS (e.g., GQ1b with Fisher syndrome and IgG anti-GD1a with AMAN), and *C. jejuni* is associated with all three major forms of GBS. Based on this information, one would expect that *C. jejuni* associated with different forms of GBS would express the appropriate epitope in its LPS core structure. However, the limited number of GBS-associated *C. jejuni* strains that have been characterized have shown much wider variation.

Ganglioside-like epitopes have been found not only in GBS-associated *C. jejuni* strains but also in strains isolated from patients with uncomplicated enteritis (113, 116, 142, 149). Recent studies on U.S. enteritis strains showed that a significant proportion of isolates are positive for GM1-like epitopes, but that serotypes that have been associated with GBS were more likely to be positive for GM1-like epitopes than were other O serotypes (113). LPS from GBS-associated *C. jejuni* strains also mimics multiple ganglioside-like epitopes within a single strain (8, 182). Because *C. jejuni* LPS is capable of expressing different ganglioside-like structures, one might expect patients to develop mixed features characteristic of AIDP, AMAN, and/or Fisher syndrome. Indeed, some patients present with typical features of AMAN and may go on to develop tetraparesis with demyelinating electrophysiology. Furthermore, a recent study by Lu et al. found both demyelination (a prominent feature of AIDP) and periaxonal macrophages (a prominent feature of AMAN) in a sural nerve biopsy specimen, suggesting possible concurrent attack against both the myelin and the axon (96).

HOST FACTORS

Several observations point out the importance of host factors in the pathogenesis of GBS. First, some *C. jejuni* strains isolated from diarrhea patients contain GM1 ganglioside-like epitopes, yet these patients do not develop anti-ganglioside antibodies (149). Second,

GBS is a sporadic disease and is rarely found in two people within the same family or even in the same village. However, a number of individuals have a second attack, often years after their first episode. Finally, although *C. jejuni* LPS may exhibit mimicry of multiple ganglioside-like epitopes, why do some people develop one form of GBS?

Preliminary studies of the HLA typing of patients with AMAN and AIDP indicate that certain HLA alleles are overrepresented in AMAN and AIDP cases compared to controls (108). A similar finding has been reported in England by Rees et al., who found that 83% of *C. jejuni*-positive GBS patients had HLA DQB1*03 compared with 49% of *C. jejuni*-negative GBS patients ($P = 0.05$) (135). Koga et al. also found an association of HLA-B54 and Cw1 in patients with GBS and Fisher's syndrome (81). Ma et al. recently found that a significantly higher frequency of the 100-bp tumor necrosis factor (TNF-α2) allele of the TNF-α microsatellite marker, which is associated with high TNF-α production, existed in *C. jejuni*-positive GBS patients than in controls, suggesting the involvement of a genetic predisposition to high TNF-α secretion in the development of *C. jejuni*-related GBS (97).

Other investigators have studied HLA molecules in patients with GBS (1, 91, 93, 98, 135, 155). Ma et al. (98) did not find statistically significant differences in HLA DRB1 or DQB1 alleles in Japanese patients with GBS, although there was a slight increased frequency of DRB1*0803 in patients with *C. jejuni*-associated GBS. Chiba et al. (24) were unable to find HLA class I associations in patients with GBS or Miller-Fisher syndrome; however, insensitive serologic analyses for class I (A, B, C) and class II (DR, DQ) were performed. Yuki et al. (179) demonstrated an increased frequency of HLA-B35 in patients with GBS following *Campylobacter* infection; only five patients were studied. In a more recent study by Yuki et al. (180), the level of B35 was only slightly increased in GBS patients (21%) versus controls (13.9%). Gorodezky et al. (45) suggested a possible association of GBS with DR3 in Mexican patients.

ANIMAL MODELS

Experimental allergic neuritis is a T-cell-mediated disease in Lewis rats, and is considered to be the in vivo model of GBS (140). Injection of Lewis rats with proteins or peptides derived from myelin of the peripheral nervous system induces primarily a T-cell-mediated disease with pathologic features of GBS (demyelination). The model has not, however, been found to be an animal model for *Campylobacter*-induced GBS (141, 169).

Several patients in both China and Mexico have reported paralyzed chickens, dogs, or pigs on the family farm at the same time the patients developed paralysis (66a). Autopsies of these animals revealed a pathology similar to that of human AMAN cases. Based on these observations, Li et al. used a *C. jejuni* isolate from a patient with AMAN to develop an animal model of AMAN. Chickens infected with this isolate via the oral route developed paralysis. Examination of their nerves showed Wallerian-like degeneration similar to that seen in the human form of the disease (95). These preliminary studies indicate that an animal model of AMAN can be developed by using the specific strain of *C. jejuni*. Two unanswered questions are the specific targets of immune system attack on the nerve fibers and the biochemical identities of the target antigens.

THERAPY

The major reduction of mortality in GBS has been due to advances in supportive care of critically ill patients. However, an increased understanding of the immunologic basis of GBS over the past 15 years has allowed us to change the natural course of this disease. Plasmapheresis was the first therapy shown to be effective in speeding recovery (40, 161). In this procedure, a patient's blood is removed and centrifuged to separate the cellular and plasma components, and the cellular components are then reinfused into the patient. The therapeutic effect is presumably due to the removal of inciting circulating factors such as antibodies. Another effective therapy is intravenous human immunoglobulins. There have been two controlled studies showing that intravenous immunoglobulin is as effective as plasmapheresis in the treatment of GBS (124, 167). The mechanism of action of infused immunoglobulin is not clear, but one possibility is that pooled immunoglobulins contain anti-idiotypic antibodies that inactivate the disease-specific antibodies.

MICROBIOLOGIC DIAGNOSTIC CONSIDERATIONS

Details for the isolation and identification of *C. jejuni* and other species are discussed in chapter 3. Isolation of *Campylobacter* from patients with GBS will depend strongly upon the methods used, as well as whether the patient has been given antimicrobial therapy for a previous illness. Antimicrobial agents, including the fluoroquinolones and macrolides, commonly used for treating diarrheal disease have excellent activity against *Campylobacter* species. Such agents quickly clear *Campylobacter* organisms from the gastrointestinal tract, making the isolation of *Campylobacter* nearly impossible. Other antimicrobial agents used to treat seemingly unrelated illnesses may also affect the recovery of *Campylobacter* species. It is important, therefore, to elicit a history of antimicrobial use from patients with GBS, since this will have a marked impact on culture results (112).

For optimal isolation of *Campylobacter* from patients with GBS, multiple stool samples should be obtained for increased sensitivity (87, 150, 166). Only one study of GBS patients has examined this issue. Kuroki et al. (87) found that for 14 patients with GBS with positive stool cultures, culture of one stool sample detected 57%, culture of two samples detected 93% and culture of three samples detected all patients. Thus, multiple stool samples (or rectal swabs) should be obtained from GBS patients immediately upon admission to the hospital, preferably three over a 3-day period. The samples should be transported to the laboratory in a suitable transport medium such as Cary-Blair medium. Both direct-plating and enrichment methods should be used (111, 112).

Enrichment culture methods are designed to isolate *Campylobacter* organisms from samples containing small numbers of organisms. In cases of *Campylobacter*-associated GBS, we presume that the level of *Campylobacter* in the stool, if present, is likely to be lower than the concentration during the acute diarrheal illness. Thus, enrichment cultures should be included among the laboratory tests for patients with GBS. A study by Taylor et al. (159) clearly showed that enrichment cultures dramatically improved the yield of *Campylobacter* organisms when most GBS patients would be seen. An increase of as much as 31% over conventional plating techniques was seen when samples were cultured more than 20 days after the onset of the diarrheal illness. A number of enrichment culture media can be used. In our studies in northern China and elsewhere, we have had good success with Preston enrichment broth (18).

CONCLUSIONS

With the delineation of an association between *C. jejuni* and GBS, it may be possible to decrease the incidence of GBS in the future. Since poultry is one of the major sources for human infection, elimination of *C. jejuni* from poultry will result not only in a decreased incidence of *Campylobacter* enteritis but also in a decrease in the sequelae of infection. In addition, better public health measures, such as a clean water supply, hand washing, and improved handling and cooking of poultry, may help prevent the spread of *C. jejuni* to humans. The cost associated with *Campylobacter*-induced GBS is staggering, estimated to be as high as $420 million in the United States alone (22).

Based on serologic and culture evidence, the association of *Campylobacter* with the development of Guillain-Barré syndrome now appears firmly established. However, much work remains to determine how *Campylobacter* can induce this disease. A recent consensus meeting on *Campylobacter* and GBS was conducted by the National Institutes of Health and outlined several areas of research (91) for the future.

REFERENCES

1. **Adams, D., J. D. Gibson, P. K. Thomas, J. R. Batchelor, R. A. Hughes, L. Kennedy, H. Festenstein, and J. Sachs.** 1977. HLA antigens in Guillain-Barré syndrome. *Lancet* **ii:** 504–505.

2. **Adams, R. D. and M. Victor.** 1993. Diseases of the peripheral nerves, p. 1117–1169. *In* R. D. Adams and M. Victor (ed.), *Principles of Neurology.* McGraw-Hill, Inc, New York, N.Y.

3. **Albert, M. J., A. Leach, V. Asche, J. Hennessy, and J. L. Penner.** 1992. Serotype distribution of *Campylobacter jejuni* and *Campylobacter coli* isolated from hospitalized patients with diarrhea in Central Australia. *J. Clin. Microbiol.* **30:** 207–210.

4. **Apostolski, S., S. A. Sadiq, A. Hays, M. Corbo, L. Suturkova-Milosevic, P. Chaliff, K. Stefansson, R. G. LeBaron, E. Ruoslahti, A. P. Hays, and N. Latov.** 1994. Identification of Gal(β1-3)GalNAc bearing glycoproteins at the nodes of Ranvier in peripheral nerve. *J. Neurosci. Res.* **38:**134–141.

5. **Arnason, B. G. W., and B. Soliven.** 1993. Acute inflammatory demyelinating polyradiculopathy, p 1437–1497. *In* P. J. Dyck, P. K. Thomas, J. W. Griffin, P. A. Low, and J. F. Poduslo (ed.), *Peripheral Neuropathy.* The W. B. Saunders Co., Philadelphia, Pa.

6. **Arvidson, B.** 1977. Cellular uptake of exogenous horseradish peroxidase in mouse peripheral nerve. *Acta Neuropathol.* **37:**35–41.

7. **Asbury, A. K., B. G. Arnason, and R. D. Adams.** 1969. The inflammatory lesion in idiopathic polyneuritis. *Medicine* **48:**173–215.

8. **Aspinall, G. O., S. Fujimoto, A. G. McDonald, H. Pang, L. A. Kurjanczyk, and J. L. Penner.** 1994. Lipopolysaccharides from *Campylobacter jejuni* associated with Guillain-Barré syndrome patients mimic human gangliosides in structure. *Infect. Immun.* **62:**2122–2125.

9. **Aspinall, G. O., A. G. McDonald, and H. Pang.** 1994. Lipopolysaccharides of *Campylobacter jejuni* serotype O:19: structures of O antigen chains from the serostrain and two bacterial isolates from patients with Guillain-Barré syndrome. *Biochemistry* **33:**250–255.

10. **Aspinall, G. O., A. G. McDonald, H. Pang, L. A. Kurjanczyk, and J. L. Penner.** 1994. Lipopolysaccharides of *Campylobacter jejuni* serotype O:19: structures of core oligosaccharide regions from the serostrain and two bacterial isolates from patients with the Guillain-Barré syndrome. *Biochemistry* **33:**241–249.

11. **Aspinall, G. O., A. G. McDonald, T. S. Raju, H. Pang, L. A. Kurjanczyk, J. L. Penner, and A. P. Moran.** 1993. Chemical structure of the core region of *Campylobacter jejuni* serotype O:2 lipopolysaccharide. *Eur. J. Biochem.* **213:**1029–1037.

12. **Aspinall, G. O., A. G. McDonald, T. S. Raju, H. Pang, A. P. Molan, and J. L. Penner.** 1993. Chemical structures of the core regions of *Campylobacter jejuni* serotypes O:1, O:4, O:23, and O:36 lipopolysaccharides. *Eur. J. Biochem.* **213:**1017–1027.

13. **Bansil, S., F. A. Mithen, S. D. Cook, A. Sheffet, and C. Rohowsky-Kochan.** 1991. Clinical correlation with serum-soluble interleukin-2 receptor levels in Guillain-Barré syndrome. *Neurology* **41:**1302–1305.

14. **Bech, E., T. F. Orntoft, L. P. Andersen, P. Skinhoj, and J. Jakobsen.** 1997. IgM anti-GM1 antibodies in the Guillain-Barré syndrome: a serological predictor of the clinical course. *J. Neuroimmunol.* **72:**59–66.

15. **Birchem, R., F. A. Mithen, K. M. L'Empereur, and M. M. Wessels.** 1987. Ultrastructural effects of Guillain-Barré serum in cultures containing only rat Schwann cells and dorsal root ganglion neurons. *Brain Res.* **421:**173–185.

16. **Black, R. E., M. M. Levine, M. L. Clements, T. P. Hughs, and M. J. Blaser.** 1988. Experimental *Campylobacter jejuni* infections in humans. *J. Infect. Dis.* **157:**472–480.

17. **Blaser, M. J., and D. J. Duncan.** 1984. Human serum antibody response to *Campylobacter jejuni* infection as measured in an enzyme-linked immunosorbent assay. *Infect. Immun.* **44:** 292–298.

18. **Bolton, F. J., and L. Robertson.** 1982. A selective medium for isolating *Campylobacter jejuni/coli. J. Clin. Pathol.* **35:**462–467.

19. **Breman, J. G., and J. S. Hayner.** 1984. Guillain-Barré syndrome and its relationship to swine influenza vaccination in Michigan, 1976–1977. *Am. J. Epidemiol.* **119:**880–889.

20. **Briscoe, D. M., J. B. McMenamia, and N. V. O'Donahue.** 1987. Prognosis in Guillain-Barré syndrome. *Arch. Dis. Child.* **62:**733–735.

21. **Buchwald, B., K. V. Toyka, J. Zielasek, A. Weishaupt, S. Schweiger, and J. Dudel.** 1998. Neuromuscular blockade by IgG antibodies from patients with Guillain-Barré syndrome: a macro-patch-clamp study. *Ann. Neurol.* **44:** 913–922.

22. **Bazby, J. C., B. M. Mishu Allos, and T. Roberts.** 1997. The economic burden of *Campylobacter* associated Guillain-Barré syndrome. *J. Infect. Dis.* **176**(Suppl. 2):S192–S197.

23. **Campbell, A. M. G.** 1958. The aetiology of polyneuritis. *Proc. R. Soc. Med.* **51:**157–159.

24. **Chiba, A., S. Kusinoki, S. Kuwata, T. Juji, Y. Sibata, and I. Kanazawa.** 1995. HLA and anti-GQ1b IgG antibody in Miller Fisher syndrome and Guillain-Barré syndrome. *J. Neuroimmunol.* **61:**85–88.

25. **Chiba, A., S. Kusunoki, H. Obata, R. Machinami, and I. Kanazawa.** 1993. Serum anti-GQ1b antibody is associated with ophthalmoplegia in Miller Fisher syndrome and Guillain-Barré syndrome: clinical and immunohistochemical studies. *Neurology* **43:**1911–1917.

26. **Chiba, A., S. Kusunoki, T. Shimizu, and I. Kanazawa.** 1992. Serum IgG antibody to ganglioside GQ1b is a possible marker of Miller Fisher syndrome. *Ann. Neurol.* **31:**677–679.

27. **Coe, C. J.** 1989. Guillain-Barré syndrome in Korean children. *Yonsei Med. J.* **30:**81–87.

28. **Cole, G. F., and D. J. Matthew.** 1987. Progress in severe Guillain-Barré syndrome. *Arch. Dis. Child.* **62:**288–291.

29. **Constant, O. C., C. C. Bentley, A. M. Denman, J. R. Lehane, and H. E. Larson.** 1983. The Guillain-Barré syndrome following *Campylobacter* enteritis with recovery after plasmapheresis. *J. Infect.* **6:**89–91.

30. **Corbo, M., A. Quattrini, N. Latov, and A. P. Hays.** 1993. Localization of GM1 and Gal(b1-3)GalNAc antigenic determinants in peripheral nerve. *Neurology* **43:**809–814.

31. **de Jager, A. E., and H. J. Sluiter.** 1991. Clinical signs in severe Guillain-Barré syndrome: analysis of 63 patients. *J. Neurol. Sci.* **104:**143–150.

32. **Dowling, P. C.** 1981. Role of infection in Guillain-Barré syndrome: laboratory confirmation of herpesviruses in 41 cases. *Ann. Neurol.* **9:**44–55.

33. **Dowling, P. C., J. P. Menonna, and S. D. Cook.** 1977. Guillain-Barré syndrome in greater New York-New Jersey. *JAMA* **238:**317–318.

34. **Enders, U., H. Karch, K. V. Toyka, M. Michels, J. Zielasek, M. Pette, J. Heesemann, and H.-P. Hartung.** 1993. The spectrum of immune responses to *Campylobacter jejuni* and glycoconjugates in Guillain-Barré syndrome and in other neuroimmunological disorders. *Ann. Neurol.* **34:**136–144.

35. **Feasby, T. E.** 1994. Axonal Guillain-Barré syndrome. *Muscle Nerve* **17:**678–679.

36. **Feasby, T. E., J. J. Gilbert, W. F. Brown, C. F. Bolton, A. F. Hahn, W. F. Koopman, and D. W. Zochedne.** 1986. An acute axonal form of Guillain-Barré polyneuropathy. *Brain* **109:**1115–1126.

37. **Feasby, T. E., J. J. Gilbert, W. F. Brown, C. F. Bolton, A. F. Hahn, W. J. Koopman,** and **D. W. Zochodne.** 1987. Acute "axonal" Guillain-Barré polyneuropathy. *Neurology* **37:** 357. (Letter.)

38. **Feasby, T. E., A. F. Hahn, W. F. Brown, C. F. Bolton, J. J. Gilbert, and W. J. Koopman.** 1993. Severe axonal degeneration in acute Guillain-Barré syndrome: evidence of two different mechanisms? *J. Neurol. Sci.* **116:**185–192.

39. **Fisher, M.** 1956. An unusual variant of acute idiopathic polyneuritis (syndrome of ophthalmoplegia ataxia and areflexia). *N. Engl. J. Med.* **255:**57–65.

40. **French Cooperative Group on Plasma Exchange in Guillain-Barré Syndrome.** 1987. Efficacy of plasma exchange in Guillain-Barré syndrome: role of replacement fluids. *Ann. Neurol.* **22:**753–761.

41. **Gao, C. Y., T. W. Ho, G. L. Wang, G. H. Zhang, J. X. Mao, C. Y. Li, J. W. Griffin, A. K. Asbury, G. M. McKhana and D. R. Cornblath.** 1997. Electrodiagnostic studies of Guillain-Barré syndrome in northern China, p. 119–128. *In* J. Kimura and R. Kaji (ed.), *Physiology of ALS and Related Disorders.* Elsevier, Amsterdam, The Netherlands.

42. **Georges-Courbot, M. C., C. Baya, A. M. Beraud, D. M. Y. Meunier, and A. J. Georges.** 1986. Distribution and serotypes of *Campylobacter jejuni* and *Campylobacter coli* in enteric *Campylobacter* strains isolated from children in the Central African Republic. *J. Clin. Microbiol.* **23:**592–594.

43. **Glaze, D. G.** 1992. Guillain-Barré syndrome. p. 464–474. *In* R. D. Feigen and J. D. Cherry (ed.), *Pediatric Infectious Diseases.* The W. B. Saunders Co., Philadelphia, Pa.

44. **Goddard, E. A., A. J. Lastovica, and A. C. Argent.** 1997. *Campylobacter* O:41 isolation in Guillain-Barré syndrome. *Arch. Dis. Child.* **76:** 526–528.

45. **Gorodezky, C., B. Varela, L. E. Castro-Escobar, A. Chavez-Negrete, A. Escobar-Gutierrez, and J. Martinez-Mata.** 1983. HLA-DR antigens in Mexican patients with Guillain-Barré syndrome. *J. Neuroimmunol.* **4:**1–7.

46. **Gregson, N. A., S. Koblar, and R. A. Hughes.** 1993. Antibodies to gangliosides in Guillain-Barré syndrome: specificity and relationship to clinical features. *Q. J. Med.* **86:** 111–117.

47. **Gregson, N. A., J. H. Rees, and R. A. C. Hughes.** 1997. Reactivity of serum IgG anti-GM1 ganglioside antibodies with the lipopolysaccharide fractions of *Campylobacter jejuni* isolates from patients with Guillain-Barré syndrome (GBS). *J. Neuroimmunol.* **73:**28–36.

48. **Griffin, J. W., C. Y. Li, T. W. Ho, M. Tian, C. Y. Gao, P. Xue, B. Mishu, D. R. Cornblath, C. Macko, G. M. McKhann, and A. K. Asbury.** 1996. Pathology of the motor-sensory axonal Guillain-Barré syndrome. *Ann. Neurol.* **39:**17–28.

49. **Griffin, J. W., C. Y. Li, T. W. Ho, P. Xue, C. Macko, D. R. Cornblath, C. Y. Gao, C. Yang, M. Tian, B. Mishu, G. M. McKhann, and A. K. Asbury.** 1995. Guillain-Barré syndrome in northern China: the spectrum of neuropathologic changes in clinically defined cases. *Brain* **118:**577–595.

50. **Griffin, J. W., C. Y. Li, C. Macko, T. W. Ho, S.-T. Hsieh, P. Xue, F. A. Wang, D. R. Cornblath, G. M. McKhann, and A. K. Asbury.** 1996. Early nodal changes in the acute motor axonal neuropathy pattern of the Guillain-Barré syndrome. *J. Neurocytol.* **25:**33–51.

51. **Gruenwald, R., A. H. Ropper, H. Lior, J. Chan, R. Lee, and V. S. Molinaro.** 1991. Serologic evidence of *Campylobacter jejuni/coli* enteritis in patients with Guillain-Barré syndrome. *Arch. Neurol.* **48:**1080–1082.

52. **Guillain, G., G. Barré, and A. Strohl.** 1916. Sur un syndrome de radiculonebrite avec hyperalbuminose du liquide cephalo-rachidien sans reaction cellulaire. Remarques sur les caracters cliniques et graphiques des reflexes tendineux. *Bull. Soc. Med. Hop. Paris* **40:**1462.

53. **Guillain-Barré Study Group.** 1985. Plasmapheresis and acute Guillain-Barré syndrome. *Neurology* **35:**1096–1104.

54. **Hafer-Macko, C., S.-T. Hsieh, C. Y. Li, T. W. Ho, K. A. Sheikh, D. R. Cornblath, G. M. McKhann, A. K. Asbury, and J. W. Griffin.** 1996. Acute motor axonal neuropathy: an antibody-mediated attack on axolemma. *Ann. Neurol.* **40:**635–644.

55. **Hafer-Macko, C., K. A. Sheikh, C. Y. Li, T. W. Ho, D. R. Cornblath, G. M. McKhann, A. K. Asbury, and J. W. Griffin.** 1996. Immune attack on the Schwann cell surface in acute inflammatory demyelinating polyneuropathy. *Ann. Neurol.* **39:**625–635.

56. **Hao, Q., T. Saida, S. Kuroki, M. Nishimura, M. Nukina, H. Obayashi, and K. Saida.** 1998. Antibodies to gangliosides and galactocerebroside in patients with Guillain-Barré syndrome with preceding *Campylobacter jejuni* and other identified infections. *J. Neuroimmunol.* **81:**116–126.

57. **Hariharan, H., K. Naseema, C. Kumaran, J. Shanmugam, M. D. Nair, and K. Radhakrishnan.** 1996. Detection of *Campylobacter jejuni/C. coli* infection in patients with Guillain-

58. **Hartung, H. P., J. D. Pollard, G. K. Harvey, and K. V. Toyka.** 1995. Immunopathogenesis and treatment of the Guillain-Barré syndrome. *Muscle Nerve* **18:**137–153.

59. **Hartung, H. P., G. Stoll and K. V. Toyka.** 1993. Immune reactions in the peripheral nervous system, p. 418–444. *In* P. J. Dyck, P. K. Thomas, J. W. Griffin, P. A. Low, and J. F. Poduslo (ed.), *Peripheral Neuropathy.* The W. B. Saunders Co., Philadelphia, Pa.

60. **Haymaker, W., and J. W. Kernohan.** 1949. The Landry-Guillain-Barré syndrome. A clinicopathologic report of fifty fatel cases and a critique of the literature. *Medicine* **28:**59–141.

61. **Herbrink, P., H. A. M. Van den Munckhof, M. Bumkens, J. Lindeman, and W. C. Van Dijk.** 1988. Human serum antibody response in *Campylobacter jejuni* enteritis as measured by enzyme-linked immunosorbent assay. *Eur. J. Clin. Microbiol. Infect. Dis.* **7:**388–393.

62. **Ho, T. W., S.-T. Hsieh, I. Nachamkin, H. J. Willison, K. Sheikh, J. Kiehlbauch, K. Flanigan, J. C. McArthur, D. R. Cornblath, G. M. McKhann, and J. W. Griffin.** 1997. Motor nerve terminal degeneration provides a potential mechanism for rapid recovery in acute motor axonal neuropathy after *Campylobacter* infection. *Neurology* **48:**717–724.

63. **Ho, T. W., C. Y. Li, D. R. Cornblath, C. Y. Gao, A. K. Asbury, J. W. Griffin, and G. M. McKhann.** 1997. Patterns of recovery in the Guillain-Barré syndromes. *Neurology* **48:**695–700.

64. **Ho, T. W., G. M. McKhann, and J. W. Griffin.** 1998. Human autoimmune neuropathies. *Annu. Rev. Neurosci.* **21:**187–226.

65. **Ho, T. W., B. Mishu, C. Y. Li, C. Y. Gao, D. R. Cornblath, J. W. Griffin, A. K. Asbury, M. J. Blaser, and G. M. McKhann.** 1995. Guillain-Barré syndrome in northern China: relationship to *Campylobacter jejuni* infection and anti-glycolipid antibodies. *Brain* **118:**597–605.

66. **Ho, T. W., H. Willison, I. Nachamkin, C. Y. Li, J. Veitch, H. Ung, G. R. Wang, R. C. Liu, D. R. Cornblath, A. K. Asbury, J. W. Griffin, and G. M. McKhann.** 1999. Anti-GD1a antibody distinguishes axonal from demyelinating forms of Guillain-Barré syndrome. *Ann. Neurol.* **45:**168–173.

66a. **Ho, T. W., et al.** Unpublished results.

67. **Hughes, R. A. C.** 1991. *Guillain-Barré Syndrome.* Springer-Verlag, London, United Kingdom.

68. Hughes, R. A. C., and J. H. Rees. 1997. Clinical and epidemiologic features of Guillain-Barré syndrome. *J. Infect. Dis.* **176**(Suppl. 2):92–98.

69. Hurwitz, E. S., R. C. Holman, D. B. Nelson, and L. B. Schonberger. 1983. National surveillance for Guillain-Barré syndrome: January 1978–March 1979. *Neurology* **33**:150–157.

70. Ilyas, A. A., F. A. Mithen, M. C. Dalakas, Z.-W. Chen, and S. D. Cook. 1992. Antibodies to acidic glycolipids in Guillain-Barré syndrome and chronic inflammatory demyelinating polyneuropathy. *J. Neurol. Sci.* **107**:111–121.

71. Ilyas, A. A., H. J. Willison, R. H. Quarles, F. B. Jungawala, D. R. Cornblath, B. D. Trapp, D. E. Griffin, J. W. Griffin, and G. M. McKhann. 1988. Serum antibodies to gangliosides in Guillain-Barré syndrome. *Ann. Neurol.* **23**:440–447.

72. Jackson, C. E., R. J. Barohn, and J. R. Mendell. 1993. Acute paralytic syndrome in three American men. Comparison with Chinese cases. *Arch. Neurol.* **50**:732–735.

73. Jacobs, B. C., H. P. Endtz, F. G. A. van der Meche, M. P. Hazenberg, H. A. M. Actere-ekte, and P. A. van Doorn. 1995. Serum anti-GQ1b IgG antibodies recognize surface epitopes on *Campylobacter jejuni* from patients with Miller Fisher syndrome. *Ann. Neurol.* **37**:260–264.

74. Jacobs, B. C., H. P. Endtz, F. G. A. van der Meche, M. P. Hazenberg, M. A. de Klerk, and P. A. van Doorn. 1997. Humoral immune response against *Campylobacter jejuni* lipopolysaccharides in Guillain-Barré and Miller Fisher syndrome. *J. Neuroimmunol.* **79**:62–68.

75. Jacobs, B. C., P. I. M. Schmitz, and F. G. A. van der Meche. 1996. *Campylobacter jejuni* infection and treatment for Guillain-Barré syndrome. *N. Engl. J. Med.* **335**:208–209.

76. Jones, D. M., E. M. Sutcliffe, and J. D. Abbott. 1985. Serotyping of *Campylobacter* species by combined use of two methods. *Eur. J. Clin. Microbiol.* **4**:562–565.

77. Kaldor, J., H. Pritchard, A. Serpell, and W. Metcalf. 1983. Serum antibodies in campylobacter enteritis. *J. Clin. Microbiol.* **18**:1–4.

78. Kaldor, J., and B. R. Speed. 1984. Guillain-Barré syndrome and *Campylobacter jejuni*: a serologic study. *Br. Med. J.* **288**:1867–1870.

79. Kaplan, J. E., P. J. Poduska, G. C. McIntosh, R. S. Hopkins, S. W. Ferguson, and L. B. Schonberger. 1985. Guillain-Barré syndrome in Larimer County, Colorado: a high incidence area. *Neurology* **35**:581–584.

80. Khoury, S. H. 1978. Guillain-Barré syndrome: epidemiology of an outbreak. *Am. J. Epidemiol.* **107**:433–438.

81. Koga, M., N. Yuki, K. Kashiwase, K. Tado-koro, T. Juji, and K. Hirata. 1998. Guillain-Barré and Fisher's syndromes subsequent to *Campylobacter jejuni* enteritis are associated with HLA-B54 and Cw1 independent of anti-ganglioside antibodies. *J. Neuroimmunol.* **88**:62–66.

82. Koga, M., N. Yuki, M. Takahashi, K. Saito, and K. Hirata. 1998. Close association of IgA anti-ganglioside antibodies with antecedent *Campylobacter jejuni* infection in Guillain-Barré and Fisher's syndromes. *J. Neuroimmunol.* **81**:138–143.

83. Koobatian, T. J., G. S. Birkhead, M. M. Schramm, and R. L. Vogt. 1991. The use of hospital discharge data for public health surveillance of Guillain-Barré syndrome. *Ann. Neurol.* **30**:618–621.

84. Kornberg, A. J., A. Pestronk, K. Bleser, T. W. Ho, G. M. McKhann, H. S. Wu, and Z. Jiang. 1994. The clinical correlates of high-titer IgG anti-GM1 antibodies. *Ann. Neurol.* **35**:234–237.

85. Koski, C. L., D. K. H. Chou, and F. B. Jungalwala. 1989. Anti-peripheral nerve myelin antibodies in Guillain-Barre syndrome bind a neutral glycolipid of peripheral myelin and cross-react with Forssman antigen. *J. Clin. Investig.* **84**:280–287.

86. Koski, C. L., R. Humphrey, and M. L. Shin. 1985. Anti-peripheral myelin antibody in patients with demyelinating neuropathy: quantitative and kinetic determination of serum antibody by complement component 1 fixation. *Proc. Natl. Acad. Sci. USA* **82**:905–909.

87. Kuroki, S., T. Saida, M. Nukina, T. Haruta, M. Yoshioka, Y. Kobayashi, and H. Nakanishi. 1993. *Campylobacter jejuni* strains from patients with Guillain-Barré syndrome belong mostly to Penner serogroup 19 and contain B-N-acetylglucosamine residues. *Ann. Neurol.* **33**:243–247.

88. Kusunoki, S., A. Chiba, S. Hitoshi, H. Takizawa, and I. Kanazawa. 1995. Anti-Gal-C antibody in autoimmune neuropathies subsequent to mycoplasma infection. *Muscle Nerve* **18**:409–413.

89. Kuwabara, S., N. Yuki, M. Koga, T. Hattori, D. Matsuura, M. Miyake, and M. Noda. 1998. IgG anti-GM1 antibody is associated with reversible conduction failure and axonal degeneration in Guillain-Barré syndrome. *Ann. Neurol.* **44**:202–208.

90. Lane, E. M., R. Batchelor, A. L. Bourgeols, D. H. Burr, and J. G. Olson. 1987. Urine and fecal IgA responses during naturally acquired infection with *Campylobacter jejuni*. *Lancet* **i**:1141. (Letter.)

91. Lang, D. 1997. Workshop summary and recom-

mendations regarding the development of Guillain-Barré syndrome following *Campylobacter* infection. *J. Infect. Dis.* **176**(Suppl. 2):198–200.

92. **Lastovica, A. J., E. A. Goddard, and A. C. Argent.** 1997. Guillain-Barre syndrome in South Africa associated with *Campylobacter jejuni* O:41 strains. *J. Infect. Dis.* **176**(Suppl. 2): 139–143.

93. **Latovitzki, N., N. Suciu-Foca, A. S. Penn, M. R. Olarte, and A. M. Chutorian.** 1979. HLA typing and Guillain-Barré syndrome. *Neurology* **29**:743–745.

94. **Lawrenson, J. G., A. R. Reid, and G. Allt.** 1994. Molecular characterization of anionic sites on the luminal front of endoneurial capillaries in sciatic nerve. *J. Neurocytol.* **23**:29–37.

95. **Li, C. Y., P. Xue, C. Y. Gao, W. Q. Tian, R. C. Liu, and C. Yang.** 1996. Experimental *Campylobacter jejuni* infection in the chicken: an animal model of axonal Guillain-Barré syndrome. *J. Neurol. Neurosurg. Psychiatry* **61**: 279–284.

96. **Lu, J. L., K. A. Sheikh, H. S. Wu, J. Zhang, D. R. Cornblath, G. M. McKhann, A. K. Asbury, J. W. Griffin, and T. W. Ho.** Physiological-pathological correlation in Guillain-Barré syndrome. *Neurology*, in press.

97. **Ma, J. J., M. Nishimura, H. Mine, S. Kuroki, M. Nukina, M. Ohta, H. Saji, H. Obayashi, H. Kawakami, T. Saida, and T. Uchiyama.** 1998. Genetic contribution of the tumor necrosis factor region in Guillain-Barré syndrome. *Ann. Neurol.* **44**:815–818.

98. **Ma, J. J., M. Nishimura, H. Mine, S. Kuroki, M. Nukina, M. Ohta, H. Saji, H. Obayashi, T. Saida, H. Kawakami, and T. Uchiyama.** 1998. HLA and T-cell receptor gene polymorphisms in Guillain-Barré syndrome. *Neurology* **51**:379–384.

99. **Mascart-Lemone, F. O., J. R. Duchateau, J. Oosterom, J.-P. Butzler, and D. L. Delacroix.** 1987. Kinetics of anti-*Campylobacter jejuni* monomeric and polymeric immunoglobulin A1 and A2 response in serum during acute enteritis. *J. Clin. Microbiol.* **25**:1253–1257.

100. **Mato, M., S. Ookawara, M. Sugamata, and E. Aikawa.** 1984. Evidences for the possible function of the fluorescent granular perithelial cells in brain as scavengers of high molecular-weight waste products. *Experientia* **40**:399–402.

101. **McKhann, G. M., D. R. Cornblath, J. W. Griffin, T. W. Ho, C. Y. Li, Z. Jiang, H. S. Wu, G. Zhaori, Y. Liu, L. P. Jou, T. C. Liu, C. Y. Gao, J. Y. Mao, M. J. Blaser, B. Mishu, and A. K. Asbury.** 1993. Acute motor axonal neuropathy: a frequent cause of acute flaccid paralysis in China. *Ann. Neurol.* **33**:333–342.

102. **McKhann, G. M., D. R. Cornblath, T. W. Ho, C. Y. Li, A. Y. Bai, H. S. Wu, Q. F. Yei, W. C. Zhang, Z. Zhaori, Z. Jiang, J. W. Griffin, and A. K. Asbury.** 1991. Clinical and electrophysiologic aspects of acute paralytic disease of children and young adults in northern China. *Lancet* **338**:593–597.

103. **McMyne, P. M. S., J. L. Penner, R. G. Mathias, W. A. Black, and J. N. Hennessy.** 1982. Serotyping of *Campylobacter jejuni* isolated from sporadic cases and outbreaks in British Columbia. *J. Clin. Microbiol.* **16**:281–285.

104. **Mishu, B., and M. J. Blaser.** 1993. Role of infection due to *Campylobacter jejuni* in the initiation of Guillain-Barré syndrome. *Clin. Infect. Dis.* **17**:104–108.

105. **Mishu, B., A. A. Ilyas, C. L. Koski, F. Vriesendorp, S. D. Cook, F. A. Mithen, and M. J. Blaser.** 1993. Serologic evidence of previous *Campylobacter jejuni* infection in patients with Guillain-Barré syndrome. *Ann. Intern. Med.* **118**: 947–953.

106. **Mishu, B., C. M. Patton, and M. J. Blaser.** 1993. Microbiologic characteristics of *Campylobacter jejuni* strains isolated from patients with Guillain-Barré syndrome. *Clin. Infect. Dis.* **17**: 538.

107. **Molnar, G. K., J. Mertsola, and M. Erkko.** 1982. Guillain-Barré syndrome associated with *Campylobacter* infection. *Br. Med. J.* **285**:652. (Letter.)

108. **Monos, D. S., M. Papaioakim, T. W. Ho, C. Y. Li, and G. M. McKhann.** 1997. Differential distribution of HLA alleles in two forms of Guillain-Barré syndrome. *J. Infect. Dis.* **176**(Suppl. 2): S180–S182.

109. **Moran, A. P., B. J. Appelmelk, and G. O. Aspinall.** 1996. Molecular mimicry of host structures by lipopolysaccharides of *Campylobacter* and *Helicobacter* spp.: implications in pathogenesis. *J. Endotoxin Res.* **3**:521–531.

110. **Moran, A. P., E. T. Rietschel, T. U. Kosunen, and U. Zahringer.** 1991. Chemical characterization of *Campylobacter jejuni* lipopolysaccharides containing N-acetylneuraminic acid and 2,3-diamino-2,3-dideoxy-D-glucose. *J. Bacteriol.* **173**:618–626.

111. **Nachamkin, I.** 1995. *Campylobacter* and *Arcobacter*, p. 483–491. *In* P. R. Murray, E. J. Baron, M. A. Pfaller, F. C. Tenover, and R. H. Yolken (ed.), *Manual of Clinical Microbiology*, 6th ed. ASM Press, Washington, D.C.

112. **Nachamkin, I.** 1997. Microbiologic approaches for studying *Campylobacter* in patients with Guillain-Barré syndrome. *J. Infect. Dis.* **176**(Suppl. 2): S106–S114.

113. Nachamkin, I., H. Ung, A. P. Moran, D. Yoo, M. M. Prendergast, M. A. Nicholson, K. Sheikh, T. W. Ho, A. K. Asbury, G. M. McKhann, and J. W. Griffin. 1999. Ganglioside GM1 mimicry in *Campylobacter* strains from sporadic infections in the United States. *J. Infect. Dis.* **179**:1183–1189.

114. Nachamkin, I., and X. H. Yang. 1989. Human antibody response to *Campylobacter jejuni* flagellin protein and a synthetic N-terminal flagellin peptide. *J. Clin. Microbiol.* **27**:2195–2198.

115. Nachamkin, I., and X. H. Yang. 1992. Local immune responses to the *Campylobacter* flagellin in acute *Campylobacter* gastrointestinal infection. *J. Clin. Microbiol.* **30**:509–511.

115a. Nachamkin, I., et al. Unpublished results.

116. Nishimura, M., M. Nukina, S. Kuroki, H. Obayashi, H. Ohta, J. J. Ma, T. Saida, and T. Uchiyama. 1997. Characterization of *Campylobacter jejuni* isolates from patients with Guillain-Barré syndrome. *J. Neurol. Sci.* **153**:91–99.

117. Ogawa-Goto, K., N. Funamoto, T. Abe, and K. Nagashima. 1992. Myelin gangliosides of human peripheral nervous system: an enrichment of GM1 in the motor nerve myelin isolated from cauda equina. *J. Neurochem.* **59**:1844–1849.

118. Ohtsuka, K., Y. Nakamura, M. Hashimoto, Y. Tagawa, M. Takahashi, K. Saito, and N. Yuki. 1998. Fisher syndrome associated with IgG anti-GQ1b antibody following infection by a specific serotype of *Campylobacter jejuni*. *Ophthalmology* **105**:1281–1285.

119. Oomes, P. G., B. C. Jacobs, M. P. H. Hazenberg, J. R. J. Banffer, and F. G. A. van der Meche. 1995. Anti-GM1 IgG antibodies and *Campylobacter* bacteria in Guillain-Barré syndrome, evidence of molecular mimicry. *Ann. Neurol.* **38**:170–175.

120. Osler, W. 1892. *Principles and Practice of Medicine*. Appleton, New York, N.Y.

121. Patton, C. M., and I. K. Wachsmuth. 1992. Typing schemes: are current methods useful? p. 110–128. *In* I. Nachamkin, M. J. Blaser, and L. S. Tompkins (ed.), *Campylobacter jejuni: Current Status and Future Trends*. American Society for Microbiology, Washington, D.C.

122. Patton, C. M., I. K. Wachsmuth, G. M. Evins, J. A. Kiehlbauch, B. D. Plikaytis, N. Troup, L. Tompkins, and H. Lior. 1991. Evaluation of 10 methods to distinguish epidemic-associated *Campylobacter* strains. *J. Clin. Microbiol.* **29**:680–688.

123. Penner, J. L., and J. N. Hennessy. 1980. Passive hemagglutination technique for serotyping *Campylobacter fetus* subsp. *jejuni* on the basis of soluble heat-stable antigens. *J. Clin. Microbiol.* **12**:732–737.

124. Plasma Exchange/Sandoglobulin Guillain-Barré Syndrome Trial Group. 1997. Randomised trial of plasma exchange, intravenous immunoglobulin, and combined treatments in Guillain-Barré syndrome. *Lancet* **349**:225–230.

125. Poduslo, J. F., and G. L. Curran. 1994. Macromolecular permeability across the blood-nerve and blood-brain barrier. *Proc. Natl. Acad. Sci. USA* **91**:5705–5709.

126. Pollard, J. D., K. W. Westland, G. K. Harvey, S. Jung, J. Bonner, J. M. Spies, K. V. Toyka, and H. P. Hartung. 1995. Activated T cells of nonneural specificity open the blood-nerve barrier to circulating antibody. *Ann. Neurol.* **37**:467–475.

127. Prineas, J. W. 1972. Acute idiopathic polyneuritis. An electron microscope study. *Lab. Investig.* **26**:133–147.

128. Prineas, J. W. 1981. Pathology of the Guillain-Barré syndrome. *Ann. Neurol.* **9**:6–19.

129. Pryor, W. M., J. S. Freiman, M. A. Gillies, and R. R. Tuck. 1984. Guillain-Barré syndrome associated with *Campylobacter* infection. *Aust. N. Z. J. Med.* **14**:687–688.

130. Ramos-Alvarez, M., L. Bessudo, and A. Sabin. 1969. Paralytic syndromes associated with noninflammatory cytoplasmic or nuclear neuronopathy: acute paralytic disease in Mexican children, neuropathologically distinguishable from Landry-Guillain-Barré syndrome. *JAMA* **207**:1481–1492.

131. Rantala, H., M. Uhari, and M. Niemela. 1991. Occurrence, clinical manifestations, and prognosis of Guillain-Barré syndrome. *Arch. Dis. Child.* **66**:706–708.

132. Rees, J. H., N. A. Gregson, and R. A. C. Hughes. 1995. Anti-ganglioside GM1 antibodies in Guillain-Barré syndrome and their relationship to *Campylobacter jejuni* infection. *Ann. Neurol.* **38**:809–816.

133. Rees, J. H., S. E. Soudain, N. A. Gregson, and R. A. C. Hughes. 1995. *Campylobacter jejuni* infection and Guillain-Barré syndrome. *N. Engl. J. Med.* **333**:1374–1379.

134. Rees, J. H., R. D. Thompson, N. C. Smeeton, and R. A. C. Hughes. 1998. Epidemiological study of Guillain-Barre syndrome in south east England. *J. Neurol. Neurosurg. Psychiatry* **64**:74–77.

135. Rees, J. H., R. W. Vaughan, E. Kondeatis, and R. A. C. Hughes. 1995. HLA class II alleles in Guillain-Barre syndrome and Miller Fisher syndrome and their associations with preceding

Campylobacter jejuni infection. *J. Neuroimmunol.* **38**:53–57.

136. **Rhodes, K. M., and A. E. Tattersfield.** 1982. Guillain-Barré syndrome associated with *Campylobacter* infection. *Br. Med. J.* **285**:173–174.

137. **Roberts, M., H. Willison, A. Vincent, and J. Newsom-Davis.** 1994. Serum factor in Miller-Fisher variant of Guillain-Barré syndrome and neurotransmitter release. *Lancet* **343**:454–455.

138. **Ropper, A. H.** 1986. Severe acute Guillain-Barre syndrome. *Neurology* **36**:429–432.

139. **Ropper, A. H.** 1988. *Campylobacter* diarrhea and Guillain-Barré syndrome. *Arch. Neurol.* **45**:655–656.

140. **Rostami, A. M.** 1995. Guillain-Barré syndrome: clinical and immunological aspects. *Springer Semin. Immunopathol.* **17**:29–42.

141. **Rostami, A. M.** 1997. P2-reactive T cells in inflammatory demyelination of the peripheral nerve. *J. Infect. Dis.* **176**(Suppl. 2):160–163.

142. **Sack, D. A., A. J. Lastovica, S. H. Chang, and G. Pazzaglia.** 1998. Microtiter assay for detecting *Campylobacter* spp. and *Helicobacter pylori* with surface gangliosides which bind cholera toxin. *J. Clin. Microbiol.* **36**:2043–2045.

143. **Sacks, J. J., S. Lieb, L. M. Baldy, S. Berta, C. M. Patton, M. C. White, W. J. Bigler, and J. J. Witte.** 1986. Epidemic campylobacteriosis associated with a community water supply. *Am. J. Public Health* **76**:424–428.

144. **Salloway, S., L. A. Mermel, M. Seamans, G. O. Aspinall, J. E. N. Shin, A. Kurjanczyk, and J. L. Penner.** 1996. Miller-Fisher syndrome associated with *Campylobacter jejuni* bearing lipopolysaccharide molecules that mimic human ganglioside GD3. *Infect. Immun.* **64**:2945–2949.

145. **Sanders, E. A., A. C. Peters, J. W. Gratana, and R. A. C. Hughes.** 1987. Guillain-Barré syndrome after varicella-zoster infection. Report of two cases. *J. Neurol.* **234**:437–439.

146. **Sawant-Mane, S., M. B. Clark, and C. L. Koski.** 1991. In vitro demyelination by serum antibody from patients with Guillain-Barré syndrome requires terminal complement complexes. *Ann. Neurol.* **29**:397–404.

147. **Sawant-Mane, S., A. Estep, and C. L. Koski.** 1994. Antibody of patients with Guillain-Barré syndrome mediates complement-dependent cytolysis of rat Schwann cells: susceptibility to cytolysis reflects Schwann cell phenotype. *J. Neuroimmunol.* **49**:145–152.

148. **Schonberger, L. B., E. S. Hurwitz, P. Katona, R. C. Holman, and D. J. Bregman.** 1981. Guillain-Barré syndrome: its epidemiology and associations with influenza vaccination. *Ann. Neurol.* **9**:31–38.

149. **Sheikh, K. A., I. Nachamkin, T. W. Ho, H. J. Willison, J. Veitch, B. S. Ung, C. Y. Li, B.-G. Shen, D. R. Cornblath, A. K. Asbury, G. M. McKhann, and J. W. Griffin.** 1998. *Campylobacter jejuni* lipopolysaccharides in Guillain-Barré syndrome: molecular mimicry and host susceptibility. *Neurology* **51**:371–378.

150. **Sjogren, E., G. B. Lindblom, and B. Kaijser.** 1987. Comparison of different procedures, transport media, and enrichment media for isolation of *Campylobacter* species from healthy laying hens and humans with diarrhea. *J. Clin. Microbiol.* **25**:1966–1968.

151. **Sliman, N. A.** 1978. Outbreak of Guillain-Barré syndrome associated with water pollution. *Br. Med. J.* **1**:751–752.

152. **Sobue, G., M. Li, S. Terao, S. Aoki, M. Ichimura, T. Ieda, M. Doyu, T. Yasuda, Y. Hashizume, and T. Mitsuma.** 1997. Axonal pathology in Japanese Guillain-Barré syndrome: a study of 15 autopsied cases. *Neurology* **48**:1694–1700.

153. **Speed, B., J. Kaldor, and P. Cavanagh.** 1984. Guillain-Barré syndrome associated with *Campylobacter jejuni* enteritis. *J. Infect. Dis.* **8**:85–86.

154. **Speed, B. R., J. Kaldor, J. Watson, H. Newton-John, W. Tee, D. Noonan, and B. W. Dwyer.** 1987. *Campylobacter jejuni/Campylobacter coli* associated Guillain-Barré syndrome. *Med. J. Aust.* **147**:13–16.

155. **Stewart, G. J., J. D. Pollard, J. G. McLeod, and C. M. Wolnizer.** 1978. HLA antigens in the Landry-Guillain-Barré syndrome and chronic relapsing polyneuritis. *Ann. Neurol.* **4**:285–289.

156. **Sumner, A. J., K. Saida, T. Saida, D. H. Silberberg, and A. K. Asbury.** 1982. Acute conduction block associated with experimental antiserum-mediated demyelination of peripheral nerve. *Ann. Neurol.* **11**:469–477.

157. **Svedhem, A., and B. Kaijser.** 1980. *Campylobacter fetus* subspecies *jejuni*: a common cause of diarrhea in Sweden. *J. Infect. Dis.* **142**:353–359.

158. **Tauxe, R. V.** 1992. Epidemiology of *Campylobacter jejuni* infections in the United States and other industrialized nations, p. 9–19. *In* I. Nachamkin, M. J. Blaser, and L. S. Tompkins (ed.), *Campylobacter jejuni: Current Status and Future Trends.* American Society for Microbiology, Washington, D.C.

159. **Taylor, D. N., P. Echeverria, C. Pitarangsi, J. Seriwatana, L. Bodhidatta, and M. J. Blaser.** 1988. Influence of strain characteristics and immunity on the epidemiology of *Campylobacter* infections in Thailand. *J. Clin. Microbiol.* **26**:863–868.

160. **Taylor, N. S., M. A. Elenberger, P. Y. Wu, and J. G. Fox.** 1989. Diversity of serotypes of *Campylobacter jejuni* and *Campylobacter coli* isolated in laboratory animals. *Lab. Anim. Sci.* **39:** 219–221.

161. **The Guillain-Barré Syndrome Study Group.** 1985. Plasmapheresis and acute Guillain-Barré syndrome. *Neurology* **35:**1096–1104.

162. **Thornton, C. A., A. S. Latif, and J. C. Emmanuel.** 1991. Guillain-Barré syndrome associated with human immunodeficiency virus infection in Zimbabwe. *Neurology* **41:**812–815.

163. **Trojaborg, W.** 1998. Acute and chronic neuropathies: new aspects of Guillain-Barré syndrome and chronic inflammatory demyelinating polyneuropathy, an overview and an update. *Electroencephalogr. Clin. Neurophysiol.* **107:** 303–316.

164. **Tsukada, N., C. S. Koh, A. Inoue, and N. Yanagisawa.** 1987. Demyelinating neuropathy associated with hepatitis B virus infection. *J. Neurol. Sci.* **77:**203–216.

165. **Valenciano, E. N., F. Perez-Gallardo, A. Gonzales, and J. Enrech.** 1971. Outbreak of paralytic illness of unknown etiology in Albecete, Spain. *Am. J. Epidemiol.* **94:**450–456.

166. **Valenstein, P., M. Pfaller, and M. Yungbluth.** 1996. The use and abuse of routine stool microbiology: a College of American Pathologists Q-probes study of 601 institutions. *Arch. Pathol. Lab. Med.* **120:**206–211.

167. **van der Meche, F. G. A., P. I. M. Schmitz, and Dutch Guillain-Barré Study Group.** 1992. A randomized trial comparing intravenous immune globulin and plasma exchange in Guillain-Barré syndrome. *N. Engl. J. Med.* **326:** 1123–1129.

168. **Visser, L. H., F. G. van der Meche, P. A. van Doorn, J. Meulstee, B. C. Jacobs, P. G. Oomes, and R. P. Kleyweg.** 1995. Guillain-Barré syndrome without sensory loss (acute motor neuropathy). A subgroup with specific clinical, electrodiagnostic and laboratory features. Dutch Guillain-Barré Study Group. *Brain* **118:**841–847.

169. **Vriesendorp, F. J.** 1997. Insights into *Campylobacter jejuni* inducted Guillain-Barré syndrome from the Lewis rat model of experimental allergic neuritis. *Clin. Infect. Dis.* **176**(Suppl. 2): 164–168.

170. **Vriesendorp, F. J., B. Mishu, M. Blaser, and C. L. Koski.** 1993. Serum antibodies to GM1, peripheral nerve myelin, and *Campylobacter jejuni* in patients with Guillain-Barré syndrome and controls: correlation and prognosis. *Ann. Neurol.* **34:**130–135.

171. **Willison, H. J., J. Veitch, G. Patterson, and P. G. E. Kennedy.** 1993. Miller Fisher syndrome is associated with serum antibodies to GQ1b ganglioside. *J. Neurol. Neurosurg. Psychiatry* **56:**204–206.

172. **Winer, J. B., R. A. C. Hughes, and C. Osmond.** 1988. A prospective study of acute idiopathic neuropathy. 2. Antecedent events. *J. Neurol. Neurosurg. Psychiatry* **51:**613–618.

173. **Winer, S. J., and J. G. Evans.** 1993. Guillain-Barré syndrome in Oxfordshire: clinical features in relation to age. *Age Ageing* **22:**164–170.

174. **Wroe, S. J., and L. D. Blumhardt.** 1985. Polyneuritis with cranial nerve involvement following *Campylobacter jejuni* infection. *J. Neurol. Neurosurg. Psychiatry* **48:**593.

175. **Wu, H. S., T. C. Liu, Z. L. Lu, L. P. Zou, W. C. Zhang, G. Zhaori, and J. Zhang.** 1997. A prospective clinical and electrophysiologic survey of acute flaccid paralysis in Chinese children. *Neurology* **49:**1723–1725.

176. **Wu, S.-J., G. Pazzaglia, R. L. Haberberger, J. J. Oprandy, D. G. Sieckmann, D. M. Watts, and C. Hayes.** 1993. Detection of immunoglobulin A in urine specimens from children with *Campylobacter*-associated diarrhea by a chemiluminescent indicator-based western immunodot assay. *J. Clin. Microbiol.* **31:**1394–1396.

177. **Yang, L. J., C. B. Zeller, N. L. Shaper, M. Kiso, A. Hasegawa, R. E. Shapiro, and R. L. Schnaar.** 1996. Gangliosides are neuronal ligands for myelin-associated glycoprotein. *Proc. Natl. Acad. Sci. USA* **93:**814–818.

178. **Yuki, N., S. Handa, T. Tai, M. Takahashi, K. Saito, Y. Tsujino, and T. Taki.** 1995. Ganglioside-like epitopes of lipopolysaccharides from *Campylobacter jejuni* (PEN 19) in three isolates from patients with Guillain-Barré syndrome. *J. Neurol. Sci.* **130:**112–116.

179. **Yuki, N., S. Sato, S. Tsuji, T. Ohsawa, and T. Miyatake.** 1993. Frequent presence of anti-GQ1b antibody in Fisher's syndrome. *Neurology* **43:**414–417.

180. **Yuki, N., M. Takahashi, Y. Tagawa, K. Kashiwase, K. Tadokoro, and K. Saito.** 1997. Association of *Campylobacter jejuni* serotype and antiganglioside antibody in Guillain-Barré syndrome and Fisher's syndrome. *Ann. Neurol.* **42:**28–33.

181. **Yuki, N., T. Taki, F. Inagaki, T. Kasama, M. Takahashi, K. Saito, S. Handa, and T. Miyatake.** 1993. A bacterium lipopolysaccharide that elicits Guillain-Barré syndrome has a GM1 ganglioside structure. *J. Exp. Med.* **178:** 1771–1775.

182. **Yuki, N., T. Taki, M. Takahashi, K. Saito, T. Tai, T. Miyatake, and S. Handa.** 1994.

Penner's serogroup 4 of *Campylobacter jejuni* has a lipopolysaccharide that bears a GM1 ganglioside epitope as well as one that bears a GD1a epitope. *Infect. Immun.* **62:**2101–2103.

183. **Yuki, N., T. Taki, M. Takahashi, K. Saito, H. Yoshino, T. Tai, S. Handa, and T. Miyatake.** 1994. Molecular mimicry between GQ1b ganglioside and lipopolysaccharides of *Campylobacter jejuni* isolated from patients with Fishers syndrome. *Ann. Neurol.* **36:**791–793.

184. **Yuki, N., H. Yoshino, S. Sato, and T. Miyatake.** 1990. Acute axonal polyneuropathy associated with anti-GM1 antibodies following *Campylobacter* enteritis. *Neurology* **40:**1900–1902.

PATHOGENESIS OF *CAMPYLOBACTER* INFECTIONS

III

CAMPYLOBACTER TOXINS AND THEIR ROLE IN PATHOGENESIS

Carol L. Pickett

9

A common theme associated with diarrheagenic bacterial pathogens is the production of protein toxins which contribute to the pathogenesis of disease. The most well-known and well-studied example of a diarrheagenic protein toxin is cholera toxin, which is a primary *Vibrio cholerae* virulence factor and is responsible for massive fluid loss in patients. *Campylobacter jejuni* diarrheal disease symptoms, which often include a transient watery diarrhea that progresses to a more bloody diarrhea, are consistent with the idea that toxins play a role in this disease. Therefore, many investigators have looked for toxic activities produced by *C. jejuni* and other closely related *Campylobacter* spp. Most of these studies have reported on either putative enterotoxic or cytotoxic activities that affect various cultured cell lines; some studies have included assays in animal models. In spite of the large number of studies, our knowledge about *C. jejuni* toxins is still rather limited. This stems in part from the diverse nature of the studies that have been performed. Different strains grown under different conditions have been tested in a variety of assays, making direct comparisons difficult.

Nonetheless, our knowledge of *Campylobacter* toxins has progressed. Work published in the last few years has dramatically improved our understanding of one *Campylobacter* cytotoxin, cytolethal distending toxin (CDT). Other toxic activities continue to receive attention, and perhaps the next few years will bring a significant improvement in our understanding of these activities.

This chapter first summarizes our knowledge of CDT, in particular *Campylobacter* CDT, but it also includes some information about the CDTs produced by other bacterial pathogens. Then non-CDT cytotoxins and enterotoxins are discussed. Since there is a quite recent, comprehensive, and thoughtful review of *Campylobacter* toxins (42), the portions of this chapter that discuss non-CDT cytotoxins and enterotoxins will concentrate on original papers published since that review, on an overview of the activities discussed in the review (42), and on current and proposed attempts to clarify the *Campylobacter* toxin field.

CYTOLETHAL DISTENDING TOXIN

CDT production by *Campylobacter* was first reported in 1988 by Johnson and Lior (18), who abbreviated the activity CLDT. They described an apparently novel toxic activity, present in culture supernatants, that caused HeLa,

Carol L. Pickett, Department of Microbiology and Immunology, University of Kentucky, Chandler Medical Center, Lexington, KY 40536.

Campylobacter, 2nd Ed., Edited by I. Nachamkin and M. J. Blaser

Chinese hamster ovary (CHO), HEp-2, and Vero cells to slowly distend over a 3- to 4-day period and then die. The activity seemed to be effective only on freshly seeded or sparsely seeded cells; no death or distension was seen when the toxin was added to confluent monolayers. They also determined that CDT was heat labile, protease sensitive, and nondialyzable and appeared to be reproducibly produced by strains even after multiple passages. The ability of CDT to cause an increase in intracellular cyclic AMP levels was tested and found to probably not be a significant attribute of this toxin. In addition, CDT appeared not to cause a positive response in an infant-mouse assay, in a rabbit skin permeability factor assay, in an adult-rabbit-ligated-ileal-loop assay, or in the Sereñy test for invasiveness. CDT did, however, appear to be able to cause some diarrheal symptoms in a rat–ileal-loop assay.

Johnson and Lior (18) assayed over 700 *Campylobacter* strains, including 583 *C. jejuni,* 109 *C. coli,* 16 *C. lari,* and 7 *C. fetus* strains, for CDT activity. They found that roughly 40% of each of these species appeared to produce active CDT and that there was no correlation between CDT production and serotype or biotype or country of origin of the tested strains.

Work published by the same authors at about the same time documented that a CDT activity also appeared to be produced by a small number of *Escherichia coli* and *Shigella* isolates (16, 17). Figure 1 illustrates the action of CDT on HeLa cells at 72 h after the addition of CDT. The dramatic distension of these cells is readily apparent. It can also be seen that the nuclei of the distended cells are similarly enlarged. Only a small percentage of CDT-treated cells contain more than one nuclei; cells with more than two nuclei are rare. This observation clearly distinguishes the effect of CDT from that of cytotoxic necrotizing factor, which, in addition to causing cells to enlarge, causes multinucleation (22). Careful examination of cells that have been incubated in the presence of CDT for 48 h suggests that few, if any, of the cells are dividing. Cell death can occur as early as 48 h after the addition of CDT to sensitive cells but usually takes 72 to 96 h. The cells become round and appear to disintegrate. Their membrane appears to consist of small blebs, and nuclear staining can show either irregular chromatin condensation or nuclear fragmentation (Fig. 1) (44). The mechanism of cell death is under investigation, but

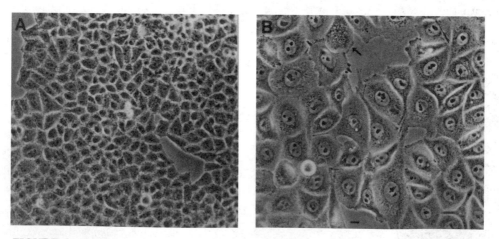

FIGURE 1 CDT-induced distension of HeLa cells. (A) HeLa cells treated with tissue culture medium. (B) HeLa cells treated with CDT. The cells have been incubated for 72 h after the additions. The CDT-treated cells are now grossly distended. Note the single nucleus in most cells. The arrow points to a cell in which the nucleus has fragmented. The bar in panel B represents 15 μm; both photographs were taken at a magnification of ×50.

at least some of the cells appear to be undergoing a programmed cell death.

Genetics

In 1996 Pickett et al. (33) reported the isolation and characterization of the *cdt* genes from *C. jejuni* 81-176. The genes were identified and isolated through the use of degenerative oligonucleotides based on conserved *cdt* sequences from two *E. coli* strains that were reported in 1994 (32, 37). CDT activity is encoded by three adjacent or slightly overlapping genes

named *cdtA, cdtB,* and *cdtC* (Fig. 2). The *C. jejuni* Cdt proteins are similar to the *E. coli* Cdt proteins but have significantly diverged amino acid sequences. The most highly conserved of the Cdt proteins is CdtB; the *E. coli* and *C. jejuni* CdtB sequences have approximately 60% amino acid similarity. All three Cdt proteins have typical leader sequences for secretion, and CdtA appears to have a consensus cleavage site for lipoproteins (34). The amino acid sequences of the Cdt proteins do not show homology to other proteins in the databases, nor

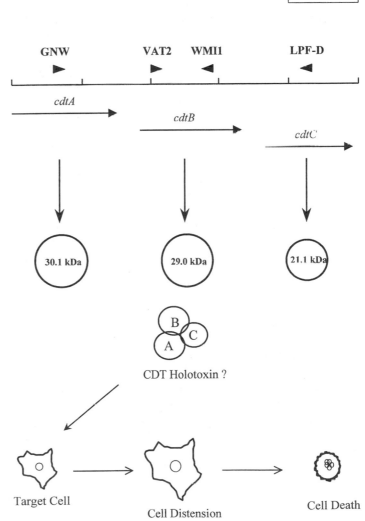

FIGURE 2 Summary of CDT genetics and action. CDT is encoded by three adjacent genes, *cdtABC*, whose location and length are indicated by the arrows underneath the line. The arrowheads shown at the top of the figure represent PCR primers that are useful for amplification of *cdt* sequences from *C. jejuni* and *C. coli* strains (8). The approximate sizes of the Cdt proteins produced by *C. jejuni* are indicated. The subunit structure of the CDT holotoxin is still not known, but it may include all three Cdt proteins. The active toxin molecule causes many sensitive cells to become slowly distended and then to die.

do the sequence data provide clues to the functions of these three proteins.

Upstream of *cdtA* is an approximately 80-bp noncoding region that was examined for typical promoter consensus sequences. No consensus sequences were found, however, and the location of the promoter awaits additional experimentation. These results may mean that the *cdt* genes do not have a typical σ^{70} promoter, but primer extension analysis or similar studies are required before this can be stated with certainty. The first open reading frame upstream of *cdtA* is on the opposite strand from *cdtA,* and its product appears to have no significant homology to known proteins. Immediately downstream of this open reading frame, and on the same strand, is the apparent *C. jejuni* gene for subunit I of cytochrome *d* oxidase. Just downstream of and slightly overlapping the end of *cdtC* is a putative rho-independent transcription termination site. The closest open reading frame downstream of *cdtC* is 180 bp away; this open reading frame encodes an L-lactate permease. Therefore, sequence data appear to indicate that the *C. jejuni cdt* genes probably exist as an operon; however, transcript analysis of these genes has not yet been presented in the literature. In addition, it is not known if the genes are constitutively expressed or if conditions exist which will up or down regulate their expression. We have tested whether iron, growth phase, or growth temperature affects the production of CDT by *C. jejuni* 81-176 and have not detected any significant differences in CDT production under these different conditions. Whether other environmental parameters affect CDT production has not been reported, but there are certainly many other conditions which could be tested, and it would be premature to conclude that expression of the *cdt* genes is not environmentally regulated.

The *C. jejuni cdt* genes are expressed in *E. coli,* apparently from their own promoter (33), although this has not been formally proven. Expression of the *cdt* genes in *E. coli* may not be very good, since the activity produced by *E. coli* cells containing the *C. jejuni cdt* putative

promoter region as well as all three *cdt* genes is not as high as that seen for a comparable number of *C. jejuni* cells containing only the chromosomal copy of the *cdt* genes. Experiments with different combinations of *cdt* clones in *E. coli* have indicated that all three genes must be expressed within the same cell to obtain active CDT (33).

Epidemiology

cdt genes appear to be universally present in *C. jejuni* strains, and they may be similarly common in at least some other *Campylobacter* spp. (9, 28, 33). CDT production may be nearly as common as the presence of the *cdt* genes in *C. jejuni* isolates. Pickett et al. (33) reported the CDT titers in 20 *C. jejuni* strains isolated from diverse geographical areas. Fourteen of these strains were isolated from humans with disease, and the remainder were isolated from cows, a goat, and a lamb. In this work, the titers were defined as the reciprocal of the highest dilution of a preparation that affected 50 to 75% of the HeLa cells in a well of a 96-well assay plate. The CDT was prepared by sonic disruption of overnight-grown cultures of the various *C. jejuni* strains. All titers were adjusted for differences in bacterial cell number (33). All 20 strains produced active toxin, although the amount of toxin produced varied for different isolates. The titers ranged from 11 to over 3,000; the significance of the different titers is not known, but it is clear that some *C. jejuni* strains consistently produce less CDT than other strains. Eyigor et al. (9) recently reported that 70 of 70 *C. jejuni* strains isolated from fresh chicken carcasses contained *cdt* sequences that could be amplified by PCR techniques. Figure 2 indicates the location of PCR primers that were used to detect *cdt* sequences in these isolates. Of the 70 strains, 69 produced active CDT, but, again, the amount of CDT produced varied from strain to strain. The differences in CDT production may be a result of inherent differences in the strains, or there may be more complex regulatory aspects of CDT production than are currently appreciated. Almost nothing is known about the *cdt* gene promoter(s): it is not known if the promoter sequences vary in different isolates, and it is not known if regulation of the expression of the *cdt* genes varies in different strains. Consequently, it is difficult to speculate about the cause of the differences in CDT production in the different isolates. Eyigor et al. (9) also determined that 35 of 35 *C. coli* strains isolated from chicken carcasses possessed *cdt* genes. However, either *C. coli cdt* genes are not expressed well under the growth conditions used or *C. coli* CDT has a substantially different specific activity on HeLa cells from *C. jejuni* CDT, since lysates of *C. coli* strains appear to only poorly intoxicate HeLa cells. Ohya et al. (28) found that CDT activity was produced by 25 of 26 *C. fetus* strains isolated from calves, suggesting that CDT production is similarly widespread in this species as well. Pickett et al. (33) also showed that at least single isolates of *C. hyointestinalis* and *C. upsaliensis* possess *cdt* genes and produce active CDT.

The *C. jejuni* and *C. coli cdt* sequences appear to be significantly diverged. Southern hybridization experiments (33) show that there is only weak cross-hybridization between the *cdtB* genes of these two species. Comparison of portions of the predicted Cdt amino acid sequences from *C. jejuni* 81-176 and *C. coli* D730 revealed numerous dissimilarities. For example, the CdtB proteins from these two species are only 68% identical. However, comparison of *cdt* sequences from other *C. jejuni* strains to the *cdt* sequences from 81-176 suggests a high degree of conservation between isolates within this species (8). Overall, the available data suggest that there is substantial identity among *cdt* sequences within *Campylobacter* species but that there is perhaps significantly less identity among the *cdt* sequences across species boundaries. Conservation of toxin sequences within a species is not at all unusual. For example, comparison of available predicted amino acid sequences of CtxA, the A subunit of cholera toxin, from four different *V. cholerae* strains, shows only two amino acid differences, and both of these represent conservative changes. Similarly, the amino acid sequences of the A

subunit of Shiga toxin from six different *E. coli* strains are available in the database; only 12 of 315 amino acids vary in these sequences, and 10 of these changes are conservative. This conservation suggests that there may be strong evolutionary pressures for maintenance of toxin sequences.

Comparison of the regions flanking the *cdt* genes of *C. jejuni* 81-176 and NCTC 11168 indicate that at least in these two strains the *cdt* genes are in identical locations, since the upstream and downstream open reading frames are conserved. Examination of the sequences within 1.5 kb upstream and downstream of the *cdt* genes in strain NCTC 11168 does not reveal any obvious IS, phage, or plasmid sequences that might indicate that the *cdt* genes were acquired relatively recently through some type of horizontal transfer. The fact that most, if not all, *C. jejuni* strains carry *cdt* genes and that the genes appear to be conserved suggests that the *cdt* genes may have evolved within *Campylobacter* spp. However, comparison to the *C. coli cdt* gene flanking regions indicates that the location of the *C. coli cdt* genes, at least in strain D730 (33), is not the same as that found in *C. jejuni*.

Mode of Action

The CDT produced by *C. jejuni* was recently shown by Whitehouse et al. (44) to cause sensitive eukaryotic cells to become blocked in the G$_2$ phase of the cell cycle. CDT preparations were applied to HeLa cells, and incubation was allowed to continue for up to 5 days. At 1 day intervals, the DNA content of the HeLa cells was examined by flow cytometry. CDT was clearly shown to cause 96% of the HeLa cells to become blocked in either the G$_2$ or early M phase within 24 h. This block appears to be permanent, since DNA content analysis at 48 and 72 h was essentially identical. After 72 h, significant numbers of the CDT-treated cells were disintegrating. A derivative of 81-176 that no longer possessed any intact *cdt* genes was used as a control in these experiments; lysates from this mutant strain had no effect on the HeLa cell cycle phase distribution. Evidence that the block was irreversible was provided by a washing experiment in which it was shown that extensive washing of the HeLa cells as soon as 20 min after the addition of CDT failed to prevent intoxication. Additional work showed that CDT-treated HeLa cells appeared to not have progressed into the M phase, since there was no evidence of chromatin condensation or tubulin reorganization typical of cells in early M phase. Control preparations showed a normal number of dividing cells. Finally, the activation state of the CDC2/cylin B1 was examined in CDT-treated HeLa cells. CDC2/cyclin B1 is the major enzymatic activity that, upon activation, will initiate entry into mitosis. Activation of CDC2/cyclin B1 involves dephosphorylation of the CDC2 subunit at a specific tyrosine residue, Tyr15. If CDC2 is not dephosphorylated at this residue, cells will not enter mitosis. The activation state of CDC2 can be ascertained in a immunoblot experiment; the dephosphorylation of CDC2 will cause a shift in the mobility of the protein on polyacrylamide gels. Therefore, HeLa cells that had been treated with CDT or control lysates for various periods were harvested and solubilized, and their total proteins were separated on polyacrylamide gels. Blots of the gels were treated with antiserum specific for CDC2 and analyzed for shifts in the mobility of CDC2 characteristic of dephosphorylation. The results of this experiment clearly showed that CDC2 in CDT-treated cells had not been dephosphorylated at Tyr15 and therefore had not been activated. This result indicates that CDT somehow prevents activation of the major kinase activity, CDC2, which must be activated for cells to enter mitosis. Thus, CDT can cause a G_2-phase-specific block in HeLa cells. There are a variety of ways in which G_2 blocks can arise, and it is not yet clear how CDT brings about the failure to activate CDC2/cyclin B1 (44).

Structure

The holotoxin structure of CDT has not yet been definitively determined. There are a number of problems associated with purification of CDT, and consequently characterization of CDT has not progressed rapidly. CDT appears to be very potent: it is possible to apply preparations of *C. jejuni* CDT with over 1,500 U of activity to polyacrylamide gels which are then silver stained and to see no protein bands. (One unit of activity is equivalent to a titer of 1, where "titer" is as defined above.) Partially purified preparations of CDT with very high activity (2,000 U/μl) will also not exhibit proteins on Coomassie blue-stained gels with sizes appropriate for the Cdt proteins. However, immunoblots of these gels, reacted with rabbit polyclonal antisera specific for His-tagged fusions of each of the Cdt proteins, clearly show that all three Cdt proteins are present.

An additional complication is the fact that over 90% of all CDT activity produced by *C. jejuni* strains is tightly associated with the membrane fraction of lysed cells. Successful purification of substantial amounts of CDT will require solubilization of the activity from the membrane. This task may be made more difficult if activity requires more than one subunit, since detergent solubilization may readily cause dissociation of multisubunit proteins.

We have not been able to find naturally soluble CDT in culture supernatants. The activity in culture supernatants does not behave as if it were soluble: it is readily pelletable at speeds that would pellet membrane vesicles, and if concentrated supernatants are applied to gel filtration columns, the activity appears in the void volume. These results are consistent with the idea that the activity in the supernatant consists of membrane particles (blebs?) that contain CDT.

Role in Pathogenesis

The role of CDT in *C. jejuni* pathogenesis has not been determined. The best method for determining a contribution of CDT to diarrheal disease would be to use an established animal model for *C. jejuni* disease, but unfortunately there are no reports in the literature of the testing of defined CDT-negative mutants in an animal model. This is probably due, at least in part, to the paucity of convenient, well-documented, widely used animal models for the study of *C. jejuni*-induced diarrheal disease.

Nonetheless, animal model studies must be done, and it is hoped that they will be done soon.

However, the activity of CDT does suggest a possible contribution of CDT to diarrheal disease. We have shown that CDT is active on Caco-2 cells (44). These cells are derived from human colonic epithelial cells and are widely used as a model for human intestinal epithelial cell functions. If CDT is similarly active on the rapidly dividing and differentiating cells in the crypts of the intestines, it may have the effect of blocking the development of the mature epithelial cells needed for absorptive functions. This could lead to a temporary disruption and erosion of the normal intestinal epithelial layer, with associated loss of function.

The CDT Family

In the past few years, it has become apparent that CDT is produced by several bacterial pathogens, including at least two that cause diseases other than gastroenteritis. Cope et al. (6) have shown that a cytotoxin produced by *Haemophilus ducreyi* is a CDT. *H. ducreyi* causes chancroid, a sexually transmitted disease characterized by genital ulcers. How CDT contributes to the pathogenesis of chancroid is not yet known but is under active investigation. In addition, an immunosuppressive activity produced by *Actinobacillus actinomycetemcomitans* has recently been shown to be a CDT. *A. actinomycetemcomitans* is a major contributor to the development of juvenile periodontitis, and it has been hypothesized that the ability of the CDT produced by this bacterium to kill T cells may play a role in promoting the chronic nature of this periodontal disease (38). In addition, other investigators have continued to study the CDTs produced by *Shigella* spp. and *E. coli* isolates. Of perhaps most relevance to this review is the finding by Okuda et al. (29) that the CDT produced by a *Shigella dysenteriae* strain was able to promote diarrheal symptoms in a dose-dependent manner in a suckling-mouse model. These investigators also showed that CDT caused necrosis and reparative hyperplasia in the descending colons of the affected animals. Recent work from several groups indicates that all of the CDTs probably have the same effect on the cell cycle of sensitive cells; i.e., the target cells become blocked in G_2 (5, 7, 38, 40).

Future Directions

The study of CDT has become fast-paced and exciting for two major reasons: (i) CDT is now known to be a family of related toxins produced by several bacterial pathogens, and (ii) the novel ability of CDT to block the eukaryotic cell cycle in the G_2 phase has created increased interest in understanding the mechanism of action of the toxin.

Current and future studies of CDT will certainly focus on discovering the specifics of its interactions with eukaryotic cells. At the same time, experiments aimed at understanding the contribution of CDT to pathogenesis will be of central importance. In addition, there are many other aspects of CDT biology which are not known. For example, the CDT holotoxin structure is not known, nor is the function of each Cdt protein. Whether one or more of the Cdt proteins have an enzymatic activity is not known. The *C. jejuni* CDT appears to have a specific receptor protein(s) on CHO and HeLa cells (3), but the nature and identity of this protein has not been published, nor has work describing a CDT receptor for the other CDT-producing bacteria been presented. In addition, studies of the expression of the *cdt* genes are very limited, and it is not clear if the expression of the genes is regulated in response to some environmental signal. However, work presented in the past few years has provided the basis for being able to answer these questions and hence to understand this fascinating cytotoxin and its role in pathogenesis.

NON-CDT CYTOTOXINS

The literature is full of reports on an apparent variety of cytotoxic activities attributed to various *Campylobacter* isolates. With a few notable exceptions, it is impossible to determine from simply reading this literature whether these reports are of the same or different activities. This section first provides an overview of reports of cytotoxic activities produced by *Campylobacter* spp. published prior to 1997, then discusses more recent reports of two activities, CLRT and a porin-lipopolysaccharide activity.

CHO/HeLa Cell Cytotoxin

In addition to CDT, Wassenaar grouped *Campylobacter* cytotoxic activities into five theoretically distinguishable cytotoxins. This overview will follow her classification scheme. One of the cytotoxic activities was called the 70-kDa cytotoxin, since several of the reports of this activity suggested that it was in the range of 30 to 70 kDa (12, 15). Most reports indicate that this 70-kDa activity is heat and trypsin sensitive and is active on CHO cells and HeLa cells but not on Vero cells. Affected cells become rounded and die; the reported titers vary considerably, and are sometimes quite low. For example, Guerrant et al. (12) reported on a cytotoxic activity found in the supernatants of polymyxin B-treated cultures. This activity was produced by several *C. jejuni* strains, but the highest titer noted for any of them (strain C31) was 8 on HeLa cells and 38 on CHO cells. Misawa et al. used CHO cell assays for detection and differentiation of *C. jejuni* cytotoxic activities present in culture supernatants (23–25). They concluded that they may be detecting three different activities based on differences in heat stability, pH sensitivity, apparent size, and activity in three different assays. However, two of these activities had titers that ranged between only 2 and 8; the third activity had a titer as high as 128. In some reports, e.g., reference 26, a CHO cell-active cytotoxin was shown to be associated with cell membranes. In summary, there are numerous reports of a *C. jejuni* cytotoxin that affects CHO and HeLa cells, that appears to be a protein, and that may be associated with the bacterial cell membrane. The typically low titer of the activity in many of the reports will make extensive characterization of the activity difficult.

Vero-Active and Shiga-Like Toxins and Hepatotoxin

There are a few reports of a cytotoxic activity that is active on Vero (and HeLa) cells (11, 15).

In common with the above 70-kDa cytotoxin, the basic response of cells to this activity is to become rounded and die. In general, the reported titers for this activity were also not high (e.g., up to 4 in reference 15), and it seems likely that furthering our understanding of this activity will require methods for improving the detection and/or increasing the production of the toxin. There is a single report of the production of a Shiga-like toxin produced by some *C. jejuni* and *C. coli* strains; however, attempts to find *C. jejuni* genes with homology to the Shiga-like toxin genes have not been successful (27), and a search of the *C. jejuni* genome did not reveal any sequences with significant homology to Shiga-like toxin sequences. Another activity, called hepatotoxin, has also been the subject of a few reports (19, 20). This activity was suggested to be responsible for a chronic hepatic disorder that develops in mice infected intragastrically with certain *C. jejuni* strains. Both infection with live *C. jejuni* and intravenous injection of partially purified hepatotoxin caused similar types of lesions in the mouse liver. These results are intriguing, and further characterization of this activity would be a useful addition to the *Campylobacter* toxin literature.

Hemolysins

Both cell-associated (contact) hemolytic activity and secreted hemolytic activities have been reported to be produced by various *C. jejuni* or *C. coli* strains (1, 14, 31, 41). A number of investigators have mentioned the presence of a contact hemolysin, yet little is known about this activity and whether the different reports are analyzing the same activity is unclear. There are two reports of a hemolytic activity present in *C. jejuni* culture filtrates, but the characterization of these activities is very preliminary. There are no reports in the literature identifying any likely hemolysin genes from *C. jejuni*. The one report of isolation of a *C. jejuni* gene which caused a hemolytic response when cloned into *E. coli* appears to have identified a protein which is probably not a true hemolysin (30), since neither cell culture supernatants from nor cell lysates of the *E. coli* strain containing the clone produced a hemolytic activity. A search of the *C. jejuni* genome's predicted proteins revealed no open reading frames with significant homology to either the *E. coli* RTX family hemolysin, HlyA (10, 43), or to the *E. coli* enterohemolysin sequences (4, 39). It is possible that the hemolysin activities reported for *C. jejuni* are the consequences of one of the already described cytotoxic activities or of the lysis in culture of older cells which are releasing some material that is toxic to erythrocytes.

CLRT and CLDT/CLRT

Hanel et al. (13) recently reported finding evidence for two *Campylobacter* cytotoxins. One was identified as CDT (called CLDT by these authors), and the other was named cytolethal rounding toxin (CLRT) based on the rounded appearance of affected CHO cells. Both toxins were reported to cause a decrease in the number of CHO cells compared to untreated cells. While, as expected, CDT appeared to cause the cells to distend and become enlarged over a 48-h period, CLRT-treated cells simply appeared rounded at 48 h. Very short incubation times (5 to 20 min) confirmed that the eventual effects of CDT can be seen with such short treatment times; however, CLRT appeared to have no effect when left in contact with the cells for such a short time. In a subsequent paper from this group (36), an additional response of cultured cells to sonic lysates from some *Campylobacter* isolates was described and named CLDT/CLRT. Lysates from CLDT/CLRT-producing strains caused a mixture of distended and rounded cells. The authors examined a variety of *Campylobacter* isolates for their ability to produce these apparently different activities and found no clear pattern of association of toxin type with the source of the isolate or the type of outbreak from which the isolates were obtained. The authors think that the CLDT/CLRT activity is really a mixture of CDT and CLRT. Whether the CLRT discussed in this paper is the same as any of the numerous reports of *Campylobacter* cytotoxins that cause cell rounding is not certain, but its basic effect on CHO cells resembles the descriptions of the effects of some of the cytotoxic activities described above.

Porin-Lipopolysaccharide

Bacon et al. (2) have reported a cytotoxic activity which appears to be associated with a porin-lipopolysaccharide complex. The HEp-2 cells treated with this activity were reported to form transient vacuoles and then to become rounded and die. The activity was seen within 24 to 48 h, depending on the dose. A purification procedure produced a 4- to 15-fold increase in specific activity (depending upon the cell culture type used for the assay) and yielded a single major band on a silver-stained polyacrylamide gel. This band was identified as the *C. jejuni* porin. The active material was also shown to contain lipopolysaccharide. Again, whether this activity is the same as one of the many activities described by other investigators is not known, but it is certainly possible.

Future Directions

While it is clear that *C. jejuni* strains make at least one cytotoxin, CDT, it is not clear how many other activities exist. The numerous reports of culture supernatants or cell extracts that cause cultured cells to become rounded and die indicates that this undoubtedly happens. However, the various reports of cytotoxic activity are quite difficult to compare, since different strains were tested and since the procedures used were often quite dissimilar. In addition, some reports did not provide data about toxin titers, making it difficult to compare these reports to the work of others or to be able to reasonably evaluate the data.

In an effort to look for non-CDT cytotoxic activities, we recently tested a CDT-negative derivative of *C. jejuni* 81-176 (33) for its ability to produce other cytotoxic activities. This strain has had most of its *cdt* coding region deleted, and it produces no CDT activity. A CDT-negative strain was chosen for this study because it appears that relatively high doses of CDT itself will cause HeLa or CHO cells to become rounded and die within 48 h. Lysates of the mutant *C. jejuni* cells grown for 48 h in brucella broth without agitation were produced by sonication (33), and culture supernatants were tested for the presence of factors that caused rounding of HeLa or CHO cells. Neither culture supernatants nor lysates of the CDT-negative mutant produced any significant level of cell rounding on HeLa cells. The first well of the dilution series sometimes contained 10 to 20% rounded cells, but any activity causing this response would have a titer of less than 2. The result on CHO cells was similar but not identical. Supernatants from the mutant strain caused 25 to 50% of the CHO cells in the first well of the dilution series to become rounded. Culture lysates caused between 75 and 100% of the cells in the first well to be rounded and about half that number in the next well, indicating a titer of 4. Controls consisted of identical preparations and assays of the parental strain, 81-176. Control supernatants had a CDT titer of 64 on HeLa cells; control lysates had a CDT titer of 128 on HeLa cells. Some cell rounding and death was visible in the first one or two wells of the dilution series of the control culture supernatants on HeLa and CHO cells; cell lysates caused dead and rounded cells through the third well of the two-fold dilution series. The control materials had significantly lower CDT titers on CHO-K1 cells, confirming our earlier observations that HeLa cells appear to be more sensitive to *C. jejuni* CDT than CHO cells do.

Overall, these results suggest that whatever is causing the cell rounding is slightly more toxic to CHO cells than to HeLa cells. However, the titers are quite low, and consequently this cell-rounding activity is probably not caused by a specific toxin but may instead be a nonspecific effect caused by some component or combination of components present in the preparations.

It would be interesting to test CDT-negative derivatives of additional *C. jejuni* strains for the presence of other toxic activities. In particular, if CDT-negative derivatives of some of the strains used by different investigators could be made, it would be possible to deter-

mine if some of the toxic effects attributed to various cytotoxins were actually caused by CDT.

In addition, it might be of interest to test CDT-negative derivatives for other potential virulence capabilities, such as colonization and invasion. These kinds of studies have not been reported.

ENTEROTOXINS

Since the clinical picture for *C. jejuni* disease can include watery diarrhea, it is reasonable to hypothesize that *C. jejuni* makes some sort of enterotoxin. Numerous reports in the literature have concluded that at least some *C. jejuni* strains can make an enterotoxic activity (see, e.g., reference 35), and other investigators have suggested that an enterotoxin with antigenic relatedness to cholera toxin is produced by *C. jejuni* (21). Nonetheless, the existence of such a *C. jejuni* enterotoxin has not been proven, and the subject remains controversial. At the center of the controversy are two key points. First, a number of laboratories have been unable to demonstrate any enterotoxic activity associated with *C. jejuni* strains, and second, genes encoding a cholera-like *C. jejuni* enterotoxin have not been discovered.

Both the data supporting an entertoxic activity and the data that have led to the controversy have been recently and thoroughly reviewed by Wassenaar (42) and are not repeated here. An answer to the question whether there is a *C. jejuni* activity with similarities to cholera toxin will require either purification and characterization of the toxin, including a demonstration of the enterotoxic activity of the purified material, or isolation of the genes encoding the activity. Neither of these events has occurred. However, the *C. jejuni* genome has been sequenced, and no cholera-like enterotoxin genes were found. This seems to indicate that there is not a cholera-like enterotoxic activity produced by *C. jejuni*. Presumably, some other toxic activity or capability of *C. jejuni* causes the watery diarrhea seen in *C. jejuni* illness. There is still the possibility that some strains of *C. jejuni* produce a cholera-like enterotoxin, but acceptance of this idea will require direct proof.

CONCLUDING REMARKS

The most rewarding aspect of *Campylobacter* toxin research has been the realization that the toxins produced by this genus are not going to be a repeat of already well-known and characterized diarrheagenic toxins. Instead, it appears that *Campylobacter* toxic acivities represent new varieties of toxins, and the continued study of these agents should yield new and exciting information not only about *Campylobacter* pathogenesis but also about paradigms of host-pathogen interactions.

REFERENCES

1. **Arini, S. M., R. W. A. Park, and C. R. Fricker.** 1990. Study of haemolytic activity of some *Camylobacter* spp. on blood agar plates. *J. Appl. Bacteriol.* **69:**384–389.
2. **Bacon, D. J., W. M. Johnson, and F. G. Rodgers.** 1999. Identification and characterisation of a cytotoxic proin-lipopolysaccharide complex from *Campylobacter jejuni. J. Med. Microbiol.* **48:**139–148.
3. **Bag, P. K., T. Ramamurthy, and U. B. Nair.** 1993. Evidence for the presence of a receptor for the cytolethal distending toxin (CLDT) of *Campylobacter jejuni* on CHO and HeLa cell membranes and development of a receptor-based enzyme-linked immunosorbent assay for detection of CLDT. *FEMS Microbiol. Lett.* **114:**285–292.
4. **Beutin, L., U. H. Stroher, and P. A. Manning.** 1993. Isolation of enterohemolysin (Ehly2)-associated sequences encoded on temperate phages of *Escherichia coli. Gene* **132:**95–99.
5. **Comayras, C., C. Tasca, S. Y. Peres, B. Cucommun, E. Oswald, and J. De Rycke.** 1997. *Escherichia coli* cytolethal distending toxin blocks the HeLa cell cycle at the G_2/M transition by preventing cdc2 protein kinase dephosphorylation and activation. *Infect. Immun.* **65:**5088–5095.
6. **Cope, L. D., S. Lumbley, J. L. Latimer, J. Klesney-Tait, M. K. Stevens, L. S. Johnson, M. Purven, R. S. Munson, Jr., T. Lagergard, J. D. Radolf, and E. J. Hansen.** 1997. A diffusible cytotoxin of *Haemophilus docreyi. Proc. Natl. Acad. Sci. USA* **94:**4056–4061.
7. **Cortes-Bratti, X., E. Chaves-Olarte, T. Lagergard, and M. Thelestam.** 1999. The cytolethal distending toxin from the chancroid bacterium Haemophilus ducreyi induces cell-cycle arrest in the G2 phase. *J. Clin. Investig.* **103:**107–115.
8. **Eyigor, A., K. A. Dawson, B. E. Langlois, and C. L. Pickett.** 1999. Cytolethal distending toxin genes in *Campylobacter jejuni* and *Campylobacter coli* isolates: Detection and analysis by PCR. *J. Clin. Microbiol.* **37:**1646–1650.
9. **Eyigor, A., K. A. Dawson, B. E. Langlois, and C. L. Pickett.** 1999. Detection of cytolethal distending toxin activity and *cdt* genes in *Campylobacter* spp. isolated from chicken carcasses. *Appl. Environ. Microbiol.* **65:**1501–1505.
10. **Felmlee, T., S. Pellett, and R. A. Welch.** 1985. Nucleotide sequence of an *Escherichia coli* chromosomal hemolysin. *J. Bacteriol.* **163:**94–105.
11. **Florin, I., and F. Antillon.** 1992. Production of enterotoxin and cytotoxin in *Campylobacter jejuni* strains in Costa Rica. *J. Med. Microbiol.* **37:**22–29.
12. **Guerrant, R. L., C. A. Wanke, R. A. Pennie, L. J. Barrett, A. A. M. Lima, and A. D. O'Brien.** 1987. Production of a unique cytotoxin by *Campylobacter jejuni. Infect. Immun.* **55:** 2526–2530.
13. **Hanel, I., F. Schulze, H. Hotzel, and E. Schubert.** 1998. Detection and characterization of two cytotoxins produced by *Campylobacter jejuni* strains. *Zentbl. Bakteriol.* **288:**131–143.
14. **Hossain, A., D. E. S. Stewart-Hull, and J. H. Freer.** 1993. Heat-labile and heat-stable haemolysis of *C. jejuni.* FEMS Immun. *Med. Microbiol.* **6:** 331–340.
15. **Johnson, W. M., and H. Lior.** 1986. Cytotoxic and cytotonic factors produced by *Campylobacter jejuni, Campylobacter coli,* and *Campylobacter laridis. J. Clin. Microbiol.* **24:**275–281.
16. **Johnson, W. M., and H. Lior.** 1987. Production of Shiga toxin and a cytolethal distending toxin (CLDT) by serogroups of *Shigella* spp. *FEMS Microbiol. Lett.* **48:**235–238.
17. **Johnson, W. M., and H. Lior.** 1988. A new heat-labile cytolethal distending toxin (CLDT) produced by *Escherichia coli* isolates from clinical material. *Microb. Pathog.* **4:**103–113.
18. **Johnson, W. M., and H. Lior.** 1988. A new heat-labile cytolethal distending toxin (CLDT) produced by *Campylobacter* spp. *Microb. Pathog.* **4:** 115–126.
19. **Kita, E., F. Nishikawa, N. Kamikaidou, A. Nakano, N. Katsui, and S. Kashiba.** 1992. Mononuclear cell response in the liver of mice infected with hepatotoxigenic *Campylobacter jejuni. J. Med. Microbiol.* **37:**326–331.
20. **Kita, E., D. Oku, A. Hamuro, F. Nishikawa, M. Emoto, Y. Yagyn, N. Datsui, and S. Kashiba.** 1990. Hepatotoxic activity of *Campylobacter jejuni. J. Med. Microbiol.* **33:**171–182.
21. **Klipstein, F. A., and R. F. Engert.** 1985. Immunological relationship of the B subunits of

Campylobacter jejuni and *Escherichia coli* heat-labile enterotoxins. *Infect. Immun.* **48**:629–633.

22. **Lerm, M., J. Selzer, A. Hoffmeyer, U. R. Rapp, K. Aktories, and G. Schmidt.** 1999. Deamidation of Cdc42 and Rac by *Escherichia coli* cytotoxic necrotizing factor 1: activation of c-Jun N-terminal kinase in HeLa cells. *Infect. Immun.* **67:** 496–503.

23. **Misawa, N., T. Ohnishi, K. Itoh, and E. Takahashi.** 1994. Development of a tissue culture assay system for *Campylobacter jejuni* cytotoxin and the influence of culture conditions on cytotoxin production. *J. Med. Microbiol.* **41**:224–230.

24. **Misawa, N., T. Ohnishi, K. Itoh, and E. Takahashi.** 1995. Cytotoxin detection in *Campylobacter jejuni* strains of human and animal origin with three tissue culture assay systems. *J. Med. Microbiol.* **43**:354–359.

25. **Misawa, N., T. Ohnishi, K. Itoh, and E. Takahashi.** 1996. Detection of serum-dependent cytotoxic activity of *Campylobacter jejuni* and its characteristics. *J. Vet. Med. Sci.* **58**:91–96.

26. **Mizuno, K., K. Takama, and S. Suzuki.** 1994. Characteristics of cytotoxin produced by *Campylobacter jejuni* strains. *Microbios* **78**:215–228.

27. **Moore, M. A., M. J. Blaser, G. I. Perez-Perez, and A. D. O'Brien.** 1988. Production of a shiga-like cytotoxin by *Campylobacter*. *Microb. Pathog.* **4**:455–462.

28. **Ohya, T., K. Tominaga, and M. Nakazawa.** 1993. Production of cytolethal distending toxin (CLDT) by *Campylobacter fetus* subsp. *fetus* isolated from calves. *J. Vet. Med. Sci.* **55**:507–509.

29. **Okuda, J., M. Fukumoto, Y. Takeda, and M. Nishibuchi.** 1997. Examination of diarrheagenicity of cytolethal distending toxin: suckling mouse response to the products of the *cdtABC* genes of *Shigella dysenteriae*. *Infect. Immun.* **65**: 428–433.

30. **Park, S. F., and P. T. Richardson.** 1995. Molecular characterization of a *Campylobacter jejuni* lipoprotein with homology to periplasmic siderophore-binding proteins. *J. Bacteriol.* **177:** 2259–2264.

31. **Pickett, C. L., T. Auffenberg, E. C. Pesci, V. L. Sheen, and S. S. D. Jusuf.** 1992. Iron acquisition and hemolysin production by *Campylobacter jejuni*. *Infect. Immun.* **60**:3872–3877.

32. **Pickett, C. L., D. L. Cottle, E. C. Pesci, and G. Bikah.** 1994. Cloning, sequencing, and expression of the *Escherichia coli* cytolethal distending toxin genes. *Infect. Immun.* **62**: 1046–1051.

33. **Pickett, C. L., E. C. Pesci, D. L. Cottle, G. Russell, A. N. Erdem, and H. Zeytin.** 1996. Prevalence of cytolethal distending toxin production in *Campylobacter jejuni* and relatedness of *Campylobacter cdtB* genes. *Infect. Immun.* **64:** 2070–2078.

34. **Pugsley, A. P.** 1993. The complete general secretory pathway in gram-negative bacteria. *Microbiol. Rev.* **57:**50–108.

35. **Ruiz-Palacios, G. M., J. Torres, N. I. Torres, E. Escamilla, B. R. Ruiz-Palacios, and J. Tamayo.** 1983. Cholera-like enterotoxin produced by *Campylobacter jejuni*. *Lancet* **ii**:250–253.

36. **Schulze, F., I. Hanel, and E. Borrmann.** 1998. Formation of cytotoxins by enteric *Campylobacter* in humans and animals. *Zentbl. Bakteriol.* **288:** 225–236.

37. **Scott, D. A., and J. B. Kaper.** 1994. Cloning and sequencing of the genes encoding *Escherichia coli* cytolethal distending toxin. *Infect. Immun.* **62:** 244–251.

38. **Shenker, B. J., T. McKay, S. Datar, M. Miller, R. Chowhan, and D. Demuth.** 1999. *Actinobacillus actinomycetemcomitans* immunosuppressive protein is a member of the family of cytolethal distending toxins capable of causing a G arrest in human T cells. *J. Immunol.* **162:**4773–4780.

39. **Stroher, U. H., L. Bode, L. Beutin, and P. A. Manning.** 1993. Characterization and sequence of a 33-kDa enterohemolysin (Ehly 1)-associated protein in *Escherichia coli*. *Gene* **132:** 89–94.

40. **Sugai, M., T. Kawamoto, S. Y. Peres, Y. Ueno, H. Komatsuzawa, T. Fujiwara, H. Kurihara, H. Suginaka, and E. Oswald.** 1998. The cell cycle-specific growth-inhibitory factor produced by *Actinobacillus actinomycetemcomitans* is a cytolethal distending toxin. *Infect. Immun.* **66:** 5008–5019.

41. **Tay, S. T., S. Devi, S. Puthucheary, and I. M. Kautner.** 1995. Detection of haemolytic activity of *Campylobacters* by agarose haemolysis and microphate assay. *J. Med. Microbiol.* **42:**175–180.

42. **Wassenaar, T. M.** 1997. Toxin production by *Campylobacter* spp. *Clin. Microbiol. Rev.* **10:** 466–476.

43. **Welch, R. A.** 1991. Pore-forming cytolysins of Gram-negative bacteria. *Mol. Microbiol.* **5:** 521–528.

44. **Whitehouse, C. A., P. B. Balbo, E. C. Pesci, D. L. Cottle, P. M. Mirabito, and C. L. Pickett.** 1998. *Campylobacter jejuni* cytolethal distending toxin causes a G_2-phase cell cycle block. *Infect. Immun.* **66**:1934–1940.

INTERACTIONS OF *CAMPYLOBACTER* WITH EUKARYOTIC CELLS: GUT LUMINAL COLONIZATION AND MUCOSAL INVASION MECHANISMS

Lan Hu and Dennis J. Kopecko

10

Campylobacter spp. are small, spiral, gram-negative bacteria with polar flagella; they are microaerophilic, a diagnostic requisite that both delayed their recognition as pathogens and probably hampers accurate measure of their true incidence in human disease today. *C. jejuni* and *C. coli* are major causes of diarrheal diseases in the world and as few as 5 to 500 organisms given orally can cause human diarrheal illness (6, 111). With the ubiquitous carriage of campylobacters by some domestic animals, combined with its low infectious dose for humans, it is not surprising that *Campylobacter* surpasses *Salmonella* in incidence as a diarrheagenic pathogen. Infection with *C. jejuni* is often associated with the onset of diarrhea, crampy abdominal pain, malaise, myalgia, headache, fever, and/or the presence of blood and leukocytes in stool (6, 7). In addition, *Campylobacter* infection has been infrequently reported to be secondarily associated with cases of meningitis, pseudoappendicitis, pancreatitis, nephritis, urinary tract infection, and reactive arthritis (5, 122), among other sequelae. Very importantly, certain serotypes of *C. jejuni* have been re-ported to be primarily responsible for cases of post-diarrheal Guillian-Barré paralysis (8).

The mechanisms by which *C. jejuni* and *C. coli* induce disease are not well understood. Skirrow and Blaser (121) have aptly noted that *Campylobacter* infection in developing countries tends to result in watery, noninflammatory diarrhea while similar infections in developed countries typically result in acute inflammatory enteritis. Despite these important generalizations, a spectrum of disease symptoms can be triggered by *Campylobacter* infection. At least three mechanisms by which *Campylobacter* may induce illness can be postulated on the basis of clinical syndromes: (i) intestinal adherence of ingested organisms and production of bacterial enterotoxins, inducing secretory diarrhea; (ii) bacterial invasion and proliferation within the intestinal mucosa, inducing cell damage and an inflammatory response clinically manifested as inflammatory diarrhea with fecal leukocytes and/or dysentery; and (iii) extraintestinal translocation, in which the organisms cross the intestinal mucosa and migrate via the lymphatic system to various extraintestinal sites, leading to meningitis, cholecystitis, urinary tract infection, mesenteric adenitis, etc. (114). It seems reasonable to presume that *Campylobacter* pathogenesis is determined by the relative susceptibility of the host and the relative virulence of

Lan Hu and Dennis J. Kopecko, Laboratory of Enteric and Sexually Transmitted Diseases, FDA Center for Biologics Evaluation and Research, Bldg. 29/420, NIH Campus, Bethesda, MD 20892.

Campylobacter, 2nd Ed., Edited by I. Nachamkin and M. J. Blaser
© 2000 American Society for Microbiology, Washington, D.C.

the infecting strain. While it has been proposed that host susceptibility may be the most important factor in determining disease progression and expression (66), it is not at all clear if different *Campylobacter* strains harbor different virulence traits which also influence the type of disease symptoms experienced.

Bacterial diseases are typically the result of a complex set of interactions between the offending bacteria and the host. In the process of evolution, humans have developed a variety of ways to protect themselves from pathogenic organisms (e.g., the mucin barrier of the gut, the organized monolayer of the absorptive epithelial mucosa, nonspecific and specific immune defenses, gut peristalsis). At the same time, bacteria have evolved ways to circumvent these host defenses (e.g., motility to penetrate the mucin barrier, gut adherence mechanisms, and epithelial-cell internalization processes). It is now well accepted that bacterial virulence is multifactorial. Proposed components of *C. jejuni* virulence include toxins (such as enterotoxin and various cytotoxins), adherence, motility, iron acquisition ability, and bacterial invasion, among other properties (67, 132).

A cholera-like enterotoxic activity has been reported for certain *C. jejuni* strains (71, 72, 114). However, the responsible gene sequences have not been detected with cholera toxin or heat-labile toxin DNA probes (99, 104). Furthermore, analysis of fecal filtrates from persons with *C. jejuni* enteritis has not revealed soluble enterotoxic activity (19), and unlike persons infected with *Vibrio cholerae* or enterotoxigenic *Escherichia coli,* affected persons do not produce serum antibodies to the putative toxin. Thus, 15 years after its initial description, there is no definitive proof of whether a cholera-like enterotoxin of *C. jejuni* exists or contributes to disease pathogenesis. There are many reports of cytotoxins in campylobacters (19, 51, 65, 67). A cytolethal distending toxin has been found in many *C. jejuni* strains and has been reported to lock target eukaryotic cells in the G_2 phase (136). A minority of *Campylobacter* strains produce a cy-

totoxin that is specifically neutralized by antiserum to *E. coli* Shiga-like toxin 1 (93). Hemolysin has also been mentioned as a possible pathogenic factor (2). The relationship of any these toxins to disease remains undefined.

The results of intestinal biopsies of patients (128), infected primates (116), and several other experimental model animals (4, 96, 112, 113, 120, 135, 139) have demonstrated that gut cell invasion by *Campylobacter* spp. occurs in vivo and support the importance of bacterial invasiveness as a virulence factor. The ability of *Campylobacter* to invade host cells in vitro is now well established, but the biochemical and molecular mechanisms involved are only now being revealed. *Campylobacter* invasion in vitro is followed after 12 to 24 h by pronounced but as yet undefined cytopathic effects, which may comprise a primary mechanism for damage to the colonic mucosa, leading to inflammation and diarrhea (116).

Many bacterial pathogens interact with host mucosal surfaces resulting in disease (e.g., *Salmonella* spp., *Shigella* spp., *Neisseria gonorrheae,* and enteropathogenic *E. coli* [EPEC]). These pathogens typically exploit the host cell machinery, which contributes to their pathogenic ability. For example, upon association with human intestinal epithelial cells, *Salmonella, Shigella,* and EPEC secrete effector proteins into the eukaryotic host cell which initiate host signal transduction events that lead to cytoskeletal rearrangements and eventual intimate colonization (for EPEC) or engulfment (for *Salmonella* and *Shigella*) of the adjacent pathogen. As with other enteric bacteria, *Campylobacter* interacts intimately with host cells during disease pathogenesis. Identifying the molecular components of this interaction of campylobacters with the host will lead to an improved understanding of disease pathogenesis and the development of new potential prophylactic and therapeutic strategies.

The pathogenesis of *Campylobacter* gastroenteritis is a complex process in which adherence and invasion of host mucosal surfaces are likely to be essential early steps. This chapter gives an overview of the interaction of *C. jejuni* and

C. coli (i.e., the key agents of *Campylobacter*-related human intestinal illness) with host cells, focusing on the bacterial and host factors involved in adherence and invasion into host cells. However, it is important to note that virtually all *C. jejuni* and *C. coli* strains show cell adherence in in vitro assays but only some strains are notably invasive in cultured host cell assays. Also, only a few strains have been fed to volunteers to demonstrate their pathogenicity (6), and there is no definitive proof of involvement of toxins in disease. Thus, it is unclear if *C. jejuni* and *C. coli* strains can be minimally divided into two pathotypes (i.e., toxigenic and adherent versus invasive and inflammatory) or whether disease expression is defined mainly by host susceptibility or other factors.

ADHERENCE AND COLONIZATION

C. jejuni is part of the normal gut flora in many animals including avians, rodents, and dogs. In mice, *C. jejuni* colonizes the mucus layer and crypts of the intestinal mucosa, mainly in the colon and cecum. In other animals, different parts of the gastrointestinal tract may be preferentially colonized, depending upon the ecological microenvironment (e.g., oxygen tension, pH, and presence of host receptors) (82). Humans typically acquire campylobacters in contaminated food or water. Following passage through the stomach, these organisms colonize the ileum and colon, where they interfere with the normal absorptive capacity of the intestine.

The first visible interaction between a pathogenic enteric organism and its host entails colonization of the mucus barrier or attachment to the eukaryotic cell surface. Little is understood about the requirements for colonization of the mucus barriers; for *Campylobacter*, motility and chemotaxis appear important. However, specific adherence to or degradation of mucus components may be involved. Microbes may express alternative cellular adherence mechanisms depending upon the environmental conditions encountered at different host surfaces. In addition to bacterial colonization of the mucus layer and adherence to the mucosal cell surface, invasive bacteria appear to bind transiently to the host cell prior to internalization. Although many *Campylobacter* surface components have been studied for their involvement in adherence to human intestinal cells, little is known about which adherence functions are important in animal colonization and why, for example, chickens are susceptible to *Campylobacter* colonization but not disease.

Bacterial Factors

The ability of many pathogenic bacteria to bind to nonprofessional phagocytic cells is an important virulence determinant since it prevents the colonizing bacteria from being removed by mechanical cleansing forces such as peristalsis and fluid flow. This is particularly valuable in the intestinal and urinary tracts, where mucosal surfaces are continually bathed by fluids. Furthermore, adherent organisms are partially protected from host immune responses (63). Virtually all known bacterial pathogens have some way of attaching themselves to host cells. Bacterial adherence is most typically due to a specific interaction between molecules on the bacterial surface (i.e., adhesins) and molecules on the host surface (i.e., receptors). Two common structures used by bacteria to attach to host cells are pili (or fimbriae), which are hair-like, rod-shaped protein structures that extend out from the bacterial surface, and afimbrial adhesins, which are bacterial surface proteins that are not organized in a rodlike structure but mediate tight binding between bacteria and the host cell (118). As is the case for other intestinal pathogens, the ability of *C. jejuni* to colonize the gastrointestinal tract by binding to epithelial cells has been proposed to be essential for disease production. Fauchere et al. (35) initially reported that *C. jejuni* isolated from individuals with fever and diarrhea exhibited much greater binding to epithelial cells than did strains isolated from asymptomatic individuals, but did not examine specific adherence mechanisms.

Pili and OMPs

Numerous studies have been performed to identify and characterize potential *Campylobacter* adhesins that mediate attachment of the organism to host cells. Doig et al. (25) recently reported that growth in the bile salt deoxycholate induces the synthesis of pili in six studied strains of *C. coli* and *C. jejuni*. A nonpiliated mutant of *C. jejuni* strain 81-176, showed no reduction in adherence to or invasion of INT407 cells in vitro. Further, this mutant could colonize but caused significantly reduced disease symptoms in infected ferrets (25). Other possible reported adhesins include outer membrane proteins (OMPs), flagella, and lipopolysaccharides (LPS) (34, 88, 89). De Melo and Pechere (24) identified four *C. jejuni* proteins with apparent molecular masses of 28, 32, 36, and 42 kDa that bind to HEp-2 cells. A *C. jejuni* gene encoding a 28-kDa protein, termed PEB1, has been identified as a conserved antigen in *C. jejuni* and *C. coli* strains and was proposed to be an adhesin (101, 102). PEB1 has homology to a periplasmic binding protein involved in nutrient acquisition (45). In other studies using a similar technique, it was found that HeLa cells bound 26- and 30-kDa proteins present in outer membrane extracts of an invasive strain of *C. jejuni* (34, 35). Antiserum raised against these HeLa cell–bound proteins inhibited the adhesion of homologous *C. jejuni* to this cell line, whereas antibodies against an unrelated 90-kDa OMP were without effect (34, 35). Thus, a number of *Campylobacter* proteins have been associated with binding to various eukaryotic cells, and expression of fimbriae is required for full virulence in ferrets (25).

Many pathogenic microorganisms are capable of binding components of the extracellular matrix such as fibronectin, laminin, vibronectin, and collagen. *C. jejuni* has also been reported to bind to extracellular matrix components (66, 75, 80). Scanning electron microscopy of infected INT407 cells first indicated that *C. jejuni* binds to fibronectin. This suspected binding was confirmed and is mediated by a 37-kDa OMP which is conserved among *C. jejuni* isolates (75). The specific roles of the above-mentioned various proteins in adherence and their respective host cell ligands remain unclear. Understanding their specific involvement in disease pathogenesis is complicated by the presence of multiple adherence factors in *Campylobacter*.

Flagella

Flagella have been implicated as adhesins or carriers of adhesins because (i) nonflagellated mutant strains adhere much less efficiently to host cells than the flagellated parent strain does and (ii) isolated flagellar preparations bind to monolayers of INT407 cells (88). In *C. jejuni*, the flagellum is composed of two closely related proteins, the major subunit FlaA and the minor subunit FlaB. The *flaA* and *flaB* genes have been cloned, individually mutated, and extensively characterized (49, 52, 97, 134, 140) (see chapter 21). Studies have shown that *C. jejuni* mutants in which wild-type flagella are present but paralyzed and nonfunctional due to a mutation at *pflA* can bind to but are greatly impaired in their ability to invade INT407 cells (140). Nonflagellated mutants are impaired in their adherence to host cells, which is enhanced by bacterial centrifugation onto the monolayer (140). Also, antibodies directed against flagella do not inhibit *Campylobacter* attachment to INT407 cells (134), and sheared flagella were not effective in blocking the attachment of *C. jejuni* to INT407 cells (89). These results suggest that motility is required for optimal *Campylobacter* adherence to host cells and for invasion ability, they but do not reveal a definitive role for flagella in adherence. Nevertheless, the polar flagellum and unique characteristics of the spiral shape of campylobacters confer a distinctive motility that is particularly effective in a viscous matrix. This motility, aided by chemotactic signaling (61, 125), may allow *Campylobacter* to penetrate the mucus layer and seek host cell receptors involved in colonization or invasion of the intestinal mucosa.

LPS and LOS

LPSs (e.g., O antigen) and lipooligosaccharides (LOS) are the major surface antigens of gram-negative bacteria and play an important role in the interaction of these bacteria with their host and/or the environment. These surface polysaccharide molecules can serve as host mucosal adherence factors, and they possess binding sites for antibodies and serum factors. Hence, LPSs and LOSs are involved in host cell recognition and maintenance or elimination of bacteria by the host. Furthermore, these polysaccharides are immunostimulatory and strongly activate lymphocytes, granulocytes, and mononuclear cells (109). LPSs possess a broad spectrum of endotoxin activities (e.g., pyrogenicity and lethal toxicity), which contribute to overall bacterial virulence (94, 109). In fact, the endotoxic properties of *Campylobacter* LPS are comparable with those of other enterobacterial LPSs (95). Chemical analyses of many of the ~50 thermostable antigen serotypes representing predominant *C. jejuni* isolates have revealed that ~40% of the serotypes express classical core-linked, high-molecular-weight O antigen (103). The remainder of the serotypes have low-molecular-weight LOS molecules or other polysaccharide polymers unlinked to the core (95, 103). In some *C. jejuni* serotypes, sialylation of the terminal core oligosaccharide sugar creates structures that mimic human gangliosides (e.g. GM_1, GD_{1a}, GD_3, and GT_{1a}); antibodies raised against these mimetic molecules are suspected to play a role in the development of post-diarrheal Guillian-Barré syndrome (7, 117). The suggestion that LPS may be an important adhesin of *C. jejuni* for cellular and mucus substrates was made more than 10 years ago (89), but no direct evidence has yet been obtained. Nevertheless, the important role played by LPSs in the virulence of other enterobacteria strongly suggests the likelihood of a similar role in *C. jejuni* virulence.

Host Factors

Several studies have attempted to demonstrate a role for host membrane carbohydrates as receptors for *C. jejuni*, but these reports have so far been inconclusive (94, 95). Experiments with Chinese hamster ovary (CHO) cell mutants with defined defects in complex-carbohydrate biosynthesis revealed that oligosaccharide sequences probably play a subordinate role in *C. jejuni* attachment to eukaryotic cells (123).

The addition of simple sugars such as mannose, fucose, glucose, N-acetylglucosamine, maltose, and galactose also did not significantly alter the binding of *C. jejuni* to CHO cells (124). *C. jejuni* may interact with lipids in host cell membranes, but lipids only partially inhibit *C. jejuni* binding to CHO cells, again suggesting that multiple interactions occur between the bacteria and host cells (124). As mentioned above, components in intestinal mucus and in the extracellular matrix may serve as important receptors for colonization. However, the data are limited, and interpretation is made difficult by the multiple adherence factors of *Campylobacter*.

ENVIRONMENTAL REGULATION OF BACTERIAL GENES

A number of observations provide evidence for environmental sensing mechanisms used by campylobacters to regulate gene expression (e.g., expressing virulence genes only under certain conditions). These regulatory systems respond to different conditions (e.g., pH, osmolarity, free-iron concentration, temperature, and bacterial growth phase) encountered during bacterial propagation or host infection. For example, several factors, such as the age of the bacterial culture, affect the adherence of *Campylobacter* organisms to host cells. In older cultures, the organisms change their morphology from the typical spiral-shaped appearance to smaller coccoid forms (11). Maximal adherence of *C. jejuni* M129 to INT407 cells was observed with cultures harvested at 24 h, and a significant decrease in adherence occurred with cells grown for 72 h (76). Bacterial growth temperature also exerts an effect on adherence. Maximum adherence of *C. jejuni* M129 to INT407 cells occurred with bacteria grown at 37°C, with a 66% decrease being exhibited by cells grown at 42°C and a 91% decrease being observed with cells cultured at 30°C. Finally, bacterial surface hydrophobicity or charge, which is determined by expression of surface components, also affects adherence to host cells. Clinical isolates with a high net negative charge and a weakly hydrophobic surface showed a greater tendency to adhere to human intestinal HT-29 cells than did strains with a less negative charge and a more hydrophobic surface (131).

Similar to members of the *Enterobacteriaceae*, *C. jejuni* synthesizes new envelope-associated proteins in response to limiting free-iron conditions within the host (36). Also, Konkel et al. (79) reported that *C. jejuni* synthesizes a series of new proteins in the presence of eukaryotic cells. A ferric uptake regulator (Fur) protein has been cloned from *C. jejuni* (15, 138) and has been proposed to control the synthesis of a set of Fe^{2+}-responsive genes, similar to the situation found in other pathogens. In addition, several two-component regulatory systems have been found in *C. jejuni* (67). These systems consist of a membrane histidine kinase sensor which is activated under appropriate environmental conditions and, in turn, phosphorylates a diffusible response regulator protein that is needed to initiate the transcription of specific genes. Finally, the expression of some genes such as *flaB* is controlled by unique genetic promoter sequences (e.g., σ^{54}) that are environmentally modulated by temperature, pH, or divalent-cation levels (1). Thus, bacterial factors affecting both adherence and invasion abilities are not typically expressed in a constitutive fashion. Rather, expression is controlled by a series of different regulatory mechanisms that are modulated by environmental factors. Unfortunately, we do not yet know the appropriate growth conditions needed to optimize bacterial adherence or invasion.

INVASION

Penetration of the epithelial mucosa is now considered to be an essential virulence mechanism of several pathogenic enteric bacteria including *Salmonella, Shigella,* enteroinvasive *E. coli, Yersinia,* and *Listeria monocytogenes* (32, 40, 110, 119, 126, 127). The results of animal studies of *Campylobacter* enteritis in infant chickens (113, 120, 135), infant mice (96, 139), newborn piglets (4), and infant monkeys (116) suggest that invasion is also a key component of *Campylobacter* pathogenesis. In addition, van Spreeuwel et al. demonstrated the presence of

intracellular *C. jejuni* in colonic epithelial cells obtained from patients with documented *C. jejuni* colitis (128). Thus, *C. jejuni* infection can result in penetration of the gut epithelial mucosa, suggesting that, at least for a subgroup of strains, tissue invasion represents an important part of pathogenesis (67, 121).

Cultured eukaryotic cell invasion assay techniques have become standard experimental tools for the study of bacterial internalization mechanisms (29, 41, 70). These adherence-invasion assay procedures allow one to quantitate over time the number of bacteria attached to the surface of or internalized into cultured host cells (30, 31, 77). In combination with the use of specific biochemical inhibitors, these assays can reveal certain bacterial requirements (e.g., nascent protein synthesis) or host cell requisites (e.g., cytoskeletal elements or signal transduction pathways) for adherence or internalization. Early work by Bukholm and Kapperud (12) suggested that *Campylobacter* spp. invade cultured HEp-2 and A549 cells but only when coinfected with other enteropathogenic bacteria, such as *Salmonella* or *Shigella*. However, de Melo et al. (22) clearly demonstrated that *C. jejuni* alone could invade human tracheal epithelial HEp-2 cells and showed that invasion was enhanced in the presence of mucin. In 1989, Konkel et al. found that several *Campylobacter* species were both adherent to and invasive in HEp-2 cells (77) and also in the human colon Caco-2 cell line (81). Enhanced levels of HEp-2 cell invasion occurred when *C. jejuni* was coinfected with enteroviruses (78). In these early studies, relatively low levels of *Campylobacter* invasion were observed (generally <0.01% of the inoculum entered host cells within 2 to 3 h). More recent studies have revealed that certain *C. jejuni* strains can invade human embryonic intestinal (INT407) cells at levels 100- to >1,000-fold higher than those observed earlier and with 1 to 5% of the inoculum entering host cells within 3 h (77, 98). Thus, the current belief that *Campylobacter* spp. invade the intestinal mucosa as an important component of pathogenesis is suggested by both in vitro cell invasion assays and in vivo animal and human clinical findings. Our current conception of the mechanism(s) of *Campylobacter* invasion is a composite developed from in vivo animal studies and in vitro cell culture invasion assays, together with data from light, fluorescence, and electron microscopy studies.

Pathogenic microorganisms utilize a variety of different molecular strategies to subvert host cell machinery and hence enable these pathogens to invade susceptible host cells (32, 40, 47, 62, 63, 91), as exemplified below. Certain viruses and *Chlamydia psittaci* bind to receptors on the host cell surface and are internalized by receptor-mediated endocytosis (48, 54, 87), which does not require the overt involvement of host cell microtubules (MTs) or microfilaments (MFs). Some pathogens utilize MF-dependent entry processes which mimic phagocytosis (i.e., Fc or C3 receptor-mediated uptake [50]) but utilize different bacterial ligands and host receptors to zipper the host membrane tightly around the pathogen (e.g., *Chlamydia trachomatis* [14] and the *Yersinia enterocolitica inv* pathway [62, 91]). Some *Chlamydia* serovars then travel along MTs within the host to the perinuclear region, where pathogen maturation apparently occurs (16). Upon contact with epithelial cells, invasive *Salmonella* or *Shigella* spp. secrete diffusible effector proteins which translocate into the host cell. These effectors trigger a signal transduction cascade that induces a host actin-based cytoskeletal reorganization which leads to MF-dependent, macropinocytotic membrane engulfment of these pathogens (17, 39, 40, 44, 47, 59). In a somewhat different mechanism, *L. monocytogenes* recognizes E-cadherin as a receptor and enters host cells via an MF-dependent process (90). Interestingly, once inside a host cell and released from the endosome, cytoplasmic *Listeria* (18), *Shigella* (47), *Rickettsia* (53), and vaccinia virus (21) nucleate actin to form "tails" to move within the host cell or to adjacent host cells (i.e., they promote intercellular spread of the pathogen). In contrast to a molecular understanding of many of the processes described above, some microorganisms enter cells via yet less well characterized mechanisms that require MTs and/or MFs (e.g., *N. gonorrhoea* [86, 108], *Citrobacter freundii*, and *C. jejuni* [98]). *C. jejuni* strains have different host cytoskeletal requirements for invasion depending on the bacterial strain and host cell used (34, 74, 76, 77, 98). This has created confusion akin to that caused by finding divergent host cell requirements with different serovars of *Chlamydia* (14, 84, 85). Only a few *C. jejuni* strains have been studied in any detail for molecular mechanisms of invasion, but the results suggest that *Campylobacter* may encode separate MF-dependent and MT-dependent pathways for host invasion; some strains may encode both mechanisms (98). Recent mechanistic studies have begun to unravel the molecular events involved in bacterial internalization into the gut mucosa.

Bacterial Requirements for Invasion of Epithelial Cells

NASCENT PROTEIN SYNTHESIS—METABOLIC AND VIRULENCE FUNCTIONS

To provoke disease, invasive microorganisms must express products that bind host cell receptors and facilitate subsequent internalization, as well as survive in this changed environment. To adjust to the metabolic needs of a new environment and upregulate virulence functions, *Salmonella* undergoes gross changes in protein pattern during growth in the intracellular environment, with >30 proteins induced and ~100 proteins repressed relative to growth in the absence of host cells (10). Similarly, new proteins are induced in campylobacters upon contact with both viable and nonviable host cells, and a subset of these proteins are induced by released host cell components (80). Rabbit antiserum raised against host cell-cultivated *C. jejuni* recognized nine new *C. jejuni* proteins, relative to medium-grown bacteria. Furthermore, invasion was reduced by 98% in the presence of this antiserum, indicating a role for one or more of these proteins in invasion (76, 80). Very recently, this antiserum was used to clone a gene termed *ciaB* (i.e., *Campylobacter* invasion antigen B), which encodes a protein of ~73 kDa. CiaB has 40 to 45% amino acid similarity to the invasion ligands of *Salmonella* (i.e., SipB) and *Shigella* (i.e., IpaB) and to the *Yersinia* YopB virulence protein (80). Mutants with mutations in *ciaB* are noninvasive for INT407 cells and somehow are blocked in the secretion of at least eight *C. jejuni* F38011 proteins in the presence of INT407 cells. Furthermore, this CiaB protein was shown by immunofluorescence microscopy to translocate into infected INT407 cells. Although still preliminary, these data suggest that *C. jejuni* may encode a secretion apparatus akin to the type III system found in animal and plant pathogens (60). Presumably, contact with host cells upregulates the secretion apparatus, which, in turn, secretes diffusible effectors of invasion that translocate into host cells and initiate "invasion-specific" signal transduction events. The precise roles of these *C. jejuni* proteins in invasion await to be determined.

Nonviable campylobacters are still able to attach to host cells, indicating that de novo bacterial protein synthesis is not required for bacterial adherence to eukaryotic cells (76). In contrast, *Campylobacter* invasion does require nascent bacterial protein synthesis (76, 98), whereas blocking of host cell protein synthesis with cycloheximide does not inhibit invasion by *C. jejuni* over several hours (98).

FLAGELLA AND MOTILITY

Functional flagella are essential for the internalization of *C. jejuni* in vitro and for colonization of the mouse intestine (1, 49, 134, 139, 140). Aflagellate, nonmotile variants lose invasion ability (140). Furthermore, a paralyzed flagellar mutant with a defined insertion in *pflA,* but containing a full-length flagellum composed mainly of FlaA, demonstrated markedly reduced levels of invasion into cultured cells, which was only slightly improved by centrifugation of the mutant onto host cells (134). Thus, motility is absolutely required for *C. jejuni* invasion ability. However, centrifugation onto a host cell monolayer of Fla⁻ *C. jejuni* does not restore invasion ability, indicating that motility does not simply function to make bacteria contact host cells. It remains undetermined if the flagellum plays an additional role as an invasion-specific ligand in the entry process. Alternatively, motile *C. jejuni* may seek "preferred invasion" host membrane sites (e.g., due to basolateral sequestering of receptors or to a numerical limitation of host receptors), or bacterial invasion ligands may be located on the poles of the bacterial surface, requiring motility to initiate effective host cell contact.

IRON AND FERRITIN

The strict limitation of free iron within mammalian hosts embodies a nonspecific, host-protective mechanism, since bacteria require 10^{-6} to 10^{-7} M Fe^{2+} for survival. Bacterial pathogens have evolved mechanisms to obtain iron within the host. These bacterial pathways are maximally expressed under iron-restricted conditions, such as via negative regulation of the Fur protein (100), described above. Unlike other invasive enteric bacteria, *C. jejuni* does not produce siderophores to sequester iron. However, *Campylobacter* can bind exogenous siderophores (36), possesses an enterochelin uptake system (107), and synthesizes bacterial ferritin, which is involved in both iron storage and bacterial protection from oxidative stress (129).

CAMPYLOBACTER INVASION EFFICIENCY—STRAIN DEPENDENCE

The invasion efficiency for cultured human cells varies greatly with different *C. jejuni* strains (31, 56, 74, 76, 98). Generally, 0.5 to 5.0% of the inoculum is typically internalized into host cells during efficient *C. jejuni* entry. Recent clinical isolates tend to be more invasion proficient (31). Invasion ability is adversely affected by *C. jejuni* passage over time. Selection for motile organisms helps maintain *Campylobacter* in an efficient invasive mode. Whether some *C. jejuni* strains lack invasion determinants or have lost virulence gene expression with passage remain important unanswered questions.

TEMPERATURE AND PHASE OF GROWTH

Bacterial growth temperature (74, 115) and growth phase (56, 74) have been reported in limited studies to influence the ability of *C. jejuni* to colonize and to invade human epithelial cells. For example, the optimal growth temperature for *C. jejuni* adherence was observed to be 37°C, with a marked decrease in adherence found for bacteria grown at 30 or 42°C (74). The responsible factors are uncharacterized.

Mid-log-phase *C. jejuni* (optical density at 600 nm ≈ 0.2 to 0.6) grown in nutrient-rich broth appears to be optimal for invasion. Growth in mucin (23) or deoxycholate (26) enhances invasion ability severalfold. Early-stationary-phase *C. jejuni* 81-176 showed approximately fivefold reduction in typical invasion efficiency relative to mid-log-phase bacteria. The requirement for de novo bacterial protein synthesis for *C. jejuni* invasion (76, 98) may partially explain the reduced invasion by older bacteria. The precise mechanisms of invasion enhancement by mucin or deoxycholate are unknown.

Host Factors That Influence Invasion

CELL LINE DEPENDENCE

As mentioned above, different *C. jejuni* or *C. coli* strains exhibit distinctly different invasion efficiencies for the same host cell line (73). In contrast, the same *Campylobacter* strain can vary in invasion efficiency for different host cell lines, and this dependence appears to be host specific (74, 98). *C. jejuni* and *C. coli* can invade many cell lines (e.g., HeLa, INT407, HCT-8, Caco-2, HEp-2, HT29, A498, Vero, CHO-k1, and MDCK). However, *Campylobacter* appears to be most effectively internalized by cell lines of human origin (23, 56, 74, 98). Because of their ease of cultivation (HEp-2 or HeLa cells) or their intestinal origin (INT407, Caco-2, and HT29 cells), these human epithelial cell lines have typically been used to study *Campylobacter* invasion.

FACTORS AFFECTING THE KINETICS OF BACTERIAL ENTRY

Semiconfluent monolayers of INT407 or Caco-2 cells appear optimally susceptible to *Campylobacter* invasion. Young but fully confluent monolayers have a severalfold reduction in invasion susceptibility relative to semiconfluent monolayers of the same host cells. Furthermore, *C. jejuni* invasion efficiency into 1- to 2-week-old differentiated Caco-2 cells is reduced by ~20-fold relative to entry into semiconfluent, young Caco-2 cells (56, 57a). These observations, together with electron microscope studies showing *Campylobacter* invasion at or within host cell junctions (78, 98), suggest that host "invasion" receptors may be sequestered basolaterally over time, which might reduce the invasion level of apically added organisms.

In addition to using young semiconfluent monolayers of human intestinal cell lines, the optimal host cell invasion assay temperature has been reported to be 37°C (74). Agents which block glycolysis (e.g., iodoacetate) or the Krebs cycle (e.g., dinitrophenol) inhibit *Campylobacter* entry, indicating a host requirement for energy during bacterial internalization (23). However, cycloheximide inhibition of host cell protein synthesis did not reduce *C. jejuni* entry over 2 h, indicating that host requirements for bacterial uptake are present in sufficient quantity in competent host cells (98).

Early preliminary studies implied that simply increasing the inoculum resulted in increased *Campylobacter*-host cell adherence (74) and invasion (22). Recently, however, detailed kinetic analyses have been conducted to ascertain the effect of incubation time and bacterial concentration on maximal invasion and the actual percentage of host cells infected (56); these analyses have revealed an important host cell limitation on entry. *C. jejuni* 81-176, a well-characterized strain which causes inflammatory diarrhea in volunteers (6), was used for these analyses. Uptake into cultured INT407 cells was first analyzed over a wide range of starting multiplicities of infection (MOI) (i.e., from 0.02 to 20,000 bacteria/epithelial cell). The efficiency of internalization after 2 h was the highest at an MOI of 0.02 and decreased steadily at higher MOIs (Fig. 1A), presumably due to reported *C. jejuni* 81-176 autoagglutination at higher densities (92). Total internalized

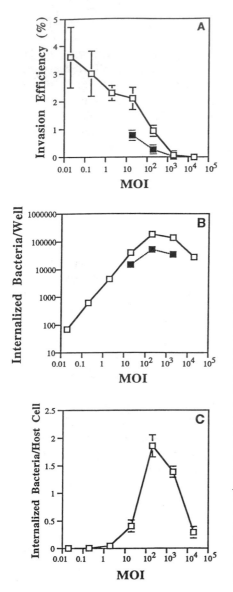

FIGURE 1 Comparative kinetic study showing the effect of varying the starting MOI or phase of bacterial growth on *C. jejuni* 81-176 invasion efficiency (i.e., percentage of the starting inoculum internalized at the end of the assay) compared to the number of bacteria internalized into INT407 cells (57). Invasion assays were conducted, as described previously (57), by testing a range of starting bacterial concentrations (expressed as MOI [added bacteria per epithelial cell]) and using a 2-h invasion period and a 2-h gentamicin kill period prior to enumeration of internalized bacteria. All assays were conducted in triplicate and were repeated on different days at least three times. Results are presented as the mean invasion efficiency and standard error. (A) Effect of varying the starting MOI and phase of bacterial growth on *C. jejuni* 81-176 invasion efficiency. (B) Effect of varying the starting MOI and phase of bacterial growth on total *C. jejuni* internalized. The total number of internalized bacteria per assay well is expressed as mean CFU per well and standard error. The CFU per well obtained at MOIs of 200 and 2,000 were significantly increased over the CFUs internalized at lower starting MOIs ($P < 0.01$). (C) Effect of varying the MOI on the resulting number of internalized bacteria averaged per epithelial cell. The total number of internalized log-phase *C. jejuni* 81-176 cells is expressed as the average number of bacteria internalized per epithelial cell (i.e., by dividing the total number of internalized bacteria by 10^5 epithelial cells in each well). Results are presented as the mean number of bacteria per epithelial cell and standard error. The resulting averaged number of bacteria per epithelial cell at MOIs of 200 or 2,000 were significantly increased over the results obtained at lower starting MOIs ($P < 0.01$). □, log-phase cells; ■, stationary-phase cells.

Campylobacter CFU (Fig. 1B) increased gradually following invasion at an MOI of 0.02 to a peak at an MOI of 200 (reaching an average of two bacteria internalized per epithelial cell [Fig. 1C]) and decreased at higher MOIs. Thus, optimal invasion efficiency (i.e., the percentage of the inoculum recovered as internalized at the end of the assay) was highest at the lowest MOI, but a maximal number of internalized *C. jejuni* was not observed until after infection at an MOI of 200. The fact that *C. jejuni* 81-176 invasion was highest at an MOI of 0.02 suggests that this organism is a highly efficient solitary invader at very low bacterial concentrations, as long as it is motile. This contrasts sharply with *S. typhi* invasion of INT407 cells (59), where invasion efficiency was suboptimal at lower and higher MOIs and reached a broad peak at an MOI of ~40. However, the maximal number of internalized *S. typhi* organisms was achieved at MOIs of 40 and above, suggesting unlike *C. jejuni,* that *S. typhi* invasion may be a cooperative process requiring the accumulation of signaling events from multiple bacteria to trigger entry.

Using the optimal MOI of 200 for *C. jejuni* 81-176, a time course of entry analysis was conducted. As shown in Table 1, bacterial invasion was first assessed by the indirect-plate-count method following a gentamicin kill period. *C. jejuni* entry was easily observed at 10 min, and the total number of internalized *C. jejuni* organisms increased at each time point up to 2 h. However, the rate of entry was optimal only for the first 90 min and then decreased. When the total number of internalized bacteria, obtained by the indirect-plate-count method, was averaged over all monolayer cells, the number of bacteria internalized per host cell steadily increased to about two (Table 1).

To assess the percentage of INT407 cells infected over time and the actual number of bacteria internalized per infected host cell, the acridine orange/crystal violet direct-visualization method (56, 59) was used. The total numbers of stained, live intracellular bacteria observed over time (Table 1) were very similar to those measured by the indirect-plate-count method. This direct viewing method revealed that an increasing number of monolayer cells were infected over time. However, after 2 h, only two-thirds of the host cells were infected, with an average of approximately two *C. jejuni* organisms per infected host cell. These internalized bacteria were typically observed as well-separated individuals (apparently as a result of two separate invasion events).

Extended time course invasion studies in which *C. jejuni* 81-176 was added at an MOI of 20 revealed that it required a 4-h invasion

TABLE 1 Kinetic analyses of *C. jejuni* 81-176 entry into INT407 cells[a]

Postinfection time (min.)	Invasion efficiency (%)[b]	% of INT407 cells infected[c]	Mean no. of internalized bacteria per host cell[d]	Mean no. of internalized bacteria per infected host cell[d]
Indirect viable-count assay				
0	0		0	
10	0.12 ± 0.04		0.18 ± 0.03	
30	0.67 ± 0.24		0.80 ± 0.17	
60	0.93 ± 0.16		1.13 ± 0.05	
90	1.36 ± 0.17		1.72 ± 0.13	
120	1.42 ± 0.18		1.76 ± 0.29	
Direct visualization assay				
0		0		0
10		10.33 ± 3.51		1.22 ± 0.00
30		22.00 ± 3.46		1.85 ± 0.17
60		51.00 ± 5.57		1.93 ± 0.12
90		66.33 ± 5.57		2.02 ± 0.18
120		68.00 ± 3.73		2.13 ± 0.23

[a] Young INT407 cells were infected with *C. jejuni* 81-176 at an MOI of ca. 200 for various times. The infected host cells were washed with Earle's balanced salt solution and incubated for an additional 2 h with fresh medium containing 100 μg of gentamicin per ml, and the internalized bacteria were enumerated by indirect bacterial counts or were observed directly by microscopic analysis of stained, infected monolayers as detailed previously (56, 59). Results shown are the mean ± standard error of at least three separate assays.

[b] Invasion efficiency represents the percentage of the inoculum internalized by the end of the assay.

[c] The direct-visualization method (i.e., acridine orange- and crystal violet-stained monolayers assessed by fluorescence microscopy [59]) was used to enumerate the actual percentage of host cells containing internalized bacteria and the number of intracellular bacteria per infected cell.

[d] The total number of bacteria internalized per well at each time point was divided by 10^5 monolayer cells or the actual number of infected host cells to determine the number of internalized bacteria averaged per host cell or the number of internalized bacteria averaged per infected host cell, respectively.

period to achieve the equivalent number of internalized bacteria as was obtained in 2 h at an MOI of 200 (56). Thus, *C. jejuni* 81-176 internalization occurs by a highly efficient and kinetically saturable process that strictly limits the number of bacteria taken up per cell (i.e., ca. two per cell) and in which the infected host cells become saturated for entry, even at higher MOIs over shorter periods. This tight restriction on entry may reflect a limited number of host cell "invasion" receptor and entry sites, a limitation of some other host biochemical requisite for entry, and/or host cell modifications during invasion that prevent further *C. jejuni* entry. In addition, as opposed to *S. typhi* invasion of 100% of INT407 cells within 1 h at an MOI of 40, the percentage of *C. jejuni*-infected INT407 cells at an MOI of 200 reached only 70% after 2 h. This number gradually increased with time to ~85% of monolayer cells infected after a 7-h invasion period, suggesting that *C. jejuni* entry may be host cell cycle dependent (56).

The above studies have demonstrated that *C. jejuni* 81-176 enters young, semiconfluent INT407 cells (and Caco-2 cells [56]) in a 2-h invasion period with typical invasion efficiencies of 1 to 4%. This level of entry is generally $>10^3$-fold higher than the level of entry of noninvasive *E. coli* strains into these same host cells. This efficient internalization of *C. jejuni* 81-176, together with the observation that the noninvasive RY213 mutant of this parent strain is decreased in invasion ability by ~2 log units (56, 141), indicates that strain 81-176 is responsible for inducing its own uptake into host cells (i.e., uptake is not a passive process for *C. jejuni*). Previous studies have shown that motility is required for *C. jejuni* invasive ability (49, 134, 141), but other invasion-essential genes or functions have not been identified for strain 81-176. It is important to note that the invasion efficiency of *C. jejuni* 81-176 is very comparable to that observed with the *Yersinia inv* system (62, 64) or *S. typhimurium* (41, 43). Thus, efficient *C. jejuni* entry equals the invasion levels obtained with other invasive enteric bacteria.

CYTOSKELETAL REQUIREMENTS AND MICROSCOPIC OBSERVATIONS

Bacterial internalization has typically been observed to involve the rearrangement of host cytoskeletal structures, resulting in endocytosis of the pathogen. The cytoskeleton of eukaryotic cells is a complex array of proteins, the most prominent of which are actin and tubulin, which comprise MFs and MTs, respectively. These filamentous structures, together with intermediate filaments, are involved in both cellular and subcellular movements, in the determination of host cell shape, and, not surprisingly, in bacterial invasion. Most invasive enteric organisms (e.g., *Salmonella*, *Shigella*, *Listeria*, and *Yersinia* [30, 39–42, 64, 70, 91]) trigger largely MF-dependent entry pathways.

Campylobacter internalization has been variously reported to require MFs (22, 73, 77), MTs (56, 98), both MFs and MTs (98), or neither (115), depending upon the host cell type used, the methods employed (often lacking appropriate controls), and the *C. jejuni* strain studied. Only a few *C. jejuni* strains have been studied in any detail for invasion mechanism, leaving the host cell cytoskeletal requirements for and the mechanism of *Campylobacter* entry into epithelial cells an open question. The available data, though very limited, suggest that *Campylobacter* may encode separate MF-dependent (74, 76) and MT-dependent (56, 98) pathways for host invasion; some strains (e.g., *C. jejuni* VC84) may encode both MT- and MF-dependent mechanisms (98).

In 1993, Oelschlaeger et al. (98) described a high-efficiency invasion process for *C. jejuni* strains and demonstrated that *C. jejuni* 81-176 entry into cultured human intestinal INT407 cells requires polymerized MTs, but is unaffected by depolymerization of MFs. Evidence for the strict MT dependence of this uptake process is strengthened by the similar behavior of a series of MT-depolymerizing agents that act at different MT sites and the finding that concurrent *Salmonella typhi* Ty2 uptake was not reduced by MT depolymerization (98). More recent studies have verified, and extended to Caco-2 cells, this strict MT dependence for

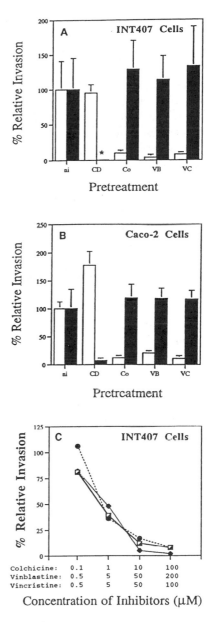

FIGURE 2 Effect of various inhibitors on *C. jejuni* 81-176 (□) internalization into INT407 (A) and Caco-2 cells (B). Data showing the concentration dependence of inhibition are also presented (C). At 1 h prior to the addition of bacteria to the monolayer, the epithelial cells were incubated with no inhibitor (ni), 2 μM cytochalasin D (CD), 10 μM colchicine (Co) (■), 50 μM vinblastine (VB) (♦), 50 μM vincristine (VC) (●), or the various inhibitor concentrations listed in panel C. Each inhibitor was maintained throughout the 2-h invasion period. The relative percent invasiveness was determined as the recovery in the presence of inhibitors divided by the recovery in the absence of inhibitors (i.e., 100% relative invasiveness). *S. typhi* Ty2W (■) served as an MF-dependent invasive control; the asterisk denotes that Ty2W internalization was decreased by >99% in the presence of CD. Results are presented as the mean and standard error of at least three separate experiments with standard error shown as bars above or below the mean (56).

entry of strain 81-176 (56). Compounds that cause depolymerization of MFs or MTs were individually used to pretreat INT407 or Caco-2 cell monolayers before and during a 2-h invasion period. As shown in Fig. 2, regardless of the cell line used, cytochalasin D pretreatment resulted in a >95% reduction of the MF-dependent invasion by the control *S. typhi* strain. In contrast, *C. jejuni* 81-176 entry into either

cell line was not inhibited by cytochalasin D. In fact, MF depolymerization actually stimulated invasion by strain 81-176 (Fig. 2B), as reported previously (98). When host cells in concomitant studies were pretreated to depolymerize MTs, the control *S. typhi* strain was not reduced in its entry ability; however, *C. jejuni* 81-176 was typically reduced more than 90% in its ability to invade either INT407 or Caco-

2 cells. Furthermore, inhibition of 81-176 invasion ability by MT depolymerization was inhibitor concentration dependent, as exemplified in Fig. 2C. Thus, *C. jejuni* 81-176, arguably the best-studied *C. jejuni* strain, enters INT407 cells via a novel mechanism that requires host cell MTs but not MFs (98). This cytoskeletal requirement for strain 81-176 invasion is readily reproducible in our assays but differs from that reported by Russell et al. (115), probably due to methodological differences. Strain 81-176 is not unique among *Campylobacter* spp. in its strong involvement of MTs during entry. Invasion by *C. coli* VC167 (98a) and other strains of *C. jejuni* (56, 57a, 98) also shows an MF-independent requirement for polymerized MTs. Nevertheless, reports of differing invasion requirements for other *C. jejuni* strains (22, 76, 98) make it likely that different *Campylobacter* strains, similar to different *Chlamydia* serovars, use different mechanisms for cell invasion.

Immunofluorescence microscopy has also been used to examine the association of *C. jejuni* 81-176 with polymerized MTs versus MFs at various times during the invasion process. INT407 cells were infected with either *C. jejuni* 81-176 or control *S. typhi* for 0.5 to 4 h prior to fixation and immunofluorescence analyses; the bacteria and the host cell MT-based cytoskeleton were differentially labeled with green or red fluorescent tags as described previously (56). Figure 3 shows black-and-white representations of fluorescent microscopic images of these *C. jejuni*-infected INT407 cells. Early in infection, *C. jejuni* was first observed interacting with the host cell at the tip of a finger-like protrusion of the cell membrane, being extended by one or a few bundled MTs (Fig. 3A). These structures suggest that initiation of invasion involves reorganization of the host cytoskeleton in response to a signal from the adjacent *C. jejuni*, since these membrane extensions were not triggered by *S. typhi* in control studies. Note that *C. jejuni* F38011 has been reported to synthesize (80) and secrete (79) novel proteins upon contact with host cells; however, the ability of

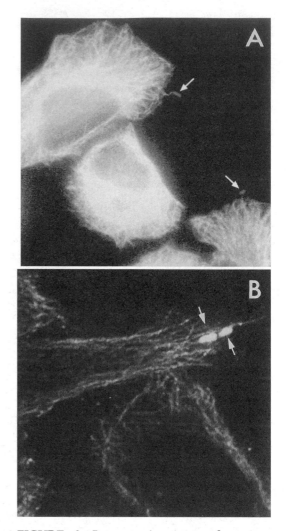

FIGURE 3 Representative immunofluorescence microscopy images of *C. jejuni*-infected INT407 cells showing bacterial interactions with MTs over time. INT407 cells infected with *C. jejuni* 81-176 for 1 h were fixed, permeabilized, and labeled with fluorescent antibodies as described previously (56). All pixels of light derived from the two different photodetection filters for either the Texas red-X (i.e., MTs) and fluorescein isothiocyanate (i.e., bacteria) fluorescent labels have been combined and are shown in white. (A) Fluorescence micrographs of *C. jejuni*-infected INT407 cells showing the overall MT cytoskeleton and MT-based, finger-like membrane protrusions with a single bacterium (see arrows) located at the tip of each of two host cell extensions. (B) Confocal fluorescence micrograph of infected INT407 cells. The MTs appear as structural skeletons outlining the cells, and the fluorescein-labeled bacteria (see arrows) appear as bright white spots along the MTs.

strain 81-176 to synthesize and secrete new proteins upon host cell contact has not yet been determined. Next, *C. jejuni* 81-176 was typically observed during the first 1 to 4 h of the invasion process to be situated in parallel with MTs and apparently associated with these structures, as exemplified in Fig. 3B. Confocal laser-scanning microscopy demonstrated a specific and tight colocalization of strain 81-176 with MTs, whereas no colocalization was observed with control *S. typhi* in infected host cells (56). During the early phases of invasion, all *C. jejuni* organisms were observed at the periphery of host cells. However, by 4 h postinfection, >50% of the bacteria had moved intracellularly to a location adjacent to the nucleus, similar to the perinuclear movement observed with a different *C. jejuni* strain (76). Similar immunofluorescence methods were used to search for any association of *C. jejuni* 81-176 with F-actin. Host membrane-bound *S. typhi,* but not *C. jejuni* 81-176, triggered actin condensation at the point of host cell contact. *C. jejuni* 81-176 showed no evidence of colocalization with MFs during invasion (56). Thus, these immunofluorescence studies revealed a tight association of *C. jejuni* with MTs but not with MFs during the invasion process.

The results of this time course analysis of the association of strain 81-176 with MTs indicated that *C. jejuni* initiates contact with the host cell through MT-based finger-like membrane extensions. The next invasion step seen in this analysis is the association of internalized bacteria in parallel with MTs and movement, over 4 h, of intracellular bacteria from the cell periphery to the perinuclear region. In related studies, neither the noninvasive mutant *C. jejuni* RY213 (141) nor *S. typhi* typically exhibited any similar physical orientation with respect to MTs and no MT-based, finger-like membrane protrusions were seen at the point of host cell contact with these control organisms (56).

Dynein is known to be responsible for MT-dependent, minus-end-directed vesicle transport from the host cell surface to the perinuclear region and might be required (i) for initial uptake of *C. jejuni* into host cells or (ii) subsequently as an MT motor in the molecular trafficking of endosomes containing *C. jejuni* to the perinuclear region. Orthovanadate, a well-described inhibitor of dynein activity (46), significantly reduced the entry of *C. jejuni* 81-176 but not control *S. typhi* into epithelial cells, suggesting a role for dynein in the initial uptake event (56). In addition, immunofluorescence microscopy studies showed that at 1 h postinfection, when invading strain 81-176 was shown to colocalize with MTs, these organisms were also observed to colocalize with dynein, suggesting a role for dynein in the intracellular molecular trafficking of strain 81-176. In contrast, invading *S. typhi* was not found to colocalize with dynein (56).

Internalization of 81-176 requires polymerized MTs but is not inhibited by stabilizing MTs with taxol, a feature that distinguishes this MT-dependent uptake mechanism from that of *Citrobacter freundii* (98). Compounds which block endosome acidification have been reported to have no effect on the invasion ability of strain 81-176 (98) or other *C. jejuni* strains (76). In contrast, inhibitors affecting coated pits (76, 98) or membrane caveolae (137) block the entry of several *C. jejuni* strains including 81-176 (filipin III has been shown to block 81-176 invasion [57]), suggesting that the host cell "invasion receptor" may reside in these related membrane structures. Recent evidence has revealed the MTs are associated at the host plasma membrane with the adenomatous polyposis coli (APC) protein (106). In preliminary experiments, monolayer pretreatment with a monoclonal antibody that recognizes a surface-exposed region of APC did not reduce *C. jejuni* internalization, failing to implicate APC as a major host cell receptor for *C. jejuni* invasion (56). Thus, the host membrane receptor(s) for *C. jejuni* invasion remains undefined.

Finally, a number of preliminary electron microscopy or immunofluorescence analyses of early interactions of several different *C. jejuni* strains with host cells have been reported (22, 35, 76, 77, 98). Two common observations that arise from these reports are as follows: (i) during invasion, *C. jejuni* appears to interact with host cells near or within the junctional space; and (ii) internalized *C. jejuni* is contained within endosomal vacuoles.

SIGNAL TRANSDUCTION EVENTS

Host cell signaling pathways are known to be induced by virtually all invasive enteric bacteria including *S. typhimurium* (9, 32, 44) and *Shigella flexneri* (47). Upon contact with host cells, these bacteria secrete effectors that translocate into the host, activating various pathways which lead to cytoskeletal rearrangements that result in bacterial internalization. *C. jejuni* F38011 has recently been reported to secrete eight proteins upon contact with host cells, and CiaB, a bacterial protein that is essential for invasive ability, translocates into the host cell (79). Although this is possibly representative of a common secretory mechanism among *Campylobacter* strains, it is yet undetermined if other *C. jejuni* strains secrete similar proteins, and the cytoskeletal requirements for F38011 invasion have not been reported.

The host "invasion" receptor(s) probably is situated in membrane invaginations (i.e., caveolae or coated pits), since inhibitors of these structures block *C. jejuni* invasion. However, it is unclear if filipin III, γ-strophantin, and monodansylcadaverine block formation of the same structures (e.g., receptors in caveolae) or if both types of membrane structures (i.e., coated and uncoated invaginations) are involved in *Campylobacter* entry.

A common signal transduction pathway in eukaryotic cells is activation of protein tyrosine kinases, which results in tyrosine phosphorylation of host proteins. Recent studies, involving the protein kinase inhibitors genistein and staurosporin (57, 58, 137) and immunoblotting with antiphosphotyrosine antibody of host proteins from infected and uninfected cells (57, 58), demonstrated that protein tyrosine kinases are activated by *C. jejuni* infection and that at least nine host proteins are specifically phosphorylated during invasion by *C. jejuni* 81-176 (57). One of the tyrosine-phosphorylated proteins has been identified as phosphoinositide 3-

kinase (PI3-kinase), through the use of wortmannin and LY294002, specific inhibitors of PI3 kinase, which dramatically block *C. jejuni* entry (57, 58, 137). Woodridge et al. (137) have also implicated heterotrimeric G proteins of the $G\alpha_s$ subfamily in the host signaling events leading to the entry of *C. jejuni* N82.

Some bacteria (e.g., *S. typhimurium* [9]) trigger transient alterations in intracellular free-Ca^{2+} levels to facilitate host cytoskeletal rearrangements for invasion. The use of Ca^{2+} chelators showed that *C. jejuni* 81-176 trigger a specific release of Ca^{2+} from intracellular stores, which is necessary for internalization (57). Although the data are limited to only a couple of strains, these results suggest that *C. jejuni* interacts with putative receptors in host membrane caveolae and/or coated pits. A signal transduction cascade is stimulated in the host cell, which results in specific tyrosine phosphorylation of at least nine proteins. Specific activation of PI3-kinase apparently leads to Ca^{2+} release from intracellular stores, which may be required for host cytoskeletal rearrangements that result in bacterial internalization. Bacterial interaction at the host membrane stimulates activation of dynein, and the bacteria move within endosomes along microtubules via dynein motors to the perinuclear region of the host cell. Strict MF dependence has not been well characterized for any *Campylobacter* strain, and signaling events for these putative MF-dependent mechanisms are yet undefined.

INTRACELLULAR SURVIVAL

Following invasion into host cells, pathogens must have the ability to survive and/or replicate intracellularly. The bacterial and host factors that determine the fate of internalized Campylobacters are not well understood. Superoxide dismutase catalyzes the breakdown of superoxide radicals and is one of major defense mechanisms of the bacterial cell against oxidative damage. Mutant *sodB C. jejuni* 81-176 shows significantly decreased survival within INT407 cells relative to the parent strain, indicating that SodB is important in intracellular survival

(105). The importance of other bacterial genes in intracellular survival, although expected, remains undefined.

Electron microscopy studies suggest that *C. jejuni* is internalized by host membrane invagination (76, 98) and is typically maintained within endosomal vacuoles inside epithelial cells (22, 35, 77, 98). The use of inhibitors that block host cell endosome acidification during the invasion period (e.g., monensin or methylamine) showed that inhibition of acidification did not markedly reduce bacterial entry (76, 98), indicating that acidification does not play a large role in recycling of internalized host receptors to the cell surface. However, longer-term use of inhibitors of endosome acidification to assess the effect on intracellular bacterial survival over many hours has not been attempted. Recent kinetic analyses of *C. jejuni* 81-176 entry suggest that following maximal invasion into INT407 cells, the internalized bacteria probably undergo one round of replication during the next 5 h. Two studies have examined longer-term intracellular survival, but of different *C. jejuni* strains and in different host cell backgrounds (22, 76). De Melo et al. (22) found that intracellular bacterial numbers began to decrease 6 h after internalization, which correlated with phagosome-lysosome fusion. The number of intracellular bacteria steadily decreased out to ~36 h, when 50 μg of gentamicin per ml was maintained in the culture medium to prevent extracellular bacterial growth (22). Konkel et al. (76) reported similar decreases in the survival of intracellular *C. jejuni* in the presence of gentamicin but found that when gentamicin was removed from the culture medium after 21 h, the numbers of intracellular bacterial increased and persisted at the higher level for >96 h. Furthermore, at 48 to 96 h postinfection, host cells were mainly detached from the culture plate, contained numerous bacteria (of which some were free in the cytoplasm), and were in an obvious state of degeneration (76). The host factors or *Campylobacter* genes involved in intracellular bacterial replication and survival or the triggering of host cell death are largely un-

defined. Intestinal epithelial cells typically survive for 4 to 6 days before being sloughed off at the intestinal lumen. Thus, the above intracellular survival times observed in vitro are considerable and would allow bacteria sufficient time to trigger mucosal abscesses (as reported clinically [121]) or allow for translocation to the lamina propria and beyond.

INTESTINAL TRANSLOCATION

Bacterial translocation entails the movement of viable bacteria across the gastrointestinal barrier, where further extraintestinal dissemination can occur. For example, after gut translocation, *S. typhi* is disseminated via macrophages/monocytes to various extraintestinal sites during typhoid fever pathogenesis. Although animal models are useful for studying intestinal translocation, polarized epithelial-cell lines provide a simple and controlled experimental alternative to animal models. Polarized human colonic carcinoma (Caco-2) cells, with differentiated apical and basolateral surfaces separated by tight junctions, express several markers characteristic of normal intestinal cells and have a well-defined brush border (41). Apical addition of *S. typhimurium* to polarized cells was initially shown to be followed by bacterial endocytosis and passage through the host cell to the basolateral domain. This transcytosis process occurred in the presence of tight cell junctions during the first few hours but caused a significant decrease in monolayer electrical resistance by 6 h (41).

Campylobacters also have been observed to translocate across a tight epithelial cell monolayer (31, 49, 81). *C. jejuni* can penetrate from the apical to the basolateral surface of polarized Caco-2 cells without disrupting transepithelial electrical resistance. Bacteria were found within vacuoles inside the Caco-2 cells and presumably pass through the monolayer while remaining within a vacuole. Translocated bacteria were observed below the cell monolayer less than 1 h after inoculation at the apical surface and continued to translocate for at least 6 h; the maximal penetration rate for *C. jejuni* was observed after 4 h. Electron microscopy studies also indicate that *Campylobacter* organisms pass between cells (81) and that some isolates appear to transcytose without invasion (31). Thus, it appears that *Campylobacter* may cross polarized epithelial cells via transcellular and paracellular routes. Unlike *Salmonella*, *C. jejuni* does not cause a loss in transepithelial electrical resistance during the first 6 h, indicating that the tight junctions between cells are not disrupted (81).

Grant et al. reported that either *C. jejuni* motility or the product of the *flaA* gene is essential for the bacterium to cross polarized monolayers, since *flaA flaB* Mot⁻ and *flaA flaB⁺* Mot⁻ mutants were unable to cross the cell barrier (49). The bacterial protein synthesis inhibitor chloramphenicol also reduced monolayer translocation of *C. jejuni* (81), suggesting that bacterial endocytosis is an important part of transcytosis. No other requirements have been defined. Translocation may be a useful marker of enhanced pathogenicity, but the role of translocation in *C. jejuni*-mediated disease requires further characterization.

INFLAMMATION AND INTERACTION WITH PHAGOCYTES

During the course of human *Campylobacter* infections, organisms elicit phagocytic cells into the intestinal lumen (7, 27) and encounter them systemically during bacteremic conditions (37, 83). Intestinal infection with *C. jejuni* is typically associated in developed counties with an inflammatory response and the presence of fecal leukocytes (6, 27, 122). Recent studies have shown that interleukin-8 (IL-8) secretion by epithelial cells may be an early signal for the acute inflammatory response following various enteric bacterial infections (20, 28, 38). Many strains of *Campylobacter* can induce secretion of IL-8 by INT407 cells. The level of IL-8 induced by *C. jejuni* appears to be comparable to those reported for *Shigella dysenteriae* and *Salmonella dublin*. Induction of IL-8 secretion requires live cells of 81-176 and is dependent on de novo bacterial protein synthesis. Studies with mutant strains suggest that inva-

sion is necessary for high-level IL-8 secretion (55).

In addition to triggering IL-8 production and an acute inflammatory response, *C. jejuni* can survive inside certain phagocytic cells. These organisms appears to be readily internalized and killed by polymorphonuclear leukocytes; without opsonization, the process was less efficient (3, 130). However, during in vitro experiments with mouse macrophages or elutriated human monocytes, *C. jejuni* was readily internalized by macrophages and monocytes (69) but was not killed rapidly following ingestion. Internalized *C. jejuni* organisms changed from the spiral to the coccal forms within 4 to 8 h and survived for 6 to 7 days in human mononuclear phagocytes (69). Monocytes, therefore, could play an important role in the dissemination of *C. jejuni* following intestinal translocation, by protecting *C. jejuni* during transit to secondary sites. The bacterial or host functions specifically involved in the above IL-8 stimulation, entry into monocytes, or survival within macrophages/monocytes remain undefined.

Current Conceptualization of Invasion
Virtually all *C. jejuni* strains analyzed have been reported to require either MTs (56, 98), MFs (22, 76), or both MTs and MFs (98) for entry into host cells. Although only a few *Campylobacter* strains have been studied in any detail for host cytoskeletal requirements for entry and most studies have been limited in scope, it appears likely that different *C. jejuni* and *C. coli* strains use several different mechanisms to enter host cells. However, only *C. jejuni* 81-176 has been studied in detail for kinetics of entry, analyses of cytoskeletal-bacterial interactions, and host signal transduction events involved in internalization. Thus, our current concept of invasion is derived mainly from studies of strain 81-176, which reveal the temporal interactions of this strain with various host cell structures and allow us to propose a coherent invasion mechanism.

Adherence of *C. jejuni* to host cell surfaces occurs even for noninvasive mutants, suggesting that cell adherence is a distinctly different process from invasion. At early times during invasion, *C. jejuni* can be observed interacting transiently with finger-like extensions of the host cell membrane containing one or a few bundled MTs. Although this is speculative, these host membrane projections may represent an early host cytoskeletal response to a diffusible signal from the nearby bacterium, as proposed for strain F38011 (79). Inhibitors affecting the formation of host membrane caveolae or coated pits block strain 81-176 internalization, suggesting that the yet undefined "invasion receptor(s)" resides in these related membrane structures, which may be sequestered to the lateral surface in older cells. Interaction of the uncharacterized bacterial invasion ligand with the putative host membrane receptor triggers protein tyrosine kinase signaling events within the host that lead to activation of dynein and PI3-kinase. PI3-kinase activation apparently results in the transient release of intracellular Ca^{2+}, which may be needed for the cytoskeletal MT rearrangements that result in bacterial internalization. Limited electron microscopy studies show internalized *C. jejuni* within endosomal vacuoles, and the dynein inhibitor orthovanadate reduces *C. jejuni* entry significantly. We hypothesize that a successful "*Campylobacter* invasion ligand-host receptor" interaction might activate dynein bound in membrane invaginations and cause this phosphorylated dynein to traverse inwardly along an MT and consequently to invaginate the dynein-bound membrane, resulting in uptake of the attached bacterium.

C. jejuni 81-176 triggers an efficient and kinetically saturable invasion of intestinal epithelial cells. Maximal entry of strain 81-176 into INT407 cells involves the uptake of two bacteria per cell. Host cell competence for *C. jejuni* entry appears to be cell cycle dependent, suggesting that receptors (or other requisites) are present at specific stages of host cell growth.

Trafficking of the endosome-contained *C. jejuni* from the cell surface to the perinuclear region involves the MT molecular motor dyncin; *C. jejuni* can be seen colocalizing with MTs and dynein during the first 4 h of entry. *C. jejuni* may undergo a change in cell shape (i.e., to coccoid) or maturation in the perinuclear region before moving to the basolateral surface for exocytosis. IL-8 is induced during bacterial infection and initiates the acute inflammatory response in the gut. Translocation of *C. jejuni* appears to occur via transcellular and paracellular routes. The bacteria released into the basolateral domain can enter and survive for several days in human monocytes, a process which could be involved in the submucosal dissemination of this pathogen.

PERSPECTIVE

Data obtained from clinical infections, experimental infections in humans and animals, and in vitro analyses of adherence and invasion in cultured human cells have now clearly demonstrated that cell invasiveness is a necessary step in *Campylobacter*-induced inflammatory diarrhea. Much progress has been made over the past decade in characterizing the *C. jejuni* and host cell requirements for invasion. We now have a solid conceptual understanding of how *C. jejuni* 81-176 is internalized into host cells. Despite these advances, many important questions await further study. Are all human-pathogenic strains of *C. jejuni* and *C. coli* invasive, or are some strains toxigenic and adherent? Identifying and cloning the responsible *C. jejuni* invasion determinants will provide appropriate probes to answer the above question. Cognate assays for invasiveness are variable and have led to the finding of different host cytoskeletal requirements for *C. jejuni* invasion. The use of assays with appropriate positive and negative invasion controls to assess the proper functioning of biochemical inhibitors will help clarify the different types of *Campylobacter* invasion mechanisms (e.g., under our assay conditions, invasion of *C. jejuni* strains, identified in other reports as MF dependent, was found to be strictly MT dependent).

The current understanding of the host cell signaling events and structural rearrangements triggered by *C. jejuni* now provides the molecular foundations on which to build a detailed molecular cell-biological model for bacterial internalization and transcytosis (and eventually for disease pathogenesis). What are the bacterial ligand(s) and host receptor(s) for *Campylobacter* uptake? Are these receptors present only on certain cell types? Do all *C. jejuni* secrete invasion effectors, as proposed by Konkel et al. (79), that trigger host signaling events? How do these signal transduction events lead to internalization of *C. jejuni,* intracellular bacterial movement, stimulation of IL-8 production, and eventual host cell death? Does *C. jejuni* encode unique mechanisms for entry into human monocytes that allow intracellular survival for several days? Finally, volunteer and animal model studies involving some defined mutants defective in, for example, invasion, translocation, or intramacrophage survival will help determine the importance of these different factors in disease pathogenesis. Improved understanding of the molecular mechanism(s) of *C. jejuni* invasion, intracellular movement, and transcytosis will aid both our knowledge of disease pathogenesis and the development of new chemotherapeutic, diagnostic, and prophylactic tools.

REFERENCES

1. **Alm, R. A., P. Guerry, and T. J. Trust.** 1993. The *Campylobacter* sigma 54 flaB flagellin promoter is subject to environmental regulation. *J. Bacteriol.* **175:**4448–4455.

2. **Arimi, S. M., R. W. Park, and C. R. Fricker.** 1990. Study of haemolytic activity of some *Campylobacter* spp. on blood agar plates. *J. Appl. Bacteriol.* **69:**384–389.

3. **Autenrieth, I. B., A. Schwarzkopf, J. H. Ewald, H. Karch, and R. Lissner.** 1995. Bactericidal properties of *Campylobacter jejuni*-specific immunoglobulin M antibodies in commercial immunoglobulin preparations. *Antimicrob. Agents Chemother.* **39:**1965–1969.

4. **Babakhani, F. K., and L. A. Joens.** 1993. Primary swine intestinal cells as a model for studying *Campylobacter jejuni* invasiveness. *Infect. Immun.* **61:**2723–2726.

5. **Berden, J. H., H. L. Muytjens, and L. B. van de Putte.** 1979. Reactive arthritis associated with *Campylobacter jejuni* enteritis. *Br. Med. J.* **1:** 380–381.

6. **Black, R. E., M. M. Levine, M. L. Clements, T. P. Hughes, and M. J. Blaser.** 1998. Experi-mental *Campylobacter jejuni* infection in humans. *J. Infect. Dis.* **157:**472–479.

7. **Blaser, M. J.** 1997. Epidemiologic and clinical features of *Campylobacter jejuni* infections. *J. Infect. Dis.* **176**(Suppl. 2):S103–S105.

8. **Blaser, M. J., D. J. Duncan, G. H. Warren, and W. L. Wang.** 1983. Experimental *Campylobacter jejuni* infection of adult mice. *Infect. Immun.* **39:**908–916.

9. **Bliska, J. B., J. E. Galan, and S. Falkow.** 1993. Signal transduction in the mammalian cell during bacterial attachment and entry. *Cell* **73:** 903–920.

10. **Buchmeier, N. A., and F. Heffron.** 1990. Induction of *Salmonella* stress proteins upon infection of macrophages. *Science* **248:**730–732.

11. **Buck, G. E., K. A. Parshall, and C. P. Davis.** 1983. Electron microscopy of the coccoid form of *Campylobacter jejuni. J. Clin. Microbiol.* **18:** 420–421.

12. **Bukholm, G., and G. Kapperud.** 1987. Expression of *Campylobacter jejuni* invasiveness in cell cultures coinfected with other bacteria. *Infect. Immun.* **55:**2816–2821.

13. **Buysse, J. M., C. K. Stover, E. V. Oaks, M. Venkatesan, and D. J. Kopecko.** 1987. Molecular cloning of invasion plasmid antigen (*ipa*) genes from *Shigella flexneri*: analysis of *ipa* gene products and genetic mapping. *J. Bacteriol.* **169:** 2561–2569.

14. **Byrne, G. I., and J. W. Moulder.** 1978. Parasite-specified phagocytosis of *Chlamydia psittaci* and *Chlamydia trachomatis* by L and HeLa cells. *Infect. Immun.* **19:**598–606.

15. **Chan, V. L., H. Louie, and H. L. Bingham.** 1995. Cloning and transcription regulation of the ferric uptake regulatory gene of *Campylobacter jejuni* TGH9011. *Gene* **164:**25–31.

16. **Clausen, J. D., G. Christiansen, H. U. Holst, and S. Birkelund.** 1997. *Chlamydia trachomatis* utilizes the host cell microtubule network during early events of infection. *Mol. Microbiol.* **25:** 441–449.

17. **Clerc, P., and P. J. Sansonetti.** 1987. Entry of *Shigella flexneri* into HeLa cells: evidence for directed phagocytosis involving actin polymerization and myosin accumulation. *Infect. Immun.* **55:**2681–2688.

18. **Cossart, P., and C. Kocks.** 1994. The actin-based motility of the facultative intracellular pathogen *Listeria monocytogenes. Mol. Microbiol.* **13:**395–402.

19. **Cover, T. L., G. I. Perez-Perez, and M. J. Blaser.** 1990. Evaluation of cytotoxic activity in fecal filtrates from patients with *Campylobacter jejuni* or *Campylobacter coli* enteritis. *FEMS Microbiol. Lett.* **58:**301–304.

20. **Crowe, S. E., L. Alvarez, M. Dytoc, R. H. Hunt, M. Muller, P. Sherman, J. Patel, Y. Jin, and P. B. Ernst.** 1995. Expression of interleukin 8 and CD54 by human gastric epithelium after *Helicobacter pylori* infection in vitro. *Gastroenterology* **108**:65–74.

21. **Cudmore, S., P. Cossart, G. Griffiths, and M. Way.** 1995. Actin-based motility of vaccinia virus. *Nature* **378**:636–638.

22. **de Melo, M. A., G. Gabbiani, and J. C. Pechere.** 1989. Cellular events and intracellular survival of *Campylobacter jejuni* during infection of HEp-2 cells. *Infect. Immun.* **57**:2214–2222.

23. **de Melo, M. A., and J. C. Pechere.** 1988. Effect of mucin on *Campylobacter jejuni* association and invasion on HEp-2 cells. *Microb. Pathog.* **5**:71–76.

24. **de Melo, M. A., and J. C. Pechere.** 1990. Identification of *Campylobacter jejuni* surface proteins that bind to eucaryotic cells in vitro. *Infect. Immun.* **58**:1749–1756.

25. **Doig, P., N. Kinsella, P. Guerry, and T. J. Trust.** 1996. Characterization of a posttranslational modification of *Campylobacter* flagellin: identification of a sero-specific glycosyl moiety. *Mol. Microbiol.* **19**:379–387.

26. **Doig, P., R. Yao, D. H. Burr, P. Guerry, and T. J. Trust.** 1996. An environmentally regulated pilus-like appendage involved in *Campylobacter* pathogenesis. *Mol. Microbiol.* **20**:885–894.

27. **Duffy, M. C., J. B. Benson, and S. J. Rubin.** 1980. Mucosal invasion in Campylobacter enteritis. *Am. J. Clin. Pathol.* **73**:706–708.

28. **Eckmann, L., M. F. Kagnoff, and J. Fierer.** 1993. Epithelial cells secrete the chemokine interleukin-8 in response to bacterial entry. *Infect. Immun.* **61**:4569–4574.

29. **Elsinghorst, E. A.** 1994. Measurement of invasion by gentamicin resistance. *Methods Enzymol.* **236**:405–420.

30. **Elsinghorst, E. A., L. S. Baron, and D. J. Kopecko.** 1989. Penetration of human intestinal epithelial cells by *Salmonella*: molecular cloning and expression of *Salmonella typhi* invasion determinants in *Escherichia coli*. *Proc. Natl. Acad. Sci. USA* **86**:5173–5177.

31. **Everest, P. H., H. Goossens, J. P. Butzler, D. Lloyd, S. Knutton, J. M. Ketley, and P. H. Williams.** 1992. Differentiated Caco-2 cells as a model for enteric invasion by *Campylobacter jejuni* and *C. coli. J. Med. Microbiol.* **37**:319–325.

32. **Falkow, S., R. R. Isberg, and D. A. Portnoy.** 1992. The interaction of bacteria with mammalian cells. *Annu. Rev. Cell Biol.* **8**:333–363.

33. **Fauchere, J. L., and M. J. Blaser.** 1990. Adherence of *Helicobacter pylori* cells and their surface components to HeLa cell membranes. *Microb. Pathog.* **9**:427–439.

34. **Fauchere, J. L., M. Kervella, A. Rosenau, K. Mohanna, and M. Veron.** 1989. Adhesion to HeLa cells of *Campylobacter jejuni* and *C. coli* outer membrane components. *Res. Microbiol.* **140**:379–392.

35. **Fauchere, J. L., A. Rosenau, M. Veron, E. N. Moyen, S. Richard, and A. Pfister.** 1986. Association with HeLa cells of *Campylobacter jejuni* and *Campylobacter coli* isolated from human feces. *Infect. Immun.* **54**:283–287.

36. **Field, L. H., V. L. Headley, S. M. Payne, and L. J. Berry.** 1986. Influence of iron on growth, morphology, outer membrane protein composition, and synthesis of siderophores in *Campylobacter jejuni. Infect. Immun.* **54**:126–132.

37. **Field, L. H., J. L. Underwood, L. M. Pope, and L. J. Berry.** 1981. Intestinal colonization of neonatal animals by *Campylobacter fetus* subsp. *jejuni. Infect. Immun.* **33**:884–892.

38. **Fierer, J., L. Eckmann, and M. Kagnoff.** 1993. IL-8 secreted by epithelial cells invaded by bacteria. *Infect. Agents Dis.* **2**:255–258.

39. **Finlay, B. B., and S. Falkow.** 1989. Common themes in microbial pathogenicity. *Microbiol. Rev.* **53**:210–230.

40. **Finlay, B. B., and S. Falkow.** 1988. Comparison of the invasion strategies used by *Salmonella cholerae-suis*, *Shigella flexneri* and *Yersinia enterocolitica* to enter cultured animal cells: endosome acidification is not required for bacterial invasion or intracellular replication. *Biochimie* **70**:1089–1099.

41. **Finlay, B. B., and S. Falkow.** 1990. *Salmonella* interactions with polarized human intestinal Caco-2 epithelial cells. *J. Infect. Dis.* **162**:1096–1106.

42. **Finlay, B. B., S. Ruschkowski, and S. Dedhar.** 1991. Cytoskeletal rearrangements accompanying salmonella entry into epithelial cells. *J. Cell Sci.* **99**:283–296.

43. **Galan, J. E., and R. Curtiss III.** 1989. Cloning and molecular characterization of genes whose products allow *Salmonella typhimurium* to penetrate tissue culture cells. *Proc. Natl. Acad. Sci. USA* **86**:6383–6387.

44. **Galan, J. E., J. Pace, and M. J. Hayman.** 1992. Involvement of the epidermal growth factor receptor in the invasion of cultured mammalian cells by *Salmonella typhimurium. Nature* **357**:588–589.

45. **Garvis, S. G., G. J. Puzon, and M. E. Konkel.** 1996. Molecular characterization of a *Campylobacter jejuni* 29-kilodalton periplasmic binding protein. *Infect. Immun.* **64**:3537–3543.

46. **Gibbons, I. R., M. P. Cosson, J. A. Evans,**

B. H. Gibbons, B. Houck, K. H. Martinson, W. S. Sale, and W. J. Tang. 1978. Potent inhibition of dynein adenosinetriphosphatase and of the motility of cilia and sperm flagella by vanadate. *Proc. Natl. Acad. Sci. USA* **75:**2220–2224.

47. Goldberg, M. B., and P. J. Sansonetti. 1993. *Shigella* subversion of the cellular cytoskeleton: a strategy for epithelial colonization. *Infect. Immun.* **61:**4941–4946.

48. Goldstein, J. L., R. G. Anderson, and M. S. Brown. 1979. Coated pits, coated vesicles, and receptor-mediated endocytosis. *Nature* **279:** 679–685.

49. Grant, C. C., M. E. Konkel, W. Cieplak, Jr., and L. S. Tompkins. 1993. Role of flagella in adherence, internalization, and translocation of *Campylobacter jejuni* in nonpolarized and polarized epithelial cell cultures. *Infect. Immun.* **61:** 1764–1771.

50. Griffin, F. M., Jr., J. A. Griffin, and S. C. Silverstein. 1976. Studies on the mechanism of phagocytosis. II. The interaction of macrophages with anti-immunoglobulin IgG-coated bone marrow-derived lymphocytes. *J. Exp. Med.* **144:** 788–809.

51. Griffiths, P. L., and R. W. Park. 1990. *Campylobacters* associated with human diarrhoeal disease. *J. Appl. Bacteriol.* **69:**281–301.

52. Guerry, P., R. A., M. E. Power, and T. J. Trust. 1992. Molecular and structural analysis of *Campylobacter jejuni*, p. 267–281. *In* I. Nachamkin, M. J. Blaser, and L. S. Tompkins (ed.), *Campylobacter jejuni: Current Status and Future Trends.* American Society for Microbiology, Washington, D.C.

53. Heinzen, R. A., S. F. Hayes, M. G. Peacock, and T. Hackstadt. 1993. Directional actin polymerization associated with spotted fever group *Rickettsia* infection of Vero cells. *Infect. Immun.* **61:**1926–1935.

54. Helenius, A., J. Kartenbeck, K. Simons, and E. Fries. 1980. On the entry of Semliki forest virus into BHK-21 cells. *J. Cell. Biol.* **84:** 404–420.

55. Hickey, T. E., S. Baqar, A. L. Bourgeois, C. P. Ewing, and P. Guerry. 1999. *Campylobacter jejuni*-stimulated secretion of interleukin-8 by INT407 cells. *Infect. Immun.* **67:**88–93.

56. Hu, L., and D. J. Kopecko. 1999. *Campylobacter jejuni* 81–176 associates with microtubules and dynein during invasion into human intestinal cells. *Infect. Immun.* **67:**4171–4182.

57. Hu, L., and D. J. Kopecko. 1999. *Campylobacter jejuni*-induced signal transduction in host intestinal epithelial cells, abstr. B/D-181, p. 64. *In Abstracts of the 99th General Meeting of the American Society for Microbiology 1999.* American Society for Microbiology, Washington, D.C.

57a. Hu, L., and D. J. Kopecko. Unpublished data.

58. Hu, L., C. Deal, J. McDaniel, and D. J. Kopecko. 1998. Host cell signal transduction events triggered by *Campylobacter jejuni*, abstr. B80, p. 70. *In Abstracts of the 98th General Meeting of American Society for Microbiology 1998.* American Society for Microbiology, Washington, D.C.

59. Huang, X. Z., B. Tall, W. R. Schwan, and D. J. Kopecko. 1998. Physical limitations on *Salmonella typhi* entry into cultured human intestinal epithelial cells. *Infect. Immun.* **66:** 2928–2937.

60. Hueck, C. J. 1998. Type III protein secretion systems in bacterial pathogens of animals and plants. *Microbiol. Mol. Biol. Rev.* **62:**379–433.

61. Hugdahl, M. B., J. T. Beery, and M. P. Doyle. 1988. Chemotactic behavior of *Campylobacter jejuni*. *Infect. Immun.* **56:**1560–1566.

62. Isberg, R. R., and S. Falkow. 1985. A single genetic locus encoded by *Yersinia pseudotuberculosis* permits invasion of cultured animal cells by *Escherichia coli* K-12. *Nature* **317:**262–264.

63. Isberg, R. R., and G. T. Van Nhieu. 1994. Two mammalian cell internalization strategies used by pathogenic bacteria. *Annu. Rev. Genet.* **28:**395–422.

64. Isberg, R. R., D. L. Voorhis, and S. Falkow. 1987. Identification of invasin: a protein that allows enteric bacteria to penetrate cultured mammalian cells. *Cell* **50:**769–778.

65. Johnson, W. M., and H. Lior. 1984. Toxins produced by *Campylobacter jejuni* and *Campylobacter coli*. *Lancet* **i:**229–230. (Letter.)

66. Ketley, J. M. 1995. The 16th C. L. Oakley Lecture. Virulence of *Campylobacter* species: a molecular genetic approach. *J. Med. Microbiol.* **42:** 312–327.

67. Ketley, J. M. 1997. Pathogenesis of enteric infection by *Campylobacter*. *Microbiology* **143:**5–21.

68. Khoramian-Falsafi, T., S. Harayama, K. Kutsukake, and J. C. Pechere. 1990. Effect of motility and chemotaxis on the invasion of *Salmonella typhimurium* into HeLa cells. *Microb. Pathog.* **9:**47–53.

69. Kiehlbauch, J. A., R. A. Albach, L. L. Baum, and K. P. Chang. 1985. Phagocytosis of *Campylobacter jejuni* and its intracellular survival in mononuclear phagocytes. *Infect. Immun.* **48:**446–451.

70. Kihlstrom, E., and L. Nilsson. 1977. Endocytosis of *Salmonella typhimurium* 395 MS and MR10 by HeLa cells. *Acta. Pathol. Microbiol. Scand. Sect. B* **85:**322–328.

71. Klipstein, F. A., and R. F. Engert. 1984.

Properties of crude *Campylobacter jejuni* heat-labile enterotoxin. *Infect. Immun.* **45:**314–319.

72. **Klipstein, F. A., and R. F. Engert.** 1984. Purification of *Campylobacter jejuni* enterotoxin. *Lancet* **i:**1123–1124. (Letter.)

73. **Konkel, M. E., and W. Cieplak, Jr.** 1992. Altered synthetic response of *Campylobacter jejuni* to cocultivation with human epithelial cells is associated with enhanced internalization. *Infect. Immun.* **60:**4945–4949.

74. **Konkel, M. E., M. D. Corwin, L. A. Joens, and W. Cieplak.** 1992. Factors that influence the interaction of *Campylobacter jejuni* with cultured mammalian cells. *J. Med. Microbiol.* **37:**30–37.

75. **Konkel, M. E., S. A. Gray, B. J. Kim, S. G. Garvis, and J. Yoon.** 1999. Identification of the enteropathogens *Campylobacter jejuni* and *Campylobacter coli* based on the *cadF* virulence gene and its product. *J. Clin. Microbiol.* **37:**510–517.

76. **Konkel, M. E., S. F. Hayes, L. A. Joens, and W. Cieplak, Jr.** 1992. Characteristics of the internalization and intracellular survival of *Campylobacter jejuni* in human epithelial cell cultures. *Microb. Pathog.* **13:**357–370.

77. **Konkel, M. E., and L. A. Joens.** 1989. Adhesion to and invasion of HEp-2 cells by *Campylobacter* spp. *Infect. Immun.* **57:**2984–2990.

78. **Konkel, M. E., and L. A. Joens.** 1990. Effect of enteroviruses on adherence to and invasion of HEp-2 cells by *Campylobacter* isolates. *Infect. Immun.* **58:**1101–1105.

79. **Konkel, M. E., B. J. Kim, V. Rivera-Amill, and S. G. Garvis.** 1999. Bacterial secreted proteins are required for the internalization of *Campylobacter jejuni* into cultured mammalian cells. *Mol. Microbiol.* **32:**691–701.

80. **Konkel, M. E., D. J. Mead, and W. Cieplak, Jr.** 1993. Kinetic and antigenic characterization of altered protein synthesis by *Campylobacter jejuni* during cultivation with human epithelial cells. *J. Infect. Dis.* **168:**948–54.

81. **Konkel, M. E., D. J. Mead, S. F. Hayes, and W. Cieplak, Jr.** 1992. Translocation of *Campylobacter jejuni* across human polarized epithelial cell monolayer cultures. *J. Infect. Dis.* **166:**308–315.

82. **Lee, A., J. O'Rourke, M. B. Phillips, and P. Barrington.** 1983. *Campylobacter jejuni as a Mucosa Associated Organism: an Ecological Study.* Public Health Laboratory Service, London, United Kingdom.

83. **Longfield, R., J. O'Donnell, W. Yudt, C. Lissner, and T. Burns.** 1979. Acute colitis and bacteremia due to *Campylobacter fetus. Dig. Dis. Sci.* **24:**950–953.

84. **Majeed, M., M. Gustafsson, E. Kihlstrom, and O. Stendahl.** 1993. Roles of Ca^{2+} and F-actin in intracellular aggregation of *Chlamydia trachomatis* in eucaryotic cells. *Infect. Immun.* **61:**1406–1414.

85. **Majeed, M., and E. Kihlstrom.** 1991. Mobilization of F-actin and clathrin during redistribution of *Chlamydia trachomatis* to an intracellular site in eucaryotic cells. *Infect. Immun.* **59:**4465–4472.

86. **Makino, S., J. P. van Putten, and T. F. Meyer.** 1991. Phase variation of the opacity outer membrane protein controls invasion by *Neisseria gonorrhoeae* into human epithelial cells. *EMBO J.* **10:**1307–1315.

87. **Matlin, K. S., H. Reggio, A. Helenius, and K. Simons.** 1981. Infectious entry pathway of influenza virus in a canine kidney cell line. *J. Cell. Biol.* **91:**601–613.

88. **McSweegan, E., D. H. Burr, and R. I. Walker.** 1987. Intestinal mucus gel and secretory antibody are barriers to *Campylobacter jejuni* adherence to INT 407 cells. *Infect. Immun.* **55:**1431–1435.

89. **McSweegan, E., and R. I. Walker.** 1986. Identification and characterization of two *Campylobacter jejuni* adhesins for cellular and mucous substrates. *Infect. Immun.* **53:**141–148.

90. **Mengaud, J., H. Ohayon, P. Gounon, R. M. Mege, and P. Cossart.** 1996. E-cadherin is the receptor for internalin, a surface protein required for entry of *L. monocytogenes* into epithelial cells. *Cell* **84:**923–932.

91. **Miller, V. L., B. B. Finlay, and S. Falkow.** 1988. Factors essential for the penetration of mammalian cells by *Yersinia. Curr. Top. Microbiol. Immunol.* **138:**15–39.

92. **Misawa, N., and M. J. Blaser.** 1997. Detection of autoagglutination activity from *Campylobacter jejuni* as virulence marker, abstr. B-518, p. 117. *In Abstracts of the 97th General Meeting of the American Society for Microbiology* 1997. American Society for Microbiology, Washington, D.C.

93. **Moore, M. A., M. J. Blaser, G. I. Perez-Perez, and A. D. O'Brien.** 1988. Production of a Shiga-like cytotoxin by *Campylobacter. Microb. Pathog.* **4:**455–462.

94. **Moran, A. P.** 1997. Structure and conserved characteristics of *Campylobacter jejuni* lipopolysaccharides. *J. Infect. Dis.* **176**(Suppl. 2):S115–S121.

95. **Moran, A. P.** 1995. Structure-bioactivity relationships of bacterial endotoxins. *J. Toxicol. Toxin Rev.* **14:**47–83.

96. **Newell, D. G., and A. Pearson.** 1984. The invasion of epithelial cell lines and the intestinal epithelium of infant mice by *Campylobacter jejuni/coli. J. Diarrhoeal Dis. Res.* **2:**19–26.

97. **Nuijten P. J. M., T. M. Wassenaar, D. G. Newell, B. A. M. Van der Zeijst.** 1992. Molecular characterization and analysis of *Campylobacter jejuni* flagellin genes and proteins, p. 282–296. *In* I. Nachamkin, M. J. Blaser, and L. S. Tompkins (ed.), *Campylobacter jejuni: Current Status and Future Trends.* American Society for Microbiology, Washington, D.C.

98. **Oelschlaeger, T. A., P. Guerry, and D. J. Kopecko.** 1993. Unusual microtubule-dependent endocytosis mechanisms triggered by *Campylobacter jejuni* and *Citrobacter freundii. Proc. Natl. Acad. Sci. USA* **90:**6884–6888.

98a. **Oelschlaeger, T. A., P. Guerry, and D. J. Kopecko.** Unpublished data.

99. **Olsvik, O., K. Wachsmuth, G. Morris, and J. C. Feeley.** 1984. Genetic probing of *Campylobacter jejuni* for cholera toxin and *Escherichia coli* heat-labile enterotoxin. *Lancet* **i:**449. (Letter.)

100. **Payne, S. M.** 1993. Iron acquisition in microbial pathogenesis. *Trends Microbiol.* **1:**66–69.

101. **Pei, Z., and M. J. Blaser.** 1993. PEB1, the major cell-binding factor of *Campylobacter jejuni,* is a homolog of the binding component in gram-negative nutrient transport systems. *J. Biol. Chem.* **268:**18717–18725.

102. **Pei, Z. H., R. T. Ellison III, and M. J. Blaser.** 1991. Identification, purification, and characterization of major antigenic proteins of *Campylobacter jejuni. J. Biol. Chem.* **266:**16363–16369.

103. **Penner, J. L., and G. O. Aspinall.** 1997. Diversity of lipopolysaccharide structures in *Campylobacter jejuni. J. Infect. Dis.* **176**(Suppl. 2): S135–S138.

104. **Perez-Perez, G. I., D. L. Cohn, R. L. Guerrant, C. M. Patton, L. B. Reller, and M. J. Blaser.** 1989. Clinical and immunologic significance of cholera-like toxin and cytotoxin production by *Campylobacter* species in patients with acute inflammatory diarrhea in the USA. *J. Infect. Dis.* **160:**460–468.

105. **Pesci, E. C., D. L. Cottle, and C. L. Pickett.** 1994. Genetic, enzymatic, and pathogenic studies of the iron superoxide dismutase of *Campylobacter jejuni. Infect. Immun.* **62:**2687–2694.

106. **Polakis, P.** 1995. Mutations in the APC gene and their implications for protein structure and function. *Curr. Opin. Genet. Dev.* **5:**66–71.

107. **Richardson, P. T., and S. F. Park.** 1995. Enterochelin acquisition in *Campylobacter coli:* characterization of components of a binding-protein-dependent transport system. *Microbiology* **141:** 3181–3191.

108. **Richardson, W. P., and J. C. Sadoff.** 1988. Induced engulfment of *Neisseria gonorrhoeae* by tissue culture cells. *Infect. Immun.* **56:**2512–2514.

109. **Rietschel, E. T., L. Brade, O. Holst, et al.** 1990. Molecular structure of bacterial enteroxin in relation to bioactivity, p. 15–32. *In* A. Nowotny, J. J. Spitzer, and E. J. Ziegler (ed.), *Endotoxin Research Series,* vol. 1, *Cellular and Molecular Aspects of Endotoxin Reactions.* Elsevier Science Publishers, Amsterdam, The Netherlands.

110. **Robins-Browne, R. M., S. Tzipori, G. Gonis, J. Hayes, M. Withers, and J. K. Prpic.** 1985. The pathogenesis of *Yersinia enterocolitica* infection in gnotobiotic piglets. *J. Med. Microbiol.* **19:**297–308.

111. **Robinson, D. A.** 1981. Infective dose of *Campylobacter jejuni* in milk. *Br. Med. J. (Clin. Res. Ed.)* **282:**1584.

112. **Ruiz-Palacios, G. M.** 1992. Pathogenesis of *Campylobacter* infection: in vitro models, p. 158–159. *In* I. Nachamkin, M. J. Blaser, and L. S. Tompkins (ed.), *Campylobacter jejuni: Current Status and Future Trends.* American Society for Microbiology, Washington, D.C.

113. **Ruiz-Palacios, G. M., E. Escamilla, and N. Torres.** 1981. Experimental *Campylobacter* diarrhea in chickens. *Infect. Immun.* **34:**250–255.

114. **Ruiz-Palacios, G. M., J. Torres, N. I. Torres, E. Escamilla, B. R. Ruiz-Palacios, and J. Tamayo.** 1983. Cholera-like enterotoxin produced by *Campylobacter jejuni.* Characterisation and clinical significance. *Lancet* **ii:**250–253.

115. **Russell, R. G., and D. C. Blake, Jr.** 1994. Cell association and invasion of Caco-2 cells by *Campylobacter jejuni. Infect. Immun.* **62:** 3773–3779.

116. **Russell, R. G., M. O'Donnoghue, D. C. Blake, Jr., J. Zulty, and L. J. DeTolla.** 1993. Early colonic damage and invasion of *Campylobacter jejuni* in experimentally challenged infant *Macaca mulatta. J. Infect. Dis.* **168:**210–215.

117. **Saida, T., S. Kuroki, Q. Hao, M. Nishimura, M. Nukina, and H. Obayashi.** 1997. *Campylobacter jejuni* isolates from Japanese patients with Guillain-Barré syndrome. *J. Infect. Dis.* **176**(Suppl. 2):S129–S134.

118. **Salyers, A. A., and D. D. Whitt.** 1994. Virulence factors that promote colonization, p. 30–46. In A. A. Salyers and D. D. Whitt (ed.), *Bacterial Pathogenesis: a Molecular Approach.* American Society for Microbiology, Washington, D.C.

119. **Sansonetti, P. J.** 1991. Genetic and molecular basis of epithelial cell invasion by *Shigella* species. *Rev. Infect. Dis.* **13**(Suppl. 4):S285–S292.

120. **Sanyal, S. C., K. M. Islam, P. K. Neogy, M. Islam, P. Speelman, and M. I. Huq.** 1984. *Campylobacter jejuni* diarrhea model in infant chickens. *Infect Immun.* **43:**931–936.

121. **Skirrow, M. B., and M. J. Blaser.** 1995. *Campylobacter jejuni,* p. 825–848. *In* M. J. Blaser,

P. D. Smith, J. I. Ravdin, H. B. Greenberg, and R. L. Guerrant (ed.), *Infections of the Gastrointestinal Tract*. Raven Press, New York, N.Y.

122. **Skirrow, M. B., D. M. Jones, E. Sutcliffe, and J. Benjamin.** 1993. *Campylobacter* bacteraemia in England and Wales, 1981–91. *Epidemiol. Infect.* **110:**567–573.

123. **Stanley, P.** 1989. Chinese hamster ovary cell mutants with multiple glycosylation defects for production of glycoproteins with minimal carbohydrate heterogeneity. *Mol. Cell. Biol.* **9:**377–383.

124. **Szymanski, C. M., and G. D. Armstrong.** 1996. Interactions between *Campylobacter jejuni* and lipids. *Infect. Immun.* **64:**3467–3474.

125. **Takata, T., S. Fujimoto, and K. Amako.** 1992. Isolation of nonchemotactic mutants of *Campylobacter jejuni* and their colonization of the mouse intestinal tract. *Infect. Immun.* **60:**3596–3600.

126. **Takeuchi, A.** 1967. Electron microscope studies of experimental *Salmonella* infection. I. Penetration into the intestinal epithelium by *Salmonella typhimurium*. *Am. J. Pathol.* **50:**109–136.

127. **Takeuchi, A., S. B. Formal, and H. Sprinz.** 1968. Experimental acute colitis in the Rhesus monkey following peroral infection with *Shigella flexneri*. An electron microscope study. *Am. J. Pathol.* **52:**503–529.

128. **van Spreeuwel, J. P., G. C. Duursma, C. J. Meijer, R. Bax, P. C. Rosekrans, and J. Lindeman.** 1985. *Campylobacter* colitis: histological immunohistochemical and ultrastructural findings. *Gut* **26:**945–951.

129. **Wai, S. N., K. Nakayama, K. Umene, T. Moriya, and K. Amako.** 1996. Construction of a ferritin-deficient mutant of *Campylobacter jejuni*: contribution of ferritin to iron storage and protection against oxidative stress. *Mol. Microbiol.* **20:**1127–1134.

130. **Walan, A., C. Dahlgren, E. Kihlstrom, O. Stendahl, and R. Lock.** 1992. Phagocyte killing of *Campylobacter jejuni* in relation to oxidative activation. *Apmis* **100:**424–430.

131. **Walan, A., and E. Kihlstrom.** 1988. Surface charge and hydrophobicity of *Campylobacter je-*

juni strains in relation to adhesion to epithelial HT-29 cells. *Apmis* **96:**1089–1096.

132. **Walker, R. I., M. B. Caldwell, E. C. Lee, P. Guerry, T. J. Trust, and G. M. Ruiz-Palacios.** 1986. Pathophysiology of *Campylobacter* enteritis. *Microbiol. Rev.* **50:**81–94.

133. **Walker, R. I., and R. L. Owen.** 1990. Intestinal barriers to bacteria and their toxins. *Annu. Rev. Med.* **41:**393–400.

134. **Wassenaar, T. M., N. M. Bleumink-Pluym, and B. A. van der Zeijst.** 1991. Inactivation of *Campylobacter jejuni* flagellin genes by homologous recombination demonstrates that *flaA* but not *flaB* is required for invasion. *EMBO J.* **10:**2055–2061.

135. **Welkos, S. L.** 1984. Experimental gastroenteritis in newly-hatched chicks infected with *Campylobacter jejuni*. *J. Med. Microbiol.* **18:**233–248.

136. **Whitehouse, C. A., P. B. Balbo, E. C. Pesci, D. L. Cottle, P. M. Mirabito, and C. L. Pickett.** 1998. *Campylobacter jejuni* cytolethal distending toxin causes a G_2-phase cell cycle block. *Infect. Immun.* **66:**1934–1940.

137. **Wooldridge, K. G., P. H. Williams, and J. M. Ketley.** 1996. Host signal transduction and endocytosis of *Campylobacter jejuni*. *Microb. Pathog.* **21:**299–305.

138. **Wooldridge, K. G., P. H. Williams, and J. M. Ketley.** 1994. Iron-responsive genetic regulation in *Campylobacter jejuni*: cloning and characterization of a *fur* homolog. *J. Bacteriol.* **176:**5852–5856.

139. **Yanagawa, Y., M. Takahashi, and T. Itoh.** 1994. The role of flagella of *Campylobacter jejuni* in colonization in the intestinal tract in mice and the cultured-cell infectivity. *Nippon Saikingaku Zasshi* **49:**395–403. (In Japanese.)

140. **Yao, R., D. H. Burr, P. Doig, T. J. Trust, H. Niu, and P. Guerry.** 1994. Isolation of motile and non-motile insertional mutants of *Campylobacter jejuni*: the role of motility in adherence and invasion of eukaryotic cells. *Mol. Microbiol.* **14:**883–893.

141. **Yao, R., D. H. Burr, and P. Guerry.** 1997. CheY-mediated modulation of *Campylobacter jejuni* virulence. *Mol. Microbiol.* **23:**1021–1031.

MOLECULAR CHARACTERIZATION OF *CAMPYLOBACTER JEJUNI* VIRULENCE DETERMINANTS

Michael E. Konkel, Lynn A. Joens, and Philip F. Mixter

11

Campylobacter jejuni is a common cause of diarrheal disease worldwide. Molecular characterization of virulence determinants has provided a better understanding of the mechanisms of *C. jejuni* pathogenicity. Recent advances include the identification and characterization of virulence factors required for *C. jejuni* binding, entry, and survival within host cells. A model is presented that includes alteration of host cell signaling pathways and induction of host cell apoptosis for *C. jejuni*-mediated enteritis. The range of symptoms manifested by individuals with *C. jejuni*-mediated enteritis can be attributed to a range in host responses and may directly correlate with the presence of bacterial virulence factors.

BACKGROUND AND HOST RESPONSE

Clinical Symptoms of Primary Infection

The clinical manifestations of *C. jejuni* infection depend on many variables including the strain of *C. jejuni*, the expression of virulence factors, and the immune status of the host. Each of these factors alone or in combination can dictate the severity of infection, degree of dissemination, and clinical outcome.

Within 2 or 3 days after ingestion of *C. jejuni*-contaminated food or water, bacteria colonize the lower gastrointestinal tract, inducing symptoms that range from mild discomfort to a characteristic bloody diarrhea lasting 5 to 7 days. Ulceration of the gastric epithelia by *C. jejuni* is associated with abdominal pain, hemorrhage, and release of blood, lymphocytes, and mucus into the stool. Infection with *C. jejuni* is often self-limiting and resolves in less than 2 weeks. In severe cases of *C. jejuni* infection, septicemia may follow intestinal colonization and sequelae may ensue.

Immune Response

Following ingestion, *Campylobacter* organisms must overcome the innate immune system by first avoiding removal by peristalsis. For successful colonization, *C. jejuni* penetrates the physical mucus barrier (100), binds to, and subsequently invades the cells lining the small intestine. Direct contact of *C. jejuni* with host cells, via outer membrane proteins with high avidity for host cell receptors, is required for colonization and disease progression (54, 82). Host cell entry allows the bacteria to evade in-

Michael E. Konkel and Philip F. Mixter, School of Molecular Biosciences, Washington State University, Pullman, WA 99164-4233. *Lynn A. Joens,* Departments of Veterinary Science and Microbiology, University of Arizona, Tucson, AZ 85721.

Campylobacter, 2nd Ed., Edited by I. Nachamkin and M. J. Blaser
© 2000 American Society for Microbiology, Washington, D.C.

nate host immune responses including complement activity and phagocytosis in naive individuals. Entry also allows *C. jejuni* to evade specific antibodies in individuals exposed previously.

With successful binding and internalization, *Campylobacter* colonizes the epithelial layer and may damage the epithelia by a number of mechanisms including host cell invasion (92, 101), toxin production (discussed elsewhere in this volume) (86, 108), and apoptosis (92). Some bacteria may translocate the epithelia and move into the lamina propria. Within this mixed environment, *Campylobacter* must avoid attack by professional phagocytes and enter the circulatory system (104). This attack by phagocytes may involve simple engulfment by phagocytosis, release of reactive oxygen intermediates, and/or secretion of cytokines (42).

In a recent review, Ketley (47) presented models proposing that immune responses leading to inflammatory damage may be key in the intestinal ulceration observed in *C. jejuni* infection. In these models, the immune response may promote infection by further perturbing the organization of the mucosal epithelia, allowing for more direct bacterial access to the lamina propria. Inflammatory lesions may provide a portal of entry. Alternatively, phagocytes recruited to these lesions may kill bacteria and provide necessary host resistance.

Humoral and Cellular Memory Responses

Infection with *C. jejuni* leads to a memory response stimulating both the cellular and humoral arms of the immune response. *Campylobacter* outer membrane proteins and lipopolysaccharides (LPS) are strongly immunogenic, stimulating the production of group-specific antisera in individuals recovering from infection. These antisera can be used to classify serovariants associated with unique disorders such as Miller-Fisher syndrome and Guillian-Barré syndrome (64, 78). Virulence factors are presumed to be immunogenic as recovering individuals produce antibodies reactive with some of these proteins (54). In patients with

previous exposure, antibodies reactive with bacterial outer membrane proteins and LPS provide a degree of immunoprotection. Mucosal anti-LPS antibodies may neutralize LPS, limiting both cytokine release in the innate response and T-independent B-cell activation. Anti-LPS antibodies may further opsonize LPS to promote LPS breakdown and clearance. Antibodies specific to outer membrane proteins will limit adhesion to and invasion of nonprofessional phagocytic cells while opsonizing the bacteria for professional phagocytes. The action of professional phagocytes is crucial for resolving *C. jejuni* infection. Any defect in an individual's ability to mount a rapid and effective memory response to the bacterial infection limits the ability to eradicate the organisms and could lead to sequelae. T-cell-dependent antibody responses help prevent the spread of *C. jejuni* infection.

Resolution and Sequelae

Individuals who develop an effective immune response, generating *C. jejuni*-specific secretory immunoglobulin A (sIgA) in the intestinal tract, frequently resolve the infection within 2 weeks. *Campylobacter*-specific sIgA is essential for preventing the immediate spread of the infection as well as preventing reinfection (104). Generally, *C. jejuni*-infected individuals make serum antibodies specific for outer membrane proteins and LPS. Antibodies bound to the surface of *C. jejuni* fix complement and augment phagocytosis by host monocytes. These monocytes may be recruited and activated by cytokines released by host epithelial and monocytic cells, including interleukin-8 (IL-8) and tumor necrosis factor (67, 71). Inflammation of the intestinal mucosa is dominated by host monocytes and recedes with time. The combination of antibodies and active professional phagocytes ultimately eradicates the bacteria from most individuals.

Disseminated *C. jejuni* infections are associated with autoimmune sequelae. *C. jejuni* has been isolated from individuals with inflammatory bowel syndromes such as Crohn's disease, but the linkage between *C. jejuni* infection and inflammatory bowel syndromes is debatable (5). Disseminated *C. jejuni* infections are associated with Reiter's syndrome, with either conjunctival or urethral inflammation (45). There is also an association between *C. jejuni* infections and reactive arthritis due to antigen mimicry and production of cross-reactive antibodies (63). Approximately 1 in every 1,000 cases of *C. jejuni* infection leads to the degenerative polyneuropathy Guillain-Barré syndrome. This tendency is linked to the structural similarity of outer O-linked sugars in certain serovariants to structures of host gangliosides. This antigen mimicry is the basis of cross-reactivity between anti-*C. jejuni* antibodies and the gangliosides, initiating damage that results in subsequent neuropathy (78). This topic is covered in detail elsewhere in this volume.

Immunodeficiency

Elements in the innate immune system, including physical barriers of the gastrointestinal mucosa and active professional phagocytes, are crucial in controlling a *Campylobacter* infection. Defects in mucosal function associated with genetic disorders or immunodeficiency may increase the susceptibility to bacterial and fungal infections, including *Campylobacter* infection (10). Individuals with impaired innate immune responses are more susceptible to infection and commonly manifest *Campylobacter*-induced sequelae.

Specific antibody responses are thought to be the critical factor in limiting dissemination (104). Any defect in either T-cell function or efficient antibody production will limit the resolution of *Campylobacter* infection. Lack of sIgA production is a common immunodeficiency, with rates estimated from 1:333 to 1:700 (18). Other immunodeficiencies (e.g. X-linked agammaglobulinemia and DiGeorge syndrome) that limit antibody production lead to increased susceptibility to all bacterial infections, including *Campylobacter* infections (12). The developing immune systems of young children are less able to mount a directed response quickly, allowing *Campylobacter* to disseminate, colonize, and persist (6, 73). Young

children may harbor the bacteria and spread it to other family members. In addition, elderly individuals may have impaired responses for a variety of reasons and are more susceptible to *C. jejuni* infection (31).

Individuals infected with human immunodeficiency virus (HIV) and manifesting impaired immune responses in the early stages of AIDS are highly susceptible to enteric infections (reviewed in reference 84). The disease resulting from infection with *Campylobacter* may be severe (reviewed in reference 2) and prognostic for the transition from latent HIV infection to the beginning of AIDS. Other *Campylobacter* spp., including *C. fetus* and *C. upsaliensis,* are prevalent in HIV-immunocompromised patients (41). In many cases, immunodeficient individuals cannot eradicate *Campylobacter* organisms and may harbor strains that are resistant to antibiotic therapy (84).

IN VIVO EXPERIMENTAL MODEL SYSTEMS FOR *C. JEJUNI* INFECTION

To elucidate the role of *C. jejuni* virulence determinants, investigators have used chickens (25, 107, 115), rodents (38, 40), rabbits (14, 102), ferrets (7, 22), pigs (3), dogs (88), macaques (92), and humans (7). Each animal model has advantages and disadvantages in terms of the disease relative to humans, ease of sample collection, and availability of reagents for analyses. In most species, colonization occurs without the bloody diarrhea common in human *Campylobacter* infections (8). This may be a result of the immunological differences between the intestinal tracts of other animals and humans (93). The removable intestinal tie adult rabbit diarrhea (RITARD) model has been used for *Campylobacter* infection studies and exhibited symptoms more closely resemble those in humans (14). Some investigators demonstrated that mixed infections with immunosuppressive effects (e.g. *Trichurius suis*) allowed greater *C. jejuni*-induced pathology (68). Larger animals used as infection models include colostrum-deprived piglets (3) and macaques (92). In these animals, the hallmarks of disease and histopathology more closely resemble those observed in human infection.

INSIGHTS INTO POTENTIAL MECHANISMS OF *C. JEJUNI* PATHOGENESIS

The ability of *C. jejuni* to cause disease is a complex, multifactorial process that requires the expression of many genes. In the past decade, in vitro assays have permitted the identification and characterization of a limited number of *C. jejuni* virulence determinants. For some of these virulence determinants, mutations have been generated in the corresponding genes and the functional roles of these proteins in *C. jejuni*-mediated enteritis have been assessed by using the in vivo infection models discussed above. In certain cases, the identification of *C. jejuni* putative virulence determinants through in vitro assays has been substantiated by in vivo models, demonstrating the usefulness of in vitro assays.

Binding of *C. jejuni* to Host Cells

The ability of *C. jejuni* to bind to the cells lining the gastrointestinal tract is essential for the development of *C. jejuni*-mediated enteritis since it prevents the organism from being swept away by mechanical cleansing forces such as peristalsis and fluid flow. In vitro adherence assays have been used extensively to characterize the interactions of *C. jejuni* with host cells and to attempt to identify the bacterial factors that mediate binding (21, 22, 24, 54, 69, 82). Fauchere et al. (24) found that *C. jejuni* strains isolated from patients with fever and diarrhea adhered to cultured cells at higher levels than did strains isolated from individuals without diarrhea or fever.

The binding of *C. jejuni* to host cells has been studied with a variety of cell lines. *C. jejuni* is capable of binding with equal efficiency to cells of both human (INT 407, HEp-2, HeLa, 293, and Caco-2) and nonhuman (Vero, CHO-K1, and MDCK) origin. The binding of *C. jejuni* to INT 407 (Henle, a human intestinal epithelial cell line) and Caco-2 (a human colonic cell line) cells has been studied exten-

sively, since these cells are reflective of the cells encountered by *C. jejuni* in vivo. Time course studies examining the kinetics of bacterial association have revealed that the binding of *C. jejuni* to INT 407 and Caco-2 cells is saturable, reaching a maximum after an incubation period of 30 min (53, 91). The adherence of *C. jejuni* to INT 407 cells is also reversible (69). Depending on the assay conditions (i.e., bacterial strain, cell line, inoculum size, and method of quantitation of adherent bacteria), the adherent proportion of the bacterial inoculum ranges from 0.5 to 2% (111, 112). Considering the differences noted between laboratories in the number of adherent bacteria for *C. jejuni* 81-176, it remains difficult to determine the significance of variations in binding for *C. jejuni* isolates in different laboratories, possibly due to subtle variations in assay procedures.

As noted in a previous study, *C. jejuni* exhibited preferential binding to discrete sites near the borders of INT 407 cells (53). This preferential binding is even more apparent upon examination of cells infected with *C. jejuni* harboring a shuttle vector with the green fluorescence protein (*gfp*) gene (Fig. 1). *C. jejuni* binds to fibronectin (54), an extracellular matrix protein, and to a wide variety of lipids including phosphatidylethanolamine, phosphatidylcholine, phosphatidylinositol, phosphatidylserine, phosphatidylglycerol, and sphingomyelin as judged by enzyme-linked immunosorbent assays (99). Szymanski and Armstrong (99) speculated that the binding of *C. jejuni* to host cell membrane lipids may act as a secondary binding site for *Campylobacter* organisms.

Bacterial Molecules Proposed To Serve as Adhesins

The binding of *C. jejuni* to host cells is mediated by constitutively synthesized products. This concept is supported by the finding that heat-killed *C. jejuni* organisms bind to cultured cells at levels equal to or greater than those at which viable, untreated *C. jejuni* organisms bind (52). Proposed *C. jejuni* adhesins include LPS, flagellin, and several outer membrane

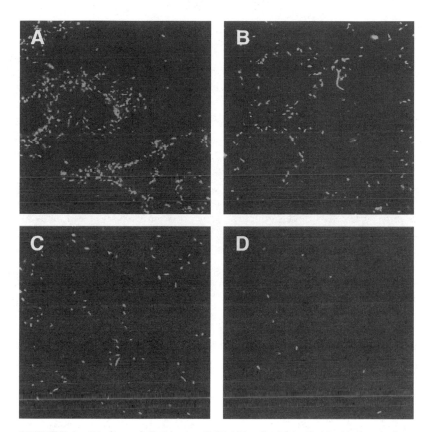

FIGURE 1 Binding of *C. jejuni* to INT 407 cells. This *C. jejuni* isolate harbors a *Campylobacter* shuttle vector containing a mutant form of the green fluorescent protein (*gfp*) gene. INT 407 cells were inoculated with 5×10^7 (A and C) and 5×10^6 (B and D) CFU of *C. jejuni*. Contact of the bacteria with the INT 407 cells was promoted by centrifugation at $600 \times g$ (A and B only). The *C. jejuni*-infected INT 407 cells were incubated for 30 min in a 5% CO_2 incubator at 37°C, and rinsed twice with phosphate-buffered saline. Bound bacteria were visualized with a Nikon inverted fluorescence microscope with a $60 \times$ objective.

proteins. Whether most of these molecules serve to promote the initial binding or facilitate more intimate contact of *C. jejuni* to host cells remains controversial.

LPS is a major antigenic molecule on the cell surface of *C. jejuni*. McSweegan and Walker (69) proposed that LPS mediated the binding of *C. jejuni* to host cells as evidenced by complete inhibition of *Campylobacter* attachment to host cells with purified LPS. However, 250 to 1,000 μg of LPS was used in these assays, which in our studies demonstrates overt toxic-

ity to host cells (results not shown). While investigators have shown that *C. jejuni* LPS binds to INT 407 cells and INT 407 membrane fractions (69, 75), additional studies are required to assess the specificity of LPS binding to target cells. With the recent identification of a number of *C. jejuni* LPS biosynthetic genes (29, 50), the role of LPS in the pathogenesis of *Campylobacter*-mediated enteritis and bacterium-host cell interactions may be addressed by using defined LPS mutants. LPS has been shown to play a role in bacterium-host cell interactions for other pathogenic bacteria including entero-pathogenic *Escherichia coli* (9), *Haemophilus influenzae* (106), *Neisseria gonorrhoeae* (95), and *Salmonella enterica* serovar Typhi (77).

Investigators have shown that purified flagellin was capable of binding to host cells and INT 407 cell membrane fractions (69, 75). In addition, the tips of the flagellin have been observed in contact with host cells in scanning electron microscopy examinations of *C. jejuni*-infected cells (53). Grant et al. (32) reported that genetically defined *C. jejuni flaA* and *flaB* mutants adhered to host cells at levels equal to those of their isogenic wild-type counterparts in a modified binding assay in which the association of the bacteria with host cells was promoted by centrifugation. However, Yao et al. (111) reported that a *flaA flaB⁺* mutant of *C. jejuni* 81-176 exhibited a 50-fold reduction in its ability to bind to cells whereas a *pflA* mutant (nonmotile or paralyzed with both FlaA and FlaB proteins) exhibited only a 2-fold reduction in binding. While these data indicate that the FlaA protein is capable of binding to host cells, the biological significance of this adhesive property is currently unclear given the requirement of motility to establish a successful infection. Wassenaar et al. (105), Grant et al. (32), and Yao et al. (111) have each reported that motility, conferred by the product of the *flaA* gene, plays a critical role in promoting the contact of *C. jejuni* with host cells and in postbinding events such as internalization and dissemination from the intestinal epithelia.

Included in the list of potential *C. jejuni* adhesins is the 43-kDa major outer membrane protein. Schröder and Moser (93a) found that the purified 43-kDa protein bound to INT 407 membrane fractions when isolated following native gel electrophoresis but not when isolated from gels in the presence of sodium dodecyl sulfate, as judged by enzyme-linked immunosorbent assay. Moser et al. (76) later reported a 15 to 20% reduction in the binding of *C. jejuni* to INT 407 cell membranes in the presence of the purified 43-kDa protein.

Significant advances have been made in the characterization of other proteins that mediate the binding of *C. jejuni* to host cells. Fauchère et al. (23a) found that two *C. jejuni* proteins, termed cell-binding factor 1 (CBF1) and cell-binding factor 2 (CBF2), bound preferentially to HeLa cells. CBF1 and CBF2 have apparent molecular masses of 27 and 29 kDa, respectively. Using a ligand-binding assay, De Melo and Pechère (21) identified four *C. jejuni* outer membrane proteins, with apparent molecular masses of 28, 32, 36, and 42 kDa, that bound to host cells. In the process of identifying *C. jejuni* proteins for the detection of *Campylobacter* organisms and candidates for vaccine development, Pei et al. (83) identified four proteins of 28, 29, 30, and 31 kDa, termed PEB1 through PEB4, respectively, in glycine-extracted material from *C. jejuni* 81-176. Pei and Blaser (81) subsequently cloned the structural gene encoding PEB1 by screening a *C. jejuni* genomic λgt11 library with a polyclonal antiserum to PEB1. This gene, designated *peb1A*, encodes a protein with a calculated molecular mass of 28,181 Da. Searches of the databases with the deduced amino acid sequence of the *peb1A* gene revealed that the protein exhibited similarity to amino acid transport proteins from other gram-negative bacteria. Most recently, two-dimensional gel electrophoresis coupled with immunoblot analysis with a rabbit antibody against CBF1 revealed that PEB1 and CBF1 were identical. Whether the 28-kDa protein identified by De Melo and Pechère (21) is the same as the CBF1/PEB1 protein is not clear. Regardless, a *C. jejuni peb1A* null mutant exhibited a 50- to 100-fold reduction in binding and a 15-fold reduction in internalization to HeLa cells compared to the *C. jejuni* parental isolate (82). The *C. jejuni peb1A* mutant also exhibited a reduction in the duration of mouse intestinal colonization compared to the parental isolate.

In addition to CBF1 (PEB1), CBF2 (PEB4) was reported to mediate the binding of *C. jejuni* to HeLa cells. However, additional studies revealed that PEB4 was not surface exposed as judged by transmission electron microscopy studies coupled with immunogold labeling with an anti-PEB4 serum (46). Kervella et al.

(46) found that purified PEB4 exhibited little binding activity to HeLa cell membranes in an adherence microassay and that antiserum against PEB4 only partially inhibited the binding of *C. jejuni* to HeLa cells. The gene encoding PEB4, *peb4A,* was cloned and sequenced by Burucoa et al. (13). The deduced amino acid sequence of the *peb4A* gene has similarity to gram-positive extracytoplasmic lipoproteins involved in processing transported proteins. Burucoa et al. (13) concluded that PEB4 may participate in the folding of secreted proteins on the outside of the cytoplasmic membrane but is unlikely to be involved in adhesion of *C. jejuni* to host cells.

Konkel et al. (54) noted that *C. jejuni* bound to the remnants of INT 407 cell adhesion plaques. *C. jejuni* also bound to fibronectin, a component of the extracellular matrix. Ligand immunoblot assays revealed that ^{125}I-labeled fibronectin bound specifically to a *C. jejuni* outer membrane protein with an apparent molecular mass of 37 kDa. Whether the 36-kDa protein identified by De Melo and Pechère (21) is the same as the 37-kDa fibronectin-binding protein is not known. The gene encoding the 37-kDa protein, designated *cadF* (for "*Campylobacter* adhesion to fibronectin"), was subsequently cloned by screening *C. jejuni* genomic libraries with a rabbit anti-37-kDa antiserum. A *C. jejuni cadF* mutant was generated. In vitro assays revealed that the *C. jejuni cadF* mutant exhibited a significant reduction in binding to fibronectin-coated coverslips (54) and to INT 407 cells (results not shown). In contrast to the *C. jejuni* parental isolate, a *C. jejuni cadF* mutant was unable to colonize orally challenged newly hatched Leghorn chickens (115). The *cadF* gene and protein are highly conserved among *C. jejuni* and *C. coli* isolates (55).

Doig et al. (22) found that *C. jejuni* produced appendages resembling pili upon growth in medium supplemented with deoxycholate (0.05%) and chenodeoxycholate (0.9%), which are major components of bile. Thus, *C. jejuni* may synthesize pili in vivo upon exposure to bile salts. To determine the role of pili in virulence, Doig et al. (22) generated a *C. jejuni*

pspA (pilus synthesis protease) null mutant. A mutation in the *pspA* gene resulted in a loss of pilus synthesis as determined by electron microscopy. In vitro assays suggested that pili do not mediate or potentiate the binding or internalization of *C. jejuni* to INT 407 cells. Pili also do not appear to be required for colonization in ferrets. However, the severity of disease symptoms in ferrets infected with a nonpilated mutant strain of *C. jejuni* 81-176 was reduced compared to that in ferrets infected with the wild-type *C. jejuni* isolate, suggesting that pili play a role in disease production. Interestingly, *C. jejuni* cultured in medium supplemented with deoxycholate and chenodeoxycholic acid exhibit an aggregative phenotype. Pili may facilitate "biofilm" formation, enabling *C. jejuni* to reach sufficient numbers to cause disease.

In summary, the binding of *C. jejuni* to host cells is reversible and motility dependent and is mediated by proteins synthesized constitutively (Fig. 2). In vitro and in vivo studies suggest that PEB1 and CadF are adhesins. The overall contribution of other *C. jejuni*-binding components, including LPS and the 43-kDa major outer membrane protein, remains to be elucidated. Pili promote an aggregative phenotype and may contribute to *C. jejuni*-mediated enteritis.

General Characteristics of Internalization

The dysentery associated with *Campylobacter* infection, coupled with the presence of *C. jejuni* in mucosal cells of infected individuals, led investigators to hypothesize that *C. jejuni* enteritis is directly related to the ability of the organism to enter the cells lining the gastrointestinal tract (6, 23). The ability of *C. jejuni* to enter, survive, and replicate in mammalian cells has been studied extensively by using tissue culture models (20, 22, 23, 56, 57, 79, 80, 82, 91, 105, 111). Typically, such model systems involve determination of the number of intracellular *C. jejuni* organisms by assaying bacterial protection from an antibiotic such as gentamicin. Gentamicin does not penetrate eukaryotic cell membranes.

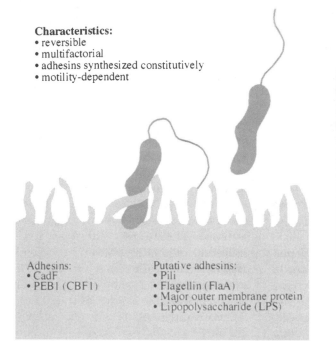

Characteristics:
• reversible
• multifactorial
• adhesins synthesized constitutively
• motility-dependent

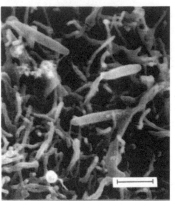

Adhesins:
• CadF
• PEB1 (CBF1)

Putative adhesins:
• Pili
• Flagellin (FlaA)
• Major outer membrane protein
• Lipopolysaccharide (LPS)

FIGURE 2 Proposed model of *C. jejuni* binding to host cells. The ability of *C. jejuni* to colonize the human gastrointestinal tract is essential for disease production. Binding to epithelial cells prevents the colonizing bacteria from being swept away by mechanical cleansing forces such as peristalsis and fluid flow. Furthermore, binding is a prerequisite for entry into host cells, where the organism may be protected from innate, humoral, and cellular immune responses. This figure shows the necessary characteristics of binding molecules and lists known and putative adhesins. Possible adhesins include outer membrane proteins and LPS.

The relative ability of *C. jejuni* to invade cultured cells appears to be strain dependent (23, 57, 79). Newell et al. (79) found that environmental isolates were much less invasive for HeLa cells than were clinical isolates as determined by immunofluorescence and electron microscopy examination of *C. jejuni*-infected cells. Everest et al. (23) observed a statistically significant difference in the level of invasion between *C. jejuni* strains from individuals with colitis and those from individuals with noninflammatory diarrhea. The differences in internalization among various *C. jejuni* isolates led investigators to hypothesize that this difference reflects separate uptake pathways. Yao et al. (111) proposed that low-level internalization is reflective of a microfilament-dependent uptake mechanism and that high-level internalization

is reflective of a microtubule-dependent pathway. The percentage of the inoculum internalized for *C. jejuni* 81-176, a highly invasive strain, has been reported to range from 0.8 to 1.8% (22, 111, 112). However, others have reported the percentage of recoverable *C. jejuni* 81-176 to be somewhat lower, ranging from $0.00537 \pm 0.0011\%$ to $0.345 \pm 0.15\%$ (82, 85). These differences in the invasive potential of one particular strain of *C. jejuni* probably reflect differences in assay conditions among laboratories, making comparisons of the invasive potential of strains among laboratories difficult. Nevertheless, quantitative comparisons among different isolates within a laboratory have proven extremely valuable in characterizing *C. jejuni* virulence determinants and host cell requirements.

Babakhani and Joens (4) found that the in vitro invasive potential of *C. jejuni* was enhanced after passage of the organism through primary intestinal cells. Based on this finding, the investigators hypothesized that invasive potential of *C. jejuni* is a regulated process. This hypothesis is further supported by two additional experimental findings: (i) the ability of *C. jejuni* to invade cells is lost after extensive in vitro passage (51), and (ii) *C. jejuni* cultured with eukaryotic cells synthesizes a subset of proteins not synthesized by organisms cultured in the absence of eukaryotic cells (52, 60).

INTERNALIZATION IS DEPENDENT ON BACTERIAL DE NOVO PROTEIN SYNTHESIS AND PROTEIN SECRETION

Pathogen-directed endocytosis requires microorganisms to synthesize molecules that mediate adherence and internalization to host cells. While the details of the mechanisms used by most invasive bacteria to enter mammalian cells are not fully known, in vitro studies have revealed that bacterial metabolic processes are required for efficient internalization of *H. influenzae* (98), *N. gonorrhoeae* (15, 89), *Rickettsia prowazekii* (103), *Salmonella typhimurium* (28), and *Shigella flexneri* (34). Some of these bacteria, including *Salmonella* and *Shigella* spp., secrete proteins via a specialized protein secretion system termed type III (reviewed in reference 39) that triggers host cell signal transduction events and that ultimately results in bacterial internalization and possibly host cell apoptosis.

The proteins that promote the entry of *C. jejuni* into host cells are probably distinct from those that facilitate binding. In support of this hypothesis, a *C. jejuni peb1* mutant displayed a 50- to 100-fold reduction in binding to HeLa cells but only a 15-fold reduction in internalization compared to the parental isolate. In contrast to bacterial adherence, the internalization of *C. jejuni* into INT 407 cells is significantly reduced in the presence of an inhibitor of bacterial protein synthesis (52, 80). Metabolic-labeling experiments revealed that *C. jejuni* cultured in the presence of epithelial cells synthesized at least 14 new proteins as judged by two-dimensional electrophoretic analysis (52, 60). These newly synthesized proteins are distinct from heat shock proteins. The synthesis of other proteins from *C. jejuni* was selectively repressed upon incubation of the organism with epithelial cells (52). These findings suggest the action of a coordinated response that results in the expression of certain genes as a response to the epithelial-cell microenvironment.

Competitive inhibition experiments with an antiserum generated by immunization of a rabbit with whole-cell *C. jejuni* cultured in the presence of INT 407 cells (Cj + INT or 1588) significantly reduced the entry of *C. jejuni* into INT 407 cells (60). The Cj + INT antiserum, in contrast to an antiserum raised against *C. jejuni* cultured in the absence of INT 407 cells (Cj − INT or 1622), reacted with several of the newly synthesized *C. jejuni* proteins. By differentially screening *C. jejuni* genomic DNA phage expression libraries with Cj + INT and Cj − INT sera, plaques that reacted only with the Cj + INT antiserum were identified. This screening resulted in the identification of a gene termed *ciaB* (for "*Campylobacter* invasion antigen B") (59). Direct sequence comparisons revealed that the deduced amino acid sequence of the 73-kDa CiaB protein exhibited a low level of similarity with *Salmonella* SipB, *Shigella* IpaB, and *Yersinia* YopB proteins. The SipB, IpaB, and YopB proteins have been shown through mutational analysis to be associated with bacterial invasion of eukaryotic cells. SipB, IpaB, and YopB are secreted proteins lacking typical signal sequences and are translocated from the bacterial cells to the eukaryotic cells via type III secretion systems (44). In vitro binding and internalization assays revealed that the *C. jejuni ciaB* null mutant bound to INT 407 cells in numbers equal to or greater than the wild-type parental isolate but exhibited a significant reduction (~100-fold) in internalization. Similar to SipB, IpaB, and YopB, CiaB does not possess an identifiable signal sequence in its amino terminus. CiaB is secreted from *C. jejuni* upon cultivation with eukaryotic cells or in medium supplemented with serum (see below) as judged by immunoblot analysis of culture supernatant fluids with an anti-CiaB antibody. CiaB also appears to be translocated into host cells, since cytoplasmic staining was observed by confocal microscopy studies with anti-CiaB antibody (59). The absence of an identifiable signal sequence from the amino terminus of the CiaB-deduced amino acid sequence suggests that *C. jejuni* may possess a type III secretion system.

Culturing *C. jejuni* in INT 407 conditioned medium results in the secretion of at least eight proteins, designated CiaA through CiaH (in order of the highest to the lowest molecular mass), into the culture medium (59). The apparent molecular masses of these eight proteins range from 12.8 to 108 kDa. Although the specific functions of the Cia secreted proteins are not currently known, the secreted Cia proteins may play a role in triggering host cell signaling events and *C. jejuni* internalization. It is important to note that inhibitors of tyrosine kinases, heterotrimeric G-proteins, and phosphatidylinositol 3-kinase (PI 3-kinase) reduce *C. jejuni* internalization (47). A hypothetical model of *C. jejuni* internalization, including the Cia proteins and altered host cell signaling, is presented in Fig. 3.

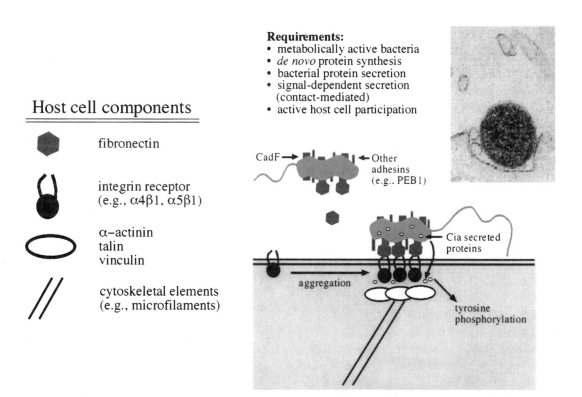

FIGURE 3 Proposed model of the uptake of *C. jejuni* by host cells. We hypothesize that intimate binding of *C. jejuni* to host cells, which is mediated by multiple adhesins including CadF and PEB1, is a requirement for *C. jejuni* internalization. We speculate that the binding of *C. jejuni* to fibronectin leads to the aggregation of host cell integrin receptors to initiate a cascade of host cell signaling events. Following contact, *C. jejuni* synthesizes a minimum of 14 new proteins, whose synthesis corresponded to a rapid increase in internalization and rearrangement of the host cell cytoskeletal components (52, 56, 60, 80). A subset of the newly synthesized proteins is secreted and translocated into the cytoplasm of target cells (59), augmenting the host cell signaling events required for *C. jejuni* uptake. Consistent with this model, inhibitors of tyrosine kinases, heterotrimeric G proteins, and phosphatidylinositol 3-kinase (PI 3-kinase) reduce *C. jejuni* internalization (47). Following binding and internalization, *C. jejuni*-infected cells release inflammatory cytokines, including IL-8 (36), that promote the recruitment of lymphocytes and professional phagocytic cells to the site of the infection. Recent studies indicate that *C. jejuni* can cause host cell-induced apoptosis, possibly promoting the survival and transmission of the organism (72).

The type III secretion system is referred to as the contact-mediated secretion system because protein secretion is triggered upon contact of an organism with eukaryotic cells. Secretion from this system can also be induced, perhaps artificially, by incubating organisms in medium containing serum (70, 114). Recent studies in our laboratory have revealed that *C. jejuni* secrete the Cia proteins upon incubation in INT 407 cell conditioned medium and in serum-supplemented tissue culture medium. Secretion of the Cia proteins can also be induced with sera from various species (e.g., human, bovine, pig, goat, sheep, rabbit, mouse, and chicken). Contact of *C. jejuni* with INT 407 cells cultured in serum-free medium also stimulates the secretion of Cia proteins. Additional work has revealed that the synthesis and secretion of the Cia proteins can be separated and that both require the presence of a stimulatory signal (90). Temporal kinetic studies have suggested a direct correlation between *C. jejuni* entry and secretion of the Cia proteins, since the Cia proteins have been detected within 30 min of incubation of *C. jejuni* in serum-supplemented medium (90).

Although the in vivo signal stimulating the synthesis of the entry-promoting proteins is not known, an adaptive response is required for *C. jejuni* to cause disease in a susceptible host. We propose that *C. jejuni* synthesizes novel proteins upon encountering the anaerobic environment of the intestinal tract. Such an adaptive response probably involves global gene regulation by a two-component regulatory system. Two-component regulatory systems consist of a sensor kinase and a response regulator. The sensors are integral membrane proteins which, in response to specific environmental signals, modulate the activity of cognate regulators by reversible phosphorylation. The regulators, whose affinity for DNA is thus modulated, act in turn as cytoplasmic gene *trans*-activator proteins. One advantage of such a global regulatory system is that it allows the simultaneous expression of unlinked genes in response to environmental stimuli.

Altered gene expression by *C. jejuni* in response to changes in temperature has been noted (11, 58). A two-component regulatory system, RacR-RacS, that is responsible for alterations in expression of at least 11 genes in response to temperature changes has been identified. The ability of a *C. jejuni racR* mutant to colonize chickens was reduced compared to that of the parental isolate (11). These findings correlate with a previous study in which a *C. jejuni dnaJ* mutant was deficient in the ability to colonize the ceca of newly hatched Leghorn chickens (58). Brás et al. (11) proposed that the *C. jejuni dnaJ* gene may be regulated by the RacR-RacS system.

In summary, the internalization of *C. jejuni* into host cells is mediated by de novo-synthesized proteins. A subset of these newly synthesized proteins are secreted and translocated into the cytoplasm of host cells, where they may alter host cell signaling pathways. The adaptive response controlling the coordinated expression of genes that encode the entry-promoting proteins may involve a two-component regulatory system.

NONPROFESSIONAL PHAGOCYTIC CELL PARTICIPATION IN INTERNALIZATION

The degree to which a particular *C. jejuni* strain is internalized is cell line dependent. Even though *C. jejuni* is capable of binding to cells of human and nonhuman origin at approximately equal levels, it is internalized much more efficiently by cells of human origin (53). Consistent with the idea that host cell participation is required for *C. jejuni* internalization, host cell microvilli have been observed in association with *C. jejuni* (53). In addition, a significant reduction in *C. jejuni* entry is noted at 4°C (53). De Melo et al. (20) reported that the internalization of *C. jejuni* by HEp-2 cells was reduced in the presence of iodoacetate and dinitrophenol. Iodoacetate and dinitrophenol inhibit glycolysis and the Krebs cycle, respectively. The inhibitory effects of these two chemicals on internalization indicate that the uptake of *C. jejuni* is an energy-dependent process.

The specific roles of the individual host cell

cytoskeletal components that participate in *C. jejuni* uptake are not yet clear due to conflicting data of various inhibitors of internalization. De Melo et al. (20) reported that cytochalasin B, an inhibitor of actin polymerization, significantly reduced the internalization of *C. jejuni* into HEp-2 cells. Konkel et al. (56) reported a similar finding by using INT 407 cells and the microfilament inhibitor cytochalasin D. Actin-like microfilaments have been observed in association with *C. jejuni* bound to HEp-2 and INT 407 cells by transmission electron microscopy and immunofluorescence microscopy (20, 56). Dense intracellular networks of actin-like microfilaments have also been observed in cells of 3.5-month-old *Macaca mulatta* experimentally infected with *C. jejuni* (92). Oelschlaeger et al. (80) found that the uptake of *C. jejuni* 81–176 by INT 407 was reduced in the presence of microtubule inhibitors (e.g., colchicine and nocodazole) whereas the uptake of *C. jejuni* VC-84 was reduced by microfilament depolymerization. Konkel et al. (56) also noted a reduction in *C. jejuni* internalization in the presence of colchicine, but the effect was not dose dependent. Russell and Blake (91) reported that microfilament and microtubule inhibitors had no effect on the internalization of *C. jejuni* 81–176 into Caco-2 cells. Konkel et al. (56) and Oelschlaeger et al. (80) both observed a significant reduction in *C. jejuni* entry into INT 407 cells in the presence of monodansylcadaverine, an inhibitor of receptor cycling and coated-pit formation. In contrast, Russell and Blake (91) concluded that coated pits are not involved in entry, given that monodansylcadaverine and δ-strophantin had no effect on the numbers of *C. jejuni* internalized with Caco-2 cells. More recently, Wooldridge et al. (110) noted a significant reduction of *C. jejuni* internalization upon pretreatment of Caco-2 cells with the sterol-binding agent filipin III. Filipin III disrupts non-clathrin-coated plasma membrane invaginations called caveolae, from which several cell signaling molecules have been localized. Wooldridge and Ketley (109) hypothesize that *C. jejuni* binds to cell receptors that colocalize with ca-

veolae, inducing cell signaling and subsequent phagocytosis via a microfilament-dependent pathway.

While host cell participation is clearly required for *C. jejuni* uptake, elucidation of the precise roles of microfilaments and microtubules in *C. jejuni* uptake and intracellular trafficking will require additional research. A particular strain of *C. jejuni* may utilize both microfilaments and microtubules for uptake or may utilize only one of these. Some aspects of cytoskeletal involvement in internalization are depicted in Fig. 3. The differential use of these cytoskeletal elements may eventually be used to segregate *C. jejuni* strains into groups with specific intracellular niches and various pathologies.

SURVIVAL IN NONPROFESSIONAL AND PROFESSIONAL PHAGOCYTIC CELLS

Ultrastructural studies of *C. jejuni*-infected HEp-2 and INT 407 nonprofessional phagocytic cells have revealed organisms within membrane-bound vacuoles shortly after inoculation (20, 56). *Campylobacter*-like organisms have also been observed within membrane-bound vacuoles upon electron microscopy examination of biopsy specimens from experimentally infected chickens (107), hamsters (40), and *M. mulatta* (92). With regard to the ability of *C. jejuni* to survive within cultured cells, De Melo et al. (20) observed a sharp decline in bacterial viability in HEp-2 cells after 9 h of incubation. Coincident within the decline in the number of intracellular bacteria, morphological evidence of phagosome-lysosome fusion was observed as judged by the presence of granules within vacuoles containing electron-dense bacteria. Based on these observations, De Melo et al. (20) concluded that *C. jejuni* is unable to survive and multiply in the hostile environment of the phagolysosome. Konkel et al. (56) also noted a marked decline in the number of viable intracellular *C. jejuni* organisms when infected INT 407 cell cultures were initially incubated with 250 μg of gentamicin per ml for 3 h to kill the extracellular bacteria and then with 50 μg of gentamicin per ml for the remainder of the assay. Removal of the antibiotic after the initial 3-h treatment period, however, resulted in a marked increase in the number of intracellular *C. jejuni* organisms over time as judged by the gentamicin protection assay. Immunofluorescence microscopy examination of these infected cells revealed *C. jejuni* within membrane-bound vacuoles clustered around the nucleus after 24 to 48 h of incubation. Prolonged infection of the cultured cells with *C. jejuni* ultimately led to deterioration of the cell monolayers, with bacteria being found in the cytoplasm of the damaged cells. While the investigators stated that it was unlikely that the increase in the number of intracellular *C. jejuni* organisms was exclusively due to intracellular replication, the data suggested that *C. jejuni* possesses the ability to survive and replicate with cultured epithelial cells. These data also suggested that gentamicin, an aminoglycosidic antibiotic that is unable to penetrate host cell membranes, may be slowly pinocytosed by nonprofessional phagocytic cells and have a bactericidal effect on intracellular organisms. *C. jejuni* has also been observed in the cytoplasm of columnar epithelial cells of infected *M. mulatta* (92). Russell et al. (92) also noted the presence of damaged cells, which were exfoliated into the lumen, that exhibited premature signs of apoptosis (see below). Collectively, the data suggest that *C. jejuni* is able to survive intracellularly and to cause death of nonprofessional phagocytic host cells.

Most pathogenic bacteria avoid the hostile environment of the phagolysosome and survive intracellularly by inhibiting endosomal acidification and/or preventing lysosome-phagosome fusion (27). Chemical agents that prevent endosomal acidification (e.g., ammonium chloride, methylamine, and monensin) have little to no effect on the internalization and short-term intracellular survival of *C. jejuni* (56, 80). Although evidence of extensive phagosome-lysosome fusion has been observed in cells infected with *C. jejuni,* it is likely that a proportion of infecting bacteria are able to avoid the inhospitable environment of the phagolyso-

some. At this point, however, additional research is required to characterize the trafficking and distinct intracellular niche where *C. jejuni* resides.

The ability of *C. jejuni* to survive for prolonged periods in both nonprofessional (56) and professional (48) phagocytic cells suggests that these bacteria synthesize proteins that facilitate their intracellular survival. Using a PCR-based approach coupled with Southern hybridization experiments, Pesci et al. (85) cloned the superoxide dismutase gene (*sodB*) from *C. jejuni*. The *sodB* gene encodes an enzyme that catalyzes the breakdown of superoxide radicals to hydrogen peroxide and dioxygen. A 12-fold reduction in the number of intracellular viable bacteria was noted upon infection of INT 407 cells with a *C. jejuni sodB* null mutant compared to that of the parental isolate. This finding suggests that SodB plays a role in the survival of *C. jejuni* within nonprofessional phagocytic cells.

Grant and Park (33) reported the cloning of the *katA* gene from *C. jejuni* by functional complementation of a catalase-deficient mutant of *E. coli*. Catalase catalyzes the degradation of hydrogen peroxide (H_2O_2) to H_2O and O_2 and, in other systems, has been shown to protect intracellular bacteria from the oxidative burst of inflammatory cells. Grant and Park (33) found that a *C. coli kat* null mutant was more sensitive to killing by H_2O_2 than was the isogenic parental strain as determined by in vitro H_2O_2 sensitivity assays. Day and Joens (19a) have also found that a *katA* mutant of *C. jejuni* is more sensitive to H_2O_2 in vitro than is the isogenic parent strain. Complementation studies of the mutant strain with a plasmid carrying the wild-type *katA* gene demonstrated that the sensitivity of the mutant strain to H_2O_2 was due to the changes in catalase expression, not to polar effects on adjacent gene expression.

Catalase appears to play an active role in promoting the survival of *C. jejuni* in professional but not in nonprofessional phagocytic cells. A significant decrease was noted in the number of viable bacteria recovered from macrophages 24 h postinfection for the *C. je-*

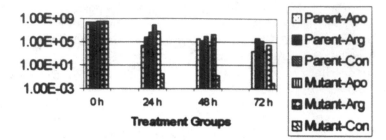

FIGURE 4 Expression of the *katA* gene encoding catalase promotes *C. jejuni* survival in macrophages. J774A.1 macrophages were infected with *C. jejuni* M129N (parent) and JD900 (*katA* null mutant), and the numbers of viable bacteria were determined over a 72-h period. In some cultures, apocynin (250 μM per well) was included to inhibit the respiratory burst, and in other cultures N^G-L-monomethyl arginine (250 μM per well) was included to inhibit nitric oxide production. Survival of *C. jejuni* was determined by using viable plate counts. Abbreviations: Apo, apocynin; Arg, N^G-L-monomethyl arginine; Con, control (untreated).

juni katA null mutant compared to the parental isolate. Furthermore, no significant differences were observed in the numbers of viable bacteria for the isogenic parental strain and the *katA* complemented mutant strain in macrophages over a 24-h period. Chemical agents that inhibit the oxidative burst (apocynin) or nitric oxide production (N^G-L-monomethyl arginine) in professional phagocytes significantly inhibit the phagolysosome from killing the internalized *C. jejuni katA* mutant, indicating that the *katA* gene is responsible for protecting the bacteria against radicals produced by the phagocyte (Fig. 4). Although the role of catalase production in infection and disease has not been examined, these in vitro studies suggest that *C. jejuni* synthesizes products that counteract host defense mechanisms and promote the intracellular survival of the bacterium.

Investigators have found that culturing *C. jejuni* in conditioned medium or exposing *C. jejuni* to epithelial cells results in de novo protein synthesis (52, 60). Galindo et al. (30) identified three de novo–synthesized outer membrane proteins, with masses of 80, 76, and 74 kDa, upon coculturing *C. jejuni* with epithelial cells. With antisera generated against these de novo-induced proteins, a seropositive clone was identified by screening a *Sau*3A I-constructed cosmid library of *C. jejuni* chromosomal DNA. This clone contained a 35-kb DNA insert. Analysis of the sequenced DNA revealed three genes with homology to *fhuA*, *fhuB*, and *fhuD* of *E. coli*. In *E. coli*, these genes are located within an operon and their products are involved in iron acquisition. Expression of the *C. jejuni fhuA* gene in *E. coli* revealed a novel protein with a mass of 80 kDa. Southern hybridization of chromosomal DNA from *C. jejuni* strains revealed a band in 60% of the samples probed with the *C. jejuni fhuA* gene. In addition, all of the DNA sequenced from the 35-kb insert had a G + C content of 70% which is foreign to the 30% G + C content of the *C. jejuni* genome. These sequence data indicate that the iron-binding operon (*fhu*) may be part of a pathogenicity island. Pathogenicity islands are blocks of foreign genes, which generally differ in their moles percent of G + C from the remainder of the chromosome, that confer a variety of virulence traits upon host bacteria (65). Regulation studies demonstrated that the presence of iron diminished the expression of the 80-kDa protein (Fig. 5), indicating that iron is an important regulatory component in the expression of *fhuA*. The role of these proteins in *C. jejuni* intracellular survival has yet to be determined.

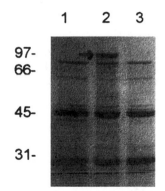

FIGURE 5 Iron depletion alters *C. jejuni* outer membrane protein profiles. *C. jejuni* outer membrane protein extracts (Sarkosyl-insoluble fractions) were separated in sodium dodecyl sulfate–12.5% polyacrylamide gels and stained with Coomassie brilliant blue R-250. Lanes: 1, *C. jejuni* incubated in iron-rich medium; 2, *C. jejuni* incubated in iron-depleted medium; 3, *C. jejuni* incubated in iron-depleted medium containing 100 μM ferric citrate. The position of FhuA from *C. jejuni* is indicated (arrow).

As noted above, expression of virulence genes in *C. jejuni* probably involves global gene regulation by two-component regulatory systems. By analogy to other pathogenic bacteria, virulence gene expression in *C. jejuni* may be affected by a variety of factors including osmolarity, pH, ion concentration, iron levels, growth phase, population density, and temperature. To date, altered virulence gene expression in *C. jejuni* cultured in medium supplemented with bile salts (22) and fetal bovine serum and in *C. jejuni* cultured with host cells in serum-free medium has been noted (90). Altered gene expression in *C. jejuni* in response to changes in temperature has also been noted (11, 58). Pathogens have maintained various environmental sensing mechanisms to conserve energy by expressing only the appropriate subset of genes in a suitable environment.

TRANSLOCATION ACROSS CELL BARRIERS

Many pathogenic bacteria have the ability to translocate, or pass across, epithelial- or endothelial-cell barriers. Such translocation is considered an important virulence attribute since it allows an organism access to underlying tissues and may permit the organism to disseminate throughout the host. Certain cell lines (e.g., Caco-2 and MDCK) form polarized cell monolayers in vitro. Polarized cells are characterized by defined apical and basolateral cell surfaces separated by tight junctions. These cell monolayers exhibit a measurable transepithelial electrical resistance, and disruption of the tight junctions between cells results in a decrease in this resistance. Investigators have used these polarized cells to assess whether bacteria are capable of translocating across epithelial cell barriers in vitro.

C. jejuni is capable of translocating across polarized Caco-2 cell monolayers (23, 61). *C. jejuni* was detected in the basolateral well 15 min after being added to the apical surface of polarized Caco-2 cell monolayers (61). This translocation continued for 6 h without a decrease in the transepithelial cell electrical resistance. This finding suggests that *C. jejuni* translocation is not dependent on degeneration of the cell monolayer or the irreversible disruption of cellular tight junctions. Everest et al. (23) noted a correlation between translocation and the clinical symptoms of *C. jejuni*-infected individuals. Translocation across polarized Caco-2 cells was observed with 86% of the *C. jejuni* strains isolated from individuals with colitis, in contrast to 48% for strains isolated from individuals with noninflammatory disease. The most convincing evidence that *C. jejuni* can translocate across a cell barrier via an endocytic pathway is that the translocation of *C. jejuni* is reduced at 20°C (61). Temperatures of 18 to 22°C preferentially inhibit eukaryotic endocytic and phagocytic processes (97). Several observations, however, indicate that *C. jejuni* can translocate across a cell monolayer by migrating between cells. Everest et al. (23) found that six noninvasive *C. jejuni* isolates, determined to be noninvasive for HeLa and Caco-2 cells by gentamicin protection assays, translocated across the polarized cell monolayers. Bacteria have also been observed in and between cells during electron microscopy examination of *C. jejuni*-infected polarized cell monolayers (61).

Collectively, these findings suggest that *C. jejuni* is capable of translocating across cell monolayers by an intracellular and paracellular route.

APOPTOSIS INDUCTION

Biopsy specimens from the intestines of *C. jejuni*-infected individuals show histopathological hallmarks of cell damage. However, the pathogenic mechanism(s) inducing this damage is unclear. The damage to intestinal epithelia could be the result of bacterial action during binding and invasion of the intestinal epithelia and/or the result of the host immune response.

Recent investigations have demonstrated that many pathogens induce cell death after target cell invasion. Cells may die by modes generally separated into two categories, necrosis and apoptosis. Cells undergoing necrosis characteristically swell until the membrane ruptures, spewing the cellular components into the interstitial space to initiate inflammation. Necrotic cell death can result from contact with toxic substances, mechanical shearing, or viral lysis. Examples of diverse pathogens that induce host cell necrosis by secretion of extracellular toxins abound (87). Some bacterial toxins can induce the host cell release of apoptosis-inducing cytokines such as tumor necrosis factor (e.g., *Pseudomonas aeruginosa* exotoxin A [94]). Recent investigations have also demonstrated apoptosis induction by diverse species of invasive bacteria. In contrast to necrosis, apoptosis is an active process requiring host cell de novo protein synthesis. Apoptosis is characterized by cellular condensation, degradation of nucleic acids, and fragmentation of the cell into apoptotic bodies with membrane integrity. Apoptotic bodies are readily phagocytized by nearby tissue macrophages, with limited recruitment of cells from the circulatory system.

Some invasive enteric bacteria induce apoptosis in epithelial cells. Kim et al. (49) noted induction of apoptosis of intestinal epithelial cells by enteroinvasive *E. coli*. Human colonic epithelial cells (e.g., T84, HT29, and Caco-2) release proinflammatory cytokines after infection with invasive, but not noninvasive, enteric bacteria (43). These data indicate that both bacterial invasion and subsequent cytokine release may play important roles in damaging the intestinal epithelia. Infection of gastric epithelial cells with enteric bacteria, including *C. jejuni*, results in cytokine release (96). It is presently unclear whether cytokines can directly cause epithelial-cell damage or whether damage is mediated indirectly by cytokine-activated inflammatory cells.

Bacterial pathogens have been postulated to cause mucosal damage by different mechanisms (26). Invasion of host cell macrophages by pathogenic enteric bacteria including *Yersinia, Salmonella,* and *Shigella* induce apoptosis in a dose-dependent and time-dependent manner (16, 74, 116). Optimal induction of host cell apoptosis after in vitro infection by *Salmonella* requires host cell contact, initiating host cell "ruffling" or cytoskeletal rearrangement, and active production and delivery of type III secretory proteins (19). *Shigella* induces apoptosis of macrophages but not intestinal epithelial cells (116). In examining *Shigella* infection of macrophages, Zychlinsky et al. (116) identified invasion plasmid antigen B (IpaB) as the factor essential for apoptosis induction. Intracellular injection of recombinant IpaB into macrophages activates interleukin-converting enzyme (also known as caspase 1), initiating the proteolytic cascade leading to apoptosis (17, 37). In addition to initiating apoptosis, the ability of IpaB to activate interleukin-converting enzyme may further enable the release of active IL-1 to promote inflammation and recruit macrophages to the site of infection (117).

Zhu et al. (113) cultured outer membrane protein extracts from *C. jejuni* or *E. coli* with chicken lymphoid tumor lines, peripheral blood lymphocytes, and purified splenic lymphocytes. Analyses of the cocultured cells indicated that extracts from *C. jejuni* induced apoptosis more often than did extracts from *E. coli* or other control preparations. The investigators postulated that the induction of lymphocyte apoptosis may enable *C. jejuni* to evade the immune response in chickens.

Epithelial Damage

Cytometric analyses of *C. jejuni*-infected INT 407 cells indicated that apoptosis induction was similar to that in mock-infected cells, regardless of the time and dose (results not shown). In contrast, parallel studies with *S. typhimurium* or *Y. enterocolitica*-infected INT 407 cells showed significant apoptosis induction. Other factors, however, may be required for the induction of epithelial-cell apoptosis by *C. jejuni* in vitro, since Russell et al. (92) noted signs of epithelial-cell apoptosis in the intestines of *C. jejuni*-infected macaques.

Apoptosis of Macrophages

Analysis of apoptosis induction in *C. jejuni*-infected J774A.1 cells revealed apoptosis levels above those in sham-infected cells, albeit lower than those in cells infected by other bacteria under similar conditions (Table 1). One possible explanation for this finding is that *C. jejuni* may not bind to murine cells to the same extent

as it binds human macrophages, minimizing invasion and limiting the induction of apoptosis to levels below those induced by other enteric bacteria. Alternatively, *C. jejuni* may bind avidly to host cell receptors but ineffectively signal the J774A.1 cells, limiting the induction of apoptosis.

C. jejuni infection of phorbol myristate acetate-stimulated human pro-myeloid THP-1 cells leads to a combination of necrosis and apoptosis. Apoptosis induction of THP-1 cells by *C. jejuni* appears to be dependent on secretion of CiaB. At multiplicity of infection of 300 for 3 h, infected THP-1 cells show increased annexin V binding and loss of membrane integrity, indicative of apoptosis and necrosis, respectively (summarized in Table 1). Parallel studies involving infection of THP-1 cells with a *C. jejuni*, CiaB-mutant resulted in no apoptosis or necrosis induction (Table 1). Future studies will focus on the mechanism of apoptosis induction in human macrophages

TABLE 1 Analysis of apoptosis induction by *C. jejuni*[a]

Organism and relevant phenotype	Induction of apoptosis or necrosis in:[b]							
	Macrophages				T cells (human Jurkat cells)			
	Murine J774A.1 (t = 3 h)		Human PMA-THP-1 (t = 3 h)		t = 3 h		t = 36 h	
	A	N	A	N	A	N	A	N
S. typhimurium SL1344 (wild type)	+ + +	±	+ + +	+	−	−	ND	ND
S. typhimurium EE638 (SipC⁻)	+	−	+	+	−	−	ND	ND
Y. enterocolitica 8081v (wild type)	+ +	−	+	−	ND	ND	ND	ND
Y. enterocolitica JP273v (InvA⁻)	−	−	−	−	ND	ND	ND	ND
C. jejuni F38011 (wild type)	±	−	+	−	−	−	+ +	−
C. jejuni (CiaB⁻)	−	−	−	−	−	−	+	−

[a] Macrophages and T-cell lines were cocultured with the indicated bacterial strains at a multiplicity of infection of 300 for 3 or 36 h. The cells were stained with annexin V–fluorescein isothiocyanate and propidium iodide for flow cytometric assessment of apoptosis and necrosis, respectively (62).

[b] Qualitative levels above those for sham-infected control cells are shown. Symbols: each +, 10% above control cells; ±, 2 to 5% above control cells; −, <2% above control cells; ND, not determined; A, apoptosis; N, necrosis.

and the potential role of macrophage apoptosis in human *C. jejuni* infection.

Induction of T-Cell Apoptosis

To determine if *C. jejuni* could induce apoptosis or necrosis of mouse peripheral blood lymphocytes, we cocultured *C. jejuni* with BALB/c splenocytes. *C. jejuni* has previously been reported to colonize mice (1). It did not readily infect or alter subpopulations of cultured mouse lymphocytes (results not shown). As noted above, species or cell preference, altered signaling, or lack of additional factors may account for this observation (53).

Due to the apparent species preference of *C. jejuni* for human cells, we further investigated its ability to induce apoptosis in human T cells by using the Jurkat leukemia cell line. A time course experiment indicated a loss in Jurkat cell viability between 12 and 24 h after infection, as defined by a size shift in cytometric scatter patterns (Fig. 6 and data not shown). Annexin V staining of the exposed phosphatidylserine residues confirmed that the Jurkat cells with decreased size were undergoing apoptosis and not necrosis (72). Apoptosis induction in *C. jejuni*-infected Jurkat cells was observed 24 h postinfection for the parental F38011 strain. However, apoptosis was delayed in the *C. jejuni* F38011 isogenic CiaB-mutant (Fig. 6), suggesting that optimal induction of human T-cell apoptosis by *Campylobacter* organisms requires the putative type III-secreted proteins.

Apoptosis induction in Jurkat cells may be induced by ligation of cell surface receptors, decreased survival signals, transmembrane delivery of proteolytic enzymes, induced stress signals, or alteration of mitochondrial oxidation states (35, 66). These signals lead to proteolytic activation of the caspase cascades leading to degradation of DNA, condensation of chromatin, and cellular fragmentation. IpaB, the CiaB homolog from *Shigella,* specifically binds and activates caspase 1 to initiate apoptosis directly, without involving caspases 2, 3, or 11 (37). CiaB could also target Caspase-1. Apoptosis can be caused by cell cycle arrest. CiaB may modulate cell cycle events in Jurkat cells, inducing apoptosis. Interestingly, *C. jejuni* cytolethal distending toxin stops the cell cycle of HeLa and Caco-2 cells (108). It is

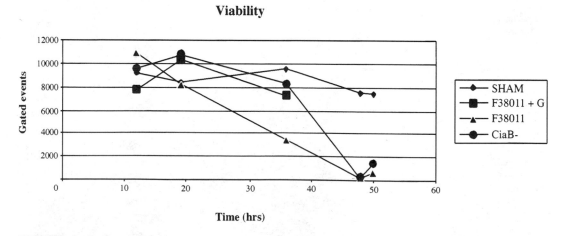

Viability

FIGURE 6 Reduced viability of *C. jejuni*-infected Jurkat cells. Jurkat cells, a human T-cell leukemia cell line, were cocultured with wild-type *C. jejuni* F38011, the isogenic CiaB⁻ mutant, or gentamicin-killed F38011 (F38011 + G) at multiplicity of infection of 100. Control cells (SHAM) were cultured in the absence of bacteria. At the time intervals noted, cells were harvested and 20,000 events were analyzed by flow cytometry. The number of events corresponding to the size and scatter properties of viable cells plotted against time of infection is shown. This figure is a composite of the results of several experiments (*n* = 3).

doubtful that CiaB causes activation-induced cell death during mitosis because the CiaB null mutant, which ineffectively induces apoptosis, possesses LPS and other components responsible for mitogenic stimulation of lymphocytes. Further examination of the mechanism of apoptosis induction in *C. jejuni*-infected T cells will further define the pathways and signals involved in this process.

CONCLUDING REMARKS

The last decade has proved to be very exciting for *Campylobacter* research with the identification of a number of *C. jejuni* virulence determinants. These virulence determinants include host cell binding, entry, and survival proteins. Some *C. jejuni* proteins also alter host cell signal transduction pathways and participate in the induction of host cell apoptosis. Advances in the areas of *C. jejuni* molecular genetics and in vivo models are enabling the analysis of the relevant functional roles of these virulence determinants. These analyses are continuing to provide new insights into the mechanism(s) of *C. jejuni*-mediated enteritis. Newfound insight into these mechanisms will lead to the development of strategies for prevention and intervention therapies for *Campylobacter*-mediated enteritis and sequelae.

ACKNOWLEDGMENTS

We thank W. Cieplak, Jr., and C. Grant for critically reviewing the manuscript. We also thank the members of our laboratories for reading the manuscript and for helpful comments. Finally, we thank Sean Gray for assistance in the preparation of figures.

MEK is supported by a grant from the NIH (DK50567-01A1). LAJ is supported by a grant from the USDA National Research Initiative Competitive Grants Program (USDA/NRICGP, grant 9802745).

REFERENCES

1. **Abimiku, A. G., and J. M. Dolby.** 1988. Cross-protection of infant mice against intestinal colonisation by *Campylobacter jejuni*: importance of heat-labile serotyping (Lior) antigens. *J. Med. Microbiol.* **26:**265–268.
2. **Angulo, F. J., and D. L. Swerdlow.** 1995. Bacterial enteric infections in persons infected with human immunodeficiency virus. *Clin. Infect. Dis.* **21**(Suppl 1):S84–S93.
3. **Babakhani, F. K., G. A. Bradley, and L. A. Joens.** 1993. Newborn piglet model for campylobacteriosis. *Infect. Immun.* **61:**3466–3475.
4. **Babakhani, F. K., and L. A. Joens.** 1993. Primary swine intestinal cells as a model for studying *Campylobacter jejuni* invasiveness. *Infect. Immun.* **61:**2723–2726.
5. **Berberian, L. S., Y. Valles-Ayoub, L. K. Gordon, S. R. Targan, and J. Braun.** 1994. Expression of a novel autoantibody defined by the VH3-15 gene in inflammatory bowel disease and *Campylobacter jejuni* enterocolitis. *J. Immunol.* **153:**3756–3763.
6. **Bhadra, R. K., P. Dutta, S. K. Bhattacharya, S. K. Dutta, S. C. Pal, and G. B. Nair.** 1992. *Campylobacter* species as a cause of diarrhoea in children in Calcutta. *J. Infect.* **24:**55–62.
7. **Black, R. E., M. M. Levine, M. L. Clements, T. P. Hughes, and M. J. Blaser.** 1988. Experimental *Campylobacter jejuni* infection in humans. *J. Infect. Dis.* **157:**472–479.
8. **Blaser, M. J., D. N. Taylor, and R. A. Feldman.** 1984. Epidemiology of Campylobacter infections, p. 143–161. *In* J. P. Butzler (ed.), *Campylobacter Infection in Man and Animals*. CRC Press, Inc., Boca Raton, Fla.
9. **Bradley, D. E., A. N. Anderson, and M. B. Perry.** 1991. Differences between the LPS cores in adherent and non-adherent strains of enteropathogenic *Escherichia coli* O119. *FEMS Microbiol. Lett.* **64:**13–17.
10. **Brandtzaeg, P., D. E. Nilssen, T. O. Rognum, and P. S. Thrane.** 1991. Ontogeny of the mucosal immune system and IgA deficiency. *Gastroenterol. Clin. North Am.* **20:**397–439.
11. **Brás, A. M., S. Chatterjee, B. W. Wren, D. G. Newell, and J. M. Ketley.** 1999. A novel *Campylobacter jejuni* two-component regulatory system important for temperature-dependent growth and colonization. *J. Bacteriol.* **181:**3298–3302.
12. **Buckley, R. H.** 1999. Primary immunodeficiencies, p. 1432–1433. *In* W. E. Paul (ed.), *Fundamental Immunology*. 4th ed. Lippincott-Raven, Philadelphia, Pa.
13. **Burucoa, C., C. Frémaux, Z. Pei, M. Tummuru, M. J. Blaser, Y. Cenatiempo, and J. L. Fauchère.** 1995. Nucleotide sequence and characterization of *peb4A* encoding an antigenic protein in *Campylobacter jejuni*. *Res. Microbiol.* **146:**467–476.
14. **Caldwell, M. B., R. I. Walker, S. D. Stewart, and J. E. Rogers.** 1983. Simple adult rabbit model for *Campylobacter jejuni* enteritis. *Infect. Immun.* **42:**1176–1182.
15. **Chen, J. C., P. Bavoil, and V. L. Clark.** 1991. Enhancement of the invasive ability of *Neisseria*

gonorrhoeae by contact with HecIB, an adenocarcinoma endometrial cell line. *Mol. Microbiol.* **5:** 1531–1538.

16. **Chen, L. M., K. Kaniga, and J. E. Galán.** 1996. *Salmonella* spp. are cytotoxic for cultured macrophages. *Mol. Microbiol.* **21:**1101–1115.

17. **Chen, Y., M. R. Smith, K. Thirumalai, and A. Zychlinsky.** 1996. A bacterial invasin induces macrophage apoptosis by binding directly to ICE. *EMBO J.* **15:**3853–3860.

18. **Clark, J. A., P. A. Callicoat, N. A. Brenner, C. A. Bradley, and D. M. Smith, Jr.** 1983. Selective IgA deficiency in blood donors. *Am. J. Clin. Pathol.* **80:**210–213.

19. **Collazo, C. M., and J. E. Galán.** 1997. The invasion-associated type III system of *Salmonella typhimurium* directs the translocation of Sip proteins into the host cell. *Mol. Microbiol.* **24:** 747–756.

19a. **Day, W. A., and L. A. Joens.** Unpublished data.

20. **De Melo, M. A., G. Gabbiani, and J.-C. Pechère.** 1989. Cellular events and intracellular survival of *Campylobacter jejuni* during infection of HEp-2 cells. *Infect. Immun.* **57:**2214–2222.

21. **De Melo, M. A., and J.-C. Pechère.** 1990. Identification of *Campylobacter jejuni* surface proteins that bind to eucaryotic cells in vitro. *Infect. Immun.* **58:**1749–1756.

22. **Doig, P., R. Yao, D. H. Burr, P. Guerry, and T. J. Trust.** 1996. An environmentally regulated pilus-like appendage involved in *Campylobacter* pathogenesis. *Mol. Microbiol.* **20:**885–894.

23. **Everest, P. H., H. Goossens, J. P. Butzler, D. Lloyd, S. Knutton, J. M. Ketley, and P. H. Williams.** 1992. Differentiated Caco-2 cells as a model for enteric invasion by *Campylobacter jejuni* and *C. coli. J. Med. Microbiol.* **37:**319–325.

23a. **Fauchère, J.-L., M. Kervella, A. Rosenau, K. Mohanna, and M. Véron.** 1989. Adhesion to Hela cells of *Campylobacter jejuni* and *C. coli* from human feces. *Res. Microbiol.* **140:**379–392.

24. **Fauchère, J.-L., A. Rosenau, M. Veron, E. N. Moyen, S. Richard, and A. Pfister.** 1986. Association with HeLa cells of *Campylobacter jejuni* and *Campylobacter coli* isolated from human feces. *Infect. Immun.* **54:**283–287.

25. **Field, L. H., V. L. Headley, J. L. Underwood, S. M. Payne, and L. J. Berry.** 1986. The chicken embryo as a model for campylobacter invasion: comparative virulence of human isolates of *Campylobacter jejuni* and *Campylobacter coli. Infect. Immun.* **54:**118–125.

26. **Finlay, B. B., and P. Cossart.** 1997. Exploitation of mammalian host cell functions by bacterial pathogens. *Science* **276:**718–725.

27. **Finlay, B. B., and S. Falkow.** 1989. Common themes in microbial pathogenicity. *Microbiol. Rev.* **53:**210–230.

28. **Finlay, B. B., F. Heffron, and S. Falkow.** 1989. Epithelial cell surfaces induce *Salmonella* proteins required for bacterial adherence and invasion. *Science* **243:**940–943.

29. **Fry, B. N., V. Korolik, J. A. ten Brinke, M. T. T. Pennings, R. Zalm, B. J. J. Teunis, P. J. Coloe, and B. A. M. van der Zeijst.** 1998. The lipopolysaccharide biosynthetic locus of *Campylobacter jejuni* 81116. *Microbiology* **144:** 2049–2061.

30. **Galindo, M., W. A. Day, and L. A. Joens.** Cloning and characterization of a Campylobacter jejuni iron-uptake island acquired by horizontal gene transfer. Submitted for publication.

31. **Gerba, C. P., J. B. Rose, and C. N. Haas.** 1996. Sensitive populations: who is at the greatest risk? *Int. J. Food Microbiol.* **30:**113–123.

32. **Grant, C. C. R., M. E. Konkel, W. Cieplak, Jr., and L. S. Tompkins.** 1993. Role of flagella in adherence, internalization, and translocation of *Campylobacter jejuni* in nonpolarized and polarized epithelial cell cultures. *Infect. Immun.* **61:** 1764–1771.

33. **Grant, K. A., and S. F. Park.** 1995. Molecular characterization of *katA* from *Campylobacter jejuni* and generation of a catalase-deficient mutant of *Campylobacter coli* by interspecific allelic exchange. *Microbiology* **141:**1369–1376.

34. **Hale, T. L., and P. F. Bonventre.** 1979. *Shigella* infection of Henle intestinal epithelial cells: role of the bacterium. *Infect. Immun.* **24:** 879–886.

35. **Hampton, M. B., B. Fadeel, and S. Orrenius.** 1998. Redox regulation of the caspases during apoptosis. *Ann. N. Y. Acad. Sci.* **854:** 328–335.

36. **Hickey, T. E., S. Baqar, A. K. Bourgeois, C. P. Ewing, and P. Guerry.** 1999. *Campylobacter jejuni*-stimulated secretion of interleukin-8 by INT407 cells. *Infect. Immun.* **67:**88–93.

37. **Hilbi, H., J. E. Moss, D. Hersh, Y. Chen, J. Arondel, S. Banerjee, R. A. Flavell, J. Yuan, P. J. Sansonetti, and A. Zychlinsky.** 1998. *Shigella*-induced apoptosis is dependent on caspase-1 which binds to IpaB. *J. Biol. Chem.* **273:** 32895–32900.

38. **Hodgson, A. E., B. W. McBride, M. J. Hudson, G. Hall, and S. A. Leach.** 1998. Experimental campylobacter infection and diarrhea in immunodeficient mice. *J. Med. Microbiol.* **47:** 799–809.

39. **Hueck, C. J.** 1998. Type III protein secretion systems in bacterial pathogens of animals and plants. *Microbiol. Mol. Biol. Rev.* **62:**379–433.

40. **Humphrey, C. D., D. M. Montag, and F.**

E. Pittman. 1985. Experimental infection of hamsters with *Campylobacter jejuni. J. Infect. Dis.* **151:**485–493.

41. **Jenkin, G. A., and W. Tee.** 1998. *Campylobacter upsaliensis*-associated diarrhea in human immunodeficiency virus-infected patients. *Clin. Infect. Dis.* **27:**816–821.

42. **Jones, S. L., F. P. Lindberg, and E. J. Brown.** 1999. Phagocytosis, p. 1011–1015. *In* W. E. Paul (ed.), *Fundamental Immunology,* 4th ed. Lippincott-Raven, Philadelphia, Pa.

43. **Jung, H. C., L. Eckmann, S. K. Yang, A. Panja, J. Fierer, E. Morzycka-Wroblewska, and M. F. Kagnoff.** 1995. A distinct array of proinflammatory cytokines is expressed in human colon epithelial cells in response to bacterial invasion. *J. Clin. Investig.* **95:**55–65.

44. **Kaniga, K., S. Tucker, D. Trollinger, and J. E. Galán.** 1995. Homologs of the *Shigella* IpaB and IpaC invasins are required for *Salmonella typhimurium* entry into cultured epithelial cells. *J. Bacteriol.* **177:**3965–3971.

45. **Keat, A., and I. Rowe.** 1991. Reiter's syndrome and associated arthritides. *Rheum. Dis. Clin. North Am.* **17:**25–42.

46. **Kervella, M., J.-M. Pagès, Z. Pei, G. Grollier, M. J. Blaser, and J.-L. Fauchère.** 1993. Isolation and characterization of two *Campylobacter* glycine-extracted proteins that bind to HeLa cell membranes. *Infect. Immun.* **61:**3440–3448.

47. **Ketley, J. M.** 1997. Pathogenesis of enteric infection by *Campylobacter. Microbiology* **143:**5–21.

48. **Kiehlbauch, J. A., R. A. Albach, L. L. Baum, and K.-P. Chang.** 1985. Phagocytosis of *Campylobacter jejuni* and its intracellular survival in mononuclear phagocytes. *Infect. Immun.* **48:**446–451.

49. **Kim, J. M., L. Eckmann, T. C. Savidge, D. C. Lowe, T. Witthöft, and M. F. Kagnoff.** 1998. Apoptosis of human intestinal epithelial cells after bacterial invasion. *J. Clin. Investig.* **102:**1815–1823.

50. **Klena, J. D., S. A. Gray, and M. E. Konkel.** 1998. Cloning, sequencing, and characterization of the lipopolysaccharide biosynthetic enzyme heptosyltransferase I gene (*waaC*) from *Campylobacter jejuni* and *Campylobacter coli. Gene* **222:**177–185.

51. **Konkel, M. E., F. Babakhani, and L. A. Joens.** 1990. Invasion-related antigens of *Campylobacter jejuni. J. Infect. Dis.* **162:**888–895.

52. **Konkel, M. E., and W. Cieplak, Jr.** 1992. Altered synthetic response of *Campylobacter jejuni* to cocultivation with human epithelial cells is associated with enhanced internalization. *Infect. Immun.* **60:**4945–4949.

53. **Konkel, M. E., M. D. Corwin, L. A. Joens, and W. Cieplak, Jr.** 1992. Factors that influence the interaction of *Campylobacter jejuni* with cultured mammalian cells. *J. Med. Microbiol.* **37:**30–37.

54. **Konkel, M. E., S. G. Garvis, S. L. Tipton, D. E. Anderson, Jr., and W. Cieplak, Jr.** 1997. Identification and molecular cloning of a gene encoding a fibronectin-binding protein (CadF) from *Campylobacter jejuni. Mol. Microbiol.* **24:**953–963.

55. **Konkel, M. E., S. A. Gray. B. J. Kim, S. G. Garvis, and J. Yoon.** 1999. Identification of the enteropathogens *Campylobacter jejuni* and *Campylobacter coli* based on the *cadF* virulence gene and its product. *J. Clin. Microbiol.* **37:**510–517.

56. **Konkel, M. E., S. F. Hayes, L. A. Joens, and W. Cieplak, Jr.** 1992. Characteristics of the internalization and intracellular survival of *Campylobacter jejuni* in human epithelial cell cultures. *Microb. Pathog.* **13:**357–370.

57. **Konkel, M. E., and L. A. Joens.** 1989. Adhesion to and invasion of HEp-2 cells by *Campylobacter* spp. *Infect. Immun.* **57:**2984–2990.

58. **Konkel, M. E., B. J. Kim, J. D. Klena, C. R. Young, and R. Ziprin.** 1998. Characterization of the thermal stress response of *Campylobacter jejuni. Infect. Immun.* **66:**3666–3672.

59. **Konkel, M. E., B. J. Kim, V. Rivera-Amill, and S. G. Garvis.** 1999. Bacterial secreted proteins are required for the internalization of *Campylobacter jejuni* into cultured mammalian cells. *Mol. Microbiol.* **32:**691–702.

60. **Konkel, M. E., D. J. Mead, and W. Cieplak, Jr.** 1993. Kinetic and antigenic characterization of altered protein synthesis by *Campylobacter jejuni* during cultivation with human epithelial cells. *J. Infect. Dis.* **168:**948–954.

61. **Konkel, M. E., D. J. Mead, S. F. Hayes, and W. Cieplak, Jr.** 1992. Translocation of *Campylobacter jejuni* across human polarized epithelial cell monolayer cultures. *J. Infect. Dis.* **166:**308–315.

62. **Koopman, G., C. P. Reutelingsperger, G. A. Kuijten, R. M. Keehnen, S. T. Pals, and M. H. van Oers.** 1994. Annexin V for flow cytometric detection of phosphatidylserine expression on B cells undergoing apoptosis. *Blood* **84:**1415–1420.

63. **Kosunen, T. U., O. Kauranen, J. Martio, T. Pitkanen, A. Ponka, L. Hortling, S. Aittoniemi, O. Mutru, O. Penttila, and S. Koskimies.** 1980. Reactive arthritis after *Campylobacter jejuni* enteritis in patients with HLA-B27. *Lancet* **i:**1312–1313.

64. **Kuroki, S., T. Saida, M. Nukina, T. Haruta,**

M. Yoshioka, Y. Kobayashi, and H. Nakanishi. 1993. *Campylobacter jejuni* strains from patients with Guillian-Barré syndrome belong mostly to Penner serogroup 19 and contain beta-N-acetylglucosamine residues. *Ann. Neurol.* **33:** 243–247.

65. Lee, C. A. 1996. Pathogenicity islands and the evolution of bacterial pathogens. *Infect. Agents Dis.* **5:**1–7.

66. Lemasters, J. J., A. L. Nieminen, T. Qian, L. C. Trost, S. P. Elmore, Y. Nishimura, R. A. Crowe, W. E. Cascio, C. A. Bradham, D. A. Brenner, and B. Herman. 1998. The mitochondrial permeability transition in cell death: a common mechanism in necrosis, apoptosis and autophagy. *Biochim. Biophys. Acta* **1366:**177–196.

67. Liebler, J. M., S. L. Kunkel, M. D. Burdick, T. J. Standford, M. W. Rolfe, and R. M. Strieter. 1994. Production of IL-8 and monocyte chemotactic peptide-1 by peripheral blood monocytes. Disparate responses to phytohemagglutinin and lipopolysaccharide. *J. Immunol.* **152:** 241–249.

68. Mansfield, L. S., and J. F. Urban, Jr. 1996. The pathogenesis of necrotic proliferative colitis in swine is linked to whipworm induced immunosuppression of mucosal immunity to resident bacteria. *Vet. Immunol. Immunopathol.* **50:**1–17.

69. McSweegan, E., and R. I. Walker. 1986. Identification and characterization of two *Campylobacter jejuni* adhesins for cellular and mucous substrates. *Infect. Immun.* **53:**141–148.

70. Ménard, R., P. Sansonetti, and C. Parsot. 1994. The secretion of the *Shigella flexneri* Ipa invasins is activated by epithelial cells and controlled by IpaB and IpaD. *EMBO J.* **13:** 5293–5302.

71. Ming, W. J., L. Bersani, and A. Mantovani. 1987. Tumor necrosis factor is chemotactic for monocytes and polymorphonuclear leukocytes. *J. Immunol.* **138:**1469–1474.

72. Mixter, P. F., V. Rivera-Amill, A. M. Siegesmund, and M. E. Konkel. *Campylobacter jejuni* induces apoptosis of human T cells in a type III-dependent manner. Unpublished data.

73. Molbak, K., N. Wested, N. Hojlyng, F. Scheutz, A. Gottschau, P. Aaby, and A. P. da Silva. 1994. The etiology of early childhood diarrhea: a community study from Guinea-Bissau. *J. Infect. Dis.* **169:**581–587.

74. Monack, D. M., J. Mecsas, N. Ghori, and S. Falkow. 1997. *Yersinia* signals macrophages to undergo apoptosis and YopJ is necessary for this cell death. *Proc. Natl. Acad. Sci. USA* **94:** 10385–10390.

75. Moser, I., W. F. K. J. Schröder, and E. Hellmann. 1992. In vitro binding of *Campylobacter jejuni/coli* outer membrane preparations to INT 407 cell membranes. *Med. Microbiol. Immunol.* **180:**289–303.

76. Moser, I., W. Schroeder, and J. Salnikow. 1997. *Campylobacter jejuni* major outer membrane protein and a 59-kDa protein are involved in binding to fibronectin and INT 407 cell membranes. *FEMS Microbiol. Lett.* **157:**233–238.

77. Mroczenski-Wildey, M. J., J. L. Di Fabio, and F. C. Cabello. 1989. Invasion and lysis of HeLa cell monolayers by *Salmonella typhi*: role of lipopolysaccharide. *Microb. Pathog.* **6:** 143–152.

78. Nachamkin, I., B. M. Allos, and T. Ho. 1998. *Campylobacter* species and Guillain-Barré syndrome. *Clin. Microbiol. Rev.* **11:**555–567.

79. Newell, D. G., H. McBride, F. Saunders, Y. Dehele, and A. D. Pearson. 1985. The virulence of clinical and environmental isolates of *Campylobacter jejuni*. *J. Hyg. Camb.* **94:**45–54.

80. Oelschlaeger, T. A., P. Guerry, and D. J. Kopecko. 1993. Unusual microtubule-dependent endocytosis mechanisms triggered by *Campylobacter jejuni* and *Citrobacter freundii*. *Proc. Natl. Acad. Sci. USA* **90:**6884–6888.

81. Pei, Z., and M. J. Blaser. 1993. PEB1, the major cell-binding factor of *Campylobacter jejuni*, is a homolog of the binding component in Gram-negative nutrient transport systems. *J. Biol. Chem.* **268:**18717–18725.

82. Pei, Z., C. Burucoa, B. Grignon, S. Baqar, X.-Z. Huang, D. J. Kopecko, A. L. Bourgeois, J.-L. Fauchere, and M. J. Blaser. 1998. Mutation in the *peb1A* locus of *Campylobacter jejuni* reduces interactions with epithelial cells and intestinal colonization of mice. *Infect. Immun.* **66:** 938–943.

83. Pei, Z., R. T. Ellison III, and M. J. Blaser. 1991. Identification, purification, and characterization of major antigenic proteins of *Campylobacter jejuni*. *J. Biol. Chem.* **266:**16363–16369.

84. Perlman, D. M., N. M. Ampel, R. B. Schifman, D. L. Cohn, C. M. Patton, M. L. Aguirre, W. L. Wang, and M. J. Blaser. 1998. Persistent *Campylobacter jejuni* infections in patients infected with the human immunodeficiency virus (HIV). *Ann. Intern. Med.* **108:** 540–546.

85. Pesci, E. C., D. L. Cottle, and C. L. Pickett. 1994. Genetic, enzymatic, and pathogenic studies of the iron superoxide dismutase of *Campylobacter jejuni*. *Infect. Immun.* **62:**2687–2694.

86. Pickett, C. L., E. C. Pesci, D. L. Cottle, G. Russell, A. N. Erdem, and H. Zeytin. 1996.

Prevalence of cytolethal distending toxin production in *Campylobacter jejuni* and relatedness of *Campylobacter* sp. *cdtB* gene. *Infect. Immun.* **64:** 2070–2078.

87. **Popoff, M. R.** 1998. Interactions between bacterial toxins and intestinal cells. *Toxicon* **36:** 665–685.

88. **Prescott, J. F., I. K. Barker, K. I. Manninen, and O. P. Miniats.** 1981. *Campylobacter jejuni* colitis in gnotobiotic dogs. *Can. J. Comp. Med.* **45:**377–383.

89. **Richardson, W. P., and J. C. Sadoff.** 1988. Induced engulfment of *Neisseria gonorrhoeae* by tissue culture cells. *Infect. Immun.* **56:**2512–2514.

90. **Rivera-Amill, V., and M. E. Konkel.** Mimicking the in vivo conditions induces the secretion of virulence determinants from *Campylobacter jejuni*. Unpublished data.

91. **Russell, R. G., and D. C. Blake, Jr.** 1994. Cell association and invasion of Caco-2 cells by *Campylobacter jejuni*. *Infect. Immun.* **62:** 3773–3779.

92. **Russell, R. G., M. O'Donnoghue, D. C. Blake, Jr., J. Zulty, and L. J. DeTolla.** 1993. Early colonic damage and invasion of *Campylobacter jejuni* in experimentally challenged infant *Macaca mulatta*. *J. Infect. Dis.* **168:**210–215.

93. **Salerno, A., and F. Dieli.** 1998. Role of gamma delta T lymphocytes in immune response in humans and mice. *Crit. Rev. Immunol.* **18:** 327–357.

93a. **Schröder, W., and I. Moser.** 1997. Primary structure analysis and adhesion studies on the major outer membrane protein of *Campylobacter jejuni*. *FEMS Microbiol. Lett.* **150:**141–147.

94. **Schumann, J., S. Angermuller, R. Bang, M. Lohoff, and G. Tiegs.** 1998. Acute hepatotoxicity of *Pseudomonas aeruginosa* exotoxin A in mice depends on T cells and TNF. *J. Immunol.* **161:**5745–5754.

95. **Schwan, E. T., B. D. Robertson, H. Brade, and J. P. van Putten.** 1995. Gonococcal *rfaF* mutants express Rd$_2$ chemotype LPS and do not enter epithelial host cells. *Mol. Microbiol.* **15:** 267–275.

96. **Sharma, S. A., M. K. R. Tummuru, G. G. Miller, and M. J. Blaser.** 1995. Interleukin-8 response of gastric epithelial cell lines to *Helicobacter pylori* stimulation in vitro. *Infect. Immun.* **63:**1681–1687.

97. **Silverstein, S. C., R. M. Steinman, and Z. A. Cohn.** 1977. Endocytosis. *Annu. Rev. Biochem.* **46:**669–722.

98. **St. Geme, J. W., III, and S. Falkow.** 1990. *Haemophilus influenzae* adheres to and enters cultured human epithelial cells. *Infect. Immun.* **58:** 4036–4044.

99. **Szymanski, C. M., and G. D. Armstrong.** 1996. Interactions between *Campylobacter jejuni* and lipids. *Infect. Immun.* **64:**3467–3474.

100. **Szymanski, C. M., M. King, M. Haardt, and G. D. Armstrong.** 1995. *Campylobacter jejuni* motility and invasion of Caco-2 cells. *Infect. Immun.* **63:**4295–4300.

101. **Van Spreeuwel, J. P., G. C. Duursma, C. J. L. M. Meijer, R. Bax, P. C. M. Rosekrans, and J. Lindeman.** 1985. *Campylobacter* colitis: histological immunohistochemical and ultrastructural findings. *Gut* **26:**945–951.

102. **Walker, R. I., E. A. Schmauder-Chock, J. L. Parker, and D. Burr.** 1988. Selective association and transport of *Campylobacter jejuni* through M cells of rabbit Peyer's patches. *Can. J. Microbiol.* **34:**1142–1147.

103. **Walker, T. S., and H. H. Winkler.** 1978. Penetration of cultured mouse fibroblasts (L cells) by *Rickettsia prowazekii*. *Infect. Immun.* **22:**200–208.

104. **Wallis, M. R.** 1994. The pathogenesis of *Campylobacter jejuni*. *Brit. J. Biomed. Sci.* **51:** 57–64.

105. **Wassenaar, T. M., N. M. Bleumink-Pluym, and B. A. van der Zeijst.** 1991. Inactivation of *Campylobacter jejuni* flagellin genes by homologous recombination demonstrates that *flaA* but not *flaB* is required for invasion. *EMBO J.* **10:** 2055–2061.

106. **Weiser, J. N.** 1992. The oligosaccharide of *Haemophilus influenzae*. *Microb. Pathog.* **13:** 335–342.

107. **Welkos, S. L.** 1984. Experimental gastroenteritis in newly-hatched chicks infected with *Campylobacter jejuni*. *J. Med. Microbiol.* **18:**233–248.

108. **Whitehouse, C. A., P. B. Balbo, E. C. Pesci, D. L. Cottle, P. M. Mirabito, and C. L. Pickett.** 1998. *Campylobacter jejuni* cytolethal distending toxin causes a G$_2$-phase cell cycle block. *Infect. Immun.* **66:**1934–1940.

109. **Wooldridge, K. G., and J. M. Ketley.** 1997. *Campylobacter*-host cell interactions. *Trends Microbiol.* **5:**96–102.

110. **Wooldridge, K. G., P. H. Williams, and J. M. Ketley.** 1996. Host signal transduction and endocytosis of *Campylobacter jejuni*. *Microb. Pathog.* **21:**299–305.

111. **Yao, R., D. H. Burr, P. Doig, T. J. Trust, H. Niu, and P. Guerry.** 1994. Isolation of motile and non-motile insertional mutants of *Campylobacter jejuni*: the role of motility in adherence and invasion of eukaryotic cells. *Mol. Microbiol.* **14:**883–893.

112. **Yao, R., D. H. Burr, and P. Guerry.** 1997. CheY-mediated modulation of *Campylobacter jejuni* virulence. *Mol. Microbiol.* **23:**1021–1031.

113. **Zhu, J., R. J. Meinersmann, K. L. Hiett, and D. L. Evans.** 1999. Apoptotic effect of outer-membrane proteins from *Campylobacter jejuni* on chicken lymphocytes. *Curr. Microbiol.* **38:** 244–249.

114. **Zierler, M. K., and J. E. Galán.** 1995. Contact with cultured epithelial cells stimulates secretion of *Salmonella typhimurium* invasion protein InvJ. *Infect. Immun.* **63:**4024–4028.

115. **Ziprin, R. L., C. R. Young, L. H. Stanker, M. E. Hume, and M. E. Konkel.** The absence of cecal colonization of chicks by a mutant of *Campylobacter jejuni* not expressing bacterial fibronectin-binding protein. *Avian Dis.* **43:** 586–589.

116. **Zychlinsky, A., M. C. Prevost, and P. J. Sansonetti.** 1992. *Shigella flexneri* induces apoptosis in infected macrophages. *Nature* **358:** 167–169.

117. **Zychlinsky, A., and P. J. Sansonetti.** 1997. Apoptosis in bacterial pathogenesis. *J. Clin. Investig.* **100:**493–495.

CAMPYLOBACTER LIPOPOLYSACCHARIDES

Anthony P. Moran, John L. Penner, and Gerald O. Aspinall

12

Lipopolysaccharides (LPSs), also termed endo-toxins, form a family of toxic phosphorylated glycolipids found in the outer membrane of gram-negative bacteria, including *Campylobacter* spp., and are essential for the physical integrity and functioning of that membrane (64). These molecules play an important role in the interaction of gram-negative bacteria with their environment and with higher organisms. In particular, LPSs possess potent immuno-modulating and immunostimulating activities, due principally to their lipid component, lipid A (33, 76); harbor binding sites for antibodies and nonimmunoglobulin serum factors (65); and contribute to bacterial virulence (64).

Interest in determining the molecular composition and chemical structures of campylobacter LPSs with the objectives of determining their role in serotyping and pathogenesis has been raised for a number of reasons. First, serotyping systems for *Campylobacter jejuni* and *Campylobacter coli* that are based on thermostable antigens, now known to be of the LPS class of molecules, were described in the 1980s (56, 57). The application of this serotyping in numerous studies has contributed to an increased understanding of the epidemiology of human infections caused by these bacteria and has led to investigations of the distribution of these organisms in animals. Moreover, serotyping of clinical isolates has confirmed an association between antecedent infections with certain serotypes of *C. jejuni* and subsequent development of the neurological disorders Guillain-Barré syndrome (GBS) and Miller-Fisher syndrome (MFS) (23, 45, 49). Second, the successful application of serotyping of *C. jejuni* and *C. coli* based on thermostable antigens has led to continued interest in its application to other *Campylobacter* spp. (13, 22, 58). Third, some immunological and biological properties of LPSs from *C. jejuni* and *Campylobacter fetus* have been assessed (30, 34, 37, 42, 54, 74), but the molecular basis for these activities was unclear. In this chapter, the biochemistry and structure of LPSs of *Campylobacter* spp., especially the relationship between molecular structure and observed activities in serotyping and pathogenesis, are reviewed.

Anthony P. Moran, Department of Microbiology, National University of Ireland Galway, University Road, Galway, Ireland. *John L. Penner,* Department of Medical Genetics and Microbiology, University of Toronto, Toronto, Ontario M5S 1A8, Canada. *Gerald O. Aspinall,* Department of Chemistry, York University, North York, Toronto, Ontario M3J 1P3, Canada.

Campylobacter, 2nd Ed., Edited by I. Nachamkin and M. J. Blaser
© 2000 American Society for Microbiology, Washington, D.C.

DEVELOPMENT OF THERMOSTABLE ANTIGEN SEROTYPING SCHEMES FOR *CAMPYLOBACTER* SPECIES

The development of serotyping systems for *C. jejuni* and *C. coli* and the rationale for the use of the passive hemagglutination (PHA) technique for determining the antigenic specificities of the strains have been reviewed in detail (43). As routinely performed in most laboratories, the serotyping procedure consists of dispensing suspensions of sheep or human erythrocytes sensitized with heat-extracted antigenic material into wells of microtiter plates containing the appropriate typing antiserum in twofold dilutions (56, 57). The PHA technique has been known for decades as a highly sensitive technique for examining the serological specificities of LPS (43, 53). The basis for the sensitization is the presence in the erythrocyte membrane of a 228-kDa lipoglycoprotein receptor that binds LPS but not homopolysaccharides, heteropolysaccharides, monosaccharides, or protein antigens of either gram-negative or gram-positive bacteria (73). Although there has been a suggestion that polysaccharides were the thermostable antigens involved in serotyping *C. jejuni* (17), this is unlikely since purified LPS inhibits PHA reactions with heat-extracted antigen (21), lipid-free polysaccharides are unable to adsorb to erythrocytes without coupling reagents (43), and application of methods to isolate lipid-containing polysaccharides (25) isolated only serologically active polysaccharides in PHA which were derived from LPSs (39).

The present schemes for serotyping (56, 57) includes 42 serostrains (serotype reference strains) for *C. jejuni* and 18 for *C. coli,* but more serotypes exist among the many nontypeable strains that have been collected since the 1980s. However, for practical purposes the schemes have not been extended to include them as new serotypes since, in most cases, antisera prepared against these strains fail to identify new specificities in heterologous strains. Nevertheless, antisera against a new group of strains have been shown to serotype a significant proportion of the clinical isolates in South Africa (24), and

these new serotypes will have to be systematically integrated into extensions of the schemes to permit serotyping to be more widely applicable. A scheme for serotyping *Campylobacter lari* has not been developed, but immunoblotting and chemical studies indicate that serotyping based on LPS structural differences should prove possible (12, 13).

The typing scheme of *C. fetus* is based on both serological and biochemical tests (15). Variations in the structure of LPSs form the basis of the thermostable antigen serotyping scheme of *C. fetus* (58), in which there are two principal serotypes, A and B (15). Serotype A contains strains of both *C. fetus* subspp. *fetus* and *venerealis,* whereas some *C. fetus* subsp. *fetus* strains belong to serotype B. Furthermore, biochemical tests can be applied to further differentiate among serotype A strains (15). As with *C. jejuni* and *C. coli,* the PHA technique can be applied to serotype *C. fetus* strains (22). Nevertheless, cross-reacting strains, designated AB, have been found under certain serological test conditions (15) and, for rationalization of the typing scheme, have required further investigation (71).

BIOCHEMICAL AND SEROLOGICAL PROPERTIES OF THE THERMOSTABLE SEROTYPING ANTIGENS OF *CAMPYLOBACTER* SPECIES

The biochemical properties of the thermostable antigens of campylobacters in PHA reflect those of LPS in their thermostability and in their ability to bind to the 228-kDa lipoglycoprotein receptor present in erythrocyte membranes (43, 73). Early electrophoretic studies of phenol-water extracts and proteinase K-treated whole cell lysates (LPS mini-preparations) with LPS-specific silver staining detected molecules of low molecular weight (M_r) (26, 31, 59). However, subsequent examination by immunoblotting of extracts from *C. jejuni* strains with serotyping antisera revealed the occurrence of two distinctly different types of molecules in this species (63). All serostrains have low-M_r molecules that resolve into a small

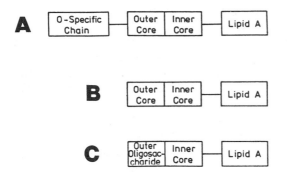

FIGURE 1 General architecture of high-M_r LPS (A), low-M_r LPS (B), and LOS (C).

number of bands similar to those of rough-form enterobacterial low-M_r LPS (39, 63, 64) (Fig. 1B) or low-M_r LPS, also termed lipooligosaccharide (LOS) characteristic of strains of *Neisseria* and *Haemophilus* spp. (45, 62) (Fig. 1C). In addition to the low-M_r molecules, some serostrains possess molecules of high M_r that band in a ladderlike pattern characteristic for smooth-form LPS molecules that have an attached O-specific polysaccharide (43, 63) (Fig. 1A). The presence of both the LPS- and LOS-like molecules in the same species is a novel feature of *C. jejuni* among gram-negative bacteria.

In contrast to the observations for *C. jejuni,* the immunoblotting of proteinase K-treated extracts from the 18 serostrains of *C. coli,* in all cases, revealed the presence of components with both low- and high-M_r molecules, reflecting the profiles of typical smooth-form enterobacterial LPS that consists of lipid A, core oligosaccharide (OS), and the O-specific polysaccharide chain (28, 64) (Fig. 1A). Interesting, however, was the finding that eight serological specificities are present among the low-M_r components; one is present in five serostrains, another is present in four, a third is present in three, a fourth is present in two, and the other four low-M_r component specificities occur in the remaining four serostrains (28). The eight low-M_r specificities among the 18 serostrains of this species represent a greater diversity than occurs in the core of *Escherichia coli,* which has only five core types, R1 to R4 and K12 (64).

However, the serological specificities of the *C. coli* low-M_r components are not detectable by PHA, indicating that *C. coli* are typed on the basis of serological specificities in the high-M_r LPS components (28). Antigenic preparations from two *C. lari* strains examined by immunoblotting in the same manner as the *C. jejuni* serostrains were found to have only low-M_r components (12, 13). More *C. lari* strains must be examined to determine if this type of thermostable antigen is characteristic of the species as a whole or if other strains, as in *C. jejuni,* also possess the high-M_r LPS components.

Unlike *C. jejuni* and *C. coli,* high-M_r molecules in proteinase K-treated extracts and LPSs of *C. fetus* strains of different serotypes and origins can be visualized by silver staining in electrophoretic gels, as well as by immunoblotting with serotyping antisera (41, 58, 59). Although the electrophoretic profiles are indicative of smooth-form LPS, resembling enterobacterial LPS (64, 65), the LPS of *C. fetus* strains exhibits profiles with clustering of high-M_r bands (41) rather than the ladderlike pattern encountered with enterobacterial smooth-form LPSs. Since the latter pattern reflects heterogeneity in the length of the O-polysaccharide chain, the profiles of *C. fetus* LPSs are thus characteristic of smooth-form LPS with O-chains of relatively homogeneous chain length. Each individual high-M_r LPS complex in electrophoresis gels consists of finely divided bands that are very closely spaced. These minor differences in relative mobility may be a consequence of incomplete sugar or O-acetyl substitution rather than a variation in the number of repeating units in the O-chain (41). A crystalline surface array (S-layer) protein is associated with virulence (16) and has been deduced to be anchored on the bacterial surface by high-M_r LPS (18). Consistent with this hypothesis, other pathogenic bacteria (e.g., *Aeromonas hydrophila* and *Aeromonas salmonicida*) that possess S-layers have LPS profiles similar to those of *C. fetus* (41), and attachment of S-layer proteins to the surface of *C. fetus* strains has been demonstrated to be serotype specific (74).

MOLECULAR STRUCTURE OF THE *CAMPYLOBACTER* LPS AND LOS-LIKE MOLECULES

In the subsequent sections, molecular structure is considered in terms of the three main regions of LPS: (i) lipid A, (ii) the core OS region, and (iii) the repetitive units of the O-antigen chain. The sugar constituents first characterized in *C. jejuni* LPSs, albeit in variable proportions, D-glucose, D-galactose, *N*-acetyl-D-galactosamine, L-*glycero*-D-*manno*-heptose (Hep), and 3-deoxy-D-*manno*-2-octulosonic acid (Kdo) (14, 46, 50), were mainly those of common occurrence in the core OS regions of low-M_r LPS in several species of the *Enterobacteriaceae* (20, 33, 64). In bacteria, such as *E. coli* and *Salmonella* spp., the serological specificities lie in the variable repeating OS units of the O-specific polysaccharide chains of high-M_r LPS (64). Upon initial examination, the rather small variations in sugar composition of low-M_r LPS or LOS of *C. jejuni* strains appeared insufficient to account for serological diversity. However, for *C. jejuni* serotypes structural differences among low-M_r isolates from various strains have now been recognized as being due to the many possible structural and stereochemical variants inherent in carbohydrate structure, not just the basic sugar constituents, but also ring size, anomeric configuration, and linkage sites for glycosyl substitution. With these variants it became clear how several structurally different OS of the same composition, but different serological specificity, could be accommodated in short OS chains (43). Similar conclusions had been reached previously for the LOS of *Neisseria* and *Haemophilus* spp. (29, 45, 62). Likewise, the LOSs of *C. lari* strains, although of similar sugar composition to those of *C. jejuni* strains, contain none of the structural features present in the outer core of *C. jejuni* strains but possess sufficient differences, within and between species, to account for serotypic variation (12, 13). On the other hand, structural differences in high-M_r LPS of *C. coli* and *C. fetus*, particularly in the O-polysaccharide chains, endow serospecificity (28, 69, 70).

CORE OLIGOSACCHARIDE COMPONENTS

Detailed structural studies on *C. jejuni* LPS began with the gel that separated from the water phase of phenol–water extraction (10). Mild-acid hydrolysis liberated soluble core OS from LPS by selective cleavage of the acid-labile glycosidic linkage between Kdo in the core OS and lipid A. The approach to analysis consisted of the stepwise degradation of the isolated core OS by enzymatic or chemical procedures which yielded a series of modified OSs, and subsequently, at each stage, sugar compositions, methylation linkage analyses to provide data on the sites of intersugar linkages, and sugar sequence analyses by mass spectrometry were performed. In addition, other features were determined by nuclear magnetic resonance spectroscopy. It must be emphasized that with branched structures and different types of linkages, in contrast to the linear sequences of monomer units in proteins and nucleic acids, several independent experimental approaches are required to obtain an unambiguous structural assignment for a complex OS.

As investigations proceeded, important aspects of LPS structure of biological and immunological significance were revealed. The first discovery was of the presence in some *C. jejuni* strains of *N*-acetylneuramimic acid (Neu5Ac) (46), a characteristic component of many mammalian glycolipids and glycoproteins. The Neu5Ac residues, like those of Kdo, are quite acid sensitive, but the mild-acid hydrolysis conditions used to cleave the Kdo–lipid A bond did not always result in complete loss of Neu5Ac from OSs. Studies on the core OSs of *C. jejuni* serostrains O:1 and O:4 showed the occurrence of a single laterally attached Neu5Ac residue (10). Recognizing the ease with which some Neu5Ac residues are removed on mild-acid treatment, methylation linkage analyses coupled with fast atom bombardment mass spectrometry were performed on O-deacylated, but otherwise intact, LOS from *C. jejuni* serostrain O:4. This analysis showed, in addition to lateral Neu5Ac, the presence of terminal Neu5Ac in the core OS of *C. jejuni* serostrain O:4 in mimicry of GD_{1a} ganglioside (11). In addition, it was shown that the termini of *C. jejuni* O:23 and O:36 core OSs are composed of the same tetrasaccharide as that present in GM_2 ganglioside, whereas the extent of mimicry of GM_2 ganglioside in *C. jejuni* serostrain O:1 is limited to a terminal trisaccharide (11). These studies represented the first complete report of ganglioside mimicry in *C. jejuni* LOSs.

Further studies on serotype O:10 and O:19 core OSs of neuropathogenic strains have shown the presence of a more extended terminal sialylated trisaccharide [Neu5Ac-α(2→8)-Neu5Ac-α(2→3)-β-D-Gal], indicating further structural resemblances between the outer regions of core OS and the outer OSs of human glycosphingolipids of the ganglioside family (8, 72). These observations have led to the recognition of the extent of molecular mimicry whereby *C. jejuni* displays the ability to synthesize molecules resident on cell surfaces of the human host (36, 45). A parallel example of molecular mimicry is that of the LOS components of *Neisseria meningitidis* and the human glycosphingolipids of the paragloboside type (45, 62).

The most complete core OS structures from seven *C. jejuni* serotypes are summarized in Fig. 2, using standard sugar shorthand abbreviations. Bearing in mind that the core OS preparations are microheterogeneous, and that truncated molecular species may occur, only the most complete chains are shown. For example, it has been estimated that >90% of the O:4 serostrain OS molecules show structural similarity to GD_{1a} and <10% to GM_1, whereas the proportions of GD1a- and GM1-like molecules of the O:19 serostrain are about equal (55). Structural studies on LPS from the seven *C. jejuni* serotypes established the presence of a rather invariable inner core region attached via Kdo to lipid A but also of serotypically distinctive terminal OSs (35, 43).

Attention is drawn to the following points (Fig. 2): (i) the conserved inner core unit, Hepα → 3Hepα1 → 5Kdo, carries a phosphate (P) or phosphorylethanolamine substituent at O-6 or O-7, and Glcβ at O-4 of the inner Hep residue; (ii) chain substitution on the outer Hep occurs at O-3 by Galβ or O-2 by Glcβ, or both, with further chain extension being more common at the former; (iii) the most extended chain termini (shown in bold type in the figure) mimic the OSs of gangliosides; and (iv) the structural variations possible in items (ii) and (iii) are sufficient to account for serotypic diversity independent of the presence or absence of Neu5Ac residues. It is noteworthy that serostrains O:1 on the one hand, and serostrains O:23 and O:36 on the other (10, 11), exhibit the same mimicry of ganglioside GM_2 but that the connections externally from the conserved inner core proceed from different sites (O-3 on the outer Hep of *C. jejuni* serostrain O:1, and O-2 on the outer Hep of *C. jejuni* serostrains O:23 and O:36) indicating structural variability. The possible significance of variations in the proportions and locations of Neu5Ac residues in those *C. jejuni* strains which have been associated with the development of the GBS and MFS is discussed below.

It should be noted that the core OSs of *C. jejuni* serostrains O:4 and O:19 are structurally identical, as are those of serostrains O:23 and O:36, but are different from those of serostrains O:4 and O:19 (8, 11). Thus, it is evident that a variety of core OS structures are present in this bacterial species, but also that strains of different serotypes may have the same OS structure. Strains with identical OSs are differentiated serologically on the basis of O-polysaccharide polymers associated with their high-M_r LPS (43).

Of those that have been studied, the LOS of only one *C. jejuni* strain (serostrain O:3) has a core OS of quite different type, containing a residue of 3-amino-3,6-dideoxy-D-glucose, quinovosamine (Qui3N), and no β-D-Gal residues able to accept Neu5Ac at O-3 (2) (Fig. 3A). Qui3N is also found in the core OS of some strains of *C. coli* (14) and, in particular, in *C. coli* serostrain O:30, where Qui3N residues in the outer core OSs carry two unusual acyl groups (6) (Fig. 3B). Other *Campylobacter* strains in which the outer core OS showed no

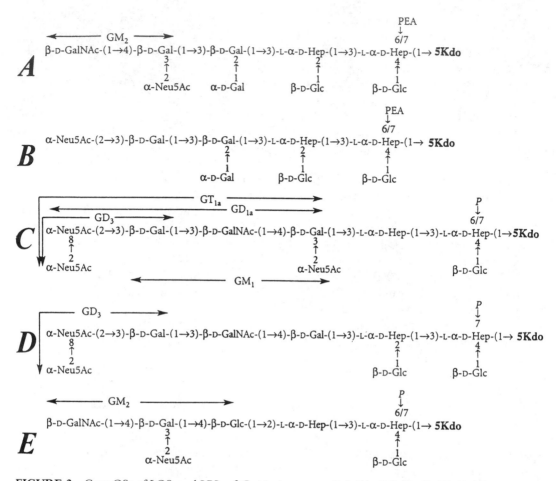

FIGURE 2   Core OSs of LOSs and LPSs of *C. jejuni* serotypes O:1 (A), O:2 (B), O:4/O:19 (C), O:10 (D), and O:23/O:36 (E). Terminal regions mimicking gangliosides are indicated with arrows. All sugars are in the pyranosidic form. *P*, phosphate; PEA, phosphoethanolamine; Kdo, 3-deoxy-D-*manno*-2-octulosonic acid; Hep, L-*glycero*-D-*manno*-heptose; Glc, glucose; Gal, galactose; GalNac, *N*-acetylgalactosamine; Neu5Ac, *N*-acetylneuraminic (sialic) acid. Unless otherwise stated, sugars are in the pyranosidic form.

similarities to those of *C. jejuni* strains were those from *C. lari* ATCC 35221 (the type strain) (12) and strain PC 637 (13) (Fig. 3C and D). As with the LOS of *C. jejuni* serostrains, they differ sufficiently from each other in detailed chemical structure to account for their recognition as distinct serotypes. Despite these structural differences in the outer core, the innermost core OSs of these four strains, one *C. jejuni*, one *C. coli*, and two *C. lari*, were indistinguishable from those of other *C. jejuni* strains. Only limited compositional data are

available on the core of *C. fetus* strains which, nevertheless, is sialylated (41).

RELATIONSHIP BETWEEN MOLECULAR STRUCTURE AND THE DEVELOPMENT OF GBS AND MFS

Special attention has focused on the LPSs and LOSs of certain *C. jejuni* strains which are associated with the subsequent development of GBS and MFS. The observation in several GBS patients in Japan of preceding *C. jejuni* infection by serotype O:19 strains, a serotype that

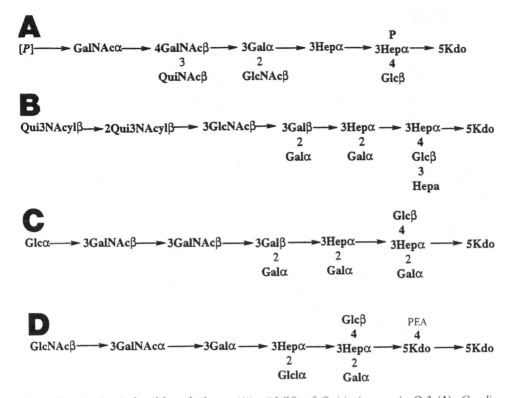

FIGURE 3 Atypical and branched core OSs of LOSs of *C. jejuni* serostrain O:3 (A), *C. coli* serostrain O:30 (B), *C. lari* PC 637 (C), and *C. lari* ATCC 35221 (D). Structures are shown in a more abbreviated form than in Fig. 1. All sugars are in the pyranosidic form and are D-enantiomers unless otherwise stated. P, phosphate; PEA, phosphoethanolamine; Kdo, 3-deoxy D *manno*-2-octulosonic acid; Hep, L-*glycero*-D-*manno*-heptose; Glc, glucose; Gal, galactose; GalNac, *N*-acetyl-galactosamine; Qui3NAc, *N*-acetylated 3-amino-3,6-dideoxyglucose (quinovosamine). The *N*-acyl substituents of Qui3NAc are 3-hydroxybutanoyl or 3-hydroxy-2,3-dimethyl-5-oxoprolyl chains.

occurs infrequently in patients with enteritis (23), prompted structural comparisons of the LOS and LPS components of such strains with those of the O:19 serostrain and those of non-neuropathogenic origin (8, 40, 75).

Figure 2 shows a composite structure of the core OS regions of the O:19 strains. In contrast to the outer core OS of the O:19 serostrain, which exhibits mimicry of GM$_1$ and GD$_{1a}$ gangliosides, the OS of two GBS-associated strains (OH 4382 and OH 4384) exhibits mimicry of a different type (1, 8). The OS of OH 4384 differs in that a disaccharide, neuraminobiose [Neu5Acα(2-8)Neu5Ac], instead of a single Neu5Ac residue, is linked to the terminal Gal residue, yielding mimicry of GT$_{1a}$ ganglioside over a hexasaccharide. On the other hand, the core OS of OH 4382 is a shorter molecule and lacks terminal Gal and GalNAc, whereby a neuraminobiose disaccharide is linked to an inner Gal residue, producing a trisaccharide with GD$_3$ mimicry. This terminal trisaccharide is a common feature of OH 4382 and 4384 core OSs (43, 55). However, analysis of other *C. jejuni* O:19 GBS-associated strains has shown mimicry of GM$_1$ and GD$_{1a}$ gangliosides by the terminal tetrasaccharides and pentasaccharides of core OSs, respectively (40, 75). Although discrepancies existed between the reported structures of the heptose region of O:19 core OS, outside the region of molecular mimicry (8, 75), these were resolved in a subsequent study (40). Furthermore, the core OSs of *C. jejuni* O:41 GBS-associated isolates are sialylated, contain a GM_1-like epitope, and structurally exhibit mimicry of GM_1 ganglioside similar to that observed in O:19 LPSs (60).

Parallel structural analyses on the LOSs of *C. jejuni* PG 836, an MFS-associated serotype O:10 isolate, and serostrain O:10 were the first performed on an MFS isolate (67, 72). Apart from small differences of unknown significance in the nature of the phosphate substituent on the inner heptose residue, no structural differences were detected between the core OSs of these two strains, which exhibited mimicry of GD_3 over their terminal trisaccharides (72) (Fig. 2). Preliminary analysis of a *C. jejuni* O:23 MFS isolate suggests structural microheterogeneity in the core OS which exhibits predominant GM_3 mimicry and minor GD_3 mimicry (3). Although the terminal disaccharide of the core OS of serostrain O:2 is found in a number of gangliosides, including GM_3 (9), no data are available on mimicry in MFS-associated *C. jejuni* serotype O:2.

Collectively, a common feature of some GBS- and MFS-associated *C. jejuni* isolates is the presence of a terminal core trisaccharide of Neu5Ac-Neu5Ac-Gal (8, 72), which is present in GD_3 and GT_{1a} gangliosides and has led to the suggestion that mimicry of this trisaccharide might play an important role in the pathogenesis of *C. jejuni*-associated neurological disease (55). Nevertheless, it is important to note that strains lacking this trisaccharide may also be associated with the development of GBS, e.g., some O:19 and O:41 strains (40, 60, 75). In brief, *C. jejuni* LPS can induce antiganglioside antibodies in animals (66, 68), and during the acute phase of illness, GBS and MFS patients with precedent *C. jejuni* infection frequently have autoantibodies to gangliosides which recognize epitopes both in gangliosides and in *C. jejuni* LPS (52, 68). Analysis with anti-GM_1 human monoclonal antibodies with

differences in fine specificities has shown the presence of GM_1-like epitopes in *C. jejuni* LPSs but also variations between LPSs in their expression of the epitopes, particularly between enteritis and GBS-associated strains (61). The relevance of mimicry of human gangliosides in the pathogenesis of *C. jejuni* has been reviewed elsewhere (36, 43, 45).

POLYSACCHARIDES AND OTHER CARBOHYDRATE POLYMERS ASSOCIATED WITH LPS EXTRACTS OF *C. JEJUNI*, *C. COLI*, AND *C. LARI*

Immunoblotting of antigenic extracts with specific homologous antisera has indicated that only a proportion of *C. jejuni* strains have electrophoretic profiles consistent with those of high-M_r LPS (63). Chemical characterization and structural analyses performed on phenol-water-extracted material from *C. jejuni*, *C. coli*, and *C. lari* have led to the finding that some strains in each of these species produce water-soluble polysaccharide polymers in addition to LPS-like or LOS-like molecules. The repeating units of these high-M_r components, which include a diverse group of glycans and phosphorylated carbohydrate polymers, are shown in Fig. 3. Whereas phenol-water extracts typically yield LPS of low and high M_r as water-insoluble gels, those of high-M_r from *Campylobacter* spp. were sometimes fully water soluble and could easily be overlooked. The polymers first analyzed were from the closely related *C. jejuni* serostrains O:23 and O:36, whose high-M_r LPS preparations showed novel features in having regular trisaccharide repeating units composed of *N*-acetylglucosamine, galactose, and one of four related heptoses (Fig. 4A), but with no evidence for or against uniformity of heptose components in individual polymer chains (4).

The O-chain polymer from high-M_r LPS of *C. jejuni* serostrain O:19 and two O:19 GBS isolates (OH 4282 and OH 4384) is a repeating structure, closely related to hyaluronic acid, with the majority of glucuronic acid residues amidated with 2-amino-2-deoxyglycerol (5)

A Closely-related repeating units

[→3)-β-D-GlcNAc-(1→3)-α-D-Gal-(1→2)-6d-α-D-*altro*-Hep-(1→]$_n$

[→3)-β-D-GlcNAc-(1→3)-α-D-Gal-(1→2)-6d-3Me-α-D-*altro*-Hep-(1→]$_n$

[→3)-β-D-GlcNAc-(1→3)-α-D-Gal-(1→2)-D-*glycero*-α-D-*altro*-Hep-(1→]$_n$

[→3)-β-D-GlcNAc-(1→3)-α-D-Gal-(1→2)-3Me-D-*glycero*-α-D-*altro*-Hep-(1→]$_n$

B [→4)-β-D-GlcA6(NGro)-(1→3)-β-D-GlcNAc-(1→]$_n$

C [→3)-L-*glycero*-α-D-*ido*-Hep-(1→4)-α-D-Gal-(1→]$_n$

D [-P→4)-α-D-Gal-(1→3)-Gro-(1→]$_n$

E [-P→5)-[6d-α-D-*talo*-Hep-(1→4)-β-D-GlcNAc-(1→3)]-Ribitol-(1→]$_n$

F [-P→3)-β-D-GlcNAc-(1→2)-6d-α-L-*gul*-Hep-(1→2)-3d-β-D-*threo*-Pen-(1→3)-6d-α-L-*gul*-Hep-(1→]$_n$

G [-P→4)-β-D-Glc-(1→5)-[6d-α-L-*gal*-Hep-(1→2)-6d-α-L-*gal*-Hep-(1→2)]-6d-α-L-*gal*-Hep*f*-(1→]$_n$

FIGURE 4 Repeating units of the high-M_r glycans and phosphorylated glycan polymers of *C. jejuni* O:23/O: 36 (A), *C. jejuni* O:19 (B), *C. jejuni* O:3 (C), *C. jejuni* O:1 (D) *C. coli* O:30 (E), *C. lari* ATCC 35221 (F), and *C. lari* PC 637 (G). Unless otherwise stated, sugars are in the pyranosidic form. *P*, phosphate; Gal, galactose; GlcNAc, *N*-acetylglucosamine; Gro, glycerol; GlcA6(NGro), glucuronic acid amidated with 2-amino-2-deoxy-glycerol; 3d-*threo*-Pen, 3-deoxy-*threo*-pentose. Note the varieties of heptoses present: 6-d-*altro*-Hep, 6-deoxy-D-*altro*-heptose; 6-d-3Me-*altro*-Hep, 6-deoxy-3-methyl-D-*altro*-heptose; *glycero*-*altro*-Hep, D-*glycero*-D-*altro*-heptose; 3Me-*glycero*-*altro*-Hep, 3-methyl-D-*glycero*-D-*altro*-heptose; *glycero*-*ido*-Hep, L-*glycero*-D-*ido*-heptose; 6d-*talo*-Hep, 6-deoxy-D-*talo*-heptose; 6d-*gulo*-Hep, 6-deoxy-L-*gulo*-heptose; 6d-*galacto*-Hep, 6-deoxy-L-*galacto*-heptose; 6d-*galacto*-Hep, 6-deoxy-L-*galacto*-heptofuranose.

(Fig. 4B). Although the observation of electrophoretic banding patterns is strongly indicative of high-M_r LPS components with regular repeating O-antigen polysaccharide chains (10, 63), definitive evidence has yet to be obtained for a covalent connection of these polysaccharides to the low-M_r LPS components. Despite this, all the O:19 strains examined express this polymer (5, 40). Of biological relevance, since mimicry of gangliosides by the core OSs of *C. jejuni* O:19 LPSs is not limited to strains that are associated with GBS, but is also present in those from individuals who develop enteritis only (40), a potential role for this hyaluronic acid–like polysaccharide in pathogenesis has been suggested (36, 45). Supporting this, a significantly greater amount of the polysaccharide

is present in strains from GBS patients than in strains from patients who develop enteritis alone (40).

Structural studies on phenol–water extracts of *C. jejuni* serostrain O:3 showed the presence of a D–Qui3NAc-containing LOS and a water-soluble glycan with a repeating disaccharide unit containing neither this sugar or typical core OS sugar constituents (2) (Fig. 4C). Hence, this polymer was concluded to be an LPS-independent polysaccharide coextracting with the LOS. Similarly, an LPS-independent polysaccharide has been purified from a *C. jejuni* O:41 isolate and is composed only of furanose sugars whose trisaccharide repeating unit contains furanose sugars of L-arabinose, 6-deoxy-D-*altro*-heptose, and L-altrose (19). The serological specificities of these polymers have not been determined, but the inability of these polysaccharides to link to the erythrocyte receptor would exclude them as participant reactants in the PHA technique (43, 73).

In addition, phosphorylated carbohydrate polymers have been isolated from a number of *Campylobacter* spp. (Fig. 4D to G). The simplest of these was obtained as a water-soluble compound from the phenol-water extracts of *C. jejuni* serostrain O:1 and is a teichoic acid-like polymer of simple repeating units with phosphoric diester linkages between galactosylglycerol units (27). Another water-soluble teichoic acid-type polymer with no apparent connection to lipid A was found in *C. coli* serotype O:30 and is a polyribitol phosphate backbone with disaccharide side chains (7). Two strains of *C. lari,* both of which had highly branched LOS structures, elaborate a different class of phosphorylated carbohydrate polymer based on a glycosylphosphateglycose connection similar to those in some capsular polysaccharides from gram-positive bacteria (12, 13).

A striking feature of carbohydrate polymers from campylobacters is the occurrence of heptose constituents of modified structure and unusual sugar ring configurations, most of which have not previously been found in nature (Fig. 3). In the absence of direct biochemical evidence, it is only possible to speculate on their origins, but with known biosynthetic pathways from hexoses to 6-deoxyhexoses, analogous pathways for the 6-deoxyheptoses would implicate the most common bacterial heptose (L-*glycero*-D-*manno*-heptose) as the most likely precursor.

O-POLYSACCHARIDES OF *C. FETUS*

As mentioned previously, the high-M_r smooth-form LPS of *C. fetus* strains can be visualized by both silver staining and immunoblotting (41, 58, 59). Initial compositional analysis of high-M_r LPSs of *C. fetus* strains of different subspecies and serotypes revealed the presence of a simple sugar composition of rhamnose, fucose, mannose, glucose, galactose, L-glycero-D-*manno*-heptose, and D-glycero-D-

manno-heptose in variable proportions in the different serotypes (41). For structural analysis, O-specific polysaccharide chains were liberated from LPS by mild-acid hydrolysis and subsequently purified by gel permeation chromatography (69). The structures of *C. fetus* O-polysaccharides are shown in Fig. 5. The serotype B O-polysaccharide of *C. fetus* subsp. *fetus* 14865 was the first analyzed and shown to be a D-rhamnan chain terminated by a residue of D-acofriose (3-O-methyl-D-rhamnose, D-Rha3Me) (69). On the other hand, the serotype A O-polysaccharide of *C. fetus* subsp. *fetus* 84−54 consists of an O-acetylated D-mannan chain (70), as does that of *C. fetus* subsp. *venerealis* 14840 (71). Thus, the structural basis for serospecificity is apparent.

Although type AB strains of *C. fetus* have been described as cross-reacting with serotype A and B typing antisera (5), the AB strain has an O-polysaccharide chain identical in structure to that of serotype B LPS (71) (Fig. 4). The latter is consistent with previous immunoblotting results (58). D-Mannose, which is present in low amounts in the liberated polysaccharides from LPS of serotypes B and AB, is not a constituent of their O chains and is a likely constituent of the LPS core (41, 71). The presence of this sugar in the core of serotype AB LPS may explain the cross-reaction of these strains with antiserum against serotype A, which possesses mannan O-chains (71).

LIPID A

Comparison of lipid A components of different gram-negative genera and families reveals that they possess a similar architectural principle (64). Three essential structural elements are present: (i) a D-hexosamine backbone, predominantly a disaccharide; (ii) substitution of the backbone by phosphate groups, which in turn may be substituted or not; and (iii) fatty acids in amide or ester linkages to the backbone (33, 76). Endotoxically active lipid A, exemplified by those of *E. coli* and *Salmonella minnesota,* contains a hydrophilic backbone of a $\beta(1\rightarrow6)$-linked D-glucosamine (GlcN) disaccharide carrying phosphate groups at positions 1 and 4′,

C. fetus fetus 84-54 (serotype A)

->3)-α-D-Man*p*2Ac-(1->

C. fetus fetus 14865 (serotype B)

α-D-Rha*p*3Me-(1->[3)-ß-D-Rha*p* –(1->2)-α-D-Rha*p*-(1->]$_n$

C. fetus venerealis 14840 (serotype A)

->3)-α-D-Man2*p*Ac-(1->

FIGURE 5 Repeating units of the O-polysaccharide chains of LPSs of *C. fetus*. Man*p*2Ac, 2-*O*-acetylated pyranosidic mannose; Rha*p*, pyranosidic rhamnose; Rha*p*Me, 3-*O*-methyl-rhamnose.

C. fetus fetus 84-94 (serotype AB)

α-D-Rha*p*3Me-(1->[3)-ß-D-Rha*p* –(1->2)-α-D-Rha*p*-(1->]$_n$

and substituted by six hydrophobic fatty acids, 12 to 14 carbons in length, in an asymmetric distribution on the backbone (33, 64, 65, 76) (Fig. 6A). Deviating backbone structures containing 2,3-diamino-2,3-dideoxy-D-glucose (GlcN3N) or D-glucosaminuronic acid have been described (33, 64, 76). In general, interbacterial species variations in lipid A structure result from the type of hexosamine present, the degree of phosphorylation, the presence of phosphate substituents, and, most notably, the nature, chain length, number, and location of fatty acyl chains (33, 64). Nevertheless, lipid A components exhibit a rather low structural variability in a given bacterial species compared with the other regions of LPS (core OS and O-polysaccharide chain). In *C. jejuni*, however, there is more variation than in most gram-negative species, since three different lipid A backbone disaccharides occur (48) (Fig. 6B).

Although initial studies reported the presence of GlcN in *C. jejuni* LPS and lipid A (14,

50, 51), more detailed investigations showed that both GlcN and GlcN3N occurred in LPSs and lipid A of a number of *C. jejuni* strains (34, 46, 47). Structural analysis of this so-called "mixed lipid A" of *C. jejuni* serostrain O:2 showed that about 73% of the lipid A molecules have a β(1→6)-linked disaccharide backbone of GlcN-GlcN3N, 15% have backbones of β(1→6)-linked GlcN3N-GlcN3N, and the remaining 12% have a β(1→6)-linked GlcN disaccharide backbone typical of enterobacterial lipid A (48). All three disaccharides are phosphorylated and acylated in the same manner; phosphate groups are present at positions 1 and 4′, and the disaccharides contain fatty acyl chains of 3-OH-14:0 at positions 2 and 3, 3-O(16:0)-14:0 or 3-O(14:0)-14:0 at position 2′, and 3-O(16:0)-14:0 at position 3′ (35, 48) (Fig. 6B). The occurrence of both GlcN and GlcN3N is a common property of all *C. jejuni* serostrains examined (34, 46). Nevertheless, preliminary structural analysis of lipid A

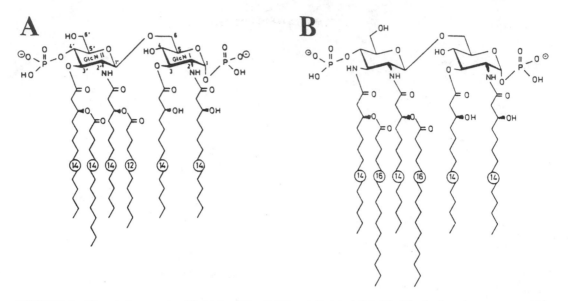

FIGURE 6 Chemical structure of lipid A of *E. coli* (A) and *C. jejuni* O:2 (B). The hydroxyl group at position 6′ on GlcN II is the attachment site of the core OS. Numbers in circles indicate the number of carbon atoms in fatty acyl chains. For *C. jejuni* lipid A, two other backbone species are present, one with a D-glucosamine disaccharide (12%) and one with a 2,3-diamino-2,3-dideoxy-D-glucose disaccharide (15%), and at position 2′, 16:0 on 3-OH-14:0 is partially (20%) replaced by 14:0.

from different *C. jejuni* serostrains has confirmed the presence of the same type of backbone structures with substitution patterns identical to those encountered in lipid A of *C. jejuni* serostrain O:2, but the relative proportions of the various backbones differed (32).

Emphasizing the specificity of lipid A structure to each bacterial species, and in contrast to *C. jejuni, C. fetus* LPS contains GlcN but not GlcN3N and has a different fatty acid composition (41). In particular, *C. fetus* lipid A has a 1,4′-bisphosphorylated β(1→6)-linked GlcN disaccharide backbone typical of enterobacterial lipid A, but is substituted by longer acyl chains (positions: 2 and 3, 3-OH-16:0 and 3-OH-14:0; 2′ and 3′, 3-O(16:0)-16:0 and 3-O(14:0)-14:0] than are encountered in enterobacterial lipid A (38).

IMMUNOLOGIC AND BIOLOGIC ACTIVITY OF *CAMPYLOBACTER* LPS

Comparisons of the biological activities and physical properties of LPSs and lipid A components with differing architectures are valuable in establishing chemicobioactivity and physicochemical relationships (33, 76). Apart from the occurrence of GlcN3N in two of the lipid A backbone disaccharides (GlcN3N-GlcN and GlcN3N-GlcN3N), including the major backbone molecular species, the architecture of lipid A of *C. jejuni* serostrain O:2 conforms with the structural principle encountered in the lipid A components of many gram-negative bacteria (33, 48, 76).

Despite the presence of GlcN3N, *C. jejuni* lipid A antigenically resembled classical enterobacterial lipid A when tested with anti-lipid A antibodies (34). This result reflects the fact that both GlcN and GlcN3N are *gluco*-configured sugars and will be recognized identically by antibodies. The only structural influence exerted by the occurrence of GlcN3N in the backbone disaccharides is the presence of a higher proportion of amide-bound 14:0(3-OH) fatty acid (75% of the total for GlcN3N-GlcN, compared with 50% for a GlcN-GlcN backbone) (35, 48). Compared with enterobacterial preparations, *C. jejuni* LPSs express slightly lower, yet comparable, endotoxic activity in biologic test systems (34). In particular, *C. jejuni* LPS possesses 50% lower lethal toxicity in mice, 30- to 50-fold lower pyrogenicity, and 100-fold lower ability to induce tumor necrosis factor secretion than does *Salmonella* spp. LPS (34). *C. jejuni* LPS and lipid A exhibit higher phase transition temperatures than do the *Salmonella* preparations, and thus *C. jejuni* preparations have lower fluidity at 37°C (34, 35). This lower fluidity of acyl chains may influence the biologic and immunologic activities of *C. jejuni* LPS. On the other hand, the states of order of the acyl chains may play a less important role in biologic activities than does the supramolecular structure of lipid A (34). The acyl chain characteristics, including the presence of a higher proportion of a longer-chain fatty acid (16:0), and the replacement of GlcN with GlcN3N may also influence the supramolecular structure of *C. jejuni* lipid A, thereby affecting biologic activities (35).

Likewise, LPS preparations from different strains of *C. fetus,* including different subspecies and serotypes, were less active than *Salmonella typhimurium* LPS in mitogenicity, *Limulus* amebocyte, lethal toxicity, and pyrogenicity assays (42). As with *C. jejuni,* this may reflect the presence of longer fatty acyl chains in *C. fetus* than enterobacterial lipid A (38). Interstrain differences in the bioactivities of *C. fetus* LPSs were observed, but no apparent correlations between lipid A composition and variations in these bioactivities existed (42). Hence, since lipid A bioactivity can be modulated by the saccharide portion of LPS (33, 64, 65) and since the polysaccharide moiety of LPS of *C. fetus* serotypes differ in composition and structure (41, 69–71), the observed biologic differences may be related to some property influenced by the composition of the polysaccharide moiety of LPS, such as solubility or lipid A conformation (42). Interestingly, the LPS of *C. fetus* subsp. *fetus* serotype A, the serotype which predominates in human infections, had the lowest biologic activity in all assays (42). Whether the lower bioactivity contributes to the pathogenesis of this serotype in humans remains an open question.

CONCLUSIONS AND CHALLENGES FOR THE FUTURE

Interesting new insights into the LPS and LOS nature of the thermostable antigens of *Campylobacter* spp. have been gained. However, the insights on serospecificity in LOS are based on a small number of serostrains, and expanded investigations are required. Moreover, the genetic basis for the production and variation of these molecules is only now becoming the focus of attention.

A critical issue for continued study in *C. jejuni* pathogenesis is the importance of molecular mimicry in LPS, compared with other contributing factors including those of the host, in the development of postinfectious neuropathies (43, 49). In particular, the number of *C. jejuni* strains that have been studied at the molecular level is small compared with the number of serotypes that have been implicated in the development of neuropathologies (36, 45). A range of gangliosides can be mimicked by *C. jejuni,* but it is not clear which of these mimicries is central in establishing postinfectious syndromes (43). Moreover, the immunological mechanisms by which tolerance to host ganglioside structures is diminished by *C. jejuni* infection also need to be determined (44). Whether the LPS of other *Campylobacter* spp. is involved in the development of neuropathy-associated infection requires evaluation, especially since *C. fetus* core OS is sialylated and its biological importance is unclear (41).

It should not be overlooked that LPS is a major surface component and toxic molecule of the outer membrane of *Campylobacter* spp. Although studies on the toxicity, immunological activity, and biologic properties of LPS preparations of *C. jejuni* and *C. fetus* have been performed (30, 34, 37, 42, 54, 74), such information on LPSs of other campylobacters is lacking. In a macromolecular context, future studies on the role of these molecules in maintaining the integrity of the outer membrane of campylobacters could prove useful in understanding their survival and interaction with their respective ecological niches.

REFERENCES

1. **Aspinall, G. O., S. Fujimoto, A. G. McDonald, H. Pang, L. A. Kurjanczyk, and J. L. Penner.** 1994. Lipopolysaccharides from *Campylobacter jejuni* associated with Guillain-Barré syndrome patients mimic human gangliosides in structure. *Infect. Immun.* **62:**2122–2125.

2. **Aspinall, G. O., C. M. Lynch, H. Pang, R. T. Shaver, and A. P. Moran.** 1995. Chemical structures of the core region of *Campylobacter jejuni* O:3 lipopolysaccharide and an associated polysaccharide. *Eur. J. Biochem.* **231:**570–578.

3. **Aspinall, G. O., A. Mainkar, M. M. Prendergast, B. Jacobs, and A. P. Moran.** 1998. Lipopolysaccharides from a neuropathy-associated infection from *Campylobacter jejuni* serotype O:23, p. 93–96. *In* A. J. Lastovica, D. G. Newell, and E. E. Lastovica (ed.), *Campylobacter, Helicobacter and Related Organisms.* Institute of Child Health and University of Cape Town, Cape Town, South Africa.

4. **Aspinall, G. O., A. G. McDonald, and H. Pang.** 1992. Structures of the O chains from lipopolysaccharides of *Campylobacter jejuni* serotypes O:23 and O:36. *Carbohydr. Res.* **231:**13–20.

5. **Aspinall, G. O., A. G. McDonald, and H. Pang.** 1994. Lipopolysaccharides of *Campylobacter jejuni* serotype O:19: structures of O antigen chains from the serostrain and two bacterial isolates from patients with the Guillain-Barré syndrome. *Biochemistry* **33:**250–255.

6. **Aspinall, G. O., A. G. McDonald, H. Pang, L. A. Kurjanczyk, and J. L. Penner.** 1993. Lipopolysaccharide of *Campylobacter coli* serotype O:30. Fractionation and structure of liberated core oligosaccharide. *J. Biol. Chem.* **268:**6263–6268.

7. **Aspinall, G. O., A. G. McDonald, H. Pang, L. A. Kurjanczyk, and J. L. Penner.** 1993. An antigenic polysaccharide from *Campylobacter coli* serotype O:30. Structure of a techoic acid-like antigenic polysaccharide associated with the lipopolysaccharide. *J. Biol. Chem.* **268:**18321–18329.

8. **Aspinall, G. O., A. G. McDonald, H. Pang, L. A. Kurjanczyk, and J. L. Penner.** 1994. Lipopolysaccharides of *Campylobacter jejuni* serotype O:19: structures of core oligosaccharide regions from the serostrain and two bacterial isolates from patients with the Guillain-Barré syndrome. *Biochemistry* **33:**241–249.

9. **Aspinall, G. O., A. McDonald, T. S. Raju, H. Pang, L. A. Kurjanczyk, J. L. Penner, and A. P. Moran.** 1993. Chemical structure of the core region of *Campylobacter jejuni* serotype O:2 lipopolysaccharide. *Eur. J. Biochem.* **213:**1029–1037.

10. **Aspinall, G. O., A. G. McDonald, T. S. Raju, H. Pang, S. D. Mills, L. A. Kurjanczyk, and J. L. Penner.** 1992. Serological diversity and chemical structures of *Campylobacter jejuni* low-molecular-weight lipopolysaccharides. *J. Bacteriol.* **174:**1324–1332.

11. **Aspinall, G. O., A. G. McDonald, T. S. Raju, H. Pang, A. P. Moran, and J. L. Penner.** 1993. Chemical structure of the core regions of *Campylobacter jejuni* serotypes O:1, O:4, O:23, and O:36 lipopolysaccharides. *Eur. J. Biochem.* **213:**1017–1027.

12. **Aspinall, G. O., M. A. Monteiro, and H. Pang.** 1995. Lipo-oligosaccharide of the *Campylobacter lari* type strain ATCC 35221. Structure of the liberated oligosaccharide and an associated extracellular polysaccharide. *Carbohydr. Res.* **279:**245–264.

13. **Aspinall, G. O., M. A. Monteiro, H. Pang, L. A. Kurjanczyk, and J. L. Penner.** 1995. Lipo-oligosaccharide of *Campylobacter lari* strain PC 637. Structure of the liberated oligosaccharide and an associated extracellular polysaccharide. *Carbohydr. Res.* **279:**227–244.

14. **Beer, W., M. Adam, and G. Seltman.** 1986. Monosaccharide composition of lipopolysaccharides from *Campylobacter jejuni* and *Campylobacter coli. J. Basic Microbiol.* **4:**201–204.

15. **Berg, R. L., J. W. Jutila, and B. D. Firehammer.** 1971. A revised classification of *Vibrio fetus. Am. J. Vet. Res.* **32:**11–22.

16. **Blaser, M. J., and Z. Pei.** 1993. Pathogenesis of *Campylobacter fetus* infections: critical role of high-molecular-weight S-layer proteins in virulence. *J. Infect. Dis.* **167:**372–377.

17. **Chart, H., J. A. Frost, A. Oza, R. Thwaites, S. Gillanders, and B. Rowe.** 1996. Heat-stable serotyping antigens expressed by strains of *Campylobacter jejuni* are probably capsular and not long-chain lipopolysaccharide. *J. Appl. Bacteriol.* **81:**635–640.

18. **Fogg, G. C., L. Yang, E. Wang, and M. J. Blaser.** 1990. Surface array proteins of *Campylobacter fetus* block lectin-mediated binding to type A lipopolysaccharide. *Infect. Immun.* **58:**2738–2744.

19. **Hannify, O. M., A. S. Shashkov, A. P. Moran, M. M. Prendergast, S. N. Senchenkova, Y. A. Knirel, and A. S. Savage.** 1999. Chemical structure of a polysaccharide from *Campylobacter jejuni* 176.83 (serotype O:41) containing only furanose sugars. *Carbohydr. Chem.* **319:**124–132.

20. **Holst, O.** Chemical structure of the core region of lipopolysaccharides. *In* H. Brade, D. C. Morrison, S. Opal, S. Vogel (ed.), *Endotoxins in Health and Disease,* in press. Marcel Dekker Inc., New York, N.Y.

21. **Jones, D. M., A. J. Fox, and J. Eldridge.** 1984. Characterization of the antigens involved in sero-

typing strains of *Campylobacter jejuni* by passive hemagglutination. *Curr. Microbiol.* **10**:105–110.

22. **Kosunen, T. U.** 1986. Serotyping of *Campylobacter fetus* subsp. *fetus* and *C. fetus* subsp. *venerealis* by passive hemagglutination technique based on soluble autoclaved antigens. *Acta Pathol. Microbiol. Immunol. Scand. Sect. B.* **94**:245–249.

23. **Kuroki, S., T. Saida, M. Nukina, T. Haruta, M. Yoshioka, Y. Kobayashi, and H. Nakanishi.** 1993. *Campylobacter jejuni* strains from patients with Guillain-Barré syndrome belong mostly to Penner serogroup 19 and contain β-*N*-acetylglucosamine residues. *Ann. Neurol.* **33**:243–247.

24. **Lastovica, A. J.** Personal communication.

25. **Liu, T.-Y., E. C. Gotschlich, E. K. Jonssen, and J. R. Wysocki.** 1971. Studies on the meningococcal polysaccharides. I. Composition and chemical properties of the group A polysaccharide. *J. Biol. Chem.* **246**:2849–2858.

26. **Logan, S. M., and T. J. Trust.** 1984. Structural and antigenic heterogeneity of lipopolysaccharides of *Campylobacter jejuni* and *Campylobacter coli*. *Infect. Immun.* **45**:210–216.

27. **MacDonald, A. G.** 1993. Lipopolysaccharides from *Campylobacter*. Ph.D. thesis. York University, Toronto, Canada.

28. **Mandatori, R., and J. L. Penner.** 1987. Structural and antigenic properties of *Campylobacter coli* lipopolysaccharides. *Infect. Immun.* **57**:3506–3511.

29. **Mandrell, R., H. Schneider, M. Apicella, W. Zollinger, P. A. Rice, and J. M. Griffiss.** 1986. Antigenic and physical diversity of *Neisseria gonorrhoeae* lipooligosaccharides. *Infect. Immun.* **54**:63–69.

30. **McSweegan, E., and R. I. Walker.** 1986. Identification and characterization of two *Campylobacter jejuni* adhesins for cellular and mucous substrates. *Infect. Immun.* **53**:141–148.

31. **Mills, S. D., W. C. Bradbury, and J. L. Penner.** 1985. Basis for serological heterogeneity of thermostable antigens of *Campylobacter jejuni*. *Infect. Immun.* **50**:284–291.

32. **Moran, A. P.** 1993. Inter-strain structural variation in the lipid A of *Campylobacter jejuni* lipopolysaccharides. *Acta Gastro-Enterol. Belg.* **56**(Suppl.):41.

33. **Moran, A. P.** 1994. Structure-bioactivity relationships of bacterial endotoxins. *J. Toxicol. Toxin Rev.* **14**:47–83.

34. **Moran, A. P.** 1995. Biological and serological characterization of *Campylobacter jejuni* lipopolysaccharides with deviating core and lipid A structures. *FEMS Immunol. Med. Microbiol.* **11**:121–130.

35. **Moran, A. P.** 1997. Structure and conserved characteristics of *Campylobacter jejuni* lipopolysaccharides. *J. Infect. Dis.* **176**(Suppl. 2):S135–S138.

36. **Moran, A. P., B. J. Appelmelk, and G. O. Aspinall.** 1996. Molecular mimicry of host structures by lipopolysaccharides of *Campylobacter* and *Helicobacter* spp.: implications in pathogenesis. *J. Endotoxin Res.* **3**:521–531.

37. **Moran, A. P., M. A. Caldwell, J. A. Houghton, A. Nolan, and D. T. O'Malley.** 1996. Effect of *Campylobacter fetus* and *Escherichia coli* LPS on bovine and human spermatozoa. *J. Endotoxin Res.* **3**(Suppl. 1):34.

38. **Moran, A. P., I. M. Helander, B. Lindner, and D. T. O'Malley.** 1996. Structural analysis of lipid A from *Campylobacter fetus* smooth-form LPS. *J. Endotoxin Res.* **3**(Suppl. 1):34.

39. **Moran, A. P., and T. U. Kosunen.** 1989. Serological analysis of the heat-stable antigens involved in serotyping *Campylobacter jejuni* and *Campylobacter coli*. *APMIS* **97**:253–260.

40. **Moran, A. P., and D. T. O'Malley.** 1995. Potential role of lipopolysaccharides of *Campylobacter jejuni* in the development of Guillain-Barré syndrome. *J. Endotoxin Res.* **2**:233–235.

41. **Moran, A. P., D. T. O'Malley, T. U. Kosunen, and I. M. Helander.** 1994. Biochemical characterization of *Campylobacter fetus* lipopolysaccharides. *Infect. Immun.* **62**:3922–3929.

42. **Moran, A. P., D. T. O'Malley, J. Vuopio-Varkila, K. Varkila, L. Pyhälä, H. Saxén, and I. M. Helander.** 1996. Biological characterization of *Campylobacter fetus* lipopolysaccharides. *FEMS Immunol. Med. Microbiol.* **15**:43–50.

43. **Moran, A. P., and J. L. Penner.** 1999. Serotyping of *Campylobacter jejuni* based on heat-stable antigens: relevance, molecular basis and implications in pathogenesis. *J. Appl. Microbiol.* **86**:361–377.

44. **Moran, A. P., and M. M. Prendergast.** 1998. Molecular mimicry in *Campylobacter jejuni* lipopolysaccharides and the development of Guillain-Barré syndrome. *J. Infect. Dis.* **178**:1549–1550.

45. **Moran, A. P., M. M. Prendergast, and B. J. Appelmelk.** 1996. Molecular mimicry of host structures by bacterial lipopolysaccharides and its contribution to disease. *FEMS Immunol. Med. Microbiol.* **16**:105–115.

46. **Moran, A. P., E. T. Rietschel, T. U. Kosunen, and U. Zähringer.** 1991. Chemical characterization of *Campylobacter jejuni* lipopolysaccharides containing *N*-acetylneuraminic acid and 2,3-diamino-2,3-dideoxy-D-glucose. *J. Bacteriol.* **173**:618–626.

47. **Moran, A. P., D. Scholz, and U. Zähringer.** 1992. Application of methylation analysis in the determination of the structure of disaccharides containing 2,3-diamino-2,3-dideoxy-D-glucose

(GlcN3N) associated with the backbone of lipid A. *Carbohydr. Res.* **231**:309–316.

48. **Moran, A. P., U. Zähringer, U. Seydel, D. Scholz, P. Stütz, and E. T. Rietschel.** 1991. Structural analysis of the lipid A component of *Campylobacter jejuni* CCUG 10936 lipopolysaccharide. Description of a lipid A containing a hybrid backbone of 2-amino-2-deoxy-D-glucose and 2,3-diamino-2,3-dideoxy-D-glucose. *Eur. J. Biochem.* **198**:459–469.

49. **Nachamkin, I., B. Mishu Allos, and T. Ho.** 1998. *Campylobacter* species and Guillain-Barré syndrome. *Clin. Microbiol. Rev.* **11**:555–567.

50. **Naess, V., and T. Hofstad.** 1984. Chemical composition and biological activity of lipopolysaccharides prepared from type strains of *Campylobacter jejuni* and *Campylobacter coli*. *Acta Pathol. Microbiol. Immunol. Scand. Sect. B* **92**:217–222.

51. **Naess, V., and T. Hofstad.** 1984. Chemical studies of partially hydrolysed lipopolysaccharides from four strains of *Campylobacter jejuni* and two strains of *Campylobacter coli*. *J. Gen. Microbiol.* **130**:2783–2789.

52. **Neisser, A., H. Bernheimer, T. Berger, A. P. Moran, and B. Schwerer.** 1997. Serum antibodies to gangliosides and *Campylobacter jejuni* lipopolysaccharides in Miller-Fisher syndrome. *Infect. Immun.* **65**:4038–4042.

53. **Neter, E., O. Westphal, O. Lüderitz, E. A. Gorzynski, and E. Eichenberger.** 1956. Studies of enterobacterial lipopolysaccharides. Effects of heat and chemicals on erythrocyte-modifying, antigenic, toxic, and pyrogenic properties. *J. Immunol.* **76**:377–385.

54. **O'Sullivan, A. M., C. J. Doré, S. Boyle, C. R. Coid, and A. P. Johnson.** 1988. The effect of campylobacter lipopolysaccharide on fetal development in the mouse. *J. Med. Microbiol.* **26**:101–105.

55. **Penner, J. L., and G. O. Aspinall.** 1997. Diversity of lipopolysaccharide structures in *Campylobacter jejuni*. *J. Infect. Dis.* **176**(Suppl. 2):S135–S138.

56. **Penner, J. L., and J. N. Hennessy.** 1980. Passive hemagglutination technique for serotyping *Campylobacter fetus* subsp. *jejuni* on the basis of soluble heat-stable antigens. *J. Clin. Microbiol.* **12**:732–737.

57. **Penner, J. L., J. N. Hennessy, and R. V. Congi.** 1983. Serotyping of *Campylobacter jejuni* and *Campylobacter coli* on the basis of thermostable antigens. *Eur. J. Clin. Microbiol.* **2**:378–383.

58. **Perez Perez, G. I., M. J. Blaser, and J. H. Bryner.** 1986. Lipopolysaccharide structures of *Campylobacter fetus* are related to heat-stable serogroups. *Infect. Immun.* **51**:209–212.

59. **Perez Perez, G. I., and M. J. Blaser.** 1985. Lipopolysaccharide characteristics of pathogenic campylobacters. *Infect. Immun.* **47**:353–359.

60. **Prendergast, M. M., A. J. Lastovica, and A. P. Moran.** 1998. Lipopolysaccharides from *Campylobacter jejuni* O:41 strains associated with Guillain-Barré syndrome exhibit mimicry of GM_1 ganglioside. *Infect. Immun.* **66**:3649–3755.

61. **Prendergast, M. M., H. J. Willison, A. J. Lastovica, and A. P. Moran.** 1998. Human monoclonal anti-GM_1 ganglioside antibodies cross-react with lipopolysaccharide of *Campylobacter jejuni* strains associated with GBS. *Ir. J. Med. Sci.* **167**(Suppl. 5):3.

62. **Preston, A., R. E. Mandrell, B. W. Gibson, and M. A. Apicella.** 1996. The lipooligosaccharides of pathogenic gram-negative bacteria. *Crit. Rev. Microbiol.* **22**:139–180.

63. **Preston, M. A., and J. L. Penner.** 1987. Structural and antigenic properties of lipopolysaccharides from serotype reference strains of *Campylobacter jejuni*. *Infect. Immun.* **55**:1806–1812.

64. **Rietschel, E. T., L. Brade, O. Holst, V. A. Kulshin, B. Lindner, A. P. Moran, U. F. Schade, U. Zähringer, and H. Brade.** 1990. Molecular structure of bacterial endotoxin in relation to bioactivity, p. 15–32. *In* A. Nowotny, J. J. Spitzer, and E. J. Ziegler (ed.), *Endotoxin Research Series*, vol. 1. *Cellular and Molecular Aspects of Endotoxin Reactions*, Elsevier Science Publishers B. V., Amsterdam, The Netherlands.

65. **Rietschel, E. T., L. Brade, U. Schade, U. Seydel, U. Zähringer, B. Lindner, A. P. Moran, V. A. Kulschin, Y. Haishima, O. Holst, E. Röhrscheidt-Andrzewski, A. J. Ulmer, H.-D. Flad, and H. Brade.** 1990. Chemical structure and biological activity of lipopolysaccharides, p. 5–18. *In* J.-D. Baumgartner, T. Calandra, and J. Carlet (ed.), *Endotoxin—from Pathophysiology to Therapeutic Approaches*. Flammarion Medecine-Sciences, Paris, France.

66. **Ritter, G., S. R. Fortunato, L. Cohen, Y. Noguchi, E. M. Bernard, E. Stockert, and L. J. Old.** 1996. Induction of antibodies reactive with GM_2 ganglioside after immunization with lipopolysaccharides from *Campylobacter jejuni*. *Int. J. Cancer* **66**:184–190.

67. **Salloway, S., L. A. Mermel, M. Seamans, G. O. Aspinall, J. E. N. Shin, L. A. Kurjanczyk, and J. L. Penner.** 1996. Miller-Fisher syndrome associated with *Campylobacter jejuni* bearing lipopolysaccharide molecules that mimic human ganglioside GD_3. *Infect. Immun.* **64**:2945–2949.

68. **Schwerer, B., A. Neisser, R. J. Polt, H. Bernheimer, and A. P. Moran.** 1995. Antibody cross-reactivities between gangliosides and lipopolysaccharides of *Campylobacter jejuni* serotypes

associated with Guillain-Barré syndrome. *J. Endotoxin Res.* **2:**395–403.

69. **Senchenkova, S. N., A. S. Shashkov, Y. A. Knirel, J. J. McGovern, and A. P. Moran.** 1996. The O-specific polysaccharide chain of *Campylobacter fetus* serotype B lipopolysaccharide is a D-rhamnan terminated with 3-O-methyl-D-rhamnose (D-acofriose). *Eur. J. Biochem.* **239:** 434–438.

70. **Senchenkova, S. N., A. S. Shashkov, Y. A. Knirel, J. J. McGovern, and A. P. Moran.** 1997. The O-specific polysaccharide chain of *Campylobacter fetus* serotype A lipopolysaccharide is a partially O-acetylated 1,3-linked α-D-mannan. *Eur. J. Biochem.* **245:**637–641.

71. **Senchenkova, S. N., A. S. Shashkov, Y. A. Knirel, J. J. McGovern, and A. P. Moran.** 1998. Structural characterization of the O-chains of *Campylobacter fetus* lipopolysaccharides: relevance to serotyping, p. 242–244. *In* A. J. Lastovica, D. G. Newell, and E. E. Lastovica (ed.), *Campylobacter, Helicobacter and Related Organisms.* Institute of Child Health and University of Cape Town, Cape Town, South Africa.

72. **Shin, J. E. N., S. Ackloo, A. S. Mainkar, M. A. Monteiro, H. Pang, J. L. Penner, and G.**

O. **Aspinall.** 1998. Lipo-oligosaccharides of *Campylobacter jejuni* serotype O:10. Structures of core oligosaccharide regions from a bacterial isolate from a patient with the Miller-Fisher syndrome and from the serotype reference strain. *Carbohydr. Res.* **305:**223–232.

73. **Springer, G. F., J. E. Adye, A. Bezkorovainy, and J. R. Murphy.** 1973. Functional aspects and nature of the lipopolysaccharide-receptor of human erythrocytes. *J. Infect. Dis.* **128**(Suppl.): S202–S212.

74. **Yang, L., Z. Pei, S. Fujimoto, and M. J. Blaser.** 1992. Reattachment of surface array proteins to *Campylobacter fetus* cells. *J. Bacteriol.* **174:** 1258–1267.

75. **Yuki, N., T. Taki, F. Inagaki, T. Kasama, M. Takahashi, K. Saito, S. Handa, and T. Miyatake.** 1993. A bacterium lipopolysaccharide that elicits Guillain-Barré syndrome has a GM1 ganglioside-like structure. *J. Exp. Med.* **178:** 1771–1775.

76. **Zähringer, U., B. Lindner, and E. T. Rietschel.** 1994. Molecular structure of lipid A, the endotoxic center of bacterial lipopolysaccharides. *Adv. Carbohydr. Chem. Biochem.* **50:** 211–276.

ANTIGLYCOSPHINGOLIPID ANTIBODIES AND GUILLAIN-BARRÉ SYNDROME

Hugh J. Willison and Graham M. O'Hanlon

13

Guillain-Barré syndrome (GBS) is an acute postinfectious paralytic illness caused by inflammatory disruption of peripheral-nerve integrity and function. It was first identified as a distinct clinical entity almost 100 years ago, and over the ensuing period considerable progress has been made in refining our knowledge of both the clinical and scientific aspects of the disease. Although GBS is now the foremost cause of acute paralysis, the incidence is relatively low at 1 to 2 per 100,000 (52), and it fortunately remains an uncommon complication of *Campylobacter* infection, occurring after only approximately 1:1,000 cases (1). However, for affected individuals it remains a serious illness, with a substantial morbidity (12% are unable to walk after 1 year) and a mortality rate of 5%. In other words, even with the optimal therapy of plasma exchange or intravenous immunoglobulin, one-fifth of patients are left severely disabled or dead. Furthermore, it commands very high health care and other economic costs, both in the acute phase of intensive management and therapy and chronically in the long-term care of those with poor recovery (13).

As discussed in detail in chapter 8 and elsewhere in this volume, GBS follows infection with only certain serostrains of *Campylobacter,* in particular the O:19 strains, which are relatively uncommonly associated with uncomplicated enteritis. In addition to *Campylobacter,* a diverse range of other infections and immunological stimuli, including most herpesviruses, respiratory viruses, mycoplasma infections, and vaccination, have been recognized as preceding the clinical onset of GBS by around 2 weeks (60). This has given rise to the working hypothesis of GBS as an autoimmune disease affecting susceptible individuals, triggered by an idiosyncratic immune reaction to infections which results in cross-reactive humoral and cytotoxic responses to components of peripheral nerve (41). *Campylobacter* was first reported as a precipitating infection for GBS almost 20 years, and the last decade, in particular, has witnessed highly significant advances toward an understanding of this complex field.

In response to the early clinical reports of GBS following *Campylobacter jejuni* and other infections, a search for antigens which might underlie a postinfectious autoimmune syndrome was undertaken. Among several lines of enquiry pursued, the most promising avenue is the possibility that antiganglioside antibodies, which are present in the acute-phase sera of

Hugh J. Willison and Graham M. O'Hanlon, University Department of Neurology, Institute of Neurological Sciences, Southern General Hospital, Glasgow G51 4TF, United Kingdom.

Campylobacter, 2nd Ed., Edited by I. Nachamkin and M. J. Blaser

GBS patients, target ganglioside-rich sites in peripheral nerve for autoimmune attack (80, 114). A strengthening of the relationship between GBS and *Campylobacter* biology emerged in the early 1990s, with the recognition that particular serostrains and isolates of *C. jejuni* bear ganglioside-like carbohydrate structures on their lipopolysaccharide (LPS) core oligosaccharides (core OSs) (6, 96, 154). This finding provided key information about the nature of the antigen(s) linking the infection and the autoimmune disease.

The merging of the two previously disparate fields of LPS structural chemistry and ganglioside immunobiology around GBS has led to a general appreciation that molecular mimicry between microbial and neural oligosaccharides is likely to be a key mediator of GBS pathogenesis, and this subject is the focus of considerable research (6, 109, 160). This chapter presents background material and current evidence about antiganglioside antibodies which both supports and contradicts this view. Other chapters in the book deal with epidemiological aspects of *C. jejuni* infection in GBS and with structural studies on LPS. Here the particular focus will therefore be on the clinical, immunological, and pathogenic aspects of antiganglioside antibodies in GBS.

GUILLAIN-BARRÉ SYNDROME: AN ENTITY EVOLVING INTO DISTINCT CLINICAL SUBTYPES

GBS has historically been considered a disease in which immune system attack principally targets the peripheral-nerve myelin sheath. Myelin is produced by Schwann cells (SCs) and comprises a spiral wrapping of multilamellar membrane, rich in glycolipids and specialized proteins, which envelopes axons in a highly controlled milieu. The junction at which adjacent SCs contact each other along the axon constitutes a structure termed the node of Ranvier. The integrity of this region, which is densely packed with ion channels, is critical for the saltatory conduction upon which rapid impulse propagation depends. Nodes of Ranvier and paranodal regions are rich in gangliosides

and are often damaged early in GBS. Because SCs can proliferate, migrate locally, and remyelinate denuded axons, the prospects for clinical recovery from demyelinating GBS have always been considered good. Historically, the pathophysiological concept of bystander or secondary axonal injury was introduced to account for the small number of GBS patients with poor long-term recovery due to permanent axonal loss and subsequent muscle atrophy due to denervation. However, in the mid-1980s, Feasby et al. first highlighted a series of GBS cases in which the axonal membrane (axolemma) itself, rather than the myelin sheath, was the primary target of immune attack. This led to the recognition of acute axonal neuropathy as a variant form of GBS (27). Although uncommon in the United States and Europe, where it represents only around 5% of GBS cases, the axonal form of GBS accounts for around 50% of the acute cases of flaccid paralysis affecting young adults and children in seasonal epidemics in rural China and is very frequently associated with *C. jejuni* enteritis (93). Other global pockets in which the frequency of this pattern of GBS is high are found in Mexico and Japan (50). The terms acute motor axonal neuropathy (AMAN) and acute motor and sensory axonal neuropathy (AMSAN) were coined to distinguish these cases from the common Western form of the disease; acute inflammatory demyelinating polyneuroapthy (AIDP) (50).

It is now appreciated that in nerve roots and trunks axonal injury can occur at the nodes of Ranvier, where the axon is relatively exposed and vulnerable to injury (37), or at the equally exposed terminal portion of the motor nerve (49). Importantly, the site of axonal injury may have a profound effect on the degree of clinical recovery: transected axons cannot locally repair themselves, but they degenerate distally and then regenerate from the site of injury to their target in order to restore functional continuity. A severe proximal axonal injury in the nerve spinal roots (potentially up to 1 m away from the target muscle) may never be able to reinnervate its target. In contrast, an equivalent injury close to the nerve terminal will produce similarly complete acute paralysis but the damaged axons can regenerate across the very short distance with relative ease. Thus, patients with AMAN can recover well or poorly depending upon both the extent and site of immune system injury, even when presenting clinically with fulminant paralysis.

In addition to categorizing GBS into demyelinating and axonal subtypes, there are important regional variants of the syndrome in which only specific nerves within the body are affected. The most common and best studied of these variants, termed Miller-Fisher syndrome (MFS), is characterized by ataxia, tendon reflex loss, and extraocular muscle paralysis (29). This produces impaired balance and an inability to move the eyes, while muscle strength in the arms and legs is entirely preserved. Many other regional variants also exist, particularly affecting cranial muscles or affecting specific nerve fiber types such as sensory or autonomic nerves (121). The importance of describing these fiber type and region-specific variants is that evidence indicates that they have distinctive immunopathologies and may be associated with particular antiganglioside antibody patterns.

GANGLIOSIDE STRUCTURE AND FUNCTION

Gangliosides are a group of over 50 structurally distinct glycosphingolipids defined by the presence of sialic acid attached to an oligosaccharide core (84, 86), and the relevant structures are shown in Table 1. Glycosphingolipids are composed of the long-chain aliphatic amine sphingosine (acylated ceramide) attached to one or more sugars (hexoses). They are amphipathic, with the hydrophobic ceramide embedded in a lipid bilayer and the hydrophilic carbohydrate structure exposed extracellularly and acting, in the context of GBS, as an antigenic determinant. Although important components of plasma membranes, glycolipids are also found in intracellular lipid compartments.

Sialic acid is a generic term for N-acylneuraminic acid; the acyl group is always acetyl in the human nervous system, as opposed to

glycolyl, which is found in other tissues and in the brains of animal species. This distinction has some relevance to the rare cases of GBS that followed "ganglioside therapy," a vogue treatment for miscellaneous diseases that is currently discredited owing to the posttreatment development of GBS in some individuals (53, 154).

Gangliosides are named according to the UIPAC-IUB commission on biochemical nomenclature (58) but are more commonly described according to the nomenclature of Svennerholm (131) by using a formula as follows: G signifies ganglio; M, D, T, and Q refer to the number of sialic acid residues (mono, di, tri, and quad, respectively); and the arabic numerals and the lowercase letters refer to the sequence of migration as determined by thin-layer chromatography. Although dependent upon the solvent system used, gangliosides tend to separate on the basis of molecular weight; those with a longer oligosaccharide core and more sialic acid migrate more slowly than the smaller gangliosides do.

Gangliosides are found throughout the body but are highly concentrated in the nervous system, particularly in neuronal cell bodies and synaptic regions of the gray matter, where the lipid-bound sialic acid comprises almost 0.1% of the wet weight of tissue (86). This is approximately 10- and 100-fold that in liver and erythrocyte membranes, respectively. In the mammalian central and peripheral nervous systems (CNS and PNS), there are four major gangliosides, GM1, GD1a, GD1b, and GT1b, and many minor gangliosides, as described in more detail below.

From a functional perspective, gangliosides regulate diverse physiological processes including modulation of neuronal and glial cell growth factor receptors, ion channels, and cell recognition/adhesion molecules. They have widespread effects on signal transduction systems, are highly enriched in synaptic regions, and modulate synaptic transmission and synaptogenesis (85, 134). They also act as receptors for a wide variety of bacterial toxins, including cholera, tetanus, and botulinum toxins and

TABLE 1 Structures of gangliosides relevant to GBS[a]

Ganglioside and glycolipid antigenic motifs	Structure[b]	Anatomical localization and immunopathological features[c]
Terminal Gal(β1–3)GalNAc-configured gangliosides	GM1, asialo-GM1, GD1b	**Glial structures:** Members of this group are present in compact myelin (20), especially small sensory fibers (103). GM1 is more abundant in VR than DR (17, 102). Areas selectively bound by ligands include Schmidt-Lanterman's incisures (95), paranodal end segments of the myelin sheath (20, 33, 34, 74, 78, 95), nodal gap (125), and abaxonal SC cytoplasm (95). **Neuronal structures:** Ligand binding was observed with motor neurons (21, 91), at the nodal axonal surface (33), at the neuromuscular junction (81, 82, 103, 104, 126, 136), and to DRG neurons (78, 91, 103, 104). **Other:** Ligand binding was observed to muscle spindles (104) and a series of Gal-GalNAc–bearing glycoproteins (3, 20, 90, 135).
Gangliosides with an (α2–8)-linked disialosyl group	GT1a, GD1b, GQ1b, GT1b, GD3, GD2	**Glial structures:** GD1b and GQ1b are enriched in the paranodal myelin (16, 70, 74, 78, 125). Anti-GD2 antibodies label the myelin sheath (162). GQ1b is enriched in the cranial nerves serving the extraocular muscle (17). **Neuronal structures:** Abundant in cultured DRG neurons (14). Antibodies bind DRG neurons (78, 91, 102, 104, 142) and are able to lyse them (105). Antibodies bind the NMJ and can disrupt normal function (11, 146). **Others:** Muscle spindles are stained strongly by an antibody to polysialylated ganglio-sides (146).

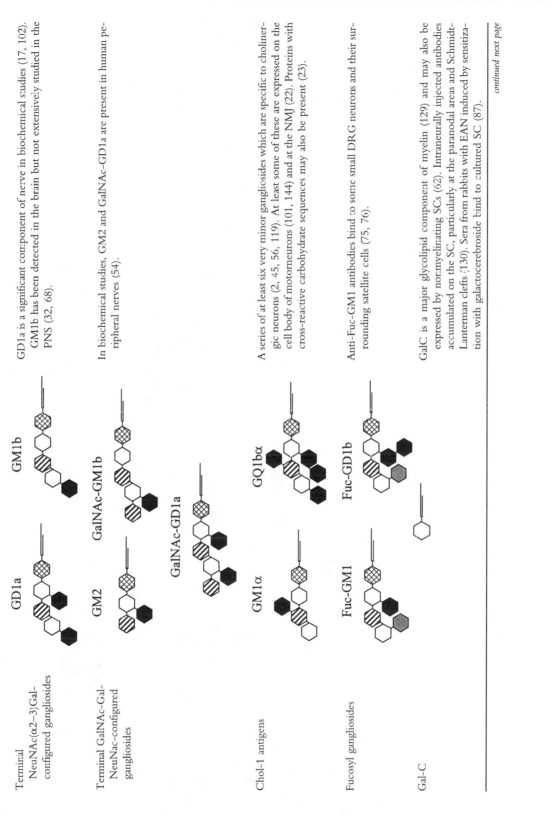

Terminal NeuNAc(α2–3)Gal-configured gangliosides

GD1a is a significant component of nerve in biochemical studies (17, 102). GM1b has been detected in the brain but not extensively studied in the PNS (32, 68).

Terminal GalNAc-Gal-NeuNac-configured gangliosides

In biochemical studies, GM2 and GalNAc-GD1a are present in human peripheral nerves (54).

Chol-1 antigens

A series of at least six very minor gangliosides which are specific to cholinergic neurons (2, 45, 56, 119). At least some of these are expressed on the cell body of motorneurons (101, 144) and at the NMJ (22). Proteins with cross-reactive carbohydrate sequences may also be present (23).

Fucosyl gangliosides

Anti-Fuc-GM1 antibodies bind to some small DRG neurons and their surrounding satellite cells (75, 76).

Gal-C

GalC is a major glycolipid component of myelin (129) and may also be expressed by normyelinating SCs (62). Intraneurally injected antibodies accumulated on the SC, particularly at the paranodal areas and Schmidt-Lanterman clefts (130). Sera from rabbits with EAN induced by sensitization with galactocerebroside bind to cultured SC (87).

continued next page

TABLE 1 (continued)

Ganglioside and glycolipid antigenic motifs	Structure[b]	Anatomical localization and immunopathological features[c]
Sulfatide		**Glial and neuronal structures:** In peripheral nerve, the most common sites in antibody binding studies include axons, resident macrophages or SC cytoplasm, especially the Schmidt-Lanterman incisures and nodes of Ranvier, and the perineuronal sheath of satellite cells in DRG (89, 99, 116). Sural biopsy specimens from patients with these antibodies show IgM and complement product C3d bound to the myelin sheaths of almost all fibers (28).
LM1		A significant component of both sensory and motor nerves (17, 105). Absent from several cranial nerves displaying CNS characteristics e.g. optic nerve (17).
SGPG/SGLPG		Neuropathy-associated antibodies cross-react with MAG (115) and the myelin proteins Po and HNK-1 (9, 12). Sural biopsy specimens from patients with these antibodies show deposits within the myelin sheath and signs of demyelination (140). SGPG and SGLPG are found by biochemical analysis in the myelin and axons of peripheral nerve (5, 19, 67). MAG is localized to regions of the myelin sheath in which the membranes are uncompacted, including the periaxonal membrane, the paranode, and Schmidt-Lanterman incisures (92, 138). Non-MAG-reactive antibodies bind at the outer surface of myelin sheaths. Faint staining is also visible at the axolemma/myelin interface, but compact myelin is not stained (150).

[a] The groupings described in this table are illustrative of cross-reactive epitopes reported in the literature but are not intended to be a definitive list. Gangliosides have common structural motifs outside of those presented here, and it should be noted that even within the presented groupings an individual ganglioside, e.g., GD1b, can fall within two or more groups. Equally, the fact that two ganglioside species appear in the same group does not necessarily imply that an antibody to one will cross-react with the others (104). Glycolipids which appear dissimilar when presented as in the table may adopt tertiary structures which display common motifs, and through the same process, similar-appearing structures may be antigenically different.

[b] Symbols:

Gal NeuNAc GalNAc Glu Fuc GlcNAc Glc UA Ceramide

[c] VR, ventral root; DR, dorsal root; MAG, myelin-associated glycoprotein.

Escherichia coli enterotoxin (30). On the cellular level, they influence cell survival, differentiation, and neuritogenesis (85, 149). It has been widely postulated, but has yet to be firmly established on an experimental level, that antiganglioside antibodies might exert some of their pathogenic effects in GBS through pharmacological effects of ganglioside-modulated functions, such as ion channel or growth factor receptor modulation, rather than solely through proinflammatory injury.

Although antiganglioside antibodies are the main focus of attention in post-*Campylobacter* GBS, antibodies to nonganglioside glycolipids including galactocerebroside (GalC), sulfatide, and sulfated glucuronyl paragloboside (SGPG), may also be important in neuropathy following other pathogenic infections (Table 1). The most structurally simple glycolipids, termed cerebrosides, comprise a single hexose linked to ceramide (i.e., monohexosyl-ceramide), of which the most abundant in humans is galacto-cerebroside (i.e., galactosyl-ceramide [GalC]). Sulfatide is GalC sulfated in the C-3 position and both are component of peripheral nerve myelin. Paragloboside is a neutral glycolipid, Gal(β1-4)GlcNAc(β1-3)Gal(β1-4)Glu(β1-1)Cer, which, when sialylated (α2-3) on the terminal galactose (i.e., sialosylparagloboside [SGP]), constitutes a major peripheral nerve glycolipid, LM1. Substitution of the terminal sialic acid of LM1 for 3-sulphated glucuronic acid forms sulfated glucuronyl paragloboside (SGPG). A higher lactosaminyl-containing homologue of SGPG, termed SGLPG, also exists. Both SGPG and SPLPG are enriched in peripheral nerve and are important antigens for neuropathy-associated antibodies (114).

ANTIGANGLIOSIDE ANTIBODIES

Antiganglioside antibodies were first found in 5 of 26 patients with GBS (19%) reported by Ilyas et al. in 1988 (55). This study was performed on the basis that anti-glycolipid antibodies had been identified in patients with chronic demyelinating polyneuropathies, particularly those associated with immunoglobulin IgM paraproteinemia (80, 114), and in patients

with multifocal motor neuropathy (112). Our knowledge of antiglycolipid antibodies in chronic neuropathies is extensive and has many interesting parallels to GBS, including possible relationships with *Campylobacter* infection (110, 139). Since then, a wealth of new information covering different aspects of this area has become available. Antibodies to a wide range of gangliosides including GM1 (163), GM1(NeuGc) (101), GM1b (77), GalNAc-GM1b (159), GD1a (161), GalNAc-GD1a (73), GD1b (145), 9-O-acetyl-GD1b (48), GD3 (145), GT1a (16, 94), GT1b (55), GQ1b (18), GQ1bα (132), LM1 (31), GalC (72), and SGPG (157) have been reported in over 200 papers on GBS and other inflammatory neuropathies, as case reports and in larger series. Analyzing this literature is not for the faint-hearted, and before we attempt an overview, we need to emphasize several points. First, antiganglioside antibodies assays, based principally on enzyme-linked immunosorbent assay methodology, are fraught with operational difficulties, with variables including antigen source and purity, timing of clinical sampling, details of assay method, and definition of normal ranges for reporting of results. Some attempts have been made to measure interlaboratory variables and to standardize methods, and they highlight these difficulties (148, 165). Second, the epidemiological patterns of antiganglioside antibodies may vary substantially among geographic regions, according to the prevalent subtypes of GBS and their relation to preceding infections. As alluded to above, the presence of antiganglioside antibodies in patients with GBS is not solely associated with *Campylobacter* infection but also occurs with other bacterial and viral infections. Furthermore, the structural mimicry between sialic acid epitopes on *Campylobacter* and gangliosides is restricted to particular serotypes with marked geographic differences in distribution. There may also be host susceptibility factors controlling the immune response to sialylated epitopes that are specifically related to individuals and/or populations with particular genetic or environmental backgrounds. In much of the literature on antiganglioside antibodies, the relation to preceding infection is not known or recorded, and clinical details of the GBS cases are sparse. Some of the most significant papers in this area have come from antiganglioside antibody analysis of sera collected as part of carefully controlled clinical studies and trials, rather than analysis of random sera collected for measurement by a referral laboratory (61, 118).

ANTIBODIES ASSOCIATED WITH PREDOMINANTLY MOTOR FORMS OF GUILLAIN-BARRÉ SYNDROME

GBS in the United States and Europe, being predominantly of the AIDP pattern, usually presents clinically with a combination of weakness and sensory symptoms, corresponding to immunopathological involvement of motor and sensory nerves, respectively. However, a proportion of patients have purely motor symptoms, and electrophysiological studies indicate exclusive or highly preferential injury to the motor system, with preservation of sensory nerves. In many of these patients, there is evidence of motor axonal dysfunction with preservation of the myelin properties of the nerve; i.e., the speed of conduction is normal but the number of functional axons is severely reduced. This pattern of GBS is referred to as purely or predominantly motor GBS, and many cases would also be classifiable as AMAN, according to the clinical and electrophysiological definition (39). The first clinical-serological association to emerge was that between anti-GM1 ganglioside antibodies and these purely motor forms of GBS with prominent axonal involvement, published initially as case reports (36, 154) and subsequently in larger series of patients. The early clinical series confirmed the presence of anti-GM1 antibodies in GBS (26, 141), and subsequent reports indicated that anti-GM1 IgG antibodies are associated with motor forms of GBS. These cases involved prominent axonal degeneration and had a severe clinical course with incomplete recovery, particularly when preceded by *Campylobacter* infection (61, 118). However, this relationship is not exclusive, since patients with anti-GM1

antibodies and precedent *Campylobacter* infection are found within an AIDP population who demonstrate good recovery. The prevalence of anti-GM1 antibodies in GBS patients varies from study to study, ranging from 0 to 80%, reflecting diverse variables including the prevalence of *Campylobacter* infection in the study population and the method used for antibody measurement. In the United States and Europe, approximately 20% of GBS patients have such antibodies. The issue of the cross-reactivity of anti-GM1 antibodies with other terminal Gal(β1-3)GalNAc-bearing glycolipids, including GA1 and GD1b, and the possible relationship of this cross-reactivity to clinical phenotype is incompletely resolved.

Anti-GD1a antibodies are also found in patients with GBS and occur in those with AMAN to a greater extent than in those with AIDP. This was first identified in case report form by Yuki et al. (164) and subsequently confirmed in larger studies (15). In a series of 138 AMAN and AIDP GBS patients from China, 60% of AMAN but only 4% of AIDP patients had anti-GD1a antibodies. Serological evidence of recent *Campylobacter* infection was present in 81% of AMAN and 50% of AIDP patients, and anti-GD1a antibodies were found in both the *Campylobacter*-infected and noninfected groups (51). In addition, antibodies to other gangliosides including GM1, GD1b, and GalNAc-GD1a were present in this patient population, including the anti-GD1a-positive AMAN patients. Notwithstanding this overlap, a strong statistical association between AMAN and anti-GD1a antibodies was observed.

In 1994, Kusonoki et al. reported that 6 of 50 GBS patients in a study had antibodies to GalNAc-GD1a (73). All these patients had post-*Campylobacter* GBS, and electrophysiological studies suggested the presence of motor axonal degeneration. The clinical outcome of these cases was variable. GalNAc-GD1a had previously been reported as a neuropathy-associated antigen in a patient with IgM paraproteinemia in which the antibody also reacted with GalNAc-GM1b and GM2, which share a terminal trisaccharide with GalNAc-GD1a (54). However, in the GBS patients reported, the IgG anti-GalNAc-GD1a antibodies did not cross-react with these other antigens, although some IgM reactivity with GM2 was observed in two of six patients. In a further series of GBS patients reported by Yuki et al. 8 of 58 had anti-GalNAc-GD1a antibodies which also reacted with GalNAc-GM1b. All these cases had preceding *Campylobacter* infection and, in the four patients where the organism was isolated from stool culture, the LPS was shown in absorption studies to contain a GalNAc-GD1a epitope (159). Although biochemical studies have shown GalNAc-GD1a, GalNAc-GM1b and GM2 to be present in the human PNS, the immunolocalization has not yet been demonstrated (54).

The minor ganglioside GM1b has also been identified as an antigen in 22 of 104 and 20 of 99 GBS patients in two series reported from Japan (77, 158, 159). Again, these cases were of the AMAN phenotype, often associated with *Campylobacter,* and the isolated organism from one patient contained the GM1b epitope, as demonstrated with an anti-GM1b monoclonal antibody. Many of these patients also had antibodies to other gangliosides including GM1, GD1a, and the minor ganglioside GM1α. The pathogenic significance of these antibodies is unknown. Such cases are likely to be very uncommon in the United States and Europe, due to the low frequency of AMAN compared with AIDP.

MILLER FISHER SYNDROME

Since the report of Chiba et al. in 1992 describing the presence of anti-GQ1b antibodies in patients with MFS (16, 18), our knowledge of this syndrome has advanced considerably, and it now stands out as the prototypic antiganglioside antibody-mediated neuropathy within the GBS spectrum. In its purest form, MFS is characterized by paralysis affecting only the extraocular muscles, and this is accompanied by ataxia and areflexia. However, many patients with MFS also have weakness of the face and bulbar muscles, and in other cases the ataxia

may be modest or absent. In addition, the condition termed Bickerstaff's brain stem encephalitis refers to an MFS-like syndrome accompanied by CNS dysfunction, including impaired consciousness or coma, and these patients may be GQ1b antibody positive (65, 153). Some cases of MFS commence typically and then proceed to a more confluent GBS-like picture with limb weakness, and the reverse pattern may also occur. Thus, some latitude is required when considering the definition of MFS, especially since all these clinical variations have in common the presence of anti-GQ1b antibodies in more than 90% of patients, an antibody absent from control populations (Fig. 1). The anti-GQ1b antibodies in MFS patients commonly cross-react with GT1a, and a further 50% demonstrate reactivity with other gangliosides containing a disialosyl epitope, such as GD3, GD1b, and occasionally GT1b (Fig. 2). As discussed below, GQ1b is enriched in extraocular nerves compared with limb nerves, and these findings provide the strongest evidence to

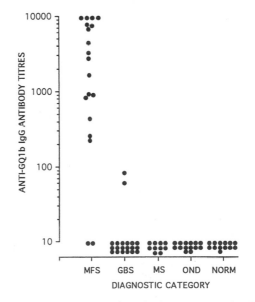

FIGURE 1 Anti-GQ1b antibodies in MFS. Of MFS patients, 90% have elevated titers of anti-GQ1b IgG antibodies. Occasionally, low titers of anti-GQ1b IgG are found in GBS patients but are absent from patients with multiple sclerosis (MS), other neurological diseases (OND), and healthy controls (NORM).

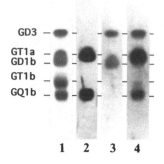

GD3

GT1a
GD1b

GT1b

GQ1b

1   2   3   4

FIGURE 2 Thin-layer chromatography immunooverlay of antiganglioside antibody-containing sera showing the typical patterns of reactivity seen in MFS. Five purified gangliosides (GD3, GT1a, GD1b, GT1b, and GQ1b) (1 μg of each per lane) were immunostained as follows: lane 1, serum (diluted 1/500) from a patient with a chronic ataxic neuropathy, which reacts with all five chromatographed gangliosides; lane 2, serum (1/200) from an MFS patient, which reacts with only GQ1b and GT1a; lane 3, serum (1/200) from a patient with acute ataxic neuropathy without ophthalmoplegia or other motor involvement, which reacts only with GD3 and GD1b; lane 4, serum (1/200) from an MFS patient, which reacts with GQ1b, GT1a, and GD3 and very weakly with GD1b and GT1b. Reprinted from reference 145 with permission.

date that the regionality of clinical syndromes is linked to the regional distribution of gangliosides (17).

Some evidence suggests that GQ1b antibodies may account for ophthalmoplegia, GT1a for bulbar paralysis, and GD1b/GD3 for ataxia, and although this is unlikely to be an absolute phenomenon, it may reflect proportional differences in the ganglioside composition of neural sites subserving these functions (64, 66, 94, 107).

MFS frequently follows *Campylobacter* enteritis but is also associated with other preceding infections including upper respiratory tract viral infections. *Campylobacter* isolates from MFS patients have been studied by spectroscopic analysis of LPS structures and by immunohistological probing with human and murine sera and monoclonal antibodies reactive with GQ1b and related structures. These stud-

ies have demonstrated that GD3- and GT1a-like OS and GQ1b cross-reactive epitopes are present in MFS-associated *Campylobacter* LPSs, again supporting a molecular-mimicry hypothesis for antibody induction (59, 123, 154).

OTHER SYNDROMES

The clinical syndrome of acute ataxic neuropathy in the absence of motor involvement is associated with anti-GD1b antibodies in some patients (145, 155). In addition, a chronic neuropathy syndrome with prominent ataxia is associated with this antibody specificity (146). Both findings correlate well with the work of Kusonoki et al., described below, in which rabbits immunized with GD1b develop clinical ataxia and pathological changes in the dorsal root and dorsal root ganglion (DRG). The minor ganglioside GQ1bα may also be an important antigen in some cases of acute ataxic neuropathy (132), consistent with its localization in lamina I and II of the thoracic dorsal horn (71), the former of which contains propriospinal fibers.

GBS ASSOCIATED WITH INFECTIONS OTHER THAN *CAMPYLOBACTER*

In patients with GBS with a precedent infection other than *Campylobacter,* associations of clinical phenotype with a particular antiganglioside antibody profile are also emerging. The association between cytomegalovirus (CMV) infection and GBS is long recognized and has recently been linked with anti-GM2 antibodies (57, 60, 98, 156). The GM2 antibodies may react with other gangliosides containing similar carbohydrate structures and fall into several patterns: reactivity with GM2, GA2, and GD2; reactivity with GM2 and GM1; and reactivity with GM2 and GalNAc-GD1a. Patients with CMV-associated GBS have prominent sensory symptoms and cranial nerve involvement which is more probably due to the nature of the infection than to the presence of anti-GM2 antibodies: however, this remains to be clarified. It is thought that the cross-reactive epitope is a GM2-like glycoprotein which may be acquired by CMV during intracellular assembly (156). *Mycoplasma pneumonia* infection preceding GBS is reported in association with anti-GalC antibodies (72). The significance of finding antibodies to Ga1C lies in the experimental demonstration that they are capable of inducing morphological and electrophysiological evidence of demyelination. To date, other infections have not been specifically linked to particular patterns of antiganglioside antibodies in case-control studies (40, 60).

MOLECULAR MIMICRY AND ANTI-GANGLIOSIDE ANTIBODY INDUCTION

Molecular mimicry between microbial and self components has been extensively promoted as a mechanism to account for the antigen and tissue specificity of immune responses in postinfectious autoimmune diseases (122). This model applies to humoral and cell-mediated antipeptide responses, in addition to antibody responses to carbohydrate structures. Since the demonstration that *Campylobacter* LPS can mimic GM1 ganglioside (7, 8, 127, 160) and the studies describing GT1a- and GD3-like LPS structures, this principle has been widely accepted as central to the pathogenesis of GBS (109, 154).

Although the data suggest that antiganglioside antibodies in post-*Campylobacter* GBS arise through molecular mimicry, other explanations remain possible. T-cell-mediated attack on peripheral nerve may lead to inflammatory destruction of neural tissue, as occurs in the principal animal model of GBS, experimental allergic neuritis, with subsequent induction of antiganglioside antibodies as a secondary event (42). It is also possible that antiganglioside antibodies, forming a component of the natural autoantibody repertoire, could be expanded nonspecifically by LPS acting as a polyclonal B-cell activator, rather than via core OS antigen-specific B-cell receptor cross-linking. This ganglioside-reactive B-cell pool might be expected to produce low-affinity IgM antibodies, since gangliosides are widely distributed throughout the body, and there should be a high degree of B-cell tolerance to ganglioside-mimicking core OS structure.

In patients with GBS, irrespective of whether anti-ganglioside antibodies are pathogenic, tolerance to self-gangliosides is broken. The mechanisms by which this occurs have not been addressed experimentally to any extent. Serum antiganglioside and anti-core OS antibodies arise 10 to 14 days postinfection and decay rapidly in the serum of GBS patients, suggestive of a primary immune response (Fig. 3). The antibodies are of IgM, IgA, and IgG classes, but are dominated by subclass-restricted IgG1 and/or IgG3. This is an uncommon subclass pattern for anticarbohydrate antibodies which (in humans) are normally IgM and, if switching occurs, IgG2 (38, 147). These features indicate dependence on T-cell help in the induction of antiganglioside antibodies in GBS, rather than a purely T-independent origin, as is usually associated with OS antigens, including LPS. Little work has been performed to date on determining the nature of the T-cell response to *Campylobacter* protein antigens that might provide this T-cell help for anticarbohydrate antibody responses or the role of lipid A in this immune system activation, either in humans or in experimental models of *Campylobacter* infection (83, 97).

GANGLIOSIDE LOCALIZATION IN THE PERIPHERAL NERVOUS SYSTEM

Gangliosides are developmentally regulated and spatially segregated, varying among different peripheral nerve types and among different species. A complete map of the ganglioside composition of human nerve and a comparison among species used for experimental modeling would be a valuable resource but is not yet available in its entirety. As indicated above, the pattern of antiganglioside activity detected in a patient's serum correlates to some extent with the clinical pattern of GBS, suggesting a differential distribution of target gangliosides throughout the PNS. However, in terms of factors which influence the development of neuropathic change, not only is the absolute distribution of target gangliosides important,

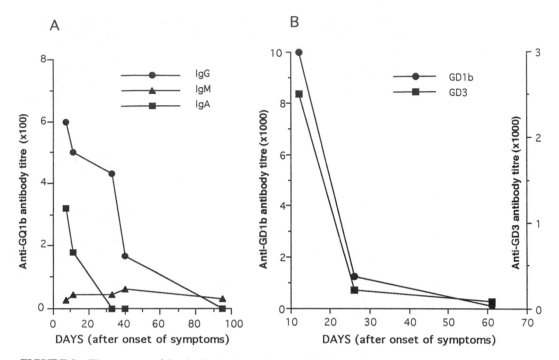

FIGURE 3 Time course of the decline in titer of antiganglioside antibodies in MFS patients. (A) Five serial samples from an MFS patient show a fall in IgA and IgG anti-GQ1b antibody titers in serum to undetectable levels over 30 and 90 days respectively. IgM anti-GQ1b antibodies were not detected. (B) Anti-GD1b and anti-GD3 IgG antibodies from a patient with acute ataxic neuropathy are highest at clinical presentation and fall concomitantly during the course of the illness. Both patients made complete and rapid clinical recoveries.

but the accessibility of those gangliosides to circulating antibodies, being protected in their neural environment by the blood–nerve barrier is also important. Certainly one explanation of the lack of CNS symptoms in GBS patients would be the protection from autoimmune attack afforded by the blood–brain barrier. It is generally assumed that the blood–nerve barrier has to be breached for the full development of GBS, which would thus allow antibody access to normally cryptic sites. This may also be mediated by antiganglioside antibodies, since it has been suggested that immunological targeting of glycolipid antigens on intraneural microvascular endothelial cells can induce the destruction or malfunction of the blood–nerve barrier (63).

In addition to localization and accessibility, ganglioside function within a given structure may influence the nature and development of antibody-mediated injury (149, 152). The calcium binding properties of gangliosides have been demonstrated in several model membrane systems, and it is possible that one function is to chelate extracellular calcium: this may be of relevance to nerve terminal injury (113). Gangliosides also affect membrane fluidity and may form microdomains in phospholipid membranes, suggesting a role in vesicle fusion. In addition, they interact with membrane proteins, including ion channels, and activate second-messenger systems (137). Thus, the pathogenic role of antiganglioside antibodies is likely to depend not only on how they affect the number and distribution of gangliosides but also on the extent to which the target gangliosides are intimately involved in modulating the function of neuronal proteins. Additionally, activated complement components may in turn affect the normal functioning of ganglioside-associated proteins. Furthermore, the relative contribution of these factors may vary from site to site, and between antiganglioside antibodies of differing reactivity.

Historically, there have been two approaches to establishing the anatomical distribution of ganglioside species, and each has its merits and limitations. First, biochemical analysis has been useful in identifying significant differences in the ganglioside composition of different nerves and can reveal subtle differences in the overall lipid composition. However, this approach is limited by the size of a structure that can be cleanly dissected from its surroundings, and no information can be obtained about the microscopic distribution of gangliosides within a tissue. In such circumstances, the second approach, that of immunohistology or other in situ ligand binding studies (e.g., with ganglioside binding bacterial toxins such as cholera toxin), can reveal fine-structure detail about ganglioside distribution on the cellular and subcellular level. With whole-serum studies such as those conducted with sera from GBS patients, the signal from non-antiganglioside antibody components of the sera complicates interpretation, and it is thus preferable to use affinity-purified antisera or monoclonal antibodies. Furthermore, many antiganglioside antibodies are not monospecific but may cross-react with structurally similar gangliosides and other glycoconjugate antigens, making interpretation of ganglioside localization difficult. The antigen density and the surrounding lipid environment can also markedly influence the ability of antiganglioside antibodies to bind; thus, failure to detect a ganglioside by immunohistology does not necessarily indicate its biochemical absence (69, 88, 111).

Both biochemical and immunohistological approaches may expose gangliosides which normally occupy cryptic sites (e.g., within compact myelin) by homogenization or tissue sectioning and can thus misrepresent the ganglioside array which would be visible to circulating antibodies in physiological environments. Furthermore, gangliosides can be heterogeneously distributed within a membrane and can form "functional rafts" into which proteins such as growth factor receptors or ion channels are specifically included or excluded (128). Such local concentrations of gangliosides may allow for good immunohistological detection, whereas a ganglioside which is evenly distributed throughout a membrane may show the same total concentration in tissue in biochemical evaluation yet not be detectable by immunohistology.

Interpretation of both biochemical and immunohistological studies thus requires caution. With this background in mind, key points about the tissue distribution of gangliosides of relevance to GBS are summarized below and in Fig. 4.

Ganglioside Composition of Motor and Sensory Nerves

The most simplistic explanation for antiganglioside antibody-associated neuropathies being confined to a motor or sensory clinical phenotype is that the two systems are composed of different gangliosides, and this issue has been addressed in several experimental studies. A comparison of total ganglioside composition of human spinal roots showed that GM1 (associated with antibodies in motor neuropathy) is relatively enriched in the ventral (motor) root compared with the dorsal (sensory) root (17, 102). Similarly, the cranial motor nerves supplying the extraocular muscles displayed a particularly high content of GQ1b, a ganglioside associated with antibodies in the ophthalmoplegia of MFS (17), compared with other cranial or spinal nerves. However, from these studies it is also apparent that key gangliosides are also present at sites unaffected by the disease process. Thus, the absolute tissue distribution of gangliosides is an insufficient explanation for the regional localization of the clinical pathology.

The Chol-1 antigen, so termed because it is specifically associated with cholinergic neurons (i.e., motor neurons but not sensory dorsal root ganglion neurons in the PNS), comprises a series of very minor gangliosides including GM1α, GD1aα, GT1aα GT1bα, GQ1bα (2,

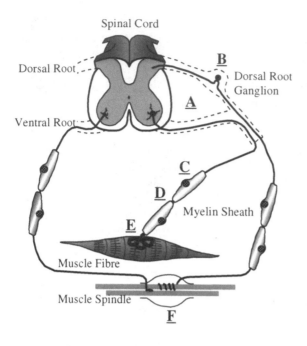

FIGURE 4 Schematic diagram of the main PNS structures and their spinal origins. Regions which are potentially vulnerable to antiganglioside antibody attack or are locations at which differential motor or sensory symptoms could be generated are indicated as follows. A, The motor and sensory systems display fundamental differences in ganglioside composition. B, DRG sensory neuron subpopulations express different carbohydrates on their surface. C, The SC surface expresses ganglioside antigens. D, Specialized structures at the node of Ranvier, of both glial and neuronal origin, have their own patterns of ganglioside expression. E, The neuromuscular junction lies outside the blood-nerve barrier, relies heavily on membrane turnover for normal functioning, and expresses ganglioside antigens. F, The muscle spindle is a sensory organelle subserving proprioception and the gamma-reflex loop. It contains both motor and sensory nerve terminals and expresses ganglioside antigens.

45, 56, 119), and, possibly, cross-reactive glycoproteins (23). At least some of these antigens are present on the neuronal cell body (100, 144) and at the neuromuscular junction (22), although their presence or absence at the nodes of Ranvier has not been noted. Evidence of developmental regulation (22) suggests a specific function for these gangliosides. In the periphery, such antigens would make strong candidates for motor-specific targets (158).

Dorsal Root Ganglion

Functional subpopulations of DRG neurons can be distinguished by the expression of lacto-series and globo-series carbohydrates on their surface, in a manner which correlates with peptide and enzymatic phenotype (24, 25). It is possible that ganglio-series antigens are distributed in a similar fashion and that differences in distribution underlie the specific nature of sensory deficits. In the rodent DRG, the GM1 ligand cholera toxin B (CTB) and anti-GM1 antibodies selectively identified a subset of DRG neurons (104). In the human DRG, CTB and GM1-reactive antibodies bound all neurons (103) (Fig. 5), and anti-GD1b antibodies bound to the vast majority (78, 91). However, an antiserum to fucosylated gangliosides was found to label a subpopulation of DRG neurons (75, 76, 151) but not components of the motor system (151), suggesting that these antigens may be an important differential marker in the human system.

Polysialylated gangliosides, especially those with an α2-8-configured disialosyl group (GD1b, GT1b, GQ1b, GD3, and GD2), were the most prominent gangliosides in cultured DRG neurons (14), and antibodies recognizing these gangliosides were able to lyse such cells (105). An anti-GD2 antibody, which when used in clinical trials as an antitumor agent was found to cause sensory neuropathy, also labeled a subpopulation of canine and rodent DRG neurons (142).

Schwann Cell Cytoplasmic Membranes

Ganglioside antigens present on the abaxonal surface of myelinating or nonmyelinating SCs may be targets for antibody-mediated damage

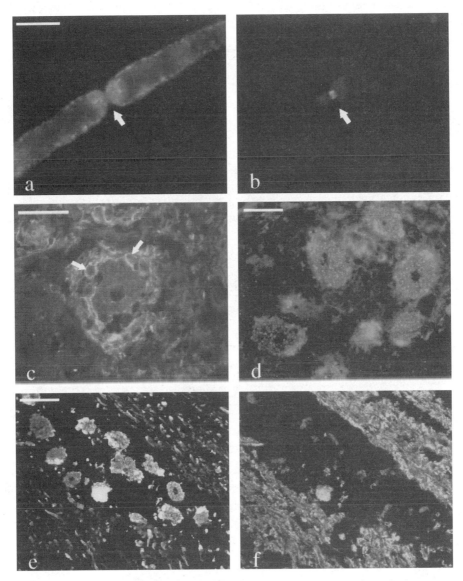

FIGURE 5 (a and b) The human anti-GM1 monoclonal antibody Wo1 displays strong binding to mouse paranodal myelin (a), with weaker labeling of the SC surface. The nodal gap (b; arrows), stained with an antibody against sodium channels in the axolemma (a gift from S. R. Levenson), is not particularly selected by Wo1. Scale bar, 10 μm. (c) The satellite cells surrounding a human DRG neuron are strongly stained by the GM1 ligand CTB (arrows), while the neuron itself displays weak cytoplasmic staining (103). Scale bar, 50 μm. Reprinted from reference 103 with permission. (d) In contrast, a human antibody reactive with polysialy-lated gangliosides (HaRCE) gives strong staining of the neuronal cytoplasm, but the satellite cells are unstained. Scale bar, 50 μm. (e and f) An anti-GM1 antibody (Br1) did not bind neurons (stained for neurofilament in panel e) but strongly stained the myelin of associated nerve fibre bundles (f) Scale bar, 100 μm.

through direct inflammatory injury or disruption of the SC physiological integrity. Weak labeling of this region was observed with CTB (33, 95, 104), but areas where the SC cytoplasm is abundant, such as the Schmidt-Lanterman's incisures and paranodal loops, were more strongly CTB reactive. The lectin peanut agglutinin, which reacts with the Gal(β1-3)GalNAc terminal structure common to asialo-GM1, GM1, and GD1b, also stained the SC surface (20). The internodal SC surface is also rich in polysialogangliosides, which could be converted to GM1 by neuraminidase treatment (34) but which were not bound by tetanus toxin (TTx), a ligand which binds primarily to GD1b and GQ1b (33).

Node of Ranvier

The node of Ranvier is a key site of injury in autoimmune neuropathy, being a highly specialized and active structure within the peripheral nerve. Autoimmune attack directed at antigenic determinants located on the paranodal SC may lead to demyelination, whereas antigens targeted to the exposed axolemma may result in axonal degeneration; both of these scenarios would result in conduction failure. Ligand binding studies have suggested that GM1 (20, 34, 95) and GD1b (74, 78, 125) are enriched in the paranodal myelin loops of peripheral nerves (Fig. 5). In oculomotor cranial nerves, GQ1b is particularly enriched at nodes of Ranvier (16, 70), but polysialylated gangliosides can be also be detected by antibody and TTx binding studies at the nodes in somatic nerves (33, 146).

With respect to neuronal components of the node of Ranvier, GM1 is present on the cytoplasmic surface of motorneurons (21) and GM1 and TTx binding gangliosides have been identified on paranodal and internodal axolemma (33) and the adaxonal membrane (95). Similarly, an antibody reactive with disialosyl gangliosides bound to the internodal axolemma and/or adaxonal SC cytoplasm (146).

In addition to the gangliosides identified above, Gal-GalNAc-bearing glycoproteins have been identified on motorneurons (90),

the paranodal region (3), and the nodal gap (3, 20) and in a biochemically isolated axonal fraction of peripheral nerve (135).

Neuromuscular Junction

The neuromuscular junction (NMJ) is also a target vulnerable to autoimmune attack in GBS since it lies outside the blood-nerve barrier, is rich in gangliosides, and is dependent upon rapid turnover of membrane for normal functioning. Many bacterial toxins that use gangliosides as ectoacceptors also act at this site. CTB is readily taken up into nerve terminals, loaded into synaptic vesicles (106), and ultimately transported back to the motor neuron cell body (46, 143), suggesting that GM1 is involved in membrane recycling. As a result of this property, enzymic conjugates of CTB are frequently used as retrograde neuronal markers (46, 143). Therefore, as expected, histological analyses demonstrated CTB and anti-GM1/GD1b antibody binding to the NMJ (81, 82, 103, 104, 126, 135) (Fig. 6). Antibodies reactive to polysialylated gangliosides also bound to the NMJ (Fig. 6) and disrupted normal function (11, 113, 146). The neurotoxic actions of botulinum toxins and TTx also depend on ganglioside binding and subsequent uptake into the NMJ (117).

As described above, at least some of the α-series gangliosides specific to cholinergic neurons (Chol-1 antigens) are expressed at the mature NMJ (22), which may make them significant targets in the generation of motor neuropathy.

Muscle Spindles

Muscle spindles are proprioceptive transducers located within the muscle, and they form an integral part of the gamma reflex loop. They contain specialized muscle fibers which have motor innervation and which are encircled by a sensory ending. Since NMJs are present in spindles, the points covered in the section above may also apply here. The neural components of spindles were labeled with CTB and GM1/GD1b-binding antibodies (104), and in addition, CTB labeled the spindle capsule (104) (Fig. 6). Furthermore, an antibody to dis-

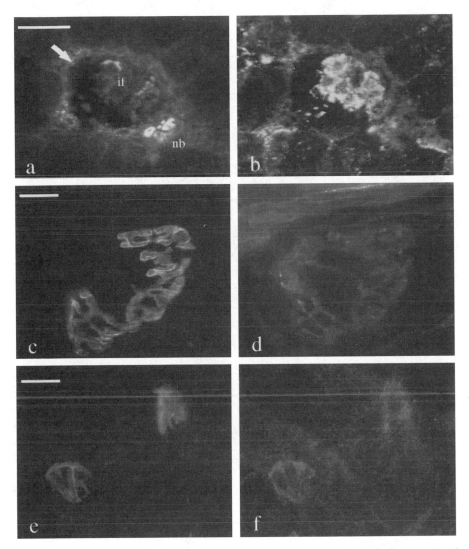

FIGURE 6 (a and b) CTB binds to the capsule of a mouse muscle spindle (a; arrow) and to neuronal structures around the intrafusal fibers (if) and the spindle-associated nerve bundle (nb). The human antibody reactive with polysialylated gangliosides, HaRCE, strongly stains the intrafusal fibres and associated neuronal structures (b). Scale bar, 25 μm. Reprinted from reference 146 with permission. (c) The mouse NMJ is delineated by α-bungarotoxin (BTx), which binds the postsynaptic terminal. (d) Both the NMJ and associated motor nerve are bound by CTB. Scale bar, 20 μm. (e and f) HaRCE (f) also binds the NMJ (labeled with BTx and an antibody against neurofilament) (e). Scale bar, 20 μm.

ialylated gangliosides which disrupted NMJ function also bound strongly to the intrafusal fibers of the spindle (146) (Fig. 6). Thus, muscle spindles may be an important target in GBS, and injury to them could account for stretch reflex changes.

PATHOGENESIS STUDIES AND ANIMAL MODELS OF GUILLAIN-BARRÉ SYNDROME

Evidence to support a direct role for antiganglioside antibodies in inflammatory neuropathy is beginning to emerge from a variety of experimental studies (146). These studies represent early steps toward generating an antiganglioside antibody-mediated animal model of GBS, to stand alongside the myelin protein-specific T-cell-mediated model of GBS termed experimental allergic neuritis (43). However, proving a role for antiganglioside antibodies in experimental models of disease has been technically difficult and controversial. In relation to anti-GM1 antibodies, passive transfer of antibody into animal nerves has been shown to cause electrophysiological abnormalities and demyelination in some studies (124) but not in others (44). Similarly, incubation of isolated nerve preparations with anti-GM1 antibodies in vitro has produced acute conduction block of myelinated nerve fibers in some studies (4, 133) but, again, not in others (47), despite deposition of anti-GM1 antibody and complement activation products at nodes of Ranvier in experimental nerves (108) (Fig. 7).

With respect to MFS syndrome, anti-GQ1b antibody-positive sera from MFS patients have been shown to cause an increase in spontaneous quantal acetylcholine release (as demonstrated by recording an increase in miniature end plate potential frequencies) at the NMJ of mouse hemidiaphragm preparations that is shortly followed by neuromuscular paralysis (120). In macro-patch clamp studies on the same preparation, the IgG fraction from an anti-GQ1b-positive MFS patient has been shown to block evoked acetylcholine release and depress the amplitude of postsynaptic potentials (10, 11). However, similar findings were observed with anti-GQ1b-negative MFS IgG, indicating that these latter electrophysiological perturbations may not be due to the antiganglioside antibody component of sera from patients with acute-phase MFS. A more recent study combining immunohistological and electrophysiological techniques has demonstrated that anti-GQ1b antibodies bind motor nerve terminals, where they induce massive quantal release of acetylcholine, eventually blocking neuromuscular transmission (113). The effect closely resembled that seen with the paralytic neurotoxin alpha latrotoxin and was clearly dependent upon complement

activation, which could be demonstrated immunohistologically (Fig. 7). In addition, anti-GQ1b antibodies cloned from mice immunized with GBS-associated strains of *C. jejuni* LPS induce identical complement-dependent electrophysiological and immunohistological abnormalities (35).

Considered collectively, these findings strongly suggest that anti-GQ1b antibodies, in conjunction with activated complement components, are the principal pathophysiological mediators of motor symptoms in patients with MFS and that the NMJ is an important site of their action. In addition to effects of anti-GQ1b antibodies at the nerve terminal, the immunohistological demonstration of GQ1b enrichment at nodes of Ranvier in extraocular nerves supports the notion that anti-GQ1b antibodies may also affect nodal conduction (16). However, it has not been possible to demonstrate this electrophysiologically in isolated mouse sciatic nerve preparations (108).

All the above pathogenesis studies have involved the exposure or passive transfer of antibodies to experimental systems. There have been no clearly positive reports of clinical neuropathy induced in experimental animals by immunization with GM1, GQ1b, or LPS species bearing cross-reactive epitopes, which would represent proof of antigen specific autoimmunity. Despite these disappointingly negative findings, an exception which provides a crucial rationale for continuing this approach is that immunization with GD1b has produced an ataxic neuropathy in rabbits with morphological changes in the dorsal roots (79). Therefore, it appears that this condition can be fulfilled for some ganglioside antigens, and this finding lends impetus to refining the immunization protocols and related immunological milieu for other ganglioside and LPS antigens.

CONCLUDING REMARKS

The last decade has seen the emergence of abundant clinical data that clearly show a disease-specific correlation between the development of post-*Campylobacter* GBS and antiganglioside antibodies. Many interesting

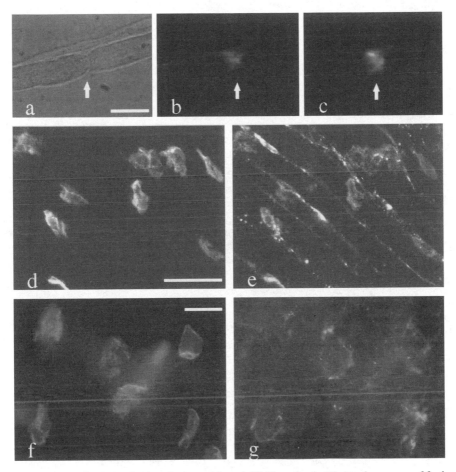

FIGURE 7 (a to c) After incubation with anti-GM1 antibody Wo1 and a source of fresh complement, a mouse node of Ranvier (a) (phase-contrast micrograph) displays immunoglobulin (b) and complement fragment C3c deposition (c). Scale bar, 20 μm. Reprinted from reference 108 with permission. (d and e) Passive transfer of a human antibody reactive with polysialylated gangliosides (HaRCE) into the mouse resulted in the accumulation of immunoglobulin (e) at the NMJ (as labeled by BTx [d]). Scale bar, 50 μm. (f and g) Treatment of a mouse hemidiaphragm with MFS reactive with polysialylated gangliosides (Smith) caused the accumulation of complement activation product C3c (g) at the NMJ (as labeled by BTx [f]). Scale bar, 20 μm. Reprinted from reference 113 with permission.

clinicoserological patterns are emerging, the strongest being between MFS and anti-GQ1b antibodies, which support the view that anti-ganglioside antibodies play a key operative role in pathogenesis. Experimental evidence obtained from animal studies is slowly beginning to support the model of post-*Campylobacter* GBS as a disease involving molecular mimicry between bacterial and neural OS. Many key issues remain unresolved across the whole

spectrum of GBS pathogenesis, ranging from the genetic and/or environmentally derived host factors that confer susceptibility to a small proportion of *Campylobacter*-infected individuals, the extent to which T-cell factors are involved in roles other than providing T-cell help to antibody production, and the nature of the immunological injury that damages the blood-nerve barrier. Once these issues have been resolved, the opportunity should arise to develop specific rationales for targeted immunotherapy, in order that we can prevent or limit the devastating injury that can result from GBS.

REFERENCES

1. **Allos, B. M.** 1997. Association between *Campylobacter* infection and Guillain-Barré syndrome. *J. Infect. Dis.* **176:**S125–S128.

2. **Ando, S., Y. Hirabayashi, K. Kon, F. Inagaki, S. Tate, and V. P. Whittaker.** 1992. A trisialoganglioside containing a sialyl α2-6 N-acetylgalactosamine residue is a cholinergic-specific antigen. Chol-1a. *J. Biochem.* **111:**287–290.

3. **Apostolski, S., S. A. Sadiq, A. Hays, M. Corbo, L. Suturkova-Milosevic, Chaliff, K. Stefansson, R. G. LeBaron, E. Ruoslahti, A. P. Hays, and N. Latov.** 1994. Identification of Gal(β1-3)GalNAc bearing glycoproteins at the nodes of Ranvier in peripheral nerve. *J. Neurosci. Res.* **38:**134–141.

4. **Arasaki, K., S. Kusunoki, N. Kudo, and I. Kanazawa.** 1993. Acute conduction block in vitro following exposure to antiganglioside sera. *Muscle Nerve* **16:**587–593.

5. **Ariga, T., T. Kohriyama, and L. Freddo.** 1987. Characterization of sulfated glucuronic acid containing glycolipids reacting with IgM M-proteins in patients with neuropathy. *J. Biol. Chem.* **262:**848–853.

6. **Aspinall, G. O., S. Fujimoto, A. G. Mcdonald, H. Pang, L. A. Kurjanczyk, and J. L. Penner.** 1994. Lipopolysaccharides from *Campylobacter jejuni* associated with Guillain-Barré syndrome patients mimic human gangliosides in structure. *Infect. Immun.* **62:**2122–2125.

7. **Aspinall, G. O., A. G. Mcdonald, T. S. Raju, H. Pang, S. D. Mills, L. A. Kurjanczyk, and J. L. Penner.** 1992. Serological diversity and chemical structures of *Campylobacter jejuni* low-molecular-weight lipopolysaccharides. *J. Bacteriol.* **174:**1324–1332.

8. **Aspinall, G. O., A. G. Mcdonald, T. S. Raju, H. Pang, A. P. Moran, and J. L. Penner.** 1993. Chemical structures of the core regions of *Campylobacter jejuni* serotypes O:1, O:4, O:23, and O:36 lipopolysaccharides. *Eur. J. Biochem.* **213:**1017–1027.

9. **Bollensen, E., A. J. Steck, and M. Schachner.** 1988. Reactivity with the peripheral myelin glycoprotein P(o) in serum from patients with monoclonal IgM gammopathy and polyneuropathy. *Neurology* **38:**1266–1270.

10. **Buchwald, B., K. V. Toyka, J. Zielasek, A. Weishaupt, S. Schweiger, and J. Dudel.** 1998. Neuromuscular blockade by IgG antibodies from patients with Guillain-Barré syndrome: a macro-patch-clamp study. *Ann. Neurol.* **44:**913–922.

11. **Buchwald, B., A. Weishaupt, K. V. Toyka, and J. Dudel.** 1998. Pre- and postsynaptic blockade of neuromuscular transmission by Miller-Fisher syndrome IgG at mouse motor nerve terminals. *Eur. J. Neurosci.* **10:**281–290.

12. **Burger, D., M. Simon, G. Perruisseau, and A. J. Steck.** 1990. The epitopes(s) recognized by HNK-1 antibody and IgM paraprotein in neuropathy is present on several N-linked oligosaccharide structures of human P0 and myelin-associated glycoprotein. *J. Neurochem.* **54:**1569–1575.

13. **Buzby, J. C., B. M. Allos, and T. Roberts.** 1997. The economic burden of *Campylobacter*-associated Guillain-Barré syndrome. *J. Infect. Dis.* **176:**S192–S197.

14. **Calderon, R. O., B. Attema, and G. H. DeVries.** 1995. Lipid composition of neuronal cell bodies and neurites from cultured dorsal root ganglia. *J. Neurochem.* **64:**424–429.

15. **Carpo, M., E. Nobileorazio, N. Meucci, M. Gamba, S. Barbieri, S. Allaria, and G. Scarlato.** 1996. Anti-GD1a ganglioside antibodies in peripheral motor syndromes. *Ann. Neurol.* **39:**539–543.

16. **Chiba, A., S. Kusunoki, H. Obata, R. Machinami, and I. Kanazawa.** 1993. Serum anti-GQ1b IgG antibody is associated with ophthalmoplegia in Miller-Fisher syndrome and Guillain-Barré syndrome: clinical and immunohistochemical studies. *Neurology* **43:**1911–1917.

17. **Chiba, A., S. Kusunoki, H. Obata, R. Machinami, and I. Kanazawa.** 1997. Ganglioside composition of the human cranial nerves, with special reference to pathophysiology of Miller Fisher syndrome. *Brain Res.* **745:**32–36.

18. **Chiba, A., S. Kusunoki, T. Shimizu, and I. Kanazawa.** 1992. Serum IgG antibody to ganglioside GQ1b is a possible marker of Miller-Fisher syndrome. *Ann. Neurol.* **31:**677–679.

19. **Chou, D. K. H., A. A. Ilyas, and J. E. Evans.** 1986. Structure of sulfated glucuronyl glycolipids in the nervous system reacting with HNK-1 antibody and some IgM paraproteins in neuropathy. *J. Biol. Chem.* **261:**11717–11725.

20. **Corbo, M., A. Quattrini, N. Latov, and A. P. Hays.** 1993. Localization of GM1 and Gal(β1-3)GalNAc antigenic determinants in peripheral nerve. *Neurology* **43:**809–814.

21. **Corbo, M., A. Quattrini, A. Lugaresi, M. Santoro, N. Latov, and A. P. Hays.** 1992. Patterns of reactivity of human anti-GM1 antibodies with spinal-cord and motor neurons. *Ann. Neurol.* **32:**487–493.

22. **Derrington, E. A., and E. Borroni.** 1990. The developmental expression of the cholinergic-specific antigen Chol-1 in the central and peripheral nervous system of the rat. *Dev. Brain Res.* **52:**131–140.

23. **Derrington, E. A., S. Kelic, and V. P. Whittaker.** 1993. A novel cholinergic-specific antigen (Chol-2) in mammalian brain. *Brain Res.* **620:**16–23.

24. **Dodd, J., and T. M. Jessell.** 1985. Lactoseries carbohydrates specify subsets of dorsal root ganglion neurons projecting to the superficial dorsal horn of rat spinal cord. *J. Neurosci.* **5:**3278–3294.

25. **Dodd, J., D. Solter, and T. M. Jessell.** 1984. Monoclonal antibodies against carbohydrate differentiation antigens identify subsets of primary sensory neurones. *Nature* **311:**469–472.

26. **Enders, U., H. Karch, K. V. Toyka, M. Michels, J. Zielasek, M. Pette, J. Heesemann, and H. P. Hartung.** 1993. The spectrum of immune-responses to *Campylobacter jejuni* and glycoconjugates in Guillain-Barré-syndrome and in other neuroimmunological disorders. *Ann. Neurol.* **34:**136–144.

27. **Feasby, T. E., J. J. Gilbert, W. F. Brown, C. F. Bolton, A. F. Hahn, W. F. Koopman, and D. W. Zochodne.** 1986. An acute axonal form of Guillain-Barré polyneuropathy. *Brain* **109:**1115–1126.

28. **Ferrari, S., M. Morbin, E. Nobile-Orazio, A. Musso, G. Tomelleri, L. Bertolasi, N. Rizzuto, and S. Monaco.** 1998. Antisulfatide polyneuropathy: antibody-mediated complement attack on peripheral myelin. *Acta Neuropathol.* **96:**569–574.

29. **Fisher, M.** 1956. An unusual variant of acute idiopathic polyneuritis (syndrome of ophthalmoplegia, ataxia and areflexia). *N. Engl. J. Med.* **255:**57–65.

30. **Fishman, P. H.** 1988. Gangliosides as cell surface receptors and transducers of biological signals. *Fidia Res. Ser.* **14:**184–201.

31. **Fredman, P., C. A. Vedeler, H. Nyland, J. A. Aarli, and L. Svennerholm.** 1991. Antibodies in sera from patients with inflammatory demyelinating polyradiculoneuropathy react with ganglioside LM1 and sulfatide of peripheral-nerve myelin. *J. Neurol.* **238:**75–79.

32. **Furuya, S., T. Hashikawa, F. Irie, A. Hasegawa, T. Nakao, and Y. Hirabayashi.** 1995. Neuronal expression of a minor monosialosyl ganglioside GM1b in rat brain: Immunochemical characterization using a specific monoclonal antibody. *Neurosci. Res.* **22:**411–421.

33. **Ganser, A. L., and D. A. Kirschner.** 1984. Differential expression of gangliosides on the surfaces of myelinated nerve fibers. *J. Neurosci. Res.* **12:**245–255.

34. **Ganser, A. L., D. A. Kirschner, and M. Willinger.** 1983. Ganglioside localization on myelinated nerve fibres by cholera toxin binding. *J. Neurocytol.* **12:**921–938.

35. **Goodyear, C. S., G. M. O'Hanion, J. J. Plomp, I. Morrison, J. Veitch, J. Conner, P. C. Molenaar, and H. J. Willison.** 1998. Anti-GQ1b ganglioside antibodies cloned from mice immunized with Miller-Fisher syndrome-associated strains of *Campylobacter jejuni* lipopolysaccharide induce neuromuscular transmission block. *Ann. Neurol.* **44:**990.

36. **Gregson, N. A., D. Jones, P. K. Thomas, and H. J. Willison.** 1991. Acute motor neuropathy with antibodies to GM1 ganglioside. *J. Neurol.* **238:**447–451.

37. **Griffin, J. W., C. Y. Li, C. Macko, T. W. Ho, S. T. Hsieh, P. Xue, F. A. Wang, D. R. Cornblath, G. M. McKhann, and A. K. Asbury.** 1996. Early nodal changes in the acute motor axonal neuropathy pattern of the Guillain-Barré syndrome. *J. Neurocytol.* **25:**33–51.

38. **Guijo, C. G., A. Garciamerino, G. Rubio, A. Guerrero, A. C. Martinez, and J. Arpa.** 1992. IgG antiganglioside antibodies and their subclass distribution in 2 patients with acute and chronic motor neuropathy. *J. Neuroimmunol.* **37:**141–148.

39. **Hadden, R. D. M., D. R. Cornblath, R. A. C. Hughes, J. Zielasek, H. P. Hartung, K. V. Toyka, and A. V. Swan.** 1998. Electrophysiological classification of Guillain-Barré syndrome: clinical associations and outcome. *Ann. Neurol.* **44:**780–788.

40. **Hao, Q., T. Saida, S. Kuroki, M. Nishimura, M. Nukina, H. Obayashi, and K. Saida.** 1998. Antibodies to gangliosides and galactocerebroside in patients with Guillain-Barré syndrome with preceding *Campylobacter jejuni* and other identified infections. *J. Neuroimmunol.* **81:**116–126.

41. **Hartung, H. P., J. D. Pollard, G. K. Harvey, and K. V. Toyka.** 1995. Immunopathogenesis and treatment of the Guillain-Barré syndrome. 1. *Muscle Nerve* **18:**137–153.

42. **Hartung, H. P., J. D. Pollard, G. K. Harvey, and K. V. Toyka.** 1995. Immunopathogenesis and treatment of the Guillain-Barré syndrome. 2. *Muscle Nerve* **18:**154–164.

43. **Hartung, H. P., H. Willison, S. Jung, M. Pette, K. V. Toyka, and G. Giegerich.** 1996. Autoimmune responses in peripheral nerve. *Springer Semin. Immunopathol.* **18:**97–123.

44. **Harvey, G. K., K. V. Toyka, J. Zielasek, R. Kiefer, C. Simonis, and H. P. Hartung.**

1995. Failure of anti-GM1 IgG or IgM to induce conduction block following intraneural transfer. *Muscle Nerve* **18**:388–394.

45. **Hirabayashi, Y., T. Nakao, F. Irie, V. P. Whittaker, K. Kon, and S. Ando.** 1992. Structural characterization of a novel cholinergic neuron-specific ganglioside in bovine brain. *J. Biol. Chem.* **267**:12973–12978.

46. **Hirakawa, M., T. McCabe, and M. Kawata.** 1992. Time-related changes in the labeling pattern of motor and sensory neurons innervating the gastrocnemius muscle, as revealed by the retrograde transport of the cholera toxin B subunit. *Cell Tissue Res.* **267**:419–427.

47. **Hirota, N., R. Kaji, H. Bostock, K. Shindo, T. Kawasaki, K. Mizutani, N. Oka, N. Kohara, T. Saida, and J. Kimura.** 1997. The physiological effect of anti-GM1 antibodies on saltatory conduction and transmembrane currents in single motor axons. *Brain* **120**:2159–2169.

48. **Hitoshi, S., S. Kusunoki, K. Kon, A. Chiba, H. Waki, S. Ando, and I. Kanazawa.** 1996. A novel ganglioside, 9-O-acetyl GD1b, is recognized by serum antibodies in Guillain-Barré syndrome. *J. Neuroimmunol.* **66**:95–101.

49. **Ho, T. W., S.-T. Hsieh, I. Nachamkin, H. J. Willison, K. Sheikh, J. Kiehlbauch, K. Flanigan, J. C. McArthur, D. R. Cornblath, G. M. McKhann, and J. W. Griffin.** 1997. Motor nerve terminal degeneration provides a potential mechanism for rapid recovery in acute motor axonal neuropathy after *Campylobacter* infection. *Neurology* **48**:717–724.

50. **Ho, T. W., G. M. McKhann, and J. W. Griffin.** 1998. Human autoimmune neuropathies. *Annu. Rev. Neurosci.* **21**:187–226.

51. **Ho, T. W., H. J. Willison, I. Nachamkin, C. Y. Li, J. Veitch, H. Ung, G. R. Wang, R. C. Liu, D. R. Cornblath, A. K. Asbury, J. W. Griffin, and G. M. McKhann.** 1999. Anti-GD1a antibody is associated with axonal but not demyelinating forms of Guillain-Barré syndrome. *Ann. Neurol.* **45**:168–173.

52. **Hughes, R. A. C., and J. H. Rees.** 1997. Clinical and epidemiologic features of Guillain-Barré syndrome. *J. Infect. Dis.* **176**:S92–S98.

53. **Illa, I., N. Ortiz, E. Gallard, C. Juarez, J. M. Grau, and M. C. Dalakas.** 1995. Acute axonal Guillain-Barré-syndrome with IgG antibodies against motor axons following parenteral gangliosides. *Ann. Neurol.* **38**:218–224.

54. **Ilyas, A. A., S. C. Li, D. K. H. Chou, Y. T. Li, F. B. Jungalwala, M. C. Dalakas, and R. H. Quarles.** 1988. Gangliosides GM2, IV⁴Gal-NAcGM1b, and IV⁴GalNAcGD1a as antigens for monoclonal immunoglobulin M in neuropa-thy associated with gammopathy. *J. Biol. Chem.* **263**:4369–4373.

55. **Ilyas, A. A., H. J. Willison, R. H. Quarles, F. B. Jungalwala, D. R. Cornblath, B. D. Trapp, D. E. Griffin, J. W. Griffin, and G. M. McKhann.** 1988. Serum antibodies to gangliosides in Guillain-Barré syndrome. *Ann. Neurol.* **23**:440–447.

56. **Irie, F., S. Kurono, Y.-T. Li, Y. Seyama, and Y. Hirabayashi.** 1996. Isolation of three novel cholinergic neuron-specific gangliosides from bovine brain and their in vitro syntheses. *Glycoconj. J.* **13**:177–186.

57. **Irie, S., T. Saito, K. Nakamura, N. Kanazawa, M. Ogino, T. Nukazawa, H. Ito, Y. Tamai, and H. Kowa.** 1996. Association of anti-GM2 antibodies in Guillain-Barré syndrome with acute cytomegalovirus infection. *J. Neuroimmunol.* **68**:19–26.

58. **IUPAC-IUB Commission on Biochemical Nomenclature (CBN).** 1977. The nomenclature of lipids. *Eur. J. Biochem.* **79**:11–21.

59. **Jacobs, B. C., H. P. Endtz, F. G. A. Vandermeche, M. P. Hazenberg, H. A. M. Achtereekte, and P. A. Vandoorn.** 1995. Serum anti-GQ1b IgG antibodies recognize surface epitopes on *Campylobacter jejuni* from patients with Miller-Fisher syndrome. *Ann. Neurol.* **37**:260–264.

60. **Jacobs, B. C., P. H. Rothbarth, F. G. A. Vandermeche, P. Herbrink, P. I. M. Schmitz, M. A. deKlerk, and P. A. Vandoorn.** 1998. The spectrum of antecedent infections in Guillain-Barré syndrome—a case-control study. *Neurology* **51**:1110–1115.

61. **Jacobs, B. C., P. A. Vandoorn, P. I. M. Schmitz, A. P. TioGillen, P. Herbrink, L. H. Visser, H. Hooijkaas, and F. G. A. Vandermeche.** 1996. *Campylobacter jejuni* infections and anti-GM1 antibodies in Guillain-Barré syndrome. *Ann. Neurol.* **40**:181–187.

62. **Jessen, K. R., L. Morgan, M. Brammer, and R. Mirsky.** 1985. Galactocerebroside is expressed by non-myelin-forming Schwann cells in situ. *J. Cell Biol.* **101**:1135–1143.

63. **Kanda, T., H. Yoshino, T. Ariga, M. Yamawaki, and R. K. Yu.** 1994. Glycosphingolipid antigens in cultured microvascular bovine brain endothelial cells: sulfoglucuronosyl paraglobo-side as a target of monoclonal IgM in demyelinative neuropathy. *J. Cell Biol.* **126**:235–246.

64. **Kashihara, K., Y. Shiro, M. Koga, and N. Yuki.** 1998. IgG anti-GT1a antibodies which do not cross react with GQ1b ganglioside in a pharyngeal-cervical-brachial variant of Guillain-Barré syndrome. *J. Neurol. Neurosurg. Psychiatry* **65**:799.

65. **Kikuchi, M., Y. Tagawa, H. Iwamoto, H.**

Hoshino, and N. Yuki. 1997. Bickerstaff's brainstem encephalitis associated with IgG anti-GQ1b antibody subsequent to *Mycoplasma pneumoniae* infection: favorable response to immunoadsorption therapy. *J. Child Neurol.* **12:** 403–405.

66. Koga, M., N. Yuki, T. Ariga, M. Morimatsu, and K. Hirata. 1998. Is IgG anti-GT1a antibody associated with pharyngeal-cervical-brachial weakness or oropharyngeal palsy in Guillain-Barré syndrome? *J. Neuroimmunol.* **86:** 74–79.

67. Kohriyama, T., S. Kusunoki, and T. Ariga. 1987. Subcellular localization of sulfated glucuronic acid-containing glycolipids reacting with anti-myelin-associated glycoprotein antibody. *J. Neurochem.* **48:**1516–1522.

68. Kotani, M., I. Kawashima, H. Ozawa, K. Ogura, I. Ishizuka, T. Terashima, and T. Tai. 1994. Immunohistochemical localization of minor gangliosides in the rat central nervous system. *Glycobiology* **4:**855–865.

69. Kremer, D. M., P. H. H. Lopez, R. K. Mizutamari, L. J. Kremer, E. A. Bacile, and G. A. Nores. 1997. Factors defining target specificity in antibody-mediated neuropathy: density-dependent binding of anti-GD1a polyclonal IgG from a neurological patient. *J. Neurosci. Res.* **47:**636–641.

70. Kusunoki, S. 1995. Antiglycolipid antibody in inflammatory neuropathy. *Clin. Neurol.* **35:** 1370–1372.

71. Kusunoki, S., A. Chiba, Y. Hirabayashi, F. Irie, M. Kotani, I. Kawashima, T. Tai, and Y. Nagai. 1993. Generation of a monoclonal antibody specific for a new class of minor ganglioside antigens, GQ1bα and GT1aα: its binding to dorsal and lateral horn of human thoracic. *Brain Res.* **623:**83–88.

72. Kusunoki, S., A. Chiba, S. Hitoshi, H. Takizawa, and I. Kanazawa. 1995. Anti-Gal-C antibody in autoimmune neuropathies subsequent to mycoplasma infection. *Muscle Nerve* **18:** 409–413.

73. Kusunoki, S., A. Chiba, K. Kon, S. Ando, K. Arisawa, A. Tate, and I. Kanazawa. 1994. *N*-Acetylgalactosaminyl GD1a is a target molecule for serum antibody in Guillain-Barré syndrome. *Ann. Neurol.* **35:**570–576.

74. Kusunoki, S., A. Chiba, T. Tai, and I. Kanazawa. 1993. Localization of GM1 and GD1b antigens in the human peripheral nervous system. *Muscle Nerve* **16:**752–756.

75. Kusunoki, S., K. Inoue, M. Iwamori, Y. Nagai, and T. Mannen. 1989. Discrimination of human dorsal root ganglion cells by anti-fucosyl GM1 antibody. *Brain Res.* **494:**391–395.

76. Kusunoki, S., K. Inoue, M. Iwamori, Y. Nagai, and T. Mannen. 1991. Fucosylated glycoconjugates in human dorsal root ganglion cells with unmyelinated axons. *Neurosci. Lett.* **126:** 159–162.

77. Kusunoki, S., M. Iwamori, A. Chiba, S. Hitoshi, M. Arita, and I. Kanazawa. 1996. GM1b is a new member of antigen for serum antibody in Guillain-Barré syndrome. *Neurology* **47:**237–242.

78. Kusunoki, S., H. Mashiko, N. Mochizuki, A. Chiba, M. Arita, S. Hitoshi, and I. Kanazawa. 1997. Binding of antibodies against GM1 and GD1b in human peripheral nerve. *Muscle Nerve* **20:**840–845.

79. Kusunoki, S., J. Shimizu, A. Chiba, Y. Ugawa, S. Hitoshi, and I. Kanazawa. 1996. Experimental sensory neuropathy induced by sensitization with ganglioside GD1b. *Ann. Neurol.* **39:**424–431.

80. Latov, N. 1994. Antibodies to glycoconjugates in neuropathy and motor-neuron disease. *Proc. Brain Res.* **101:**295–303.

81. Latov, N., A. P. Hays, P. D. Donofrio, J. Liao, H. Ito, S. McGinnis, K. Manoussos, L. Freddo, M. E. Shy, W. H. Sherman, H. W. Chang, H. S. Greenberg, J. W. Albers, A. G. Alessi, D. Keren, R. K. Yu, H. S. Rowland, and E. A. Kabat. 1988. Monoclonal IgM with unique specificity to gangliosides GM1 and GD1b and to lacto-*N*-tetraose associated with human motor neuron disease. *Neurology* **38:** 763–768.

82. Latov, N., A. P. Hays, R. K. Yu, H. Ito, and F. P. Thomas. 1988. Antibodies to glycoconjugates in human motor neuron disease. *Neurochem. Pathol.* **8:**181–187.

83. Latov, N., I. Wirguin, L. Suturkovamilosevic, and C. Briani. 1996. Mechanism of induction of anti-ganglioside antibodies in immune mediated neuropathy. *J. Neurochem.* **66:** S97.

84. Ledeen, R. W. 1985. Gangliosides of the neuron. *Trends Neurosci.* **10:**169–174.

85. Ledeen, R. W., G. S. Wu, Z. H. Lu, D. Kozireski-Chuback, and Y. Fang. 1998. The role of GM1 and other gangliosides in neuronal differentiation—overview and new findings. *Ann. N. Y. Acad. Sci.* **845:**161–175.

86. Ledeen, R. W., and R. K. Yu. 1982. Gangliosides: structure, isolation and analysis. *Methods Enzymol.* **83:**139–191.

87. Lisak, R. P., T. Saida, and P. G. E. Kennedy. 1980. EAE, EAN and galactocerebroside sera bind to oligodendrocytes and Schwann cells. *J. Neurol. Sci.* **48:**287–296.

88. Lloyd, K. O., C. M. Gordon, I. J. Thampoe,

and C. DiBenedetto. 1992. Cell surface accessibility of individual gangliosides in malignant melanoma cells to antibodies is influenced by the total ganglioside composition of the cells. *Cancer Res.* **52**:4948–4953.

89. Lopate, G., A. Pestronk, A. J. Kornberg, J. Yue, and R. Choksi. 1997. IgM anti-sulfatide autoantibodies: patterns of binding to cerebellum, dorsal root ganglion and peripheral nerve. *J. Neurol. Sci.* **151**:189–193.

90. Lugaresi, A., M. Corbo, F. P. Thomas, N. Miyatani, T. Ariga, R. K. Yu, A. P. Hays, and N. Latov. 1991. Identification of glycoconjugates which are targets for anti-Gal(β-1-3)GalNAc autoantibodies in spinal motor neurons. *J. Neuroimmunol.* **34**:69–76.

91. Maehara, T., K. Ono, K. Tsutsui, S. Watarai, T. Yasuda, H. Inoue, and A. Tokunaga. 1997. A monoclonal antibody that recognizes ganglioside GD1b in the rat central nervous system. *Neurosci. Res.* **29**:9–16.

92. Martini, R., and M. Schachner. 1986. Immunoelectron microscopic localization of neural cell adhesion molecules (L1, N-CAM, and MAG) and their shared carbohydrate epitope and myelin basic protein in developing sciatic nerve. *J. Cell Biol.* **103**:2439–2448.

93. McKhann, G. M., D. R. Cornblath, J. W. Griffin, T. W. Ho, C. Y. Li, Z. Jiang, H. S. Wu, G. Zhaori, Y. Liu, L. P. Jou, T. C. Liu, C. Y. Gao, J. Y. Mao, M. J. Blaser, B. Mishu, and A. K. Asbury. 1993. Acute motor axonal neuropathy—a frequent cause of acute flaccid paralysis in China. *Ann. Neurol.* **33**:333–342.

94. Mizoguchi, K., A. Hase, T. Obi, H. Matsuoka, M. Takatsu, Y. Nishimura, F. Irie, Y. Seyama, and Y. Hirabayashi. 1994. 2 Species of antiganglioside antibodies in a patient with a pharyngeal-cervical-brachial variant of Guillain-Barré syndrome. *J. Neurol. Neurosurg. Psychiatry* **57**:1121–1123.

95. Molander, M., C.-H. Berthold, H. Persson, K. Andersson, and P. Fredman. 1997. Monosialoganglioside (GM1) immunofluorescence in rat spinal roots studied with a monoclonal antibody. *J. Neurocytol.* **26**:101–111.

96. Moran, A. P., B. J. Appelmelk, and G. O. Aspinall. 1996. Molecular mimicry of host structures by lipopolysaccharides of *Campylobacter* and *Helicobacter* spp: Implications in pathogenesis. *J. Endotoxin Res.* **3**:521–531.

97. Moran, A. P., and M. M. Prendergast. 1998. Molecular mimicry in *Campylobacter jejuni* lipopolysaccharides and the development of Guillain-Barré syndrome. *J. Infect. Dis.* **178**:1549–1550.

98. Nakamura, K., S. Irie, N. Kanazawa, T. Saito, and Y. Tamai. 1998. Anti-GM2 antibodies in Guillain-Barré syndrome with acute cytomegalovirus infection. *Ann. N. Y. Acad. Sci.* **845**:423.

99. Nardelli, E., A. Bassi, G. Mazzi, P. Anzini, and N. Rizzuto. 1995. Systemic passive transfer studies using IgM monoclonal antibodies to sulfatide. *J. Neuroimmunol.* **63**:29–37.

100. Obrocki, J., and E. Borroni. 1988. Immunocytochemical evaluation of a cholinergic-specific ganglioside antigen (Chol-1) in the central nervous system of the rat. *Exp. Brain Res.* **72**:71–82.

101. Odaka, M., N. Yuki, H. Yoshino, T. Kasama, S. Handa, F. Irie, Y. Hirabayashi, A. Suzuki, and K. Hirata. 1998. N-Glycolylneuraminic acid-containing GM1 is a new molecule for serum antibody in Guillain-Barré syndrome. *Ann. Neurol.* **43**:829–834.

102. Ogawa-Goto, K., N. Funamoto, Y. Ohta, T. Abe, and K. Nagashima. 1992. Myelin gangliosides of human peripheral nervous system: An enrichment of GM1 in the motor nerve myelin isolated from cauda equina. *J. Neurochem.* **59**:1844–1849.

103. O'Hanlon, G. M., G. J. Paterson, J. Veitch, G. Wilson, and H. J. Willison. 1998. Mapping immunoreactive epitopes in the human peripheral nervous system using human monoclonal anti-GM1 ganglioside antibodies. *Acta Neuropathol.* **95**:605–616.

104. O'Hanlon, G. M., G. J. Paterson, G. Wilson, D. Doyle, P. McHardie, and H. J. Willison. 1996. Anti-GM1 ganglioside antibodies cloned from autoimmune neuropathy patients show diverse binding patterns in the rodent nervous system. *J. Neuropathol. Exp. Neurol.* **55**:184–195.

105. Ohsawa, T., T. Miyatake, and N. Yuki. 1993. Anti-B-series ganglioside-recognizing autoantibodies in an acute sensory neuropathy patient cause cell death of rat dorsal root ganglion neurons. *Neurosci. Lett.* **157**:167–170.

106. Oldfors, A. 1986. Cholera toxin B-subunit incorporation into synaptic vesicles of the neuromuscular junction of the rat. *Experientia* **42**:415–417.

107. O'Leary, C. P., J. Veitch, W. F. Durward, A. M. Thomas, J. H. Rees, and H. J. Willison. 1996. Acute oropharyngeal palsy is associated with antibodies to GQ1b and GT1a gangliosides. *J. Neurol. Neurosurg. Psychiatry* **61**:649–651.

108. Paparounas, K., G. M. O'Hanlon, C. P. O'Leary, E. G. Rowan, and H. J. Willison. 1999. Anti-ganglioside antibodies can bind peripheral nerve nodes of Ranvier and activate the complement cascade without inducing acute conduction block *in vitro*. *Brain* **122**:807–816.

109. **Penner, J. L., and G. O. Aspinall.** 1997. Diversity of lipopolysaccharide structures in *Campylobacter jejuni. J. Infect. Dis.* **176:**S135–S138.

110. **Pestronk, A.** 1998. Multifocal motor neuropathy: diagnosis and treatment. *Neurology* **51:**S22–S24.

111. **Pestronk, A., R. Choksi, G. Blume, and G. Lopate.** 1997. Multifocal motor neuropathy: serum IgM binding to a GM1 ganglioside-containing lipid mixture but not to GM1 alone. *Neurology* **48:**1104–1106.

112. **Pestronk, A., D. R. Cornblath, A. A. Ilyas, H. Baba, R. H. Quarles, J. W. Griffin, K. Alderson, and R. N. Adams.** 1988. A treatable multifocal motor neuropathy with antibodies to GM1 ganglioside. *Ann. Neurol.* **24:**73–78.

113. **Plomp, J. J., P. C. Molenaar, G. M. O'Hanlon, B. C. Jacobs, J. Veitch, M. R. Daha, P. A. Van Doorn, F. G. A. van der Meché, A. Vincent, B. P. Morgan, and H. J. Willison.** 1999. Miller-Fisher anti-GQ1b antibodies: α-latrotoxin-like effects on motor end plates. *Ann. Neurol.* **45:**189–199.

114. **Quarles, R. H.** 1997. The spectrum and pathogenesis of antibody-mediated neuropathies. *Neuroscientist* **3:**195–204.

115. **Quarles, R. H., A. A. Ilyas, and H. J. Willison.** 1986. Antibodies to glycolipids in demyelinating diseases of the human peripheral nervous system. *Chem. Phys. Lipids* **42:**235–248.

116. **Quattrini, A., M. Corbo, S. K. Dhaliwal, S. A. Sadiq, A. Lugaresi, A. Oliveira, A. Uncini, K. Abouzahr, J. R. Miller, L. Lewis, D. Estes, L. Cardo, A. P. Hays, and N. Latov.** 1992. Anti-sulfatide antibodies in neurological disease: binding to rat dorsal root ganglia neurons. *J. Neurol. Sci.* **112:**152–159.

117. **Raff, M. C., K. L. Fields, S. I. Hakomori, R. Mirsky, and R. M. Pruss.** 1978. Cell-type specific markers for distinguishing and studying neurons and the major classes of glial cells in culture. *Brain Res.* **174:**283–308.

118. **Rees, J. H., N. A. Gregson, and R. A. C. Hughes.** 1995. Antiganglioside GM1 antibodies in Guillain-Barré syndrome and their relationship to *Campylobacter jejuni* infection. *Ann. Neurol.* **38:**809–816.

119. **Richardson, P. J., J. H. Walker, R. T. Jones, and V. P. Whittaker.** 1982. Identification of a cholinergic-specific antigen Chol-1 as a ganglioside. *J. Neurochem.* **38:**1605–1614.

120. **Roberts, M., H. Willison, A. Vincent, and J. Newsomdavis.** 1994. Serum factor in Miller-Fisher variant of Guillain-Barré syndrome and neurotransmitter release. *Lancet* **343:**454–455.

121. **Ropper, A. H.** 1994. Miller-Fisher syndrome and other acute variants of Guillain-Barré syndrome. *Baillieres Clin. Neurol.* **3:**95–106.

122. **Rose, N. R.** 1998. The role of infection in the pathogenesis of autoimmune disease. *Semin. Immunol.* **10:**5–13.

123. **Salloway, S., L. A. Mermel, M. Seamans, G. O. Aspinall, J. E. N. Shin, L. A. Kurjanczyk, and J. L. Penner.** 1996. Miller-Fisher syndrome associated with *Campylobacter jejuni* bearing lipopolysaccharide molecules that mimic human ganglioside GD3. *Infect. Immun.* **64:**2945–2949.

124. **Santoro, M., A. Uncini, M. Corbo, S. M. Staugaitis, F. P. Thomas, A. P. Hays, and N. Latov.** 1992. Experimental conduction block induced by serum from a patient with anti-GM1 antibodies. *Ann. Neurol.* **31:**385–390.

125. **Scherer, S. S.** 1996. Molecular specializations at nodes and paranodes in peripheral nerve. *Microsc. Res. Tech.* **34:**452–461.

126. **Schluep, M., and A. J. Steck.** 1988. Immunostaining of motor nerve terminals by IgM M protein with activity against gangliosides GM1 and GD1b from a patient with motor neuron disease. *Neurology* **38:**1890–1892.

127. **Schwerer, B., A. Neisser, R. J. Polt, H. Bernheimer, and A. P. Moran.** 1995. Antibody cross-reactivities between gangliosides and lipopolysaccharides of *Campylobacter jejuni* serotypes associated with Guillain-Barré syndrome. *J. Endotoxin Res.* **2:**395–403.

128. **Simons, K., and E. Ikonen.** 1997. Functional rafts in cell membranes. *Nature* **387:**569–572.

129. **Stoffel, W., and A. Bosio.** 1997. Myelin glycolipids and their functions. *Curr. Opin. Neurobiol.* **7:**654–661.

130. **Sumner, A. J., K. Saida, and T. Saida.** 1982. Acute conduction block associated with experimental antiserum-mediated demyelination of peripheral nerve. *Ann. Neurol.* **11:**469–477.

131. **Svennerholm L.** 1963. Chromatographic separation of gangliosides. *J. Neurochem.* **10:**613–623.

132. **Tagawa, Y., F. Irie, Y. Hirabayashi, and N. Yuki.** 1997. Cholinergic neuron-specific ganglioside GQ1bα a possible target molecule for serum IgM antibodies in some patients with sensory ataxia. *J. Neuroimmunol.* **75:**196–199.

133. **Takigawa, T., H. Yasuda, R. Kikkawa, Y. Shigeta, T. Saida, and H. Kitasato.** 1995. Antibodies against GM1 ganglioside affect K^+ and Na^+ currents in isolated rat myelinated nerve fibers. *Ann. Neurol.* **37:**436–442.

134. **Tettamanti, G., and L. Riboni.** 1993. Gangliosides and modulation of the function of neural cells. *Adv. Lipid Res.* **25:**235–265.

135. **Thomas, F. P., P. H. Adapon, G. P. Goldberg, N. Latov, and A. P. Hays.** 1989. Locali-

zation of neural epitopes that bind to IgM monoclonal autoantibodies (M-proteins) from two patients with motor neuron disease. *J. Neuroimmunol.* **21:**31–39.

136. **Thomas, F. P., A. M. Lee, S. N. Romas, and N. Latov.** 1989. Monoclonal IgMs with anti-Gal(β1-3)GalNAc activity in lower motor neuron disease; identification of glycoprotein antigens in neural tissue and cross-reactivity with serum immunoglobulins. *J. Neuroimmunol.* **23:**167–174.

137. **Thomas, P. D., and G. J. Brewer.** 1990. Gangliosides and synaptic transmission. *Biochim. Biophys Acta* **1031:**277–289.

138. **Trapp, B. D., S. B. Andrews, A. Wong, M. O'Connell, and J. W. Griffin.** 1989. Co-localization of the myelin-associated glycoprotein and the microfilament components, F-actin and spectrin, in Schwann cells of myelinated nerve fibers. *J. Neurocytol.* **18:**47–60.

139. **Trojaborg, W.** 1998. Acute and chronic neuropathies: new aspects of Guillain-Barré syndrome and chronic inflammatory demyelinating polyneuropathy, an overview and an update. *Electroencephalogr. Clin. Neurophysiol.* **107:**303–316.

140. **Trojaborg, W., A. P. Hays, L. Van den Berg, D. S. Younger, and N. Latov.** 1995. Motor conduction parameters in neuropathies associated with anti-MAG antibodies and other types of demyelinating and axonal neuropathies. *Muscle Nerve* **18:**730–735.

141. **Vriesendorp, F. J., B. Mishu, M. J. Blaser, C. L. Koski, and R. A. Fishman.** 1993. Serum antibodies to GM1, GD1b, peripheral nerve myelin, and *Campylobacter jejuni* in patients with Guillain-Barré syndrome and controls: correlation and prognosis. *Ann. Neurol.* **34:**130–135.

142. **Vriesendorp, F. J., S. M. Quadri, R. E. Flynn, M. R. Malone, D. M. Cromeens, L. C. Stephens, and H. M. Vriesendorp.** 1997. Preclinical analysis of radiolabeled anti-GD2 immunoglobulin G. *Cancer* **80:**2642–2649.

143. **Wan, X. C. S., J. Q. Trojanowski, and J. O. Gonatas.** 1982. Cholera toxin and wheat germ agglutinin conjugates as neuroanatomical probes: their uptake and clearance, transganglionic and retrograde transport and sensitivity. *Brain Res.* **243:**215–224.

144. **Whittaker, V. P., and S. Kelic.** 1995. Cholinergic-specific glycoconjugates. *Neurochem. Res.* **20:**1377–1387.

145. **Willison, H. J., A. Almemar, J. Veitch, and D. Thrush.** 1994. Acute ataxic neuropathy with cross-reactive antibodies to GD1b and GD3 gangliosides. *Neurology* **44:**2395–2397.

146. **Willison, H. J., G. M. O'Hanlon, G. Paterson, J. Veitch, G. Wilson, M. Roberts, T. Tang, and A. Vincent.** 1996. A somatically mutated human antiganglioside IgM antibody that induces experimental neuropathy in mice is encoded by the variable region heavy chain gene, V1-18. *J. Clin. Investig.* **97:**1155–1164.

147. **Willison, H. J., and J. Veitch.** 1994. Immunoglobulin subclass distribution and binding characteristics of anti-GQ1b antibodies in Miller-Fisher syndrome. *J. Neuroimmunol.* **50:**159–165.

148. **Willison, H. J., J. Veitch, A. V. Swan, N. Baumann, G. Comi, N. A. Gregson, I. Illa, B. C. Jacobs, J. Zielasek, and R. A. C. Hughes.** 1999. Inter-laboratory validation of an ELISA for the determination of serum anti-ganglioside antibodies. *Eur. J. Neurol.* **6:**71–77.

149. **Wu, G. S., and R. W. Ledeen.** 1994. Gangliosides as modulators of neuronal calcium. *Proc. Brain Res.* **101:**101–112.

150. **Yamawaki, M., T. Ariga, J. W. Bigbee, H. Ozawa, I. Kawashima, T. Tai, T. Kanda, and R. K. Yu.** 1996. Generation and characterization of anti-sulfoglucuronosyl paragloboside monoclonal antibody NGR50 and its immunoreactivity with peripheral nerve. *J. Neurosci. Res.* **44:**586–593.

151. **Yoshino, H., T. Ariga, N. Latov, T. Miyatake, Y. Kushi, T. Kasama, S. Handa, and R. K. Yu.** 1993. Fucosyl-GM1 in human sensory nervous tissue is a target antigen in patients with autoimmune neuropathies. *J. Neurochem.* **61:**658–663.

152. **Yu, R. K., and T. Ariga.** 1998. The role of glycosphingolipids in neurological disorders—mechanisms of immune action. *Ann. N. Y. Acad. Sci.* **845:**285–306.

153. **Yuki, N.** 1995. Successful plasmapheresis in Bickerstaffs brain-stem encephalitis associated with anti-GQ1b antibody. *J. Neurol. Sci.* **131:**108–110.

154. **Yuki, N.** 1998. Anti-ganglioside antibody and neuropathy: review of our research. *J. Periph. Nerv. Syst.* **3:**3–18.

155. **Yuki, N., and K. Hirata.** 1998. Postinfection sensory neuropathy associated with IgG anti-GD1b antibody. *Ann. Neurol.* **43:**685–687.

156. **Yuki, N., and Y. Tagawa.** 1998. Acute cytomegalovirus infection and IgM anti-GM2 antibody. *J. Neurol. Sci.* **154:**14–17.

157. **Yuki, N., Y. Tagawa, and S. Handa.** 1996. Autoantibodies to peripheral nerve glycosphingolipids SPG, SLPG, and SGPG in Guillain-Barré syndrome and chronic inflammatory demyelinating polyneuropathy. *J. Neuroimmunol.* **70:**1–6.

158. **Yuki, N., Y. Tagawa, F. Irie, Y. Hirabayashi, and S. Handa.** 1997. Close association

of Guillain-Barré syndrome with antibodies to minor monosialogangliosides GM1b and GM1α. *J. Neuroimmunol.* **74:**30–34.

159. **Yuki, N., T. Taki, and S. Handa.** 1996. Antibody to GalNAc-GD1a and GalNAc-GM1b in Guillain-Barré syndrome subsequent to *Campylobacter jejuni* enteritis. *J. Neuroimmunol.* **71:** 155–161.

160. **Yuki, N., T. Taki, F. Inagaki, T. Kasama, M. Takahashi, K. Saito, S. Handa, and T. Miyatake.** 1993. A bacterium lipopolysaccharide that elicits Guillain-Barré syndrome has a GM1 ganglioside-like structure. *J. Exp. Med.* **178:**1771–1775.

161. **Yuki, N., M. Yamada, S. Sato, E. Ohama, Y. Kawase, F. Ikuta, and T. Miyatake.** 1993. Association of IgG anti-GD1a antibody with severe Guillain-Barré syndrome. *Muscle Nerve* **16:** 642–647.

162. **Yuki, N., M. Yamada, Y. Tagaawa, and H. Takahashi.** 1997. Pathogenesis of the neurotoxicity caused by anti-GD2 antibody therapy. *J. Neurol. Sci.* **149:**127–130.

163. **Yuki, N., H. Yoshino, S. Sato, and T. Miyatake.** 1990. Acute axonal polyneuropathy associated with anti-GM1 antibodies following *Campylobacter* enteritis. *Neurology* **40:**1900–1902.

164. **Yuki, N., H. Yoshino, S. Sato, K. Shinozawa, and T. Miyatake.** 1992. Severe acute axonal form of Guillain-Barré syndrome associated with IgG anti-GD1a antibodies. *Muscle Nerve* **15:**899–903.

165. **Zielasek, J., G. Ritter, S. Magi, H. P. Hartung, and K. V. Toyka.** 1994. A comparative trial of anti-glycoconjugate antibody-assays—IgM antibodies to GM1. *J. Neurol.* **241:**475–480.

ANIMAL MODELS OF
CAMPYLOBACTER INFECTION

Vincent B. Young, David B. Schauer, and James G. Fox

14

A brief overview of naturally occurring enteric campylobacteriosis and the use of selected animal models for the study of this disease is provided in this chapter to alert the investigator to their potential value in his or her research.

DEFINITION AND SELECTION OF APPROPRIATE IN VIVO MODELS

Several papers have been published on the importance of selecting the proper animal model to study a particular human disease (21, 52, 61). Criteria for selection of the animal model suggested by these authors include the following: (i) it reproduces the pathology of the disease being studied; (ii) it is readily available commercially in sufficient numbers; (iii) it can be easily transported or exported; (iv) it is easy to maintain and handle in laboratories; (v) it is well characterized biologically; (vi) its disease status is established; and (vii) it has a sufficient life span for the study in question (70, 115).

It is also important to exploit diseases that occur naturally in a variety of animal species and that closely mimic similar diseases in humans. In addition, issues such as cost, animal welfare, public concern, and animal legislation regarding the use of certain species may in part dictate the selection of a given species for a particular study (70, 115).

Since the recognition of the *Campylobacter* species as important causes of gastroenteritis in the 1970s, there have been numerous publications by investigators attempting to establish appropriate models for the study of enteric campylobacteriosis. Although investigators have successfully established intestinal colonization of several species of animals with *Campylobacter jejuni* and *Campylobacter coli,* few studies have reproduced the clinical diarrheal disease associated with acute *C. jejuni* infection in humans. These colonization models have been important in the development of candidate vaccines for *Campylobacter,* which is discussed elsewhere in this volume (chapter 15).

In selecting animal models for *Campylobacter* research, it is imperative that the species chosen has no preexisting colonization by *Campylobacter* species in the gastrointestinal tract; equally importantly, the immune status of the animal to previous or current *Campylobacter* infection must be quantified. In selecting the appropriate model, the availability of immune reagents (e.g., conjugated immunoglobulins,

Vincent B. Young, Division of Bioengineering and Environmental Health, Massachusetts Institute of Technology (MIT), Cambridge, MA 02139, and Infectious Diseases Unit, Department of Medicine, Massachusetts General Hospital, Boston, MA 02114. *David B. Schauer and James G. Fox,* Division of Bioengineering and Environmental Health and Division of Comparative Medicine, MIT, Cambridge, MA 02139.

Campylobacter, 2nd Ed., Edited by I. Nachamkin and M. J. Blaser
© 2000 American Society for Microbiology, Washington, D.C.

assays for secretory immunoglobulin A [IgA], and monoclonal antibodies to lymphocyte subclasses) is an important consideration when studies require monitoring of some aspect of the immune system response of the animal. The overall immune status of the animal can influence susceptibility to infection and can influence disease manifestations. For example, the use of mice with altered immune systems has been crucial in eliciting specific clinical syndromes in various model systems of infection with gastrointestinal pathogens including *Campylobacter* and *Helicobacter* species (20, 49, 58, 65).

When screening animals for enteric campylobacteriosis, it is important not only to identify various campylobacters to the species level but also to identify newly recognized enterohepatic *Helicobacter* species (29). These organisms have been demonstrated to be gastrointestinal pathogens in humans and a variety of animals (29, 35, 59, 101, 108). Many of these organisms appear to occupy the same ecological niche as *Campylobacter* spp., and they share many of the same phenotypic traits, which has resulted in their misidentification as *Campylobacter*-like organisms (5, 105). In addition, their presence in the intestines of animals may interfere with immunological profiles being proposed for the species in question (63).

Other microbial agents in the test animal, as well as environmental variables, may also interfere with the model system. Prior knowledge of the health status of the animals being selected, routine health surveillance, and the use of commercially reared and barrier-maintained animals will help determine the ultimate success of the model being used. Not only can intercurrent pathogens cause clinical disease, but also host defenses may be altered or compromised. Insidious or latent infections may affect immunological parameters or other biological systems. For example, a synergistic effect has been postulated between *C. jejuni* and other enteropathogens such as enteroinvasive *Salmonella* spp., *Shigella* spp., *Escherichia coli* (17), and *Cryptosporidium parvum*. One study showed a significant increase in *C. jejuni* inva-

sion of HEp-2 cells preinfected with enteroviruses such as echovirus type 7 and coxsackievirus B3, whereas poliovirus and swine enterovirus had no effect on *C. jejuni* invasive properties in the same in vitro system (57).

NATURAL COLONIZATION AND PREVALENCE OF ENTERIC CAMPYLOBACTERS IN ANIMALS

Successful *C. jejuni* or *C. coli* colonization of several species of laboratory animals is not surprising, given the number of domestic and wild animals and birds that are naturally colonized by a variety of enteric *Campylobacter* species (13, 48, 66, 71, 74, 87, 92, 93). Indeed, *C. jejuni* milk-borne infection in humans, associated with foil-capped milk bottles that had been delivered to residences and had been pecked open by birds with beaks contaminated with *C. jejuni*, provide an example of the variety and importance of animals and birds as *Campylobacter* reservoirs (50).

C. jejuni intestinal colonization of chickens and, to a lesser extent, turkeys, with subsequent contamination of the carcasses of the birds, accounts for the greatest single risk of infection in humans in the United States (100). Other domestic food animals are colonized with *Campylobacter* species, although it appears that contamination of food products derived from these animals presents lower risk than from poultry (106, 107). *C. fetus* subsp. *venerealis* and *fetus* are important causes of septic abortion in cattle and other large domesticated animals, but a discussion of this subject is beyond the scope of this chapter.

Dogs and cats also present zoonotic risk to pet owners and animal technicians; this happens particularly with younger animals, with and without diarrhea, when they shed *C. jejuni*, *C. coli*, *C. helveticus*, or *C. upsaliensis* in their feces (13, 22, 31, 34, 39, 42, 48, 69, 104, 111).

Lagomorphs and rodents, particularly hamsters (from certain vendors but not others) commonly shed *C. jejuni*, *C. coli*, and *C. hyointestinalis* in their feces, sometimes for protracted periods and without showing clinical signs of disease (45–47, 87, 109). Hamsters have been shown to be a reservoir for *H. cinaedi* and have been linked to zoonotic infections in humans (29, 46).

Various nonhuman primates, including Old World species such as macaques, patas, and baboons, as well as New World monkeys, marmosets, and squirrel and owl monkeys, commonly shed campylobacters, particularly during quarantine; newly captured primates routinely become infected while being housed at trapping stations in their country of origin (16, 73, 112–114). Endemic enteric campylobacteriosis is also commonly observed, as pointed out by Russell et al., in captive-primate colonies, where constant reinfection and colonization by *Campylobacter* species occurs (96–98). Endemic campylobacteriosis also occurs when other laboratory animal species, such as dogs, ferrets, and cats, are housed in groups in environments where fecal contamination occurs frequently (31, 32, 34, 37, 40). Colonization with multiple Penner serotypes of *C. jejuni* and *C. coli* is also common (34, 74, 98).

Members of the genus *Campylobacter* are not thought to be normal inhabitants of the human gastrointestinal tract. However, a recent study has demonstrated the presence of rRNA gene sequences corresponding to an as yet uncultured and previously unrecognized *Campylobacter* species in the stool and saliva of asymptomatic human volunteers (60). *Campylobacter rectus* has been isolated as a chronic colonizer in the oral cavity of humans, where it is associated with periodontal disease (89).

IN VIVO CAMPYLOBACTERIOSIS MODELS

The rapid progress of in vivo models of enteric campylobacteriosis in defining the pathophysiology of *C. jejuni* and *C. coli* has been severely curtailed by the lack of an animal model that fulfills the criteria mentioned above. As pointed out by Fox in the previous edition of this volume (30), many different species have been used in an attempt to establish a model system that would mimic the enteric disease in humans. Examination of animal species in which natural *C. jejuni*/*C. coli*-associated diarrhea has been documented provides an insight into species in which experimental infections with *C. jejuni* and *C. coli* have succeeded in producing diarrheal illness (32, 37, 38, 69, 97, 112).

Poultry

Since ingestion of contaminated poultry products is considered the major route of infection with *C. jejuni* in developed countries, a number of studies have investigated the dynamics of colonization of poultry flocks in order to develop methods of decreasing the rates of carriage (102, 118). In vivo studies designed to decrease *C. jejuni* colonization have been done with chickens, in experiments involving either defined competitive exclusion bacteria (100) or oral vaccines (91). Experiments with chickens have also demonstrated the importance of flagella as a colonization factor for *C. jejuni* (75, 120). More recently, chickens have been used not to study *C. jejuni*-induced gastroenteritis but, rather, as a model of experimental paralytic neuropathy in an attempt to develop an animal model of post-*C. jejuni* Guillain-Barré syndrome (64). A more extensive review of the study of *Campylobacter* species in poultry is provided elsewhere in this volume (chapter 26).

Dogs and Cats

In many cases cats and dogs are asymptomatic carriers of *Campylobacter* spp.; the clinical syndrome, when present, occurs most frequently in dogs younger than 6 months. *Campylobacter*-associated diarrhea has a wide clinical spectrum in dogs as well as humans, ranging from loose feces to watery diarrhea to bloody mucoid diarrhea (38, 40). Acute campylobacteriosis that develops in pups and some adult dogs is manifested by mucus-laden, watery, or bile-streaked diarrhea (with or without blood and leukocytes) lasting 5 to 15 days, partial anorexia, and occasional vomiting. Elevated temperature and leukocytosis may also be present (37, 38, 40, 69). In certain cases, diarrhea can be chronic for 2 weeks or more, intermittent, or, in some cases, present for several months (22). *C. jejuni* has also been infrequently isolated from the livers of infected, symptomatic dogs (81).

Experimental dosing with *C. jejuni* in random-source kittens and pups resulted in minimal clinical signs of diarrhea, even though the strain caused diarrhea in the researcher, who unintentionally infected himself (88). Similar results have been noted in other studies involving pups and adult dogs (67, 80). These findings have led some researchers to suggest that *C. jejuni/coli* either are primary pathogens or, together with predisposing factors such as virus infections, act as secondary pathogens (80, 99). However, the high prevalence of subclinical *Campylobacter* colonization in dogs may provide acquired immunity (79) and provide the host with the ability to resist experimental infection. To guard against this possibility, Prescott et al. successfully produced mild diarrhea in gnotobiotic pups by oral inoculation of *C. jejuni* (86). At necropsy 43 h postinoculation, the colons of two animals were congested and edematous and contained fluid. Microscopically, the colons and ceca showed decreases in epithelial cell height, brush borders, and numbers of goblet cells; hyperplasia of epithelial glands resulted in a thickened mucosa. Subepithelial congestion, hemorrhage, and inflammatory infiltrate were also seen (86). However, cost and lack of gnotobiotic facilities limit extensive use of germfree dogs.

Mustelids

Mink raised commercially are known to develop severe *C. jejuni/C. coli*-associated colitis (51). The ferret, another carnivore belonging to the family Mustelidae, is being used increasingly in biomedical research. Ferrets reared commercially and sold for research purposes commonly shed *C. jejuni* in their feces (32). Young weanling ferrets have *C. jejuni*-associated mucoid diarrhea, sometimes bloody or watery, lasting 5 to 10 days. This model has been used to study *C. jejuni*-induced diarrhea and its relationship to acquired and maternal immunity (9, 10, 33). In this model, self-limiting diarrhea can be produced consistently. As shown in the primate model of Russell et al.

(94) and the removable-intestinal-tie-adult-rabbit-diarrhea (RITARD) model (82), acquired immunity is characterized by the development of serum antibodies and provides at least partial resistance to infection, manifested mainly by shortened periods of *C. jejuni* colonization. Thus, antibodies do not prevent colonization by *C. jejuni* but do provide immunity against diarrheal illness (9, 10). A mild colitis is seen histologically in infected ferrets (10, 33). However, concurrent cryptosporidiosis, although reported to be nonpathogenic in ferrets, makes interpretation of the lesions more difficult in some *C. jejuni*-infected ferrets (90). Although raising germfree ferrets is possible, it is costly and time-consuming (68). The commercial availability of specific-pathogen-free ferrets, without prior exposure to *C. jejuni* and free of intercurrent infection, is needed before this model can be fully utilized (68). Ferrets are also naturally infected with *Helicobacter* species, and commercially available *Helicobacter*-free animals are also needed (41).

Mice

Laboratory mice are not naturally colonized with *C. jejuni*. As mentioned above, this may be due to competition with enterohepatic *Helicobacter* species, which have been recently recognized as murine commensals and pathogens (29). However, mice (and, to a lesser extent, rats) have been used in numerous experiments involving *C. jejuni,* because of their availability commercially, ease of housing and handling, defined microbial flora, and, in many cases, prescribed genetic traits (70). Also, the recent introduction of a varied and seemingly endless array of genetically manipulated mouse models offers a unique opportunity to study the influence of host genotype on the expression of diseases (53, 54).

With few exceptions, oral dosing of mice of different strains (both inbred and outbred) with *C. jejuni* results in intestinal colonization and in some cases bacteremia, but the organism usually does not cause clinical diarrhea (1, 2, 12, 25). Pretreatment with oral antibiotics can prolong the colonization. Continued debate focuses on whether *C. jejuni* in the mouse intestine colonizes the mucus in intestinal crypts or whether adherence to mucus epithelial cells also occurs (62, 77, 78). The mouse model also has highlighted the essential nature of the flagella in colonization of the intestinal mucosa (1, 2, 23, 72, 77). This was also verified in *C. jejuni* colonization studies with hamsters (3). More recently, mutations in a *C. jejuni* cell-binding factor, *peb1A*, were shown to significantly reduce the rate and duration of colonization of mice by *C. jejuni* 81-176 (83).

Since most strains of mice can be experimentally colonized with *C. jejuni*, they have been used in a number of studies of naturally acquired and vaccine-induced immunity developed to this bacterium. Investigators have demonstrated protection against colonization in offspring of female mice immunized with the homologous strain of *C. jejuni*, via immunity conferred through IgG antibodies in the milk of the dam (1, 2). Similarly, 39 of 68 offspring of female mice vaccinated with a particular Lior serotype (57%) were protected from intestinal colonization when challenged orally with a heterologous strain. In contrast, none of the infant mice challenged with a strain carrying the same heat-stable antigen (i.e., of the same Penner serotype as the vaccine strain) were afforded protection against colonization (1, 2). Interestingly, the use of passive immunization with monoclonal antibodies was not protective when directed against flagellar antigens (76).

Mice have been to used to test the immunogenicity and protective efficacy of a killed whole-cell *Campylobacter* vaccine (6). Oral administration of a 1 : 1 mixture of heat- and formalin-inactivated *C. jejuni* 81-176 and an adjuvant (*E. coli* heat-labile enterotoxin) resulted in the generation of significant levels of secretory IgA. Moreover, vaccinated animals were protected from colonization and systemic spread when orally challenged with *C. jejuni* 81-176 (6). No clinical disease was observed during the course of this experiment. The same authors also tested vaccine efficacy by using an intranasal challenge model with *C. jejuni* 81-176

(7). Intranasal challenge of BALB/c mice with 5×10^9 CFU of *C. jejuni* 81-176 resulted in mortality in 70 to 80% of infected animals. Other strains of mice (C3H/Hej and CBA/CAJ) exhibited a lower mortality rate (30 to 50%) in the setting of the same intranasal dose of bacteria, and the C58/J strain of mice exhibited no mortality with this challenge dose (7). Vaccination with heat-killed and/or formalin-fixed *C. jejuni* 81-176, as well as intranasal challenge with sublethal doses of this strain, protected mice from colonization and death.

Some authors have been successful in developing diarrhea in infant mice dosed intragastrically (55). One of three strains of *C. jejuni* caused severe diarrhea in 36 of 42 mice after virulence enhancement of the organisms (in iron dextran) by serial intraperitoneal passage in mice. Intraperitoneal injection of mice with 10^6 CFU of *C. jejuni* produced a self-limiting diarrhea, characterized by soft mucoid stools, blood, and fecal leukocytes, in outbred Swiss mice or inbred BALB/c mice (103). Higher doses ($>10^9$ CFU) killed the mice in 48 h. Although this model was proposed for virulence studies of *C. jejuni*, further studies have not been published.

Because infection of immunocompromised human patients with *C. jejuni* is associated with more severe clinical disease and prolonged carriage (84, 110), it is understandable why several investigators have used immunocompromised mice for infection studies. Athymic, germfree nude mice are effectively colonized by *C. jejuni* when challenged orally (123, 124). In these studies, *C. jejuni* colonized the epithelial surface of the intestine. Infected mice developed "transient diarrhea" when infected with a mouse-adapted *C. jejuni* strain (124). Cecal shrinkage was noted in infected mice, and histopathologically there was marked edema in the lamina propria, congestion, goblet cell loss, and a cellular infiltrate consisting of neutrophils, eosinophils, and a few lymphocytes. The epithelial layer remained intact. The colons had similar histopathology but with less edema and fewer inflammatory cells. In addition, frequent neutrophil-filled crypt abscesses were noted in the glandular mucosa. Euthymic, germfree mice of the same genetic background (BALB/c) did not develop diarrhea or histopathology, although they were also consistently colonized. Of interest is the finding that colonization of these C. jejuni monoassociated mice with a complex mouse fecal microflora eliminated viable C. jejuni from the ceca (123).

More recently, Hodgson et al. have described the development of diarrhea in C.B.-17-scid-Beige mice inoculated intragastrically with clinical isolates of C. jejuni (49). Diarrhea developed in about 10 to 20% of inoculated mice, and histopathologic examination of these mice revealed large-intestine pathology characterized by mucosal thickening and focal areas of infiltration of the lamina propria by polymorphonuclear lymphocytes, macrophages, and small mononuclear cells. A laboratory-passaged strain of C. jejuni colonized these immunocompromised mice but did not produce clinical signs of disease.

We have also exploited the use of fresh clinical isolates of Campylobacter to induce pathology in immunocompromised mice (122). Four-week old Tac:Icr:Ha(ICR)-scid mice were challenged with a fresh clinical isolate of C. fetus by oral gavage, for a total of three doses on alternating days. Mice were monitored for colonization by culture and Campylobacter-specific PCR of feces. The mice were examined by necropsy at 1 week, 3 weeks, and 3 months after infection, and the gastrointestinal tract was subjected to histopathologic examination. At all time points, the mice were colonized with the challenge C. fetus organism. Although C. fetus was detected by culture and PCR of stomach tissue and feces, diarrhea was not noted in any of the mice. At necropsy, large clusters of argyrophilic spiral organisms, with a morphology consistent with Campylobacter, were seen in the glandular mucosa of the stomach. These organisms were luminal and often closely opposed to the epithelium. The stomachs of the infected animals exhibited a progressive hyperplasia and a persistent active inflammatory response characterized by large numbers of infiltrating neutrophils and eosinophils. These

histopathologic changes were confined to the gastric antrum at the two early time points (1 and 3 weeks after challenge), but by 3 months they had spread to involve the gastric fundus as well. Additionally, the histopathology involving the fundus was characterized by loss of parietal cells. Despite positive isolation of C. fetus from the large intestine, colonic lesions were not noted. Importantly, culture and PCR for Helicobacter species were negative. In a follow-up study, ICR-scid mice as well as wild-type ICR mice were challenged with this C. fetus isolate and the gastric mucosa of both types of animals was consistently colonized. In wild-type mice, however, the anatomic extent of colonization was more limited, and the degree of inflammation and epithelial alterations was significantly less than observed in infected scid mice. To our knowledge, this is the first report of C. fetus-associated gastritis in any animal model. Yrios and Balish (123, 124) reported chronic gastric colonization of germfree nude mice with C. fetus, but they found no gastric pathology. We are currently investigating the role of potential Campylobacter virulence factors in this model system.

Also of interest is the finding of hepatitis in mice 1 to 2 months after oral dosing with C. jejuni (41, 42). Tissue culture studies with mouse hepatocytes demonstrated that low concentrations of factors isolated from whole-cell lysates of C. jejuni and purified by column chromatography caused the release of hepatic enzymes and that higher concentrations induced cytolysis (42). These effects were neutralized by antisera to the factor but not by antisera to lipopolysaccharide of C. jejuni or heat-labile enterotoxin of E. coli (42). Unfortunately, information on whether C. jejuni-infected mice (or mice used for antisera) were also infected by other pathogens that invaded their livers, particularly mouse hepatitis virus, was not provided (59). In addition, since these reports appeared in the literature, it has become clear that infection with Helicobacter hepaticus and H. bilis is common among many mouse colonies (101), and infection with this organisms results in chronic hepatitis (36, 43,

44, 119, 121). It is possible that these mice had a coinfection with *H. hepaticus* or *H. bilis*.

Rabbits

The RITARD model, has proved very useful in studies of intestinal colonization and development of immunization strategies (116, 117). Like the mouse model, the rabbit model, through oral-challenge studies, has shown the importance of cross-strain protection (by using the Lior serotype), thus implicating the flagellum as a protective antigen. In contrast, *C. jejuni*-immunized rabbits challenged with matched Penner-unmatched Lior strains showed little protection (82). Furthermore, an aflagellated mutant of *C. jejuni* failed to colonize rabbits, regardless of the route of administration. A single feeding of this aflagellated strain did not protect rabbits against challenge with the parent strain, but three feedings of the mutant strain did, indicating that antigens not located on the flagella can also produce protection against homologous flagellated strains (82). The model is also very useful in measuring the secretory IgA response to *C. jejuni* oral inoculation (18, 19). Other studies with the RITARD model have also demonstrated that the M cell, an important antigen-processing cell found in the epithelial layer over intestinal Peyer's patches, is a probable route for systemic spread of *C. jejuni* (117).

In experimental studies conducted with human volunteers, *C. jejuni* 81-176 caused higher attack rates and a greater number and volume of stools than did *C. jejuni* A 3249 (11). However, similar clinical outcomes were noted when the two strains were inoculated into RITARD rabbits (i.e., illness in all animals, with three deaths in each test group). This suggests that the two strains were of equal virulence or, alternatively, that the RITARD rabbit model was relatively insensitive to strain differences (11). Perhaps the age and source of the rabbit, as well as the in vitro growth conditions of the *C. jejuni* strain, also may affect the clinical course of the disease in individual experiments. Also, because rabbits are susceptible to a variety of infectious enteropathies, the source, health status, and housing conditions of the rabbits will also influence the success of this model when used by other investigators.

In spite of the potential benefits of the RITARD model, it has not been widely employed as a system with which to study *Campylobacter* pathogenesis since the previous edition of this volume. Perhaps since it is a surgical model, it requires more time and resources than are readily available to some researchers. Still, it is probably a useful model in which to test the role of the expanding numbers of potential virulence factors that are being studied in vitro and described elsewhere in this volume (chapters 20 and 23).

Nonhuman Primates

The nonhuman primate, albeit the most expensive of the models and limited in supply, has many of the clinical and epidemiological features noted in naturally occurring human campylobacteriosis, particularly for patients suffering from the disease in third-world countries. As with other species maintained in communal environments, where fecal-oral contamination is frequent, nonhuman primates in many colonies are infected with *Campylobacter* (16, 28, 73, 96, 97, 112–114). Although detailed epidemiologic data for these species are lacking, episodes of *Campylobacter*-associated diarrhea or asymptomatic infection have been documented in *Macaca mulatta, M. fascicularis,* Patas monkeys, and marmosets. In a study of the epidemiology of diarrhea in colony-born *M. nemestrina,* 205 neonates and infants in an infant research laboratory, plus 248 neonates, juveniles, and adolescents up to 4 years of age in a different facility were commonly diagnosed with *Campylobacter, Shigella,* and *Cryptosporidium* infections (96). Chronic diarrhea was noted in 10% of the animals. More recently, Russell et al. explored the prevalence of *Campylobacter* spp. in infant *M. nemestrina* animals, with and without diarrhea, housed in a nursery under hyperendemic conditions. They determined by using serotyping, DNA hybridization, and polyacrylamide gel electrophoresis that during a 12-month period, multiple reinfections with different strains of *C. jejuni* and *C. coli* occurred (98). The duration of infection with a particular strain averaged 3 to 4 weeks; *C. jejuni* and *C. coli* infection correlated with diarrhea in infants from 1 to 4 months of age. The 3- to 4-week course of infection with a particular strain is similar to the course of infection with a particular strain in susceptible humans and in experimentally infected infant *M. nemestrina* animals (14, 94). Also, isolation of multiple serotypes over time was similar to that found in children during a 12-week study in Thailand. Infant primates were infected at an early age, particularly if their mothers had nursed them. Infants raised in the nursery in isolettes did not become infected until moved into single cages in a holding room. Finger contact and aerosolization of feces during cleaning probably accounted for fecal-oral transmission in this setting. Interestingly, in this study, infants were also infected with nalidixic acid-resistant campylobacters; the duration of infection with those strains was only 1 ± 1.4 weeks. These isolates have been subsequently identified as *C. fetus* subsp. *fetus, C. hyointestinalis,* and *Aroobacter butzleri* (56, 95). Their significance as a cause of primary diarrhea in *Macaca* species requires further analysis.

Earlier experimental studies with *Macaca* species suggested that these animals were susceptible to both colonization with campylobacters and, in some cases, diarrhea following inoculation of the organism. Three *M. fascicularis* animals inoculated orally with thermophilic campylobacters isolated from diarrheic nonhuman primates did not develop diarrhea but had either partial or complete anorexia 1 week postinoculation. Two of the animals shed the organism for 5 and 6 weeks (113). These studies were followed by a more controlled and detailed study, in which eight young rhesus monkeys (*M. mulatta*) were infected orally with a human strain of *C. jejuni* (26). The disease induced was mild, with inappetence and diarrhea of short duration, but prolonged intermittent excretion of the bacteria in the feces occurred. Bacteremia generally was present for 2 to 3 days, and later the organisms were local-

ized in the liver and gallbladder. When challenged with the same strain, animals that had recovered showed no clinical symptoms and no bacteremia and excreted the organisms in the feces for only 3 days. At necropsy, no lesions attributable to *C. jejuni* were observed in any portion of the gastrointestinal tract (26).

More recently, a well-controlled and -designed study with infant *M. nemestrina* animals demonstrated the usefulness of this model in studying enteric campylobacteriosis (94). The experiment is particularly relevant, given that the strain used, 81-176 (Penner serotype 23/36), was isolated initially during an outbreak of milk-borne campylobacteriosis in Minnesota and later used in experimental infections of humans (11). Four infant pigtail macaques, 3.5 to 4 months old and specific pathogen (i.e., *Campylobacter* and *Shigella*) free, developed acute diarrheal illness, lasting approximately 7 to 11 days, when inoculated with strain 81-176 (3×10^{11} CFU). The illness was characterized by fluid diarrhea, bloody feces, and fecal leukocytes. Histologically, the animals had an acute colitis but no small intestine abnormalities. The *C. jejuni* strain was present 2 to 4 weeks postchallenge. Infants also developed IgG, IgA, and IgM titers to *C. jejuni* after experimental challenge. Partial protective immunity was noted by the appearance of mild diarrhea after rechallenge of the infants with the homologous strain or with a heterologous *C. jejuni* strain, 79-168. Four 1-year-old *M. nemestrina* animals, which had previously experienced several infections with *Campylobacter* species and preexisting *C. jejuni* antibody titers, did not develop diarrhea when dosed with *C. jejuni* 81-176 (94).

Interestingly, infant *M. nemestrina* animals have also been recently used as a model to study diarrheal disease caused by the enterohepatic *Helicobacter* species *H. cinaedi* and *H. fennelliae* (27). Both organisms caused acute watery diarrhea and bacteremia 3 to 7 days postinoculation in 12- to 25-day-old macaques. Rectal biopsy specimens were obtained in five of the animals and were normal in four. The remaining specimen was notable for acute mucosal inflammation. One monkey inoculated with *H. cinaedi* was euthanized. Histopathologic evaluation of the small intestinal and colonic mucosa gave normal results, and there was no evidence of either acute mucosal inflammation or of adherent microorganisms. After resolution of clinical signs, the stools were positive for the organism for >3 weeks postinoculation.

Rhesus monkeys have been used to determine the safety and immunogenicity of the *Campylobacter* whole-cell vaccine described in the section on mouse models (6, 8). Oral administration of *Campylobacter* whole-cell vaccine with *E. coli* heat-labile enterotoxin as an adjuvant resulted in the generation of *Campylobacter*-specific serum IgA and IgG responses (8).

In addition to being used as models of gastroenteritis, nonhuman primates have been studied as models of periodontal disease. Various nonhuman primates including *M. nemestrina* (85) and *M. mulatta* (24), are colonized with the periodontal pathogen *C. rectus,* and colonization appears to correlate with the presence of periodontal disease. There have not been any reports of experimental infection of nonhuman primates with *C. rectus* in an effort to induce periodontal disease. However, *C. rectus* has been shown to induce bone loss in an experimental mouse model of periodontal disease that involves injection of organisms into the subcutaneous tissues overlying the calvaria of normal mice (125).

CONCLUSIONS

Results of in vivo studies of rodents, lagomorphs, carnivores, and nonhuman primates have established several important criteria necessary for enteric colonization of *C. jejuni* in mammalian hosts. Although other virulence factors are poorly defined, the requirement for flagella on *C. jejuni* for colonization has been clearly documented. Also, flagellin plays a major antigenic role during colonization and development of colonization resistance to subsequent rechallenge with *C. jejuni* in both the rabbit and mouse models. Therefore, it is important for investigators to know the Lior and Penner serotype in designing in vivo challenge

studies. Also, other surface antigens, such as the cell-binding factor *peb1A,* probably play a role in developing immunity.

Thus far, *M. nemestrina* and perhaps the ferret offer useful models for studies of host-organism interaction, development of intestinal lesions, and conferred immunity. Both of these models, however, need development of species-specific immunological reagents, as well as the widespread commercial availability of specific-pathogen-free animals. As noted by Russell et al., additional studies are required to characterize the mechanisms of *C. jejuni*-induced colitis and to define the mucosal immunity to *C. jejuni* infection (94). Also, the importance of flagellin antigen in effecting protective immunity in the primate and ferret must be documented. The use of these models, however, may be limited by the cost of maintaining the animals.

Until recently, mouse models of *Campylobacter* infection have been limited to colonization models. Although these models have provided useful information about requirements for colonization by *Campylobacter,* they have not represented fully validated disease models. The finding that immunocompromised mice can develop significant pathology when challenged with *Campylobacter* represents a potentially important advance in the use of rodent models. Further work is required to characterize and utilize these models to test potential virulence factors.

Future in vivo experiments should include careful characterization of the infecting strain and, possibly, more general use of well-characterized *C. jejuni* strains, such as strain 81-176, previously validated in human experimental trials and other in vivo models (11, 94). However, the use of fresh clinical isolates that have undergone minimal passage in the laboratory may have advantages, including a greater likelihood of producing pathology that resembles infection in humans. Additionally, as other members of the genus *Campylobacter* such as *C. upsaliensis* (15) are recognized as important pathogens, in vivo studies on these organisms will have to be performed. The ability to sufficiently characterize clinical isolates may require the use of molecular techniques such as DNA probes or PCR-based assays for potential virulence factors. The determination of the complete *C. jejuni* genome sequence (4) should further accelerate the need for in vivo pathogenesis studies. Hopefully, by the judicious use of animal models in the next decade, further progress can be made in our understanding of the pathogenesis of and the prospects of a protective vaccine for this important enteric pathogen.

REFERENCES

1. **Abimiku, A. G., and J. M. Dolby.** 1988. Cross-protection of infant mice against intestinal colonisation by *Campylobacter jejuni:* importance of heat-labile serotyping (Lior) antigens. *J. Med. Microbiol.* **26**:265–268.

2. **Abimiku, A. G., J. M. Dolby, and S. P. Borriello.** 1989. Comparison of different vaccines and induced immune response against *Campylobacter jejuni* colonization in the infant mouse. *Epidemiol. Infect.* **102**:271–280.

3. **Aguero-Rosenfeld, M. E., X. H. Yang, and I. Nachamkin.** 1990. Infection of adult Syrian hamsters with flagellar variants of *Campylobacter jejuni. Infect. Immun.* **58**:2214–2219.

4. **Anonymous.** 1999. Genomic sequence of *C. jejuni* NTCC 11168. Sanger Center website, 6 October 1999. http://www.sanger.ac.uk/Projects/C_jejuni/

5. **Atabay, H. I., J. E. Corry, and S. L. On.** 1998. Identification of unusual *Campylobacter*-like isolates from poultry products as *Helicobacter pullorum. J. Appl. Microbiol.* **84**:1017–1024.

6. **Baqar, S., L. A. Applebee, and A. L. Bourgeois.** 1995. Immunogenicity and protective efficacy of a prototype *Campylobacter* killed whole-cell vaccine in mice. *Infect. Immun.* **63**:3731–3735.

7. **Baqar, S., A. L. Bourgeois, L. A. Applebee, A. S. Mourad, M. T. Kleinosky, Z. Mohran, and J. R. Murphy.** 1996. Murine intranasal challenge model for the study of *Campylobacter* pathogenesis and immunity. *Infect. Immun.* **64**:4933–4939.

8. **Baqar, S., A. L. Bourgeois, P. J. Schultheiss, R. I. Walker, D. M. Rollins, R. L. Haberberger, and O. R. Paviovskis.** 1995. Safety and immunogenicity of a prototype oral whole-cell killed *Campylobacter* vaccine administered with a mucosal adjuvant in non-human primates. *Vaccine* **13**:22–28.

9. **Bell, J. A., and D. D. Manning.** 1990. A do-mestic ferret model of immunity to *Campylobacter jejuni*-induced enteric disease. *Infect. Immun.* **58**:1848–1852.

10. **Bell, J. A., and D. D. Manning.** 1991. Evaluation of *Campylobacter jejuni* colonization of the domestic ferret intestine as a model of proliferative colitis. *Am. J. Vet. Res.* **52**:826–832.

11. **Black, R. E., M. M. Levine, M. L. Clements, T. P. Hughes, and M. J. Blaser.** 1988. Experimental *Campylobacter jejuni* infection in humans. *J. Infect. Dis.* **157**:472–479.

12. **Blaser, M. J., D. J. Duncan, G. H. Warren, and W. L. Wang.** 1983. Experimental *Campylobacter jejuni* infection of adult mice. *Infect. Immun.* **39**:908–916.

13. **Blaser, M. J., F. M. LaForce, N. A. Wilson, and W. L. Wang.** 1980. Reservoirs for human campylobacteriosis. *J. Infect. Dis.* **141**:665–669.

14. **Blaser, M. J., R. B. Parsons, and W. L. Wang.** 1980. Acute colitis caused by *Campylobacter fetus ss. jejuni. Gastroenterology* **78**:448–453.

15. **Bourke, B., V. L. Chan, and P. Sherman.** 1998. *Campylobacter upsaliensis:* waiting in the wings. *Clin. Microbiol. Rev.* **11**:440–449.

16. **Bryant, J. L., H. F. Stills, R. H. Lentsch, and C. C. Middleton.** 1983. *Campylobacter jejuni* isolated from patas monkeys with diarrhea. *Lab. Anim. Sci.* **33**:303–305.

17. **Bukholm, G., and G. Kapperud.** 1987. Expression of *Campylobacter jejuni* invasiveness in cell cultures coinfected with other bacteria. *Infect. Immun.* **55**:2816–2821.

18. **Burr, D. H., M. B. Caldwell, A. L. Bourgeois, H. R. Morgan, R. Wistar, Jr., and R. I. Walker.** 1988. Mucosal and systemic immunity to *Campylobacter jejuni* in rabbits after gastric inoculation. *Infect. Immun.* **56**:99–105.

19. **Burr, D. H., D. T. Kerner, C. S. Blanco, A. L. Bourgeois, and R. Wistar, Jr.** 1987. Gastric lavage: a simple method to obtain IgA-rich intestinal secretions from the rabbit. *J. Immunol. Methods* **99**:277–281.

20. **Cahill, R. J., C. J. Foltz, J. G. Fox, C. A. Dangler, F. Powrie, and D. B. Schauer.** 1997. Inflammatory bowel disease: an immunity-mediated condition triggered by bacterial infection with *Helicobacter hepaticus. Infect. Immun.* **65**:3126–3131.

21. **Cheville, N. F.** 1980. Criteria for development of animal models of diseases of the gastrointestinal system. *Am. J. Pathol.* **101**(Suppl.):S67–S76.

22. **Davies, A. P., C. J. Gebhart, and S. A. Meric.** 1984. *Campylobacter*-associated chronic diarrhea in a dog. *J. Am. Vet. Med. Assoc.* **184**:469–471.

23. **Diker, K. S., G. Hascelik, and S. Diker.** 1992. Colonization of infant mice with flagellar

variants of *Campylobacter jejuni. Acta Microbiol. Hung.* **39:**133–136.

24. **Eke, P. I., L. Braswell, R. Arnold, and M. Fritz.** 1993. Sub-gingival microflora in *Macaca mulatta* species of rhesus monkey. *J. Periodontal Res.* **28:**72–80.

25. **Field, L. H., J. L. Underwood, L. M. Pope, and L. J. Berry.** 1981. Intestinal colonization of neonatal animals by *Campylobacter fetus subsp. jejuni. Infect. Immun.* **33:**884–892.

26. **Fitzgeorge, R. B., A. Baskerville, and K. P. Lander.** 1981. Experimental infection of Rhesus monkeys with a human strain of *Campylobacter jejuni. J. Hyg.* **86:**343–351.

27. **Flores, B. M., C. L. Fennell, L. Kuller, M. A. Bronsdon, W. R. Morton, and W. E. Stamm.** 1990. Experimental infection of pig-tailed macaques (*Macaca nemestrina*) with *Campylobacter cinaedi* and *Campylobacter fennelliae. Infect. Immun.* **58:**3947–3953.

28. **Fox, J. G.** 1982. Campylobacteriosis—a "new" disease in laboratory animals. *Lab. Anim. Sci.* **32:**625–637.

29. **Fox, J. G.** 1997. The expanding genus of *Helicobacter:* pathogenic and zoonotic potential. *Semin. Gastrointest. Dis.* **8:**124–141.

30. **Fox, J. G.** 1992. In vivo models of enteric campylobacteriosis: natural and experimental infections, p. 131–138. *In* I. Nachamkin, M. J. Blaser, and L. S. Tompkins (ed.), *Campylobacter jejuni: Current Status and Future Trends.* American Society for Microbiology, Washington, D.C.

31. **Fox, J. G., J. A. Ackerman, and C. E. Newcomer.** 1985. The prevalence of *Campylobacter jejuni* in random-source cats used in biomedical research. *J. Infect. Dis.* **151:**743–744. (Letter.)

32. **Fox, J. G., J. I. Ackerman, and C. E. Newcomer.** 1983. Ferret as a potential reservoir for human campylobacteriosis. *Am. J. Vet. Res.* **44:**1049–1052.

33. **Fox, J. G., J. I. Ackerman, N. Taylor, M. Claps, and J. C. Murphy.** 1987. *Campylobacter jejuni* infection in the ferret: an animal model of human campylobacteriosis. *Am. J. Vet. Res.* **48:**85–90.

34. **Fox, J. G., M. C. Claps, N. S. Taylor, K. O. Maxwell, J. I. Ackerman, and S. B. Hoffman.** 1988. *Campylobacter jejuni/coli* in commercially reared beagles: prevalence and serotypes. *Lab. Anim. Sci.* **38:**262–265.

35. **Fox, J. G., F. E. Dewhirst, Z. Shen, Y. Feng, N. S. Taylor, B. J. Paster, R. L. Ericson, C. N. Lau, P. Correa, J. C. Araya, and I. Roa.** 1998. Hepatic *Helicobacter* species identified in bile and gallbladder tissue from Chileans with chronic cholecystitis. *Gastroenterology* **114:**755–763.

36. **Fox, J. G., F. E. Dewhirst, J. G. Tully, B. J. Paster, L. Yan, N. S. Taylor, M. J. Collins, Jr., P. L. Gorelick, and J. M. Ward.** 1994. *Helicobacter hepaticus* sp. nov., a microaerophilic bacterium isolated from livers and intestinal mucosal scrapings from mice. *J. Clin. Microbiol.* **32:**1238–1245.

37. **Fox, J. G., S. Krakowka, and N. S. Taylor.** 1985. Acute-onset *Campylobacter*-associated gastroenteritis in adult beagles. *J. Am. Vet. Med. Assoc.* **187:**1268–1271.

38. **Fox, J. G., K. O. Maxwell, and J. I. Ackerman.** 1984. *Campylobacter jejuni* associated diarrhea in commercially reared beagles. *Lab. Anim. Sci.* **34:**151–155.

39. **Fox, J. G., K. O. Maxwell, N. S. Taylor, C. D. Runsick, P. Edmonds, and D. J. Brenner.** 1989. "*Campylobacter upsaliensis*" isolated from cats as identified by DNA relatedness and biochemical features. *J. Clin. Microbiol.* **27:**2376–2378.

40. **Fox, J. G., R. Moore, and J. I. Ackerman.** 1983. *Campylobacter jejuni*-associated diarrhea in dogs. *J. Am. Vet. Med. Assoc.* **183:**1430–1433.

41. **Fox, J. G., B. J. Paster, F. E. Dewhirst, N. S. Taylor, L. L. Yan, P. J. Macuch, and L. M. Chmura.** 1992. *Helicobacter mustelae* isolation from feces of ferrets: evidence to support fecal-oral transmission of a gastric *Helicobacter. Infect. Immun.* **60:**606–611. (Erratum, **60:**4443.)

42. **Fox, J. G., N. S. Taylor, J. L. Penner, B. Shames, R. V. Gurgis, and F. N. Tomson.** 1989. Investigation of zoonotically acquired *Campylobacter jejuni* enteritis with serotyping and restriction endonuclease DNA analysis. *J. Clin. Microbiol.* **27:**2423–2425.

43. **Fox, J. G., L. Yan, B. Shames, J. Campbell, J. C. Murphy, and X. Li.** 1996. Persistent hepatitis and enterocolitis in germfree mice infected with *Helicobacter hepaticus. Infect. Immun.* **64:**3673–3781.

44. **Fox, J. G., L. L. Yan, F. E. Dewhirst, B. J. Paster, B. Shames, J. C. Murphy, A. Hayward, J. C. Belcher, and E. N. Mendes.** 1995. *Helicobacter bilis* sp. nov., a novel *Helicobacter* species isolated from bile, livers, and intestines of aged, inbred mice. *J. Clin. Microbiol.* **33:**445–454.

45. **Fox, J. G., S. Zanotti, and H. V. Jordan.** 1981. The hamster as a reservoir of *Campylobacter fetus* subspecies *jejuni. J. Infect. Dis.* **143:**856.

46. **Gebhart, C. J., C. L. Fennell, M. P. Murtaugh, and W. E. Stamm.** 1989. *Campylobacter cinaedi* is normal intestinal flora in hamsters. *J. Clin. Microbiol.* **27:**1692–1694.

47. **Gebhart, C. J., G. E. Ward, K. Chang, and H. J. Kurtz.** 1983. *Campylobacter hyointestinalis*

(new species) isolated from swine with lesions of proliferative ileitis. *Am. J. Vet. Res.* **44:**361–367.

48. **Hald, B., and M. Madsen.** 1997. Healthy puppies and kittens as carriers of *Campylobacter* spp., with special reference to *Campylobacter upsaliensis*. *J. Clin. Microbiol.* **35:**3351–3352.

49. **Hodgson, A. E., B. W. McBride, M. J. Hudson, G. Hall, and S. A. Leach.** 1998. Experimental campylobacter infection and diarrhoea in immunodeficient mice. *J. Med. Microbiol.* **47:**799–809.

50. **Hudson, S. J., N. F. Lightfoot, J. C. Coulson, K. Russell, P. R. Sisson, and A. O. Sobo.** 1991. Jackdaws and magpies as vectors of milkborne human *Campylobacter* infection. *Epidemiol. Infect.* **107:**363–372.

51. **Hunter, D. B., J. F. Prescott, D. M. Hoover, G. Hlywka, and J. A. Kerr.** 1986. *Campylobacter* colitis in ranch mink in Ontario. *Can. J. Vet. Res.* **50:**47–53.

52. **Jones, T. C.** 1980. The value of animal models. *Am. J. Pathol.* **101**(Suppl.)**:**S3–S9.

53. **Kaufmann, S. H.** 1994. Bacterial and protozoal infections in genetically disrupted mice. *Curr. Opin. Immunol.* **6:**518–525.

54. **Kaufmann, S. H., and C. H. Ladel.** 1994. Application of knockout mice to the experimental analysis of infections with bacteria and protozoa. *Trends Microbiol.* **2:**235–242.

55. **Kazmi, S. U., B. S. Roberson, and N. J. Stern.** 1984. Animal-passed, virulence-enhanced *Campylobacter jejuni* causes enteritis in neonatal mice. *Curr. Microbiol.* **11:**159–164.

56. **Kiehlbauch, J. A., D. J. Brenner, M. A. Nicholson, C. N. Baker, C. M. Patton, A. G. Steigerwalt, and I. K. Wachsmuth.** 1991. *Campylobacter butzleri* sp. nov. isolated from humans and animals with diarrheal illness. *J. Clin. Microbiol.* **29:**376–385.

57. **Konkel, M. E., and L. A. Joens.** 1990. Effect of enteroviruses on adherence to and invasion of HEp-2 cells by *Campylobacter* isolates. *Infect. Immun.* **58:**1101–1105.

58. **Kullberg, M. C., J. M. Ward, P. L. Gorelick, P. Caspar, S. Hieny, A. Cheever, D. Jankovic, and A. Sher.** 1998. *Helicobacter hepaticus* triggers colitis in specific-pathogen-free interleukin-10 (IL-10)-deficient mice through an IL-12- and gamma interferon-dependent mechanism. *Infect. Immun.* **66:**5157–5166.

59. **Kusters, J. G., and E. J. Kuipers.** 1998. Nonpylori *Helicobacter* infections in humans. *Eur. J. Gastroenterol. Hepatology* **10:**239–241.

60. **Lawson, A. J., D. Linton, and J. Stanley.** 1998. 16S rRNA gene sequences of "*Candidatus* *Campylobacter hominis*," a novel uncultivated species, are found in the gastrointestinal tract of healthy humans. *Microbiology* **144:**2063–2071.

61. **Leader, R. W., and G. A. Padgett.** 1980. The genesis and validation of animal models. *Am. J. Pathol.* **101**(Suppl.)**:**S11–S16.

62. **Lee, A., J. L. O'Rourke, P. J. Barrington, and T. J. Trust.** 1986. Mucus colonization as a determinant of pathogenicity in intestinal infection by *Campylobacter jejuni:* a mouse cecal model. *Infect. Immun.* **51:**536–546.

63. **Lee, A., M. W. Phillips, J. L. O'Rourke, B. J. Paster, F. E. Dewhirst, G. J. Fraser, J. G. Fox, L. I. Sly, P. J. Romaniuk, T. J. Trust, and S. Kouprach.** 1992. *Helicobacter muridarum* sp. nov., a microaerophilic helical bacterium with a novel ultrastructure isolated from the intestinal mucosa of rodents. *Int. J. Syst. Bacteriol.* **42:**27–36.

64. **Li, C. Y., P. Xue, W. Q. Tian, R. C. Liu, and C. Yang.** 1996. Experimental *Campylobacter jejuni* infection in the chicken: an animal model of axonal Guillain-Barré syndrome. *J. Neurol. Neurosurg. Psychiatry* **61:**279–284.

65. **Li, X., J. G. Fox, M. T. Whary, L. Yan, B. Shames, and Z. Zhao.** 1998. SCID/NCr mice naturally infected with *Helicobacter hepaticus* develop progressive hepatitis, proliferative typhlitis, and colitis. *Infect. Immun.* **66:**5477–5484.

66. **Luechtefeld, N. W., R. C. Cambre, and W. L. Wang.** 1981. Isolation of *Campylobacter fetus* subsp. *jejuni* from zoo animals. *J. Am. Vet. Med. Assoc.* **179:**1119–1122.

67. **Macartney, L., R. R. Al-Mashat, D. J. Taylor, and I. A. McCandlish.** 1988. Experimental infection of dogs with *Campylobacter jejuni*. *Vet. Rec.* **122:**245–249.

68. **Manning, D. D., and J. A. Bell.** 1990. Derivation of gnotobiotic ferrets: perinatal diet and hand-rearing requirements. *Lab. Anim. Sci.* **40:**51–55.

69. **McOrist, S., and J. W. Browning.** 1982. Carriage of *Campylobacter jejuni* in healthy and diarrhoeic dogs and cats. *Aust. Vet. J.* **58:**33–34. (Letter.)

70. **Migaki, G., and C. C. Capen.** 1984. Animal models in biomedical research, p. 667–695. *In* J. G. Fox, B. J. Cohen, and F. M. Loew (ed.), *Laboratory Animal Medicine.* Academic Press, Inc., Orlando, Fla.

71. **Moreno, G. S., P. L. Griffiths, I. F. Connerton, and R. W. Park.** 1993. Occurrence of campylobacters in small domestic and laboratory animals. *J. Appl. Bacteriol.* **75:**49–54.

72. **Morooka, T., A. Umeda, and K. Amako.** 1985. Motility as an intestinal colonization factor for *Campylobacter jejuni*. *J. Gen. Microbiol.* **131:**1973–1980.

73. **Morton, W. R., M. Bronsdon, G. Mickelsen, G. Knitter, S. Rosenkranz, L. Kuller, and D. Sajuthi.** 1983. Identification of *Campylobacter jejuni* in *Macaca fascicularis* imported from Indonesia. *Lab. Anim. Sci.* **33:**187–188.

74. **Munroe, D. L., J. F. Prescott, and J. L. Penner.** 1983. *Campylobacter jejuni* and *Campylobacter coli* serotypes isolated from chickens, cattle, and pigs. *J. Clin. Microbiol.* **18:**877–881.

75. **Nachamkin, I., X. H. Yang, and N. J. Stern.** 1993. Role of *Campylobacter jejuni* flagella as colonization factors for three-day-old chicks: analysis with flagellar mutants. *Appl. Environ. Microbiol.* **59:**1269–1273.

76. **Newell, D. G.** 1986. Monoclonal antibodies directed against the flagella of *Campylobacter jejuni:* production, characterization and lack of effect on the colonization of infant mice. *J. Hyg.* **96:** 131–141.

77. **Newell, D. G., H. McBride, and J. M. Dolby.** 1985. Investigations on the role of flagella in the colonization of infant mice with *Campylobacter jejuni* and attachment of *Campylobacter jejuni* to human epithelial cell lines. *J. Hyg.* **95:**217–227.

78. **Newell, D. G., and A. Pearson.** 1984. The invasion of epithelial cell lines and the intestinal epithelium of infant mice by *Campylobacter jejuni/coli. J. Diarrhoeal Dis. Res.* **2:**19–26.

79. **Newton, C. M., D. G. Newell, M. Wood, and M. Baskerville.** 1988. *Campylobacter* infection in a closed dog breeding colony. *Vet. Rec.* **123:**152–154.

80. **Olson, P., and K. Sandstedt.** 1987. *Campylobacter* in the dog: a clinical and experimental study. *Vet. Rec.* **121:**99–101.

81. **Oswald, G. P., D. C. Twedt, and P. Steyn.** 1994. *Campylobacter jejuni* bacteremia and acute cholecystitis in two dogs. *J. Am. Anim. Hosp. Assoc.* **30:**165–169.

82. **Pavlovskis, O. R., D. M. Rollins, R. L. Haberberger, Jr., A. E. Green, L. Habash, S. Strocko, and R. I. Walker.** 1991. Significance of flagella in colonization resistance of rabbits immunized with *Campylobacter* spp. *Infect. Immun.* **59:**2259–2264.

83. **Pei, Z., C. Burucoa, B. Grignon, S. Baqar, X. Z. Huang, D. J. Kopecko, A. L. Bourgeois, J. L. Fauchere, and M. J. Blaser.** 1998. Mutation in the *peb1A* locus of *Campylobacter jejuni* reduces interactions with epithelial cells and intestinal colonization of mice. *Infect. Immun.* **66:** 938–943.

84. **Perlman, D. M., N. M. Ampel, R. B. Schifman, D. L. Cohn, C. M. Patton, M. L. Aguirre, W. L. Wang, and M. J. Blaser.** 1988. Persistent *Campylobacter jejuni* infections in patients infected with the human immunodeficiency virus (HIV). *Ann. Intern. Med.* **108:** 540–546.

85. **Persson, G. R., L. D. Engel, B. J. Moncla, and R. C. Page.** 1993. *Macaca nemestrina:* a nonhuman primate model for studies of periodontal disease. *J. Periodontal Res.* **28:**294–300.

86. **Prescott, J. F., I. K. Barker, K. I. Manninen, and O. P. Miniats.** 1981. *Campylobacter jejuni* colitis in gnotobiotic dogs. *Can. J. Comp. Med.* **45:**377–383.

87. **Prescott, J. F., and C. W. Bruin-Mosch.** 1981. Carriage of *Campylobacter jejuni* in healthy and diarrheic animals. *Am. J. Vet. Res.* **42:** 164–165.

88. **Prescott, J. F., and M. A. Karmali.** 1978. Attempts to transmit campylobacter enteritis to dogs and cats. *Can. Med. Assoc. J.* **119:** 1001–1002. (Letter.)

89. **Rams, T. E., D. Feik, and J. Slots.** 1993. *Campylobacter rectus* in human periodontitis. *Oral Microbiol. Immunol.* **8:**230–235.

90. **Rehg, J. E., F. Gigliotti, and D. C. Stokes.** 1988. Cryptosporidiosis in ferrets. *Lab. Anim. Sci.* **38:**155–158.

91. **Rice, B. E., D. M. Rollins, E. T. Mallinson, L. Carr, and S. W. Joseph.** 1997. *Campylobacter jejuni* in broiler chickens: colonization and humoral immunity following oral vaccination and experimental infection. *Vaccine* **15:**1922–1932.

92. **Rosef, O., B. Gondrosen, G. Kapperud, and B. Underdal.** 1983. Isolation and characterization of *Campylobacter jejuni* and *Campylobacter coli* from domestic and wild mammals in Norway. *Appl. Environ. Microbiol.* **46:**855–859.

93. **Rosef, O., G. Kapperud, S. Lauwers, and B. Gondrosen.** 1985. Serotyping of *Campylobacter jejuni, Campylobacter coli,* and *Campylobacter laridis* from domestic and wild animals. *Appl. Environ. Microbiol.* **49:**1507–1510.

94. **Russell, R. G., M. J. Blaser, J. I. Sarmiento, and J. Fox.** 1989. Experimental *Campylobacter jejuni* infection in *Macaca nemestrina. Infect. Immun.* **57:**1438–1444.

95. **Russell, R. G., J. A. Kiehlbauch, C. J. Gebhart, and L. J. DeTolla.** 1992. Uncommon *Campylobacter* species in infant *Macaca nemestrina* monkeys housed in a nursery. *J. Clin. Microbiol.* **30:**3024–3027.

96. **Russell, R. G., L. Krugner, C. C. Tsai, and R. Ekstrom.** 1988. Prevalence of *Campylobacter* in infant, juvenile and adult laboratory primates. *Lab. Anim. Sci.* **38:**711–714.

97. **Russell, R. G., S. L. Rosenkranz, L. A. Lee, H. Howard, R. F. DiGiacomo, M. A. Bronsdon, G. A. Blakley, C. C. Tsai, and W. R. Morton.** 1987. Epidemiology and etiol-

ogy of diarrhea in colony-born *Macaca nemestrina*. *Lab. Anim. Sci.* **37**:309–316.

98. **Russell, R. G., J. I. Sarmiento, J. Fox, and P. Panigrahi.** 1990. Evidence of reinfection with multiple strains of *Campylobacter jejuni* and *Campylobacter coli* in *Macaca nemestrina* housed under hyperendemic conditions. *Infect. Immun.* **58**:2149–2155.

99. **Sandstedt, K., and M. Wierup.** 1981. Concomitant occurrence of *Campylobacter* and parvoviruses in dogs with gastroenteritis. *Vet. Res. Commun.* **4**:271–273.

100. **Schoeni, J. L., and A. C. Wong.** 1994. Inhibition of *Campylobacter jejuni* colonization in chicks by defined competitive exclusion bacteria. *Appl. Environ. Microbiol.* **60**:1191–1197.

101. **Shames, B., J. G. Fox, F. Dewhirst, L. Yan, Z. Shen, and N. S. Taylor.** 1995. Identification of widespread *Helicobacter hepaticus* infection in feces in commercial mouse colonies by culture and PCR assay. *J. Clin. Microbiol.* **33**:2968–2972.

102. **Shanker, S., A. Lee, and T. C. Sorrell.** 1990. Horizontal transmission of *Campylobacter jejuni* amongst broiler chicks: experimental studies. *Epidemiol. Infect.* **104**:101–110.

103. **Stanfield, J. T., B. A. McCardell, and J. M. Madden.** 1987. *Campylobacter* diarrhea in an adult mouse model. *Microb. Pathog.* **3**:155–165.

104. **Stanley, J., A. P. Burnens, D. Linton, S. L. On, M. Costas, and R. J. Owen.** 1992. *Campylobacter helveticus sp. nov.*, a new thermophilic species from domestic animals: characterization, and cloning of a species-specific DNA probe. *J. Gen. Microbiol.* **138**:2293–2303.

105. **Stanley, J., D. Linton, A. P. Burnens, F. E. Dewhirst, S. L. On, A. Porter, R. J. Owen, and M. Costas.** 1994. *Helicobacter pullorum sp. nov.*—genotype and phenotype of a new species isolated from poultry and from human patients with gastroenteritis. *Microbiology* **140**:3441–3449.

106. **Stanley, K. N., J. S. Wallace, J. E. Currie, P. J. Diggle, and K. Jones.** 1998. The seasonal variation of thermophilic campylobacters in beef cattle, dairy cattle and calves. *J. Appl. Microbiol.* **85**:472–480.

107. **Stanley, K. N., J. S. Wallace, J. E. Currie, P. J. Diggle, and K. Jones.** 1998. Seasonal variation of thermophilic campylobacters in lambs at slaughter. *J. Appl. Microbiol.* **84**:1111–1116.

108. **Steinbrueckner, B., G. Haerter, K. Pelz, S. Weiner, J. A. Rump, W. Deissler, S. Breswill, and M. Kist.** 1997. Isolation of *Helicobacter pullorum* from patients with enteritis. *Scand. J. Infect. Dis.* **29**:315–318.

109. **Stills, H. F., Jr., R. R. Hook, Jr., and D. A. Kinden.** 1989. Isolation of a *Campylobacter*-like organism from healthy Syrian hamsters (*Mesocricetus auratus*). *J. Clin. Microbiol.* **27**:2497–2501.

110. **Tee, W., and A. Mijch.** 1998. *Campylobacter jejuni* bacteremia in human immunodeficiency virus (HIV)-infected and non-HIV-infected patients: comparison of clinical features and review. *Clin. Infect. Dis.* **26**:91–96.

111. **Torre, E., and M. Tello.** 1993. Factors influencing fecal shedding of *Campylobacter jejuni* in dogs without diarrhea. *Am. J. Vet. Res.* **54**:260–262.

112. **Tribe, G. W., and M. P. Fleming.** 1983. Biphasic enteritis in imported cynomolgus (*Macaca fascicularis*) monkeys infected with *Shigella, Salmonella* and *Campylobacter* species. *Lab. Anim.* **17**:65–69.

113. **Tribe, G. W., and A. Frank.** 1980. *Campylobacter* in monkeys. *Vet. Rec.* **106**:365–366.

114. **Tribe, G. W., P. S. Mackenzie, and M. P. Fleming.** 1979. Incidence of thermophilic *Campylobacter* species in newly imported simian primates with enteritis. *Vet. Rec.* **105**:333. (Letter.)

115. **Van Citters, R.** 1973. *The Role of Animal Research in Clinical Medicine*, p. 3–8. U.S. Department of Health, Education, and Welfare publication. NIH 72-333. National Institutes of Health, Bethesda, Md.

116. **Walker, R. I., M. B. Caldwell, E. C. Lee, P. Guerry, T. J. Trust, and G. M. Ruiz-Palacios.** 1986. Pathophysiology of *Campylobacter* enteritis. *Microbiol. Rev.* **50**:81–94.

117. **Walker, R. I., E. A. Schmauder-Chock, J. L. Parker, and D. Burr.** 1988. Selective association and transport of *Campylobacter jejuni* through M cells of rabbit Peyer's patches. *Can. J. Microbiol.* **34**:1142–1147.

118. **Wallace, J. S., K. N. Stanley, and K. Jones.** 1998. The colonization of turkeys by thermophilic campylobacters. *J. Appl. Microbiol.* **85**:224–230.

119. **Ward, J. M., M. R. Anver, D. C. Haines, and R. E. Benveniste.** 1994. Chronic active hepatitis in mice caused by *Helicobacter hepaticus*. *Am. J. Pathol.* **145**:959–968.

120. **Wassenaar, T. M., B. A. van der Zeijst, R. Ayling, and D. G. Newell.** 1993. Colonization of chicks by motility mutants of *Campylobacter jejuni* demonstrates the importance of flagellin A expression. *J. Gen. Microbiol.* **139**:1171–1175.

121. **Whary, M. T., T. J. Morgan, C. A. Dangler, K. J. Gaudes, N. S. Taylor, and J. G. Fox.** 1998. Chronic active hepatitis induced by *Helico-*

bacter hepaticus in the A/JCr mouse is associated with a Th1 cell-mediated immune response. *Infect. Immun.* **66**:3142–3148.

122. **Young, V. B., C. A. Dangler, J. G. Fox, and D. B. Schauer.** 1999. Experimental gastritis in scid mice experimentally infected with *Campylobacter fetus,* abstr. DB-68, p. 86. *In Abstracts of the 99th General Meeting of the American Society for Microbiology,* 1999. American Society for Microbiology, Washington, D.C.

123. **Yrios, J. W., and E. Balish.** 1986. Colonization and infection of athymic and euthymic germfree mice by *Campylobacter jejuni* and *Campylobacter fetus* subsp. *fetus. Infect. Immun.* **53:** 378–383.

124. **Yrios, J. W., and E. Balish.** 1986. Pathogenesis of *Campylobacter* spp. in athymic and euthymic germfree mice. *Infect. Immun.* **53:**384–392.

125. **Zubery, Y., C. R. Dunstan, B. M. Story, L. Kesavalu, J. L. Ebersole, S. C. Holt, and B. F. Boyce.** 1998. Bone resorption caused by three periodontal pathogens in vivo in mice is mediated in part by prostaglandin. *Infect. Immun.* **66**:4158–4162.

PROTECTION AGAINST
CAMPYLOBACTER INFECTION AND
VACCINE DEVELOPMENT

Daniel A. Scott and David R. Tribble

15

RATIONALE FOR *CAMPYLOBACTER* VACCINE DEVELOPMENT

Campylobacter species, predominantly *Campylobacter jejuni,* are a common cause of diarrheal illness worldwide. The incidence of disease (cases/100,00 population) varies widely, generally falling into one of three different three epidemiologic scenarios: (i) hyperendemic levels (40,000/100,000 children younger than 5 years) in developing regions (20, 21, 31, 51–53, 112, 122); (ii) endemic levels (25/100,000 population), occurring most commonly as sporadic disease in young adults and infants, in developed countries (20, 21, 35, 120, 122) and (iii) traveler's diarrhea (TD) in persons from industrialized countries visiting regions of hyperendemic infection (20, 21, 29, 80, 96, 115, 120, 122, 123). Studies of these at-risk populations have contributed knowledge about *Campylobacter*-acquired immunity and the viability of developing an effective *Campylobacter* vaccine. Epidemiologic studies of children in the developing world have provided evidence of protective immunity through investigations of disease incidence, clinical presentation, stool microbiology, and *Campylobacter*-specific immunology (20–22, 26, 31,

51–53, 78, 112, 114, 122, 124, 125). Children (typically younger than 2 years) with *Campylobacter*-associated illness present with a less severe clinical course than do affected individuals in regions with a lower incidence of campylobacterioses (21, 27, 53, 67, 70, 118, 122, 124). Patients with *Campylobacter* enteritis presenting for care in industrialized regions more commonly exhibit moderate to severe symptoms and signs of an inflammatory diarrhea or dysentery (such as fevers and bloody diarrhea) consistent with a naive or semi-immune status. The clinical outcomes do not appear to be related to regional strain differences, since travelers visiting these areas experience patterns of clinical illness similar to those for *Campylobacter*-associated disease in industrialized countries (96, 115).

In addition to these clinical observations, studies including microbiologic surveillance in children in the developing world have documented a shift in illness-to-infection ratio accompanied by an apparent development of colonization resistance, in children between 2 and 5 years old (52, 122, 124, 125). Coincident with the increasing proportion of asymptomatic infections, there is a shortened excretion period during convalescence and a gradual increase in *Campylobacter*-specific serology (20, 21, 122, 125, 125). Cross-sectional and cohort

Daniel A. Scott and David R. Tribble, Enteric Diseases Program, Naval Medical Research Institute, 8901 Wisconsin Ave., Bethesda, MD 20889-5607.

Campylobacter, 2nd Ed., Edited by I. Nachamkin and M. J. Blaser
© 2000 American Society for Microbiology, Washington, D.C.

studies of age-related *C. jejuni*-specific serology demonstrate a progressive rise in the levels of all isotypes during the first 2 years of life followed by continued increases in immunoglobulin A (IgA) titers (possibly indicative of frequent exposure and subsequent mucosal immunity), declines in IgG titers, and plateauing of IgM titers in age group prevalence surveys (20, 21, 78). More direct evidence of immune system correlates with clinical outcome derives from studies of breast-fed Mexican infants (younger than 6 months) (100). A lower incidence of *Campylobacter*-associated diarrhea occurred in infants whose mothers had colostral *Campylobacter*-specific secretory IgA antibodies in breast milk.

The frequency and magnitude of exposure in industrialized regions is severalfold lower than the experience of children in the developing world. Observational studies in selected populations originating in lower-incidence regions but experiencing periods of more frequent exposure provide indirect evidence of acquired immunity (24, 25). This situation has been observed in reduced *C. jejuni*-associated diarrheal attack rates and increased *Campylobacter*-specific antibody levels in chronic raw-milk consumers on dairy farms compared to individuals with first-time exposure to raw milk. Expatriate residents in Thailand were observed to have reduced prevalence rates of *Campylobacter*-associated diarrheal illness related to the duration of residency: 8 of 47 (17%) for persons resident for less than 1 year versus 2 of 58 (3%) for persons resident for more than 1 year (49). In addition to epidemiologic evidence, experimental *C. jejuni* infection studies in humans documented short-term protection from illness caused by the homologous strain at 1 to 2 months following the initial infection (17, 19). Experimental-infection studies at the University of Maryland demonstrated infection-induced serologic and intestinal antibody responses, higher prechallenge *C. jejuni*-specific (acid-extracted protein) levels of IgA in serum and jejunal fluid in noninfected than infected subjects, and increased levels of IgA in jejunal fluid during rechallenge in subjects re-

maining well on the second exposure. Homologous rechallenge provided complete protection from illness; however, colonization resistance following this second *C. jejuni* exposure (10^9 CFU challenge dose) was observed in only two of the seven subjects (29%). Our investigative team at the U.S. Naval Medical Research Center (NMRC) and the U.S. Army Medical Research Institute of Infectious Diseases (USAMRIID) has undertaken recent studies reassessing the *C. jejuni* experimental model (126). These studies have provided confirmation of complete homologous protection from *Campylobacter*-associated illness as seen in the University of Maryland study. Subjects receiving rechallenge with a 10^9 CFU infectious dose approximately 1 month after initial infection were all protected from illness and 38% demonstrated resistance to colonization. Observational and experimental studies provide ample evidence of acquired immunity developing in humans exposed to *C. jejuni*, lending support to the concept of vaccine development. Prevention and control strategies for enterically transmitted *Campylobacter* infections involve a multifaceted approach including reduction and avoidance of *C. jejuni* contamination across critical control points along the farm-to-table food chain as well as immunoprophylaxis for at-risk populations.

POTENTIAL TARGET POPULATIONS FOR VACCINE APPLICATION

Campylobacter vaccine development strategy must integrate basic scientific knowledge of pathogenesis and immunity and appreciation of the antigens and host responses most strongly associated with the development of protective immunity. More practical concerns include the need to optimize vaccine production methods, delivery methods, and regimen selection followed by an assessment of vaccine safety, immunogenicity, and efficacy in target populations. Field site development for vaccine testing also requires risk assessment and feasibility evaluation in at-risk populations early in the development process. Issues to consider include such areas as the multiple serotypes of *C. jejuni* associated with disease, protective epitopes, immune correlates of protection, the duration and cross-serotypic nature of protective responses, and numerous pragmatic considerations related to the target population demographics, period of risk, and vaccination method.

Children in the Developing World

As stated above, *C. jejuni*-associated disease occurs commonly in three settings: children (0 to 4 years old) in the developing world, persons in industrialized nation (the highest rates are in infants and young adults), and naive or semi-immune travelers to the developing world. There are several concerns and possible limitations regarding *C. jejuni* vaccine development for children in the developing world. The frequency and magnitude of exposure in this hyperendemic environment, 0.4 infectious episode annually over the first 4 to 5 years of the child's life, would require vaccination during the initial 6 months of life to decrease the diarrheal disease burden during this vulnerable period (122). Challenges to the vaccine's effectiveness in this population include frequent and possibly high-level exposures to virulent organisms, exposures to multiple strains age-related differences in immune system development (total IgA levels are approximately 80% of the adult levels by 8 years of age) (34), coexistent non-*Campylobacter*-associated diarrheal disease and/or malnutrition, and potential difficulties encountered in delivering an oral immunization to young infants. An effective vaccination program during infancy may lead to a modification of the at-risk age range by shifting disease onset to older children, who would probably tolerate diarrheal illness with less morbidity and mortality. A vaccine strategy may involve repeated booster doses in a population with anticipated ongoing exposures; alternatively the repeated exposures themselves may serve to solidify protective immunity, as observed in epidemiologic studies, with less overall risk of serious disease.

Individuals in Industrialized Countries

The major impact of diarrheal disease in industrialized countries such as the United States relates to short-term morbidity and economic burden. Diarrhea-related mortality typically is limited to populations at the extremes of age, particularly the elderly. Overall case-fatality rates in the United States are far lower than rates seen within the most at-risk population (children younger than 5 years) in developing countries, 0.014 and 13.6 deaths per 1,000 persons/year respectively (108). *C. jejuni* has been estimated to be the most common bacterial etiology of diarrhea in industrialized nations (2, 35, 95). A full appreciation of diarrheal disease in the United States is lacking due to the usually self-limited nature of the disease, infrequent medical evaluation, lack of diagnostic work-up, and incomplete reporting and passive-surveillance systems. The Centers for Disease Control and Prevention has formed a food-borne disease evaluation program called FoodNet as part of its Emerging Infections Program (35). The objectives of this program are to more precisely assess the burden of food-borne disease, determine the relative proportion of specific etiologic agents contributing to disease episodes, and develop the infrastructure needed to respond to emerging food-borne threats. The program is a population-based active-surveillance system in clinical microbiology laboratories in certain states. A population survey in 1997 of 10,000 residents within the surveillance area found an 11% diarrhea rate within the preceding month, which would yield an annual rate of 1.4 episodes/person. Of these affected persons, only 8% sought medical advice, and when they did, only 20% of practitioners obtained a stool specimen for analysis. It is somewhat intuitive and certainly clear through this survey that active surveillance based in clinical microbiology laboratories represents only a small fraction of diarrheal illnesses and detects the more severe and/or prolonged cases. FoodNet surveillance from 1997 found *C. jejuni* to be the most commonly encountered bacterial enteropathogen (24.9/100,000 population). Sporadic cases were most typical, with increased rates observed in children younger than 1 year (57/100,000) (35). The predominance of *Campylobacter* infections as the leading food-borne pathogen has also been observed in European surveillance systems. The incidence and the resultant morbidity, however, are not high enough to warrant broad application of a *Campylobacter* vaccine to the general population. Targeting subpopulations at extremely high risk (e.g., chronically immunosuppressed patients) may be more reasonable.

Travelers to Areas of Hyperendemic Infection

Naïve or semi-immune travelers to regions of hyperendemic *Campylobacter* infection constitute a moderate- to high-risk population that is most amenable to vaccination. This diverse population consists of business, leisure, and military travelers, as well as expatriates residing in developing regions. The naïve or semi-immune traveler leaving a relatively low-risk environment to travel to an area where bacterial enteropathogens are hyperendemic has an approximately 40% diarrhea risk (16, 33, 45, 116). In most TD series in tourists and the military, enterotoxigenic *Escherichia coli* (ETEC) is the most commonly identified agent, representing between 5 and 40% of cases (16, 33, 45, 116). *C. jejuni* (3 to 45%), *Shigella* spp. (2 to 10%), and nontyphoidal *Salmonella* spp. (2 to 10%) are other commonly identified etiologic agents, with regional and seasonal variability affecting the relative agent-specific distribution (16, 33, 45, 80, 116). In certain regions, such as Thailand, *Campylobacter* has consistently been the most common enteropathogen isolated from patients with TD in deployed military populations (72, 86, 96). "Typical" TD represents a spectrum of illness from a fleeting mild diarrhea without associated symptoms or activity limitation to a serious dehydrating and/or febrile dysentery requiring hospitalization. Most commonly, TD consists of a self-limited diarrheal illness lasting 3 to 5 days (45, 48, 68). The mean duration of symptoms without treatment is approximately 4 days (median, 2 days). The duration of *C. jejuni* illness exceeds 1 week in up to 20 to 25% of affected individuals, as seen in follow-up studies of out-

breaks and sporadic disease (23, 66, 82). A study of Finnish travelers to Morocco demonstrated a more severe clinical illness with *C. jejuni* than with ETEC (79). The patients with *Campylobacter*-associated cases had an increased frequency of diarrheal stools on the follow-up visits (days 2 and 3) as well as more fevers, myalgias, abdominal cramps, and nausea or vomiting. In addition to a relatively more severe clinical course, the management of *Campylobacter*-associated TD is further complicated by an increasing level of antimicrobial resistance. Since 1990, ciprofloxacin-resistant *Campylobacter* strains have been found in numerous locations (50, 59, 99, 104, 113). In Thailand from 1990 to the present, ciprofloxacin-resistant *C. jejuni/coli* strains have increased from 0 to >85% of isolates (72, 86, 96). Macrolide (erythromycin and azithromycin)-resistant organisms also were observed in 9 (31%) of 54 patients during a 1-month military deployment in 1994 (86).

Consideration of a *Campylobacter* vaccine must be addressed in the context of a combined TD vaccine, taking into account other common bacterial enteropathogens such as ETEC and *Shigella* spp. An effective TD vaccine should contain a *Campylobacter* component based on the relative contribution of *C. jejuni* as a major bacterial enteropathogen, increasing antimicrobial resistance noted against first-line TD empirical antibiotics, and the relatively increased clinical severity of *C. jejuni*-associated TD compared to TD due to other major enteropathogens (primarily ETEC).

CONSIDERATIONS FOR VACCINE DEVELOPMENT
Properties of the Bacterium

Despite the importance of *Campylobacter* spp. as human enteropathogens, relatively little is known about the mechanisms of *Campylobacter* pathogenesis or the development of protective immunity. Until recently, the lack of experimental genetic systems, compared to those available for the study of other enteric pathogens, has slowed progress in defining the pathogenesis of infection (121). However, our knowledge base is growing, with some data suggesting that given the variety of symptoms associated with *Campylobacter* infections, there may be multiple mechanisms of pathogenesis, similar to those of diarrheagenic *E. coli*.

Campylobacter organisms exhibit rapid, darting motility. This motility appears to play an important role in pathogenesis, since nonmotile and nonchemotacic strains are unable to colonize experimental animals or volunteers (17, 89). Motility and chemotaxis are also necessary for invasion of epithelial cells in vitro (54, 130, 133, 134). Motility is imparted by a single polar flagellum that is composed of two highly related protein subunits, FlaA and FlaB. By using a mutation in a gene required for function of the flagellar motor, it has been shown that immobilized flagella can mediate some adherence but that this adherence in the absence of motility does not lead to invasion (133). Thus, motility, rather than the presence of the FlaA or FlaB protein, is necessary for invasion. Flagellin has also been shown to be an immunodominant protein (78, 131).

Other than motility, the best-studied virulence factor is cytolethal distending toxin (CDT). Initially found in diarrheagenic *E. coli*, CDT is detected in most strains of *C. jejuni* and has also been found in *Shigella* spp., *Haemophilus ducreyi,* and *Actinobacillus actinomycetemcomitans* (41, 61, 63, 97, 117). CDT has profound effects on a variety of eukaryotic cell lines, including CHO, HeLa, Vero, HEp-2, and lymphocytes (4, 62, 63, 111). The primary morphologic change in epithelial cells is marked cellular distension without the multinucleation caused by cytotoxic necrotizing factor (32). The growth of cells exposed to either *E. coli* or *C. jejuni* CDT is arrested in the G_2 phase of the cell cycle (40, 94, 132), an effect which is associated with cyclin-dependent kinase 2 (cdc2). However, the role of CDT in diarrheal disease is not clear. CDT mutants of *C. jejuni* 81-176 are still able to cause disease in the ferret diarrheal-disease model. Nothing is known about the role of CDT or the immune response to this protein in humans.

Several strains have been reported to be invasive in vitro (54, 69, 87, 133), but there is considerable variation in their ability to invade intestinal epithelial cells. For example, *C. jejuni* 81-176 invades at a much higher level than do most clinical isolates. In volunteer feeding studies, *C. jejuni* 81-176 caused a more severe disease in humans than did *C. jejuni* A3249, which is noninvasive (i.e. less invasive than *E. coli* K-12) (55). Mutants of 81-176 which are defective in invasion in vitro are also nonvirulent in the mouse intranasal model and the ferret disease model. However, invasion is not understood at the molecular level, and therefore it is difficult to exploit this properly for vaccine development.

Recently, a new surface structure required for virulence in the ferret model was described (44). Growth of *Campylobacter* in the presence of several bile salts induces expression of peritrichous pilus-like appendages. Electron microscopy indicates that the pili are 4 to 7 nm in diameter and longer than 1 μm and are often seen in bundles. While the pilin subunit has not been characterized, two accessory genes required for biosynthesis or assembly of pili have been identified in *C. jejuni* 81-176. Site-specific mutation of either of these genes results in loss of ability to synthesize pili; these nonpiliated mutants are significantly reduced in virulence in the ferret model.

Great strides in defining *Campylobacter* pathogenesis and vaccine development may come from genomics. The Sanger Center in the United Kingdom has sequenced the 1.7-Mb genome of *C. jejuni* NCTC 11168 (http://www.sanger.ac.uk/Projects/C_jejuni). Examination of an annotated version of this sequence has failed to reveal any striking homology to known virulence genes of other pathogens. However, approximately 25% of the genome is *Campylobacter* specific, and many of these genes are likely to be involved in virulence.

Animal Models

The paucity of simple animal models that mimic human gastrointestinal disease has also slowed pathogenesis and vaccine development efforts. Campylobacters naturally colonize numerous animal species, but usually without symptoms. However, experimental infection of nonhuman primates (*Macaca nemestrina*) with virulent *C. jejuni* closely mimics human disease with the same strain (101, 102). *Campylobacter* enteritis also appears to be an important cause of diarrheal diseases in primate colonies. Data from both challenge studies and epidemiologic studies in primate colonies indicate that prior infection provides protection against illness upon rechallenge (101). These data suggest that nonhuman primates would serve as a useful model for vaccine testing. However, the expense of primate models has limited their application.

Small-animal models of diarrheal disease include ferrets, newborn piglets, and a surgical rabbit model (7, 13, 28, 128, 129). Gnotobiotic and newborn colostrum-deprived piglets both develop diarrhea when challenged orally with *C. jejuni* (7, 128). The disease affects mainly the colon and is similar histopathologically to that seen in humans. However, the requirement for newborn animals makes this a logistically difficult and expensive model for most laboratories. It also means the model is not useful for testing the efficacy of vaccines.

In the removable intestinal tie adult rabbit diarrhea (RITARD) model, the cecum is ligated to prevent reabsorption of fluid and a reversible tie is placed below the bacterial inoculum to impede normal bowel motility and improve bacterial attachment and colonization. When young rabbits are challenged in this manner with live motile *C. jejuni* organisms, most animals become bacteremic and develop diarrhea (129). For pathogenesis research, the surgical nature of the RITARD model limits its usefulness. Older rabbits challenged by the RITARD procedure become colonized but do not develop diarrhea. Therefore, this model cannot be used to measure protection against disease offered by vaccine candidates. However, young rabbits can be orally immunized with either live strains or vaccines and then, approximately 30 days later, challenged by the RITARD procedure with either the same

strain or a heterologous organism to measure protection against colonization. Protection against colonization in this model seems to be Lior serotype specific. Thus, immunization with one strain of *Campylobacter* protects against other strains of the same Lior serogroup but not strains of other Lior serogroups (1, 89).

Unlike most small mammals, young ferrets develop diarrhea when they are naturally or experimentally infected with *C. jejuni* via the orogastric route. Adult ferrets that have been intragastrically inoculated with at least some strains of live *Campylobacter* (e.g., *C. jejuni* 81-176) develop enteric symptoms lasting up to 3 days and remain colonized for up to 8 days. The disease is characterized by mild to moderate diarrhea containing mucus, fecal leukocytes, and occasionally frank blood (13). Ferrets that have been immunized in this manner do not develop disease when rechallenged with the same strain. However, colonization resistance does not develop until after several additional exposures. This is similar to human volunteer studies, where protection against disease developed before resistance to colonization. These characteristics make the ferret an excellent model for studying pathogenesis and highly promising for studying *Campylobacter* immunity and the efficacy of candidate vaccines by using protection against diarrhea rather than resistance to colonization as the criterion.

Several nondiarrheal murine models have also been used in vaccine development. Mice immunized or challenged via the orogastric route have been used to study the safety and immunogenicity of oral vaccines and the induction of *Campylobacter* colonization resistance against oral challenge. An oral/intranasal-immunization–intranasal-challenge murine model has been adapted from its original use in studies of *Shigella* immunity (10,77). Naive mice infected intranasally with virulent strains of *Campylobacter* develop pulmonary disease accompanied by weight loss and other signs of illness including ruffled fur, hunched back, dehydration, and lethargy, and some of them die (10). Following intranasal infection, most

Campylobacter strains colonize the intestine and some strains disseminate to the liver, spleen, and other organs. This model of oral/intranasal immunization followed by intranasal challenge appears to be useful in measuring the immune response and protective efficacy as measured by protection against pulmonary disease, intestinal colonization, and disseminated disease. However, correlation to protection in humans has not been established.

Serotypes

Development of a vaccine may be complicated by the tremendous antigenic diversity of the organism and the fact that the protective epitopes are not clearly defined. The most common typing schemes are the Lior system, which has 108 serotypes, and the Penner system, which has more than 60 serotypes (76, 88, 93). The Penner or O serotyping system is based on lipopolysaccharide and lipooligosaccharide antigens; the serodeterminant of the Lior scheme is a heat-labile antigen, which was originally thought to be flagellin. Genetic analyses with site-specific flagellin mutants, however, have indicated that in most serotypes examined, flagellin is not the Lior serodeterminant (3). Animal studies have indicated that protection against intestinal colonization in at least one animal model is Lior serotype specific (1, 89). The lack of specific information on the nature of the Lior serodeterminant and the large numbers of serotypes complicate vaccine development. However, several studies indicate that a limited number of Lior serotypes predominate in different regions of the world (88). For example, in Thailand, approximately 75% of all isolates belong to one of five Lior serotypes.

Immune Responses

Our understanding of what constitutes a protective immune response to *Campylobacter* infection is also fairly rudimentary. As noted above, the level of *Campylobacter*-specific secretory IgA and serum IgA antibodies correlates with protection against disease. However, all of the studies that support these conclusions used very crude, complex antigens such as glycine extracts. There is very little data on antigen-specific immune responses. The role of cellular immunity is also very poorly defined.

Safety

A major consideration in the development of any vaccine is safety. For *Campylobacter,* this includes symptoms that may be caused by a vaccine in the first 24 to 72 h, as well as the potential for postvaccination sequelae 2 to 4 weeks after immunization. Like *Salmonella, Shigella,* and *Yersinia, Campylobacter* enteritis has been associated with the development of a reactive arthritis/arthropathy (RA) (14, 15, 30, 46, 47, 58, 60, 74, 127). Studies of outbreaks and case series have found an incidence of rheumatic complaints ranging from about 1 to 14% in subjects with evidence of *C. jejuni* infection. However, these studies did not use a consistent definition of RA and included patients with joint symptoms that in some cases lasted only 3 to 7 days (60). In the majority of reported cases, symptoms have resolved completely.

A less common but potentially more devastating complication of *Campylobacter* infection is Guillain-Barré syndrome (GBS) (71, 83, 84). The association between GBS and *Campylobacter* infection is supported by both serologic and culture data and is discussed elsewhere in this volume (chapter 8). The pathogenesis of GBS is thought to be related to the fact that some strains of *C. jejuni* have structures in their LPS core that mimic human gangliosides (5, 6, 85, 105).

The impact of vaccination on the incidence of postinfectious sequelae is not clear. Epidemiologic studies to determine whether prior exposure to *Campylobacter* will increase or decrease the risk of RA or GBS after a subsequent infection are lacking. An effective vaccine will, by definition, prevent the clinical syndrome of *Campylobacter* enteritis, but it may not prevent colonization. Volunteer studies have clearly shown that colonization without disease can induce both local intestinal and serum antibody responses (19), which could potentially trigger postinfectious sequelae. However, if illness and intestinal tissue damage are required for the development of RA and GBS, a vaccine that prevents illness would decrease the risk of these sequelae. If the bacterial structures involved in inducing GBS can be clearly delineated, it may be possible to construct even live attenuated vaccines that could be given without a risk of causing GBS. No bacterial factors have been identified in the pathogenesis of RA.

CAMPYLOBACTER VACCINE STRATEGIES

For a vaccine to be effective against an enteric pathogen, most experts believe that it must be able to stimulate intestinal immunity (80a). For this reason, the oral route of immunization has been the preferred approach for candidate Campylobacter vaccines. Oral immunization takes advantage of the tremendous amounts of lymphoid tissue in the oropharynx and intestine and is simpler than parenteral immunization. A number of strategies could be used in the development of such a vaccine, and research efforts in each of these areas are under way.

Live Attenuated Vaccines

Several live attenuated oral vaccines have been shown to effectively stimulate mucosal immunity and provide excellent protection in field or volunteer challenge studies. These include vaccines attenuated by serial passage (oral polio vaccine) (103), chemical mutagenesis (the Ty21A vaccine strain of Salmonella typhi) (18), and targeted deletion of genes encoding for important virulence factors (cholera toxin A subunit-deleted cholera vaccine CVD 103HgR) (64, 65). A genetic approach to developing a living attenuated Campylobacter vaccine would allow the inclusion of the full complement of antigens. Challenge studies have clearly shown that infection with a wild-type strain produces solid protective immunity in volunteers, and so it is reasonable to expect that a live attenuated vaccine could produce similar results. The paucity of information on the pathogenesis and physiology of the organism complicates this ap-

proach. In addition, the association between campylobacter infection and GBS makes the development of a safe live attenuated vaccine difficult. GBS appears to be associated with specific LPS serotypes in which structures in the LPS mimic human gangliosides such as GM1, GQ1b, and GD1a. Detailed studies of C. jejuni 81-176, a well-characterized strain that could be used in vaccine constructs, have shown no ganglioside mimicry, making it a candidate strain for modification to produce a safe live vaccine.

Several mutants which are attenuated in animal models and could serve as the basis of a live attenuated vaccine have been described. Studies have shown that a mutant of the C. jejuni 81-176 diploid for the chemotaxis gene cheY is nonadherent and noninvasive in in vitro assays compared to the wild-type organism (134). This mutant is able to colonize mice but, more importantly, was attenuated in the ferret diarrhea model.

C. jejuni 81-176 produces peritrichous pilus-like structures that are induced by growth in the presence of bile acids (44). Although the pilin subunit gene has not been identified, nonpiliated mutants of C. jejuni 81-176 carrying a mutation in a pilin biosynthesis gene have been constructed. They are motile and able to colonize ferrets but are attenuated in the ferret diarrhea model. With the completion of the C. jejuni genomic sequence, construction of auxotrophic mutants may also be possible.

Unlike other enteric pathogens, C. jejuni is naturally transformable. The inclusion of a recA mutation (57) would preclude reversion to the wild type. Mutants of 81-176 that are nonvirulent in the ferret model are currently being evaluated in our laboratories for their protective efficacy in animal models. However, in addition to the attenuation of the organism, more must be learned about the mechanisms by which Campylobacter is able to induce reactive arthropathy or GBS before the large-scale use of a live attenuated strain would be practical.

Subunit Vaccines

A subunit vaccine would probably consist of a recombinant protein given alone, in combination with an adjuvant, or expressed in carrier vaccine strain such as live attenuated *Salmonella, Shigella,* or *Vibrio*. Such a vaccine would pose significantly less risk of postinfectious sequelae than a live attenuated vaccine. Two campylobacter antigens, flagellin and PEB1, have been suggested as potential subunit vaccine candidates.

Campylobacters possess a single polar flagellum at one or both ends, which is thought to be essential for motility and virulence. The flageller subunit protein, flagellin, is the predominant protein antigen and appears immunodominant. Flagellin has long been recognized as an immunodominant antigen recognized during infection, and numerous studies have suggested that it plays a role in protection (78, 131). The overall structure of *Campylobacter* flagellins is similar to that of the flagellins in members of the *Enterobacteriaceae,* in that the amino- and carboxy-terminal ends, which function in the transport and assembly of the monomers into the filament, are highly conserved among different *Campylobacter* strains and the central region appears antigenically diverse (98). Power et al. (98) have studied the antigenicity of *C. coli* VC167 flagellin in detail and have shown that the major immune response seems to reside in the highly conserved amino and carboxy-terminal ends of the protein, areas which are not surface exposed in the flagellar filament. In fact, the only surface-exposed epitopes identified were those which react with antibodies directed against posttranslational glycosyl modifications (43, 98). Moreover, a mutant defective in the ability to synthesize these glycosyl modifications loses the ability to protect against strains of the same Lior serotype in the RITARD model, suggesting a role in the protective immune response for the modified flagellin but not the unmodified primary amino acids (56). The antigenic diversity of campylobacter flagellins, coupled with the fact that these eubacterial proteins are glycosylated, seemed to make the development of flagellin subunit-based vaccines highly problematic. However recent studies with a truncated recombinant flagellin (discussed in chapter 20) in

which a highly conserved region of FlaA was fused to *E. coli* maltose binding protein showed that it conferred broad protection in an animal model (73). These data suggest that recombinant flagellin has promise as a subunit vaccine.

PEB1 is a highly immunogenic protein conserved among *C. jejuni* strains (90). It plays an important role in epithelial cell interactions and colonization in mice (90, 91). A recombinant form of the PEB1 protein, expressed and purified from *E. coli,* was found to induce protection against illness and colonization in the mouse intranasal-challenge model (8). These data suggest that PEB should be evaluated further as a candidate vaccine antigen.

As more is understood about pathogenesis of *Campylobacter* spp., it is likely that additional subunit target proteins which are conserved among strains with the same mechanisms of pathogenesis will be identified. One such candidate is likely to be the pilin subunit proteins, although the antigenic diversity of pili remains to be determined. As noted above peritrichous pili are expressed during growth in the presence of bile salts. It is known from volunteer challenge studies that *C. jejuni* initially colonizes the upper small intestine before causing disease in the colon. Presumably these pilus structures are induced by the growth in the presence of bile acids in the upper small intestine and may serve an important function in the initial adherence and colonization of the intestine, making them good candidate vaccine antigens. However, a pilin subunit gene has not yet been identified. The recently completed genomic sequence of *C. jejuni* NCTC 11168 contains pilin synthesis genes but does not contain an identifiable pilin subunit gene. However, this strain does produce pili, and so efforts to identify the pilin subunit gene are under way.

CDT may be important in pathogenesis and, if so, could be an important protective antigen. The *cdt* genes have now been sequenced from three *C. jejuni* strains, and the predicted amino acid sequences are identical in each of the three strains (81, 97). If this protein is immunogenic, this degree of conservation suggests that it will provide heterologous protection.

Killed Whole-Cell Vaccines

Inactivated microorganisms offer several advantages as potential vaccines for mucosal immunization. Physically, they are natural microparticles, which should enhance interactions between their surface and mucosal lymphoid tissues. As vaccines, they are inexpensive to produce and possess multiple antigens, which can be important for protection. Formulations can be modified to offer protection against prevalent serotypes over time or in different geographic regions, as is done for influenza vaccines. Presentation of multiple antigens may be particularly important for pathogens, such as *Campylobacter,* for which protective antigens are not known or not available in recombinant forms. Although less appealing for parenteral administration, these whole-cell preparations are generally safe for mucosal immunization.

Several killed whole-cell oral vaccines are currently under development and are being marketed in Europe. The best studied is an oral inactivated cholera vaccine composed of heat- and formalin-killed *Vibrio cholerae* whole cells, of different biotypes and serotypes, plus the nontoxic B subunit (BS-B subunit purified from *V. cholerae*) of cholera toxin (WC/BS vaccine). A randomized, double-blind, placebo-controlled field trial involving 63,000 individuals in rural Bangladesh established the safety, immunogenicity, and efficacy of the WC/BS vaccine against cholera (36–39). Two or three doses of the WC/BS vaccine conferred 85% protection against cholera for the first 6 months in all age groups tested and 51% overall protection after 3 years. No adverse effects attributable to the vaccine were reported. More recently, a new formulation of the WC/BS cholera vaccine, containing a recombinant cholera toxin B-subunit (WC/rBS) was also found to be safe and to give high levels of protection (protective efficacy = 86%) against symptomatic cholera in Peruvian military recruits (106, 107). The same WC/rBS vaccine provided 86% protection against ETEC diar-

rhea in Finnish travelers (92). Although not as immunogenic as live attenuated *V. cholerae* strains (75, 119), these vaccines have proven the concept that an orally administered whole-cell vaccine can be safe and can provide reasonable protection against an enteric pathogen.

The Enterics Program at NMRC has studied the hypothesis that a killed whole-cell vaccine against *Campylobacter* could be safe and immunogenic and could protect against disease, particularly if combined with an effective mucosal adjuvant such as *E. coli* heat-labile toxin (LT). Initial studies with *C. coli* VC167 showed that when sonicated cells were combined with 25 mg of LT and give orally to mice, the mucosal immune response was equal to that for live infection with the same strain (12). The duration of intestinal colonization after live-organism challenge could also be significantly shortened in mice or rabbits immunized with sonicates plus LT but not by immunization with sonicates alone.

More recent work with a mixture of heat- and formalin-killed *C. jejuni* 81-176 in mice has shown that LT enhances the mucosal immune response over a wide range of vaccine doses (9). Mice were orally immunized with three doses (48-h intervals) of either 10^5, 10^7, or 10^9 *C. jejuni* whole cells (CWC) alone or in combination with 25 mg of LT. Significant levels of *Campylobacter*-specific IgA and low levels of IgG were detected in intestinal lavage fluid only after immunization with vaccine plus adjuvant. In contrast, whole cells with or without LT stimulated similar levels of *Campylobacter*-specific serum antibody. The optimal secretory immune response was induced following vaccination with the formulation containing 10^7 CWC plus LT, suggesting that the ratio of adjuvant to inactivated cells may be important. When challenged orally with live *C. jejuni* 81-176, mice immunized with either 10^5, 10^7, or 10^9 CWC plus LT showed colonization resistance whereas only the highest dose of CWC alone (10^9 cells) gave comparable protection. Both vaccine formulations provided similar levels of protection against systemic spread of challenge organisms (9).

In follow-on experiments, the relative protective efficacy and duration of immunity induced by CWC or CWC-LT vaccines were compared in an oral immunization-intranasal challenge model (77). Both CWC and CWC-LT formulations provided protection against illness and intestinal colonization for up to 4 months after completion of the two-dose primary immunization series (14-day intervals). However, the preparation containing adjuvant appeared superior to formalin-inactivated CWC alone in that immunity in this vaccination group was still evident in mice at 8 months postimmunization (8). In vitro T-cell proliferative responses to *C. jejuni* antigens were also measurably enhanced by the addition of LT (8).

Two doses of orally administered CWC vaccine with or without LT were well tolerated in rhesus monkeys (11). Elevated *Campylobacter*-specific IgA- and IgG antibody-secreting cells (ASCs) were detected in the peripheral blood of most animals after vaccination, but the IgA antibody-secreting cell response was significantly enhanced in a dose-dependant manner, by coadministration of LT. LT also significantly enhanced the *Campylobacter*-specific IgA and IgG responses in serum.

These results suggest that both killed CWC alone and preparations containing LT adjuvant are promising oral *Campylobacter* vaccine candidates. The addition of LT in different animal models enhances the mucosal and serum immune response as well as Th1-type cell-mediated immune responses to *Campylobacter* antigens, enhances the protective efficacy of the CWC at lower vaccine doses, and prolongs the duration of immunity compared to CWC alone. The disadvantage of LT is its enterotoxic activity. However, all of the immunomodulating effects of LT are seen when CWC is combined with the LTR192G, which has a mutation in the A subunit cleavage site that makes it less toxic in mice and humans (8, 42, 109). Given these data, our laboratory concluded that a CWC vaccine plus adjuvant warranted further evaluation in human volunteers.

Currently, we are studying a monovalent, formalin-inactivated, CWC vaccine made from *C. jejuni* 81-176 (Penner serotype 23/36; Lior serogroup 5). This strain is invasive in cell culture (87) and was originally isolated from the feces of a 9-year-old girl with diarrhea who became ill during a milk-borne outbreak in Minnesota (70). In 1984, the strain was used in a human volunteer study at the Center for Vaccine Development, University of Maryland, as described above (17). The organism used to make the vaccine was recovered from a challenged volunteer with diarrhea. The vaccine was prepared by the Walter Reed Army Institute of Research, Department of Biologics Research, and Antex Biologics, Gaithersburg, Md. The cells used for vaccine preparation were grown under conditions that attempted to maximize motility, flagellum expression, and ability to invade eukaryotic cells in vitro and was inactivated with 0.2% formalin. The final preparation was shown to have intact flagella by electron microscopy and to retain its ability to agglutinate in Lior 5 antisera.

Phase I safety and immunogenicity studies of this vaccine have recently been completed. In this study, the vaccine was well tolerated and moderately immunogenic (110). Studies investigating the safety and immunogenicity of a range of CWC doses combined with LTR192G and a vaccine challenge study have recently been completed (126).

REFERENCES

1. **Abimiku, A. G., and J. M. Dolby.** 1988. Cross-protection of infant mice against intestinal colonization by *Campylobacter jejuni*: importance of heat-labile serotyping (Lior) antigens. *J. Med. Microbiol.* **26:**265–268.
2. **Allos, B. M., and M. J. Blaser.** 1995. *Campylobacter jejuni* and the expanding spectrum of related infections. *Clin. Infect. Dis.* **20:**1092–1099.
3. **Alm, R. A., P. Guerry, M. E. Power, H. Lior, and T. J. Trust.** 1991. Analysis of the role of flagella in the heat-labile Lior serotyping scheme of thermophilic campylobacters by mutant allele exchange. *J. Clin. Microbiol.* **29:**2438–2445.
4. **Aragon, V., K. Chao, and L. A. Dreyfus.** 1997. Effect of cytolethal distending toxin on F-actin assembly and cell division in Chinese hamster ovary cells. *Infect. Immun.* **65:**3774–3780.

5. **Aspinall, G. O., S. Fujimoto, A. G. McDonald, H. Pang, L. A. Kurjanczyk, and J. L. Penner.** 1994. Lipopolysaccharides from *Campylobacter jejuni* associated with Guillain-Barré syndrome patients mimic human gangliosides in structure. *Infect. Immun.* **62:**2122–2125.

6. **Aspinall, G. O., A. G. McDonald, and H. Pang.** 1994. Lipopolysaccharides of *Campylobacter jejuni* serotype O:19: structures of O antigen chains from the serostrain and two bacterial isolates from patients with the Guillain-Barré syndrome. *Biochemistry* **33:**250–255.

7. **Babakhani, F. K., G. A. Bradley, and L. A. Joens.** 1993. Newborn piglet model for campylobacteriosis. *Infect. Immun.* **61:**3466–3475.

8. **Baqar, S.** Unpublished data.

9. **Baqar, S., L. A. Applebee, and A. L. Bourgeois.** 1995. Immunogenicity and protective efficacy of a prototype *Campylobacter* killed whole-cell vaccine in mice. *Infect. Immun.* **63:** 3731–3735.

10. **Baqar, S., A. L. Bourgeois, L. S. Applebee, A. S. Mourad, M. T. Kleinosky, Z. Mohran, and J. R. Murphy.** 1996. Murine intranasal challenge model for the study of *Campylobacter* pathogenesis and immunity. *Infect. Immun.* **64:** 4933–4939.

11. **Baqar, S., A. L. Bourgeois, P. J. Schultheiss, R. I. Walker, D. M. Rollins, R. L. Haberberger, and O. R. Pavlovskis.** 1995. Safety and immunogenicity of a prototype oral whole-cell killed *Campylobacter* vaccine administered with a mucosal adjuvant in non-human primates. *Vaccine* **13:**22–28.

12. **Baqar, S., N. D. Pacheco, and F. M. Rollwagen.** 1993. Modulation of mucosal immunity against *Campylobacter jejuni* by orally administered cytokines. *Antimicrob. Agents Chemother.* **37:** 2688–2692.

13. **Bell, J. A., and D. D. Manning.** 1990. A domestic ferret model of immunity to *Campylobacter jejuni*-induced enteric disease. *Infect. Immun.* **58:** 1848–1852.

14. **Bengtsson, A., F. D. Lindstrom, and B. E. Normann.** 1983. Reactive arthritis after *Campylobacter jejuni* enteritis. A case report. *Scand. J. Rheumatol.* **12:**181–182.

15. **Berden, J. H., H. L. Muytjens, and L. B. van de Putte.** 1979. Reactive arthritis associated with *Campylobacter jejuni* enteritis. *Br. Med. J.* **1:** 380–381.

16. **Black, R. E.** 1990. Epidemiology of travelers' diarrhea and relative importance of various pathogens. *Rev. Infect. Dis.* **12**(Suppl. 1):S73–S79.

17. **Black, R. E., M. M. Levine, M. L. Clements, T. P. Hughes, and M. J. Blaser.** 1988. Experimental *Campylobacter jejuni* infection in humans. *J. Infect. Dis.* **157:**472–479.

18. **Black, R. E., M. M. Levine, C. Ferreccio, M. L. Clements, C. Lanata, J. Rooney, and R. Germanier.** 1990. Efficacy of one or two doses of Ty21a *Salmonella typhi* vaccine in enteric-coated capsules in a controlled field trial. Chilean Typhoid Committee. *Vaccine* **8:**81–84.

19. **Black, R. E., D. Perlman, M. L. Clements, M. M. Levine, and M. J. Blaser.** 1992. Human volunteer studies with *Campylobacter jejuni,* p. 201–215. *In* I. Nachamkin, M. J. Blaser, and L. S. Tompkins (ed.), *Campylobacter jejuni: Current Status and Future Trends.* American Society for Microbiology, Washington, D. C.

20. **Blaser, M. J.** 1997. Epidemiologic and clinical features of *Campylobacter jejuni* infections. *J. Infect. Dis.* **176**(Suppl. 2):S103–S105.

21. **Blaser, M. J., I. D. Berkowitz, M. LaForce, J. Cravens, L. B. Reller, and W. I. Wang.** 1979. *Campylobacter* enteritis clinical and epidemiologic features. *Ann. Intern Med.* **91:**179–185.

22. **Blaser, M. J., R. E. Black, D. J. Duncan, and J. Amer.** 1985. *Campylobacter jejuni*-specific serum antibodies are elevated in healthy Bangladeshi children. *J. Clin. Microbiol.* **21:**164–167.

23. **Blaser, M. J., P. Checko, C. Bopp, A. Bruce, and J. M. Hughes.** 1982. *Campylobacter* enteritis associated with foodborne transmission. *Am. J. Epidemiol.* **116:**886–894.

24. **Blaser, M. J., D. J. Duncan, M. T. Osterholm, G. R. Istre, and W. L. Wang.** 1983. Serologic study of two clusters of infection due to *Campylobacter jejuni. J. Infect. Dis.* **147:**820–823.

25. **Blaser, M. J., E. Sazie, and L. P. J. Williams.** 1987. The influence of immunity on raw milk–associated *Campylobacter* infection. *JAMA* **257:**43–46.

26. **Blaser, M. J., D. N. Taylor, and P. Echeverria.** 1986. Immune response to *Campylobacter jejuni* in a rural community in Thailand. *J. Infect. Dis.* **153:**249–254.

27. **Blaser, M. J., J. G. Wells, R. A. Feldman, R. A. Pollard, and J. R. Allen.** 1983. Campylobacter enteritis in the United States. A multicenter study. *Ann. Intern. Med.* **98:**360–365.

28. **Boosinger, T. R., and T. A. Powe.** 1988. *Campylobacter jejuni* infections in gnotobiotic pigs. *Am. J. Vet. Res.* **49:**456–458.

29. **Bourgeois, A. L., C. H. Gardiner, S. A. Thornton, R. A. Batchelor, D. H. Burr, J. Escamilla, P. Echeverria, N. R. Blacklow, J. E. Herrmann, and K. C. Hyams.** 1993. Etiology of acute diarrhea among United States military personnel deployed to South America and west Africa. *Am. J. Trop. Med. Hyg.* **48:** 243–248.

29a. **Boyaka, P. N., M. Marinaro, J. L. Vancott, I. Takahashi, K. Fujihashi, M. Yamamoto, F. W. Van Ginkel, R. J. Jackson, H. Kiyono, and J. R. McGhee.** 1999. Strategies for mucosal vaccine development. *Am. J. Trop. Med. Hyg.* **60**(4):35–45.

30. **Bremell, T., A. Bjelle, and A. Svedhem.** 1991. Rheumatic symptoms following an outbreak of *Campylobacter* enteritis: a five year follow up. *Ann. Rheum. Dis.* **50**:934–938.

31. **Calva, J. J., G. M. Ruiz-Palacios, A. B. Lopez-Vidal, A. Ramos, and R. Bojalil.** 1988. Cohort study of intestinal infection with *Campylobacter* in Mexican children. *Lancet* **i**:503–506.

32. **Caprioli, A., V. Falbo, F. M. Ruggeri, L. Baldassarri, R. Bisicchia, G. Ippolito, E. Romoli, and G. Donelli.** 1987. Cytotoxic necrotizing factor production by hemolytic strains of *Escherichia coli* causing extraintestinal infections. *J. Clin. Microbiol.* **25**:146–149.

33. **Castelli, F., and G. Carosi.** 1995. Epidemiology of traveler's diarrhea. *Chemotherapy* **41**(Suppl. 1)**1**:20–32.

34. **Cejka, J., D. W. Mood, and C. S. Kim.** 1974. Immunoglobulin concentrations in sera of normal children: quantitation against an international reference preparation. *Clin. Chem.* **20**:656–659.

35. **Centers for Disease Control and Prevention.** 1998. Incidence of foodborne illnesses—FoodNet, 1997. *Morbid. Mortal. Weekly Rep.* **47**:782–786.

36. **Clemens, J. D., D. A. Sack, J. R. Harris, J. Chakraborty, M. R. Khan, B. F. Stanton, B. A. Kay, M. U. Khan, M. Yunus, W. Atkinson, et al.** 1986. Field trial of oral cholera vaccines in Bangladesh. *Lancet* **ii**:124–127.

37. **Clemens, J. D., D. A. Sack, J. R. Harris, J. Chakraborty, P. K. Neogy, B. Stanton, N. Huda, M. U. Khan, B. A. Kay, M. R. Khan, et al.** 1988. Cross-protection by B subunit-whole cell cholera vaccine against diarrhea associated with heat-labile toxin-producing enterotoxigenic *Escherichia coli*: results of a large-scale field trial. *J. Infect. Dis.* **158**:372–377.

38. **Clemens, J. D., D. A. Sack, J. R. Harris, F. van Loon, J. Chakraborty, F. Ahmed, M. R. Rao, M. R. Khan, M. Yunus, N. Huda, et al.** 1990. Field trial of oral cholera vaccines in Bangladesh: results from three-year follow-up. *Lancet* **335**:270–273.

39. **Clemens, J. D., D. A. Sack, M. R. Rao, J. Chakraborty, M. R. Khan, B. Kay, F. Ahmed, A. K. Banik, F. P. van Loon, M. Yunus, et al.** 1992. Evidence that inactivated oral cholera vaccines both prevent and mitigate *Vibrio cholerae* O1 infections in a cholera-endemic area. *J. Infect. Dis.* **166**:1029–1034.

40. **Comayras, C., C. Tasca, S. Y. Peres, B. Ducommun, E. Oswald, and J. De Rycke.** 1997. *Escherichia coli* cytolethal distending toxin blocks the HeLa cell cycle at the G_2/M transition by preventing cdc2 protein kinase dephosphorylation and activation. *Infect. Immun.* **65**:5088–5095.

41. **Cope, L. D., S. Lumbley, J. L. Latimer, J. Klesney-Tait, M. K. Stevens, L. S. Johnson, M. Purven, R. S. Munson, Jr., T. Lagergard, J. D. Radolf, and E. J. Hansen.** 1997. A diffusible cytotoxin of *Haemophilus ducreyi*. *Proc. Natl. Acad. Sci. USA* **94**:4056–4061.

42. **Dickinson, B. L., and J. D. Clements.** 1995. Dissociation of *Escherichia coli* heat-labile enterotoxin adjuvanticity from ADP-ribosyltransferase activity. *Infect. Immun.* **63**:1617–1623.

43. **Doig, P., N. Kinsella, P. Guerry, and T. J. Trust.** 1996. Characterization of a posttranslational modification of *Campylobacter* flagellin: identification of a serospecific glycosyl moiety. *Mol. Microbiol.* **95**:379–387.

44. **Doig, P., R. Yao, D. H. Burr, P. Guerry, and T. J. Trust.** 1996. An environmentally regulated pilus-like appendage involved in *Campylobacter* pathogenesis. *Mol. Microbiol.* **20**:885–894.

45. **DuPont, H. L.** 1995. Traveler's diarrhea, p. 299–310. *In* M. J. Blaser, P. D. Smith, J. I. Ravdin, H. B. Greenberg, and R. L. Guerrant (ed.), *Infections of the Gastrointestinal Tract*. Raven Press, New York, N.Y.

46. **Eastmond, C. J., J. A. Rennie, and T. M. Reid.** 1983. An outbreak of *Campylobacter* enteritis—a rheumatological followup survey. *J. Rheumatol.* **10**:107–108.

47. **Ebright, J. R., and L. M. Ryan.** 1984. Acute erosive reactive arthritis associated with *Campylobacter jejuni*-induced colitis. *Am. J. Med.* **76**:321–323.

48. **Ericsson, C. D., and H. L. DuPont.** 1993. Travelers' diarrhea: approaches to prevention and treatment. *Clin. Infect. Dis.* **16**:616–624.

49. **Gaudio, P. A., P. Echeverria, C. W. Hoge, C. Pitarangsi, and P. Goff.** 1996. Diarrhea among expatriate residents in Thailand: correlation between reduced *Campylobacter* prevalence and longer duration of stay. *J. Travel Med.* **3**:77–79.

50. **Gaunt, P. N., and L. J. Piddock.** 1996. Ciprofloxacin resistant *Campylobacter* spp. in humans: an epidemiological and laboratory study. *J. Antimicrob. Chemother.* **37**:747–757.

51. **Gedlu, E., and A. Aseffa.** 1996. *Campylobacter* enteritis among children in north-west Ethiopia:

a 1-year prospective study. *Ann. Trop. Paediatr.* **16:**207–212.

52. **Georges-Courbot, M. C., A. M. Beraud-Cassel, I. Gouandjika, and A. J. Georges.** 1987. Prospective study of enteric *Campylobacter* infections in children from birth to 6 months in the Central African Republic. *J. Clin. Microbiol.* **25:**836–839.

53. **Glass, R. I., B. J. Stoll, M. I. Huq, M. J. Struelens, M. Blaser, and A. K. Kibriya.** 1983. Epidemiologic and clinical features of endemic *Campylobacter jejuni* infection in Bangladesh. *J. Infect. Dis.* **148:**292–296.

54. **Grant, C. C., M. E. Konkel, W. Cieplak, Jr., and L. S. Tompkins.** 1993. Role of flagella in adherence, internalization, and translocation of *Campylobacter jejuni* in nonpolarized and polarized epithelial cell cultures. *Infect. Immun.* **61:**1764–1771.

55. **Guerry, P.** Unpublished data.

56. **Guerry, P., P. Doig, R. A. Alm, D. H. Burr, N. Kinsella, and T. J. Trust.** 1996. Identification and characterization of genes required for post-translational modification of *Campylobacter coli* VC167 flagellin. *Mol. Microbiol.* **19:**369–378.

57. **Guerry, P., P. M. Pope, D. H. Burr, J. Leifer, S. W. Joseph, and A. L. Bourgeois.** 1994. Development and characterization of *recA* mutants of *Campylobacter jejuni* for inclusion in attenuated vaccines. *Infect. Immun.* **62:**426–432.

58. **Gumpel, J. M., C. Martin, and P. J. Sanderson.** 1981. Reactive arthritis associated with campylobacter enteritis. *Ann. Rheum. Dis.* **40:**64–65.

59. **Hoge, C. W., J. M. Gambel, A. Srijan, C. Pitarangsi, and P. Echeverria.** 1998. Trends in antibiotic resistance among diarrheal pathogens isolated in Thailand over 15 years. *Clin. Infect. Dis.* **26:**341–345.

60. **Johnsen, K., M. Ostensen, A. C. Melbye, and K. Melby.** 1983. HLA-B27-negative arthritis related to *Campylobacter jejuni* enteritis in three children and two adults. *Acta Med. Scand.* **214:**165–168.

61. **Johnson, W. M., and H. Lior.** 1987. Production of Shiga toxin and a cytolethal distending toxin (CLDT) by serogroups of *Shigella* spp. *FEMS Microbiol. Lett.* **48:**235–238.

62. **Johnson, W. M., and H. Lior.** 1987. Response of Chinese hamster ovary cells to a cytolethal distending toxin (CDT) of *Escherichia coli* and possible misinterpretation as heat-labile (LT) enterotoxin. *FEMS Microbiol. Lett.* **43:**19–23.

63. **Johnson, W. M., and H. Lior.** 1988. A new heat-labile cytolethal distending toxin (CLDT) produced by *Escherichia coli* isolates from clinical material. *Microb. Pathog.* **4:**103–113.

64. **Kaper, J. B., H. Lockman, M. M. Baldini, and M. M. Levine.** 1984. A recombinant live oral cholera vaccine. *Bio/Technology* **2:**345–349.

65. **Kaper, J. B., H. Lockman, M. M. Baldini, and M. M. Levine.** 1984. Recombinant non-toxinogenic *Vibrio cholerae* strains as attenuated cholera vaccine candidates. *Nature* **308:**655–658.

66. **Kapperud, G., J. Lassen, S. M. Ostroff, and S. Aasen.** 1992. Clinical features of sporadic *Campylobacter* infections in Norway. *Scand. J. Infect. Dis.* **24:**741–769.

67. **Karmali, M. A., and P. C. Fleming.** 1979. Campylobacter enteritis in children. *J. Pediatr.* **94:**527–533.

68. **Katelaris, P. H., and M. J. Farthing.** 1995. Traveler's diarrhea: clinical presentation and prognosis. *Chemotherapy* **41**(Suppl. 1):40–47.

69. **Konkel, M. E., and L. A. Joens.** 1989. Adhesion to and invasion of HEp-2 cells by *Campylobacter* spp. *Infect. Immun.* **57:**2984–2990.

70. **Korlath, J. A., M. T. Osterholm, L. A. Judy, J. C. Forfang, and R. A. Robinson.** 1985. A point-source outbreak of campylobacteriosis associated with consumption of raw milk. *J. Infect. Dis.* **152:**592–596.

71. **Kuroki, S., T. Haruta, M. Yoshioka, Y. Kobayashi, M. Nukina, and H. Nakanishi.** 1991. Guillain-Barré syndrome associated with *Campylobacter* infection. *Pediatr. Infect. Dis. J.* **10:**149–151.

72. **Kuschner, R. A., A. F. Trofa, R. J. Thomas, C. W. Hoge, C. Pitarangsi, S. Amato, R. P. Olafson, P. Echeverria, J. C. Sadoff, and D. N. Taylor.** 1995. Use of azithromycin for the treatment of *Campylobacter* enteritis in travelers to Thailand, an area where ciprofloxacin resistance is prevalent. *Clin. Infect. Dis.* **21:**536–541.

73. **Lee, L. H., E. Burg, S. Baqar, A. L. Bourgeois, D. H. Burr, C. P. Ewing, T. J. Trust, and P. Guerry.** Unpublished data.

74. **Leung, F. Y., G. O. Littlejohn, and C. Bombardier.** 1980. Reiter's syndrome after *Campylobacter jejuni* enteritis. *Arthritis Rheum.* **23:**948–950.

75. **Levine, M. M., and J. B. Kaper.** 1993. Live oral vaccines against cholera: an update. *Vaccine* **11:**207–212.

76. **Lior, H., D. L. Woodward, J. A. Edgar, L. J. Laroche, and P. Gill.** 1982. Serotyping of *Campylobacter jejuni* by slide agglutination based on heat-labile antigenic factors. *J. Clin. Microbiol.* **15:**761–768.

77. **Mallett, C. P., L. VanDeVerg, H. H. Collins, and T. L. Hale.** 1993. Evaluation of *Shi-*

gella vaccine safety and efficacy in an intranasally challenged mouse model. *Vaccine* 11:190–196.

78. **Martin, P. M., J. Mathiot, J. Ipero, M. Kirimat, A. J. Georges, and M. C. Georges-Courbot.** 1989. Immune response to *Campylobacter jejuni* and *Campylobacter coli* in a cohort of children from birth to 2 years of age. *Infect. Immun.* 57:2542–2546.

79. **Mattila, L.** 1994. Clinical features and duration of traveler's diarrhea in relation to its etiology. *Clin. Infect. Dis.* 19:728–734.

80. **Mattila, L., A. Siitonen, H. Kyronseppa, I. Simula, P. Oksanen, M. Stenvik, P. Salo, and H. Peltola.** 1992. Seasonal variation in etiology of traveler's diarrhea. Finnish-Moroccan Study Group. *J. Infect. Dis.* 165:385–388.

81. **McVeigh, A. L., P. Guerry, R. E. Michielutti, G. Borchert, and D. A. Scott.** Unpublished data.

82. **Millson, M., M. Bokhout, J. Carlson, L. Spielberg, R. Aldis, A. Borczyk, and H. Lior.** 1991. An outbreak of *Campylobacter jejuni* gastroenteritis linked to meltwater contamination of a municipal well. *Can. J. Public Health* 82:27–31.

83. **Mishu, B., and M. J. Blaser.** 1993. Role of infection due to Campylobacter jejuni in the initiation of Guillain-Barré syndrome. *Clin. Infect. Dis.* 17:104–108.

84. **Mishu, B., A. A. Ilyas, C. L. Koski, F. Vriesendorp, S. D. Cook, F. A. Mithen, and M. J. Blaser.** 1993. Serologic evidence of previous *Campylobacter jejuni* infection in patients with the Guillain-Barré syndrome. *Ann. Intern. Med.* 118:947–953.

85. **Moran, A. P., B. J. Appelmelk, and G. O. Aspinall.** 1996. Molecular mimicry of host structures by lipopolysaccharides of *Campylobacter* and *Helicobacter* spp.: implication in pathogenesis. *J. Endotoxin Res.* 3:521–531.

86. **Murphy, G. S., P. Echeverria, L. R. Jackson, M. K. Arness, C. LeBron, and C. Pitarangsi.** 1996. Ciprofloxacin- and azithromycin-resistant *Campylobacter* causing traveler's diarrhea in U.S. troops deployed to Thailand in 1994. *Clin. Infect. Dis.* 22:868–869.

87. **Oelschlaeger, T. A., P. Guerry, and D. J. Kopecko.** 1993. Unusual microtubule-dependent endocytosis mechanisms triggered by *Campylobacter jejuni* and *Citrobacter freundii*. *Proc. Natl. Acad. Sci. USA* 90:6884–6888.

88. **Patton, C. M., and I. K. Wachsmuth.** 1992. Typing schemes: are current methods useful? p. 110–130. *In* I. Nachamkin, M. J. Blaser, and L. S. Tompkins (ed.), *Campylobacter jejuni: Current Status and Future Trends.* American Society for Microbiology, Washington, D.C.

89. **Pavlovskis, O. R., D. M. Rollins, R. L. Haberberger, Jr., A. E. Green, L. Habash, S. Strocko, and R. I. Walker.** 1991. Significance of flagella in colonization resistance of rabbits immunized with *Campylobacter* spp. *Infect. Immun.* 59:2259–2264.

90. **Pei, Z., and M. J. Blaser.** 1993. PEB1, the major cell-binding factor of *Campylobacter jejuni,* is a homolog of the binding component in gram-negative nutrient transport systems. *J. Biol. Chem.* 268:18717–18725.

91. **Pei, Z., C. Burucoa, B. Grignon, S. Baqar, X. Z. Huang, D. J. Kopecko, A. L. Bourgeois, J. L. Fauchere, and M. J. Blaser.** 1998. Mutation in the *peb1A* locus of *Campylobacter jejuni* reduces interactions with epithelial cells and intestinal colonization of mice. *Infect. Immun.* 66:938–943.

92. **Peltola, H., A. Siitonen, H. Kyrönseppä, I. Simula, L. Mattila, P. Oksanen, M. J. Kataja, and M. Cadoz.** 1991. Prevention of travellers' diarrhoea by oral B-subunit/whole-cell cholera vaccine. *Lancet* 338:1285–1289.

93. **Penner, J. L., and J. N. Hennessy.** 1980. Passive hemagglutination technique for serotyping *Campylobacter fetus* subsp. *jejuni* on the basis of soluble heat-stable antigens. *J. Clin. Microbiol.* 12:732–737.

94. **Peres, S. Y., O. Marches, F. Daigle, J. P. Nougayrede, F. Herault, C. Tasca, J. De Rycke, and E. Oswald.** 1997. A new cytolethal distending toxin (CDT) from *Escherichia coli* producing CNF2 blocks HeLa cell division in G_2/M phase. *Mol. Microbiol.* 24:1095–1107.

95. **Peterson, M. C.** 1994. Clinical aspects of *Campylobacter jejuni* infections in adults. *West. J. Med.* 161:148–152.

96. **Petruccelli, B. P., G. S. Murphy, J. L. Sanchez, S. Walz, R. DeFraites, J. Gelnett, R. L. Haberberger, P. Echeverria, and D. N. Taylor.** 1992. Treatment of traveler's diarrhea with ciprofloxacin and loperamide. *J. Infect. Dis.* 165:557–560.

97. **Pickett, C. L., E. C. Pesci, D. L. Cottle, G. Russell, A. N. Erdem, and H. Zeytin.** 1996. Prevalence of cytolethal distending toxin production in *Campylobacter jejuni* and relatedness of *Campylobacter* sp. *cdtB* genes. *Infect. Immun.* 64:2070–2078.

98. **Power, M. E., P. Guerry, W. D. McCubbin, C. M. Kay, and T. J. Trust.** 1994. Structural and antigenic characteristics of *Campylobacter coli* FlaA flagellin. *J. Bacteriol.* 176:3303–3313.

99. **Reina, J., N. Borrell, and A. Serra.** 1992. Emergence of resistance to erythromycin and fluoroquinolones in thermotolerant *Campylo-*

bacter strains isolated from feces 1987–1991. *Eur. J. Clin. Microbiol. Infect. Dis.* **11**:1163–1166.

100. **Ruiz-Palacios, G. M., J. J. Calva, L. K. Pickering, Y. Lopez-Vidal, P. Volkow, H. Pezzarossi, and M. S. West.** 1990. Protection of breast-fed infants against *Campylobacter* diarrhea by antibodies in human milk. *J. Pediatr.* **116**: 707–713.

101. **Russell, R. G.** 1992. *Campylobacter jejuni* colitis and immunity in primates: epidemiology of natural infection, p. 148–157. *In* I. Nachamkin, M. J. Blaser, and L. S. Tompkins (ed.), *Campylobacter jejuni: Current Status and Future Trends.* American Society for Microbiology, Washington, D.C.

102. **Russell, R. G., M. J. Blaser, J. I. Sarmiento, and J. Fox.** 1989. Experimental *Campylobacter jejuni* infection in *Macaca nemestrina. Infect. Immun.* **57**:1438–1444.

103. **Sabin, A. B.** 1965. Oral poliovirus vaccine. *JAMA* **194**:872–876.

104. **Sack, R. B., M. Rahman, M. Yunus, and E. H. Khan.** 1997. Antimicrobial resistance in organisms causing diarrheal disease. *Clin. Infect. Dis.* **24**(Suppl. 1):S102–S105.

105. **Salloway, S., L. A. Mermel, M. Seamans, G. O. Aspinall, J. E. Nam Shin, L. A. Kurjanczyk, and J. L. Penner.** 1996. Miller-Fisher syndrome associated with *Campylobacter jejuni* bearing lipopolysaccharide molecules that mimic human ganglioside GD3. *Infect. Immun.* **64**: 2945–2949.

106. **Sanchez, J. L., A. F. Trofa, D. N. Taylor, R. A. Kuschner, R. F. DeFraites, S. C. Craig, M. R. Rao, J. D. Clemens, A. M. Svennerholm, and J. C. Sadoff.** 1993. Safety and immunogenicity of the oral, whole cell/recombinant B subunit cholera vaccine in North American volunteers. *J. Infect. Dis.* **167**: 1446–1449.

107. **Sanchez, J. L., B. Vasquez, R. E. Begue, R. Meza, G. Castellares, C. Cabezas, D. M. Watts, A. M. Svennerholm, J. C. Sadoff, and D. N. Taylor.** 1994. Protective efficacy of oral whole-cell/recombinant-B-subunit cholera vaccine in Peruvian military recruits. *Lancet* **344**: 1273–1276.

108. **Savarino, S. J. and A. L. Bourgeois.** 1993. Diarrhoeal disease: current concepts and future challenges. Epidemiology of diarrhoeal diseases in developed countries. *Trans. R. Soc. Trop. Med. Hyg.* **87**(Suppl. 3):7–11.

109. **Scott, D. A.** 1995. Evaluation of *E. coli* heat-labile toxin (LT) as an oral mucosal adjuvant for enteric vaccines. *IBC International Conference on Mucosal Immunization.* International Business Communications, Southborough, Mass.

110. **Scott, D. A.** 1999. Unpublished data.

111. **Shenker, B. J., T. McKay, S. Datar, M. Miller, R. Chowhan, and D. Demuth.** 1999. *Actinobacillus actinomycetemcomitans* immunosuppressive protein is a member of the family of cytolethal distending toxins capable of causing a G2 arrest in human T cells. *J. Immunol.* **162**: 4773–4780.

112. **Simango, C., and M. Nyahanana.** 1997. Campylobacter enteritis in children in an urban community. *Cent. Afr. J. Med.* **43**:172–175.

113. **Sjögren, E., B. Kaijser, and M. Werner.** 1992. Antimicrobial susceptibilities of *Campylobacter jejuni* and *Campylobacter coli* isolated in Sweden: a 10-year follow-up report. *Antimicrob. Agents Chemother.* **36**:2847–2849.

114. **Sjögren, E., G. Ruiz-Palacios, and B. Kaijser.** 1989. *Campylobacter jejuni* isolations from Mexican and Swedish patients, with repeated symptomatic and/or asymptomatic diarrhoea episodes. *Epidemiol. Infect.* **102**:47–57.

115. **Speelman, P., M. J. Struelens, S. C. Sanyal, and R. I. Glass.** 1983. Detection of *Campylobacter jejuni* and other potential pathogens in travellers' diarrhoea in Bangladesh. *Scand. J. Gastroenterol. Suppl.* **84**:19–23.

116. **Steffen, R.** 86. Epidemiologic studies of travelers' diarrhea. Severe gastrointestinal infections, and cholera. *Rev. Infect. Dis.* **8**(Suppl. 2): S122–S130.

117. **Sugai, M., T. Kawamoto, S. Y. Peres, Y. Ueno, H. Komatsuzawa, T. Fujiwara, H. Kurihara, H. Suginaka, and E. Oswald.** 1998. The cell cycle-specific growth-inhibitory factor produced by *Actinobacillus actinomycetemcomitans* is a cytolethal distending toxin. *Infect. Immun.* **66**:5008–5019.

118. **Svedhem, A., and B. Kaijser.** 1980. *Campylobacter fetus* subspecies *jejuni*: a common cause of diarrhea in Sweden. *J. Infect. Dis.* **142**:353–359.

119. **Tacket, C. O., G. Losonsky, J. P. Nataro, S. J. Cryz, R. Edelman, A. Fasano, J. Michalski, J. B. Kaper, and M. M. Levine.** 1993. Safety and immunogenicity of live oral cholera vaccine candidate CVD 110, a delta *ctxA* delta zot delta ace derivative of El Tor Ogawa *Vibrio cholerae. J. Infect. Dis.* **168**:1536–1540.

120. **Tauxe, R. V.** 1992. Epidemiology of *Campylobacter jejuni* infections in the United States and other industrialized nations, p. 9–19. *In* I. Nachamkin, M. J. Blaser, and L. S. Tompkins (ed.), *Campylobacter jejuni: Current Status and Future Trends.* American Society for Microbiology, Washington, D.C.

121. **Taylor, D. E.** 1992. Genetics of *Campylobacter* and *Helicobacter. Annu. Rev. Microbiol.* **46**:35–64.

122. **Taylor, D. N.** 1992. *Campylobacter* infections in developing countries, p. 20–30. *In* I. Nacham-

kin, M. J. Blaser, and L. S. Tompkins (ed.), *Campylobacter jejuni: Current Status and Future Trends*. American Society for Microbiology, Washington, D.C.

123. **Taylor, D. N., and P. Echeverria.** 1986. Etiology and epidemiology of travelers' diarrhea in Asia. *Rev. Infect. Dis.* **8**(Suppl. 2):S136–S141.

124. **Taylor, D. N., P. Echeverria, C. Pitarangsi, J. Seriwatana, L. Bodhidatta, and M. J. Blaser.** 1988. Influence of strain characteristics and immunity on the epidemiology of *Campylobacter* infections in Thailand. *J. Clin. Microbiol.* **26**:863–868.

125. **Taylor, D. N., D. M. Perlman, P. D. Echeverria, U. Lexomboon, and M. J. Blaser.** 1993. *Campylobacter* immunity and quantitative excretion rates in Thai children. *J. Infect. Dis.* **168**:754–758.

126. **Tribble, D. R.** Unpublished data.

127. **van de Putte, L. B., J. H. Berden, M. T. Boerbooms, W. H. Muller, J. J. Rasker, A. Reynvaan-Groendijk, and S. M. van der Linden.** 1980. Reactive arthritis after *Campylobacter jejuni* enteritis. *J. Rheumatol.* **7**:531–535.

128. **Vitovec, J., B. Koudela, J. Sterba, I. Tomancova, Z. Matyas, and P. Vladik.** 1989. The gnotobiotic piglet as a model for the pathogenesis of *Campylobacter jejuni* infection. *Int. J. Med. Microbiol.* **271**:91–103.

129. **Walker, R. I., D. M. Rollins, and D. H. Burr.** 1992. Studies of *Campylobacter* infection in the adult rabbit, p. 139–147. *In* I. Nachamkin, M. J. Blaser, and L. S. Tompkins (ed.), *Campylobacter jejuni: Current Status and Future Trends*. American Society for Microbiology, Washington, D.C.

130. **Wassenaar, T. M., N. M. Bleumink-Pluym, and B. A. van der Zeijst.** 1991. Inactivation of *Campylobacter jejuni* flagellin genes by homologous recombination demonstrates that *flaA* but not *flaB* is required for invasion. *EMBO J.* **10**:2055–2061.

131. **Wenman, W. M., J. Chai, T. J. Louie, C. Goudreau, H. Lior, D. G. Newell, A. D. Pearson, and D. E. Taylor.** 1985. Antigenic analysis of *Campylobacter* flagellar protein and other proteins. *J. Clin. Microbiol.* **21**:108–112.

132. **Whitehouse, C. A., P. B. Balbo, E. C. Pesci, D. L. Cottle, P. M. Mirabito, and C. L. Pickett.** 1998. *Campylobacter jejuni* cytolethal distending toxin causes a G_2-phase cell cycle block. *Infect. Immun.* **66**:1934–1940.

133. **Yao, R., D. H. Burr, P. Doig, T. J. Trust, H. Niu, and P. Guerry.** 1994. Isolation of motile and non-motile insertional mutants of *Campylobacter jejuni*: the role of motility in adherence and invasion of eukaryotic cells. *Mol. Microbiol.* **14**:883–893.

134. **Yao, R., D. H. Burr, and P. Guerry.** 1997. CheY-mediated modulation of *Campylobacter jejuni* virulence. *Mol. Microbiol.* **23**:1021–1031.

PATHOGENESIS OF *CAMPYLOBACTER FETUS* INFECTIONS

Stuart A. Thompson and Martin J. Blaser

16

Campylobacter fetus has been recognized as a significant pathogen of livestock for nearly a century. In 1909, McFaydean and Stockman cultured an unnamed vibrioid organism and identified it as the etiologic agent of abortion in sheep and cattle (58). In 1919, the organism was cultured by Theobald Smith from aborted bovine fetal fluids (86) and was named *Vibrio fetus* due to its morphologic resemblance to *V. cholerae*. It was first recognized as a pathogen of humans in a case of infectious abortion with bacteremia in France in 1947 (99). As with many bacteria, the nomenclature of *V. fetus* changed substantially with increased study of the organism (summarized in Table 1). In 1963, Sebald and Veron noted that the guanosine-plus-cytosine content of *V. fetus* (32 to 35% G + C) was quite unlike that of other members of the genus *Vibrio* (47% G + C). With the additional distinction that *V. fetus* did not ferment sugars, it was suggested that *V. fetus* should define a novel genus, and the name *Campylobacter* was proposed (81). Antigenic typing was added to Bryner's biotyping scheme by Berg et al. (6), resulting in the classification

of *C. fetus* that currently is in use (97). Serogroup A-1 had heat-stable antigen A and the biochemical characteristics of biotype I. Similarly, groups A-1 and A-2 had heat-stable antigen A but were subtype I and II, respectively. Group B consisted only of biotype II organisms but with heat-stable antigen B. Group C organisms differed, since they had heat-stable antigen C, and they also were distinguished from groups A and B by their growth at 42°C. *C. fetus* strains of serogroup C were eventually reclassified as *C. jejuni* and *C. coli* (85). Subspecies of *C. fetus* now have been designated based on Berg's typing. *C. fetus* subsp. *fetus* and *C. fetus* subsp. *venerealis,* while sharing many characteristics, have important biological differences and are responsible for different diseases in mammalian hosts.

C. FETUS INFECTIONS IN ANIMALS

Both *C. fetus* subsp. *fetus* and *C. fetus* subsp. *venerealis* can cause disease in cattle; however, their niches are different, and it is *C. fetus* subsp. *venerealis* that causes the majority of problems. *C. fetus* subsp. *venerealis* infection of cattle is a sexually transmitted disease and is the primary cause of campylobacterial bovine infertility (bovine veneral campylobacteriosis [BVC]). The reservoir for *C. fetus* subsp. *venerealis* is the penile prepuce of the bull, where the organism

Stuart A. Thompson, Department of Biochemistry and Molecular Biology, Medical College of Georgia, Augusta, GA 30912-2100. *Martin J. Blaser,* Division of Infectious Diseases, Vanderbilt University School of Medicine, Nashville, TN 37232-2605.

Campylobacter, 2nd Ed., Edited by I. Nachamkin and M. J. Blaser
© 2000 American Society for Microbiology, Washington, D.C.

TABLE 1 Classification of *C. fetus* and related *Campylobacter* species

Current designation (97)	Previous designations			
	Mohanty et al. (60)	Bryner et al. (18)	Berg et al. (6)	Smibert (85)
C. fetus subsp. *venerealis*	I	Biotype 1	A-1	*C. fetus* subsp. *fetus*
C. fetus subsp. *venerealis*	III	Biosubtype 1	A-sub 1	*C. fetus* subsp. *fetus*
C. fetus subsp. *fetus*	II	Biotype 2	A-2	*C. fetus* subsp. *intestinalis*
C. fetus subsp. *fetus*	II	Biotype 2	B	*C. fetus* subsp. *intestinalis*
C. jejuni			C	*C. fetus* subsp. *jejuni*
C. coli			C	*C. fetus* subsp. *jejuni*

is maintained predominantly within epithelial crypts, although it also can be recovered from the glans penis and distal urethra (85). Young bulls are relatively resistant to infection and may clear an established infection without intervention. Older bulls are highly susceptible to colonization, and once established, infection is lifelong. The increased incidence of *C. fetus* subsp. *venerealis* infection in older bulls correlates with an increase in the size and number of epithelial crypts in the prepuce, which may provide the organism with both the required microaerobic atmosphere for growth and a sequestered site from the host immune response. Since *C. fetus* subsp. *venerealis* is present in preputial fluids and semen, it is transmitted to cows during coitus. In cows and heifers, *C. fetus* subsp. *venerealis* infects the vagina, cervix, uterus, and oviducts (85) in an ascending infection (22). Bacteremia is not recognized but may occur transiently. The infection is usually contained by the bovine immune response but often persists for several months. Temporary immunity to reinfection occurs following resolution of the first infection—this immunity is longer-lasting in the uterus than in the vagina.

Infection in cows results primarily in infertility due to failure of implantation secondary to endometritis; abortion is less common. Over several months, the cow develops an immunoglobulin G (IgG) response—this allows the cow to clear the infection from the uterus, but vaginal colonization persists. Thus, an infected cow can become pregnant even while being a vaginal carrier. Prolonged vaginal carriage is beneficial to *C. fetus* since it allows the organism to be transmitted to other animals in the herd, especially to new bulls. Shortly after infection, cows develop secretory IgA in the vaginal mucus, which is long-lasting and is diagnostic for previous exposure to *C. fetus* subsp. *venerealis*. Since BVC is typically a subclinical infection, it is not usually suspected until low calving rates are noted within a herd and losses have already occurred. Consequently, BVC has been called the "quiet profit-taker."

The distribution of BVC is worldwide (50). There is little information on the carriage of *C. fetus* subsp. *venerealis* in cattle herds around the world and therefore little data on the economic impact of BVC. However, *C. fetus* infection in bulls remains widespread in South Africa (67), and campylobacteriosis is still a significant problem in Australia (50), the United Kingdom (3), Nigeria (5), Nepal (85), Argentina (34), Jamaica (43), and parts of the United States (34) as well. For example, in a study of beef herds in New South Wales, Australia (1989 to 1991), BVC was present on 35% of farms and was suspected to be present on another 11%. A total of 25% of herds were endemically infected, and an estimated 5% of herds acquired infections each year. The annual economic loss from BVC in New South Wales was estimated at 60 million dollars, a significant source of loss for the industry (50).

The continued problems with BVC occur despite the availability of an effective vaccine, which has been available since 1973. Vaccination of cows and bulls with killed *C. fetus* subsp. *venerealis* cells in oil adjuvant results in a vigorous systemic and mucosal IgG response which prevents infection by *C. fetus* subsp. *venerealis* and also rapidly eradicates a previously existing infection (22). The continued prevalence of BVC is due to failure to properly vaccinate herds, especially prior to the introduction of new (unvaccinated) bulls. In regions where it is practiced, artificial insemination with semen from vaccinated, disease-free bulls has greatly limited BVC (84).

C. *fetus* subsp. *fetus* causes a different spectrum of disease in cattle and is a less frequent problem than *C. fetus* subsp. *venerealis*. In contrast to *C. fetus* subsp. *venerealis*-mediated disease, in both cattle and sheep *C. fetus* subsp. *fetus* causes sporadic abortions but is not usually associated with infertility. Abortions due to *C. fetus* also have been found in goats, pigs, and horses (84). *C. fetus* subsp. *fetus* is not spread via sexual intercourse but, rather, is transmitted via contaminated food and water. After oral ingestion of *C. fetus* subsp. *fetus*, a transient bacteremia occurs. In pregnant cows or ewes, the organism may localize to the placenta, resulting in abortion. *C. fetus* subsp. *fetus* is able to live in the bovine or ovine intestinal tract and can be isolated from the feces and bile of infected animals. *C. fetus* subsp. *fetus* can be recovered from the liver, hepatic lymph nodes, gallbladders, and intestines of infected sheep; persistent biliary carriage may occur. Acute *C. fetus* subsp. *fetus* infection leads to abortion during the last trimester of ovine pregnancy, and bacteria can be recovered from the placenta, chorion, cotyledons, and allantoic fluid. *C. fetus* subsp. *fetus* also can infect other animals such as reptiles and birds, and infected birds may play a significant role in the spread of *C. fetus* subsp. *fetus* by contaminating drinking water. The organism also can be transmitted on the boots or clothing of farm workers.

C. FETUS INFECTIONS IN HUMANS

C. *fetus* is an uncommon and opportunistic pathogen of humans, although its incidence is almost certainly underestimated and probably increasing (7). Nearly all *C. fetus* infections in humans are due to *C. fetus* subsp. *fetus* rather than *C. fetus* subsp. *venerealis* (70, 85). Several

cases of *C. fetus* subsp. *venerealis*-mediated vaginosis in Sweden have been documented (34), paralleling bovine carriage, although this type of infection seems to be rare. The majority of patients with significant *C. fetus* subsp. *fetus* infection either are pregnant or have an underlying illness such as alcoholism, cirrhosis, neoplasm, diabetes, hematological malignancies, cardiovascular diseases, or infection with human immunodeficiency virus. Although diarrhea is sometimes reported as a symptom of *C. fetus* subsp. *fetus* infection, especially in previously healthy hosts, it is much less likely to cause diarrhea than is *C. jejuni* (1). Instead, most *C. fetus* subsp. *fetus* infections of humans are systemic or have a systemic component (Fig. 1). The mode of transmission of most cases of *C. fetus* subsp. *fetus* to humans is uncertain but is likely to be similar to that for livestock, i.e., by ingestion of contaminated food. Cases of diarrheal illness due to *C. fetus* subsp. *fetus* after ingestion of raw milk underscores this point (53, 89). *C. fetus* also can be transmitted

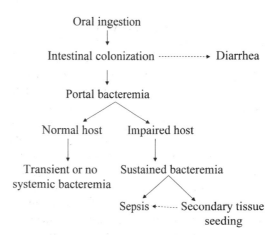

FIGURE 1 Model for *C. fetus* subsp. *fetus* disease of humans (7). *C. fetus* subsp. *fetus* is ingested in contaminated food and then colonizes the intestinal tract. Bacteremia can occur, but in normal hosts it is limited by the immune system. In compromised hosts, the bacteremia may be prolonged due in part to bacterial virulence factors such as its S-layer, which allows secondary infection of additional anatomical sites. These may subsequently serve as a source of bacteria for sustained or renewed sepsis. Reprinted from reference 7 with permission.

via alternative therapies for malignancies ("nutritional therapy"), in which raw calf's liver is the source of the inoculum (45). Following colonization of the intestinal tract, a transient bacteremia can occur, which may be symptomatic but often is not. In compromised hosts, sustained bacteremia is one of the more common detectable manifestations of *C. fetus* disease (16, 48, 64, 76, 98). Other conditions such as meningitis (48, 76, 96), pericarditis (64, 98), aortic aneurism (56), abortion, thrombophlebitis (48, 74, 76), cellulitis (51), pneumonia, pleuritis, septic arthritis, and peritonitis occur, but these are likely to be preceded by dissemination of *C. fetus* subsp. *fetus* through the bloodstream. The fact that most systemic *C. fetus* illness occurs in debilitated hosts underscores the importance of normal host defenses in resisting invasiveness by *C. fetus* beyond the gastrointestinal tract. The localization of *C. fetus* subsp. *fetus* in secondary anatomical sites can result in a sequestered focus for renewed sepsis, which can be chronic and difficult to treat (66).

C. FETUS METABOLISM AND STRUCTURE

Like other campylobacters, *C. fetus* are spiral, gram-negative rods, with a single polar flagellum at one or both ends of the cell. They lack alkaline phosphatase activity and do not hydrolyze DNA or sodium hippurate. The inability to hydrolyze hippurate distinguishes *C. fetus* from the majority of *C. jejuni* strains (49). Most but not all strains of *C. fetus* are unable to grow at 42°C. They are microaerophilic, requiring less oxygen (5 to 6%) than that found in ambient air. *C. fetus* does not grow well anaerobically and may be missed by blood culture detection systems since it is neither an aerobe nor an anaerobe (102). Oxygen toxicity may be lessened by superoxide dismutase, which is present as two bands following gel electrophoresis (85). Chemically defined media that support *C. fetus* growth are available. Importantly, *C. fetus* neither utilizes nor ferments carbohydrates (85).

Iron is an essential nutrient for bacteria, and they therefore have developed high-affinity uptake systems for its acquisition. Limited studies have been done on the Fe uptake systems of *C. fetus* (46). All 24 *C. fetus* strains grown under Fe-limiting conditions produced a 75-kDa Fe-repressed protein that cross-reacted with proteins of similar size in *C. fetus, C. coli,* and *C. lari.* Antibodies to this protein were found in convalescent-phase sera, indicating its expression in vivo. Since similarly sized Fe-repressed proteins are often outer membrane receptors for extracellular Fe-sequestering proteins (siderophores) in other bacteria, this protein may play such a role in a *C. fetus* Fe uptake system. However, the 75-kDa *C. fetus* protein did not cross-react with antibodies against the enterobactin and aerobactin receptors from *Escherichia coli,* and *C. fetus* chromosomal DNA did not hybridize with DNA probes derived from the *E. coli* systems. The *C. fetus* Fe uptake system therefore seems to be distinct from those in *E. coli.*

C. fetus shows variable resistance to quinolone antibiotics. *C. fetus* is highly resistant to nalidixic acid, in contrast to *C. jejuni.* Resistance to nalidixic acid is typically determined by sequences in the DNA gyrase (GyrA) protein. Although the sequences of the *C. fetus* and *C. jejuni* GyrA proteins are known, there were no obvious amino acid differences that would explain the innate resistance of *C. fetus* to nalidixic acid (87). Although cross-resistance to ciprofloxacin is not typical for *C. fetus* subsp. *fetus,* it can occur due to a D91 → Y mutation in the GyrA protein (59, 87). Tremblay and Gaudreau reported that 27% of *C. fetus* strains were resistant to tetracycline (93). Although the mechanism is unknown, it may be related to plasmid-borne tetracycline resistance that can be transmitted among campylobacters (88).

The genome of *C. fetus* is relatively small but is variable in size among the different strains of *C. fetus* examined (78). Salama et al. used pulsed-field gel electrophoresis (PFGE) to investigate differences in genome size and found that the *C. fetus* subsp. *fetus, C. fetus* subsp. *venerealis,* and *C. fetus* subsp. *intermedius* chromosomes were 1.1, 1.3, and 1.5 Mb, respectively

(78). These differences allow PFGE to be used in conjunction with biochemical and immunological tests in the typing of *C. fetus* subspecies. Another study reported that the genome of *C. fetus* subsp. *fetus* strain TK(+) was considerably larger, at 2.0 Mb (40). The reason for this apparent discrepancy is unknown.

Dunn et al. used two-dimensional gel electrophoresis to characterize cell envelope proteins of *C. fetus* (27). The most abundant proteins were seen at 45 to 47, 63, and 100 kDa. The 100-kDa protein was easily extractable with acidic glycine, although it was somewhat labile and tended to degrade under these conditions. It stained with periodic acid, indicating that it was a glycoprotein. The proteins that migrated at 45 to 47 kDa were the major porins. Although typically these were present in single isomeric forms, in some cases minor isomeric forms of the 47-kDa porin existed. The 63-kDa protein was the flagellar subunit. It consisted not of a single discrete entity but, rather, of a charge train. This suggests heterogeneity in the charge on flagellar subunits, which could be related to posttranscriptional modification analogous to the observations for *C. coli* (2).

C. FETUS LIPOPOLYSACCHARIDE

An important molecule possessed by all gram-negative bacteria is lipopolysaccharide (LPS), which is composed of two major portions. The interior portion of LPS is the lipid A moiety, which is widely conserved and, in effect, a modified form of the outer leaflet of the outer membrane. In addition to its essential structural role in the outer membrane, lipid A is a bioreactive molecule that is responsible for the acute biological reactions leading to endotoxic shock (61); in pathogenic bacteria, LPS can be a major determinant of disease outcome due to LPS-mediated interactions with the host. Although *C. fetus* LPS has features that are conserved for all bacterial LPS, it also has unique characteristics that contribute to the biology and virulence of *C. fetus*.

LPS from *C. fetus* has extremely low biological activity, and as in other bacteria, this is due to lipid A. Moran et al. (63) purified LPS from *C. fetus* subsp. *venerealis* (serotype A) and from *C. fetus* subsp. *fetus* (serotypes A and B) and tested their bioactivities including mitogenicity, pyrogenicity, and lethal toxicity. In all assays, *C. fetus* LPS preparations had significantly lower biological activities than did LPS purified from *Salmonella*. This might have been due to the presence of longer fatty acid chains in *C. fetus* lipid A than in *Salmonella*. Among *C. fetus* LPS preparations, LPS from a serotype A *C. fetus* subsp. *fetus* strain consistently had lower activity than did those from other *C. fetus* serotypes. Although the exact composition of lipid A (e.g., phosphorylation) may influence biological activity, there appeared to be no correlation between the lower activity of *C. fetus* subsp. *fetus* serotype A LPS and interstrain differences in lipid A composition. The structure of the polysaccharide moiety also can have a modulating effect on LPS activity, and interstrain differences in this portion of LPS might be responsible for the different *C. fetus* LPS activities. Since these organisms achieve persistent colonization of hosts, LPS of low biological activity may have been selected.

External to lipid A is a polysaccharide that can be subdivided into two regions, the core oligosaccharide and the O antigen. The core oligosaccharide often contains 2-keto-3-deoxyoctanate (KDO), and its presence in the *C. fetus* core is unremarkable (62, 71). Cross-reactive antiserum against the LPS core region of *C. fetus* demonstrated the presence of conserved antigens among serum-sensitive *C. fetus* subsp. *fetus* strains, but these epitopes were not accessible in serum-resistant strains (73). The core epitopes did not cross-react with those of *C. jejuni* LPS.

More external on the bacterial cell surface is the O antigen. As with other bacteria, the O antigen harbors many of the epitopes to which the host immune system responds. Early studies defined three heat-stable serotypes (A, B, and AB) in a slide agglutination test (6), and these were subsequently shown to be based on epitopes in the *C. fetus* O antigen (72). Characterization of purified LPS from the different serotypes showed that *C. fetus* strains that were originally characterized as type AB had LPS profiles distinct from type A and indistinguishable from type B (72). Therefore, *C. fetus* is probably composed of two main serotypes (A and B), with the AB serotype being a minor variant of serotype B.

In general, LPS recovered from serum-resistant *C. fetus* is smooth and relatively constant in size. The "ladder" effect representing variability in the number of saccharide repeat units in LPS from members of the *Enterobacteriaceae* was different in LPS from *C. fetus,* which contained very few "rungs," indicating a relatively low diversity in the number of repeat units. These results indicated probable constraints on the length and variability of the O–antigen side chains, which may be critical for its interactions with the surface layer (see below) (62, 71). In contrast, LPS isolated from serum-sensitive *C. fetus* strains was rough, suggesting that longer O–antigen side chains are associated with serum resistance (71). In addition to the length and immunogenicity of the O antigen, there are obvious additional chemical differences among the LPS from different strains. Several different methods have been used to obtain satisfactory recovery of LPS from different strains; no single method works well for all strains, and this is probably due to differences in the LPS molecules themselves (62, 71). Furthermore, chemical differences among LPS are not synonymous with serotypes and therefore represent heterogeneity in addition to that detected immunologically (62).

In a compositional analysis, all *C. fetus* LPS were found to contain L-rhamnose, L-fucose, D-mannose, D-galactose, and L- and D-glycero-D-mannoheptose (62). Two strains (type B and AB) contained the unique sugar 3-O-methyl-L-rhamnose (L-acofriose, later reported to actually be D-acofriose [83]). LPS from all strains had aminoacetylneuraminic (sialic) acid and D-galactosamine. It is unknown whether the presence of sialic acid on the LPS contributes to the serum resistance of *C. fetus* strains, as occurs with *Neisseria gonorrhoeae*.

C. fetus LPS has significant differences from

that of *C. jejuni*. The lipid A of *C. fetus* contains no 2,3-diamino-2,3-dideoxy-D-glucose and therefore has a backbone different from *C. jejuni* LPS. In addition, the inner core of *C. fetus* LPS contains both L- and D-glyero-D-mannoheptose whereas *C. jejuni* contains the L isomer only (62).

Two main differences were found in the LPS constitutions of different serotypes of *C. fetus*. First, the molar ratio of rhamnose was much higher in LPS from serotype B and AB strains than from type A strains (62). Second, the unique sugar D-acofriose was found only in LPS from types B and AB strains and was absent from type A LPS, confirming the observations of Pérez-Pérez et al. on the high similarity of type B and AB strains (72). The component of type AB LPS that cross-reacts with type A serum is currently unknown.

The precise structures of the O antigens of type A and B *C. fetus* LPS were subsequently determined by ^{1}H- and ^{13}C-nuclear magnetic resonance spectroscopy and gas chromatography-mass spectrometry (82, 83). Confirming previous data, type A and type B O antigens were distinct. The type A O antigen was composed of a partially O-acetylated D-mannan chain of 10 to 12 residues of a monosaccharide unit of [→3)-α-D-Manp2Ac-(1→] (82). In contrast, the type B O antigen consisted of a D-rhamnan chain containing a disaccharide repeat of [→3)-β-D-Rhap-(1→2)-α-D-Rhap-(1→], terminated by a single residue of D-acofriose (83). Clearly, these chemical differences are an important cause of the differing immunological properties of these molecules.

Although two main serotypes of LPS could be identified by both biochemical and immunological techniques, there also was interstrain variability in LPS profiles within individual serotypes. Variation in mobility, staining, and banding patterns of LPS molecules in sodium dodecyl sulfate-polyacrylamide gel electrophoresis demonstrated that structural differences existed (62). Further evidence of LPS differences was exemplified by the varying chemical extraction of LPS molecules into aqueous and organic phases during hot-phenol extraction of LPS from *C. fetus,* and can be observed both among strains and within a single strain. LPS molecules that partitioned into the aqueous phase tended to be slightly larger (M_r = 8,850 to 9,824) than those that were extracted in the phenol phase (M_r = 7,270 to 8,550). In addition to the slight size differences, the variable extraction reflects the nonstoichiometric presence of sugars among LPS molecules, different levels of substitution of the sugars, and differences in hydrophobicity. Interstrain variation in the level of phosphorylation also was substantial (62).

In summary, *C. fetus* has LPS that in many ways is typical of gram-negative bacterial LPS. It contains lipid A, KDO, and a polysaccharide O antigen. The lipid A portion of *C. fetus* LPS has low biological activity compared to members of the *Enterobacteriaceae.* In contrast to the rough LPS isolated from serum-sensitive *C. fetus,* LPS from serum-resistant strains is long and relatively constant in size, suggesting selection for the maintenance of smooth LPS and serum resistance. The O antigens of type A and type B strains are quite different and are responsible for the *C. fetus* serotyping scheme.

THE *C. FETUS* SURFACE LAYER

For bacterial pathogens, the interaction of the cell surface with the host often is a critical determinant of virulence. The structures on the cell surface can either promote virulence or serve as targets for the host immune response in reducing virulence. For example, outer membrane proteins can mediate attachment of bacteria to host cells, mediate transfer of toxins into the extracellular space or directly into host cells, or induce blocking antibodies that prevent an effective immune response against important bacterial surface structures. The cell surface also contains most of the antigens to which an effective immune response is generated and is the site of complement deposition that, when productive, leads to cell lysis or phagocytosis. Similarly, the *C. fetus* cell surface also is critical for its virulence. However, with *C. fetus* it is not the components of the outer membrane but, rather, an external structure

that is the prime virulence factor of this organism. This structure is the proteinaceous surface layer (S-layer).

Early observations on the virulence of *C. fetus* were that (i) *C. fetus* were resistant to phagocytosis by mononuclear cells (23) and (ii) persistence of *C. fetus* in cattle was accompanied by variation of surface antigens (80). In 1971, Myers isolated a 135-kDa protein from *C. fetus* broth culture supernatants (65). In seminal work toward the understanding of *C. fetus* virulence, McCoy et al. purified and characterized this superficial antigen that was responsible for both of these traits (57). This antigen, which was termed antigen [a], could easily be removed from the cell surface of wild-type *C. fetus* 23D by treatment with 0.2 M glycine (pH 2.2). Antigen [a] was proteinaceous and was reported to have a low level of glycosylation. When present on the cell surface, antigen [a] blocked agglutination with O antiserum. In contrast, O antiserum agglutinated either 23D cells from which antigen [a] had been removed or cells of a spontaneous mutant (23B) that had lost the production of antigen [a]. Electron microscopy with negative staining of *C. fetus* cells showed a distinct outer structural layer in the antigen [a]-producing 23D that was absent in the mutant 23B (Fig. 2). This structure was designated the *C. fetus* "microcapsule." The strong binding of cationized ferritin to this structure indicated that it was acidic. Finally, and importantly, in the absence of immune serum, the presence of the antigen [a] "microcapsule" inhibited the uptake of 23D cells by macrophages. Phagocytosis of 23B cells, which lack the microcapsule, was efficient. If the 23D cells were preopsonized with [a] antiserum, phagocytosis was able to proceed efficiently. Therefore, McCoy et al. (57) showed that *C. fetus* has an acidic outer layer (microcapsule) that covers LPS epitopes and resists phagocytosis.

Antigen [a], purified from culture supernatants of strain 23D and subjected to biochemical analysis, was found to be 98 kDa (105), rich in glycine, alanine, and aspartic acid, and poor in cysteine, histidine, and tryptophan (105). When membrane vesicles were prepared, anti-

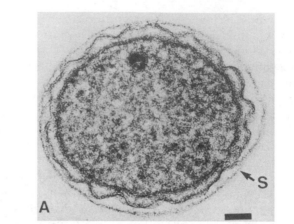

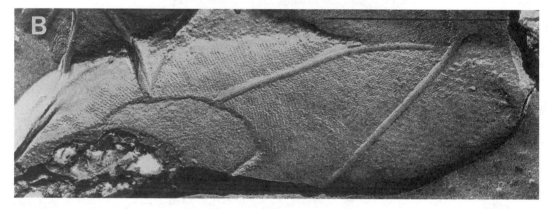

FIGURE 2 Electron microscopy of the *C. fetus* S-layer. (A) Shown in ultra-thin cross-section (26), the S-layer appears as a ring-like structure external to the outer membrane (arrow). (B) In freeze-etch preparations of the cell surface (38), it appears as either regular tetragonal (left side) or hexagonal (right side) arrays. This micrograph demonstrates the ability of a single cell to express more than one type of S-layer. Reprinted from references 26 (A) and 38 (B) with permission.

gen [a] was complexed with LPS, although this association could be disrupted with EDTA. Incubation of free antigen [a] with strain 23B in the presence of 10 mM $CaCl_2$ allowed the reassembly of a microcapsule around those cells. Because of the chemical and structural similarities of the microcapsule to the S-layer of *Aquaspirillum serpens* (19), it was suggested that the *C. fetus* microcapsule formed an analogous structure.

In addition to phagocytosis resistance, another explanation for the disproportionate number of human systemic infections caused by *C. fetus* subsp. *fetus* relative to other campylobacters (11, 77) was that *C. fetus* was more

resistant to the bactericidal effects of human serum and was therefore more likely to disseminate via the bloodstream. A comparison of the serum susceptibilities of *C. fetus, C. coli,* and *C. jejuni* strains subsequently showed this to be true. In a serum bactericidal assay, all *C. coli* and *C. jejuni* strains were susceptible to killing while all *C. fetus* strains were completely resistant despite high serum concentrations, prolonged incubations, or the use of immune serum (10, 12). The killing of *C. coli* and *C. jejuni* was mediated by both complement and antibody; neither of these components promoted the killing of *C. fetus*.

What was the molecular basis for the ability

of *C. fetus* to resist killing by serum? A collection of 38 *C. fetus* subsp. *fetus* strains isolated either from feces or from systemic sites were used to investigate whether certain proteins were associated with serum resistance (10). All of the serum-resistant strains expressed cross-reactive surface proteins of approximately 100 or 125 kDa, and these were absent in serum-sensitive strains. Furthermore, spontaneous laboratory-passaged mutants of two serum-resistant strains lost the production of their 100-kDa protein and had become serum sensitive. Therefore, *C. fetus* subsp. *fetus* serum resistance was associated with expression of the 100- or 125-kDa surface proteins, presumably components of the S-layer (10).

To directly study the function of the S-layer in serum resistance, encapsulated (S+) and serum-resistant and nonencapsulated (S−) and serum-sensitive *C. fetus* subsp. *fetus* were examined for their abilities to bind and be killed by components of the complement system (13). While a copious amount of complement factor C3 was bound to S− *C. fetus,* very little C3 was bound by S+ bacteria (Fig. 3), and these small amounts were in a degraded (nonfunc-

tional) form. The difference in C3 binding led to greater consumption of the components of the complement membrane attack complex (C5 and C9) by S− but not S+ cells. The low abundance of C5 and C9 on the cell surfaces of encapsulated bacteria was shown to be due to the direct inhibition of the S-layer on the binding of complement factor C3b, thereby eliminating formation of the C5 convertase and all downstream events that normally would lead to cell lysis. In other experiments, S+ *C. fetus* cells were found not to activate the alternative pathway of complement, explaining the small amount of C3b deposited (103).

The low binding of C3b by the S+ *C. fetus* strains rendered them resistant to phagocytic killing by polymorphonuclear leukocytes, which exhibited minimal uptake of these bacteria and generated a minimal chemiluminescent response (9). However, if S+ bacteria were preopsonized with immune rabbit serum (either containing or not containing anticapsule antibodies), they were efficiently killed by polymorphonuclear leukocytes. Therefore, the presence of the *C. fetus* S-layer makes these bacteria resistant to the complement system,

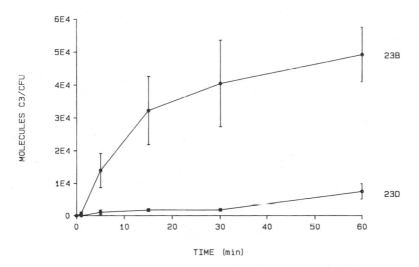

FIGURE 3 Inhibition of complement factor C3 binding by *C. fetus.* ^{125}I-labeled C3 was incubated with either *C. fetus* 23D (S+) or 23B (S−), and the amount of bound C3 was determined. The S-layer in 23D prevents significant C3 binding. Reprinted from reference 13 with permission.

either by complement-mediated cell lysis or by phagocytic killing stimulated by cell-bound C3b. Antibody-mediated opsonophagocytosis remains effective in killing S⁺ bacteria.

These in vitro results were extended by using a mouse model of *C. fetus* infection (68). Outbred HA/ICR mice challenged with S⁺ or S⁻ *C. fetus* strains differed widely in their rates of bacteremia and death. The S⁻ strain was a spontaneous mutant derived from extensive laboratory passage of the S⁺ strain. Mice challenged intraperitoneally with the S⁺ *C. fetus* strain showed a much higher mortality than did those challenged with the S⁻ strain. After oral inoculations, no mortality was observed for either strain; however, the S⁺ strain caused an immediate and high-grade bacteremia that persisted for 5 days. Bacteremia was not detected in mice given the S⁻ strain. Protection against bacteremia by the S⁺ strain was observed when mice were passively immunized with rabbit antiserum against the purified 100-kDa S-layer protein expressed by this *C. fetus* strain. The S-layer protein (SLP) itself was not toxic to mice but could be reattached to S⁻ *C. fetus* cells, regenerating increased virulence in mice. These results were not due to artifacts arising from the laboratory passage history of the S⁻ strain, since similar results were obtained with bacteria that had been made S⁻ by removal of the S-layer by pronase treatment of S⁺ cells (9). Together these studies provided direct evidence, in an animal model, of the conclusions drawn from in vitro studies: the S-layer is critical for inhibition of complement binding, serum and phagocytosis resistance, and virulence.

Subsequently, two groups purified and characterized the proteins that comprised the S-layer (26, 69). The 131-kDa SLP of type B strain VC119 and the 100-, 127-, and 149-kDa SLPs from type A strain 23D were removed from the cell surface by treatment with acidic glycine or proteinase K or by rinsing the cells in water. These proteins were similar in composition, were surface exposed, were the predominant antigens recognized by antiserum generated against whole *C. fetus* cells (26, 69),

and appeared identical to antigen [a] (105). The proteins were relatively hydrophobic (37 to 39% hydrophobicity), and, like the microcapsule of McCoy, contained large amounts of aspartic acid, threonine, glycine, leucine, valine, and alanine. Histidine and cysteine were undetected. They were heat stable and relatively acidic (isoelectric points of 6.35 for the VC119 SLP and 4.1 to 4.3 for the 23D SLPs), and were refractory to digestion by trypsin or chymotrypsin. The amino acid sequences of the amino termini of the SLPs derived from type A strains were identical to each other but different from the amino terminus of the type B-derived SLP. To determine whether the SLPs were glycoproteins, the purified proteins were subjected to a variety of techniques including Schiff staining, periodate oxidation, and lectin affinity chromatography and trifluoromethanesulfonic acid treatment. Unlike previous results (57), glycosylation of the S-layer protein could not be detected by any of these techniques (26, 69). Most probably earlier reports of glycosylation of the SLP were due to contamination with minor amounts of LPS, with which the SLPs tend to associate.

Electron microscopy provided further insight into the *C. fetus* S-layer and showed that variant SLPs produced by *C. fetus* cells give rise to S-layers with different structures (26, 38, 39). In strain VC119, the S-layer was arranged as a linear (or possibly tetragonal) array of 131-kDa SLP subunits with 8.75 nm center-to-center spacing that completely covered the cell surface (26). In strain TK, both tetragonal and hexagonal structures were seen (38). Cells that expressed 98-kDa SLPs had hexagonally arrayed S-layers, with 24-nm center-to-center spacing. In contrast, those that expressed 127- or 149-kDa SLPs possessed tetragonal S-layers with 8-nm center-to-center spacing. Based on these results and the relative paucity of S-layers with linear symmetry, it is likely that the observation of a linear array (8.75-nm spacing) generated by the 131-kDa SLP in strain VC119 was due to an artifact of the electron microscopy shadowing technique (as suggested by Dubreuil et al. [26]) and that the structure is in fact tetragonal. The 98-, 127-, and 149-kDa SLPs, while having unique antigenic determinants, also have immunologic epitopes in common that are detectable both by polyclonal serum (10, 44, 69, 101) and monoclonal antibodies (101).

The reattachment of SLPs to the *C. fetus* cell surface was investigated in vitro by using SLPs that had been removed from S$^+$ bacteria by extractions with water (106). SLPs could be reattached to the exteriors of cells made S$^-$ by mutation or by removal of the S-layer by water extraction in a manner that was dependent on the presence of divalent cations; neither monovalent nor trivalent cations supported reattachment. Binding of SLPs to the cell was serotype specific: SLPs purified from type A strains could be reattached only to type A (not type B) cells and vice versa. A recombinant 98-kDa SLP and truncated amino-terminal 65- and 50-kDa fragments thereof also were able to bind to S$^-$ cells. These data indicated that LPS-binding ability was contained in the amino-terminal half of the protein and that *C. fetus* post translational modification of the SLP was not required for LPS binding. Quantitative enzyme-linked immunosorbent assay showed the copy number of SLPs to be at least 10^5/*C. fetus* cell.

Lectins were used to detect the presence of the S-layer and to differentiate between different serotypes of LPS (37). Lectins from *Bandeiraea simplicifolia* II (BS-II), *Helix pomatia* (HPA), and wheat germ agglutinin (WGA) specifically bound to the O-antigen side chains of type A (*C. fetus*) LPS, but not to LPS from type B (*C. fetus*) or type C (*C. jejuni*) LPS. However, binding to type A *C. fetus* did not occur in the presence of the S-layer, suggesting that the entirety of the LPS molecule is shielded by the S-layer.

Characterization of *sap* Genes

A gene encoding a subunit of the S-layer was first cloned and sequenced from serotype A strain 23D by Blaser and Gotschlich (8). This gene was designated *sapA* (for "Surface Array Protein type A"). The *sapA* gene was 2,802 nucleotides in length and predicted an acidic (pI = 4.55) 933-amino-acid protein of 97 kDa. The amino terminus of the protein predicted from the DNA sequence exactly matched the amino-terminal sequence of the purified protein, and the initiating methionine was not processed. This, together with visual inspection of the DNA sequence, showed that despite its ultimate extracellular localization, SapA lacked an amino-terminal signal sequence that would direct its secretion to the cell surface. Prior to this, the only SLP that lacked a signal sequence was that of *Caulobacter crescentus* (36). All other SLPs had amino-terminal signal sequences, suggesting that their secretion was mediated by the general (*sec* dependent) secretory pathway (17, 75). Another notable characteristic of the SapA protein was its single cysteine residue, suggesting that intramolecular disulfide bonds were not required for maintaining the secondary structure of this protein. Because the cloned DNA terminated just upstream of the *sapA* open reading frame (ORF), no predictions about promoter sequences upstream of *sapA* could be made (8). However, a putative transcriptional terminator was located just downstream of *sapA*, suggesting that *sapA* was not cotranscribed with downstream genes.

Subsequently, an additional two SLP-encoding genes from type A strains (32, 95) and two genes from type B strains (20, 33) were sequenced. Not surprisingly, these genes had conserved and divergent characteristics, consistent with both the common functions and the antigenic differences of the encoded proteins (Fig. 4). Comparison of the three *sapA* alleles (*sapA, sapA1,* and *sapA2*) revealed highly conserved DNA sequences at the 5′ end of each gene. The conservation began 74 bp prior to the ATG translational initiation codon and continued 552 to 654 bp into the ORF (8, 32, 94, 95). Contained within the 74-bp conserved *sapA* upstream sequences were several features of note. First, each of the genes contains a sequence that has 7-of-8-bp identity to the χ site (32, 95), which in *E. coli* serves as a signal for RecBCD enzyme to initiate homologous recombination (54). Immediately following the putative χ site is a pentameric sequence

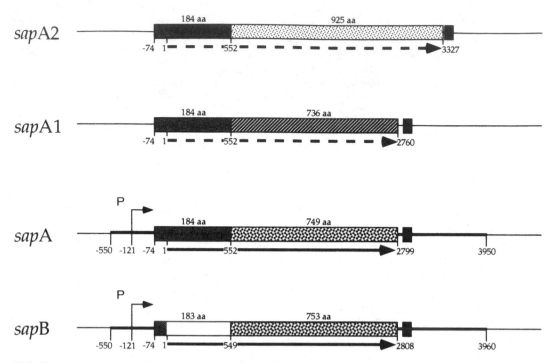

FIGURE 4 Schematic representation of genes encoding type A and type B SLPs. The conserved 5' regions of each gene are indicated by large black (type A) or white (type B) rectangles, and the 3' conserved regions are indicated by small black rectangles. Stippled and hatched boxes indicate the divergent 3' regions of each *sapA* homolog. Solid and broken arrows denote expressed and nonexpressed genes, respectively. aa, amino acids. Reprinted from reference 29 with permission.

(ATTTT) that is repeated three times consecutively (32, 95). Finally, a 7-bp inverted repeat overlapping the ribosome-binding site and terminating immediately upstream of the ATG initiation codon was found in all three genes (8, 32, 95). In contrast to the high conservation at the 5' ends of the *sapA* genes, the 3' ends of the ORFs were divergent. Consequently, downstream of the 5' conserved regions, the *sapA* gene had only limited nucleotide identity to the *sapA1* and *sapA2* genes (8, 32, 95), and this was reflected in significant differences in the encoded proteins (see below). Immediately downstream of each of *sapA, sapA1,* and *sapA2* were additional conserved sequences of approximately 50 bp. In each case, these conserved sequences also contained putative transcriptional terminators. A repeated 10-nucleotide sequence (TTTTAAATTT) was present numerous times downstream of *sapA2*

(32) and to a lesser extent downstream of *sapA* and *sapA1* (8, 95).

The *sapB* and *sapB2* genes were organized in a manner parallel to their *sapA* counterparts (20, 33). Conserved sequences were found at the 5' ends of the *sapB* and *sapB2* genes (20), although these conserved sequences were different from those at the 5' ends of *sapA* homologs (33). Divergence at the 3' ends of the *sapB* and *sapB2* genes was noted, similar to that seen at the 3' ends of the *sapA* homologs. Similar to the conserved regions upstream of *sapA* homologs, pentameric ATTTT repeats were found upstream of the *sapB* and *sapB2* genes (20, 33). However, the putative χ sites and inverted repeats found upstream of *sapA* genes were absent from the corresponding locations of the *sapB* genes (20, 33).

Several studies have addressed the genetic organization of *sap* genes (32, 40, 79, 95). In two separate genome maps (40, 79), genes encoding SLPs were clustered. Hybridization studies performed during the cloning of *sapA* homologs also revealed the presence of clustering of multiple *sapA* genes (32, 95). Finally, Southern hybridization was used to conduct a survey of 27 *C. fetus* strains for the genetic organization of SLP-encoding genes (42). A probe derived from the conserved region of *sapA* was used in experiments showing that all 23 of the type A strains contained *sapA*-homologous sequences. Predictably, due to the divergence of the *sapB* DNA sequence in the region of this probe, none of the non-type A strains hybridized. In each type A strain, there were at least six copies of *sapA* genes. Furthermore, hybridization experiments with PFGE showed that in every strain the genes were located within a small region of the chromosome (≤90 kb), suggesting that clustering of these genes is highly conserved.

The characteristics of the proteins predicted from the *sapA* and *sapB* genes characterized thus far are summarized in Table 2. These proteins range in size from 95 to 113 kDa and have isoelectric points of 4.2 to 4.6. Although they did not possess amino-terminal signal sequences, the SLPs isolated from a given serotype had nearly identical amino termini. For type A proteins, the amino-terminal 184 amino acids were more than 98% identical to each other; a similar relationship was found among the amino termini of type B proteins. However, the amino termini of type A proteins were completely different from those of type B proteins. The remainders of the type A and type B *C. fetus* SLPs diverged significantly within each family (Table 2). Regions of similarity and divergence in type A and B SLPs are represented graphically in Fig. 5A and B. At first glance, the extreme carboxy-terminal segments of each of these proteins appeared to have little sequence conservation. However, later experimentation revealed that not only must significant carboxy-terminal sequence and/or structural conservation exist but that also such conserved features are important for the function of these proteins (see below).

With the exception of the 184 amino acids at the amino termini of SapA and SapB, these proteins were nearly identical (Fig. 5C) and can therefore be considered equivalent proteins within their respective serotypes. SapA2 and SapB2 shared a similar relationship, although the presence of a region of divergence at the carboxy terminus of these proteins suggests that although closely related to SapA2, SapB2 might actually be allelic with another yet uncharacterized SapA homolog.

The high similarity of the amino termini of SLPs within a serotype, in contrast to the divergence between serotypes, suggested a role of the amino terminus in binding to homologous LPS. To test this hypothesis, deletions were made from the 3′ end of the *sapA2* gene, yielding progressively shorter amino-terminal frag-

TABLE 2 Biochemical properties of *C. fetus* S-layer proteins

Protein	No. of amino acids	Mass (kDa)	pI	% Amino acid similarity to SapA or SapB				No. of cysteine residues	Reference
				Similarity to SapA at positions:		Similarity to SapB at positions:			
				1–184	185–end	1–184	185–end		
Type A									
SapA	933	97	4.55	100	100	35.8	89.3	1	8
SapA1	920	95	4.36	98.9	44.2	35.8	48.0	1	95
SapA2	1,109	112	4.22	99.4	28.1	35.8	28.3	0	32
Type B									
SapB	936	96	4.40	35.8	89.3	100	100	0	33
SapB2	1,112	113	4.24	35.8	26.4	98.9	23.6	0	20

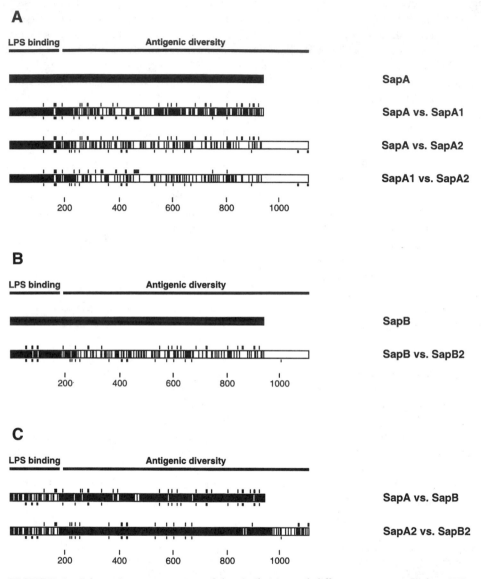

FIGURE 5 Schematic representation of the similarities and differences among *C. fetus* SLPs. Regions of amino acid similarity are shown as vertical black lines within the rectangles representing the SLPs. Short vertical lines above and below the proteins denote gaps generated in the alignment of the two proteins. The LPS-binding and antigenic variability domains are indicated. (A and B) Comparisons of proteins within serotypes A (A) and B (B). LPS-binding domains are conserved within serotypes, but the remainders of the proteins diverge, endowing the proteins with individual antigenic and structural characteristics. (C) Comparison of allelic proteins between serotypes. Although the LPS-binding domains are quite different (e.g., between SapA and SapB), the remainder of the proteins are homologous, suggesting conserved function in the two serotypes. The sizes of the proteins (in amino acids) are indicated by the scale at the bottom of each panel.

ments of the SapA2 protein (32). These recombinant proteins then were tested for their abilities to attach to *C. fetus* cells. As expected, none of the type A proteins was able to attach to type B LPS. In contrast, SapA2 derivatives containing large carboxy-terminal deletions retained the ability to bind to type A cells. These results localized the LPS-binding domain to the first 189 amino acids of the type A protein. The poor immunogenicity of SapA2 peptides shorter than 189 amino acids prevented their testing for proficiency in LPS binding. Similarly, the analogous region of SapB was responsible for serospecific binding to homologous type B LPS (33).

In summary, the genes encoding *C. fetus* SLPs are monocistronic and contain conserved DNA sequences at both the 5′ and 3′ ends of the genes. The presence of conserved DNA outside of the ORFs predicts that this DNA homology has functions other than simply encoding identical proteins. Among the encoded SLPs were important conserved features, as well as features that impart unique type- and protein-specific characteristics to these molecules. Highly conserved regions at the amino termini of *C. fetus* SLPs are responsible for binding to LPS. The remainder of each protein has divergent amino acid sequences, which endows each protein with individual immunologic and structural characteristics.

Antigenic Variation of *C. fetus* SLPs

Early observations of experimentally infected cattle indicated that *C. fetus* exhibited antigenic variation of its surface antigens during infection (24, 80). This was subsequently shown to be due to variations in the expression of the S-layer protein (25, 44, 95, 101). Antigenic variation of surface structures is a common theme in bacterial pathogenesis, although the mechanisms involved vary among bacteria.

Observations made during the cloning of *sapA* genes were important for understanding the mechanisms by which the expression and antigenic variation of the encoded proteins are controlled. First, all of the genes that were cloned were complete and could express a full-

length product in *E. coli*. This indicated that antigenic variation occurred by a mechanism different from that of *Neisseria gonorrhoeae* pilin, which uses partial gene copies recombined into an expression locus. Second, most of the cloned genes were not situated downstream of recognizable promoters, suggesting that each was not expressed from its own promoter but instead requiring that each gene be brought into the context of a promoter for its expression. To understand how SLP-encoding genes were expressed, the region upstream of an expressed *sapA* gene was characterized (94). Primer extension with total cellular RNA and a *sapA*-specific primer identified a single transcriptional initiation site 114 bp upstream of the *sapA* initiation codon and downstream of a sequence that resembled an *E. coli* σ^{70} promoter. This promoter was present in a single copy on the *C. fetus* 23D chromosome. In three unrelated laboratory-passaged strains, the promoter was deleted, resulting in nonexpression of SLPs and an S⁻ phenotype (41, 94). This suggests both that *sapA* expression is controlled by a single promoter and that spontaneous deletion of this promoter is common in vitro.

To investigate whether genetic changes accompanied the switch from one antigenic form of SapA protein expressed to another, two *C. fetus* strains were chosen (95). One was a laboratory-passaged strain (23D-11) derived from the other, the wild-type strain 23D. 23D expressed predominantly a 97-kDa SapA protein but had switched to producing a 127-kDa protein in 23D-11. Southern hybridization with several probes encompassing the *sapA* locus showed that accompanying the switch in SLP production was a reciprocal exchange of DNA between the loci encoding the 97- and 127-kDa proteins. This exchange resulted in the placement of the *sapA* gene encoding the 127-kDa protein downstream of the *sapA* promoter in strain 23D-11, thereby allowing its expression. In this strain, the remaining *sapA* genes were intact, indicating that the genetic changes that had resulted in the switch between two *sapA* homologs did not involve wholesale rearrangements of additional *sapA* genes.

The *sapA* gene was mutagenized by the insertion of a kanamycin resistance (*aphA*) cassette (14). The mutation generated a predominant, truncated 50-kDa SapA protein, indicating that the *sapA* gene was downstream of the active *sapA* promoter. The 50-kDa truncated SapA protein was not exported by *C. fetus*, implicating the carboxy-terminal region of SapA as containing sequences necessary for its secretion (see below). However, preparations of these cells also contained minor amounts of SLPs of 96 to 149 kDa. These data suggested that cells arising from a progenitor mutant that contained an interrupted *sapA* gene had undergone phenotypic reversion at extremely high frequency ($\sim 10^{-3}$) to the expression of alternate, full-length SLPs. Selection based on serum resistance of strains expressing the full-length but not the truncated *sapA* homolog confirmed the high frequency of the reversion events. The reversion events were accompanied by the reacquisition of other phenotypes associated with the S-layer: poor complement binding and bacteremia in mice. Revertants contained DNA rearrangements that had recombination endpoints in the conserved regions at the 5' ends of *sapA* homologs, and resulted in the movement of complete alternate *sapA* gene copies to a location downstream of the *sapA* promoter. Importantly, the kanamycin resistance cassette was not lost during these reversion events, indicating that the genetic exchanges were due to reciprocal recombination (bidirectional) rather than to gene conversion (unidirectional). Similar findings were reported for *C. fetus* subsp. *venerealis* in experimental infections in cattle (44). A *C. fetus* subsp. *venerealis* strain that expressed a 110-kDa SLP was inoculated into the vagina of a 9-month-old heifer. Protein profiles of the *C. fetus* subsp. *venerealis* isolates recovered weekly showed progressive switching between SLPs of sizes ranging from 110 to 160 kDa. The variation in SLP expression also was accompanied by genetic rearrangements detectable by DNA

hybridization with a probe specific for the 5' end of the *sapA* coding region. Therefore, both in vitro and in vivo, the antigenic variation of SLPs occurs at high frequency and is due to reciprocal recombination among *sapA* genes.

Molecular Mechanism of SLP Antigenic Variation

Questions remained about the expression and antigenic variation of SLPs. First, is the expression of SLPs dependent on the single promoter upstream of *sapA*? Several lines of evidence suggested that it was, including primer extension, Southern and Northern hybridization, and the lack of SLP expression in mutant 23B, in which a deletion of the known *sapA* promoter had occurred (14, 94). However, the presence of additional promoters upstream of other *sapA* homologs could not be excluded. Second, what exactly was the nature of the recombinational events that resulted in altered expression of *sapA* genes? Further investigations of these questions were performed by introducing a promoterless *aphA* cassette into either the *sapA* or the *sapA2* locus of wild-type strain 23D (28). Since the cassette lacked its own promoter, kanamycin resistance resulted only when the copy of *sapA* containing the *aphA* gene was present downstream of the *sapA* promoter. In strains containing either of these constructs (*aphA* in *sapA* or in *sapA2*), when kanamycin resistance was selected, no expression of SLPs was observed. This was in contrast to previous results with an *aphA* cassette containing its own promoter, when simultaneous selection of kanamycin resistance and expression of SLPs was detected (14). This result suggested that only a single *sapA* promoter existed and that when it was positioned to drive kanamycin resistance, it was unavailable for the expression of SLPs. This hypothesis was tested further by placing kanamycin-resistant cells into human serum. As stated previously, survival of *C. fetus* in human serum requires the presence of an S-layer (10). Therefore, exposure to serum provides a strong selection for the detection of an S-layer.

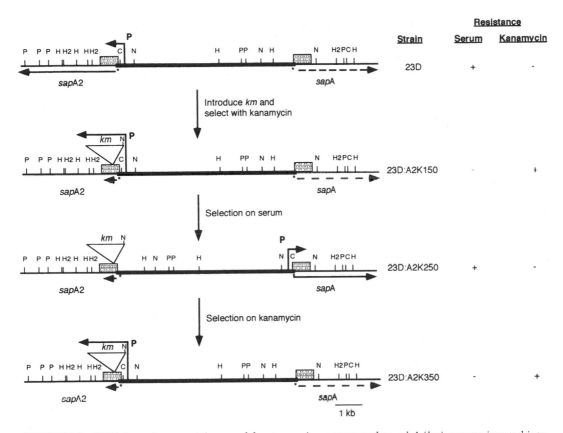

FIGURE 6 DNA inversion events in a model system, using a promoterless *aphA* (*km*) cassette inserted into the wild-type *sapA2* locus (top line). When the *sapA* promoter is positioned in the proper orientation, resistance to kanamycin results in S⁻ bacteria at a frequency of 10^{-4} (second line). When kanamycin-resistant cells are removed from kanamycin selection and subjected to serum selection, S⁺ (serum-resistant), kanamycin-sensitive cells arise at a frequency of 10^{-4} (third line). Solid arrows represent expressed genes, and broken arrows represent silent (unexpressed) genes. The stippled boxes represent the 600-bp conserved regions at the 5′ ends of *sapA* genes, and asterisks show the positions of the embedded inverted repeats that may play a role in the inversion process. The heavy line is the 6.2-kb invertible region. Reprinted from reference 28 with permission.

When strains in which *aphA* was present within *sapA* or *sapA2* were grown on kanamycin and then subjected to serum selection, only cells in which the *sapA* promoter had been moved upstream of a gene encoding a native SLP would be able to survive (Fig. 6). The opposing kanamycin and serum selections then were used to isolate a series of variants that had undergone recombination events to alter the expression of *sapA* homologs. The original *sapA-aphA* and *sapA2-aphA* strains were first selected on kanamycin, as described above, and SLP expression was undetectable. However, incubation of these bacteria in serum followed by plating on medium lacking kanamycin allowed the identification of bacteria that had switched to the expression of an S-layer and therefore survived serum selection. These S⁺ bacteria were recovered at a frequency of 10^{-4} and were kanamycin sensitive, as expected. Plating of these S⁺ cells on medium containing kanamycin allowed the recovery of kanamycin resistance (with concomitant serum sensitivity), again at a frequency of 10^{-4}. The inability to express both the *sapA-aphA* construct (resulting in kanamycin resistance) and another *sapA* homolog (resulting in an S-layer and serum-resistance) verified that a single *sapA* promoter existed.

Chromosomal DNA from these variants was subjected to Southern hybridization with probes specific for the *sapA* promoter or *aphA* gene. These experiments were used to map the locations of the *sapA* promoter in relation to the *aphA* gene and to other *sapA* genes and to correlate this with the expression state of the given genes. The hybridization results predicted the model shown in Fig. 6, which indicates inversion of a DNA segment containing the promoter. All inversion events have in common a 6.2-kb segment of DNA that contains the unique outward-facing *sapA* promoter flanked by *sapA* homologs (Fig. 6). With endpoints in the 600-bp conserved regions at the 5′ ends of each *sapA* homolog, this region can invert, now orienting the *sapA* promoter such that it initiates the expression of the alternate flanking *sapA* gene. This model provides a means for the alternating expression of the two *sapA* genes that flank the 6.2-kb invertible region.

However, wild-type *C. fetus* strains have multiple SLP-encoding genes: strain 23D has eight (94) and strain TK has seven (40). These genes are clustered on the chromosome rather than dispersed, and this tight arrangement is conserved among *C. fetus* strains (32), suggesting that this genetic organization has been selected for the recombination events resulting in the expression of alternate *sapA* homologs. To investigate the expression of *sapA* homologs other than *sapA* and *sapA2,* an inversion reporter system similar to that described above was constructed (30). A strain was isolated that contained insertions of promoterless chloramphenicol (*cat*) and kanamycin (*aphA*) resistance genes in the *sapA* and *sapA2* genes, respectively. Selection of resistance to either antibiotic resulted in recovery of cells (at a frequency of 10^{-4}) in which the *sapA* promoter was upstream and driving the expression of the relevant antibiotic resistance gene. In this manner,

antibiotic resistance could be used to assay simple inversion events, exactly as described above. However, if serum resistance was selected in this strain, it required that a gene that did not originally flank the invertible region be brought downstream of the *sapA* promoter (Fig. 7). Surprisingly, this type of inversion event occurred at a frequency similar to that of simple inversions (approximately 10^{-4}). These experiments also provided strong evidence for the utilization of extremely large inversion events such that any of the clustered *sapA* homologs potentially could be expressed.

All of the inversion events detected in these experiments involved recombination between the 600 bp conserved regions at the 5′ ends of the *sapA* homologs (Fig. 6 and 7). To investigate *trans*-acting factors involved in the inversion, the *C. fetus recA* gene was cloned and a *recA* mutant was constructed (31). RecA is a ubiquitous protein found in essentially all bacteria and is a critical component of the homologous recombination system. As such, it might be predicted to be essential for the types of recombination events leading to *sapA* promoter inversion. The putative χ sites upstream of *sapA* homologs are further suggestions of the involvement of homologous recombination. However, previously characterized inversion systems operated independently of RecA and instead required site-specific invertases. Nevertheless, in a *C. fetus recA* mutant *sapA* promoter inversion was undetectable. Thus, homologous recombination is required to be able to detect *C. fetus* SLP antigenic variation. It should be noted that while RecA appears to be necessary for inversion, it has not been shown to be sufficient. The possibility still exists that other proteins are required for initiating inversion events by generating site-specific DNA strand breaks. The potential roles of the putative χ sites and inverted repeats remain to be shown, since the *sapB* genes lack these features.

An area that has not yet been investigated is the potential role of homologous recombination in generating novel *sapA* genes. With DNA homology both upstream and downstream of each *sapA* gene, there exists the possi-

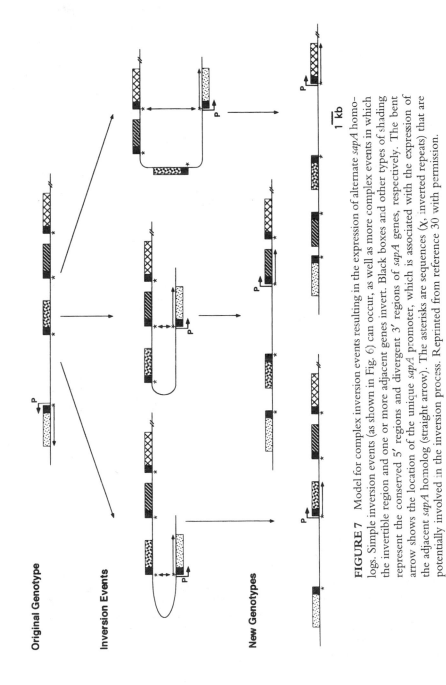

FIGURE 7 Model for complex inversion events resulting in the expression of alternate *sapA* homologs. Simple inversion events (as shown in Fig. 6) can occur, as well as more complex events in which the invertible region and one or more adjacent genes invert. Black boxes and other types of shading represent the conserved 5′ regions and divergent 3′ regions of *sapA* genes, respectively. The bent arrow shows the location of the unique *sapA* promoter, which is associated with the expression of the adjacent *sapA* homolog (straight arrow). The asterisks are sequences (χ, inverted repeats) that are potentially involved in the inversion process. Reprinted from reference 30 with permission.

bility for either homologous recombination or gene conversion events between directly repeated genes, not involving the *sapA* promoter. These types of events would not result in changes in *sapA* expression but, rather, would create chimeric *sapA* homologs that would have novel antigenic determinants. Reassortment of antigenic domains occurs in this manner in gonococcal opacity proteins (21). Such an increase in the arsenal of SLP antigens would enhance the "immune avoidance" capabilities of *C. fetus* during infections.

In summary, the importance of the *C. fetus* S-layer is evident by the substantial segment of the small *C. fetus* genome that is devoted to the expression of SLPs and by the complexity with which SLP-encoding genes can be rearranged. SLPs are expressed from a family of multiple, complete genes by using a single, highly active promoter. An inverting segment of DNA, ranging in size from a minimum of 6.2 kb to an undetermined maximum of perhaps 20 to 30 kb, contains an outward-facing unique *sapA* promoter. The inversion of this segment occurs at a frequency of 10^{-4} and places the promoter in a position to express any of a family of *sapA* genes. Unlike previously characterized inversion systems, the *C. fetus* SLP system requires RecA and homologous recombination for its high frequency inversion events. Recent data suggest that RecA-independent inversion may be occurring at much lower frequency (47).

Secretion of *C. fetus* SLPs

A more recent development in understanding the biogenesis of the *C. fetus* S-layer relates to the secretion of the S-layer subunits prior to assembly at the cell surface. In a study initiated as an attempt to understand *sapA* promoter inversion in greater detail, Thompson et al. characterized the 6.2-kb minimal invertible region from both type A strain 23D and type B strain 84–107 (92). The DNA sequences of the invertible regions from the two strains were virtually identical, again underscoring the high degree of conservation among the factors controlling the biogenesis of the S-layer. The invertible region of the type A strain was studied in the greatest detail, but due to the high similarity of the type B segment at both the DNA and predicted protein levels, the conclusions reached for the type A sequence are certainly going to be true for the type B segment as well. Subtle differences between the type A and type B invertible region sequences are mentioned below.

As stated above, the minimal type A invertible region is 6.2 kb. The 74-bp sequences at either end of the type A invertible region are inverted repeats of each other. These comprise the 5′ ends of the 600-bp "conserved boxes" that serve as the sites of homologous recombination during the inversion events that result in SLP antigenic variation (28, 32, 95) (Fig. 6 and 7). Internal to the inverted repeats and at

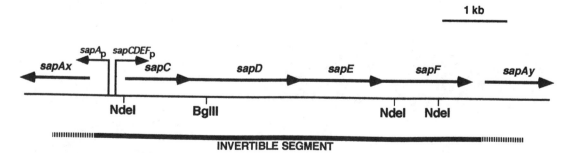

FIGURE 8 Genetic organization of the 6.2-kb invertible region. Bold arrows indicate genes contained within the invertible region. Bent arrows represent the divergent *sapA* and *sapCDEF* promoters. The hatched lines denote the conserved 5′ regions of the flanking *sapA* homologs, indicated here as *sapAx* and *sapAy*. Reprinted from reference 92 with permission.

one end is the outward-facing *sapA* promoter, which allows expression of the *sapA* homolog that is located immediately downstream (Fig. 8). Features of the 114-bp 5′ untranslated region (UTR) of the *sapA* mRNA (inverted 7-bp repeats, repeated pentameric sequences, and χ site) were found as previously described (see above). Adjacent to the *sapA* promoter, but positioned in the opposite orientation, are several potential promoter sequences that would direct the transcription of an operon of four genes (*sapCDEF*) that occupies the remainder of the invertible region. Initial primer extension studies aimed at precisely mapping the *sapCDEF* transcriptional start site were unable to detect this mRNA (91). In contrast to the abundance of cellular *sapA* mRNA, the steady-state level of *sapCDEF* mRNA apparently is extremely low.

Downstream of the *sapCDEF* promoter region begin the *sapCDEF* genes. These genes are 1.0, 1.8, 1.3, and 1.3 kb in size, respectively, and each overlaps the adjacent gene. The predicted SapC protein is a 39.7-kDa protein with a pI of 9.3. The predicted SapC protein currently has no homologies in GenBank to suggest its function. A homology search of the finished but unpublished version of the Sanger Centre *C. jejuni* genome-sequencing project (http://www.sanger.ac.uk/Projects/C_jejuni/) suggests that *C. jejuni* does not contain a *sapC* homolog. Since *C. jejuni* is thought not to possess an S-layer, it is possible that the function of SapC is in some way related to the expression of S-layers by *Campylobacter* species. Whether this gene is present in S-layer-producing campylobacters other than *C. fetus* (such as *C. rectus*) is currently unknown. Potential roles for SapC in the regulation of intracellular SapA accumulation are being investigated.

In contrast to the lack of SapC-homologous proteins, database searches indicated that the *sapDEF* genes predicted proteins that constituted the three components of a type I protein secretion apparatus. The use of a type I transporter for the secretion of *C. fetus* SLPs was suggested by previous observations on the SLPs themselves. First, none of the characterized *C. fetus* SLPs had an amino-terminal secretion signal, unlike most other bacterial SLPs (8, 17, 20, 32, 33, 95). Second, SapA derivatives in which the carboxy terminus of the protein had been deleted were secretion deficient, suggesting that the carboxy terminus of the protein was required for its extracellular transport (14). Carboxy-terminal secretion signals are typical of type I-secreted proteins. Recently, the use of type I transporters in SLP secretion has been reported for two other bacterial species, *Caulobacter crescentus* and *Serratia marcescens* (4, 52). The *C. rectus* SLP lacks an amino-terminal signal sequence and may be secreted by a similar pathway (100).

Based on studies of type I transporters in other bacteria, the model shown in Fig. 9 can be predicted for the *C. fetus* SLP transporter. SapD is a 64-kDa protein and by homology is an inner membrane protein and a member of the large ATP-binding cassette (ABC) superfamily of transport proteins. These proteins use the binding and hydrolysis of ATP to energize the movement of molecules across bacterial membranes (15). SapE (47.9 kDa) is another inner membrane protein, which belongs to the membrane fusion protein family. SapF (49.4 kDa) is an outer membrane protein, which may serve as a pore as the outermost component of the transport apparatus. The interaction of the *C. fetus* SLP secretion signal with SapD probably initiates the sequential recruitment of SapE and SapF protein (trimers?) to assemble the intact SLP transporter, which contains a pore bridging the inner and outer membranes (55, 90). The initial event in translocation of SapA by the SapDEF type I transporter probably is recognition of the SapA secretion signal by SapD. Unlike *sec*-dependent protein secretion, which utilizes amino-terminal signal sequences, type I secreted proteins typically have carboxy-terminal secretion signals (75). Careful inspection of the carboxy-terminal 100 amino acids of each of the characterized *C. fetus* SLPs reveals conserved residues that may play a role in the secretion process (92). The relative

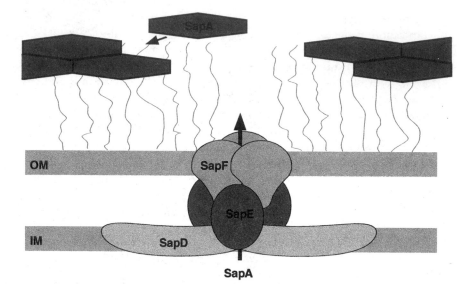

FIGURE 9 Model for secretion and assembly of the S-layer. A hypothetical structure of the *C. fetus* SLP transporter is shown, based on similarities to other type I transporters. The putative stoichiometry of the SapE and SapF proteins in the assembled transport apparatus is based on data gathered for the *E. coli* HlyA transporter (90). Recognition of the SapA carboxy-terminal secretion signal is mediated by the SapD protein. The SapA-SapD complex initiates the sequential assembly of SapE and SapF trimers, resulting in a contiguous pore through which SapA is secreted. SapA then may attach to LPS and be added to the growing S-layer.

simplicity of the type I secretion apparatus facilitates its study. The *C. fetus* invertible region cloned into *E. coli* is functional and can mediate the secretion of SapA from *E. coli* into the culture medium (92). This will permit the study of factors important in the SapA secretion process, using more complex genetics than currently are available for *C. fetus*.

The lack of a recognizable transcriptional terminator downstream of *sapF* raises the question whether a *sapA* homolog correctly positioned at the end of the invertible region opposite the *sapA* promoter could be expressed from the *sapCDEF* promoter. However, the *sapCDEF* operon appears to be transcribed at a very low level (see above). Furthermore, it is possible that *C. fetus* transcriptional terminators do not resemble those of *E. coli* and that sequences downstream of *sapF* in fact function to cause the cessation of transcription. Similar to this, *Helicobacter pylori* lacks-inverted repeat-type

(rho-independent) transcriptional terminators downstream of the operons predicted by the genomic sequence (104). For both of these reasons, a minimal contribution of *sapCDEF* transcription to the expression of alternate *sapA* homologs is expected.

Is the production of SLPs by *C. fetus* regulated? SLPs are among the most abundant proteins produced by *C. fetus* and as such represent a major burden to the metabolic machinery of the call. Furthermore, it is possible that SLPs accumulating intracellularly will exert a toxic effect on the cell. It therefore would seem beneficial for the cell to have a mechanism to repress the accumulation of these proteins, and this may be linked to the rate of their secretion. For some proteins that are secreted via type I systems, mutations involving the transport apparatus lead to the inability to detect the nontransported protein within the cell (92). Although not addressed experimentally, this has been assumed to be due simply to proteolytic degradation of the protein within the cell. General or specific degradation of these proteins certainly would be one means of preventing an intracellular buildup of aberrantly nonsecreted proteins. However, a second possibility is that there may be a specific regulatory mechanism that prevents further synthesis of proteins once the intracellular pool of these proteins surpasses an acceptable level. An example of this type of regulation occurs with the S-layer-producing bacterium *Thermus thermophilus* (35). The mRNA from which its SLP (SlaA) is translated contains a 127-bp 5′ UTR. During conditions of intracellular accumulation of SLPs, this 5′ UTR serves as a binding site for SlaA. The binding of SlaA to its own mRNA prevents further translation of the mRNA, and the rate of SlaA synthesis is decreased. Whether the 114-bp 5′ UTR of the *C. fetus sapA* mRNA performs a similar function is under current investigation.

In summary, the following model of S-layer expression, variation, and biogenesis has emerged from these studies. Within both type A and type B strains, SLPs are encoded by families of *sap* genes. The *sap* genes encode serotype-specific SLPs that have highly conserved amino termini. The conserved amino termini of these proteins are responsible for the binding of the SLPs to homologous LPS and therefore allow adherence of the S-layer to the cell surface. The remainder of each protein is divergent, and this bestows structural, antigenic, and possibly functional differences among S-layers constructed from the individual SLPs.

Each *sap* gene is complete and contains all the information needed to encode a functional SLP. However, only one of these genes is expressed at a given time, and its expression requires that the unique *sap* promoter be present immediately upstream of the expressed gene. The movement of the *sap* promoter upstream of a *sap* gene involves novel high-frequency DNA inversion events mediated by homologous recombination. This recombination is strongly promoted by RecA protein and probably by the conserved homologous DNA sequences found at the 5′ ends of each *sap* gene. Other *cis*-acting features (putative χ sites, direct and inverted repeats, and conserved 3′ homology) also may be required. Factors that are responsible for the secretion of SLPs to the cell surface are encoded on the invertible element, and these comprise a type I protein secretion system (SapDEF) that is different from the secretion systems by which most SLPs are transported. The role of SapC is unknown.

REFERENCES

1. **Allos, B. M., A. J. Lastovica, and M. J. Blaser.** 1995. Atypical Campylobacters and related microorganisms, p. 849–865. *In* M. J. Blaser, J. I. Ravdin, H. B. Greenberg, and R. L. Guerrant (ed.), *Infections of the Gastrointestinal Tract.* Raven Press, New York, N.Y.

2. **Alm, R. A., P. Guerry, M. E. Power, and T. J. Trust.** 1992. Variation in antigenicity and molecular weight of *Campylobacter coli* VC167 flagellin in different genetic backgrounds. *J. Bacteriol.* **174:**4230–4238.

3. **Atabay, H. I., and J. E. Corry.** 1998. The isolation and prevalence of campylobacters from dairy cattle using a variety of methods. *J. Appl. Microbiol.* **84:**733–740.

4. **Awram, P., and J. Smit.** 1998. The *Caulobacter crescentus* paracrystalline S-layer protein is secreted by an ABC transporter (type I) secretion apparatus. *J. Bacteriol.* **180:**3062–3069.

5. **Bawa, E. K., J. O. Adekeye, E. O. Oyedipe, and J. U. Omoh.** 1991. Prevalence of bovine campylobacteriosis in indigenous cattle of three states in Nigeria. *Trop. Anim. Health Prod.* **23:**157–160.

6. **Berg, R. L., J. W. Jutila, and B. D. Firehammer.** 1971. A revised classification of *Vibrio fetus. Am. J. Vet. Res.* **32:**11–22.

7. **Blaser, M. J.** 1998. *Campylobacter fetus*—emerging infection and model system for bacterial pathogenesis at mucosal surfaces. *Clin. Infect. Dis.* **27:**256–258.

8. **Blaser, M. J., and E. C. Gotschlich.** 1990. Surface array protein of *Campylobacter fetus.* Cloning and gene structure. *J. Biol. Chem.* **265:**14529–14535.

9. **Blaser, M. J., and Z. Pei.** 1993. Pathogenesis of *Campylobacter fetus* infections: critical role of high-molecular-weight S-layer proteins in virulence. *J. Infect. Dis.* **167:**372–377.

10. **Blaser, M. J., P. F. Smith, J. A. Hopkins, I. Heinzer, J. H. Bryner, and W. L. Wang.** 1987. Pathogenesis of *Campylobacter fetus* infections: serum resistance associated with high-mo-

lecular-weight surface proteins. *J. Infect. Dis.* **155:**696–706.

11. **Blaser, M. J., P. F. Smith, and P. A. Kohler.** 1985. Susceptibility of *Campylobacter* isolates to the bactericidal activity in human serum. *J. Infect. Dis.* **151:**227–235.

12. **Blaser, M. J., P. F. Smith, and P. F. Kohler.** 1985. Susceptibility of *Campylobacter* isolates to the bactericidal activity of human serum. *J. Infect. Dis.* **151:**227–235.

13. **Blaser, M. J., P. F. Smith, J. E. Repine, and K. A. Joiner.** 1988. Pathogenesis of *Campylobacter fetus* infections. Failure of encapsulated *Campylobacter fetus* to bind C3b explains serum and phagocytosis resistance. *J. Clin. Investig.* **81:**1434–1444.

14. **Blaser, M. J., E. Wang, M. K. Tummuru, R. Washburn, S. Fujimoto, and A. Labigne.** 1994. High-frequency S-layer protein variation in *Campylobacter fetus* revealed by *sapA* mutagenesis. *Mol. Microbiol.* **14:**453–462.

15. **Blight, M. A., and I. B. Holland.** 1990. Structure and function of haemolysin B, P-glycoprotein and other members of a novel family of membrane translocators. *Mol. Microbiol.* **4:**873–880.

16. **Bokkenheuser, V.** 1970. *Vibrio fetus* infection in man. I. Ten new cases and some epidemiologic observations. *Am. J. Epidemiol.* **91:**400–409.

17. **Boot, H. J., and P. H. Pouwels.** 1996. Expression, secretion and antigenic variation of bacterial S-layer proteins. *Mol. Microbiol.* **21:**1117–1123.

18. **Bryner, J. H., A. H. Frank, and P. A. O'Berry.** 1962. Dissociation studies of Vibrios from the bovine genital tract. *Am. J. Vet. Res.* **23:**32–41.

19. **Buckmire, F. L., and R. G. Murray.** 1973. Studies on the cell wall of *Spirillum serpens*. II. Chemical characterization of the outer structured layer. *Can. J. Microbiol.* **19:**59–66.

20. **Casadémont, I., D. Chevrier, and J. L. Guesdon.** 1998. Cloning of a *sapB* homologue (*sapB2*) encoding a putative 112-kDa *Campylobacter fetus* S-layer protein and its use for identification and molecular genotyping. *FEMS Immunol. Med. Microbiol.* **21:**269–281.

21. **Connell, T. D., W. J. Black, T. H. Kawula, D. S. Barritt, J. A. Dempsey, K. Kverneland, Jr., A. Stephenson, B. S. Schepart, G. L. Murphy, and J. G. Cannon.** 1988. Recombination among protein II genes of *Neisseria gonorrhoeae* generates new coding sequences and increases structural variability in the protein II family. *Mol. Microbiol.* **2:**227–236.

22. **Corbeil, L. B.** 1999. Immunization and diagnosis in bovine reproductive tract infections. *Adv. Vet. Med.* **41:**217–239.

23. **Corbeil, L. B., R. R. Corbeil, and A. J. Winter.** 1975. Bovine venereal vibriosis: activity of inflammatory cells in protective immunity. *Am. J. Vet. Res.* **36:**403–406.

24. **Corbeil, L. B., G. G. D. Schurig, P. J. Bier, and A. J. Winter.** 1975. Bovine venereal vibriosis: antigenic variation of the bacterium during infection. *Infect. Immun.* **11:**240–244.

25. **Dubreuil, J. D., M. Kostrzynska, J. W. Austin, and T. J. Trust.** 1990. Antigenic differences among *Campylobacter fetus* S-layer proteins. *J. Bacteriol.* **172:**5035–5043.

26. **Dubreuil, J. D., S. M. Logan, S. Cubbage, D. N. Eidhin, W. D. McCubbin, C. M. Kay, T. J. Beveridge, F. G. Ferris, and T. J. Trust.** 1988. Structural and biochemical analyses of a surface array protein of *Campylobacter fetus*. *J. Bacteriol.* **170:**4165–4173.

27. **Dunn, B. E., M. J. Blaser, and E. L. Snyder.** 1987. Two-dimensional gel electrophoresis and immunoblotting of *Campylobacter* outer membrane proteins. *Infect Immun.* **55:**1564–1572.

28. **Dworkin, J., and M. J. Blaser.** 1996. Generation of *Campylobacter fetus* S-layer protein diversity utilizes a single promoter on an invertible DNA segment. *Mol. Microbiol.* **19:**1241–1253.

29. **Dworkin, J., and M. J. Blaser.** 1997. Molecular mechanisms of *Campylobacter fetus* surface layer protein expression. *Mol. Microbiol.* **26:**433–440.

30. **Dworkin, J., and M. J. Blaser.** 1997. Nested DNA inversion as a paradigm of programmed gene rearrangement. *Proc. Natl. Acad. Sci. USA* **94:**985–990.

31. **Dworkin, J., O. L. Shedd, and M. J. Blaser.** 1997. Nested DNA inversion of *Campylobacter fetus* S-layer genes is *recA* dependent. *J. Bacteriol.* **179:**7523–7529.

32. **Dworkin, J., M. K. Tummuru, and M. J. Blaser.** 1995. A lipopolysaccharide-binding domain of the *Campylobacter fetus* S-layer protein resides within the conserved N terminus of a family of silent and divergent homologs. *J. Bacteriol.* **177:**1734–1741.

33. **Dworkin, J., M. K. Tummuru, and M. J. Blaser.** 1995. Segmental conservation of *sapA* sequences in type B *Campylobacter fetus* cells. *J. Biol. Chem.* **270:**15093–15101.

34. **Eaglesome, M. D., and M. M. Garcia.** 1992. Microbial agents associated with bovine genital tract infections and semen. I. *Brucella abortus, Leptospira, Campylobacter fetus* and *Tritrichomonas foetus*. *Vet. Bull.* **62:**743–775.

35. **Fernandez-Herrero, L. A., G. Olabarria, and J. Berenguer.** 1997. Surface proteins and a novel transcription factor regulate the expression of the S-layer gene in *Thermus thermophilus* HB8. *Mol. Microbiol.* **24:**61–72.

36. **Fisher, J. A., J. Smit, and N. Agabian.** 1988. Transcriptional analysis of the major surface array gene of *Caulobacter crescentus. J. Bacteriol.* **170:** 4706–4713.

37. **Fogg, G. C., L. Y. Yang, E. Wang, and M. J. Blaser.** 1990. Surface array proteins of *Campylobacter fetus* block lectin-mediated binding to type A lipopolysaccharide. *Infect. Immun.* **58:** 2738–2744.

38. **Fujimoto, S., A. Takade, K. Amako, and M. J. Blaser.** 1991. Correlation between molecular size of the surface array protein and morphology and antigenicity of the *Campylobacter fetus* S layer. *Infect Immun.* **59:**2017–2022.

39. **Fujimoto, S., A. Umeda, A. Takade, K. Murata, and K. Amako.** 1989. Hexagonal surface layer of *Campylobacter fetus* isolated from humans. *Infect. Immun.* **57:**2563–2565.

40. **Fujita, M., and K. Amako.** 1994. Localization of the *sapA* gene on a physical map of *Campylobacter fetus* chromosomal DNA. *Arch. Microbiol.* **162:**375–380.

41. **Fujita, M., T. Moriya, S. Fujimoto, N. Hara, and K. Amako.** 1997. A deletion in the *sapA* homologue cluster is responsible for the loss of the S-layer in *Campylobacter fetus* strain TK. *Arch. Microbiol.* **167:**196–201.

42. **Fujita, M., T. Morooka, S. Fujimoto, T. Moriya, and K. Amako.** 1995. Southern blotting analyses of strains of *Campylobacter fetus* using the conserved region of *sapA. Arch. Microbiol.* **164:**444–447.

43. **Garcia, M. M., M. D. Eaglesome, C. F. Hawkins, and F. C. Alexander.** 1980. Campylobacteriosis in Jamaican cattle. *Vet. Rec.* **106:**287–288.

44. **Garcia, M. M., C. L. Lutze-Wallace, A. S. Denes, M. D. Eaglesome, E. Holst, and M. J. Blaser.** 1995. Protein shift and antigenic variation in the S-layer of *Campylobacter fetus* subsp. *venerealis* during bovine infection accompanied by genomic rearrangement of *sapA* homologs. *J. Bacteriol.* **177:**1976–1980.

45. **Ginsberg, M. M., M. A. Thompson, C. R. Peter, D. G. Ramras, and J. Chin.** 1981. *Campylobacter* sepsis associated with "nutritional therapy"—California. *Morbid. Mortal. Weekly Rep.* **30:**294–295.

46. **Goossens, H., R. van den Abbeele, J. P. Butzler, and P. Williams.** 1989. Study of iron uptake in *Campylobacter fetus* and *C. jejuni,* p. 414–415. *In* G. M. Ruiz-Palacios, E. Calva, and B. R. Ruiz-Palacios (ed.), *Campylobacter V.* Instituto Nacional de la Nutricion, Mexico City, Mexico.

47. **Grogono-Thomas, R., J. Dworkin, M. J. Blaser, R. M. Woodland, and D. G. Newell.** 1997. The role of surface-layer proteins in ovine *Campylobacter* abortion, abstr. H9. *In 9th International Workshop on Campylobacter, Helicobacter and Related Organisms.*

48. **Guerrant, R. L., R. G. Lahita, W. C. Winn, and R. B. Roberts.** 1978. Campylobacteriosis in man: pathogenic mechanisms and review of 91 bloodstream infections. *Am. J. Med.* **65:** 584–592.

49. **Hébert, G. A., D. G. Hollis, R. E. Weaver, M. A. Lambert, M. J. Blaser, and C. W. Moss.** 1982. 30 years of campylobacters: biochemical characteristics and a biotyping proposal for *Campylobacter jejuni. J. Clin. Microbiol.* **15:** 1065–1073.

50. **Hum, S.** 1996. Bovine venereal Campylobacteriosis, p. 355–358. *In* D. G. Newell, J. M. Ketley, and R. A. Feldman (ed.), *Campylobacters, Helicobacters, and Related Organisms.* Plenum Press, New York, N.Y.

51. **Ichiyama, S., S. Hirai, T. Minami, Y. Nishiyama, S. Shimizu, K. Shimokata, and M. Ohta.** 1998. *Campylobacter fetus* subspecies *fetus* cellulitis associated with bacteremia in debilitated hosts. *Clin. Infect. Dis.* **27:**252–255.

52. **Kawai, E., H. Akatsuka, A. Idei, T. Shibatani, and K. Omori.** 1998. *Serratia marcescens* S-layer protein is secreted extracellularly via an ATP-binding cassette exporter, the Lip system. *Mol. Microbiol.* **27:**941–952.

53. **Klein, B. S., J. M. Vergeront, M. J. Blaser, P. Edmonds, D. J. Brenner, D. Janssen, and J. P. Davis.** 1986. *Campylobacter* infection associated with raw milk. An outbreak of gastroenteritis due to *Campylobacter jejuni* and thermotolerant *Campylobacter fetus* subsp. *fetus. JAMA* **255:** 361–364.

54. **Kowalczykowski, S. C., D. A. Dixon, A. K. Eggleston, S. D. Lauder, and W. M. Rehrauer.** 1994. Biochemistry of homologous recombination in *Escherichia coli. Microbiol. Rev.* **58:** 401–465.

55. **Létoffé, S., P. Delepelaire, and C. Wandersman.** 1996. Protein secretion in Gram-negative bacteria: assembly of the three components of ABC protein-mediated exporters is ordered and promoted by substrate binding. *EMBO J.* **15:**5804–5811.

56. **Marty, A. T., T. A. Webb, K. G. Stubbs, and R. R. Penkava.** 1983. Inflammatory abdominal aortic aneurysm infected by *Campylobacter fetus. JAMA* **249:**1190–1192.

57. **McCoy, E. C., D. Doyle, K. Burda, L. B. Corbeil, and A. J. Winter.** 1975. Superficial antigens of *Campylobacter (Vibrio) fetus:* characterization of an antiphagocytic component. *Infect. Immun.* **11:**517–525.

58. **McFaydean, J., and S. Stockman.** 1909. *Report of the Department Committee Appointed by the Board of Agriculture and Fisheries to Inquire into Epizootic Abortion,* vol. 3. His Majesty's Stationery Office, London, United Kingdom.

59. **Meier, P. A., D. P. Dooley, J. H. Jorgensen, C. C. Sanders, W. M. Huang, and J. E. Patterson.** 1998. Development of quinolone-resistant *Campylobacter fetus* bacteremia in human immunodeficiency virus-infected patients. *J. Infect. Dis.* **177:**951–954.

60. **Mohanty, S. B., G. J. Plumer, and J. E. Faber.** 1962. Biochemical and colonial characteristics of some bovine vibrios. *Am. J. Vet. Res.* **23:**554–557.

61. **Moran, A. P.** 1995. Structure-bioreactivity relationships of bacterial endotoxins. *J. Toxicol. Toxin Rev.* **14:**47–83.

62. **Moran, A. P., D. T. O'Malley, T. U. Kosunen, and I. M. Helander.** 1994. Biochemical characterization of *Campylobacter fetus* lipopolysaccharides. *Infect. Immun.* **62:**3922–3929.

63. **Moran, A. P., D. T. O'Malley, J. Vuopio-Varkila, K. Varkila, L. Pyhala, H. Saxen, and I. M. Helander.** 1996. Biological characterization of *Campylobacter fetus* lipopolysaccharides. *FEMS Immunol. Med. Microbiol.* **15:**43–50.

64. **Morrison, V. A., B. K. Lloyd, J. K. Chia, and C. U. Tuazon.** 1990. Cardiovascular and bacteremic manifestations of *Campylobacter fetus* infection: case report and review. *Rev. Infect. Dis.* **12:**387–392.

65. **Myers, L. L.** 1971. Purification and partial characterization of a *Vibrio fetus* immunogen. *Infect. Immun.* **3:**562–566.

66. **Neuzil, K. M., E. Wang, D. W. Haas, and M. J. Blaser.** 1994. Persistence of *Campylobacter fetus* bacteremia associated with absence of opsonizing antibodies. *J. Clin. Microbiol.* **32:** 1718–1720.

67. **Pefanis, S. M., S. Herr, C. G. Venter, L. P. Kruger, C. C. Queiroga, and L. Amaral.** 1988. Trichomoniasis and campylobacteriosis in bulls in the Republic of Transkei. *J. S. Afr. Vet. Assoc.* **59:**139–140.

68. **Pei, Z., and M. J. Blaser.** 1990. Pathogenesis of *Campylobacter fetus* infections. Role of surface array proteins in virulence in a mouse model. *J. Clin. Investig.* **85:**1036–1043.

69. **Pei, Z., R. T. Ellison III, R. V. Lewis, and M. J. Blaser.** 1988. Purification and characterization of a family of high molecular weight surface-array proteins from *Campylobacter fetus. J. Biol. Chem.* **263:**6416–6420.

70. **Penner, J. L.** 1988. The genus *Campylobacter:* a decade of progress. *Clin. Microbiol. Rev.* **1:** 157–172.

71. **Pérez-Pérez, G. I., and M. J. Blaser.** 1985. Lipopolysaccharide characteristics of pathogenic campylobacters. *Infect. Immun.* **47:**353–359.

72. **Pérez-Pérez, G. I., M. J. Blaser, and J. H. Bryner.** 1986. Lipopolysaccharide structures of *Campylobacter fetus* are related to heat-stable serogroups. *Infect. Immun.* **51:**209–212.

73. **Pérez-Pérez, G. I., J. A. Hopkins, and M. J. Blaser.** 1985. Antigenic heterogeneity of lipopolysaccharides from *Campylobacter jejuni* and *Campylobacter fetus. Infect. Immun.* **48:**528–533.

74. **Pönkä, A., R. Tilvis, J. Helle, and T. U. Kosunen.** 1984. Infection with *Campylobacter fetus. Scand. J. Infect. Dis.* **16:**127–128.

75. **Pugsley, A. P.** 1993. The complete general secretory pathway in gram-negative bacteria. *Microbiol. Rev.* **57:**50–108.

76. **Rettig, P. J.** 1979. *Campylobacter* infections in human beings. *J. Pediatr.* **94:**855–864.

77. **Riley, L. W., and M. J. Finch.** 1985. Results of the first year of national surveillance of *Campylobacter* infections in the United States. *J. Infect. Dis.* **151:**956–959.

78. **Salama, S. M., M. M. Garcia, and D. E. Taylor.** 1992. Differentiation of the subspecies of *Campylobacter fetus* by genomic sizing. *Int. J. Syst. Bacteriol.* **42:**446–450.

79. **Salama, S. M., E. Newnham, N. Chang, and D. E. Taylor.** 1995. Genome map of *Campylobacter fetus* subsp. *fetus* ATCC 27374. *FEMS Microbiol. Lett.* **132:**239–245.

80. **Schurig, G. D., C. E. Hall, K. Burda, L. B. Corbeil, J. R. Duncan, and A. J. Winter.** 1973. Persistent genital tract infection with *Vibrio fetus intestinalis* associated with serotypic alteration of the infecting strain. *Am. J. Vet. Res.* **34:** 1399–1403.

81. **Sebald, M., and M. Véron.** 1963. Teneur en bases de l'ADN et classification des vibrions. *Ann. Inst. Pasteur* **105:**897–910.

82. **Senchenkova, S. N., A. S. Shashkov, Y. A. Knirel, J. J. McGovern, and A. P. Moran.** 1997. The O-specific polysaccharide chain of *Campylobacter fetus* serotype A lipopolysaccharide is a partially O-acetylated 1,3-linked alpha-D-mannan. *Eur. J. Biochem.* **245:**637–641.

83. **Senchenkova, S. N., A. S. Shashkov, Y. A. Knirel, J. J. McGovern, and A. P. Moran.** 1996. The O-specific polysaccharide chain of *Campylobacter fetus* serotype B lipopolysaccharide is a D-rhamnan terminated with 3-O-methyl-D-rhamnose (D-acofriose). *Eur. J. Biochem.* **239:** 434–438.

84. **Skirrow, M. B.** 1994. Diseases due to *Campylobacter, Helicobacter* and related bacteria. *J. Comp. Pathol.* **111:**113–149.

85. **Smibert, R. M.** 1978. The genus *Campylobacter*. *Annu. Rev. Microbiol.* **32:**673–709.

86. **Smith, T., and M. Taylor.** 1919. Some morphological and biological characters of the spirilla (*Vibrio fetus*, n. sp.) associated with disease of the fetal membranes in cattle. *J. Exp. Med.* **30:** 299–311.

87. **Taylor, D. E., and A. S. Chau.** 1997. Cloning and nucleotide sequence of the *gyrA* gene from *Campylobacter fetus* subsp. fetus ATCC 27374 and characterization of ciprofloxacin-resistant laboratory and clinical isolates. *Antimicrob. Agents Chemother.* **41:**665–671.

88. **Taylor, D. E., R. S. Garner, and B. J. Allan.** 1983. Characterization of tetracycline resistance plasmids from *Campylobacter jejuni* and *Campylobacter coli*. *Antimicrob. Agents Chemother.* **24:** 930–935.

89. **Taylor, P. R., W. M. Weinstein, and J. H. Bryner.** 1979. *Campylobacter fetus* infection in human subjects: association with raw milk. *Am. J. Med.* **66:**779–783.

90. **Thanabalu, T., E. Koronakis, C. Hughes, and V. Koronakis.** 1998. Substrate-induced assembly of a contiguous channel for protein export from *E. coli*: reversible bridging of an inner-membrane translocase to an outer membrane exit pore. *EMBO J.* **17:**6487–6496.

91. **Thompson, S. A., K. C. Ray, and M. J. Blaser.** Unpublished data.

92. **Thompson, S. A., O. L. Shedd, K. C. Ray, M. H. Beins, J. P. Jorgensen, and M. J. Blaser.** 1998. *Campylobacter fetus* surface layer proteins are transported by a type I secretion system. *J. Bacteriol.* **180:**6450–6458.

93. **Tremblay, C., and C. Gaudreau.** 1998. Antimicrobial susceptibility testing of 59 strains of *Campylobacter fetus* subsp. *fetus*. *Antimicrob. Agents Chemother.* **42:**1847–1849.

94. **Tummuru, M. K., and M. J. Blaser.** 1992. Characterization of the *Campylobacter fetus sapA* promoter: evidence that the *sapA* promoter is deleted in spontaneous mutant strains. *J. Bacteriol.* **174:**5916–5922.

95. **Tummuru, M. K., and M. J. Blaser.** 1993. Rearrangement of *sapA* homologs with conserved and variable regions in *Campylobacter fetus*. *Proc. Natl. Acad. Sci. USA* **90:**7265–7269.

96. **Ullmann, U., H. Langmaack, and C. Blas-**
ius. 1982. Campylobacteriosis in humans caused by subspecies intestinalis and fetus. Six new diseases. *Infection* **10**(Suppl. 2):S64–S66.

97. **Véron, M., and R. Chatelain.** 1973. Taxonomic study of the genus *Campylobacter* Sebald and Véron and designation of the neotype strain for the type species *Campylobacter fetus* (Smith and Taylor) Sebald and Véron. *Int. J. Syst. Bacteriol.* **23:**122–134.

98. **Verresen, L., M. Vrolix, J. Verhaegen, and R. Lins.** 1985. *Campylobacter* bacteraemia. Report of 2 cases and review of the literature. *Acta Clin. Belg.* **40:**99–104.

99. **Vinzent, R., J. Dumas, and N. Picard.** 1947. Septicemie grave au cours de la grossesse due a un vibrion: avortment consecutif. *Bull. Acad. Natl. Med.* **131:**90–93.

100. **Wang, B., E. Kraig, and D. Kolodrubetz.** 1998. A new member of the S-layer protein family: characterization of the *crs* gene from *Campylobacter rectus*. *Infect. Immun.* **66:**1521–1526.

101. **Wang, E., M. M. Garcia, M. S. Blake, Z. Pei, and M. J. Blaser.** 1993. Shift in S-layer protein expression responsible for antigenic variation in *Campylobacter fetus*. *J. Bacteriol.* **175:** 4979–4984.

102. **Wang, W. L., and M. J. Blaser.** 1986. Detection of pathogenic *Campylobacter* species in blood culture systems. *J. Clin. Microbiol.* **23:**709–714.

103. **Washburn, R. G., N. C. Julian, E. Wang, and M. J. Blaser.** 1991. Inhibition of complement by surface array proteins from *Campylobacter fetus*, abstr. 1328. *In Program and Abstracts of the 31st Interscience Conference on Antimicrobial Agents and Chemotherapy*. American Society for Microbiology, Washington, D.C.

104. **Washio, T., J. Sasayama, and M. Tomita.** 1998. Analysis of complete genomes suggests that many prokaryotes do not rely on hairpin formation in transcription termination. *Nucleic Acids Res.* **26:**5456–5463.

105. **Winter, A. J., E. C. McCoy, C. S. Fullmer, K. Burda, and P. J. Bier.** 1978. Microcapsule of *Campylobacter fetus*: chemical and physical characterization. *Infect. Immun.* **22:**963–971.

106. **Yang, L. Y., Z. H. Pei, S. Fujimoto, and M. J. Blaser.** 1992. Reattachment of surface array proteins to *Campylobacter fetus* cells. *J. Bacteriol.* **174:**1258–1267.

MOLECULAR
GENETICS

IV

TB be
clonal to differ from ancestors
only by the accumulation of mutations
without interclonal recombinant shorts

POPULATION GENETICS AND GENEALOGY OF *CAMPYLOBACTER JEJUNI*

Richard J. Meinersmann

17

BACTERIAL POPULATION GENETICS PARADIGMS

Population genetics is the study of gene flow in and between populations. For bacteria, this is often reduced to the question, "Is this species/type clonal?" To be clonal is to differ from ancestors only by the accumulation of mutations, without interclonal recombinant events (9). A mutation, in this respect, is any nonrecombinant event that changes the primary DNA sequence. The original paradigm for bacterial reproduction is by asexual binary fission. In this model, each progeny is exactly like the parent, grandparent, and so on, except for the accumulation of mutations. For the first part of this discussion, assume that binary fission and random mutation are the only contributions to *Campylobacter* population structure. The history of *Campylobacter* is represented in Fig. 1 up to the point labeled "Current Diversity." For the phylogenist, the left-hand apex represents the very first *Campylobacter* organism, perhaps millions of years ago. For the population geneticist, the left-hand apex represents the first member of a new clone, perhaps days, months, or years ago. The triangle represents the expansion of the population. The vertical

bar at the right side of the triangle represents the entire population, with the shaded gradient representing the current diversity in the population due to the accumulation of mutations. The degree of variation is a function of the frequency of mutations and time from the origin of the population.

This simple paradigm does not depict the complete "real-world" picture. Barriers or bottlenecks, i.e., anything that keeps some proportion of the population from reproducing, can occur. They include both purely chance events (selectively neutral) unrelated to the fitness of the strain, such as random transmission from one host to the next, and selective events, such as exposure to an antibiotic or some environmental stress that destroys the portion of the population that is not fit. Adding the barriers, the history of *Campylobacter* is then represented by the whole of Fig. 1. Clones are members of a subpopulation that are descended from a single ancestor with distinct characteristics in the species. Still assuming asexual reproduction, the members of each subpopulation will be the same as the parents that made it through the bottlenecks, except for the accumulation of new mutations. The differences from one subpopulation to the next will depend on two factors. The first factor is the impact or frequency of the barriers, which determines how

Richard J. Meinersmann, Poultry Processing and Meat Quality Research Unit, USDA Agricultural Research Service, P.O. Box 5677, Athens, GA 30604.

Campylobacter, 2nd Ed., Edited by I. Nachamkin and M. J. Blaser

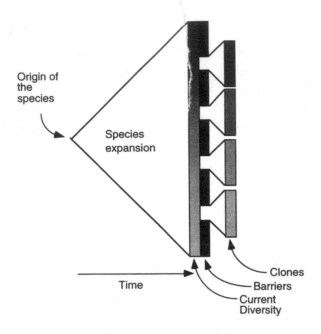

Origin of
the
species

Species
expansion

Time

Clones
Barriers
Current
Diversity

FIGURE 1 Model of asexual bacterial population growth. The left-hand apex of the triangle represents the single individual from which the species arose. During species expansion, mutations accumulate, and diversity is represented by the shade gradient. The solid vertical bars represent barriers to portions of the population; these barriers are penetrated by clones that grow into new clones that reflect the diversity of the individuals that crossed the barriers.

many individuals contribute to the next generation. If the barriers had been selective pressures, it is easy to see that a given subpopulation that is adapted will reflect a given niche. However, even if the bottlenecks are chance events, the subpopulations will reflect their niche. This is because it is unlikely that the same chance event will occur twice. Therefore, different subpopulations, or clones, will prevail after different chance events and will survive in different niches. In either case, fitness selection or random chance, the subpopulations will have undergone a "selective purification" and the diversity within that subpopulation of alleles for all the genes will be reduced (4).

The second factor that defines a clone is the number of mutations that accumulated before the barriers arose. Mutations are (mostly) independent events. Mutations in characterized bacterial species occur at a rate of approximately 10^{-11} to 10^{-9} per base pair site per generation. If *Campylobacter* organisms have the same mutation rate, with a genome of 1.7 million bp there will only be one mutation of a random base pair for every 600 to 60,000 new individuals. According to the neutral theory of evolution, most mutations are either deleterious or neutral (28). The deleterious mutations are rapidly purged from the population and are rarely available for sampling; therefore, they are rarely seen. Whether a neutral mutation becomes prevalent or fixed (occurring in all the members) is completely a random phenomenon. The mutations that occur in one niche are not likely to be the same as the ones that occur elsewhere. It is not possible to have enough mixing of organisms between niches in order to have the entire diversity instantaneously represented at any given place at a given time. Therefore, for instance, the subpopulations isolated in Colorado should be different from those in Georgia.

The model presented so far is still incomplete, because bacteria are not strictly asexual; they do exchange DNA and recombine their chromosomes into new individuals. The exchange of DNA between subpopulations will drive toward homogenization of genomes and return to a state in which the subpopulations become indistinguishable (4). The rate of this homogenization depends on the effective recombination rate (ERR), which is expressed as $4Nc$ (24), where c is the recombination rate per site on the genome per generation and is dependent on the biology of the organism and *N* is the effective population size, i.e., the number of individuals within a population that can and do participate in genetic exchange. Participating individuals must have both ability (i.e., must have the mechanisms for incorporating the DNA and must not be impeded by recombination barriers) and availability (i.e., must be in the right place at the right time). Also, the pair of organisms involved in effective recombination must be different from each other in order for the product to be something new and different that can be detected.

The effective population size is also affected by the migration rate of the organism, since this affects its availability for recombination. If an organism and its progeny remain in a single niche, it is less likely to participate in recombination events in other niches. Since the migration rate and the recombination rate are both time dependent, even with rapid recombination rates, typing of organisms can be epidemiologically useful information. *Campylobacter* clearly can cross between different niches. The major source of human infection has been found to be poultry products, and the organism grows well in chickens (78). Population genetics studies will help describe migration pathways of the global population of *Campylobacter*.

ERR can be estimated from studies of the population-genetic structures of an organism. $4Nc$ is estimated to be approximately 10^{-7} for *Escherichia coli* (4). Experimental data have shown that *E. coli* has clonal associations with its niches (92). That is to say, members in a subpopulation found in a particular niche arose from a single parent. On the other hand, experimental evidence reviewed here shows that *Campylobacter* is unclear in its clonal associations with niches. Cohan (4) has mathematically demonstrated that $4Nc$ must be greater than 10^{-5} to dilute the clonal association with niches. If *Campylobacter* is not clonal, it can be concluded that ERR is at least 100-fold greater for *Campylobacter* than it is for *E. coli*. This could mean that there are many more *Campylobacter* organisms in the world than there are *E. coli* organisms or that *Campylobacter* organisms

are much more active in interstrain recombination events, or both.

To be clonal or nonclonal is not a black-and-white issue; there are shades of gray, as illustrated by the concept of clonal frameworks or meroclones described by Milkman and Bridges (42). In the meroclone structure, the preponderance of the genome is inherited through a direct lineage and portions of the genome are mixed between clones. The threshold of when an organism is called clonal is dependent on the genotypic test that is used and the assumptions used for that test. *C. jejuni* appears to fit the clonal-framework model, but the proportion of the genome that is inherited through a direct lineage is probably smaller than that seen with *E. coli* or with most serovars of *Salmonella enterica* (36).

Phylogeny is "the historical relationships among lineages of organisms or their parts" (23). Some authors reserve the term "phylogeny" for the evolution of species and use the term "genealogy" for lineages of genes without consideration of the genesis of new species (77). Most molecular phylogeny studies, including essentially all those done for *Campylobacter*, use descriptive data of contemporary individuals to statistically reconstruct historical relationships based on assumptions of the changes the organisms can make and how those changes are brought about over time. Thus, this chapter also considers the evolution of some characteristics of *C. jejuni* and the mechanisms of how those changes may have occurred.

POPULATION GENETICS DATA

Much of the data useful for population genetic analyses may be imperfect for phylogenetic analyses. There are several criteria that have to be satisfied by character states (see below) that are analyzed for the phylogenetic analyses to be accurate. One criterion that is difficult to realize, especially for bacteria, is that the rate of change has to be consistent over the entire set being analyzed throughout the history being reconstructed (76). The rRNA sequences are one set of data that are considered to fulfill the rate criterion and have been widely analyzed (50). Through rRNA sequence analyses, the taxonomic classification of the *Campylobacter* species has been confirmed, and the genus *Campylobacter* has been placed in the epsilon subdivision of the *Proteobacteria,* which also includes *Helicobacter, Arcobacter,* and *Wolinella* (80, 83). However, the rate of change of rRNA is generally too slow to be helpful in distinguishing subpopulations and deducing their histories. One interesting observation is that strains of *C. jejuni* have variability in transcribed spacers (83). The population genetics implications of this observation have not yet been determined.

Another important difference between phylogenetic analyses and population genetics is that ancestral types are usually extinct in phylogeny and usually radiated into only two new species at a given time. In population genetics, the ancestral types may still be extant and several lineages may link to an ancestral type that is still extant (18). The ancestral types may or may not be on their way to extinction, and in sexual species more than one ancestral type may still be extant. Any organism that exchanges DNA is considered sexual in this context, and *Campylobacter* appears to obey this rule. *Campylobacter* organisms are known to be naturally transformable (86), and the analyses discussed here appear to show that they do incorporate foreign DNA into their chromosomes in the wild.

Most descriptive data of *C. jejuni* genotypes have been generated for epidemiological investigations. This has influenced the types of assays that have been done and the makeup of the populations that have been tested. Most tested *C. jejuni* strains have been from human infections or suspected sources of human infection. The number of *C. jejuni* strains associated with humans is probably only a small proportion of the global population. This means that the bulk of the studies for which population structure conclusions can be drawn have a heavy bias that may not represent the real global situation. Population genetics also requires determination of multiple distinct characteristics for each

individual that is assayed. For sequence data, each base position is handled as a distinct character that is scored according to the nucleotide that occurs in that base position. Gel band methods, such as pulsed-field gel electrophoresis (PFGE), use each band position as a distinct character that is scored by the presence of absence of the band (7). The score for each characteristic is known as the "character state" (34, 76). Ideally, for phylogenetic inferences, the character state for each characteristic should be independent of the character state for any other characteristic (76). This criterion is frequently violated, which is probably the main reason why population structure of *C. jejuni* remains confusing. This chapter should help the reader become aware of the limitations in inferences that can be made with current data in the population genetics of *C. jejuni.*

All methods that are valid for phylogenetic reconstruction should give the same results for a given population (9, 75). In other words, the phylogenetic trees should be the same, within statistical limits. Apart from errors in analyses, such as poor sampling of members of the test population or lack of independence of the tested traits, a method may give trees that are phylogenetically invalid because of random recombinant events. Strong selective pressures on the traits being assayed can bias the analyses as well. Strong selective pressures may lead to an increase in the number of individuals in a population that have either mutations or recombinant events (67). Host immune reactions constitute an especially important selective barrier (44). For this reason, potential targets of immune responses are usually not used for phylogenetic reconstruction. However, the methods used for phylogenetic analyses can give clues to the mechanisms used to generate diversity.

Epidemiologists are interested in tracing an organism as it flows through a host of interest. They usually are only tracing a particular genotype, a phenotype, or a set of phenotypes against the background of the remainder of the genomic makeup. Hopefully, the phenotype represents a specific genetic type, as opposed to an induced state. Groupings based on phenotypes that do not reflect phylogeny are called phenetic. A study can be valid for epidemiological purposes without being informative with respect to the population genetics of the organism. Hunter (25) has promoted discriminatory power as being the most important criterion for epidemiological investigations. Discriminatory power is an estimate of the ability of the test to differentiate between two unrelated strains. It is desirable to be able to identify a particular strain wherever it occurs and to distinguish it from other strains. On the other hand, it is not helpful if every isolate is different and the association of each strain cannot be determined. Discrimination is reliant on rates of genetic changes, i.e., rates of gene flow. Changes have to occur fast enough to generate new types but not so fast that new types develop by the time the specimens are sampled (35).

There have been many studies of methods to subtype *Campylobacter,* and all show a tremendous diversity. A total of 57 antisera are used for heat-stable (O–antigen) typing, and 55 antisera are used for heat-labile (HL) antigen typing (58). More than one O or HL type may occur on a given isolate of *Campylobacter.* However, only five O serotypes and six HL serotypes accounted for about half of 298 isolates from patients with sporadic cases in the United States (58). It is not known how many genes affect the HL serotype of *Campylobacter.* At least some of the serotypes may represent a single epitope (48) that would be an allele for a single gene. However, most HL serotypes are not as clearly defined.

An entire operon is necessary for the construction of O polysaccharides (62); therefore, the O serotype represents a polygenic allele. Since the makeup of the operon controlling the construction of a specific O serotype is more likely to be coinherited rather than brought together in recombination events, it is a plausible assumption that members of an O serotype are members of a clone. Powerful support for this assumption comes from the study by Jackson et al. (26) that showed a highly

significant linkage of O and HL serotypes among several thousand random, sporadic isolates of *Campylobacter* from the United Kingdom.

However, the members of serogroups are not homogeneous (14, 58). In a subset of 15 isolates that were serovar O 23/HL 5, Jackson et al. (26) found eight biotypes, three phage types (including nontypeable), and three ribotypes. Also, the serotypes were not found in exclusive associations of O and HL types. *Campylobacter* serotypes are not species specific; some types have been found in both *C. jejuni* and *C. coli* (43, 61). There is currently insufficient information to determine if this is due to recombinant exchange between the species, convergent evolution, or incidental cross-reactivity between complex antigens.

PFGE analysis of chromosomal DNA has been suggested as a method for discriminating strains of *Campylobacter* (13, 51, 74). In fact, it is rare to find independently collected strains of *Campylobacter* that have the same PFGE profile. Unfortunately, PFGE has not contributed to an understanding of the population genetics of *Campylobacter.* This may be overcome in the future with the development of better algorithms for analysis, but the determination may be forever confounded by the high rate of gene order shuffling that appears to occur in *C. jejuni* (88) (see also chapter 18). Any of the methods used to analyze the gross structure of the *Campylobacter* genome will be susceptible to the same problems found with PFGE, but this will occur to differing degrees that cannot be currently predicted.

Total–protein analysis evaluates the presence or absence of bands in an electrophoresis gel. Total–protein electrophoresis analysis is often criticized because many of the proteins that are observed may represent only induced states (76). There are several reasons why a protein may be absent, such as gene suppression under certain growth conditions, a deletion, a premature stop mutation, or a mutation in a regulator. The protein analysis does not give information on what reason accounts for an absence, and there also is no information on allelic varia-

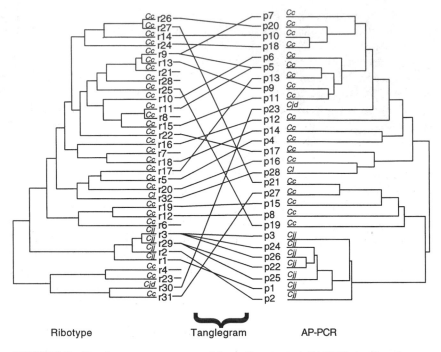

Ribotype   Tanglegram   AP-PCR

FIGURE 2 Dendrograms reconstructed from ribotype and AP-PCR data in reference 21 and a tanglegram to link isolates used in the two analyses. Individuals are identified by the type name that was assigned (prefix 'r' for ribotypes, and prefix 'p' for AP-PCR types). The species of each type are identified as follows: *Cc, C. coli; Cjj, C. jejuni* subsp. *jejuni; Cjd, C. jejuni* subsp. *doylei; Cl, C. lari.* The tanglegram in the center links individuals in each dendrogram (some types had more than one member that separated in the alternate method, and some isolates were not typed by AP-PCR, leaving some ribotypes without links).

tion of the bands that are present. All this being said, there have been studies of electrophoretic protein patterns that show distinction between species-specific groups of *Campylobacter* and discrimination of variants within the species (5, 54, 84). Comparison of the relationships developed by the protein electropherograms with relationships developed by comparison of rRNA sequences (83) or DNA-DNA hybridization analysis (3, 53, 66) shows that the protein electropherograms do not properly reconstruct phylogenetic relationships.

Several points about the population genetics of *Campylobacter* can be made with the data presented by Hernandez et al. (21), in which isolates were typed by ribotyping and arbitrary-primer PCR (AP-PCR, another name for random-amplified polymorphic DNA [RAPD]).

The results are reproduced in Fig. 2. The "tanglegram" is a term that was coined by Page (57) for the comparison of two dendrograms that are linked to show individuals grouped by two different methods. This method is used to compare the evolution of species that depend on each other, such as a host and a pathogen. It is also used, as it is in this case, to compare the apparent genealogy of different genes or different methods of collecting data. The branch orders of the trees were swapped to give the least complex tanglegram. This results in trees that look dramatically different from those published by Hernandez et al. (21) but in fact have almost identical information. One exception was the placement of the p28 AP-PCR type. This was a single isolate of *C. lari*, which in the analyses presented here falls within a cluster mostly populated with *C. coli* whereas in the original analysis this isolate was seen as an independent strain. The single strain of *C. jejuni* subsp. *doylei* (p23) also placed within a cluster of *C. coli*. The results for the ribotyping experiments have similar problems in that some *C. coli* strains are more distant from the bulk of the *C. coli* strains than the cluster containing all the *C. jejuni* subsp. *jejuni*. Thus, it appears that neither the ribotyping nor the AP-PCR results are phylogenetically accurate, at least at the species level. The crossing of the lines in the tanglegram show that the two methods are not measuring the same thing and that at least one of the methods must be phylogenetically inaccurate. This could be a result of recombination events that place markers into a background with a different ancestry. However, the cluster containing r3, r29, r2, and r1 may be clonal, since there is little change in that part of the dendrogram between the two methods.

Even if it is decided that the data are not phylogenetically accurate, they can still be phenetically useful. With the evaluation of enough characteristics, it would be unlikely to have a pair of organisms with identical phenotype that are not related to each other, and, thus, epidemiologic investigations can be based on phenotype. It is plausible that a particular phenotype is required for survival in a specific niche, although this has not yet been noted for *Campylobacter*. However, the likelihood that isolates with similar phenotypic characteristics had recent ancestors in common should be interpreted with caution. A common mistake is to inspect a phenogram and designate clusters by the density of branching rather than by the depth (or time) at which the branches occur. The population used in Fig. 2 was divided into three clusters by both methods (21). A principal-component analysis (PCA) is an alternative nonphylogenetic cluster analysis that might be more helpful in designating groups (65). The data used to generate Fig. 2 were reanalyzed, and the results of a PCA are presented in Fig. 3. The "factors" are scores of the variance that are found in the three most influential dimensions of a multidimensional coordinate system (the number of dimensions that are produced equals the number of variables that are sampled,

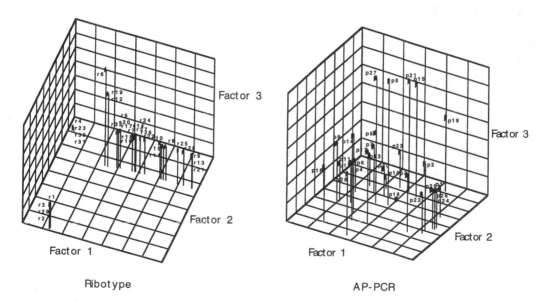

Ribotype   AP-PCR

FIGURE 3 PCA of ribotype and AP-PCR data in reference 21. See the text for an explanation. The scales of the factors are not relevant and are left out to avoid confusion. Spots represent individual types and are labeled with the type name that was assigned.

and the values of the factors are numbers that can be used for plotting but have no further physical meaning). Each point represents a specific isolate. It can be concluded from the ribotype data that there are two small clusters and one large group, but it is also justified to conclude that the large group actually consists of four or five small clusters. The PCA of the AP-PCR data may be showing one or two small clusters, but most of the isolates appear to be randomly associated. Thus, more accurate groupings can be made by the PCA without drawing inappropriate phylogenetic conclusions.

MUTILOCUS ENZYME ELECTROPHORESIS ANALYSIS

Multilocus enzyme electrophoresis (MLEE) is a method of simultaneously evaluating the genetic makeup of many parts of the genome (69). Several enzymes that have low selective pressure for variability are analyzed for different allotypes based on changes in electrophoretic properties that have occurred due to amino acid substitutions. The allotype of each enzyme is determined for several strains and analyzed to determine if allotype linkage occurs. Simply, linkage is a measure of how often a particular allotype of one enzyme is found to occur with a particular allotype of another enzyme (90). This is compared to the predicted results if the allotypes were totally randomly associated (so-called linkage equilibrium) or to the predicted results if there is always an association of allotypes of one enzyme with those of another enzyme (so-called linkage disequilibrium). A high level of linkage disequilibrium is indicative of clonal populations (36).

A search of the literature revealed three published studies of *Campylobacter* that include MLEE analyses (1, 12, 59). A study has also been completed in our laboratory (40). The studies by Fraser et al. (12) and Patton et al. (59) focused on comparing the discrimination ability of MLEE with that of other molecular methods for the purpose of epidemiological studies. MLEE was more discriminatory than serotyping, biotyping, phage typing, ribotyping, and plasmid profiling and was equally discriminatory to restriction digest analysis (59).

Aeschbacher and Piffaretti (1) analyzed populations of *C. jejuni* and *C. coli* collected in Switzerland for allotype distribution of 10 enzymes: malate dehydrogenase, adenlyate kinase, L-phenylalanyl-L-leucine peptidase, isocitrate dehydrogenase, aconitase, malic enzyme, fumarase, alkaline phosphatase, threonine dehydrogenase, and catalase. Using the same set of enzymes plus phenylalanyl-proline peptidase, we analyzed 156 isolates of 11 species and subspecies from disparate sources (40). Almost all the isolates clustered into species-specific groups. The diversity scores, which are the odds of randomly selected pairs of strains being different from one another, were high in both studies, corroborating that the members of the *Campylobacter* genera are very diverse (Table 1). The mean number of alleles per locus was also large in the MLEE studies of *Campylobacter* (Table 1). Several alleles appeared to be shared by multiple species, but this is difficult to prove since different alleles can comigrate in the gels

TABLE 1 Statistics derived from MLEE results for *Campylobacter* spp.

Species	Mean genetic diversity	Mean no. of alleles/locus	I_A (mean $\pm$ SE)
All *Campylobacter* spp.	0.797	11.9	3.19 ± 0.135
C. jejuni subsp. *jejuni*	0.504	5.3	1.29 ± 0.212
C. jejuni subspp. *jejuni* and *doylei*	0.570	6.3	1.85 ± 0.202
C. coli	0.450	4.3	0.85 ± 0.249
C. lari	0.372	2.3	-0.03 ± 0.306
Other *Campylobacter* spp.			3.2

and appear as one. However, the number of shared alleles for each locus did not correlate with the total number of alleles for that locus. Given a single common ancestor for species pairs, a shared allele between the species can exist without any special mechanisms of genetic exchange between the two species. However, if a locus has multiple shared alleles between a pair of species, there was either misidentification of alleles or mechanisms to share those alleles. There were several instances of sharing alleles at a single locus by pairs of species in the MLEE studies. Since the sharing of multiple alleles did not correlate with the total number of alleles in each locus, misidentification of alleles due to comigration seems unlikely.

Such sharing of multiple alleles across species is a homoplasy, which is a similarity of a locus that cannot be attributed to common ancestry (34). The processes responsible for homoplasy include convergent, parallel, and reverse evolution. In the absence of selective pressure, the most likely mechanisms to result in homoplasies are recombination events, in which genes from differing ancestry are brought together. The consistency index (CI) is a measure of the number of homoplasies in a population study (34). The maximum possible value of 1.0 is achieved when there is no homoplasy. Analysis of the CI for each locus in our MLEE study showed that the differing loci had greatly differing contributions to the overall CI. The CI ranged from 0.75 for adenylate kinase to as low as 0.26 for catalase. It is possible that catalase has strong selective pressures associated with the host-parasite relationship that selects for diversity, but the second-lowest locus CI, at 0.33, was for aconitase, an enzyme that should not reflect selection for diversity.

The range of CI values for the loci suggests that some loci are more stable than other loci. Linkage analyses were performed to determine if this was true. The index of association (I_A) values published by Maynard-Smith et al. (36) were determined for the total population and each subpopulation (Table 1). I_A values approaching zero are indicative of very little linkage between alleles for different loci as a result of widespread sharing of DNA in recombinant events within the species. I_A values seen for *C. jejuni* and *C. coli* were significantly greater than zero in both our study (40) and the study by Aeschbacher and Piffaretti (1), indicating clonal development in these species. However, it can be concluded from the data that *C. lari* is not clonal. Frequent recombination between members of a population is expected to result in homogenization of the alleles (4, 92). This may be why only 2.3 alleles per locus were observed for *C. lari* (Table 1).

A pairwise linkage analysis of loci, the Q statistic of Hedrick and Thomson (20), was performed in our study and revealed the mosaic nature of the *Campylobacter* genome. *C. coli* had 15 pairs of loci that were significantly linked to each other and 13 pairs that were not linked. *C. jejuni* (subspecies *jejuni* and *doylei*) had 46 pairs of linked loci and 9 pairs that were not linked. Malic enzyme, phenylalanyl-proline peptidase, threonine dehydrogenase, and isocitrate dehydrogenase were also statistically linked to the source of the isolate. We proposed that the data for *C. jejuni* support a meroclonal structure, such as the framework suggested by Milkman and Bridges (42) for *E. coli*.

MULTIPLE-SEQUENCE ANALYSES

Multiple-sequence analyses have been performed on six genes from *C. jejuni*: *flaA* (11, 19, 37), *flaB* (38), *flgE* (33), a putative GTPase gene (85), *ompH1* (22), and *peb1A* (22). Additionally, Studer et al. (73) have published multiple-sequence data on part of the intervening sequence between *flaA* and *flaB*. The conclusions of these studies are mixed, and more work is needed to understand the processes that increase the diversification of *Campylobacter* genes. The *fla* gene products and the *flgE* product (flagellar hook protein) are exposed to the host immune response and show evidence of pressure for diversification. The three genes (*flaA*, *flaB*, and *flgE*) all show hypervariable regions that probably correspond to surface-exposed parts of the proteins. Figure 4 shows an overlay of a window analysis of the variability of the amino acid sequence of *flaA* (derived

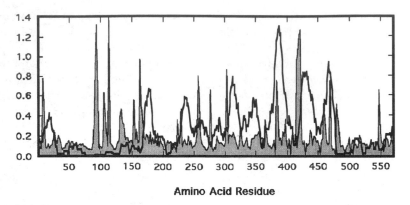

Amino Acid Residue

FIGURE 4 Amino acid sequence variability and epitope analysis of flagellin from *C. jejuni*. The horizontal axis represents the position of the amino acid sequence. The solid line illustrates the sequence variability among the flagellins in 15 strains of *C. jejuni* (37). The higher the line, the more variability within that segment of the gene. The line bounding the shaded region illustrates the results of epitope analyses (46). Synthesized epitopes were probed with antibodies from human patients who had recovered from campylobacteriosis. The shaded peaks represent segments of the flagellin product that bind antibody.

from data in reference 37) with the results of an epitope analysis of antibody reactivity to segments of flagellin (46). It can be seen that with the exception of epitopes in the region of amino acids 80 to 150, the reactive epitopes are in portions of the flagellin with greatest diversity.

flaA and *flaB* are members of a gene family, which means that they probably arose from a duplication event of a single gene. It has been hypothesized that the second copy of *fla* serves as a potential donor for reassortment and recombination of the DNA as a mechanism for creating new antigenic variants for immune avoidance (2, 15). Wassenaar et al. (87) supported this hypothesis by selecting a variant in which *flaB* apparently replaced a defective *flaA*. *flaA* and *flaB* differ within a strain by about 2 to 5%. However, between strains, the *flaA* genes may differ by as much as 30%. Using cloned fragments of the flagellin gene as hybridization probes. Thornton et al. (81) recognized that the middle portion of the flagellin genes was hypervariable. This was confirmed by multiple-sequence analyses (11, 37). The sequence variability of the flagellin genes is sufficiently high that PCR products of the flagellin gene, of just over 1,700 bp, yield a discriminatory method of typing *Campylobacter* when digested with appropriate restriction endonucleases (45, 55). A remarkable observation was that the hypervariable region that varies the most between strains is the same portion of the gene that is the most highly conserved within a strain (38). In comparisons among seven strains, only one nonsynonymous base pair difference was found between the *flaA* and *flaB* sequences in the region that was the hypervariable region between strains (synonymous base changes are substitutions that do not change the amino acid translation, whereas nonsynonymous base changes result in a change in the amino acid translation [23]). Such conservation of sequence within members of a gene family within a clone is called concerted evolution.

The mechanisms of concerted evolution are uncertain; two major mechanisms have been proposed (32). The first, in which there is some form of editing of a gene based on the sequence of another copy, is called gene conversion. The second occurs by some form of recombinant event. The most common form of recombination associated with concerted evolution is unequal crossing over. Unequal crossing over usually causes changes in the copy number. Chan (3a) has reported finding a third copy of *fla* but has not published this result. If the third copy of *fla* is involved in unequal crossing over, it would be predicted that it would not be found in all strains and may be only temporary in those that do contain the gene.

There is convincing evidence that recombination of segments of the *fla* genes occurs between strains (19). This is based on patterns of base substitutions that are most probably explained by recombination. Recombination can increase diversity, not only by bringing together fragments from different branches of evolution but also from the errors that occur at the recombination junction. These errors are often insertion or deletion events (commonly called indels, since it normally cannot be distinguished whether an alignment gap was due to an insertion in one lineage or a deletion in the other). Indels occur in the hypervariable region of the *fla* genes, but there is little evidence for recombination that can be gathered from the substitution pattern that supports recombination between strains in this part of the genes. However, the high substitution rate in the hypervariable region may mask the patterns that are needed to statistically reveal the likelihood of recombination.

Further analysis has shown that a second variable region, the short variable region (SVR), is separated by a short conserved region 5' to the major variable region. A recently completed unpublished study of multiple-sequence analysis of the SVR showed that populations of *Campylobacter* may be segregated (41). There was a cluster of alleles that did not include any isolates recovered from chickens. This means that there is a subpopulation of the *Campylobacter fla* gene that does not traffic through chickens and does not participate in recombinant events with strains that do traffic through chickens, at least for that portion of the genome. This could mean that that segment is not active in recombination or that there is no opportunity for certain groups of *Campylobacter* to acquire DNA from some other groups. If some groups of *Campylobacter* had restriction modification barriers to uptake of DNA, there could be transitory sharing of niches without the opportunity for recombination events. Alternatively, the subpopulations may never share a niche or, if they do, one or both strains from the different groups may not survive to pass on their genes. The separation of the clusters of the SVR sequences was ancient and thus cannot be due to modern methods of raising chickens. Representatives from both major groups of *Campylobacter* segregated by the SVR sequence were isolated from humans.

flgE is the gene encoding the flagellar hook protein (33). Since this protein is a surface-exposed protein, it is no surprise that *flgE* also has a high degree of variability. Like the *fla* genes, the variability is most pronounced in central regions of the *flgE* gene. Using the sequence from the *Campylobacter* genomic sequencing project plus the sequences for *Campylobacter flgE* obtained from GenBank in Sawyer's test for recombination (68), there was significant evidence that recombination played a role in the ancestry of the gene. Also, there are numerous indels in the sequence alignments. Unlike *fla,* there appears to be only one copy of *flgE* in the *C. jejuni* genome. Therefore, even if concerted evolution plays a role in the generation of diversity in the *fla* gene, it cannot be so with the *flgE* gene, although this gene has an equivalent amount of variability.

ompH1 and *pebIA* are an interesting pair of genes that have also been subjected to multiple-sequence analyses. *peb1A* was first described by Pei and Blaser (60) and was analyzed because of its apparent role in adherence of *C. jejuni* to mammalian cell lines. *ompH1* was analyzed by Meinersmann et al. (39) because it is expressed differently in a strain of *C. jejuni* that was a poor colonizer of chickens and in a congenic strain that was an efficient colonizer. The amino acid sequences of both genes have significant similarity (greater than 56%) to the glutamine-binding protein (the *glnH* product) of *Bacillus stearothermophilus* and close to the same similarity to each other (approximately 54%). The products of both of these genes appear to be surface exposed on the bacteria, but there does not seem to be the selection for diversity seen with *fla* and *flgE*. The average pairwise nucleotide difference for *peb1A* in multiple strains was 0.88%, and the average pairwise nucleotide difference for *ompH1* in the same strains was 1.35%. The pattern of nucleotide substitutions in this pair of genes is uniform, without any apparent hot spots for mutation. The number of synonymous substitutions is similar in *ompH1* and *peb1A,* suggesting that the genes were acquired by *Campylobacter* at about the same time (10, 70). The rate of nonsynonymous changes in *ompH1* was higher than that in *peb1A,* suggesting that there is less pressure against diversification on *ompH1*. When phylograms were constructed from sequence data for *ompH1* and *peb1A* from the same group of strains, there were changes in the branching order in the trees. This indicates that the two genes had different ancestral lineages. The most likely manner in which this would happen is by recombination between clones bringing variants together.

A study of the multiple alignment of the *flaA-flaB* intervening sequence in 48 strains published by Studer et al. (73) gives several interesting lessons. There were several indels, occurring in some strains immediately 3' of the *flaA* stop codon. There was insufficient sequence information to determine if recombination is likely to be between clones in this segment, but the indels indicate that recombination is likely at least within clones. The larger indels were 12, 19, and 27 bases. Two of these are multiples of a 3-base codon, but there is insufficient information to know if this is significant. Within the 78 bp of intergenic sequence that was published, there was a 21-bp segment that was conserved in all the strains (18 bp in the alignment used in reference 73). The conserved segment had a G + C content of approximately 32%, whereas the remaining intergenic region had only 20% G + C. Like the conservation of G or C use in codons noted below in the discussion of G + C content, this is another instance of apparent favoritism for conservation of G or C. It is possible that the conserved sequence is important for regulation of expression or regulation of recombinant events (like the chi sequence [91]).

The multiple-sequence analysis of a portion of the putative GTPase gene discovered by van Doorn et al. (85) revealed significant distinction of the thermophilic *Campylobacter* species (*C. lari, C. coli, C. upsaliensis,* and *C. jejuni*), enough that a oligonucleotide hybridization assay that was highly specific in identifying the species could be developed. The fragment that was sequenced was only 153 bp, which cannot be expected to be fully informative in recombination analyses. However, the degree of the segregation of the species probably rules out interspecies recombination in recent history. On the other hand, *C. upsaliensis* was clustered in a manner that was not consistent with relationships developed by comparison of rRNA sequence (83) or DNA-DNA hybridization analysis (3, 53, 66). This could be due to sharing of the GTPase alleles long ago but after speciation, and since then barriers to the sharing of this gene have arisen.

G + C CONTENT AND CODON BIAS

All *Campylobacter* species have a low G + C content. *C. jejuni* averages about 34% G + C. I have noted (unpublished) that the G + C content of structural genes tends to be slightly higher, as much as 37%. The 23S rRNA genes in GenBank have a G + C content of about 43%, and the 16S rRNA genes of *C. jejuni* are approximately 50% G + C. The intergenic segments can have an extremely low G + C content, as low as 19%. Codon usage tables for all the species that have sequences in GenBank can be found on the World Wide Web at http://www.kazusa.or.jp/codon/ *C. jejuni* clearly has a codon bias to allow the infrequent use of guanisine and cytosine. The bias is most pronounced at the third codon base position, which has an overall G + C content of about 19%. An example of the codon bias is the use of codons for proline, in which CCT and CCA are used at about 10 times the frequency of CCC and CCG. Since most third codon base changes are synonymous, there is little selective pressure at the protein level for the G + C content at that base position. The second codon position is also biased in *C. jejuni,* with about 35% G + C. The codon translation table shows a greater redundancy in codons with G or C as the middle base than is seen with A or T as the middle base. This minimizes the selective pressure at the protein level for G + C content in the second base. Accounting for the codon bias when designing degenerate primers will dramatically improve the performance of the primers. *C. jejuni* essentially uses a reduced set of synonymous codons.

What drives the selection toward the lower G + C content? Biochemically, mutations from a pyrimidine to a pyrimidine base or from a purine to a purine base (transitions) are more favored than mutations from a pyrimidine to a purine base or vice versa (transversions) (32). In most species, transitions exceed transversions 3- to 10-fold (32). This would actually favor drift toward a 50% G + C content. With *ompH1* and *peb1A,* which have an average difference between strains of less than 1.5%, the transition-to-transversion ratio was about 8 : 1, which is consistent with most species (22). However, the *fla* and *flgE* genes, which have an average distance of about 15% (*fla*) to 20% (*flgE*), had transition-to-transversion ratios close to 1 : 1 (unpublished observation).

The most likely explanation for codon bias has to do with efficiency of translation (71). Certain codons may be more efficiently translated for a variety of reasons, such as abundance of tRNA for the codon or affinity to the tRNA wobble base. The wobble-base fidelity may be more important because of the higher temperature preference displayed by *C. jejuni*. In *E. coli,* more highly expressed structural genes have a stronger codon bias (71). Such analysis has not been done for *Campylobacter*. Since ribosomal genes do not depend on translation for selection, it would be expected that they would have a G + C content more closely approaching 50%, which they do in *Campylobacter*. However, intergenic segments that have been studied have a greatly reduced G + C content, even though they are also not translated. Another possible reason for low G + C content is

that DNA repair mechanisms may favor insertions of A or T into a mismatch. It has also been my observation that G and C bases are more likely to be conserved across multiple *Campylobacter* strains. This might suggest that mutations from A or T to G or C are fixed by mismatch repair mechanisms and mutations from G or C to A or T are lost by functional selection. Answers to many of these questions might be obtained from analyses of the genomic sequence.

Segments of DNA that differ from the remainder of the chromosome in codon bias and G + C content have been found in several species of bacteria. These are believed to be relatively recent cross-species acquisitions by the species (29). Pathogenicity islands, which are segments of DNA that are rich in virulence genes, are often recognizable because of changes in the codon preference and G + C content from the remainder of the genome (17, 31). However, no reports of pathogenicity islands have been made for *Campylobacter*.

MECHANISMS OF GENOTYPIC CHANGE

The mechanisms responsible for the generation of diversity among *Campylobacter* species are almost completely unknown. We have seen the effects of the processes, but we have little information on how they come about. Lederberg (30) summarized interclonal and intraclonal processes that can lead to genetic evolution among infectious agents. Phase variation has also been suggested to play a role in the expression of flagellin in *C. jejuni* (6, 16, 49) and has been proven to occur for surface layer proteins for *C. fetus* (8). Phase variations are reversible changes that usually involve a systematic rearrangement of regulatory elements on the chromosome. The classic model for phase variation is the control of the phase 1 and phase 2 flagellin genes in *Salmonella,* which switch expression by the inversion of a promoter-containing fragment of the chromosome (72). It is not known how often such mechanisms play a role in *Campylobacter,* but if segmental inversions of the chromosome are common, genomic variations will be seen without a real change in the clonal structure.

Campylobacter organisms have plamids that are transmissible (79). Attempts to exchange plasmids between some strains of *Campylobacter* have been unsuccessful, and this may be due to restriction modification systems that limit the incorporation of foreign DNA (89). However, a plasmid has been found in *C. coli* that had an *aphA3* kanamicin resistance gene that was identical to a gene found in *Streptococcus* and nearly identical to one found in *Staphylococcus* (82).

Chromosomal acquisition of heterologous DNA also has been noted. An *aphA1* kanamicin resistance gene nearly identical to the Tn*903* antibiotic resistance gene was found in an isolate of a "*Campylobacter*-like organism" (52). This gene was found adjacent to a fragment of DNA that was homologous to IS*15Δ*, but no other parts of a transposon were found. Richardson and Park (64) also found a strain-specific fragment of DNA in *C. jejuni* that was flanked by direct repeats of 45 bp. There was an open reading frame between the repeats, but the function of this gene is unknown and there were no other features of a transposon. To my knowledge, there remains no report of a functional transposon in *Campylobacter*. Richardson and Park (63) also found that nonreplicating plasmids could donate heterologous DNA to apparently random chromosomal sites at a low rate (about 5×10^{-13} per generation) in a strain of *C. coli*. To date, there have been no published reports of pathogenicity islands in *Campylobacter*. Phages are well known in *Campylobacter* and are used for subtyping. However, there have been no reports of transducing or lysogenic phages within *Campylobacter*.

CONCLUSIONS

Selection occurs at the level of the gene, not the organism, and this is enhanced whenever there is a mechanism for genetic exchange. This is demonstrated by the observation that the flagellin gene DNA sequence for two isolates of *C. coli* did not segregate from sequences

analyzed for the same gene from *C. jejuni* (37). Genes that are physically linked to those that have selective pressure may be pulled along in recombinant events. This may account for the low CI of aconitase in the MLEE study. The converse may also be seen. Portions of the genome that are of necessity more highly conserved may be flanked by genes that are more highly conserved than otherwise expected. In a study by Owen et al. (56) that included 54 PFGE types of *Campylobacter,* there were only 15 patterns for 16S rRNA gene-specific probe binding. This probably means that the regions of the chromosome that bear the rRNA codon are more highly conserved than the chromosome as a whole. Readers interested in the mechanisms used by bacteria to generate diversity should read the review by Moxon et al. (44). However, virtually none of the mechanisms they discuss have been documented for *Campylobacter,* although none can be ruled out.

If the bulk of the biomass of *C. jejuni* is non-human and if human isolates represent only a small sampling, the phylogenetic conclusions that can be reached will be largely affected by the routes by which humans are infected and the fitness of isolates for exploiting those routes. The quantity of data is insufficient to be conclusive, but analyses of phylogenetic trees for patterns of sequence divergence by the methods described by Nee et al. (47) indicate that the total population size of *Campylobacter* has been stable. This means that modern technology has not affected the development of the size of the *Campylobacter* population. Outbreaks of campylobacteriosis are relatively infrequent, and the rate of human-to-human transmission of *Campylobacter* appears to be low (78). The types observed in humans represent only the types that are transmitted to humans. However, it currently appears that humans are subject to infection with any type of *Campylobacter* but that they do not appear to be the preferred host and do not serve as a bridge from one host to another. The observation by MLEE that *Campylobacter* strains may be linked to their source and the SVR sequence data showing that there is segregation of isolates found in chickens lead to the provocative hypothesis that humans appear to be not only an accidental host but also a dead-end host; i.e., humans do not appear to pass *Campylobacter* back to animal sources. This means that any selective pressure that is exerted within the human ecosystem does not shape further generations. This also means that the pathogenic mechanisms used by *Campylobacter* did not evolve to exploit the human enteric niche. Verification of this hypothesis could sharply change the study of the genesis of pathogenic traits among *C. jejuni*.

REFERENCES

1. **Aeschbacher, M., and J. C. Piffaretti.** 1989. Population genetics of human and animal enteric *Campylobacter* strains. *Infect. Immun.* **57:** 1432–1437.

2. **Alm, R. A., P. Guerry, and T. J. Trust.** 1993. Distribution and polymorphism of the flagellin genes from isolates of *Campylobacter coli* and *Campylobacter jejuni. J. Bacteriol.* **175:**3051–3057.

3. **Belland, R. J., and T. J. Trust.** 1982. Deoxyribonucleic acid sequence relatedness between thermophilic members of the genus *Campylobacter. J. Gen. Microbiol.* **128:**2515–2222.

3a.**Chan, V.** Personal communication.

4. **Cohan, F. M.** 1996. The role of genetic exchange in bacterial evolution. *ASM News* **62:**631–636.

5. **Costas, M., R. J. Owen, and P. J. H. Jackman.** 1987. Classification of *Campylobacter sputorum* and allied campylobacters based on numerical analysis of electrophoretic protein patterns. *Syst. Appl. Microbiol.* **9:**125–131.

6. **Diker, K. S., G. Hascelik, and M. Akan.** 1992. Reversible expression of flagella in *Campylobacter* spp. *FEMS Microbiol. Lett.* **78:**261–264.

7. **Dowling, T. E., C. Moritz, J. D. Palmer, and L. H. Rieseberg.** 1996. Nucleic acids III: analysis of fragments and restriction sites, p. 249–320. *In* D. M. Hillis, C. Moritz, and B. K. Mable (ed.), *Molecular Systematics,* 2nd ed. Sinauer Associates, Inc., Sunderland, Mass.

8. **Dworkin, J., and M. J. Blaser.** 1997. Molecular mechanisms of *Campylobacter fetus* surface layer protein expression. *Mol. Microbiol.* **26:**433–440.

9. **Dykhuizen, D. E., and L. Green.** 1991. Recombination in Escherichia coli and the definition of biological species. *J. Bacteriol.* **173:**7257–7268.

10. **Eyre-Walker, A., and M. Bulmer.** 1995. Synonymous substitution rates in enterobacteria. *Genetics* **140:**1407–1412.

11. **Fischer, S. H., and I. Nachamkin.** 1991. Common and variable domains of the flagellin gene, *flaA*, in *Campylobacter jejuni. Mol. Microbiol.* **5:** 1151–1158.

12. **Fraser, A. D., B. W. Brooks, M. M. Garcia, and H. Lior.** 1992. Molecular discrimination of *Campylobacter coli* serogroup 20 biotype I (Lior) strains. *Vet. Microbiol.* **30:**267–280.

13. **Gibson, J., E. Lorenz, and R. J. Owen.** 1997. Lineages within *Campylobacter jejuni* defined by numerical analysis of pulsed-field gel electrophoretic DNA profiles. *J. Med. Microbiol.* **46:**157–163.

14. **Gibson, J. R., C. Fitzgerald, and R. J. Owen.** 1995. Comparison of PFGE, ribotyping and phage-typing in the epidemiological analysis of *Campylobacter jejuni* serotype HS2 infections. *Epidemiol. Infect.* **115:**215–225.

15. **Guerry, P., R. A. Alm, M. E. Power, S. M. Logan, and T. J. Trust.** 1991. Role of two flagellin genes in *Campylobacter* motility. *J. Bacteriol.* **173:**4757–4764.

16. **Guerry, P., S. M. Logan, S. Thornton, and T. J. Trust.** 1990. Genomic organization and expression of *Campylobacter* flagellin genes. *J. Bacteriol.* **172:**1853–1860.

17. **Hacker, J., G. Blum-Oehler, I. Muhldorfer, and H. Tschape.** 1997. Pathogenicity islands of virulent bacteria: structure, function and impact on microbial evolution. *Mol. Microbiol.* **23:** 1089–1097.

18. **Harding, R. M.** 1996. New phylogenies: an introductory look at the coalescent, p. 15–22. *In* P. H. Harvey, A. J. Leigh-Brown, J. Maynard-Smith, and S. Nee (ed.), *New Uses for New Phylogenies.* Oxford University Press, Oxford, United Kingdom.

19. **Harrington, C. S., F. M. Thomson-Carter, and P. E. Carter.** 1997. Evidence for recombination in the flagellin locus of *Campylobacter jejuni:* implications for the flagellin gene typing scheme. *J. Clin. Microbiol.* **35:**2386–2392.

20. **Hedrick, P. W., and G. Thomson.** 1986. A two-locus neutrality test: applications to humans, *E. coli* and lodgepole pine. *Genetics* **112:**135–156.

21. **Hernandez, J., A. Fayos, J. L. Alonso, and R. J. Owen.** 1996. Ribotypes and AP-PCR fingerprints of thermophilic campylobacters from marine recreational waters. *J. Appl. Bacteriol.* **80:** 157–164.

22. **Hiett, K. L., and R. J. Meinersmann.** Phylogenetic analysis of the *Campylobacter jejuni* chromosomal genes *ompH1* and *peb1A*. Submitted for publication.

23. **Hillis, D. M., C. Moritz, and B. K. Mable (ed.).** 1996. *Molecular Systematics,* 2nd ed. Sinauer Associates, Inc., Sunderland, Mass.

24. **Hudson, R. R.** 1987. Estimating the recombination parameter of a finite population model without selection. *Genet. Res.* **50:**245–250.

25. **Hunter, P. R.** 1990. Reproducibility and indices of discriminatory power of microbial typing methods. *J. Clin. Microbiol.* **28**:1903–1905.

26. **Jackson, C. J., A. J. Fox, D. M. Jones, D. R. A. Wareing, and D. N. Hutchinson.** 1998. Associations between heat-stable (O) and heat-labile (HL) serogroup antigens of *Campylobacter jejuni:* evidence for interstrain relationships within three O/HL serovars. *J. Clin. Microbiol.* **36:** 2223–2228.

27. **Khawaja, R., K. Neote, H. L. Bingham, J. L. Penner, and V. L. Chan.** 1992. Cloning and sequence analysis of the flagellin gene of *Campylobacter jejuni* TGH9011. *Curr. Microbiol.* **24:** 213–221.

28. **Kimura, M.** 1983. *The Neutral Theory of Molecular Evolution.* Cambridge University Press, Cambridge, United Kingdom.

29. **Lawrence, J. G., and H. Ochman.** 1997. Amelioration of bacterial genomes: rates of change and exchange. *J. Mol. Evol.* **44:**383–397.

30. **Lederberg, J.** 1997. Infectious disease as an evolutionary paradigm. *Emerg. Infect. Dis.* **3:**417–423.

31. **Lee, C. A.** 1996. Pathogenicity islands and the evolution of bacterial pathogens. *Infect. Agents Dis.* **5:**1–7.

32. **Li, W.-H.** 1997. *Molecular Evolution,* p. 309–334. Sinauer Associates, Inc., Sunderland, Mass.

33. **Luneberg, E., E. Glenn-Calvo, M. Hartmann, W. Bar, and M. Frosch.** 1998. The central, surface-exposed region of the flagellar hook protein FlgE of *Campylobacter jejuni* shows hypervariability among strains. *J. Bacteriol.* **180:** 3711–3714.

34. **Maddison, W. P. and D. R. Maddison.** 1992. *MacClade: Analysis of Phylogeny and Character Evolution,* version 3. Sinauer Associates, Inc., Sunderland, Mass.

35. **Maslow, J. N., M. E. Mulligan, and R. D. Arbeit.** 1993. Molecular epidemiology: application of contemporary techniques to the typing of microorganisms. *Clin. Infect. Dis.* **17:**153–164.

36. **Maynard-Smith, J., N. H. Smith, M. O'Rourke, and B. G. Spratt.** 1993. How clonal are bacteria? *Proc. Natl. Acad. Sci. USA* **90:** 4384–4388.

37. **Meinersmann, R. J., L. O. Helsel, P. I. Fields, and K. L. Hiett.** 1997. Discrimination of *Campylobacter jejuni* isolates by *fla* gene sequencing. *J. Clin. Microbiol.* **35:**2810–2814.

38. **Meinersmann, R. J., and K. Hiett.** Concerted evolution of duplicate fla genes in Campylobacter. Submitted for publication.

39. **Meinersmann, R. J., K. L. Hiett, and A. Tarplay.** 1997. Cloning of an outer membrane protein gene from *Campylobacter jejuni. Curr. Microbiol.* **34:**360–366.

40. **Meinersmann, R. J., C. M. Patton, G. M. Evin, B. D. Plikaytis, I. K. Wachsmuth, and P. I. Fields.** Unpublished data.

41. **Meinersmann, R. J., N. J. Stern, K. L. Hiett, J. S. Bailey, and P. F. Cray.** Unpublished data.

42. **Milkman, R., and M. M. Bridges.** 1990. Molecular evolution of the *Escherichia coli* chromosome. III. Clonal frames. *Genetics* **126:**505–517.

43. **Mills, S. D., R. V. Congi, J. N. Hennessy, and J. L. Penner.** 1991. Evaluation of a simplified procedure for serotyping *Campylobacter jejuni* and *Campylobacter coli* which is based on the O antigen. *J. Clin. Microbiol.* **29:**2093–2098.

44. **Moxon, E. R., P. B. Rainey, M. A. Nowak, and R. E. Lenski.** 1994. Adaptive evolution of highly mutable loci in pathogenic bacteria. *Curr. Biol.* **4:**24–33.

45. **Nachamkin, I., K. Bohachick, and C. M. Patton.** 1993. Flagellin gene typing of *Campylobacter jejuni* by restriction fragment length polymorphism analysis. *J. Clin. Microbiol.* **31:**1531–1536.

46. **Nachamkin, I., and X.-H. Yang.** 1992. Immune response to *Campylobacter* flagellin, p. 216–222. *In* I. Nachamkin, M. J. Blaser, and L. S. Tompkins (ed.), *Campylobacter jejuni: Current Status and Future Trends.* ASM Press, Washington, D.C.

47. **Nee, S., E. C. Holmes, A. Rambaut, and P. H. Harvey.** 1996. Inferring population history from molecular phylogenies, p. 66–80. *In* P. H. Harvey, A. J. Leigh-Brown, J. Maynard-Smith, and S. Nee (ed.), *New Uses for New Phylogenies.* Oxford University Press, Oxford, United Kingdom.

48. **Newell, D. G.** 1986. Monoclonal antibodies directed against the flagella of *Campylobacter jejuni:* cross-reacting and serotypic specificity and potential use in diagnosis. *J. Hyg. (Camb.)* **96:**377–384.

49. **Nuijten, P. J., L. Marquez-Magana, and B. A. van der Zeijst.** 1995. Analysis of flagellin gene expression in flagellar phase variants of *Campylobacter jejuni* 81116. *Antonie Leeuwenhoek* **67:** 377–383.

50. **Olsen, G. J., C. R. Woese, and R. Overbeek.** 1994. The winds of (evolutionary) change: breathing new life into microbiology. *J. Bacteriol.* **176:**1–6.

51. **On, S. L. W.** 1998. In vitro genotypic variation of *Campylobacter coli* documented by pulsed-field gel electrophoretic DNA profiling: implications for epidemiological studies. *FEMS Microbiol. Lett.* **165:**341–346.

52. **Ouellette, M., G. Gerbaud, T. Lambert, and P. Courvalin.** 1987. Acquisition by a *Campylobacter*-like strain of aphA-1, a kanamycin resistance determinant from members of the family *Entero-*

bacteriaceae. Antimicrob. Agents Chemother. **31:** 1021–1026.

53. **Owen, R. J.** 1983. Nucleic acids in the classification of *Campylobacters. Eur. J. Clin. Microbiol.* **2:** 367–377.

54. **Owen, R. J., M. Costas, L. Sloss, and F. J. Bolton.** 1988. Numerical analysis of electrophoretic protein patterns of *Campylobacter laridis* and allied thermophilic campylobacters from the natural environment. *J. Appl. Bacteriol.* **65:**69–78.

55. **Owen, R. J., A. Fayos, J. Hernandez, and A. Lastovica.** 1993. PCR-based restriction fragment polymorphism analysis of DNA sequence diversity of flagellin genes of *Campylobacter jejuni* and allied species. *Mol. Cell. Probes* **7:**471–480.

56. **Owen, R. J., K. Sutherland, C. Fitzgerald, J. Gibson, P. Borman, and J. Stanley.** 1995. Molecular subtyping scheme for serotypes HS1 and HS4 of *Campylobacter jejuni. J. Clin. Microbiol.* **33:**872–877.

57. **Page, R. D. M.** 1995. *TreeMap 1.0.* A program available from http://evolve.zps.ox.ac.uk/packages/treemap.

58. **Patton, C. M., M. A. Nicholson, S. M. Ostroff, A. A. Ries, I. K. Wachsmuth, and R. V. Tauxe.** 1993. Common somatic O and heat-labile serotypes among *Campylobacter* strains from sporadic infections in the United States. *J. Clin. Microbiol.* **31:**1525–1530.

59. **Patton, C. M., I. K. Wachsmuth, G. M. Evins, J. A. Kiehlbauch, B. D. Plikaytis, N. Troup, L. Tompkins, and H. Lior.** 1991. Evaluation of 10 methods to distinguish epidemic-associated *Campylobacter* strains. *J. Clin. Microbiol.* **29:**680–688.

60. **Pei, Z., and M. J. Blaser.** 1993. PEB1, the major cell-binding factor of *Campylobacter jejuni,* is a homolog of the binding component in Gram-negative nutrient transport systems. *J. Biol. Chem.* **268:** 18717–18725.

61. **Penner, J. L., J. N. Hennessy, and R. V. Congi.** 1983. Serotyping of *Campylobacter jejuni* and *Campylobacter coli* on the basis of thermostable antigens. *Eur. J. Clin. Microbiol.* **2:**378–383.

62. **Raetz, C. R. H.** 1996. Bacterial lipopolysaccharides: a remarkable family of bioactive macroamphiphiles, p. 1035–1063. *In* F. C. Neidhardt, R. Curtiss III, J. L. Ingraham, E. C. C. Lin, K. B. Low, B. Magasanik, W. S. Reznikoff, M. Riley, M. Schaechter, and H. E. Umbarg (ed.), *Escherichia coli and Salmonella: Cellular and Molecular Biology,* 2nd ed. ASM Press, Washington, D.C.

63. **Richardson, P. T., and S. F. Park.** 1997. Integration of heterologous plasmid DNA into multiple sites on the genome of *Campylobacter coli* following natural transformation. *J. Bacteriol.* **179:** 1809–1812.

64. **Richardson, P. T., and S. F. Park.** 1998. Molecular characterization of a strain-specific sequence in *Campylobacter jejuni. Lett. Appl. Microbiol.* **26:**113–117.

65. **Rohlf, F. J.** 1997. *NTSYSpc: Numerical Taxonomy and Multivariate Analysis System,* version 2.00. Exeter Software, Setauket, N.Y.

66. **Roop, R. M., R. M. Smibert, J. L. Johnson, and N. R. Krieg.** 1984. Differential characteristics of catalase-positive campylobacters correlated with DNA homology groups. *Can. J. Microbiol.* **30:**938–951.

67. **Saunders, J. R.** 1995. Population genetics of phase variable antigens. *Symp. Soc. Gen. Microbiol.* **52:**247–268.

68. **Sawyer, S.** 1989. Statistical tests for detecting gene conversion. *Mol. Biol. Evol.* **6:**526–538.

69. **Selander, R. K., D. A. Caugant, H. Ochman, J. M. Musser, M. N. Gilmour, and T. S. Whittam.** 1986. Methods of multilocus enzyme electrophoresis for bacterial population genetics and systematics. *Appl. Environ. Microbiol.* **51:** 873–884.

70. **Sharp, P. M.** 1991. Determinants of DNA sequence divergence between Escherichia coli and Salmonella typhimurium: codon usage, map position, and concerted evolution. *J. Mol. Evol.* **33:** 23–33.

71. **Sharp, P. M., M. Stenico, J. F. Peden, and A. T. Lloyd.** 1993. Codon usage: mutational bias, translational selection, or both? *Biochem. Soc. Trans.* **21:**835–841.

72. **Silverman, M., J. Zieg, M. Hilment, and M. Simon.** 1979. Phase variation in *Salmonella:* genetic analysis of a recombinational switch. *Proc. Natl. Acad. Sci. USA* **76:**391–395.

73. **Studer, E., M. Domke, B. Wegmuller, J. Luthy, S. Schmid, and U. Candrian.** 1998. RFLP and sequence analysis of *Campylobacter jejuni* and *Campylobacter coli* PCR products amplified directly from environmental samples. *Lebensm.-Wiss. Technol.* **31:**537–545.

74. **Suzuki, Y., M. Ishihara, M. Funabashi, R. Suzuki, S. Isomura, and T. Yokochi.** 1993. Pulsed-field gel electrophoretic analysis of *Campylobacter jejuni* DNA for use in epidemiological studies. *J. Infect.* **27:**39–42.

75. **Swofford, D. L.** 1991. When are phylogeny estimates from molecular and morphological data incongruent, p. 295–333. *In* M. M. Miyamoto and J. Cracraft (ed.), *Phylogenetic Analysis of DNA Sequences.* Oxford University Press, New York, N.Y.

76. **Swofford, D. L., G. J. Olsen, P. J. Waddell, and D. M. Hillis.** 1996. Phylogenetic inference, p. 407–514. *In* D. M. Hillis, C. Moritz, and B. K.

Mable (ed.), *Molecular Systematics,* 2nd ed. Sinauer Associates, Inc., Sunderland, Mass.

77. **Takahata, N.** 1990. A simple genealogical structure of strongly balanced allelic lines and transspecies evolution of polymorphism. *Proc. Natl. Acad. Sci. USA* **87:**2419–2423.

78. **Tauxe, R. V.** 1992. Epidemiology of *Campylobacter jejuni* infections in the United States and other industrialized nations, p. 9–19. *In* I. Nachamkin, M. J. Blaser, and L. S. Tompkins (ed.), *Campylobacter jejuni: Current Status and Future Trends.* ASM Press, Washington, D.C.

79. **Taylor, D. E., S. A. DeGrandis, M. A. Karmali, and P. C. Fleming.** 1981. Transmissible plasmids from *Campylobacter jejuni. Antimicrob. Agents Chemother.* **19:**831–835.

80. **Thompson, L. M., III, R. M. Smibert, J. L. Johnson, and N. R. Krieg.** 1988. Phylogenetic study of the genus *Campylobacter. Int. J. Syst. Bacteriol.* **38:**190–200.

81. **Thornton, S. A., S. M. Logan, T. J. Trust, and P. Guerry.** 1990. Polynucleotide sequence relationships among flagellin genes of *Campylobacter jejuni* and *Campylobacter coli. Infect. Immun.* **58:**2686–2689.

82. **Trieu-Cuot, P., G. Gerbaud, T. Lambert, and P. Courvalin** 1985. In vivo transfer of genetic information between gram-positive and gram-negative bacteria. *EMBO J.* **4:**3583–3587.

83. **Trust, T. J., S. M. Logan, C. E. Gustafson, P. J. Romaniuk, N. W. Kim, V. L. Chan, M. A. Ragan, P. Guerry, and R. R. Gutell.** 1994. Phylogenetic and molecular characterization of a 23S rRNA gene positions the genus *Campylobacter* in the epsilon subdivision of the *Proteobacteria* and shows that the presence of transcribed spacers is common in *Campylobacter* spp. *J. Bacteriol.* **176:**4597–4609.

84. **Vandamme, P., B. Pot, and K. Kersters.**

1991. Differentiation of campylobacters and *Campylobacter*-like organisms by numerical analysis of the one-dimensional electrophoretic protein patterns. *Syst. Appl. Microbiol.* **14:**57–66.

85. **van Doorn, L. J., A. Verschuuren-van Haperen, A. Burnens, M. Huysmans, P. Vandamme, B. A. J. Giesendorf, M. J. Blaser, and W. G. V. Quint.** 1999. Rapid identification of thermotolerant *Campylobacter jejuni, Campylobacter coli, Campylobacter lari,* and *Campylobacter upsaliensis* from various geographic locations by a GTPase-based PCR-reverse hybridization assay. *J. Clin. Microbiol.* **37:**1970–1796.

86. **Wang, Y., and D. E. Taylor.** 1990. Natural transformation in *Campylobacter* species. *J. Bacteriol.* **172:**949–955.

87. **Wassenaar, T. M., B. N. Fry, and B. A. M. Vanderzeijst.** 1995. Variation of the flagellin gene locus of *Campylobacter jejuni* by recombination and horizontal gene transfer. *Microbiology* **141:**95–101.

88. **Wassenaar, T. M., B. Geilhausen, and D. G. Newell.** 1998. Evidence of genomic instability in *Campylobacter jejuni* isolated from poultry. *Appl. Environ. Microbiol.* **64:**1816–1821.

89. **Waterman, S. R., J. Hackett, and P. A. Manning.** 1993. Isolation of a restriction-less mutant and development of a shuttle vector for the genetic analysis of *Campylobacter hyointestinalis. Gene* **125:**19–24.

90. **Weir, B. S.** 1996. Intraspecific differentiation, p. 385–405. *In* D. M. Hillis, C. Moritz, and B. K. Mable (ed.), *Molecular Systematics,* 2nd ed. Sinauer Associates, Inc., Sunderland, Mass.

91. **West, S. C.** 1992. Enzymes and molecular mechanisms of genetic recombination. *Annu. Rev. Biochem.* **61:**603–640.

92. **Whittam, T. S.** 1995. Genetic population structure and pathogenicity in enteric bacteria. *Symp. Soc. Gen. Microbiol.* **52:**217–245.

GENOTYPING AND THE CONSEQUENCES OF GENETIC INSTABILITY

Trudy M. Wassenaar, Stephen L. W. On, and Richard J. Meinersmann

18

In this chapter the hypothetical and practical consequences of genetic instability to the application of genetic typing methods for *Campylobacter* spp. are discussed. The genotyping methods applied to *Campylobacter* are only briefly outlined here, since a more detailed description is given in chapter 2. This chapter concentrates on whether and how the outcome of any genetic typing method will be influenced by instability of the genome or of genetic loci and how to interpret the resulting changes in genotype. Part of this discussion is theoretical, since some mechanisms leading to genetic instability are proposed but not yet proven to occur in *Campylobacter*. The experimental or epidemiological evidence available on genetic instability is discussed. The issue of genetic instability partly overlaps that of population genetics, which is covered in chapter 17. The background provided here may help the reader to recognize and interpret changes or deviations of genotypic characteristics that are caused by genetic instability.

Trudy M. Wassenaar, Institute of Medical Microbiology and Hygiene, Johannes Gutenberg University, Hochhaus am Augustusplatz, D-55101 Mainz, Germany. *Stephen L. W. On,* Danish Veterinary Laboratory, Bülowsvej 27, DK 1790 Copenhagen V, Denmark. *Richard J. Meinersmann,* Poultry Processing and Meat Research Unit, USDA Agricultural Research Service, P.O. Box 5677, Athens, GA 30604.

GENOTYPING METHODS

The genotyping methods applied to *Campylobacter* spp. on a more or less routine basis to date are flagellin typing, randomly amplified polymorphic DNA (RAPD), pulsed-field gel electrophoresis of chromosomal DNA (PFGE), and ribotyping. Other methods that have been described are not generally used at present. A brief description of each method is given below. For a more detailed review and for literature citations, the reader is referred to chapter 2.

Flagellin typing is a PCR-based restriction fragment length polymorphism (RFLP) analysis of the flagellin gene locus. The retrieved genetic information is present on a single locus of the genome, with either *flaA* or the combination of *flaA* and *flaB* as the target genes for a PCR. A segment of these genes is amplified with the use of conserved primers, and strain-to-strain variation is reflected by differences in restriction enzyme recognition sites present in the less highly conserved regions of the PCR amplicons.

RAPD is a PCR-based fingerprinting technique. Arbitrarily designed primers are used to amplify fragments derived from random loci all over the genome. The PCR products obtained result in a banding pattern of stronger and weaker bands of variable length. Strain-to-strain variation is caused by the presence, num-

Campylobacter, 2nd Ed., Edited by I. Nachamkin and M. J. Blaser
© 2000 American Society for Microbiology, Washington, D.C.

ber, distance, and mismatch fidelity of the sites to which the primers anneal. The efficiency of primer annealing to sites present on the genome is dependent on the T_m of the primer and on the experimental conditions such as Mg^{2+} concentration and annealing temperature.

PFGE is a typing method based on the presence of restriction enzyme recognition sites. The enzymes of choice cut so infrequently that large (20- to 200-kbp) fragments are formed, which are separated by using special electrophoretic conditions. The strain-to-strain variation depends on the presence of the restriction sites (generally 5 to 20 in total) on the chromosome.

Ribotyping depends on restriction enzyme recognition sites flanking the three rRNA genes generally present on the genome of *C. jejuni*. All three ribosomal gene loci are analyzed together by Southern blot hybridization with a probe specific for rRNA genes. Strain-to-strain variation depends on the distribution of restriction enzymes around the three rRNA genes.

It is clearly desirable that a genotype of a given strain be stable. However, there are a number of phenomena described for *Campylobacter* that can, theoretically, alter the genotype of a given strain as detected by one or more of these techniques. Indeed, evidence has been obtained in some instances of unstable genotypes. No data are available yet on the frequency of such events, since genotyping methods have been applied only recently, and the deviations of the expected genotype may have been unnoticed, ignored, or misinterpreted. Hopefully, this contribution increases public awareness of the problem, so that in the near future more data will become available and the mechanisms can be studied in more detail.

DEFINITION OF GENETIC INSTABILITY

Genetic instability is defined here as a single event, or series of events, leading to a change in the genetic organization of a given bacterial strain. The mechanisms leading to such changes are outlined below. The term is not intended to describe mutations occurring at a natural rate during replication, which is given as 10^{-11} to 10^{-9} per base pair per cell per generation for bacteria in general. The latter (called "genetic drift") can result in a heterogeneous bacterial population, since most mutations are neutral, i.e., give neither a selective advantage nor a selective disadvantage, as discussed in chapter 17. However, in instances where point mutations can alter the genotype of a strain, as determined by methods dependent on restriction enzymes, such as PFGE and *fla* typing, the consequences of such mutations are discussed.

Point Mutations in Restriction Sites

Point mutations that alter restriction sites used for PFGE analysis will lead to differences in genetic fingerprints. It has been noted for other bacteria that PFGE profiles of outbreak strains sometimes differed somewhat from each other. Tenover et al. (40) reviewed the effect of various genetic phenomena on PFGE profiles and provided a much-needed set of interpretative guidelines for molecular epidemiologists using this method. However, the authors stated that the guidelines were intended for investigating outbreaks due to species whose PFGE profiles comprised more than 10 DNA fragments. In these respects, the guidelines could be described as inapplicable to PFGE-based epidemiological studies of *Campylobacter* spp., since the most commonly used enzyme for PFGE typing (*Sma*I) usually results in profiles containing just 8 to 10 fragments. However, where profiles are changed by point mutations in a restriction site, the aforementioned interpretative guidelines may apply. In these circumstances, a single-base substitution can lead to the deletion of a restriction site or the creation of a new one. A restriction site deletion results in the loss of one fragment and a size increase in another; in a restriction site creation, a fragment is lost and two smaller fragments appear, the sum of which is equivalent to that of the first. The simplest way to confirm that an aberrant PFGE pattern stems from a point mutation is to use an alternative restriction enzyme which will not be affected by the point mutation. An example of this strategy applied to *C. sputorum* has been published (28). In this way it is easy to differentiate between point mutations and recombinations involving large DNA segments, which may also result in band differences of the type described above. Recombinations of large DNA segments are more likely to be detected by more than one restriction enzyme. Finally, to identify two isolates with different PFGE patterns as being derived from the same parent strain, any epidemiological data should be carefully considered, and other typing methods, either phenotypic or genotypic, should be applied as well.

Point mutations in the flagellin genes can result in gain or loss of restriction sites and consequently change the banding pattern derived by *fla* typing. It is common practice to define strains with any difference in banding patterns as belonging to different genotypes, and this practice is needed to give the method sufficient discriminatory power. The consequence of this, i.e., that point mutations in the flagellin region can result in new *fla* genotypes despite the clonal origin of isolates, cannot be avoided.

Genetic Instability, Fidelity, and Strain Identity

A change in genotype as a consequence of genetic instability should not be confused with genotypic variation detected as a result of shortcomings of the method applied (e.g., poor reproducibility). Moreover, the triggers for the mechanisms leading to genetic instability, if these exist, have not been identified. Genotypic stability or instability as determined under laboratory conditions may be different under more natural conditions.

It is generally accepted that a phenotypic characteristic of a strain can be unstable. Loss of a given phenotype (e.g., toxin production) does not alter the identity of the strain altogether. Instability of a given genotype should also be interpreted in this way. The alteration of one genetic characteristic may be detected by a certain method, but the strain may still be correctly identified by other methods. Phenotypic and genotypic changes do not have to be correlated: a loss of phenotype may or may not be detected by genetic methods, and, similarly, a change in genotype does not necessarily lead to detectable phenotypic differences. For instance, one point mutation may alter expression patterns of one gene or a group of genes, which may be detected on a phenotypic level. Depending on the method, the mutation can also be detected by genotyping.

MECHANISMS LEADING TO GENETIC INSTABILITY

The following processes can lead to a drastic change in genetic organization: (i) insertions or deletions of DNA fragments due to the activity of mobile elements, such as bacteriophages, transposons, and insertion sequences; (ii) recombinations of DNA segments in either a "programmed" or a "random" manner; (iii) high-frequency mutations at so-called hot spots; and/or (iv) incorporation of "foreign" DNA after natural transformation.

Each of these mechanisms can in theory be applied to *Campylobacter,* but for some of them evidence is limited (Table 1). The proposed mechanisms of genetic instability are discussed here, with examples given whenever genotypic variation has been observed. There is a fundamental difference between mechanisms (i) and (iv) as opposed to (ii) and (iii): recombinations and mutations do not result in an overall change in the genetic makeup of the organism, unless there are errors at the junction of recombinant fragments; however, they may severely change the detected genotype of a given strain. In contrast, DNA uptake by natural transformation or by the activity of mobile elements does change the genetic content of a strain. All of these events can easily result in misidentification of bacterial strains unless one is aware of such processes and knows how to interpret the results.

Mobile Elements

Several elements are known to be involved in bacterial chromosome plasticity (16), and some of these have been described for *Campylobacter.* Transposons and insertional elements, or rem-

TABLE 1 Proposed mechanisms leading to genetic instability in *Campylobacter* spp.

Mechanism	Genotypic method to detect instability	Reference(s)[a]
Bacteriophage activity	PFGE, possibly ribotyping, RAPD	43
Programmed DNA recombinations	RFLP of locus involved, possibly RAPD	7
DNA recombinations on a genomic scale	PFGE, ribotyping	11, 28, 36, 43
Recombinations within the *fla* locus	*fla* typing, less likely for a combined *flaA*-plus-*flaB* typing method	12
DNA transformation	*fla* typing, possibly RAPD, PFGE, ribotyping	12, 37

[a] Genetic instability as observed by PFGE in poultry meat isolates was possibly attributed to bacteriophage activity (43). The *sap* locus of *C. fetus* has been shown to undergo programmed DNA rearrangements; however no data about the extent to which this influences the genotype as determined by RAPD or other methods are available (7). Genetic instability was observed by PFGE during extensive subculturing of *C. jejuni* strains in vivo (28). PFGE analysis of *C. jejuni* isolates derived from a single patient over an extended period showed minor but significant changes in genotype which may have been caused by recombinations (36). PFGE analysis of *C. jejuni* strains before and after chicken colonization showed differences in genotype, which correlated with changes in ribotype (11). *fla* typing of *C. jejuni* strains from an epidemiological investigation over a 2-year period showed evidence for recombinations and gene transfer within the flagellin locus of a natural bacterial population (12). *C. jejuni/coli* isolates from ostriches displayed different PFGE patterns which, due to their epidemiological relationship, were attributed to natural transformation (37).

nants thereof, have been observed in *Campylobacter* (8, 20, 29, 31), but transposition activity has not been reported. The frequency of transposition is believed to be too low to be of importance to genetic instability; however, this remains to be tested. More than 170 bacteriophages have been described to be infective to *Campylobacter*, but there are no data available about chromosomal insertion of phage DNA or whether phage activity has left its footprints on the chromosome (32). Several typing schemes have been developed for *C. jejuni* based on the sensitivity to bacteriophages (9, 13, 33), and the extended use of these typing schemes has led to some interesting observations. For example, occasionally a strain will lose its sensitivity for a single phage (rendering the isolate nontypeable in this scheme), and this can coincide with other phenotypic alterations (see below). Such changes may be reflected by changes on the chromosome and consequently could be detected by genetic methods. One such case has been studied in detail (42), as discussed below.

Programmed Recombinations of DNA Segments

Recombinations of specific DNA segments in a number of bacteria have been described to occur within genetic loci where more than one homologous gene or gene fragment is present. In such instances, recombinations resulting in gene or promoter inversion cause a switch of gene expression from one gene homologue to another and are a genetic basis for antigenic variation. There is evidence that at least some of the chromosomal rearrangements observed in *Campylobacter* spp. fit this type of antigenic variation. Dworking and Blaser (7) described the inversion of a 6.2-kb promoter-bearing segment of DNA that regulates the expression of the *sap* gene in *C. fetus*. Multiple copies of the *sap* gene are present, and one of these is combined with the promoter by recombination. As a result, expression of the antigen varies with time. The promoter inversion is similar to the regulation of flagellin phase variation in *Salmonella* (34). The *Salmonella* invertible sequence is 950 bp, is flanked by inverted repeats, and carries a gene for a site-specific recombinase that catalyzes the inversion. A site-specific recombinase has yet to be described for *C. fetus*. Although such recombinations are referred to as "programmed," the choice of which *sap* gene is sequentially expressed is more or less random. A genotyping method has been developed for *C. fetus* based on the *sap* locus (6); however, the occurrence and high frequency of recombinations make this locus less suitable as a target for genetic typing. Other observations suggesting programmed DNA rearrangements were made by Guerry et al. (10), who described a reversible change in Southern blot patterns with restriction enzyme-treated genomes from a strain of *C. coli* induced to undergo flagellin phase variation. The blots were probed with DNA from *S. typhimurium*, and the hybridized genes were not identified. A similar observation of antigenic variation in *C. jejuni* was made by Mills et al. (22), who described changes in somatic lipopolysaccharide antigenic side chain changes; however, a genetic basis for this variation could not be detected by restriction enzyme analysis.

Recombinations of this type are not likely to be detected by PFGE, since the DNA segments involved are rather small. However, recombination could influence RAPD patterns if this area of the genome contains recognition sites for the primers used. To date, genotyping data for *C. fetus* are not available to indicate which methods can detect genotypic instability associated with antigenic changes. However, differences in RAPD fingerprints observed in *C. jejuni* isolates from chickens that were epidemiologically related have been suggested to be the result of genetic instability (1).

The finding that two highly similar flagellin genes are present in tandem in *C. jejuni* and *C. coli* (3) led to early speculations that programmed recombinations may occur between them, as is the case in *Salmonella*. However, different from the flagellin genes of *Salmonella*, each *fla* gene of *Campylobacter* contains its own promoter, and gene inversion has never been demonstrated. Nevertheless, recombinations between parts of *flaA* and *flaB* can occur, as discussed in a later section.

Random Recombinations of Large DNA Segments

Chromosomal maps have been constructed for a limited number of *C. jejuni* strains by means of PFGE and Southern blot analysis (14, 25, 39). When these maps are compared, striking differences in the positions of some of the mapped genes are apparent. The maps of *C. jejuni* TGH9011 (14) and 81116 (25) are reconstructed in Fig. 1, along with a map of strain NCTC 11168, constructed from the *C. jejuni* Genomic Sequencing Project (5). Even though the data are limited and the resolution of PFGE is questionable, differences in gene order are detected. Gene order plasticity is virtually unknown among the members of the *Enterobacteriaceae*, especially within any given species (17, 26). However, changes in gene order have been observed with *Salmonella typhi* (18, 19) and *Helicobacter pylori* (12). For *S. typhi*, it has been shown that the seven rRNA gene loci (*rrn*) are the sites of recombination; the order of the genes on the chromosome segments between *rrn* genes is relatively conserved. In contrast, *C. jejuni* has only three *rrn* genes, and the positions of genes mapped between these do differ between strains (Fig. 1). In this respect, the genome plasticity of *C. jejuni* resembles that of *H. pylori*. Interestingly, the high plasticity of

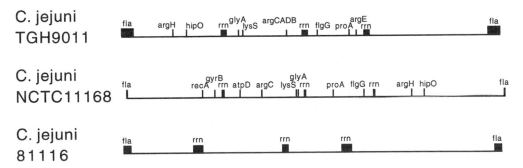

FIGURE 1 Genomic maps made from PFGE analysis of *C. jejuni* TGH9011 (14) and *C. jejuni* 81116 (25) and from the Genomic Sequencing Project for *C. jejuni* NCTC 11168 (5). Circular maps are made linear, with the *fla* gene being used as the reference point for the beginning and end.

H. pylori has been suggested to result from long-term carriage of a single strain in a limited number of individuals or families. This does not in general apply to *C. jejuni*.

An accurate estimate of how often rearrangements of gene order occur in *Campylobacter* or whether these events are regulated cannot be made from current data. Also, there are no data to tell if rearrangements occur within an individual organism or if transfer of DNA to a second individual is required. In either case, despite a resulting change in gene order and possibly in gene expression, there will not be a change in the overall genetic content of the strain if the rearrangement occurs within the clone, unless the cutting and splicing at the ends of the recombinant unit is error prone. The most likely error to be seen in that case would be duplications or deletions.

Random rearrangements would be detectable by PFGE but would most probably not be detected by RAPD or ribotyping because of the small size of the bands generated by these methods. In several cases, variations in the PFGE patterns of *Campylobacter* spp. were observed, which may well have been caused by such recombinations of large DNA segments. Three examples are listed here.

(i) In an attempt to determine the stability of PFGE profiles during subculturing, six *C. coli* strains were maintained under continuous subculture for up to 50 passages (27). In four of the six strains, notable differences were observed between subculture profiles obtained with each of the three restriction enzymes used (*Sma*I, *Sal*I, and *Bam*HI); of these four strains, two gave different patterns after 20 subcultures. The most significant changes were obtained between 20 and 40 passages. Large-scale genomic rearrangement was the most plausible explanation for the changes seen in this study, since there was no opportunity for the acquisition of exogenous foreign DNA under the conditions used. Moreover, certain features in between-subculture profiles suggested an evolution in the genotype of a given strain, a reasonable presumption since DNA samples were prepared from plate cultures that had not been derived from single colonies. Interestingly, the genome size of certain strains diminished after extended periods of subculture (27), suggesting the loss of plasmid DNA (the presence or absence of which was not checked in this study) or perhaps of DNA coding for a function that became redundant after continued maintenance under artificial culture conditions.

(ii) During an epidemiological study, clinical isolates from short- and long-term-infected patients were typed (35). In one case (from a total of 49 cases), a variation in PFGE genotype was detected in case-related strains. Two isolates of *C. jejuni* obtained from a patient at an interval of 1 month were different in PFGE genotype for four bands. Although it could not be ruled out that the patient had originally suffered a double infection with two strains or had been reinfected with a different strain (the isolates were not compared by other typing methods than PFGE), it is quite possible that the isolates were derived from one strain undergoing DNA recombination during the infection.

(iii) In a study determining the PFGE genotypes of poultry strains, variation in banding patterns was observed between single-colony isolates obtained within one batch of poultry meat (42). The variation was striking because the banding patterns were all similar but significantly different, and in total 14 genotypes were recognized for 21 isolates. Since these isolates were found to be identical by several other typing methods, such as flagellin typing, serotyping, biotyping, and phage typing (but see below), it was concluded that all isolates were originally derived from the same parental strain and that the variation in PFGE genotype was most likely to be the result of mosaic rearrangements of large (>20-kbp) chromosomal DNA segments. A second interesting observation in this study was that minor variation was detected in the biotypes of some of the isolates. This often coincided with the loss of phage type, suggesting that phage activity can be the trigger for the observed variation in biotype and possibly in PFGE genotype. However, more research is needed to test this hypothesis.

Instability of PFGE Genotype by Natural Transformation

Both *C. jejuni* and *C. coli* are known to be naturally competent, although this trait appears to be more prevalent in the latter species (37, 38). Both chromosomal and plasmid DNAs are accepted, although not with equal efficiencies, and strain differences in levels of competence do exist (43). Plasmid DNA bearing no significant sequence similarity to genomic DNA can be acquired by *C. coli* by natural transformation and can integrate into multiple sites on the chromosome by illegitimate recombination (30).

Acquisition of exogenous DNA may affect a PFGE profile in several ways. A plasmid which is not integrated into the chromosome will appear as an additional band in the PFGE profile. If the plasmid contains a single restriction site, this band will electrophorese true to size. More than one restriction site will result in several extra bands, assuming that they are resolved under the electrophoresis conditions used. These differences assume the plasmid is present in sufficient quantities to be visualized in the samples under investigation. An indication for the presence of plasmids is a stronger or weaker ethidium bromide staining of a single band or several bands due to nonstoichiometric concentrations. The extra band of ca. 98 kb seen in a few *C. sputorum* bv. *paraureolyticus* cattle herd strains (28) may represent an example of a plasmid containing a single *Sma*I site.

Integration of exogenous DNA into the chromosome may result in less predictable changes in a PFGE profile. Assuming that the foreign DNA contains no restriction sites for the endonuclease chosen for genotyping and that its integration does not result in the loss or gain of a restriction site, a simple band shift (i.e., increased size of a fragment) will be the only change in a PFGE profile. However, integration of exogenous DNA resulting in the loss or gain of a restriction site will cause more drastic changes. The identification of strain relationships in such cases becomes extremely challenging. An indication for integration of exogenous DNA is a change in the total genome size of suspected related strains without loss of stoichiometric staining of all bands. When this is observed, a plausible epidemiological hypothesis can be made only if appropriate additional information is available. For example, an outbreak investigation of *C. coli*-associated hepatitis in ostriches identified the outbreak strain among farms with known trade connections but described one unusual strain profile from a farm with no declared relationship with the other flocks (36). Although a close resemblance between these *C. coli* types was evident, the distinct profile contained several discrepant bands and demonstrated an increased genome size compared with the outbreak strain. Further information indicated differences in chemical and antibiotic resistance characteristics between the outbreak strain and the distinct *C. coli* strain. The authors proposed that these types were related and that the acquisition of exogenous DNA may have resulted in the observed phenotypic and genotypic differences (36). The fact that these strains are also highly similar in terms of their amplified fragment length polymorphism (AFLP) profiles (15) supports an epidemiological relationship.

Instability of the Flagellin Gene Locus by Natural Transformation

To date, the flagellin locus is the only locus on the *Campylobacter* genome proven to be sufficiently heterogeneous between strains to serve as a target for RFLP analysis. The presence of highly conserved parts of the flagellin genes between strains furthermore has enabled the development of primers that permit nearly 100% typeability for *C. jejuni* and *C. coli*. However, the flagellin genes can be subject to recombinations, so that this locus may not be completely stable in each strain. Moreover, the flagellin locus of a strain can be completely or partly replaced by a different variant by integration of DNA taken up via natural transformation, as was shown to occur under laboratory conditions (2, 44). In these experiments, an antibiotic resistance gene had been introduced in the flagellin locus of the donor strain to monitor and select for recombinants. Further experimental evidence showed that exchange of flagellin gene loci can occur between strains and even between the species *C. jejuni* and *C. coli* (2, 43). The superficial induction of competence under experimental conditions (41) is not required for exchange of flagellin loci, since doubly resistant recombinants were generated during cocultivation of isogenic mutants bearing two different resistance markers (44). In this case, the donor and acceptor strains were mutants derived from the same parental strain, and thus limitations due to restriction modification systems were absent.

Since flagellin loci (or parts thereof) can be shared between strains under laboratory conditions, it is important to know whether this can also take place under natural conditions. One ecological niche where *Campylobacter* is likely to meet other members of the species is the avian cecum, where colonization levels can be very high and free DNA is likely to be abundant due to the rapid turnover of bacteria. When the above-mentioned isogenic mutants, which had been shown to exchange their flagellin gene locus during cocultivation in vitro, were tested in a chicken colonization model, no transformants were detected, despite the high colonization levels obtained for both mutants during cocolonization (42). These data suggest that natural transformation does not occur in the chicken gut under the conditions of the colonization model applied. This could be due to lack of competence or to rapid degradation of extracellular DNA. Clearly, more data are needed to assess the risk of horizontal gene transfer during avian colonization under natural or farming conditions. Data obtained in a long-term epidemiological study in which flagellin typing was applied do suggest that exchange of (parts of) flagellin genes between strains does occur under natural conditions (11). This is discussed in more detail in chapter 17. As a consequence, the sole use of flagellin typing for strain identification of field isolates should be interpreted with care, since it may be that an individual flagellin locus rather than a bacterial strain is being detected.

Instability of the Flagellin Genes by Recombinations within the Locus

In addition to locus exchange by natural transformation, the flagellin genes can be subject to

recombinations within an individual genome. Experimental evidence was obtained that internal parts of *flaA* and *flaB* can be exchanged (3, 44). Also in this instance, the recombination was detected because of the presence of an antibiotic resistance marker, which had originally been introduced in *flaA* and was found to be present in *flaB* after the spontaneous recombination. The crossover positions that had led to this recombinant could be mapped to a small portion of the gene, and it was found that a segment of 160 bp identical between *flaA* and *flaB* was sufficient for the recombination to occur (44). Recombinational events of this type have also been observed for isolates in an epidemiological study (11). These observations and their implications for epidemiology and bacterial populations genetics are discussed in more detail in chapter 17.

Differences in Sensitivity of *fla* Typing Methods to Recombinations

Do the present *fla* typing methods detect recombinations between *flaA* and *flaB* of one strain? To answer this question, the level of conservation between *flaA* and *flaB* within one strain must be considered. When the sequences of two genes within strains were compared, a striking identity was detected for the six strains studied (21). The two genes are near to identical, but for three regions (see chapter 17). This is corroborated by the observation, that approximately only 10% of the *C. jejuni* isolates tested are different in RFLP patterns for *flaA* and *flaB* (23, 24). As a consequence of this high identity and because of the positions of the primers used for *fla* typing, only recombinations exchanging the middle variable region are likely to be detected by *fla* typing (Fig. 2).

The 5′ portions of the *flaA* and *flaB* genes differ considerably within one strain, and it is to this segment that *flaA*-specified primers have been designed (45). In two typing systems, a combination of two primers which are specific for *flaA* and *flaB*, respectively, is used, and these primers are combined with a reversed primer which recognizes both genes (4, 23). With the choice of these three primers, most recombina-

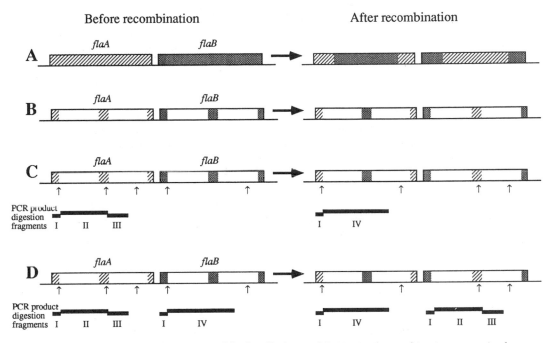

FIGURE 2   (A) Schematic representation of the flagellin locus of *C. jejuni* and recombinations occurring between *flaA* and *flaB* within this locus. (B) Only the parts of the genes in which *flaA* and *flaB* actually differ are shaded. (C) PCR products derived with a primer set specific for *flaA* sequences only. Before recombination, the PCR product results in restriction fragments I, II, and III when digested with an enzyme cutting at the sites represented by the arrows. After recombination, PCR digestion products I and IV are obtained. (D) PCR products of a PCR based on *flaA* and *flaB*. When these products are digested and analyzed together, the obtained banding pattern will be identical before and after recombination, since bands I, II, III, and IV will be obtained in both cases.

tions will not be detected as long as the fragments derived from *flaA* and *flaB* are digested and analyzed together (Fig. 2). Only in exceptional cases will recombinations result in a change of genotype in this method. One such exception would be when the crossing over occurs between two restriction enzyme sites that both differ between *flaA* and *flaB*. This will not occur frequently, in view of the strong conservation of these two genes within one strain. The other exception is when errors are introduced at the recombination junctions, leading to small insertions or deletions. On the basis of these considerations, it is expected that a typing scheme determining combined *flaA* and *flaB* RFLPs (by using three primers) will be less strongly influenced by recombinations of the type described here than will a typing scheme based on *flaA* only. Since such genetic exchange events do not significantly alter the

nature of a given strain, it could be argued that a typing scheme missing these events is still valid for strain identification.

A different situation arises when recombinations in the *fla* locus occur after takeup of foreign DNA. Such events would most probably be detected by *fla* typing since they would probably introduce changes in the restriction sites present. Such recombinations could take place in either *flaA* or *flaB*. The addition of *flaB* to the typing scheme renders this system sensitive to the latter event as well.

CONCLUSIONS

Several mechanisms have been proposed to result in genetic instability. Most genotypic methods are sensitive to at least one of the genetic phenomena that *Campylobacter* spp. display. In general, the use of a single genotyping

TABLE 2 Protocols for interpreting and confirming genotypic data that may indicate the occurrence of genetic instability

---

PFGE

    Observation: Isolates A and B have overall similar banding patterns, but some bands differ in size and/or extra bands are present while others are missing.

    Recommendation: Use a second restriction enzyme to compare isolates A and B.

    • If all isolates are identical with a second enzyme, the first enzyme most probably detected minor (point) mutations. A and B are likely to be genetically related. Confirm this by an independent typing method.

    • If differences similar to the original observation are observed with a second enzyme, genomic plasticity most probably occurred or DNA was taken up by natural transformation. Identify the genetic relationship by other methods.

    • If the second enzyme results in completely different patterns, the two isolates are most probably not closely related. The first enzyme of choice may have too low a discrimination power for this set of strains.

fla **typing**

    Observation: Different *flaA* types are found in two isolates of assumed common identity.

    Recommendation: Determine the identity of the two isolates by other typing methods available. Possibly the *fla* genotype has changed due to transformation, recombination, or a point mutation.

    • When of interest, a combined *flaA* + *flaB* PCR or two separate reactions the *flaA*- and *flaB*-specific primers can be done to determine if recombinations between *flaA* and *flaB* have occurred.

    Observation: Identical *fla* types are found in isolates of assumed different identity.

    Recommendation: Use alternative restriction enzymes for the RFLP. Different enzymes may have a different resolution with subsets of strains.

    • If alternative enzymes also give identical patterns, the discriminatory power of *fla* typing may be too low for these strains. Different strains can share identical *fla* genes. Alternative methods are required to confirm the assumed difference in identity.

RAPD

    Observation: Differences in RAPD patterns are observed between isolates of presumed common identity.

    Recommendation: Confirm that the differences are not due to poor reproducibility. If this is not the case, confirm the presumed identity by other methods.

    • RAPD patterns may differ due to point mutations or genome plasticity when these events affect the annealing sites of the primer.

Ribotyping

    Observation: Differences in ribotypes are observed between isolates of presumed common identity.

    Recommendation: Use alternative restriction enzymes to exclude the possibility that point mutations resulted in the observed changes.

    • If the differences are confirmed, alternative methods are required to determine the presumed identity. The ribotypes may differ between closely related strains due to genome plasticity. Since this may also affect PFGE pattern, this method is not a suitable alternative.

    Observation: Identical ribotypes are observed between isolates of presumed different identity.

    Recommendation: Use alternative restriction enzymes for the ribotyping. Different enzymes may have different resolution with subsets of strains.

    • If the ribopatterns remain identical, confirm the presumed difference in identity by other methods. The resolution of ribotyping may not be high enough for this subset of strains.

---

method is not sufficient to determine the bacterial lineage. Examples of observations that may be indicative of genetic instability and the experimental approaches that could be used to confirm this, are given in Table 2. The use of a combination of methods for strain identification is strongly recommended. The choice of methods will depend on availability, expertise, costs etc. However, any combination of a single-locus genotypic method and one determining multiple loci of the genome (e.g., PFGE, RAPD, and ribotyping) will be sufficient to correctly identify genetic processes of the type discussed. Alternatively, a combination of a genotypic method with at least one phenotypic method can be used, provided that the latter has a sufficiently high discriminatory power. Genetic instability may complicate the interpretation of genetic typing methods; however, a better understanding of these processes will facilitate interpretation of the data for epidemiological studies.

ACKNOWLEDGMENTS

We thank Diane Newell and Clare Harrington for useful discussions.

REFERENCES

1. **Aarts, H. J. M., L. A. J. T. Van Lith, and W. F. Jacobs-Reitsma.** 1995. Discrepancy between Penner serotyping and polymerase chain reaction fingerprinting of *Campylobacter* isolated from poultry and other animal sources. *Lett. Appl. Microbiol.* **20:**371–374.

2. **Alm, R. A., P. Guerry, M. E. Power, and T. J. Trust.** 1992. Variation in antigenicity and molecular weight of *Campylobacter coli* VC167 flagellin in different genetic backgrounds. *J. Bacteriol.* **174:**4230–4238.

3. **Alm, R. A., P. Guerry, and T. J. Trust.** 1993. Significance of duplicated flagellin genes in *Campylobacter. J. Mol. Biol.* **230:**359–363.

4. **Ayling, R. D., M. J. Woodward, S. Evans, and D. G. Newell.** 1996. Restriction fragment length polymorphism of polymerase chain reaction products applied to the differentiation of poultry campylobacters for epidemiological investigations. *Res Vet. Sci.* **60:**168–172.

5. **Barrell, B., et al.** 1999. The *Campylobacter jejuni* genome website. http://microbiosl.mds.qmw.ac.uk/camplobacter/index.html.

6. **Denes, A. S., C. L. Lutze-Wallace, M. L. Cormier, and M. M. Carcia.** 1997. DNA fingerprinting of *Campylobacter fetus* using cloned constructs of ribosomal RNA and surface array protein genes. *Vet. Microbiol.* **54:**185–193.

7. **Dworkin, J., and M. J. Blaser.** 1997. Molecular mechanisms of *Campylobacter fetus* surface layer protein expression. *Mol. Microbiol.* **26:**433–440.

8. **Gibreel, A., and O. Skold.** 1998. High-level resistance to trimethoprim in clinical isolates of *Campylobacter jejuni* by acquisition of foreign genes (*dfr1* and *dfr9*) expressing drug-insensitive dihydrofolate reductases. *Antimicrob. Agents Chemother.* **42:**3059–3064.

9. **Grajewski, R. A., J. W. Kusek, and H. M. Gelfand.** 1985. Development of a bacteriophage typing system for *Campylobacter jejuni* and *Campylobacter coli. J. Clin. Microbiol.* **22:**13–18.

10. **Guerry, P., S. M. Logan, and T. J. Trust.** 1988. Genomic rearrangements associated with antigenic variation in *Campylobacter coli. J. Bacteriol.* **170:**316–319.

11. **Harrington, C., F. M. Thomson-Carter, and P. E. Carter.** 1997. Evidence for recombination in the flagellin locus of *Campylobacter jejuni:* implications for the flagellin gene typing scheme. *J. Clin. Microbiol.* **35:**2386–2392.

12. **Jiang, Q., K. Hiratsuka, and D. E. Taylor.** 1996. Variability of gene order in different *Helicobacter pylori* strains contributes to genome diversity. *Mol. Microbiol.* **20:**833–842.

13. **Khakhria R., and H. Lior.** 1992. Extended phage-typing scheme for *Campylobacter jejuni* and *Campylobacter coli. Epidemiol. Infect.* **108:**403–414.

14. **Kim, N. W., R. Lombardi, H. Bingham, E. Hani, D. Louie, D. Ng, and V. L. Chan.** 1993. Fine mapping of the three rRNA operons on the updated genomic map of *Campylobacter jejuni* TGH9011 (ATCC 43431). *J. Bacteriol.* **175:**7468–7470.

15. **Kokotovic, B., and S. L. W. On.** 1999. High-resolution genomic fingerprinting of *Campylobacter jejuni* and *Campylobacter coli* by analysis of amplified fragment length polymorphisms. *FEMS Microbiol. Lett.* **173:**77–84.

16. **Kolsto, A.-B.** 1997. Dynamic bacterial genome organization. *Mol. Microbiol.* **24:**241–248.

17. **Liu, S. L., A. Hessel, and K. E. Sanderson.** 1993. Genomic mapping with I-Ceu I, an intron-encoded endonuclease specific for genes for ribosomal RNA, in *Salmonella* spp., *Escherichia coli,* and other bacteria. *Proc. Natl. Acad. Sci. USA* **90:**6874–6878.

18. **Liu, S. L., and K. E. Sanderson.** 1995. Rearrangements in the genome of the bacterium *Salmonella typhi. Proc. Natl. Acad. Sci. USA* **92:**1018–1022.

19. **Liu, S. L., and K. E. Sanderson.** 1996. Highly plastic chromosomal organization in *Salmonella typhi. Proc. Natl. Acad. Sci. USA* **93:**10303–10308.

20. **Manavathu, E. K., K. Hiratsuka, and D. E. Taylor.** 1988. Nucleotide sequence analysis and expression of a tetracyclin-resistance gene from *Campylobacter jejuni. Gene* **62:**17–26.

21. **Meinersmann, R. J., L. O. Helsel, P. I. Fields, and K. L. Hiett.** 1997. Discrimination of Campylobacter jejuni isolates by *fla* gene sequencing. *J. Clin. Microbiol.* **35:**2810–2814.

22. **Mills, S. D., L. A. Kurjanczyk, B. Shames, J. N. Hennessy, and J. L. Penner.** 1991. Antigenic shifts in serotype determinants of *Campylobacter coli* are accompanied by changes in the chromosomal DNA restriction endonuclease digestion pattern. *J. Med. Microbiol.* **35:**168–173.

23. **Mohran, Z. S., P. Guerry, H. Lior, J. R. Murphy, A. M. El-Gendy, M. M. Mikhail, and B. A. Oyofo** 1996. Restriction fragment length

polymorphism of flagellin genes of *Campylobacter jejuni* and/or *C. coli* isolated from Egypt. *J. Clin. Microbiol.* **34:**1216–1219.

24. **Newell, D. G.** Unpublished data.

25. **Nuijten, P. J. M., C. Bartels, N. M. C. Bleu-mink-Pluym, W. Gaastra, and B. A. M. van der Zeijst.** 1990. Size and physical map of the *Campylobacter jejuni* chromosome. *Nucleic Acids Res.* **18:**6211–6214.

26. **Ochman, H., and U. Bergthorsson.** 1995. Genome evolution in enteric bacteria. *Curr. Opin. Genet. Dev.* **5:**734–738.

27. **On, S. L. W.** 1998. In vitro genotypic variation of *Campylobacter coli* documented by pulsed-field gel electrophoretic DNA profiling: implications for epidemiological studies. *FEMS Microbiol. Lett.* **165:**341–346.

28. **On, S. L. W., H. I. Atabay, and J. E. L. Corry.** 1999. Clonality of *Campylobacter sputorum* bv. *paraureolyticus* determined by macrorestriction profiling and biotyping, and evidence for long-term persistence in cattle. *Epidemiol. Infect.* **122:**175–182.

29. **Ouellette, M., G. Gerbaud, T. Lambert, and P. Courvalin.** 1987. Acquisition by a *Campylobacter*-like strain of *aphA-1*, a kanamycin resistance determinant from members of the family *Enterobacteriaceae. Antimicrob. Agents Chemother.* **31:**1021–1026.

30. **Richardson, P. T., and S. F. Park.** 1997. Integration of heterologous plasmid DNA into multiple sites on the genome of *Campylobacter coli* following natural transformation. *J. Bacteriol.* **179:**1809–1812.

31. **Richardson, P. T., and S. F. Park.** 1998. Molecular characterization of a strain-specific sequence in *Campylobacter jejuni. Lett. Appl. Microbiol.* **26:**113–117.

32. **Sails, A. D., R. A. Wareing, F. J. Bolton, A. J. Fox, and A. Curry.** 1998. Characterisation of 16 *Campylobacter jejuni* and *Campylobacter coli* typing bacteriophages. *J. Med. Microbiol.* **47:**123–128.

33. **Salama, S. M., F. J. Bolton, and D. N. Hutchinson.** 1990. Applications of a new phage typing scheme to campylobacters isolated during outbreaks. *Epidemiol. Infect.* **104:**405–411.

34. **Silverman, M., J. Zieg, M. Hilmen, and M. Simon.** 1979. Phase variation in *Salmonella*: genetic analysis of a recombinational switch. *Proc. Natl. Acad. Sci. USA* **76:**391–395.

35. **Steinbrueckner, B., F. Ruberg, and M. Kist.** 1998. The stability of genetic fingerprints of *Campylobacter jejuni* and *Campylobacter coli* in vivo, p. 70–71. *In* A. J. Lastovica, D. G. Newell, and E. E. Lastovica (ed.), *Campylobacter, Helicobacter and Related Organisms.* Institute of Child Health, University of Cape Town, Cape Town, South Africa.

36. **Stephens, C. P., S. L. W. On, and J. A. Gibson.** 1998. An outbreak of infectious hepatitis in commercially reared ostriches associated with *Campylobacter coli* and *Campylobacter jejuni. Vet. Microbiol.* **61:**183–190.

37. **Taylor, D. E.** 1992. Genetic analysis of *Campylobacter* spp. p. 255–266. *In* I. Nachamkin, M. J. Blaser, and L. S. Tompkins (ed.), *Campylobacter jejuni: Current Status and Future Trends.* American Society for Microbiology, Washington, D.C.

38. **Taylor, D. E.** 1992. Genetics of *Campylobacter* and *Helicobacter. Annu. Rev. Microbiol.* **46:**35–64.

39. **Taylor, D. E., E. M. Eaton, W. Yan, and N. Chang.** 1992. Genome maps of *Campylobacter jejuni* and *Campylobacter coli. J. Bacteriol.* **174:**2332–2337.

40. **Tenover, F. C., R. D. Arbeit, R. V. Goering, P. A. Mickelsen, B. E. Murray, D. H. Persing, and B. Swaminathan.** 1995. Interpreting chromosomal DNA restriction patterns produced by pulsed-field gel electrophoresis: criteria for bacterial strain typing. *J. Clin. Microbiol.* **33:**2233–2239.

41. **Wang, Y., and D. Taylor.** 1990. Natural transformation in *Campylobacter* species. *J. Bacteriol.* **172:**949–955.

42. **Wassenaar, T. M., B. Geilhausen, and D. G. Newell.** 1998. Evidence of genomic instability in *Campylobacter jejuni* isolated from poultry meat. *Appl. Environm. Microbiol.* **64:**1816–1821.

43. **Wassenaar, T. M., B. N. Fry, and B. A. M. van der Zeijst.** 1993. Genetic manipulation of *Campylobacter*: evaluation of natural transformation and electro-transformation. *Gene* **132:**131–135.

44. **Wassenaar, T. M., B. N. Fry, and B. A. M. van der Zeijst.** 1995. Variation of the flagellin gene locus of *Campylobacter jejuni* by recombination and horizontal gene transfer. *Microbiology* **141:**95–101.

45. **Wassenaar, T. M., and D. G. Newell.** 2000. The genotyping of *Campylobacter* spp. *Appl. Environ. Microbiol.* **66:**1–9.

GENETICS OF *CAMPYLOBACTER* LIPOPOLYSACCHARIDE BIOSYNTHESIS

Benjamin N. Fry, Neil J. Oldfield, Victoria Korolik,
Peter J. Coloe, and Julian M. Ketley

19

Campylobacter jejuni is the causative agent of human enterocolitis and is the most common cause of bacterial diarrhea in many countries (59). *C. jejuni* is a commensal in the intestine of birds (10, 56), but human infection most frequently results in acute abdominal pain and inflammatory diarrhea, often with fever (14). Bacteremia may accompany enteric disease, although this is usually during the initial stages of infection or in immunocompromised patients. Most *C. jejuni* strains are highly serum sensitive, but in the absence of opsonization some strains are resistant to phagocytic killing (69). *C. jejuni* is also involved in a significant proportion of cases of the neuropathological autoimmune diseases Guillain-Barré and Miller-Fisher syndromes (44). However, the bacterial determinants, particularly surface polysaccharide structures, involved in *C. jejuni* intestinal colonization, inflammatory diarrhea, and the induction of autoimmune disease remain poorly characterized.

Lipopolysaccharides (LPS) are an abundant surface component of the outer membrane of gram-negative bacteria. The LPS molecule consists of three distinct regions. Anchored in the outer membrane is the lipid A moiety, which is the endotoxic part of the LPS molecule. Attached to lipid A by ketodeoxyoctulosonic acid (Kdo) is a branched-chain core oligosaccharide with an inner and an outer region. Specific for the inner core is the presence of Kdo and heptose residues, which are not present in the outer core. Attached to the core and extending from the cell surface is the O-chain, a repeat of 10 to 30 sugar subunits generally composed of one to five sugars (54). The O-chain protects the organism against complement and other serum components (24, 30) and is involved in resistance to polymorphonuclear leukocytes (57).

In *E. coli* and *Salmonella* spp., lipid A and core oligosaccharide are synthesized together as one unit on the inner membrane. The O-chain subunits are synthesized on a lipid carrier, undecaprenol phosphate, on the inner face of the cytoplasmic membrane. The first sugar residue is transferred to the lipid carrier by the WbaP (previously called RfbP) glycosyltransferase, and subsequently, other specific glycosyltransferases link additional sugar residues to the growing subunit (50). The completed sub-

Benjamin N. Fry and Peter J. Coloe, Department of Applied Biology and Biotechnology, RMIT University, GPO Box 2476V, Melbourne 3001, Australia. *Neil J. Oldfield and Julian M. Ketley,* Department of Genetics, University of Leicester, University Road, Leicester LE1 7RH, United Kingdom. *Victoria Korolik,* School of Health Science, Griffith University, Gold Coast, PMB 50, Gold Coast Mail Centre, Queensland, Australia.

Campylobacter, 2nd Ed., Edited by I. Nachamkin and M. J. Blaser
© 2000 American Society for Microbiology, Washington, D.C.

unit is transported to the periplasmic face of the inner membrane by the O-subunit flippase, Wzx (RfbX), and is then linked to other subunits by the Wzy (Rfc) polymerase to form an O-chain polymer. The number of subunits that are polymerized into the O-chain is controlled by the Wzz (Cld) protein. The completed O-chain is then ligated to the lipid A-core complex by the WaaL (RfaL) ligase. Finally, an ATP-binding cassette (ABC) transporter translocates the complete LPS molecule from the cytoplasmic membrane to the outer membrane. Most of the genes encoding the proteins involved in O-chain synthesis are clustered on the bacterial chromosome. A variant of the LPS molecule, seen in bacterial genera such as *Neisseria, Haemophilus,* and *Bordetella,* is the lipooligosaccharide (LOS) molecule; this molecule lacks the O-chain polymer.

C. jejuni strains synthesize LPS molecules with or without an O-chain-like polysaccharide repeat (49). The LPS molecules of *Campylobacter* spp. have endotoxic properties (12, 42, 45). Furthermore, they have been reported to be important as adhesins (40) and may play a role in antigenic variation, since the bacteria have the ability to change the LPS antigenic composition (41).

The sugar compositions and structures of the core oligosaccharides from several *C. jejuni* strains, belonging to nine serotypes, have been analyzed and are described in chapter 12. For many bacteria the core structure is highly conserved within a genus (18, 29). However, the core oligosaccharide structure of *C. jejuni* is variable, although the sugar composition is not very different between strains. Limited variability has also been observed for the core oligosaccharides from *Neisseria* and *Haemophilus* spp. (38), but not to the extent seen in *C. jejuni*. This variability in the *Campylobacter* LPS cores explains the ability of the Penner serotyping system (46) to discriminate between strains with LOS-type LPS.

The O-chain repeats of three *C. jejuni* strains have been analyzed so far (4–6) and have been found to consist of only two or three sugars. The position on the core oligosaccharide

to which the O-chain is attached has not been determined, but the inner core heptose-KDO region has been suggested (5). Non-LPS-core-linked O-chain has been described for serotype O:3, where the polysaccharide consists of a disaccharide repeat of L-*glycero*-D-*ido*-heptose1β-4Gal covalently linked to a lipid (4), and in O:41, where a polysaccharide repeat structure may be independent of LPS core (47).

The metabolic pathways and enzymes required to synthesize LPS molecules have not yet been characterized in *C. jejuni*. Rapid progress in the study of LPS synthesis in other bacteria has been made by a genetic approach in combination with knowledge of the structure of LPS. Understanding LPS genetics for *Campylobacter* spp. will provide an insight into the role of LPS in infection and colonization through the ability to create specific mutants. Moreover, it would enable a better understanding of the level of structural variation and the mechanism of LPS synthesis in *Campylobacter* spp.

ISOLATION OF THE DNA REGION INVOLVED IN LPS SYNTHESIS

The genetic study of LPS biosynthesis in *Campylobacter* arose from studies to isolate and define genetic regions coding for major surface antigens of *C. hyoilei* (33). A genomic cosmid library was screened by using antiserum raised to the parent *C. hyoilei* strain, and restriction endonuclease analysis of four positive recombinant plasmids showed unique but overlapping inserts that expressed small immunoreactive molecules. These molecules were proteinase K resistant, indicating a glycolipid antigen. To further investigate the nature of these molecules, an LPS extraction was done on the cosmid clones, and the LPS was analyzed by Western blotting. *C. hyoilei* antiserum reacted with the extracted expressed antigens, indicating that they were LPS associated. The minimum DNA insert size required for expression of *C. hyoilei* LPS antigens in *Escherichia coli* was 11.8 kb. This region was subcloned into pBR322, and partial sequencing of the 11.8-kb region showed two open reading frames (ORFs), des-

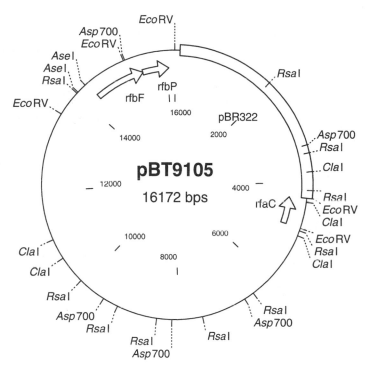

FIGURE 1 Structure of plasmid pBT9105 showing the genes found in the sequenced parts. The single line indicates the 11.7-kb insert; the open bar indicates the vector pBR322. The arrows indicate the putative genes *rfbF* and *rfbP*. The available part of the *rfaC* gene is also indicated.

ignated *ddhA* (*rfbF*) and *wbaP* (*rfbP*), with homology to the *ddhA* gene from *Serratia marcescens* and the *wbaP* gene from *Salmonella typhimurium*. Both genes are involved in LPS synthesis. The region also contained a sequence homologous to the *waaC* (*rfaC*) gene of *E. coli* and *S. typhimurium,* which is involved in core oligosaccharide synthesis (Fig. 1).

The study of the genetics of LPS synthesis was continued with *C. jejuni* 81116, which belongs to the Penner 6 serogroup (LPS type), and then extended to include strain NCTC 11168 (the Penner 2 strain used for genomic sequencing [60]) and NCTC 11351 (Penner 23). A cosmid library of the genome of *C. jejuni* 81116 was constructed in cosmid vector pLA2917. Five clones, designated pBT9502 to pBT9506, were isolated that hybridized with the 11.8-kb DNA region from *C. hyoilei* containing the LPS-associated genes. Three clones (pBT9502, pBT9505, and pBT9506) containing overlapping inserts (Fig. 2) were tested for expression of *Campylobacter* antigens. Both *E. coli*(pBT9502) and *E. coli*(pBT9506) reacted

with Penner 6 antiserum in a Western blot analysis.

LPS ANALYSIS

LPS was isolated from *E. coli*(pBT9502), *E. coli*(pBT9505), and *E. coli*(pBT9506). The isolated LPS was resolved by Tricine-sodium dodecyl sulfate-polyacrylamide gel electrophoresis (SDS-PAGE) and analyzed by silver staining and Western blotting (Fig. 3). The silver-stained *C. jejuni* 81116 LPS showed one band of 6 kDa (this and subsequent size estimations were made with protein markers [35]). This size is in accordance with LPS isolated from other *Campylobacter* strains. The *E. coli* strains carrying recombinant cosmids showed different LPS profiles when stained with silver. *E. coli*(pBT9505) LPS demonstrated the same pattern as the control *E. coli*(pLA2917) LPS. *E. coli*(pBT9502) and *E. coli*(pBT9506) LPS showed identical patterns with additional bands of 4.5, 6.5, 7.5, and 8 kDa [LPS from *E. coli*(pBT9502) is shown in Fig. 3] compared to *E. coli*(pLA2917). The

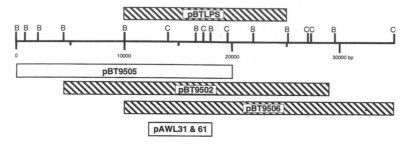

FIGURE 2 Restriction map of the genomic region of *C. jejuni* 81116 encoding the synthesis of LPS. The inserts of cosmids pBT9502, pBT9505, and pBT9506 are shown as bars. The inserts of plasmids pBTLPS, pAWL31, and pAWL61 are also shown. Striped bars indicate expression of LPS in *E. coli*. C and B are abbreviations for *Cla*I and *Bgl*II, respectively.

changed LPS pattern indicated that the cloned DNA region is involved in LPS synthesis.

Western blotting with Penner 6 antiserum showed that *C. jejuni* 81116 LPS extract contained a complete high–molecular-mass LPS O–chain-specific ladder pattern, between 6 and 40 kDa (Fig. 3). LPS isolated from *E. coli*(pBT9502) and *E. coli*(pBT9506) (data not

shown) gave identical profiles, i.e., an LPS O–chain-like ladder pattern with the immunoreactive bands situated between 10 and 45 kDa and a lipid A–core complex of 9 kDa. This complex appears to have a higher molecular mass than that of *C. jejuni* 81116. Possibly the lipid A–core complex of *E. coli* is used and the *Campylobacter* LPS subunits are coupled onto it. The *Campylobacter* O–chain-like polysaccharide repeats expressed in *E. coli* do not stain with silver. E. coli(pBT9505) did not react with Penner 6 antiserum.

Partial cleavage of pBT9502 and cloning into pBR322 resulted in a series of clones, of which the smallest insert still being able to express *Campylobacter* LPS was 16 kb. The plasmid containing this insert was named pBTLPS (Fig. 3 and 4). To exclude possible complementation of the *E. coli* HB101 LPS genes by *Campylobacter* genes, pBT9502 and pBTLPS were also expressed in *E. coli* Sφ874, a strain lacking all genes involved in O–chain synthesis. LPS isolated from these Sφ874 strains showed the same O–chain-like ladder pattern reacting with Penner 6 antiserum.

DNA SEQUENCE ANALYSIS

The insert of pBTLPS was subcloned into sequencing vectors, and the complete 16-kb region was sequenced. A probe derived from the 16-kb region was used to identify LPS biosynthesis genes from chromosomal libraries of a

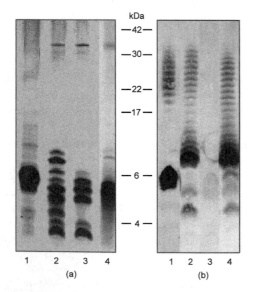

FIGURE 3 LPS profiles in Tricine–SDS-PAGE. (a) Silver-stained samples. (b) Western blots reacted with Penner 6 antiserum. Lanes: 1, *C. jejuni* 81116; 2, *E. coli* HB101(pBT9502); 3, *E. coli* HB101(pLA2917); 4, *E. coli* HB101(pBTLPS).

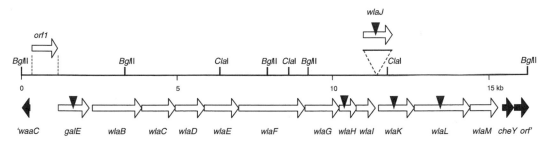

FIGURE 4 The 16-kb region containing the *wla* cluster (open arrows) and flanking genes of *C. jejuni* 81116. The additional genes that are found in strain 11168 are presented above the center line. The *waaC* and *orf* genes are incompletely present.

further two *C. jejuni* strains (Fig. 2) (68). An insert of 7 kb from NCTC 11168 (Penner 2; LOS type) formed pAWL61, and an insert of 6.5 kb from NCTC 11351 (Penner 23; LPS type) formed pAWL31; both inserts were completely sequenced.

Analysis of the DNA sequence of the insert from pBTLPS showed that it contains 13 ORFs and 2 incompletely present ORFs (Fig. 4). Comparison with the sequence of pAWL31 showed that this part was identical to that found in pBTLPS. In contrast, pAWL61 contained an additional gene (*wlaJ*) not present in pBTLPS (Fig. 5). Of the 13 complete ORFs from 81116, 12 showed homology to genes involved in LPS synthesis (Table 1) and were named *galE* and *wlaB* to *wlaM* (*wla* genes), according to the newly proposed bacterial polysaccharide gene nomenclature (51). The extra gene found in strain NCTC 11168 was named *wlaJ* (formerly *orfE* [68]). The remaining complete ORF was that of the chemotaxis gene *cheY* from *C. jejuni* (31, 70), which is not thought to be involved in LPS synthesis. At the 3′ end, an incomplete ORF without homology was found. The incomplete ORF at the 5′ terminus, transcribed in a direction opposite to that of the other genes (Fig. 4), is similar to *waaC* genes and was therefore named *waaC*. *galE* and *wlaB* to *wlaM* are very closely spaced, with most of the designated ORFs showing overlap; this seems to be a common feature of the *C. jejuni* genome (60). The largest spacing between two ORFs, of 97 bp, was found be-

tween genes *wlaI* and *wlaK*, which, in NCTC 11168, contained the *wlaJ* ORF. All these genes have the same transcriptional direction, and therefore it is likely that they are transcribed as a single operon. All ORFs possessed a G + C content between 28 and 34%, which is consistent with the low G + C content of *Campylobacter* spp. (30%) (31). The characteristics of the genes within the analyzed region of all three strains are discussed in the order in which they are present, starting with the *waaC* gene (Table 1).

waaC

The deduced partial protein sequence has similarity to the amino-terminal regions of lipopolysaccharide heptosyltransferases I, which transfer a heptose residue to the Kdo molecule, initiating the synthesis of the inner core. In strain 81116, at least four other genes adjacent to *waaC* seem to be involved in polysaccharide synthesis; however, there is some variation in gene content in this region in other strains (data not shown). Therefore, the *waaC* ortholog may be the first of a gene cluster involved in inner core synthesis. Klena et al. (32) have recently shown that the *waaC* gene from *C. coli* can complement an *S. typhimurium waaC* mutant as judged by novobiocin sensitivity, LPS-specific phage sensitivity, and PAGE-resolved LPS profiles. This suggests that the *C. coli waaC* gene is a functional orthologue of the *S. typhimurium waaC* gene and encodes a product with heptosyltransferase I activity.

```
WlaB-Cj  KYLFKNLNINIKKGEKIAFIGESGCGKSTLVDLIIGLLKPKEGQIIIDKQELNASNAKNYRQKIGYIPQNIYLFNDSIAKN  442
HetA-An  NLVLNNITLTIERCKTTALVGASGAGKTTLADLIPRFYDPTEGQIIVDGLDVQYFEINSIRRKMAVVSQDTFIFNTSIRDN  457
ValA-Fn  HKVLSGVSVDIKAGQTVAFVGKSGSGKTTLTSIISRFYTQHKGEIILDGVDTRELTLENISHLSIVSQNVHLFDDTVYNN   422
MsbA-Ec  VPALRNINLKIPAGKTVALVGRSGSGKSTIASLITRFYDIDEGEILMDGHDLREYTLASIRNQVALVSQNVHLFNDTVANN  436
HlyB-Ec  PVILDNINLSIKQGEVIGIVGRSGSGKSTLTKLIQRFYIPENGQVLIDGHDLALADPNWIRRQVGVVLQDNVLLNRSIIDN  562
HlyB-Ac  PVILNDVNLSIQQGEVIGIVGRSGSGKSTLTKLIQRFYIPENGQVLIDGHDLALADPNWIRRQVGVVLQDNVLLNRSIRDN  562
                           G----GKS
                              A
                              T

WlaB-Cj  ITFGD--AVDEEKLNKVIKQANLEHFIKNLPQGVQTKVGDCGSNLSGGQQRIAIARAIYLEPEITVLDEATSALDTQSEA  521
HetA-An  IAYGT-SGASEAEIREVARLANALQFIEEMPEGFDTKLGDRGVRLSGGQRQRIAIARAILRDPEILIDEATSALDSVSER  537
ValA-Fn  IAFGLSREVSEDEVIDALKRANAYEFVQELSDGIHTNICMNGSKLSGGQRQRISIARAILKNAPVLIFDEATSALDNESER 503
MsbA-Ec  IAYARTEQYSREQIEEAARMAYAMDFINKMDNGLDTVICENGVLSGGQRQRIAIARAILRDSPILIFDEATSALDTESER  517
HlyB-Ec  ISLAN-PGMSVEKVIYAAKLAGAHDFISELREGYNTIVGEQGAGLSGGQRQRIAIARAIVNNPKILIFDEATSAIDYESEH 642
HlyB-Ac  IALAD-PGMPMEKIVHAAKLAGAHEFISELREGYNTIVGEQGAGISGGQRQRIAIARAIVNNPKILIFDEATSALDYESEH 642
                                               1S2GxxxK34x56

WlaB-Cj  KIMDEIYKISKDKTMIITAHRLSTITQCDKVYRLEHGKLKEEK--------------  564
HetA-An  LIQESIEKLSVGRTVIAIAHRLSTIAKADKVVVMEQGRIVEQGNYQEFLEQRGKLWKYHQMQHESGQTNS  607
ValA-Fn  VVQQALESLTESCTTIVIAHRLSTVENADKIVVMDGGKVVESGKHQEFLEQGGLYTGSINRDFNSTYAR-  572
MsbA-Ec  AIQAALDELQKNRTSVIAHRLSTIEKADEIVVVEDGVIVERGTHNDLLEHRGVYAQLHKMQFGQ-----  582
HlyB-Ec  VIMRNMHKICKGRTVIIAHRLSTVKNADRIIVMEKGKIVEQGKHKELLSEPESLYSYLYQLQSD------  707
HlyB-Ac  IIMRNMHQICKGRTVIIAHRLSTVKNADRIIVMEKGQIVEQGKHKELLADPNGLYHYLHQLQSE------  707
```

FIGURE 5 Alignment of the carboxyl-terminal part of WlaB with homologous proteins. Identical amino acids within all six sequences are inversed. The ATP-binding-site motif and the ABC transporter family signature (underlined) are presented below the alignment. When multiple amino acids are possible in one of the positions of the ABC transporter family signature, numbers are inserted: 1, LIVMFY; 2, SAG; 3, RKA; 4, LIVMYA; 5, LIVMF; 6, SAG. Cj, *C. jejuni*; An, *Anabaena* sp.; Fn, *Francisella novicida*; Ec, *E. coli*; Ac, *Actinobacillus pleuropneumoniae*.

TABLE 1 Deduced proteins present in the *C. jejuni wla* region and their homologues

C. jejuni protein	Similar protein	Organism	Function	% Identity/ similarity	Database accession
WaaC[a]	RfaC	*Escherichia coli*	Heptosyltransferase I	28.6/51.2	P24173
	RfaC	*Neisseria gonorrhoeae*	Heptosyltransferase I	28.6/51.2	S60783
	RfaC	*Bordetella pertussis*	Heptosyltransferase I	28.6/48.8	X90711
	RfaC	*Salmonella typhimurium*	Heptosyltransferase I	26.2/52.4	P26469
Orfl					
GalE	GalE	*Haemophilus influenzae*	UDP-glucose 4-epimerase	37.5/52.4	A64063
	GalE	*Neisseria meningitidis*	UDP-glucose 4-epimerase	36.3/53.1	S39638
	GalE	*Escherichia coli*	UDP-glucose 4-epimerase	36.0/52.2	P09147
WlaB	HetA	*Anabaena* sp.	Polysaccharide involvement	30.1/48.7	P22638
	HlyB	*Escherichia coli*	Export of hemolysin	30.1/46.2	P08716
	HlyB	*Actinobacillus pleuropneumoniae*	Export of hemolysin	27.5/44.0	P26760
	MsbA	*Escherichia coli*	Export[a]	24.3/43.3	P27299
	ValA	*Francisella novicida*	Secretion of LPS	23.4/41.5	L17003
WlaC	TrsD	*Yersinia enterocolitica*	Glycosyltransferase[b]	28.8/47.0	S51263
	AmsD	*Erwinia amylovora*	Glycosyltransferase[b]	27.4/44.8	S52144
	EpsG	*Streptococcus thermophilus*	Glycosyltransferase[b]	26.8/40.8	U40830
WlaD	Orf8.7	*Yersinia pseudotuberculosis*	Abequosyltransferase[b]	27.2/38.9	L01777
	TrsB	*Yersinia enterocolitica*	Glycosyltransferase[b]	23.3/42.4	S51261
	EpsI	*Streptococcus thermophilus*	Glycosyltransferase[b]	23.0/38.8	U40830
	SpsA	*Bacillus subtilis*	Polysaccharide synthesis	22.2/41.0	P39621
WlaE	AmsD	*Erwinia amylovora*	Glycosyltransferase[b]	25.1/41.3	S52144
	TrsD	*Yersinia enterocolitica*	Glycosyltransferase[b]	24.9/40.5	S51263
	TrsE	*Yersinia enterocolitica*	Glycosyltransferase[b]	25.6/40.1	S51264
	CapH	*Staphylococcus aureus*	Glycosyltransferase[b]	23.1/37.8	U10927
WlaF	STT-3	*Caenorhabditis elegans*	Oligosaccharyl-transferase	19.5/35.9	P46975
	Wzy (Rfc)	*Escherichia coli*	O-antigen polymerase	18.8/39.7	P37748
	STT-3	*Saccharomyces cerevisiae*	Oligosaccharyl-transferase	16.3/34.5	JC4355
WlaG	CpsF	*Proteus mirabilis*	Glycosyltransferase[b]	30.8/48.1	L36873
	RfbF	*Serratia marescens*	Galactantransferase[b]	27.1/41.2	L34167
	RfpB	*Shigella dysenteriae*	Galactosyltransferase	26.6/44.7	S27671
	RfbF	*Klebsiella pneumoniae*	Galactantransferase	26.1/41.5	L31762
WlaH	WbaP (RfbP)	*Salmonella enterica*	Galactosyltransferase first step	39.5/55.5	P26406
	WbaP (RfbP)	*Haemophilus influenzae*	Galactosyltransferase[b]	38.5/53.0	B64099
	EpsE	*Streptococcus thermophilus*	Galactosyltransferase first step[b]	36.0/53.0	U40830
	ExoY	*Rhizobium* sp.	Galactosyltransferase first step	36.0/52.0	X16704
WlaI	NeuD	*Escherichia coli*	Polysialic acid capsule synthesis	28.1/45.8	U05248
	LpxD	*Salmonella enterica*	Acyltransferase	26.6/44.3	P18482
	LpxD	*Yersinia enterocolitica*	Acyltransferase	26.1/42.0	P32203
	LpxD	*Escherichia coli*	Acyltransferase	25.1/43.8	P21645
WlaJ					
WlaK	RfbE	*Vibrio cholorae*	Perosamine synthetase[b]	32.2/51.2	S28471
	DegT	*Bacillus stearothermophilus*	Transamination	29.0/44.4	P15263
	FlaA2	*Caulobacter crescentus*	Motility/polysaccharide	25.9/44.0	U27301
	SpsC	*Bacillus subtilis*	Polysaccharide synthesis	25.4/43.0	P39623
WlaL	CapD	*Staphylococcus aureus*	Capsule synthesis	38.5/55.6	P39853
	TrsG	*Yersinia enterocolitica*	Acetylgalactosamine synthesis[b]	37.5/51.7	S51266
	WpbM	*Pseudomonas aeruginosa*	LPS B-band synthesis	34.4/53.2	U44089
WlaM	AcfB	*Vibrio cholerae*	Accessory colonization factor	26.9/48.2	L25660

[a] Incompletely present.
[b] Putative function.

orf1

In NCTC 11168 there is a deduced ORF between *waaC* and *galE* that encodes 269 residues, whereas in strain 81116 (20) minor sequence differences disturb the ORF. *orf1* shows no similarity to any known LPS biosynthesis gene. Nevertheless, it may form the first gene in an operon of up to 14 genes. Deduced amino acid sequence similarity was observed with a hypothetical protein from *Helicobacter pylori* (HP0688/689), and low levels of similarity to a large number of DNA polymerases were found. The significance of the lack of *orf1* in strain 81116 for the LPS phenotype has yet to be determined, and the status of the ORF in other strains is not known.

galE

The protein encoded by *galE* has sequence similarity to UDP-galactose-4-epimerase (GalE), an enzyme catalyzing the interconversion between UDP-Glc and UDP-Gal. Gal is a component of the LPS core structure of *E. coli* and *S. typhimurium*. Defects in *galE* result in a truncated LPS molecule. In *Neisseria meningitidis* a mutated *galE* gene results in truncation of the LOS chain by deletion of the outer core (25). The amino-terminal region of the predicted GalE protein possesses the consensus NAD-binding domain (GxxGxxG) (37) commonly present in epimerases. All known *Campylobacter* LPS structures contain both Gal and Glc, and we have recently shown by functional analysis that the *galE* gene encodes a UDP-galactose-4-epimerase (see below).

wlaB

The protein product of the *wlaB* gene contains an ATP-binding site and the signature for ABC transporters (26), suggesting that this protein is involved in transport across the cytoplasmic membrane. The protein contains six potential transmembrane segments, which are also seen in other membrane transport molecules (11). Sequence conservation with other transport proteins is located mainly in the C-terminal part, where the ATP-binding site and the ABC transporter family motif are located (Fig. 5). Comparison of the hydrophobicity plots of these proteins indicated that the six transmembrane segments were located at identical positions (data not shown). WlaB most probably has a signal peptide, which is cleaved between amino acids 45 and 46. The similarities described above suggest that the WlaB protein from *C. jejuni* is involved in the transport of LPS molecules across the cytoplasmic membrane.

wlaC, wlaD, and wlaE

The protein products of *wlaC*, *wlaD*, and *wlaE* all possess one or two putative transmembrane segments. All three deduced proteins are similar to putative glycosyltransferases. TrsD and TrsE from *Yersinia enterocolitica*, which show amino acid sequence similarity to WlaC and WlaE, are putative galactosaminyltransferases or *N*-acetylgalactosaminyltransferases involved in outer core synthesis (55). WlaC and WlaE are closely related, with 30.2% identical amino acids and 43.6% similar amino acids. All three proteins seem to be glycosyltransferases, and WlaC and WlaE may link Gal or GalNAc to the growing polysaccharide chain.

wlaF

wlaF is the largest gene found in the cluster and encodes a predicted protein of 82.2 kDa. This protein is similar to the transmembrane oligosaccharyltransferases (STT3) from eukaryotes and the O-chain polymerase from *E. coli*. The STT3 protein from yeast is possibly involved in the transfer of an oligosaccharide from a lipid precursor to a protein (71). The amino-terminal part of WlaF contains 12 putative transmembrane segments. The carboxy-terminal part is hydrophilic. These last two characteristics are also seen in the STT3 protein. The Wzy (Rfc) polymerase often is also highly hydrophobic, containing 12 putative transmembrane segments. Therefore, by amino acid sequence comparison and hydrophobicity profile, we would speculate that the *C. jejuni* WlaF protein is involved in the transfer of oligosaccharides, possibly from a lipid carrier onto the lipid A-core complex.

wlaG

The whole of the deduced *wlaG* amino acid sequence shows similarity to galactosyltransferases. The *rfbF* gene products of *Klebsiella pneumoniae* and *Serratia marcescens* transfer the disaccharide β-D-Gal*f*-1β3-α-D-Gal*p,* representing a single repeating unit of D-galactan I to the GlcNAc-containing lipid intermediate (15, 58). The WbbP (RfpB) protein of *Shigella dysenteriae* transfers a single Gal residue to a GlcNAc-containing lipid (22). Unlike the WbbP (RfpB) protein of *S. dysenteriae* and the CpsF protein of *Proteus mirabilis* (23), the predicted WlaG protein of *C. jejuni* is probably not membrane bound, since it has no significant hydrophobic regions. However, the DdhA (RfbF) protein of *Klebsiella pneumoniae* is also not membrane bound. Since galactose residues are present in the LPS molecules of all *C. jejuni* strains analyzed, we suggest that the WlaG protein functions as a galactosyltransferase.

wlaH

WlaH shows similarity to enzymes (WbaP) involved in transferring the first sugar of the subunits of O-chain to the lipid precursor undecaprenol phosphate. This first sugar differs between bacterial species and strains, but in most cases Gal is the first sugar with which O-chain synthesis is initiated. The proteins showing highest similarity to WlaH transfer a Gal residue. Like other WbaP proteins, WlaH contains a hydrophobic domain required for the interaction with the undecaprenol phosphate lipid carrier (Fig. 6). Some WbaP-like proteins are bifunctional, with the above-mentioned transferase activity assigned to the C-terminal domain. Recently it has been proposed that the amino-terminal domain of the WbaP protein of *Salmonella enterica* is involved in the release of undecaprenol pyrophosphate-linked galactose from WbaP (65) and does not have a flippase function as earlier reported (66). When WlaH is compared to WbaP from *S. enterica* and *Haemophilus influenzae* (Fig. 6), the amino acid sequence alignment shows that the N-terminal domain is missing and thus WlaH probably possesses only the transferase activity.

wlaJ

The 203-amino-acid product of *wlaI* is most similar to the 207-amino-acid NeuD protein

from *E. coli*, an enzyme involved in the synthesis of the K1 polysaccharide (3), a β-2,8-linked linear polymer of about 200 sialic acid (NeuNAc) residues. The NeuD protein is suggested to be involved in NeuNAc transfer (3). The carboxy-terminal part of the WlaI protein is also similar, although to a lesser extent, to the 340-amino-acid UDP-*N*-acetylglucosamine acyltransferases (LpxD) of *Escherichia coli, Salmonella enterica,* and *Yersinia enterocolitica,* which play a role in lipid A synthesis (16, 27, 64). *lpxD*-like genes have been found in several gene clusters involved in LPS O-chain synthesis including *wlbB* (*bplB*) in *Bordetella pertussis* (1) and *wbpD* in *Pseudomonas aeruginosa* (13), which both encode acetyltransferases. The *wlaI* deduced protein sequence also shows amino acid sequence similarity to this group of transferases.

A hexapeptide motif, also termed the isoleucine patch (17), is present in some transferases (62). Each motif starts with an isoleucine, leucine, or valine residue and often contains a glycine in the second position. The repeating motif is present (Fig. 7) in the WlaI protein of *C. jejuni* as well as in the LpxD-like proteins described above. We propose a function for the WlaI protein as a NeuNAc transferase, since the NeuD protein from *E. coli* shows the highest similarity. The NeuD protein, like the WlaI protein, is small, containing only 207 amino acids, whereas all known LpxD proteins contain around 340 amino acids. The presence of NeuNAc residues in seven of the eight analyzed *C. jejuni* LPS molecules indicates the need for such an enzyme activity.

wlaJ

The *wlaJ* gene is present in NCTC 11168 but not in 81116 or NCTC 11351 (see below). The protein does not have significant similarity to any other protein, and thus the function of WlaJ in *C. jejuni* remains unclear. Further analysis of the gene (see below) indicates that its presence may affect the production of the O-chain ladder.

wlaK

The predicted protein designated WlaK shows the highest similarity to the Per (RfbE) protein

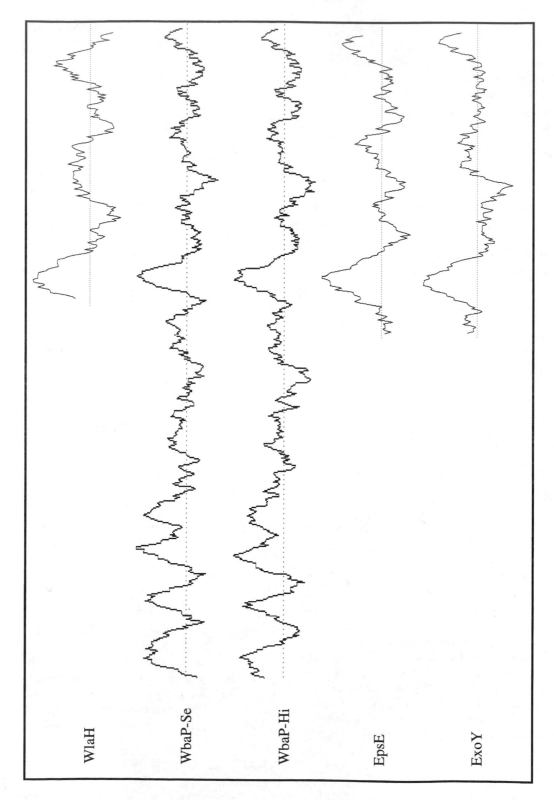

WlaH

WbaP-Se

WbaP-Hi

EpsE

ExoY

```
WlaI_Cj   115   KAK IEKGVI INTSSV IEHECV IGEFSH VSVGAK CAGNVK   153
NeuD_Ec   116   DTR IHDAVV INTRSL IEHGNE IGCCSN ISTNVV LNGDVS   154
LpxD_Se   221   DTV IGNGVI IDNQCQ IAHNVV IGDNTA VAGGVI MAGSLK   259
LpxD_Ec   221   DTI IGNGVI IDNQCQ IAHNVV IGDNTA VAGGVI MAGSLK   259
LpxD_Ye   221   NTI IGNGVI IDNQCQ IAHNVV IGDNTA VAGGVI MAGSLK   259
                    ..  *  ..* ...  *.*. **  . .... .*...

WlaI_Cj   154   IGKNCF LGINSC VLPNLS LADDSI LGGGAT LVKSQNEKG   192
NeuD_Ec   155   VGEETF VGSVTV VNGQLK LGSKSI IGSGSV VIRNIPSNV   193
LpxD_Se   260   IGRYCM IGGASV INGHME ICDKVT VTGMGM VMRPITEPG   298
LpxD_Ec   260   IGRYCM IGGASV INGHME ICDKVT VTGMGM VMRPITEPG   298
LpxD_Ye   260   VGRYCM IGGASV INGHME ICDKVT ITGMGM VMRPITEPG   298
                .*  . .*.    ...  . .. ... . ...
```

FIGURE 7 Protein sequences of WlaI and homologous proteins (see Table 1). The first residues of the isoleucine patch are boxed and bold. Glycine residues in second position are also shown in bold. Asterisks indicate identical amino acids, and dots indicate conserved substitutions. Cj, *C. jejuni;* Ec, *E. coli;* Se, *Salmonella enterica;* Ye, *Yersinia enterocolitica.*

from *Vibrio cholerae,* a putative perosamine synthetase (39). Similarity to DegT from *Bacillus stearothermophilus* was also found. This protein is required in the pathway to synthesize 2,6-, 3,6- and 4,6-dideoxyhexoses and is thought to be an enzyme for transaminations leading to amino sugars (61). The SpsC protein from *Bacillus subtilis* (21), also belonging to the DegT family and involved in spore coat polysaccharide biosynthesis, is also similar to the *C. jejuni* WlaK protein. The *Caulobacter crescentus flmB* (formerly *flaA2*) gene product, involved in flagellin synthesis (34), is also similar to WlaK, and thus the polysaccharide may be involved in flagellum biogenesis. The WlaK protein of *C. jejuni* is probably also involved in the synthesis of an amino sugar, possibly GalNAc or NeuNAc, which are both common components of the *Campylobacter* LPS molecule. *Neisseria gonorrhoeae,* however, uses exogenous NeuNAc to sialylate its LOS by an outer membrane-bound NeuNAc transferase, which has been detected in the outer membrane (38). Preliminary analysis of the NCTC 11168 genome sequence (60) indicates that there are at least three loci that may be involved in NeuNAc biosynthesis.

wlaL

The WlaL protein is homologous throughout the entire protein to the CapD, WbpM, and TrsG proteins from *Staphylococcus aureus, Pseudomonas aeruginosa,* and *Yersinia enterocolitica,* respectively (13, 36, 55). All these proteins contain five hydrophobic domains in the amino-terminal part, which are predicted to be transmembrane segments. The central part contains an NAD-binding site and is homologous to UDP-glucose-4-epimerases. The function of the CapD protein is not known, but the TrsG protein is thought to be involved in the biosynthesis of acetylgalactosamine or acetylfucosamine and the WbpM protein is possibly a dehydrogenase or epimerase needed for the biosynthesis of a 2-acetamido-2,6-dideoxy-D-galactose residue. A putative signal peptide has been found in WlaL, which is probably cleaved at position 29. We suggest that the WlaL protein is involved in the synthesis of an amino sugar, for example, GalNAc or NeuNAc.

wlaM

The *wlaM* gene product shows a low level of similarity to an accessory colonization factor,

FIGURE 6 Hydrophobicity plots of WlaH and homologous proteins (see Table 1). Se, *Salmonella enterica;* Hi, *Haemophilus influenzae.*

AcfB (19), which contains a methyl-accepting chemotaxis motif (2). However, the similarity of AcfB to WlaM was confined to the amino-terminal region, which does not contain this motif. Like WlaF, WlaM is also a hydrophobic protein containing six putative transmembrane regions, and therefore WlaM could also function as a flippase or a polymerase.

The sequence data show that the 16-kb region contains 11 genes, whose deduced protein sequence shows homology to proteins involved in LPS synthesis in other bacteria. On the basis of the observed similarity of deduced Wla proteins to proteins involved in LOS synthesis, especially synthesis of the outer core of *Yersinia enterocolitica* and *Bordetella pertussis* (1, 55), it is likely that the *wla* gene cluster of *C. jejuni* is involved in the synthesis of the O-chain-like polysaccharide as well as of the outer core but not of the inner core.

GENE DISTRIBUTION AND ORGANIZATION

Variation in the LPS composition and structure within a species is often reflected by gene insertions, deletions, or mutations within the biosynthesis locus (54). Southern blot analysis showed that strain 81116 carries only one copy of the *waaC*-to-*wlaL* region, and Southern blot analysis and genome sequencing (60) confirms this to be also true for strain NCTC 11168. Variation at the putative LPS biosynthesis locus of *C. jejuni* was investigated by using ORF-specific primers in a PCR-based approach. Amplification was performed from a reverse anchor primer to each of a series of forward primers for other genes. This approach was applied to 36 strains of *C. jejuni* including 81116, NCTC 11168, and NCTC 11351 (Table 2). With respect to the region spanning *waaC* through *wlaM,* no variation in gene content or organization was observed other than the presence or absence of *wlaJ* (Fig. 4). Of the tested strains, 17 produced a PCR profile (confirmed by Southern hybridization [data not shown]) indicating the presence of *wlaJ* and 19 strains lacked *wlaJ* (Table 2). The presence or absence of *wlaJ* did not correlate with serotype

TABLE 2 Genetic distribution of *wlaJ* in different *C. jejuni* strains[a]

wlaJ[b]	Serotype[c]	Phenotype[c,d]	No. of strains[e]
Present	1, 2, 4	LOS	7
	19	LPS	1
	11, 5, 50	NK	3
	UT	NK	4
	ND	NK	2
Absent	1, 2, 41	LOS	6
	6, 23, 23/36	LPS	4
	5, 11, 15, 28	NK	4
	UT	NK	3
	ND	NK	2

[a] Adapted from reference 68.
[b] Presence of *wlaJ* determined by PCR assay.
[c] ND, not done; UT, untypeable; NK, not known.
[d] Phenotype predicted from that reported for each O serotype.
[e] Number of strains with genotype-phenotype combination.

or LPS/LOS phenotype. Seven strains from patients with Guillain-Barré syndrome were included in the screening; four contained *wlaJ,* and three did not. Preliminary data indicate that substantial variation in LPS biosynthesis gene content is present upstream of the locus described here (unpublished results).

ANALYSIS OF LPS BIOSYNTHESIS GENES

To begin to associate LPS biosynthetic function with specific ORFs, mutations were constructed by insertion of antibiotic resistance cassettes by homologous recombination (63) into the chromosomal loci of *C. jejuni* 81116 or NCTC 11168. Each mutation was confirmed by PCR and Southern hybridization before the LPS biosynthesis phenotype of each mutant was assessed. NCTC 11351 could not be transformed, and consequently no mutants were constructed for this strain.

Analysis of the *galE* Gene

To confirm the function of the putative *galE* gene from *C. jejuni,* a plasmid containing this gene was transferred into SL761 (an *S. typhimurium galE* mutant strain). To test for complementation, the parent *S. typhimurium* wild-type strain and the transformants were first grown on modified MacConkey agar. In contrast to SL761, wild-type *S. typhimurium* strains ferment galactose in the LeLoir pathway, resulting in the production of acid, which is detected on modified MacConkey agar medium. Complementation of the *S. typhimurium galE* mutation by the *C. jejuni galE* gene was detected by acidification of the modified MacConkey agar medium.

Complementation of UDP-glucose epimerase activity was also assessed. UDP-glucose epimerase activity in *S. typhimurium* was induced by galactose, whereas the mutant strain SL761 did not show any UDP-glucose epimerase activity with or without the addition of galactose. SL761 containing the *C. jejuni galE* gene showed epimerase activity with and without galactose (Fig. 8), showing that the *galE* gene from *C. jejuni* encodes a UDP-glucose epimerase.

The inactivation of the *galE* gene in *S. typhi-*

murium results in the expression of a truncated LPS molecule lacking the O-chain. To investigate if the *C. jejuni galE* gene can restore the expression of the complete LPS molecule in strain SL761, LPS was isolated from the parent *S. typhimurium* strain, SL761, and from SL761 containing the *C. jejuni galE* gene and analyzed by Tricine-SDS-PAGE followed by silver staining. The presence of the *C. jejuni galE* in SL761 resulted in the production of a complete O-chain similar to that seen in wild-type *S. typhimurium* (Fig. 9).

To deduce the function of the *galE* gene in *C. jejuni*, a *galE* mutant strain was constructed. Inverse PCR was used to delete part of the *galE* gene and permit the insertion of a kanamycin resistance cassette. Two 81116 *galE* mutants containing the kanamycin resistance cassette in both orientations with respect to the *galE* gene were produced (*galE*a and *galE*b).

The effect of the *galE* mutation on LPS synthesis was investigated by analyzing LPS by Tricine-SDS-PAGE followed by silver staining

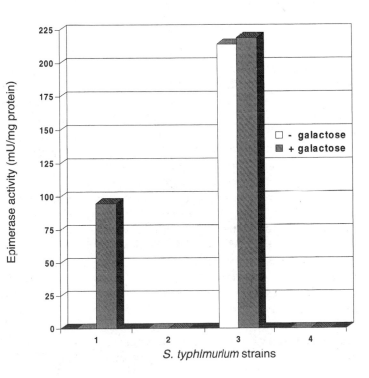

FIGURE 8 UDP-galactose epimerase activity, given as milliunits per milligram of protein for *S. typhimurium* (bars 1), mutant SL761 (bars 2), complemented mutant SL761 (pBF84And47) (bars 3), and control SL761(pBl) (bars 4). The activity was measured for these strains grown on media with and without 1% galactose.

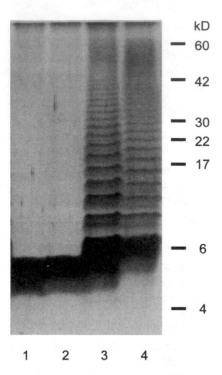

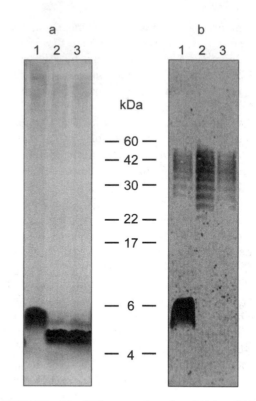

FIGURE 9 LPS analysis by Tricine-SDS–PAGE of LPS prepared from *S. typhimurium* strains. LPS was visualized by silver staining. Lanes: 1, SL761; 2, control SL761(pBl); 3, SL761(pBF84And47); 4, parent strain SL696.

FIGURE 10 LPS separation by Tricine-SDS–PAGE. (a) Silver-stained LPS samples. (b) Immunoblot with *C. jejuni* 81116 LPS antiserum. Lanes: 1, parent *C. jejuni*; 2, *galE*a; 3, *galE*b.

and Western blotting (Fig. 10). The silver staining showed that the parent strain expressed a lipid A-core molecule of around 5.5 kDa whereas the *galE* mutant strains expressed a molecule of 4.5 kDa. This is consistent with the loss of galactose-containing units from the core. The Western blot showed that the lipid A-core complex expressed by the *galE* mutant strain no longer reacted with antiserum raised against strain 81116. These results indicate that the core molecule expressed by the *galE* mutant strain is truncated and that this modification removes core-specific epitopes that react with the anti-81116 antiserum. However, the O-chain-like structure was present in the *galE* mutant strain. Therefore, we can conclude that the O-chain-like structure either is attached to the inner part of the LPS molecule or is not part of the LPS molecule. It is unlikely that the

observed phenotypic changes are due to polar effects since the kanamycin cassette does not contain a transcription terminator and the kanamycin cassette can be inserted in both orientations. In addition, the gene downstream of the *galE* gene (*wlaB*) seems to be essential (unpublished data).

Mutational Analysis of *wlaK*, *wlaL*, and *wlaH*

A *wlaK* mutation was also constructed by an inverse PCR approach and the insertion of a kanamycin resistance cassette. The LPS phenotype of *wlaK* mutants in both strains 81116 and NCTC 11168 was determined by silver staining and Western blotting with the specific serotyping serum for each strain. Silver staining of the mutants showed no consistent alteration of the LPS. Mutation of *wlaK* altered the reactiv-

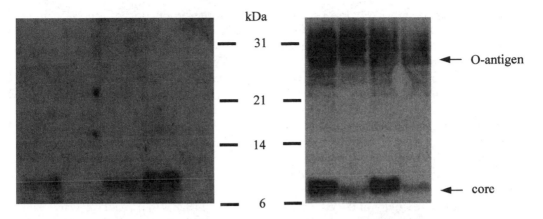

FIGURE 11 Mutant *C. jejuni* LPS and LOS profiles (68). LPS and LOS samples were electrophoresed on an SDS-PAGE gel by using the Tricine-SDS-PAGE system and subsequently detected by Western blotting with O:2 antiserum against NCTC 11168 and its mutants (left) and O:6 antiserum against 81116 and its mutants (right). In both panels, the lanes show, from left to right, *C. jejuni* wild type, *wlaK* mutant, *wlaL* mutant, *wlaJ* mutant, and large deletion mutant.

ity of the core molecule to antiserum (Fig. 11), but no effect on O-chain production was detected by Western blotting of the *wlaK* mutant of 81116. The *wlaK* mutant did, however, demonstrate an altered cell morphology compared with the wild type; the mutants were shorter and wider than their parents (Fig. 12). The reduced reactivity of antiserum with the core of the LPS and LOS molecules indicates that WlaK may be involved in core biosynthesis, perhaps affecting the sialyation of the core due to lack of synthesis of NeuNAc.

A *wlaL* mutation was introduced into both strains 81116 and NCTC11168 as described above. Mutation of *wlaL* had no detectable effect on the LOS or LPS profiles of mutants constructed for either strain (Fig. 11), and no change in cell morphology was observed. The inability to detect any phenotypic alteration when mutating *wlaL* may be due to the use of a polyclonal antiserum in the Western blot that does not detect minor changes in the structure of the LPS. Another possibility is the presence of compensating genes in another locus; however, we have no evidence of a second *capD* ortholog (see below). Cryptic LPS biosynthesis genes have been found in *Neisseria* (48, 52) and *Haemophilus influenzae* (28), both of which pro-

duce LOS but not LPS. Insertional mutagenesis of several genes from both these species failed to alter their LOS profiles.

Attempts were also made to mutate the *wbaP* homologue, *wlaH*, but no transformants

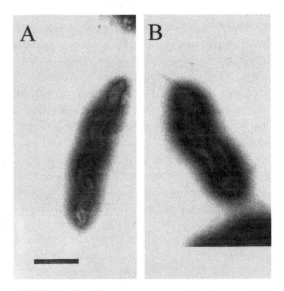

FIGURE 12 Electron micrograph of negatively stained NCTC 11168 (A) and *wlaK* mutant (B), illustrating that the mutation results in a change in morphology to shorter and wider cells. Bar, 1 μm.

were obtained with either *C. jejuni* strain. Nevertheless, it proved possible to create a large deletion, which removed the sequence between the 3′ end of *wlaF* and the 5′ end of *wlaK*. One possible explanation is the toxic buildup of a pathway intermediate when *wlaH* alone is mutated. The ability to produce the larger deletion would therefore suggest that *wlaF, wlaG, wlaI,* or *wlaK* acts as a suppressor mutation for the disruption of *wlaH*. The large deletion mutant had a phenotype identical to that seen with the *wlaK* mutant. The mutants showed a change of reactivity of the core with serotyping serum in a Western blot, but there was no change in the ability to produce the O-chain ladder in the 81116 background. The large deletion mutant also showed the alteration in morphology.

Mutational Analysis of *wlaJ*

A *wlaJ* mutation was constructed only in NCTC 11168 since the ORF is not present in strain 81116. Mutation of *wlaJ* in NCTC 11168 did not alter the LOS profile of this strain (Fig. 11). The effect of the mutation of *wlaJ* on the production of the O-chain could not be determined since wild-type NCTC 11168 does not produce the O-chain and is also dependent on the use of O:2 antiserum. A strategy was therefore designed to insert *wlaJ* into an LPS producer to analyze the effect of adding *wlaJ* into this strain (Fig. 13). The intact *wlaJ* ORF derived from NCTC 11168 was inserted into 81116 together with a chloramphenicol resistance cassette (CAT). The LPS from 81116 (*wlaJ* absent), NCTC 11168 (*wlaJ* present), and the mutant 81116 containing *wlaJ* [NCTC 11828::(*wlaJ*+CAT)] were analyzed by Western blotting with O:6 antiserum (Fig. 14, lanes 1, 5, and 3, respectively). The LPS of the mutant strain consistently showed no alteration in serospecificity, but the O-chain was no longer detectable (lane 3).

wlaJ was subsequently disrupted in the 81116::(*wlaJ*+CAT) mutant by using a kanamycin cassette insertion (KAN). The production of O-chain was not detected in 81116::(*wlaJ*::KAN)+CAT (Fig. 14, lane 4). To determine the effect of the CAT cassette alone on LPS phenotype at the position of insertion

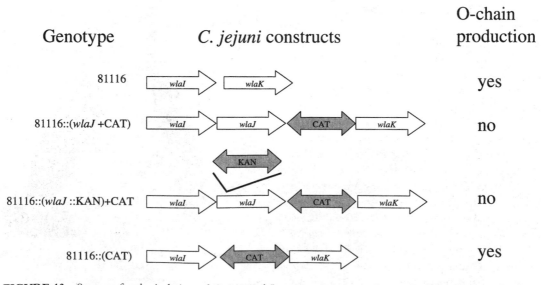

Genotype	*C. jejuni* constructs	O-chain production
81116	*wlaI* / *wlaK*	yes
81116::(*wlaJ* +CAT)	*wlaI* / *wlaJ* / CAT / *wlaK*	no
81116::(*wlaJ* ::KAN)+CAT	*wlaI* / *wlaJ* / CAT / *wlaK* (KAN)	no
81116::(CAT)	*wlaI* / CAT / *wlaK*	yes

FIGURE 13 Strategy for the isolation of *C. jejuni wlaJ* mutants. Schematic diagrams of the *wlaI to wlaK* region and all mutant constructs are shown. The position and orientation (double-headed arrows illustrate that both orientations were constructed) of the antibiotic resistance cassette in *wlaJ* and the *wlaI to wlaK* intergenic region are shown. Strain genotypes are indicated on the left, and O-chain production phenotype are shown on the right.

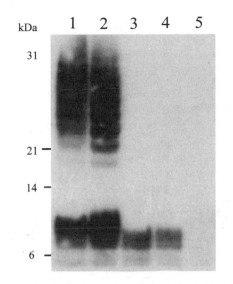

FIGURE 14 LPS and LOS profiles of *C. jejuni* 81116 with the *wlaJ* mutations (68). LPS and LOS samples were electrophoresed on a Tricine-SDS-PAGE system and subsequently detected by Western blotting with O:6 antiserum. Lanes: 1, *C. jejuni* 81116; 2, *C. jejuni* 81116::(CAT); 3, *C. jejuni* 81116::(*wlaJ* + CAT); 4, *C. jejuni* 81116::(*wlaJ*::Kan) + CAT; 5, *C. jejuni* NCTC 11168.

of *wlaJ* into 81116, a mutant in which the CAT cassette was inserted between *wlaI* and *wlaK* was created. The 81116::(CAT) mutant was found to have a detectable O-chain (lane 2).

Given that the locus may be involved in core oligosaccharide biosynthesis, interpretation of our data is complicated by the fact that the O-chain is no longer visible after the insertion of *wlaJ* into 81116. Disruption of this gene by insertion of a KAN cassette does not restore the O-chain; however, the presence of the CAT cassette alone did not affect O-chain biosynthesis. Therefore, it is a change associated with the presence of *wlaJ* sequence (*wlaJ* or *wlaJ*::KAN) and not the disruption of the operon at this position that is of importance.

Given that changes associated with the insertion of *wlaJ* into the chromosome of 81116 can have an effect on O-chain production, we would have expected to see a correlation between the presence of *wlaJ* and the LOS phe-

notype. The absence of such a correlation (Table 2) might reflect the complexity of O-chain biosynthesis, where the presence or absence of many other genes will also affect the production of O-chain and strains of a particular serotype may not have identical O-chain structure. Alternatively, if *C. jejuni* produces capsule-like polysaccharides that are not attached to lipid A-core structures (see below), the presence or absence of *wlaJ* might affect the attachment of the O-chain to different lipids.

GENERAL COMMENTS

Cell-associated polysaccharide structures, including LPS and LOS, are candidate virulence determinants for several stages and aspects of *Campylobacter* gastrointestinal disease. The role played by ganglioside-like epitopes in LPS and LOS in the etiology of *Campylobacter*-associated neuropathies is widely accepted but still requires confirmation by using defined structural variants and an appropriate animal model. A genetic strategy to investigate the role of *Campylobacter* LPS and LOS in human disease is now possible, given the identification of a chromosomal locus containing a cluster of genes associated with LPS and LOS biosynthesis. Deduced amino acid sequence comparisons of the genes in the locus and the genetic analysis of *waaC, galE, wlaJ,* and *wlaK* have confirmed the involvement of members of the cluster in LPS and LOS biosynthesis. The only genetic variation in the region between *waaC* and *wlaM* appears to be associated with *orf1* and *wlaJ*. However, variation in core structure and serotype would be expected to also depend upon the variation in gene content noted upstream of *waaC* (unpublished data).

DEVELOPING A MODEL FOR LPS AND LOS BIOSYNTHESIS IN CAMPYLOBACTERS

Genes in the *waaC* to *wlaM* region may be involved in core biosynthesis. Although the function of only *waaC* and *galE* have been confirmed, deduced amino acid sequence similarities support a role for several other genes in

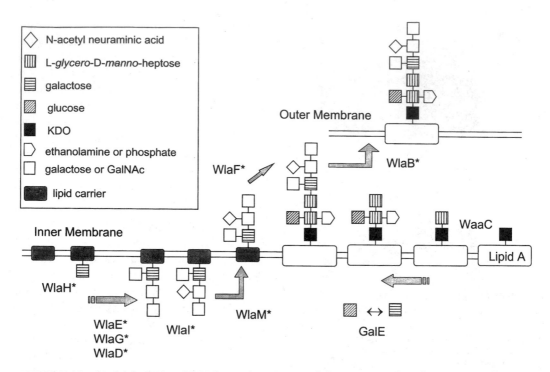

FIGURE 15 Model for LPS and LOS biosynthesis in campylobacters. Asterisks indicate putative functions of proteins. ACL, acyl lipid carrier.

this region in core biosynthesis. Based on comparisons and complementation data, a preliminary model to provide testable predictions about gene function in core biosynthesis can be developed. The model illustrated in Fig. 15 presents the biosynthesis of a non-strain-specific LOS structure in *C. jejuni* and is based on the functions predicted for the genes in the *waaC* to *wlaM* cluster.

Three genes involved in the biosynthesis of sugars are present in the *waaC* to *wlaM* cluster. The presence of *galE,* converting Glc to Gal, is predictable, since all known outer-core molecules of *C. jejuni* contain Gal residues. The *wlaK* and *wlaL* genes are probably involved in the synthesis of amino sugars, such as GalNAc and NeuNAc, that are found in core molecules of several *C. jejuni* strains.

The *C. jejuni* outer-core molecule is probably synthesized on a lipid carrier independent of the inner-core lipid A structure. Such a bio-synthetic pattern is supported by the presence of the *wlaH* gene, which most probably encodes a galactosyltransferase linking a Gal residue to the lipid carrier, and the observation that almost all analyzed outer-core molecules from *C. jejuni* start with a Gal residue. A similar pattern of outer-core oligosaccharide synthesis has also been suggested for the outer core of *Yersinia enterocolitica,* where a Gal–lipid carrier transferase gene was also found to be present in the outer core synthesis gene cluster (55). The biosynthesis of the inner-core lipid A molecule is not likely to involve the *wla* genes. The product of the *waaC* gene attaches the first heptose to the Kdo-lipid A molecule, and the remaining inner-core heptoses are likely to be attached by products of genes flanking the region described here.

The proposed sugar transferases within the *wla* gene cluster consist of the Gal or GalNAc transferases, WlaC and WlaE, an unknown transferase, WlaD, a Gal transferase, WlaG, a Gal-to-lipid carrier transferase, WlaH, and a NeuNAc transferase, WlaI. If, as suggested above, the outer core is synthesized on a lipid carrier, WlaH probably initiates the synthesis of the outer core by transferring a Gal residue onto the lipid carrier. All but one of the known core molecules of *C. jejuni* contain a GalNAc residue bound to a backbone Gal residue. The proposed function of WlaC and WlaE as Gal-NAc transferases would predict the presence of a GalNAc residue in the outer core of strain 81116. However, the LPS molecule of strain NCTC 11168 does not contain a GalNac residue, whereas this strain does carry the *wlaC* and *wlaE* genes. All backbone Gal residues in the outer-core molecules of *C. jejuni* are branched with a NeuNAc residue, for which WlaI is the proposed transferase.

Three transport steps have been observed during LPS synthesis of *E. coli* and *Salmonella* spp. The first is transport of an oligosaccharide subunit attached to a lipid carrier across the inner membrane. The second is transfer of saccharide structures from a lipid carrier to the lipid A-core complex. The third is transport of the complete LPS molecule from the inner membrane to the outer membrane. We assume that the outer-core molecule in *C. jejuni* is synthesized at the cytoplasmic side of the inner membrane, like an LPS O-chain subunit. After completion, it has to be "flipped" to the periplasmic side of the inner membrane; this could occur before or after it has been ligated to the lipid A–inner-core complex. It is possible that WlaM is involved in the flippase process and that WlaF functions as a polymerase linking the flipped outer core to the lipid A–inner-core complex. The complete LOS molecule might then be translocated across the inner membrane to the outer membrane by WlaB.

ATTACHMENT OF O-CHAIN STRUCTURES

The observation that campylobacters produce LPS containing a lipid A-core and repeating O-chain-like structures suggests that some strains synthesize "classical" LPS, where the O-chain is attached to the outer-core oligosaccharide. The structural disruption of the outer core of *C. jejuni* LPS, as might result from the removal of galactose residues, is therefore predicted to affect O-chain attachment. However, the mutation of *galE* resulted in core changes without any associated effect on O-chain production. Therefore, the position or actuality of linkage of O-chain-like structures to the lipid A-core structures in *C. jejuni* can be questioned.

Polysaccharides that are not attached to lipid A-core structures have been found in *C. jejuni* (4, 47). It is possible, therefore, that *C. jejuni* also contains genes that encode enzymes involved in the production of another polysaccharide(s) and produce a lipid-linked polysaccharide rather than LPS. Interestingly, part of an ABC transporter system with closest similarity to genes involved in capsular polysaccharide biosynthesis has been identified in *C. jejuni* (30a); the mutation of these genes also has an effect on the production of O-chain in *C. jejuni*. It is possible that in some *C. jejuni* strains (for example, those without *wlaJ*), the polysaccharide is also added to lipid A-core. Such a structure would be analogous to the lipid A-core-linked enterobacterial common antigen (ECA$_{LPS}$) and lipid A-core-linked K antigen (K$_{LPS}$) (67).

The phenotype associated with the *galE* mutant supports our previous suggestion (20, 68) that the O-chain-like structure from *C. jejuni* is not linked to the LPS molecule and therefore resembles capsular polysaccharide or enterobacterial common antigen, as found in *E. coli*, and not LPS O-chain. This may imply that campylobacters are LOS producers, with some strains also containing an additional polysaccharide structure that is independent of core oligosaccharide. Inspection of the NCTC 11168 genome sequence (60) does not reveal the presence of genes encoding O-chain-specific enzymes like O-chain ligase, flippase, or chain length determinant (unpublished data). However, the fact that this strain does not produce an O-chain-like repeat might account for the absence of these genes.

FUTURE PERSPECTIVES

The processes of LPS and LOS biosynthesis gene identification and the analysis of the functions of these genes are now well under way for *C. jejuni*. The work will enable the construction of specific defined mutations with predicted effects on LPS and LOS structure and the subsequent determination of any role in colonization, invasion, or inflammation. Defined mutants will be particularly important for the study of the mechanisms involved in LPS-induced neuropathies such as Guillain-Barré syndrome. The role of molecular mimicry between NeuNAc-containing LPS epitopes and gangliosides could be investigated by the inactivation of NeuNAc transferases. Clearly, the identification of determinants necessary for the production of epitopes involved in molecular mimicry could form the basis of a predictive test for patients with *Campylobacter*-associated food-borne disease to determine the risk of neurological complications.

The variation found in polysaccharides including LOS forms the basis for the Penner serotyping system, and therefore the composition and arrangement of all the genes responsible for such polysaccharides could form a DNA-based approach to strain typing. In addition, the presence of certain genes within the clusters might be used for diagnostic purposes in a rapid species-specific test for campylobacters. The understanding of the genetic basis for LPS biosynthesis will also facilitate the design of strategies for the prevention of *Campylobacter*-mediated food-borne disease. If *Campylobacter* LPS and LOS is important in disease pathology but not intestinal colonization, any preventive strategy involving a probioticum in farm animals could take advantage of specific LPS and LOS mutants. Probioticum strains that express LPS and LOS structures that both attenuate virulence in humans and remove any subsequent risk of neurological complication could be constructed. Finally, vaccine strategies based on subunits or whole cells may need to include any protective LPS and LOS-based antigens, avoiding the specific epitopes involved in molecular mimicry of gangliosides.

ACKNOWLEDGMENTS

This work was funded by RMIT University, the Australian Chicken Meat Research and Development Corporation, the U.K. Department of Health, and the Biotechnology and Biological Sciences Research Council.

REFERENCES

1. **Allen, A., and D. Maskell.** 1996. The identification, cloning and mutagenesis of a genetic locus required for lipopolysaccharide biosynthesis in *Bordetella pertussis. Mol. Microbiol.* **19**:37–52.
2. **Alley, M. R., J. R. Maddock, and L. Shapiro.** 1992. Polar localization of a bacterial chemoreceptor. *Genes Dev.* **6**:825–836.
3. **Annunziato, P. W., L. F. Wright, W. F. Vann, and R. P. Silver.** 1995. Nucleotide sequence and genetic analysis of the *neuD* and *neuB* genes in region 2 of the polysialic acid gene cluster of *Escherichia coli* K1. *J. Bacteriol.* **177**:312–319.
4. **Aspinall, G. O., C. M. Lynch, H. Pang, R. T. Shaver, and A. P. Moran.** 1995. Chemical structures of the core region of *Campylobacter jejuni* O:3 lipopolysaccharide and an associated polysaccharide. *Eur. J. Biochem.* **231**:570–578.
5. **Aspinall, G. O., A. G. McDonald, and H. Pang.** 1994. Lipopolysaccharides of *Campylobacter jejuni* serotype O:19: structures of O antigen chains from the serostrain and two bacterial isolates from patients with the Guillain-Barré syndrome. *Biochemistry* **33**:250–255.
6. **Aspinall, G. O., A. G. McDonald, and H. Pang.** 1992. Structures of the O chains from lipopolysaccharides of *Campylobacter jejuni* serotypes O:23 and O:36. *Carbohydr. Res.* **231**:13–30.
7. Reference deleted
8. Reference deleted
9. Reference deleted
10. **Blaser, M. J., and L. B. Reller.** 1981. *Campylobacter* enteritis. *N. Engl. J. Med.* **305**:1444–1452.
11. **Blight, M. A., and I. B. Holland.** 1990. Structure and function of haemolysin B, P-glycoprotein and other members of a novel family of membrane translocators. *Mol. Microbiol.* **4**:873–880.
12. **Branquinho, M. R., C. S. Alviano, and I. D. Ricciardi.** 1983. Chemical composition and biological action of lipopolysaccharide (LPS) of *Campylobacter fetus* ss. *jejuni. Rev. Microbiol.* **14**:90–96.
13. **Burrows, L. L., D. F. Charter, and J. S. Lam.** 1996. Molecular characterization of the Pseudomonas aeruginosa serotype O5 (PAO1) B-band li-

popolysaccharide gene cluster. *Mol. Microbiol.* **22:** 481–495.

14. **Butzler, J. P., and M. B. Skirrow.** 1979. *Campylobacter* enteritis. *Clin. Gastroenterol.* **8:** 737–765.

15. **Clarke, B. R., D. Bronner, W. J. Keenleyside, W. B. Severn, J. C. Richards, and C. Whitfield.** 1995. Role of Rfe and RfbF in the initiation of biosynthesis of D-galactan I, the lipopolysaccharide O antigen from *Klebsiella pneumoniae* serotype O1. *J. Bacteriol.* **177:**5411–5418.

16. **Dicker, I. B., and S. Seetharam.** 1991. Cloning and nucleotide sequence of the *firA* gene and the *firA200*(Ts) allele from *Escherichia coli. J. Bacteriol.* **173:**334–344.

17. **Dicker, I. B., and S. Seetharam.** 1992. What is known about the structure and function of the *Escherichia coli* protein FirA? *Mol. Microbiol.* **6:** 817–23.

18. **Di Padova, F. E., H. Brade, G. R. Barclay, I. R. Poxton, E. Liehl, E. Schuetze, H. P. Kocher, G. Ramsay, M. H. Schreier, D. B. McClelland, and E. T. Rietschel.** 1993. A broadly cross-protective monoclonal antibody binding to *Escherichia coli* and *Salmonella* lipopolysaccharides. *Infect. Immun.* **61:**3863–3872.

19. **Everiss, K. D., K. J. Hughes, M. E. Kovach, and K. M. Peterson.** 1994. The *Vibrio cholerae acfB* colonization determinant encodes an inner membrane protein that is related to a family of signal-transducing proteins. *Infect. Immun.* **62:** 3289–3298.

20. **Fry, B. N., V. Korolik, J. A. ten Brinke, M. T. Pennings, R. Zalm, B. J. Teunis, P. J. Coloe, and B. A. van der Zeijst.** 1998. The lipopolysaccharide biosynthesis locus of *Campylobacter jejuni* 81116. *Microbiology* **144:**2049–2061.

21. **Glaser, P., F. Kunst, M. Arnaud, M. P. Coudart, W. Gonzales, M. F. Hullo, M. Ionescu, B. Lubochinsky, L. Marcelino, I. Moszer, et al.** 1993. *Bacillus subtilis* genome project: cloning and sequencing of the 97 kb region from 325 degrees to 333 degrees. *Mol. Microbiol.* **10:**371–384.

22. **Gohmann, S., P. A. Manning, C. A. Alpert, M. J. Walker, and K. N. Timmis.** 1994. Lipopolysaccharide O-antigen biosynthesis in *Shigella dysenteriae* serotype 1: analysis of the plasmid-carried *rfp* determinant. *Microb. Pathog.* **16:**53–64.

23. **Gygi, D., M. M. Rahman, H. C. Lai, R. Carlson, J. Guard-Petter, and C. Hughes.** 1995. A cell-surface polysaccharide that facilitates rapid population migration by differentiated swarm cells of *Proteus mirabilis. Mol. Microbiol.* **17:**1167–1175.

24. **Hackett, J., P. Wyk, P. Reeves, and V. Mathan.** 1987. Mediation of serum resistance in *Salmonella typhimurium* by an 11-kilodalton polypeptide encoded by the cryptic plasmid. *J. Infect. Dis.* **155:**540–549.

25. **Hammerschmidt, S., C. Birkholz, U. Zahringer, B. D. Robertson, J. van Putten, O. Ebeling, and M. Frosch.** 1994. Contribution of genes from the capsule gene complex (*cps*) to lipooligosaccharide biosynthesis and serum resistance in *Neisseria meningitidis. Mol. Microbiol.* **11:** 885–896.

26. **Higgins, C. F., S. C. Hyde, M. M. Mimmack, U. Gileadi, D. R. Gill, and M. P. Gallagher.** 1990. Binding protein-dependent transport systems. *J. Bioenerg. Biomembr.* **22:**571–592.

27. **Hirvas, L., P. Koski, and M. Vaara.** 1990. Primary structure and expression of the Sac-protein of *Salmonella typhimurium. Biochem. Biophys. Res. Commun.* **173:**53–59.

28. **Hood, D. W., M. E. Deadman, T. Allen, H. Masoud, A. Martin, J. R. Brisson, R. Fleischmann, J. C. Venter, J. C. Richards, and E. R. Moxon.** 1996. Use of the complete genome sequence information of *Haemophilus influenzae* strain Rd to investigate lipopolysaccharide biosynthesis. *Mol. Microbiol.* **22:**951–965.

29. **Jansson, P. E., A. A. Lindberg, B. Lindberg, and R. Wollin.** 1981. Structural studies on the hexose region of the core in lipopolysaccharides from *Enterobacteriaceae. Eur. J. Biochem.* **115:** 571–577.

30. **Joiner, K. A., N. Grossman, M. Schmetz, and L. Leive.** 1986. C3 binds preferentially to long-chain lipopolysaccharide during alternative pathway activation by *Salmonella montevideo. J. Immunol.* **136:**710–715.

30a. **Karlyshev, A.** Personal communication.

31. **Ketley, J. M.** 1997. Pathogenesis of enteric infection by *Campylobacter. Microbiology* **143:**5–21.

32. **Klena, J. D., S. A. Gray, and M. E. Konkel.** 1998. Cloning, sequencing, and characterization of the lipopolysaccharide biosynthetic enzyme heptosyltransferase I gene (*waaC*) from *Campylobacter jejuni* and *Campylobacter coli. Gene* **222:** 177–185.

33. **Korolik, V., B. N. Fry, M. R. Alderton, B. A. van der Zeijst, and P. J. Coloe.** 1997. Expression of *Campylobacter hyoilei* lipo-oligosaccharide (LOS) antigens in *Escherichia coli. Microbiology* **143:**3481–3489.

34. **Leclerc, G., S. P. Wang, and B. Ely.** 1998. A new class of *Caulobacter crescentus* flagellar genes. *J. Bacteriol.* **180:**5010–5019.

35. **Lesse, A. J., A. A. Campagnari, W. E. Bittner, and M. A. Apicella.** 1990. Increased resolution of lipopolysaccharides and lipooligosaccharides utilizing tricine-sodium dodecyl sulfate-polyacrylamide gel electrophoresis. *J. Immunol. Methods* **126:**109–117.

36. **Lin, W. S., T. Cunneen, and C. Y. Lee.** 1994. Sequence analysis and molecular characterization of genes required for the biosynthesis of type 1 capsular polysaccharide in *Staphylococcus aureus*. *J. Bacteriol.* **176:**7005–7016.

37. **Macpherson, D. F., P. A. Manning, and R. Morona.** 1994. Characterization of the dTDP-rhamnose biosynthetic genes encoded in the *rfb* locus of *Shigella flexneri*. *Mol. Microbiol.* **11:**281–292.

38. **Mandrell, R. E., and M. A. Apicella.** 1993. Lipo-oligosaccharides (LOS) of mucosal pathogens: molecular mimicry and host-modification of LOS. *Immunobiology* **187:**382–402.

39. **Manning, P. A., U. H. Stroeher, L. E. Karageorgos, and R. Morona.** 1995. Putative O-antigen transport genes within the *rfb* region of *Vibrio cholerae* O1 are homologous to those for capsule transport. *Gene* **158:**1–7.

40. **McSweegan, E., and R. I. Walker.** 1986. Identification and characterization of two *Campylobacter jejuni* adhesins for cellular and mucous substrates. *Infect. Immun.* **53:**141–148.

41. **Mills, S. D., B. Kuzniar, B. Shames, L. A. Kurjanczyk, and J. L. Penner.** 1992. Variation of the O antigen of *Campylobacter jejuni* in vivo. *J. Med. Microbiol.* **36:**215–219.

42. **Moran, A. P.** 1995. Biological and serological characterization of *Campylobacter jejuni* lipopolysaccharides with deviating core and lipid A structures. *FEMS Immunol. Med. Microbiol.* **11:**121–130.

43. Reference deleted

44. **Nachamkin, I., B. M. Allos, and T. Ho.** 1998. *Campylobacter* species and Guillain-Barré syndrome. *Clin. Microbiol. Rev.* **11:**555–567.

45. **Naess, V., and T. Hofstad.** 1984. Chemical composition and biological activity of lipopolysaccharides prepared from type strains of *Campylobacter jejuni* and *Campylobacter coli*. *Acta Pathol. Microbiol. Immunol. Scand. Sect. B* **92:**217–222.

46. **Penner, J. L., and J. N. Hennessy.** 1980. Passive hemagglutination technique for serotyping *Campylobacter fetus* subsp. *jejuni* on the basis of soluble heat-stable antigens. *J. Clin. Microbiol.* **12:**732–737.

47. **Prendergast, M. M., A. J. Lastovica, and A. P. Moran.** 1998. Lipopolysaccharides from *Campylobacter jejuni* O:41 strains associated with Guillain-Barré syndrome exhibit mimicry of GM1 ganglioside. *Infect. Immun.* **66:**3649–3655.

48. **Preston, A., R. E. Mandrell, B. W. Gibson, and M. A. Apicella.** 1996. The lipooligosaccharides of pathogenic Gram-negative bacteria. *Crit. Rev. Microbiol.* **22:**139–180.

49. **Preston, M. A., and J. L. Penner.** 1987. Structural and antigenic properties of lipopolysaccharides from serotype reference strains of *Campylobacter jejuni*. *Infect. Immun.* **55:**1806–1812.

50. **Reeves, P. R.** 1994. Biosynthesis and assembly of lipopolysaccharide, p. 281–317. *In* J.-M. Ghuysen and R. Hakenbeck (ed.), *Bacterial Cell Wall*. Elsevier Science, Amsterdam, The Netherlands.

51. **Reeves, P. R., M. Hobbs, M. A. Valvano, M. Skurnik, C. Whitfield, D. Coplin, N. Kido, J. Klena, D. Maskell, C. R. H. Raetz, and P. D. Rick.** 1996. Bacterial polysaccharide synthesis and gene nomenclature. *Trends Microbiol.* **4:**495–503.

52. **Robertson, B. D., M. Frosch, and J. P. van Putten.** 1994. The identification of cryptic rhamnose biosynthesis genes in *Neisseria gonorrhoeae* and their relationship to lipopolysaccharide biosynthesis. *J. Bacteriol.* **176:**6915–6920.

53. Reference deleted

54. **Schnaitman, C. A., and J. D. Klena.** 1993. Genetics of lipopolysaccharide biosynthesis in enteric bacteria. *Microbiol. Rev.* **57:**655–682.

55. **Skurnik, M., R. Venho, P. Toivanen, and A. al-Hendy.** 1995. A novel locus of *Yersinia enterocolitica* serotype O:3 involved in lipopolysaccharide outer core biosynthesis. *Mol. Microbiol.* **17:**575–594.

56. **Stern, N. J., J. S. Bailey, L. C. Blankenship, N. A. Cox, and F. McHan.** 1988. Colonization characteristics of *Campylobacter jejuni* in chick ceca. *Avian Dis.* **32:**330–334.

57. **Stinavage, P., L. E. Martin, and J. K. Spitznagel.** 1989. O antigen and lipid A phosphoryl groups in resistance of *Salmonella typhimurium* LT-2 to nonoxidative killing in human polymorphonuclear neutrophils. *Infect. Immun.* **57:**3894–3900.

58. **Szabo, M., D. Bronner, and C. Whitfield.** 1995. Relationships between *rfb* gene clusters required for biosynthesis of identical D-galactose-containing O antigens in *Klebsiella pneumoniae* serotype O1 and *Serratia marcescens* serotype O16. *J. Bacteriol.* **177:**1544–1553.

59. **Tauxe, R. V.** 1992. Epidemiology of *Campylobacter jejuni* infections in the United States and other industrialized nations, p. 9–19. *In* I. Nachamkin, M. J. Blaser, and L. S. Tompkins (ed.), *Campylobacter jejuni: Current Status and Future Trends*. American Society for Microbiology, Washington, D.C.

60. **The Sanger Centre—*Campylobacter jejuni*.** 26 January 1999, revision date. [Online.] http://www.sanger.ac.uk/Projects/C_jejuni/. [1 June 1999, last date accessed.]

61. **Thorson, J. S., S. F. Lo, and H.-W. Liu.** 1993. Biosynthesis of 3,6-dideoxyhexoses: new mechanistic reflections upon 2,6-dideoxy, 4,6-dideoxy, and amino sugar construction. *J. Am. Chem. Soc.* **115:**6993–6994.

62. **Vaara, M.** 1992. Eight bacterial proteins, includ-

ing UDP-*N*-acetylglucosamine acyltransferase (LpxA) and three other transferases of *Escherichia coli*, consist of a six-residue periodicity theme. *FEMS Microbiol Lett.* **76:**249–254.

63. **van Vliet, A. H. M., K. G. Wooldridge, and J. M. Ketley.** 1998. Iron-responsive gene regulation in a *Campylobacter jejuni fur* mutant. *J. Bacteriol.* **180:**5291–5298.

64. **Vuorio, R., T. Harkonen, M. Tolvanen, and M. Vaara.** 1994. The novel hexapeptide motif found in the acyltransferases LpxA and LpxD of lipid A biosynthesis is conserved in various bacteria. *FEBS Lett.* **337:**289–292.

65. **Wang, L., D. Liu, and P. R. Reeves.** 1996. C-terminal half of *Salmonella enterica* WbaP (RfbP) is the galactosyl-1-phosphate transferase domain catalyzing the first step of O-antigen synthesis. *J. Bacteriol.* **178:**2598–2604.

66. **Wang, L., and P. R. Reeves.** 1994. Involvement of the galactosyl-1-phosphate transferase encoded by the *Salmonella enterica rfbP* gene in O-antigen subunit processing. *J. Bacteriol.* **176:**4348–4356.

67. **Whitfield, C., P. A. Amor, and R. Koplin.** 1997. Modulation of the surface architecture of gram-negative bacteria by the action of surface polymer:lipid A-core ligase and by determinants of polymer chain length. *Mol. Microbiol.* **23:**629–638.

68. **Wood, A. C., N. J. Oldfield, C. A. O'Dwyer, and J. M. Ketley.** 1999. Cloning, mutation and distribution of a putative lipopolysaccharide biosynthesis locus in *Campylobacter jejuni*. *Microbiology* **145:**379–388.

69. **Wooldridge, K. G., and J. M. Ketley.** 1997. Campylobacter-host cell interactions. *Trends Microbiol.* **5:**96–102.

70. **Yao, R., D. H. Burr, and P. Guerry.** 1997. CheY-mediated modulation of *Campylobacter jejuni* virulence. *Mol. Microbiol.* **23:**1021–1031.

71. **Yoshida, S., Y. Ohya, A. Nakano, and Y. Anraku.** 1995. *STT3,* a novel essential gene related to the PKC1/STT1 protein kinase pathway, is involved in protein glycosylation in yeast. *Gene* **164:**167–172.

STRUCTURE, FUNCTION, AND ANTIGENICITY OF *CAMPYLOBACTER* FLAGELLA

Patricia Guerry, Richard Alm, Christine Szymanski, and Trevor J. Trust

20

Researchers have been intrigued by the single polar flagellum of *Campylobacter* spp. from the earliest descriptions of the genus. The rapid darting motility of *Campylobacter* spp. is unusual and can be used to presumptively diagnose the organism in wet mounts of stools. Moreover, motility is absolutely necessary for campylobacters to colonize animals and ultimately to cause disease. Campylobacters, unlike other enteric pathogens, show enhanced motility in highly viscous solutions, such as mucus, that immobilize peritrichously flagellated bacteria (20, 77). Moreover, campylobacters appear to swim in markedly different patterns in media of low viscosity from those used in media of high viscosity (73, 77). Studies by Ferrero and Lee (20) with freshly prepared scrapings of mouse intestines showed that *C. jejuni* can swim very actively in mucus-filled crypts without any evidence of direct attachment to epithelial cells (66). This motility, as discussed below, is key to initial colonization of intestinal tracts by campylobacters. Moreover, the flagellin subunit is the immunodominant antigen recognized during human and animal infection and has been suggested to be an epithelial cell adhesin (51) and a protective antigen (49). This chapter reviews the current data on the structure, function, and antigenicity of campylobacter flagella and analyzes the genetics of flagellar biogenesis.

FLAGELLIN STRUCTURAL GENES

The flagella of *Campylobacter* spp. are complex, being composed of two related subunits, FlaA and FlaB. These two flagellins, both of which have an approximate predicted M_r of 59,000 and are >93% homologous to each other, are encoded by genes which are adjacent on the chromosome but regulated by distinct promoters. The *flaA* gene is regulated by the classical flagellin promoter, σ^{28}, and the *flaB* gene, like some flagellin genes from *Caulobacter crescentus*, is regulated by a σ^{54} promoter (26, 61). In *C. coli* VC167, the two genes are expressed concomitantly, but under normal laboratory conditions, *flaA* is expressed at much higher levels than *flaB* (27). Mutation of *flaA* in VC167 resulted in the synthesis of a truncated flagellar filament, composed exclusively of FlaB. This truncated flagellar filament conferred greatly reduced motility compared to that of a wild-type flagellum. Mutation of *flaB* in VC167 resulted in a flagellar filament which was indistinguishable from the wild-type filament in length and with motility that was re-

Patricia Guerry and Christine Szymanski, Enteric Diseases Program, Naval Medical Research Center, National Naval Medical Center, 8901 Wisconsin Ave., Bethesda, MD 20889-5607. *Richard Alm and Trevor J. Trust,* Astra Research Center Boston, 128 Sidney St., Cambridge, MA 02139-4239.

Campylobacter, 2nd Ed., Edited by I. Nachamkin and M. J. Blaser
© 2000 American Society for Microbiology, Washington, D.C.

duced only slightly compared to that of a wild-type cell. Thus, expression of both flagellins appears to be necessary for maximal motility. Similar results have been reported for *C. jejuni* 81116, but in that organism, no *flaB*-specific mRNA was detected except in a *flaA* background, causing Wassenaar et al. (83) to conclude that *flaB* is not normally expressed in *C. jejuni*. An alternative explanation is that the low levels of *flaB*-specific mRNA were not detected experimentally.

It appears that all strains of *C. jejuni* and *C. coli* have two flagellin genes (6). However, the reasons why campylobacters maintain two highly related flagellin genes in a tandem and, one would predict, unstable configuration are speculative. The σ^{54} promoter of *flaB*, like σ^{54} promoters in other bacteria, has been shown to be environmentally regulated by using gene fusions to a promoterless chloramphenicol resistance gene (5). Thus, the levels of FlaB in the filament may be modulated according to growth conditions, subsequently affecting the level of motility. In addition, *flaB* appears able to serve as a "backup" gene copy of flagellin. Alm et al. (7) reported the isolation of revertants of a *flaA* mutant of *C. coli* VC167 in which the *flaB* information had recombined into the adjacent *flaA* gene which had been insertionally inactivated with a kanamycin resistance gene. The resulting Km^s, fully motile revertants expressed a hybrid flagellin composed of the N terminus of FlaA fused to the carboxy end of FlaB, under the control of the *flaA* σ^{28} promoter. Similar results were subsequently reported in *C. jejuni* (84).

MUTATIONAL ANALYSIS OF OTHER FLAGELLAR GENES

Surprisingly few genes necessary for flagellar biogenesis or regulation have been studied in campylobacters. However, the limited data available suggest some important distinctions from the flagella systems of the family *Enterobacteriaceae*. The genes, other than the flagellin structural genes, which have been characterized experimentally to date are summarized below.

The rotation of the flagellar filament is driven by a complex motor located within the cell envelope which is connected to the filament through an axial coupling structure, the flagellar hook. The 105- by 24-nm campylobacter hook, which is one of the longest bacterial hooks described, displays a conical protrusion at the proximal end, a concave cavity at the distal end, and helically arranged subunits. The average apparent subunit molecular weight of the campylobacter hook subunit protein as determined by sodium dodecyl sulfate polyacrylamide gel electrophoresis (SDS-PAGE) is 92,500, which is significantly larger than that of other bacterial hook proteins. The hook proteins of *Helicobacter pylori* and *H. mustelae* are 78,000 Da (65), while those of other bacteria range from 42,000 to 70,000 Da (2, 16, 40). The large sizes of both the hook subunit and the hook structure may reflect the need for campylobacters to be motile in the thick mucous blanket of the intestine. Several studies have suggested that the flagellar hook, which protrudes from the surface of the cell, contributes to the serological diversity of campylobacters (33, 45, 54, 70). The *flgE* gene, encoding the hook protein, has been cloned from both *C. coli* VC167 (37) and several strains of *C. jejuni* (24). The gene is regulated by a σ^{54} promoter, which, interestingly, has a different putative upstream enhancer sequence from the σ^{54} promoter of *flaB* and appears to be transcribed at higher levels than *flaB* (36). The amino and carboxy ends of FlgE proteins are conserved among different campylobacter strains (37, 47, 70), and the central region, which presumably contains the surface-exposed, serospecific epitopes, is hypervariable, much like the structure of the flagellin subunits. Mutational analyses have indicated that the carboxy terminus of FlgE is necessary for assembly of the hook structure but not for secretion of FlgE (36). Additionally, in a *flgE* background, flagellin accumulates intracellularly in *Campylobacter* (36). This is consistent with the lack of a FlgM homolog in campylobacter (see below) and represents a major distinction between the flagellar regulatory cascades of *Campylobacter* spp. and the *Enterobacteriaceae.*

The *flhA* gene, originally designated *flbA,* was cloned by Miller et al. (53) based on homology to the LcrD/FlbF family of proteins involved in flagellar transport and type III secretion. Mutation of this gene in *C. jejuni* 81-176 resulted in loss of motility with no intracellular accumulation of flagellin.

The *pflA* gene (for "paralyzed flagella") was initially identified by selection for noninvasive mutants (reference 88 and see below). Strains with mutations in this gene synthesized a nonfunctional flagellar filament of the same length as that of the wild type but with slight morphological differences observed in the basal region of the flagellum by electron microscopy (88). The PflA protein, which is predicted to be a membrane associated protein with an M_r of 90,997, is likely to be involved in motor function.

A gene encoding a putative GTP-binding protein required for flagellar biogenesis has been identified in *C. jejuni* 81-176 (38). Interestingly, homologs of this gene, called *flhF,* are found in *Bacillus subtilis, Treponema pallidum, Borrelia burgdorferi,* and *H. pylori* but not in members of the *Enterobacteriaceae.* Mutants of strain 81-176 defective in *flhF* fail to synthesize either the flagellin subunits or hook protein, suggesting a flagellar regulatory cascade which affects both the σ^{28} and σ^{54} promoters.

OTHER FLAGELLAR GENES OF *CAMPYLOBACTER* SPP.

As summarized above, only a handful of genes involved in flagellar biosynthesis and function have been experimentally characterized in *C. jejuni,* unlike *Escherichia coli,* where 50 genes have been identified (48) (Table 1). *E. coli* MG1655 protein sequences (GenBank accession no. U00096) were used to identify the orthologous genes involved in flagellar biosynthesis and function from the recently completed *C. jejuni* NCTC 11168 genome (http://www.sanger.ac.uk/Projects/C. jejuni). There were 11 genes in *E. coli* for which orthologs could not be identified in *C. jejuni.* The precise

functions of five of these genes in *E. coli* remain unknown. Significantly, *C. jejuni* does not contain the anti-sigma factor FlgM, which binds to the α^{28} factor (FliA) and prevents it from binding to the α^{28}-specific promoters (class 3), or the FliT protein, which regulates FlgM export (90). This finding supports the experimental evidence mentioned above that *C. jejuni* mutants with mutations in the flagellar hook gene (*flgE*) still produce intracellular, unassembled flagellin (37). This lack of regulation in the flagellar hierarchy of *C. jejuni* is also evidenced by the absence of the FlhC and FlhD orthologs, which, in *E. coli,* combine to produce a DNA-binding complex which regulates the expression of class 2 flagellar genes (43). The remaining two *E. coli* proteins absent in *C. jejuni* NCTC 11168 are the CheY phosphatase (CheZ) and the FliK protein, which controls the length of the flagellar hook (Table 1). Analysis of the *C. jejuni* NCTC 11168 genome sequence has identified 12 additional genes associated with flagellar biogenesis which are not found in *E. coli* (Table 1). The products of two of these, PflA and FlhF, have been shown experimentally to be involved in flagellar function, as mentioned above, whereas the others show homology to proteins involved in flagellar biogenesis in other bacterial species. Most of these proteins display homology to proteins of unknown function, although CJ0285 encodes a CheV homolog. The CheV protein possesses a CheW domain fused to a response regulator domain of the CheY family, and the CheA-dependent phosphorylation of CheV is predicted to play a role in adaptation (72).

Significantly, all of the genes identified in *C. jejuni* which are absent in *E. coli,* except CJ0720, have orthologs in the closely related species *H. pylori.* The flagellar biogenesis system of *H. pylori,* with its complex flagellar filament made up of two distinct flagellin species (FlaA and FlaB), is very similar to that of *C. jejuni,* although the two *H. pylori* flagellin genes are not tandemly arranged. *H. pylori* lacks the same 11 genes as *C. jejuni* compared to *E. coli,* and, of all the *C. jejuni* genes in Table 1, there

TABLE 1 *C. jejuni* proteins involved in flagellar biosynthesis and function

Protein	Function	Protein no. (length in amino acids) in:	
		E. coli	*C. jejuni*
E. coli flagellar proteins			
FlgN	Unknown	1070 (138)	—[a]
FlgM	Anti-sigma factor	1071 (97)	—
FlgA	P-ring assembly protein	1072 (219)	769 (220)
FlgB	Cell-proximal portion of basal-body rod	1073 (138)	528 (143)
FlgC	Cell-proximal portion of basal-body rod	1074 (134)	527 (164)
FlgD	Hook cap, scaffold (initiation of hook assembly)	1075 (231)	42 (294)
FlgE[c]	Hook protein	1076 (402)	1729 (865)
FlgF	Cell-proximal portion of basal-body rod	1077 (251)	697 (270)
FlgG	Cell-distal portion of basal-body rod	1078 (260)	698 (263)
FlgH	Basal-body L ring	1079 (232)	687 (232)
FlgI	Basal-body P ring	1080 (365)	1462 (348)
FlgJ	Unknown	1081 (313)	—
FlgK	Hook-filament junction protein	1082 (547)	1466 (608)
FlgL	Hook-filament junction protein	1083 (317)	887 (750)
FlhE	Unknown	1878 (130)	—
FlhA[c]	Export apparatus	1879 (692)	82 (724)
FlhB	Unknown	1880 (382)	35 (362)
CheZ	Che Y phosphatase	1881 (214)	—
CheY[c]	Switch regulator	1882 (129)	1118 (130)
CheB	Methylesterase	1883 (349)	924 (184)
CheR	Methyltransferase	1884 (286)	923 (262)
Tap	Dipeptide MCP	1885 (533)	MCP[d]
Tar	Aspartate MCP	1886 (553)	MCP[d]
CheW	CheA-positive regulator	1887 (167)	283 (178)
CheA	CheY/CheB kinase	1888 (654)	284 (769)
MotB	Motor rotation	1889 (308)	336 (247)
MotA	Motor rotation	1890 (295)	337 (258)
FlhC	Positive regulation of gene expression	1891 (192)	—
FlhD	Positive regulation of gene expression	1892 (119)	—
FliA[c]	Sigma factor (σ^{28})	1922 (239)	61 (238)
FliC[c]	Flagellin subunit	1923 (498)	1339&1338 (572)
FliD	Filament cap protein	1924 (468)	548 (642)
FliS	Filament elongation protein	1925 (136)	549 (128)
FliT	Negative regulation of FlgM export	1926 (121)	—
FliE	Basal-body protein (possibly at MS-ring–rod junction)	1937 (104)	526 (98)
FliF	Basal-body MS-ring and collar protein	1938 (552)	318 (560)
FliG	Motor switch and energizing protein	1939 (331)	319 (343)
FliH	Export apparatus?	1940 (235)	320 (276)
FliI	Export apparatus?	1941 (457)	195 (461)
FliJ	Unknown	1942 (147)	—
FliK	Hook length control	1943 (375)	—
FliL	Unknown	1944 (154)	1408 (178)
FliM	Motor switch and energizing protein	1945 (334)	60 (359)
FliN	Motor switch and energizing protein	1946 (137)	351 (103)
FliO	Unknown	1947 (101)	—
FliP	Export apparatus?	1948 (245)	820 (244)
FliQ	Export apparatus?	1949 (89)	1675 (89)
FliR	Export apparatus?	1950 (261)	1179 (255)
Tsr	Serine MCP	4355 (551)	MCP[d]
Trg	Ribose and galactose MCP	1421 (546)	MCP[d]

Continued

TABLE 1 *(continued)*

Protein	Function	Designation (length in amino acids) in: E. coli	Designation (length in amino acids) in: C. jejuni
C. jejuni-specific proteins			
—[e]	Unknown	—[a]	950 (144)
PflA[e]	Motor switch and energizing protein	—[a]	1565 (788)
—[e]	Unknown	—[a]	176 (43)
—[f]	Motor switch and energizing protein	—[a]	59 (280)
FlhF[c]	Unknown	—[a]	64 (484)
—[g]	Unknown	—[a]	547 (121)
FlbA★[h]	Unknown	—[a]	1313 (157)
—[c]	Unknown	—[a]	371 (201)
[i]	Unknown	—[a]	848 (93)
—[j]	Unknown	—[a]	43 (545)
CheV	Chemotaxis (CheW–CheY fusion)	—[a]	285 (318)
—[h]	Unknown	—[a]	720 (249)

[a] —, ortholog not found.
[b] Homology JHP1370, with homology to P-ring assembly protein (FlgA).
[c] Proteins encoded by genes shown experimentally to be involved in flagellar biosynthesis and function. The two structural genes in *C. jejuni* are called *flaA* and *flaB*, not *fliC* as in *E. coli*.
[d] Several proteins contain the conserved motif found in methyl-accepting chemotaxis proteins. They are (lengths in parentheses) 1506 (701), 144 (660), 1564 (663), 262 (666), 1190 (475), 1110 (430), 448 (366), 19 (593), 951 (225), and 246 (376).
[e] Has homology to *H. pylori* proteins shown phenotypically to be involved in motility.
[f] Has homology to the *B. subtilis* FliY/CheD protein.
[g] Has homology to the FlaG protein from *P. aeruginosa* and *A. salmonicida*.
[h] Has homology to the *C. crescentus* FlaG/FlbA protein.
[i] Has homology in the C-terminal domain of FlhB.
[j] Has similarity to FlgE (hook) proteins of several species.
[k] Has similarity to flagellin subunit genes.

are only 3 which do not have orthologs in either of the sequenced *H. pylori* strains (8, 80). These encode CheR and CheB, enzymes which add methyl groups to or remove methyl groups from, respectively, the methyl-chemoaccepting proteins (MCPs), precisely modulating the chemotactic response, suggesting that the chemotaxis observed in *H. pylori* may occur by a CheB- and CheR-independent mechanism, similar to that seen in CheB and CheR mutants of *E. coli* (76). The other gene found in *C. jejuni* but not in *H. pylori* is CJ0720, which encodes a 249-amino-acid protein with significant homology to the structural flagellin subunits and was previously called *flaC* (GenBank accession no. U85622). In addition, while *C. jejuni* possesses only one CheV homolog, both sequenced *H. pylori* genomes contain a paralogous CheV family consisting of three members.

Apart from the differences discussed above, the flagellar systems of *C. jejuni* and *H. pylori*

appear the same and contain several unique proteins, including PflA (CJ1565 or JHP1195), discussed above. Additionally, both *H. pylori* and *C. jejuni* contain a protein, JHP0844 and CJ0043, respectively, which is predicted to be located in the basal-body complex. These proteins have homology to several other proteins which are located in the basal-body complex, including FlgE, FlgG, FlgF, and FlgK. It should be mentioned that three genes are identified in *C. jejuni* as flagellar genes because of homology to unique *H. pylori* genes which have been phenotypically associated with motility in that organism (64) (Table 1).

PHYSICAL ORGANIZATION OF FLAGELLAR GENES

The 50 flagellar biogenesis genes in *E. coli* whose products are listed in Table 1 are located in six distinct clusters. Region I (proteins 1070 to 1083) contains the majority of the structural genes for the basal-body complex, whereas region II (bases 1878 to 1892) largely contains genes involved in regulation and function (*mot* and *che*). The final two clusters, regions IIIa (bases 1922 to 1926) and IIIb (bases 1937 to 1950), are separated by approximately 6.6 kb and appear to contain many of the genes involved in the flagellar export apparatus, as well as the flagellar filament structural gene (FliC) and the flagellar sigma factor (FliA). Two of the MCP genes, *tsr* and *trg*, are located as single genes. In contrast to this highly organized physical arrangement of flagellar genes in *E. coli*, the 48 genes in *C. jejuni* are scattered across the genome at 32 individual loci. There are several smaller gene clusters, some of which contain adjacent genes in the same physical arrangement as found in *E. coli* whereas others are made up of genes from distinct *E. coli* regions. The largest gene cluster with a common arrangement between the two species is that containing the *fliF, fliG,* and *fliH* genes. Other common gene arrangements are the *flgF* and *flgG* genes as well as the *motA* and *motB* genes, which in *C. jejuni* lie adjacent to the *flhB* gene (Table 1). The *flgB* and *flgC* genes, encoding two of the basal-body rod proteins, are adjacent in both *E. coli* and *C. jejuni*, although in *C. jejuni* they are linked to the *fliE* gene, which also encodes a basal-body structural protein. *C. jejuni* has two clusters of *che* genes similar to the arrangement in *E. coli*; *cheB* and *cheR* are adjacent, as are *cheW* and *cheA*, which in *C. jejuni* are linked to *cheV*. There are three additional gene clusters which involve genes not found in *E. coli*. These are *fliD* and *fliS* linked to CJ0547; *fliA, fliM,* and CJ0059; and *flgD* and CJ0043 (Table 1). Significantly, most of the clusters of genes in *C. jejuni* are also conserved in arrangement in *H. pylori*. These include *fliE, flgB,* and *flgC; fliF, fliG,* and *fliH; fliA, fliM,* and the CJ0059 ortholog; *fliD, fliS,* and the CJ0547 ortholog; and *cheW* and *cheA* genes linked to one of the *cheV* paralogs. While *motA* and *motB* are linked in *H. pylori*, they are not adjacent to the *flhB* gene.

METHYL CHEMOACCEPTING GENES

The four MCPs identified in *E. coli* are all between 533 and 553 amino acids in length, and contain a highly conserved signaling domain which lies between the two methylating helices (MH1 and MH2). This conserved signaling domain has been also found in other bacterial proteins which are probably involved in signal transduction pathways other than chemotaxis, such as fimbria-mediated twitching motility in *Pseudomonas aeruginosa* (15), cell aggregation to form fruiting bodies in *Myxococcus xanthus* (50), or hemolysin secretion in *Vibrio cholerae* (9). Analysis of the *C. jejuni* NCTC 11168 genomic sequence identified 10 proteins which contained strong similarity to the MCP signaling domain (Table 1). It is not known how many of these are involved in flagellar chemotaxis or whether some are involved in other cellular processes. However, they appear to fall into three clusters based on their size. Five of them (CJ0019, CJ0144, CJ0262, CJ1506, and CJ1564) are between 593 and 701 amino acid residues, whereas the others are smaller. In contrast, *H. pylori* contains only four proteins with this characteristic MCP signaling motif, and these proteins range in size from 433 to 675 amino acids.

FLAGELLAR PHASE VARIATION

The ability of some strains of *C. jejuni* to turn the expression of flagella on and off in vitro at relatively high frequencies has been termed phase variation (13). Nuijten et al. showed that *flaA* was not transcribed in such nonmotile phase variants (62), although the FlaB protein could be detected (63). They also reported that the hook and basal bodies were not synthesized in phase variants (63), although no molecular mechanisms were suggested. Surprisingly, these studies remain the only molecular characterizations of phase variation. Wenman et al. found that a nonmotile phase variant of *C. jejuni* lost the ability to be serotyped in the heat-labile serotyping scheme of Lior (86). This led to the still widely held misconception that flagellin is the serodeterminant of the Lior scheme. However, using site-specific mutations of the flagellin genes in multiple strains of eight different Lior serotypes, Alm et al. (3) showed that a *flaA* mutant of a Lior 4 strain became nontypeable but that mutants with similar site-specific mutations in the other seven serotypes retained their ability to be serotyped. This indicated first that the Lior serodeterminant varies among different serotypes and second that in most cases the serodeterminant is not flagellin. Thus, the observations of Wenman et al. (86) that a spontaneously isolated nonmotile phase variant lost the ability to be serotyped would suggest that phase variation may affect additional genes beyond flagellin, including, at least in some strains, the Lior serodeterminants. It is an intriguing possibility that virulence gene expression is also coordinately regulated with motility genes, similar to systems described in better-characterized pathogens (66).

ASSOCIATION OF FLAGELLA WITH VIRULENCE

It has long been recognized that motility is necessary for intestinal colonization of campylobacters in animals. Nonmotile (56) and actively motile but nonchemotactic (79) mutants of *C. jejuni* made by chemical mutagenesis could not colonize animal intestinal tracts. Nonmotile phase variants became fully motile when fed to rabbits (13) or hamsters (1); also, Black et al. (11) showed that a mixture of motile and nonmotile cells became fully motile when fed to human volunteers. Subsequent work with site-specific flagellin mutants indicated that nonflagellated strains showed defects in colonization in both rabbits (67) and chickens (58, 85).

Motility also appears necessary for campylobacters to adhere to and invade tissue culture cells in vitro. Independent work by Grant et al. (25) and Wassenaar et al. (83) showed that *flaA* mutants but not *flaB* mutants of *C. jejuni* 81116 were noninvasive for epithelial cells in vitro. However, these data could not distinguish a need for motility per se from a requirement for the FlaA protein. Yao et al. (88) re-

ported on a fully flagellated but nonmotile (paralyzed) mutant of 81-176 mutated in a gene described above (*pflA*). This mutant adhered to INT407 cells at approximately 40% of the levels of wild-type 81-176 but invaded at only about 1% the level of the parent strain. These data suggested that immobilized campylobacter flagellin might function as an adhesin but could not mediate subsequent internalization into the INT407 cells. This is consistent with earlier work of McSweegan and Walker, who showed that purified campylobacter flagellin could bind to INT407 cells but could not block the subsequent adherence of living bacteria (51). Thus, flagellin may function as one of multiple adhesins reported for *Campylobacter* (39, 68), but the functional significance of this adhesin in vivo is unknown.

Modulation of the levels of the CheY protein, a signal transducer involved in chemotaxis, can also affect adherence and invasion (89). A *cheY* mutant of 81-176 adhered to and invaded INT407 cells at approximately three times the level of wild-type 81-176, similar to results reported for *cheY* mutants of *Salmonella typhimurium* (34, 35). However, a *cheY* mutant of 81-176 was unable to colonize mice, again emphasizing the importance of motility and chemotaxis for campylobacter survival in vivo (89). When a second copy of the *cheY* gene was introduced into wild-type 81-176 on a shuttle plasmid in *trans* or inserted into the nonessential arylsulfatase gene (90) on the chromosome, the resulting strains adhered to and invaded at 5 to 10% of the levels of the parental strain (89). This effect of CheY levels on adherence and invasion again suggests the possibility of coordinate regulation of motility and virulence determinants.

Interestingly, this association of motility and virulence has now been extended to the ability of *C. jejuni* to induce cytokines in vitro, a newly recognized aspect of campylobacter pathogenesis. Adherence and/or invasion also appears to be associated with the ability of live *C. jejuni* to induce the release of interleukin-8 (IL-8) from INT407 cells (30). Thus, mutations in a flagellar gene (*flaA* or *pflA*) or the putative adhesin gene *peblA* (68) resulted in significant reductions in the ability of 81-176 to induce the release of IL-8. Moreover, the effects of *cheY* copy number on adherence and/or invasion were also reflected in IL-8 induction levels. Thus, in experiments reported by Hickey et al. (30), wild-type strain 81-176 induced the release of 652 ± 34 pg of IL-8 per ml from INT407 cells. An isogenic *cheY* mutant induced 1,482 ± 78 pg of IL-8 per ml ($P <$ 0.001), and a strain with a second chromosomal copy of *cheY* produced only 194 ± 24 pg of IL-8 per ml ($P < 0.001$). Thus, the ability of live *C. jejuni* cells to induce IL-8 release from INT-407 cells appears to be directly related to its ability to adhere to and/or invade these eukaryotic cells, which is in turn modulated by motility and chemotaxis.

FLAGELLAR ANTIGENIC VARIATION AND POSTTRANSLATIONAL MODIFICATIONS

In numerous early studies on campylobacter flagella, flagellin was often observed as a broad, diffusely staining band in SDS-PAGE or in immunoblots, suggesting the presence of flagellins with different subunit molecular weights. In some strains, two distinct flagellin bands were observed (29, 36). In strains of the Lior 8 serogroup, these two bands were ultimately shown to represent antigenic variants (29). Cultivation of the progeny of a single colony of *C. coli* VC167, which was originally the type strain of the Lior 8 serogroup, in the presence of an antiserum which recognized one antigenic type of flagellin enabled the isolation of cells producing the second antigenic type. This variation was reversible, since subsequent growth of this second antigenic type in a specific serum allowed reisolation of the original antigenic type of flagellin. Cells producing the antigenic type 1 (T1) flagellin produced a flagellin with an apparent M_r on SDS-PAGE gels of 61,500, which was reactive with the type 1-specific serum (LAH1) but not with the type 2-specific serum (LAH2). Cells expressing the antigenic type 2 (T2) flagellin produced a fla-

gellin with an apparent M_r of 59,500, which was LAH1$^-$ LAH2$^+$. When nonimmune rabbits were infected with antigenic T1 cells, campylobacters isolated from the feces of these animals initially produced the M_r 61,500 LAH1$^+$ LAH2$^-$ flagellin, but over the course of the infection, the antigenic type gradually changed such that all isolates eventually produced the M_r 59,500 LAH1$^-$ LAH2$^+$ flagellin. Rabbits which were infected with antigenic T2 cells shed campylobacters producing the M_r 59,500 LAH1$^-$ LAH2$^+$ flagellin throughout the infection (44). These data suggest that cells producing the antigenic T2 flagellin have an in vivo advantage.

The mechanism of this antigenic variation did not involve changes in the amounts of FlaA or FlaB in the filament or changes in primary amino acid sequences within the flagellin gene products (27, 46). Rather, a number of lines of evidence suggested that campylobacter flagellins are posttranslationally modified and that the differences between T1 and T2 flagellin were due to changes in these posttranslational modifications as follows. (i) Numerous blocked amino acids in campylobacter flagellin were identified by N-terminal amino acid sequencing of internal peptides, and subsequent DNA sequence analysis indicated that all of these blocked amino acids were serines (46). (ii) When the flagellin gene from T1 was put into a T2 genetic background, the apparent M_r of the flagellin changed to that of T2 and the flagellin became LAH2$^+$; thus, the variation was dependent on the host background rather than the primary amino acid sequence of the flagellin (4). (iii) Power et al. (71) characterized numerous antiflagellin antibodies in terms of their ability to bind to synthetic overlapping amino acids of the complete FlaA sequence of VC167 T2 and to bind to the surface of the flagellar filament by immunogold electron microscopy. Their results indicated that none of the antibodies which bound to primary amino acids were surface exposed in the flagellar filament. The only antiserum which bound to the surface of the flagellar filament was LAH2, and LAH2 antiserum did not bind to any of the synthetic

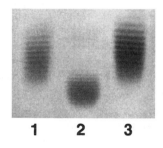

FIGURE 1 Isoelectric focusing gels of campylobacter flagellins. Purified flagellins were separated in gels made with ampholytes of pH 4 to 6 as described previously (19). Lanes: 1, VC167 T2; 2, VC167 T2 *ptmB*; 3, VC156 T2.

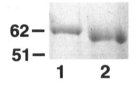

FIGURE 2 Coomassie blue-stained profile of 81-176 flagellin which has been electrophoresed on an SDS-PAGE gel (8.25% polyacrylamide). Lane 1, untreated flagellin; 2, flagellin chemically deglycosylated with TFMS (78). Molecular weight markers (in thousands) are indicated to the left.

peptides. These results indicated that LAH2 recognized either conformational epitopes or a posttranslational modification. (iv) Campylobacter flagellins display multiple charge trains in isoelectric focusing gels, which is characteristic of glycoproteins (19, 28, 59). An example of this is shown in Fig. 1 (also see below).

CAMPYLOBACTER FLAGELLINS ARE GLYCOPROTEINS

The first direct proof that campylobacter flagellins were glycosylated came from biochemical studies described by Doig et al. (19) in which flagellins from *C. jejuni, C. coli,* and *C. fetus* were shown to be sensitive to oxidation with periodate, indicating the presence of carbohydrates. Moreover, these flagellins also reacted with a lectin from *Limax flavus* (LFA) which recognizes terminal sialic acids regardless of linkage. Treatment of purified VC167 T1 and T2 flagellins with as little as 1 mM periodate eliminated their reactivity with LAH1 and LAH2 antisera, respectively. LFA also competitively inhibited LAH1 and LAH2 binding in an enzyme-linked immunosorbent assay. Thus, flagellin is the second major surface antigen of campylobacters shown to be sialylated, the other being the lipopolysaccharide (LPS) core. Moreover, these surface-exposed posttranslational modifications confer serospecificity on the flagellar filament, since the LAH antisera react with flagellins from all strains of the Lior 8 serogroup but not with flagellins from other serogroups (4). Thus, even though flagellin is not the Lior serodeterminant of the Lior 8 serogroup (3), flagellar epitopes are highly conserved within Lior 8 strains and perhaps within other serogroups.

Additional evidence that campylobacter flagellin is a glycoprotein is shown in Fig. 2. Flagellin from *C. jejuni* 81-176 was treated with trifluoromethanesulfonic acid (TFMS), which chemically deglycosylates glycoproteins without damaging the protein backbone. This deglycosylated flagellin shows a difference in apparent M_r from that of glycosylated flagellin on SDS-PAGE. The glycosylated flagellin migrates with an apparent M_r of approximately 62,000, while the chemically deglycosylated flagellin migrates with an apparent M_r of approximately 60,000. The predicted M_r of flagellin from 81-176 is 59,240 (42).

GENES INVOLVED IN BIOSYNTHESIS OF THE POSTTRANSLATIONAL MODIFICATIONS OF CAMPYLOBACTER FLAGELLINS

Two sets of genes involved in biosynthesis of the posttranslational modifications to campylobacter flagellin have been identified. The first set, called *ptm* genes (for "posttranslational modification"), were initially described in *C. coli* VC167. These genes were originally mapped by genetic transformation experiments to a region near to the flagellin structural genes (4) and subsequently cloned by chromosome walking (28). Mutation of either *ptmA* or *ptmB* results in loss of LAH1 reactivity in the VC167 T1 background or LAH2 reactivity in the

VC167 T2 background. Moreover, there are changes in the apparent M_r of the flagellins isolated from the *ptmA* or *ptmB* mutants on SDS-PAGE and changes in the glycoform patterns on isoelectric focusing gels, as shown in Fig. 1. The glycoform pattern of flagellin purified from VC167 T2 cells (Fig. 1, lane 1) is markedly different from that of flagellin isolated from the *ptmB* mutant of VC167 T2 (lane 2). Lane 3 shows that the glycoform pattern of flagellin isolated from another Lior 8 strain, *C. jejuni* VC156 T2 (LAH2$^+$), is identical to that of flagellin from *C. coli* VC167 T2.

The *ptmA* gene encodes a predicted protein with an M_r of 28,486, which shows significant sequence similarity to a family of alcohol-polyol dehydrogenases, including enzymes involved in the biotransformation of cholic and chenodeoxycholic acids to deoxycholic and lithocholic acids, respectively, by *Eubacterium* spp. in the intestine. The *ptmB* gene encodes a protein which has significant sequence similarity to CMP-sialic acid (CMP-NeuNAc) synthetases from *E. coli* K1 and *Neisseria meningitidis*. Specifically, CMP-NeuNAc synthetase activates sialic acid to CMP-sialic acid, which serves as the substrate for a sialyltransferase to generate the polysialic acid capsule found on the surface of both of these neuropathogens. CMP-NeuNAc synthetase activity is present in VC167 and is subsequently lost in the *ptmB* mutant (28). The involvement of this homolog of a sialic acid capsule gene, as well as additional homologs of sialic acid biosynthetic genes (26), in synthesis of the posttranslational modification of flagellin is consistent with the biochemical data of Doig et al. (19), which indicated that the flagellin protein is sialylated. The chemical structure of the posttranslational modifications on VC167 flagellin is currently being determined.

A second set of genes involved in biosynthesis of posttranslational modifications has been described in *C. jejuni* 81-176; these genes are called *pgl* (for "protein glycosylation") in the nomenclature used for genes required for glycosylation of *Neisseria* pilin (reference 32 and see below). These genes, summarized in

Table 2, were originally described as genes involved in the biosynthesis of LPS based on their high homology to such genes from other bacteria (see below and Table 2) and the data of Fry et al. (22). These workers showed that a region of 16 kb which includes homologs of these genes and six additional genes from *C. jejuni* 81116 (Penner or O serotype 6), when cloned into *E. coli* HB101, synthesized O side chains which were immunoreactive with O:6 antiserum. However, no mutational data on any of these genes in either *E. coli* or *C. jejuni* was reported, and so the specific genes required for O-antigen synthesis were not determined. However, Wood et al. (87) have recently reported the isolation of a subset of these genes from two other strains of *C. jejuni*. Although mutation of some of these genes in *C. jejuni* resulted in reduced core reactivity with the appropriate O typing sera, there were no difference in either core mobility or O-antigen biosynthesis in the mutants (87). Szymanski et al. (78) have more fully characterized six of these genes in *C. jejuni* 81-176 (O:23,36) and failed to demonstrate any role in LPS core or O side chain biosynthesis. Indeed, mutation of each of these six genes in 81-176 resulted in LPS cores and O side chains which were indistinguishable from those from wild-type cells. Instead, there were major changes in the immunoreactivity of various proteins in these mutants, including flagellin, when immunodetected with O:23 and O:36 antisera. An example of this is shown in Fig. 3. As seen in Fig. 3A the Coomassie stained profile of glycine extracted proteins from wildtype 81-176 (lane 1) and a *pglB* mutant (lane 2) appear similar. However, when these protein preparations were immunodetected with O typing sera, there were major differences in immunoreactivity. Figure B and C show the results of immunodetection with O:23 and O:36 antisera, respectively. In both cases, there are more bands reacting in the wild-type 81-176 (lane 1) than in the *pglB* mutant (lane 2), although there are differences in the profiles with the two antisera and differences among the different mutants (78). For example, the differences in immuno-

TABLE 2 Homology comparisons of the Pgl proteins in *C. jejuni* 81–176

Protein	Homolog/organism	% Identity/similarity	Function (accession no.)
PglB[a]	WlaF/*Campylobacter jejuni*	92/92	Putative LPS biosynthesis (Y11648, AF001497, AF001498)[b]
	hypothetical/*Methanobacterium thermoautotrophicum*	19/17	Putative oligosaccharide transferase (AE000942)
	STT3/*Saccharomyces cerevisiae*	15/30	Oligosaccharide transferase in N-linked protein glycosylation (P39007); transfer of Glc3Man9GlcNAc2 from lipid carrier to asparagine residues
PglA	WlaG/*Campylobacter jejuni*	98/98	Putative LPS biosynthesis (AF001498, Y11648, AF001497)[b]
	RfbF/*Campylobacter hyolei*	82/88	Putative LPS biosynthesis (X91081)
	PglA/*Neisseria meningitidis*	27/46	Pilin glycosyltransferase (U73942); transfer of α1–3Gal to 2,4-diacetamido-2,4.6-trideoxyhexose
Pg1C	WlaH/*Campylobacter jejuni*	100/100	Putative LPS biosynthesis (Y11648, AF001497, AF001498)[b]
	RfbP/*Campylobacter hyolei*	96/97	Putative LPS biosynthesis (X91081)
	galactosyltransferase/*Actinobacillus actinomycetemcomitans*	16/23	Capsular antigen biosynthesis (AB002668)
PglD	WlaI/*Campylobacter jejuni*	100/100	Putative LPS biosynthesis (Y11648, AF001498, AF001497)[b]
	NeuD/*Escherichia coli* K1	25/46	Acetyltransferase required for polysialic acid capsular biosynthesis (I55145)
PglE	WlaK/*Campylobacter jejuni*	98/98	Putative LPS biosynthesis (Y11648, AF001498, AF001497)[b]
	Hypothetical/*Bacillus subtilis*	49/67	Putative spore coat polysaccharide biosynthesis (Z71928)
	RfbE/*Escherichia coli* O157:H7	32/53	Perosamine synthetase in LPS O-side chain biosynthesis (S83460)
	FlmB/*Caulobacter crescentus*	25/46	Glycosylation of flagellin (U27301)
PglF	WlaL/*Campylobacter jejuni*	98/98	Putative LPS biosynthesis (Y11648, AF001498, AF001497)[b]
	RfbU/*Vibrio cholerae*	33/50	LPS O-side chain biosynthesis (Y07788)
	TsrG/*Yersinia enterocolitica*	33/48	Outer core LPS biosynthesis (S51266)
	FlmA/*Caulobacter crescentus*	15/27	Glycosylation of flagellin (U27301)
PglG	WlaM/*Campylobacter jejuni*	98/99	Putative LPS biosynthesis (Y11648)[b]
	HP0158/*Helicobacter pylori*	38/60	Unknown (AE000536)
	JHP0146/*Helicobacter pylori*	37/58	Unknown (AE001453)

[a] Truncated.

[b] The percent identity/similarity is given for the gene products published by Fry et al. (22) under accession no. Y11648. Similar genes from *C. jejuni* NCTC 11168 and NCTC 11351 have been described by Wood et al. under accession no. AF001497 and AF001498, respectively (87).

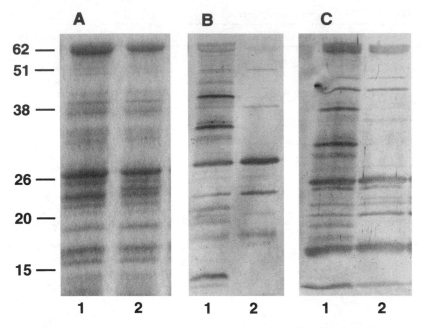

FIGURE 3 Comparison of glycine extracted proteins of 81-176 (lane 1) and an isogenic *pglB* mutant (lanes 2) separated on an SDS-PAGE gel (12.5% polyacrylamide). (A) Coomassie blue stain; (B) immunodetection with O:23 antiserum (1:400 dilution); (C) immunodetection with O:36 antiserum (1:400 dilution). Molecular weight markers (in thousands) are indicated to the left.

reactivity with flagellin, which is the major band in Fig. 3A at an apparent M_r of 62,000, are obvious in the *pglB* mutant when detected with O:23 but not when detected with O:36. Interestingly, immunodetection with O:23 resolves 81-176 flagellin into two bands, reminiscent of antigenic variation (29). Similar differences in the immunoreactivity of numerous proteins between wild-type 81-176 and the pgl mutants were also observed when soluble and membrane fractions of the cells were used (78). Moreover, treatment of these protein preparations from wild-type 81-176 cells with TFMS resulted in changes in immunoreactivity with the same subset of proteins whose immunoreactivity was affected in the *pgl* mutants. Thus, these antisera appear to be recognizing carbohydrate moieties on numerous cellular proteins, including flagellin. Most of the proteins affected in these mutants, with the exception of flagellin, are present at relatively low concentrations as judged by staining with Coomassie blue. The strong immunoreactivity and relatively low concentration of these proteins suggests that the carbohydrate moieties are immunodominant and that they may function to mask the primary amino acids from the host immune response. It should be clarified that the Penner typing sera are generated against live, whole cells of the serotype strains of *Campylobacter* injected intravenously into rabbits and that they are not cross-absorbed (69). Thus, the typing sera contain antibodies to protein antigens and to LPS antigens. Since the Penner scheme is a passive slide agglutination assay, it is these latter LPS-specific antibodies which react with LPS bound to the erythrocytes via lipid A and which are responsible for the passive agglutination of the erythrocytes (74).

Glycosylation of proteins was once thought to be a eukaryotic phenomenon, but increasing numbers of prokaryotic glycoproteins have now been identified. These include *N. menin-*

gitidis pilin (75, 82), bacterial cellulases (10), numerous *Mycobacterium* antigens (18, 21, 23), S-layer proteins (52), the type 4 pili of *Pseudomonas aeruginosa* (14), and flagellins from *Azospirillum brasilense* (55), *P. aeruginosa* (12), and *Caulobacter crescentus* (41). It is interesting that three of the 81-176 *pgl* genes encode proteins which show significant homology to proteins involved in glycosylation of some of these other prokaryotic proteins, as summarized in Table 2. PglE and PglF show significant homology to FlmB and FlmA, respectively, which were recently found to be involved in the temporally regulated glycosylation of flagellin in *C. crescentus* (41). PglA of *C. jejuni* shows significant homology to PglA of *N. meningitidis,* from which the gene nomenclature was adapted. This protein in *Neisseria* is predicted to function as a galactosyltransferase in the biosynthesis of a trisaccharide modification to pilin (32). In addition, *pglB* encodes a protein identified in the genomic sequence of *Methanobacterium thermoautotrophicum* which has significant similarity to an enzyme involved in the general protein glycosylation pathway of *Saccharomyces cerevisiae.*

IS FLAGELLIN A PROTECTIVE ANTIGEN?

The immunodominance of flagellin during human and experimental animal infections led to early speculation about its possible role in protection. Early animal experiments indicated that some antiflagellin monoclonal antibodies could protect mice against colonization with *C. jejuni* (60, 81). Epidemiologic studies, moreover, suggested that the development of antibodies against flagellin correlated with the development of protection against disease (49).

For flagellin to be an effective vaccine, it would have to elicit protection against strains of multiple serotypes. Studies on the antigenicity of campylobacter flagellin have shown that, as in the *Enterobacteriaceae,* there are conserved and variable regions. The conserved, cross-reacting epitopes are predominantly in the amino and carboxy ends of the protein, the regions which have been shown in *Salmonella* to be required for transport and assembly of the monomers into the filament (31). However, Power et al. (71) have shown by immunogold electron microscopy that antibodies to these regions of campylobacter flagellin, just as in flagellins of the *Enterobacteriaceae,* are not surface exposed in the intact flagellar filament and therefore do not represent good vaccine targets. The central region of the molecule, which lacks functional constraints, is hypervariable. This is again similar to the flagellins of the *Enterobacteriaceae,* in which this central region of flagellin, which is surface exposed, is responsible for H-antigen serospecificity. Although there is no H serotyping scheme for campylobacters, differences within the primary sequences of flagellins have been examined by a number of investigators using restriction fragment length polymorphisms and have been shown to be very extensive (6, 57). Moreover, the presence of serospecific posttranslational modifications on the surface of the filament increases the likelihood of extensive variation of the surface-exposed epitopes on flagellin. The role of the posttranslational modifications in protection against colonization has been examined in one study by using the removable-intestinal-tie adult rabbit diarrhea (RITARD) model (28). In this model, oral infection of rabbits with *Campylobacter* spp. protects against subsequent infection with both the homologous strain and heterologous strains of the same Lior serotype but not strains of other Lior serotypes. Thus, immunization with *C. coli* VC167 (Lior 8) protects against subsequent colonization with VC167, as well as two other *C. jejuni* Lior 8 strains, VC156 and VC159 (67). However, immunization with a *ptmA* mutant of VC167 results in protection against the homologous strain, VC167, but in greatly reduced protection against VC156 and VC159, suggesting that the posttranslational modification on flagellin is a major factor in this heterologous protection. This is consistent with the previously described conservation of the posttranslational modification on the flagellin proteins among Lior 8 strains, as measured by cross-reactivity with the LAH antisera (4).

Recent studies also suggest the immuno-dominance of the modifications during natural infection. Antisera from experimentally infected ferrets and human volunteers showed stronger immunoreactivity with glycosylated flagellins directly purified from campylobacters than with recombinant, unglycosylated campylobacter flagellin overexpressed and purified from *E. coli* (42). Nonetheless, immune sera do recognize epitopes on the unglycosylated recombinant flagellin, albeit at much lower dilutions. Moreover, studies with an adjuvanted (17), truncated, recombinant protein in which a highly conserved part of FlaA from VC167 was fused to the maltose-binding protein of *E. coli* have suggested that nonglycosylated flagellin can show broader protection than can the native glycosylated flagellin (42). These data again suggest that the immunodominance of the posttranslational modifications may mask other primary amino acid epitopes and that removal of the modification in the recombinant flagellin protein facilitates antibody formation against the normally less immunodominant but highly conserved amino acid residues.

ACKNOWLEDGMENTS

We thank Ben King and Cheryl Pratt Ewing.

This work was supported by Naval Medical Research and Development Command Work no. 61102A3M161102BS13 AK.111.

REFERENCES

1. **Aguero-Rosenfeld, M. E., X. H. Yang, and I. Nachamkin.** 1990. Infection of adult syrian hamsters with flagellar variants of *Campylobacter jejuni*. *Infect. Immun.* **58:**2214–2219.

2. **Aizawa, S.-I., G. E. Dean, C. J. Jones, R. M. Macnab, and S. Yamaguchi.** 1985. Purification and characterization of the flagellar hook-basal body complex of *Salmonella typhimurium*. *J. Bacteriol.* **161:**836–849.

3. **Alm, R. A., P. Guerry, M. E. Power, H. Lior, and T. J. Trust.** 1991. Analysis of the role of flagella in the heat-labile Lior serotyping scheme of thermophilic campylobacters by mutant allele exchange. *J. Clin. Microbiol.* **29:**2438–2445.

4. **Alm, R. A., P. Guerry, M. E. Power, and T. J. Trust.** 1992. Variation in antigenicity and molecular weight of *Campylobacter coli* VC167 flagellin in different genetic backgrounds. *J. Bacteriol.* **174:**4230–4238.

5. **Alm, R. A., P. Guerry, and T. J. Trust.** 1993. The *Campylobacter* sigma^{54} flagellin promoter is subject to environmental regulation. *J. Bacteriol.* **175:**4448–4455.

6. **Alm, R. A., P. Guerry, and T. J. Trust.** 1993. Distribution and polymorphism of the flagellin genes among isolates of *Campylobacter coli* and *Campylobacter jejuni*. *J. Bacteriol.* **175:**3051–3057.

7. **Alm, R. A., P. Guerry, and T. J. Trust.** 1993. Significance of duplicated flagellin genes in *Campylobacter*. *J. Mol. Biol.* **230:**359–363.

8. **Alm, R. A., L. L. Ling, D. T. Moir, B. L. King, E. D. Brown, P. C. Doig, D. R. Smith, B. Noonan, B. C. Guild, B. L. deJonge, G. Carmel, P. J. Tummino, A. Caruso, M. Uria-Nickelsen, D. M. Mills, C. Ives, R. Gibson, D. Merberg, S. D. Mills, Q. Jiang, D. E. Taylor, G. F. Vovis, and T. J. Trust.** 1999. Genomic sequence comparison of two unrelated strains of the human gastric pathogen *Helicobacter pylori*. *Nature* **397:**176–180.

9. **Alm, R. A., and P. A. Manning.** 1990. Characterization of the *hlyB* gene and its role in the production of the El Tor haemolysin of *Vibrio cholerae* O1. *Mol. Microbiol.* **4:**413–425.

10. **Bisaria, V. X., and S. Mishra.** 1989. Regulatory aspects of cellulase biosynthesis and secretion. *Crit. Rev. Biotechnol.* **9:**61–104.

11. **Black, R. E., M. M. Levine, M. L. Clements, T. P. Hughes, and M. J. Blaser.** 1988. Experimental *Campylobacter jejuni* infections in humans. *J. Infect. Dis.* **157:**472–479.

12. **Brimer, C. D., and T. C. Montie.** 1998. Cloning and comparison of *fliC* genes and identification of glycosylation in the flagellin of *Pseudomonas aeruginosa* a-type strains. *J. Bacteriol.* **180:**3209–3217.

13. **Caldwell, M. B., P. Guerry, E. C. Lee, J. P. Burans, and R. I. Walker.** 1985. Reversible expression of flagella in *Campylobacter jejuni*. *Infect. Immun.* **50:**941–943.

14. **Castric, P.** 1995. *pilO*, a gene required for glycosylation of *Pseudomonas aeruginosa* 1244 pilin. *Microbiology* **141:**1247–1254.

15. **Darzins, A.** 1994. Characterization of a *Pseudomonas aeruginosa* gene cluster involved in pilus biosynthesis and twitching motility: sequence similarity to the chemotaxis proteins of enterics and the gliding bacterium *Myxococcus xanthus*. *Mol. Microbiol.* **11:**137–153.

16. **DePamphilis, M. L., and J. Adler.** 1971. Fine structure and isolation of the hook-basal body complex of flagella from *Escherichia coli* and *Bacillus subtilis*. *J. Bacteriol.* **105:**384–395.

17. **Dickenson, B. L., and J. D. Clements.** 1995. Dissociation of *Escherichia coli* heat-labile enterotoxin adjuvanticity from ADP-ribosyltransferase activity. *Infect. Immun.* **63:**1617–1623.

18. **Dobos, K. M., K.-H. Khoo, K. M. Swiderek, P. J. Brennen, and J. T. Belisle.** 1996. Definition of the full extent of glycosylation of the 45-kilodalton glycoprotein of *Mycobacterium tuberculosis*. *J. Bacteriol.* **178:**2498–2506.

19. **Doig, P., N. Kinsella, P. Guerry, and T. J. Trust.** 1996. Characterization of a posttranslational modification of *Campylobacter* flagellin: identification of a serospecific glycosyl moiety. *Mol. Microbiol.* **19:**379–387.

20. **Ferrero, R. L., and A. Lee.** 1988. Motility of *Campylobacter jejuni* in a viscous environment: comparison with conventional rod-shaped bacteria. *J. Gen. Microbiol.* **134:**53–59.

21. **Fifis, T., C. Costopoulos, A. J. Radford, A. Bacic, and P. R. Wood.** 1991. Purification and characterization of major antigens from a *Mycobacterium bovis* culture filtrate. *Infect. Immun.* **59:**800–807.

22. **Fry, B. N., V. Korolik, J. A. ten Brinke, M. T. T. Pennings, R. Zalm, B. J. J. Teunis, P. J. Coloe, and B. A. M. van der Zeijst.** 1998. The lipopolysaccharide biosynthesis locus of *Campylobacter jejuni* 81116. *Microbiology* **144:**2049–2061.

23. **Garbe, T., D. Harris, M. Vordermeier, R. Lathigra, J. Ivanyi, and D. Young.** 1993. Expression of the *Mycobacterium tuberculosis* 19-kilodalton antigen in *Mycobacterium smegmatis*-immunological analysis and evidence for glycosylation. *Infect. Immun.* **61:**260–267.

24. **Glenn-Calvo, E., W. Bar, and M. Frosch.** 1994. Isolation and characterization of the flagellar hook of *Campylobacter jejuni*. *FEMS Microbiol. Lett.* **123:**299–304.

25. **Grant, C. C. R., M. E. Konkel, W. Cieplak, Jr., and L. S. Tompkins.** 1993. Role of flagellin in adherence, internalization and translocation of *Campylobacter jejuni* in non polarized and polarized epithelial cell cultures. *Infect. Immun.* **61:**1764–1771.

26. **Guerry, P.** Unpublished data.

27. **Guerry, P., R. A. Alm, M. E. Power, S. M. Logan, and T. J. Trust.** 1991. Role of two flagellin genes in *Campylobacter* motility. *J. Bacteriol.* **173:**4757–4764.

28. **Guerry, P., P. Doig, R. A. Alm, D. H. Burr, N. Kinsella, and T. J. Trust.** 1996. Identification and characterization of genes required for posttranslational modification of *Campylobacter coli* VC167 flagellin. *Mol. Microbiol.* **19:**369–378.

29. **Harris, L. A., S. M. Logan, P. Guerry, and T. J. Trust.** 1987. Antigenic variation of *Campylobacter* flagella. *J. Bacteriol.* **169:**5066–5071.

30. **Hickey, T., S. Baqar, A. L. Bourgeois, C. P. Ewing, and P. Guerry.** 1999. *Campylobacter jejuni*-mediated stimulation of interleukin-8 by INT407 cells. *Infect. Immun.* **67:**88–93.

31. **Homma, M., H. Fujita, S. Yamaguchi, and T. Iino.** 1987. Regions of *Salmonella typhimurium* flagellin essential for its polymerization and excretion. *J. Bacteriol.* **169:**291–296.

32. **Jennings, M. P., M. Virji, D. Evans, V. Foster, Y. N. Srikhanta, L. Steeghs, P. van der Ley, and E. R. Moxon.** 1998. Identification of a novel gene involved in pilin glycosylation in *Neisseria meningitidis*. *Mol. Microbiol.* **29:**975–984.

33. **Jin, T., and J. L. Penner.** 1988. Role of the 92.5-kilodalton outer membrane protein of *Campylobacter jejuni* in serological reactions. *J. Clin. Microbiol.* **26:**2480–2483.

34. **Jones, B. D., C. A. Lee, and S. Falkow.** 1992. Invasion by *Salmonella typhimurium* is affected by the direction of flagellar rotation. *Infect. Immun.* **60:**2475–2480.

35. **Khoramian-Falsafi, T., S. Harayama, K. Kutsukake, and J. C. Pechere.** 1990. Effect of motility and chemotaxis on the invasion of *Salmonella typhimurium* into Hela cells. *Microb. Pathog.* **9:**47–53.

36. **King, V., and C. L. Clayton.** 1991. Genomic investigation of phenotypic variation of *Campylobacter jejuni* flagellin. *FEMS Microbiol. Lett.* **68:**107–111.

37. **Kinsella, N., P. Guerry, J. Cooney, and T. J. Trust.** 1997. The *flgE* gene of *Campylobacter coli* is under the control of the alternative sigma factor σ54. *J. Bacteriol.* **179:**4647–4653.

38. **Kinsella, N., P. Guerry, P. Doig, R. Yao, and T. J. Trust.** Unpublished data.

39. **Konkel, M. E., S. G. Garvis, S. L. Tipton, D. E. Anderson, Jr., and W. Cieplak, Jr.** 1997. Identification and molecular cloning of a gene encoding a fibronectin-binding protein (CadF) from *Campylobacter jejuni*. *Mol. Microbiol.* **24:**953–963.

40. **Lagenaur, C., M. DeMartini, and N. Agabian.** 1987. Isolation and characterization of *Caulobacter crescentus* flagellar hooks. *J. Bacteriol.* **136:**795–798.

41. **LeClerc, G., S. P. Wang, and B. Ely.** 1998. A new class of *Caulobacter crescentus* flagellar genes. *J. Bacteriol.* **180:**5010–5019.

42. **Lee, L. H., E. Burg III, S. Baqar, A. L. Bourgeois, D. H. Burr, C. P. Ewing, T. J. Trust, and P. Guerry.** 1999. Evaluation of a truncated recombinant flagellin subunit vaccine against *Campylobacter jejuni*. *Infect. Immun.* **67:**5799–5805.

43. **Liu, X., and P. Matsumura.** 1994. The FlhD/FlhC complex, a transcriptional activator of the *Escherichia coli* flagellar class II operons. *J. Bacteriol.* **176:**7345–7351.

44. **Logan, S. M., P. Guerry, D. M. Rollins, D. H. Burr, and T. J. Trust.** 1989. In vivo antigenic variation of *Campylobacter* flagellin. *Infect. Immun.* **57:**2583–2585.

45. **Logan, S. M. and T. J. Trust.** 1983. Molecular identification of surface protein antigens of *Campylobacter jejuni. J. Bacteriol.* **168**:739–745.

46. **Logan, S. M., T. J. Trust, and P. Guerry.** 1989. Evidence for posttranslational modification and gene duplication of *Campylobacter* flagellin. *J. Bacteriol.* **171**:3031–3038.

47. **Luneberg, E., E. Glenn-Calvo, M. Hartmann, W. Bar, and M. Frosch.** 1998. The central, surface-exposed region of the flagellar hook protein FlgE of *Campylobacter jejuni* shows hypervariability among strains. *J. Bacteriol.* **180**: 3711–3714.

48. **MacNab, R.** 1996. Flagella and motility, p. 123–145. *In* F. C. Neidhardt, R. Curtiss III, J. L. Ingraham, E. C. C. Lin, K. B. Low, B. Magasanik, W. S. Reznikoff, M. Riley, M. Schaechter, and H. E. Umbarger (ed.), *Escherichia coli and Salmonella: Cellular and Molecular Biology,* 2nd ed. American Society for Microbiology, Washington, D.C.

49. **Martin, P. M., J. Mathiot, J. Ipero, M. Kirimat, A. J. Georges, and M. C. Georges-Courbot.** 1989. Immune response to *Campylobacter jejuni* and *Campylobacter coli* in a cohort of children from birth to 2 years of age. *Infect. Immun.* **57**:2542–2546.

50. **McBride, M. J., T. Kohler, and D. R. Zusman.** 1992. Methylation of FrzCD, a methyl-accepting taxis protein of *Myxococcus xanthus,* is correlated with factors affecting cell behavior. *J. Bacteriol.* **174**:4246–4257.

51. **McSweegan, E., and R. I. Walker.** 1986. Identification and characterization of two *Campylobacter jejuni* adhesins for cellular and mucous substrates. *Infect. Immun.* **53**:141–148.

52. **Messner, P., and U. B. Sleytr.** 1991. Bacterial surface layer glycoproteins. *Glycobiology* **1**: 545–551.

53. **Miller, S., E. C. Pesci, and C. L. Pickett.** 1993. A *Campylobacter jejuni* homolog of the LcrD/FlbF family of proteins is necessary for flagellar biogenesis. *Infect. Immun.* **61**:2930–2936.

54. **Mills, S. D., and W. C. Bradbury.** 1988. Human antibody response to outer membrane proteins of *Campylobacter jejuni* during infection. *Infect. Immun.* **43**:739–743.

55. **Moens, S., K. Michiels, and J. Vanderleyden.** 1995. Glycosylation of the flagellin of the polar flagellum of *Azospirillum brasilense,* a Gram-negative nitrogen-fixing bacterium. *Microbiology* **141**: 2651–2657.

56. **Morooka, T., A. Umeda, and K. Amako.** 1985. Motility as an intestinal colonization factor for *Campylobacter jejuni. J. Gen. Microbiol.* **131**: 1973–1980.

57. **Nachamkin, I., K. Bohachick, and C. M. Patton.** 1993. Flagellin gene typing of *Campylobacter jejuni* by restriction fragment length polymorphism analysis. *J. Clin. Microbiol.* **31**:1531–1536.

58. **Nachamkin, I., X. H. Yang, and N. J. Stern.** 1993. Role of *Campylobacter jejuni* flagella as colonization factors for three-day-old chicks: analysis with flagellar mutants. *Appl. Environ. Microbiol.* **59**: 1269–1273.

59. **Nachamkin, I., and X. H. Yang.** 1988. Isoelectric focusing of *Campylobacter jejuni* flagellin: microheterogeneity and restricted antigenicity of charged species with a monoclonal antibody. *FEMS Microbiol. Lett.* **49**:235–238.

60. **Newell, D. G.** 1986. Monoclonal antibodies directed against the flagella of *Campylobacter jejuni:* production, characterization and lack of effect on the colonization of infant mice. *J. Hyg.* **96**: 131–141.

61. **Ninfa, A. J., D. A. Mullin, G. Ramakrishnan, and A. Newton.** 1989. *Escherichia coli* σ^{54} RNA polymerase recognizes *Caulobacter crescentus flbG* and *flaN* flagellar gene promoters in vitro. *J. Bacteriol.* **171**:383–391.

62. **Nuijten, P. J., N. M. Bleumink-Pluym, W. Gaatra, and B. A. van der Zeijst.** 1989. Flagellin expression in *Campylobacter jejuni* is regulated at the transcriptional level. *Infect. Immun.* **57**: 1084–1088.

63. **Nuijten, P. J., L. Marquez-Magana, and B. A. van der Zeijst.** 1995. Analysis of flagellin gene expression in flagellar phase variants of *Campylobacter jejuni* 81116. *Antonie Leeuwenhoek* **67**: 377–383.

64. **Odenbreit, S., M. Till, and R. Haas.** 1996. Optimized BlaM-transposon shuttle mutagenesis of *Helicobacter pylori* allows the identification of novel genetic loci involved in bacterial virulence. *Mol. Microbiol.* **20**:361–373.

65. **O'Toole, P. W., M. Kostrynska, and T. J. Trust.** 1994. Non-motile mutants of *Helicobacter pylori* and *Helicobacter mustelae* defective in flagellar hook production. *Mol. Microbiol.* **14**:691–703.

66. **Ottemann, K. M. and J. F. Miller.** 1997. Roles for motility in bacterial-host interactions. *Mol. Microbiol.* **24**:1109–1117.

67. **Pavlovskis, O. R., D. M. Rollins, R. L. Haberberger, Jr., A. E. Green, L. Habash, S. Stroko, and R. I. Walker.** 1991. Significance of flagella in colonization resistance of rabbits immunized with *Campylobacter* spp. *Infect. Immun.* **59**:2259–2264.

68. **Pei, Z., C. Burucoa, B. Grignon, S. Baqar, X.-Z. Huang, D. J. Kopecko, A. L. Bourgeois, and M. J. Blaser.** 1998. Mutation in the *peb1A* locus of *Campylobacter jejuni* reduces interactions with epithelial cells and intestinal colonization of mice. *Infect. Immun.* **66**:938–943.

69. **Penner, J. L., and J. N. Hennessy.** 1980. Passive hemagglutination technique for serotyping *Campylobacter fetus* subsp. *jejuni* on the basis of soluble heat-stable antigens. *J. Clin. Microbiol.* **12**: 732–737.

70. **Power, M. E., R. A. Alm, and T. J. Trust.** 1992. Biochemical and antigenic properties of the *Campylobacter* flagellar hook protein. *J. Bacteriol.* **174:**3874–3883.

71. **Power, M. E., P. Guerry, W. D. McCubbin, C. M. Kay, and T. J. Trust.** 1994. Structural and antigenic characteristics of *Campylobacter coli* FlaA flagellin. *J. Bacteriol.* **176:**3303–3313.

72. **Rosario, M. M., K. L. Fredrick, G. W. Ordal, and J. D. Helmann.** 1994. Chemotaxis in *Bacillus subtilis* requires either of two functionally redundant CheW homologs. *J. Bacteriol.* **176:** 2736–2739.

73. **Shigematsu, M., A. Umeda, S. Fujimoto, and K. Amako.** 1998. Spirochaete-like swimming mode of *Campylobacter jejuni* in a viscous environment. *J. Med. Microbiol.* **47:**521–526.

74. **Springer, G. F., J. C. Adye, A. Bezkorovainy, and J. R. Murthy.** 1973. Functional aspects and nature of the lipopolysaccharide-receptor of human erythrocytes. *J. Infect. Dis.* **128:** S202–S212.

75. **Stimson, E., M. Virji, S. Barker, M. Panico, I. Blench, J. Saunders, G. Payne, E. R. Moxon, A. Dell, and H. R. Morris.** 1996. Discovery of a novel protein modification: alpha-glycerophosphate is a substituent of menigococcal pilin. *Biochem. J.* **316:**29–33.

76. **Stock, J., G. Kersulis, and D. E. Koshland, Jr.** 1985. Neither methylating nor demethylating enzymes are required for bacterial chemotaxis. *Cell* **42:**683–690.

77. **Szymanski, C. M., M. King, M. Haardt, and G. D. Armstrong.** 1995. *Campylobacter jejuni* motility and invasion of Caco-2 cells. *Infect. Immun.* **63:**4295–4300.

78. **Szymanski, C. M., R. Yao, C. P. Ewing, T. J. Trust, and P. Guerry.** 1999. Evidence for a system of general protein glycosylation in *Campylobacter jejuni*. *Mol. Microbiol.* **32:**1022–1030.

79. **Takata, T., S. Fujimoto, and K. Amako.** 1992. Isolation of nonchemotactic mutants of *Campylobacter jejuni* and their colonization of the mouse intestinal tract. *Infect. Immun.* **60:** 3596–3600.

80. **Tomb, J.-F., O. White, A. R. Kerlavage, R. A. Clayton, G. G. Sutton, R. D. Fleischmann, K. A. Ketchum, H. P. Klenk, S. Gill, B. A. Dougherty, K. Nelson, J. Quackenbush, L. Zhou, E. F. Kirkness, S. Peterson, B. Loftus, D. Richardson, R. Dodson, H. G. Khalak, A. Glodek, K. McKenney, L. M. Fitzegerald, N. Lee, M. D. Adams, E. K. Hickey, D. E. Berg, J. D. Gocayne, T. R. Utterback, J. D. Peterson, J. M. Kelley, M. D. Cotton, J. M. Weidman, C. Fujii, C. Bowman, L. Watthey, E. Wallin, W. S. Hayes,** M. Borodovsky, P. D. Karp, H. O. Smith, C. M. Fraser, and J. C. Venter. 1997. The complete genome sequence of the gastric pathogen *Helicobacter pylori*. *Nature* **388:**539–542.

81. **Ueki, Y., A. Umeda, S. Fujimoto, M. Misuyama, and K. Amako.** 1987. Protection against *Campylobacter jejuni* infection in suckling mice by anti-flagellar antibody. *Microbiol. Immunol.* **31:** 1161–1171.

82. **Virji, M.** 1997. Post-translational modifications of meningococcal pili. Identification of common substituents: glycans and α-glycerophosphate—a review. *Gene* **192:**141–147.

83. **Wassenaar, T. M., N. M. C. Bleumink-Pluym, and B. A. M. van der Zeijst.** 1991. Inactivation of *Campylobacter jejuni* flagellin genes by homologous recombination demonstrates that *flaA* but not *flaB* is required for invasion. *EMBO J.* **10:**2055–2061.

84. **Wassenaar, T. M., B. N. Fry, and B. A. M. van der Zeijst.** 1995. Variation of the flagellin gene locus of *Campylobacter jejuni* by recombination and horizontal gene transfer. *Microbiology* **141:** 95–101.

85. **Wassenaar, T. M., B. A. M. van der Zeijst, R. Ayling, and D. G. Newell.** 1993. Colonization of chicks by motility mutants of *Campylobacter jejuni* demonstrates the importance of flagellin A expression. *J. Gen. Microbiol.* **139:**1171–1175.

86. **Wenman, W. M., J. Chai, T. J. Louie, C. Goudreau, H. Lior, D. G. Newell, A. D. Pearson, and D. E. Taylor.** 1985. Antigenic analysis of *Campylobacter* flagellar protein and other proteins. *J. Clin. Microbiol.* **21:**108–112.

87. **Wood, A. C., N. J. Oldfield, C. A. O'Dwyer, and J. M. Ketley.** 1999. Cloning, mutation and distribution of a putative lipopolysaccharide biosynthesis locus in *Campylobacter jejuni*. *Microbiology* **145:**379–388.

88. **Yao, R., D. H. Burr, P. Doig, T. J. Trust, H. Niu, and P. Guerry.** 1994. Isolation of motile and non-motile insertional mutants of *Campylobacter jejuni* defective in invasion of eukaryotic cells: the role of flagella in invasion. *Mol. Microbiol.* **14:**883–893.

89. **Yao, R., D. H. Burr, and P. Guerry.** 1997. CheY-mediated modulation of *Campylobacter jejuni* virulence. *Mol. Microbiol.* **23:**1021–1032.

90. **Yao, R., and P. Guerry.** 1996. Molecular cloning and site-specific mutagenesis of a gene involved in arylsulfatase synthesis in *Campylobacter jejuni*. *J. Bacteriol.* **178:**3335–3338.

91. **Yokoseki, T., T. Iino, and K. Kutsukae.** 1996. Negative regulation by *fliD*, *fliS*, and *fliT* of the export of the flagellum-specific anti-sigma factor, FlgM, in *Salmonella typhimurium*. *J. Bacteriol.* **178:** 899–901.

ENVIRONMENTAL REGULATORY GENES

Simon F. Park

21

Compared to other food-borne bacterial pathogens, *Campylobacter jejuni* and *Campylobacter coli* have limited capacity for growth in the environment. Accordingly, the organisms are microaerophilic, have minimum growth temperatures between 32 and 36°C, and have complex nutritional requirements. However, despite these growth limitations, the pathogens are frequently isolated from the gastrointestinal tracts of animals all over the world and from a wide range of other environmental sources including food and surface waters. The ability of campylobacters to initiate adaptive survival responses to this diverse range of environments and the corresponding stresses is cardinal to the infective and contamination cycle of these pathogens.

To colonize the gastrointestinal tract, for instance, campylobacters must be able to compete successfully in a complex and dynamic environment for nutrients, such as iron. In contrast, these organisms must also be able to survive for extended periods in environments of low osmolarity containing few or no nutrients, such as surface waters. Furthermore, to cause infection in the human host, campylobacters must be able to tolerate a series of environmental insults ranging from acid stress in the stomach to the conditions encountered during invasion of epithelial cells. Although the organisms do not grow below 30°C, campylobacters will also encounter fluctuations in the temperature of the environment and must be able to respond to these. For example, they colonize the gastrointestinal tracts of birds, which have a body temperature of 42°C, and humans, which have a body temperature of 37°C. In addition, human infection is frequently acquired following the consumption of undercooked poultry, a process during which the organism will encounter heat stress.

Many bacteria, including enteric pathogens, are capable of surviving diverse environmental conditions. The ability to respond rapidly to changes in the environment is essential for the success of the bacterium and requires that it be able to sense its surroundings and modify its physiology accordingly. Pathogens, in particular, must be able to recognize the environmental cues which signal their entry into the host and to respond by inducing the expression of virulence determinants. In the absence of a host-specific effector, human pathogens are able to recognize a variety of varied environmental parameters which are likely to be encountered within the human body, such as iron limitation and temperature.

Simon F. Park, School of Biological Sciences, University of Surrey, Guildford GU2 5XH, United Kingdom.

Campylobacter, 2nd Ed., Edited by I. Nachamkin and M. J. Blaser
© 2000 American Society for Microbiology, Washington, D.C.

Knowledge of the global regulatory systems that exist to enable the growth and survival of bacteria under different conditions has been derived mainly from studies on *Escherichia coli, Salmonella typhimurium,* and *Bacillus subtilis.* Many complex networks of multigene systems which respond to various stimuli, including nutrient limitation, oxidative stress, temperature stress, and osmotic pressure, are found in these bacteria. However, until recently and before the availability of the *C. jejuni* genome sequence, our knowledge of the mechanisms governing the environmental regulation of gene expression in campylobacters and their response to the environment was very limited. Despite this, it is clear that campylobacters are able to recognize and respond to a number of stresses inducing environmental stresses. In this context, a number of proteins have been shown to be induced by heat stress (27, 62, 63, 73). Campylobacters are also known to modulate gene expression in response to iron limitation, as demonstrated in early work by Field et al. (14). More recent studies have demonstrated that gene expression in *C. jejuni* can be modulated by the presence of bile (13).

The aim of this chapter is to summarize our current understanding of the mechanisms of differential gene expression in campylobacters in response to the environment. While we know little of the response of these bacteria to many environmental stresses, a number of recent studies have provided considerable insight into their adaptive responses to iron limitation, oxidative stress, and heat shock. This chapter therefore discusses the regulatory aspects of these inducible stress tolerance mechanisms. The completion of the sequencing project for the *C. jejuni* genome has led to the expectation that the study of the complex physiological processes of adaptation in this pathogen will be facilitated by analysis of the enormous gene and protein database that has been generated. In this context, the capacity for the environmental regulation of gene expression in campylobacters is also discussed in light of the information emerging from the genome sequence of *C. jejuni* NCTC 11168 (http://www.medmicro. mds.qmw.ac.uk/campylobacter).

IDENTIFICATION AND CHARACTERIZATION OF ENVIRONMENTALLY REGULATED GENE EXPRESSION

To characterize environmentally regulated gene expression in a bacterium and hence its capacity to respond to environmental stress, it is first necessary to identify the shifts in gene expression which occur in response to changes in environmental conditions. This can be achieved by monitoring for variation at the transcriptional level or by assessing changes in the level of protein synthesis. In this context, a variety of methods have been used to identify differential gene expression in campylobacters.

Reporter Gene Systems for Monitoring Environmental Gene Expression

The placement of transcriptionally silent reporter genes under the control of a promoter sequence, and the subsequent generation of a quantifiable marker response, has proved to be an extremely powerful tool in elucidating many aspects of bacterial physiology. In particular, reporter genes are especially suitable for the identification and characterization of environmentally regulated genes when no assay for a particular gene product exists. Furthermore, when the product of the reporter gene produces a readily detectable phenotype, whose expression can be detected in complex environments, reporter gene systems can be used to monitor the actual changes in gene expression that occur in vivo or in complex natural environments.

Typically, three groups of reporter genes are used to generate marker gene fusions, and these encode either antibiotic resistance determinants, enzymes involved in the production of chromogenic changes, or fluorescent proteins or luciferase enzymes. To date, however, only a limited number of promoter probes, through which marker gene fusions can be constructed, have been developed for use in campylobacters (1, 11, 39, 46, 71).

The use of *cat* markers, encoding chloramphenicol transacetylase, has allowed the environmental regulation of expression of FlaB, a constituent of the *Campylobacter* flagellin, to be monitored in detail (1) and has permitted the isolation of *Campylobacter* promoters (11). Many different chromogenic systems have found application as bioreporters, perhaps the most widely used being *lacZ* fusions. A shuttle promoter probe vector, pMW10, which utilizes a promoterless *lacZ* gene, has been constructed for use in *C. jejuni*. Using this vector, Wosten et al. (71) were able to isolate and characterize a number of *Campylobacter* promoter sequences and thereby derive a consensus sequence for a *C. jejuni* promoter. A recent innovation in systems for monitoring the regulation of gene expression in *C. coli* is the use of a *hipO* reporter gene. Hippuricase, the product of the *hipO* gene (20), acts to cleave *N*-benzoylglycine (hippurate) into the constituent products glycine and benzoic acid. Since glycine formation can be readily detected by using a ninhydrin-based system (39), HipO expression serves as a convenient reporter of gene expression in *C. coli*, which, unlike *C. jejuni*, does not naturally possess the *hipO* gene, and has been used to monitor iron-dependent changes in the expression of catalase and differential expression of the *flaA* and *flaB* genes (39).

Another and potentially very useful class of bioreporters is made up of *lux* fusions. The product of the *luxAB* genes, bacterial luciferase, catalyzes a mixed-function oxidation requiring flavin mononucleotide ($FMNH_2$), oxygen, and a long-chain fatty aldehyde, which results in the production of blue-green light. The versatility of bacterial luciferase renders it suitable for incorporation into systems for the study of gene expression and for bacterial detection (58). In this context, bacterial luciferase has proved a sensitive real-time monitor of gene expression in campylobacters (46).

Physical Methods for Characterizing Environmental Gene Expression

Changes in the mRNA content of a bacterial cell, with particular relevance to differential gene expression in response to the environment, can also be investigated by using more direct methods of analysis. PCR-based protocols, such as differential-display PCR and RNA arbitrarily primed PCR, have recently found application in the identification of differentially expressed genes in a number of prokaryotes, the latter having recently been used to identify a heat-inducible gene in *C. jejuni* (63). However, the analysis of differential gene expression in *C. jejuni* is likely to enter a new era following the completion of the *C. jejuni* genome sequence. This information, together with the emergence of technology that enables the production of high-density gridded arrays of DNA representing an entire genome in a small area, now allows gene expression in *C. jejuni* to be characterized, for the first time, in a panoramic manner by using transcriptosome analysis (54).

Ultimately, the phenotype of a bacterium under a particular set of conditions, and in part its resistance to the stress imposed by these, is governed by its ability to differentially modulate the expression of proteins. Consequently, a powerful technique for characterizing environmentally modulated gene expression in bacteria is based on the determination of the subset of proteins expressed under a particular set of conditions by polyacrylamide gel electrophoresis. To date, this technology has seen somewhat limited application in campylobacters, although both one-dimensional and two-dimensional polyacrylamide gel electrophoresis have been used to characterize changes in gene expression in response to iron limitation (2, 14, 65) and various stresses including heat shock (27, 73). However, with advances in the analysis of protein expression based on two-dimensional gel electrophoresis and the emergence of powerful new technologies for the identification of proteins, it is inevitable that such approaches will see widespread application in the study of environmental adaptation in campylobacters.

IRON-RESPONSIVE GENE EXPRESSION

Iron is essential for the growth of nearly all microorganisms studied to date, including campylobacters. During their life cycle, campylobacters are likely to encounter widely fluctuating levels of this essential element and therefore must maintain iron homeostasis through the differential expression of iron uptake and storage systems in order to survive.

In the human host, high-affinity iron-binding proteins which are found in serum and at mucosa surfaces serve to maintain free iron at levels that are too low for the growth of most bacteria. As a response to the nutritional restriction imposed by iron limitation, many pathogens have evolved highly efficient systems for sequestering iron. A strategy for iron sequestration used by many microorganisms comprises the secretion of highly specific chelators for ferric ions, termed siderophores, followed by their reinternalization via a cognate high-affinity transport system and the subsequent release of iron into the cytoplasm. Alternatively, some pathogenic bacteria are able to obtain iron from host-derived iron-containing compounds. *E. coli,* for example, has eight different iron uptake systems (68). In contrast to *E. coli,* campylobacters have a smaller number of iron uptake systems. To date, only systems for enterochelin uptake (41, 48), a putative hemin uptake system (44), and a transporter for an unidentified siderophore (18) have been characterized.

Although iron is an essential nutrient, its presence within a bacterial cell can be problematical since it can participate in the production of free radicals. Consequently, iron homeostasis must be carefully balanced by the strict regulation of iron uptake and storage. In many bacteria, iron-regulated gene expression is transcriptionally controlled by Fur (for "a ferric uptake regulator"). Above a certain concentration threshold, iron (Fe^{2+}) can complex with Fur and mediate the formation of a dimer that is able to bind to a palindromic control sequence which overlaps the promoters of Fur-regulated genes. Thus, during growth under iron-replete conditions, the Fur protein binds to the promoter regions of Fur-regulated genes and thereby prevents transcription.

Iron-responsive protein expression was first identified in campylobacters some time ago (14). However, it was not until much later that a Fur-like iron-responsive genetic regulator was first identified in *C. jejuni* (9, 69). Although the Fur-like protein from *C. jejuni* is significantly divergent from that of other *Proteobacteria,* it performs a similar function. Inactivation of the gene encoding the Fur homologue by allelic exchange has confirmed that this protein plays a key role in iron-responsive gene regulation in *C. jejuni* (65). A comparison of the protein profiles of the parental strain and a Fur-deficient mutant has demonstrated that the expression of at least seven proteins is iron responsive and regulated by Fur. The identity of a number of these proteins has been attributed to components of the CeuBCDE transport system for enterochelin (41, 48); ChuABCD, a putative hemin transporter (44, 65); and CfrA, a component of a putative siderophore transporter (18, 65).

Compared to other pathogens, the number of proteins regulated by Fur in *C. jejuni* is small. In *Pseudomonas aeruginosa,* for example, there are at least 20 Fur-regulated genes (38). Nevertheless, it is clear that Fur plays an important role in controlling gene expression in campylobacters in response to iron limitation and in a manner analogous to that in other bacteria. Thus, during iron starvation, in order to maintain iron homeostasis within the cell, campylobacters induce the expression of a number of systems for transporting iron, in the form of siderophores and iron-containing host-derived compounds, and this is mediated by Fur at the transcriptional level.

REGULATION OF GENE EXPRESSION IN RESPONSE TO OXIDATIVE STRESS

Exposure to oxygen, while inevitable for most bacterial pathogens, leads to the formation of reactive oxygen intermediates as harmful by-products that are capable of damaging nucleic acids, proteins, and membranes. Consequently, as a response to distinct reactive oxygen intermediate excess, many prokaryotic cells are able induce the synthesis of antioxidant enzymes. As an example, the *soxRS* regulon coordinates the induction of at least 12 genes, including that encoding Mn-superoxide dismutase (Mn-SOD), in response to superoxide or nitric oxide in *E. coli* (10). Furthermore, treatment of *E. coli* cells with low doses of hydrogen peroxide results in the induction of 30 proteins and resistance to killing by higher doses of hydrogen peroxide. The expression of nine of these hydrogen peroxide-inducible proteins, including catalase, glutathione reductase, and alkyl hydroperoxide reductase, is controlled by the positive regulator OxyR (60). The appropriate regulation of genes involved in oxidative stress resistance also enables pathogens to adapt to the intracellular environment of the host and, accordingly, can confer on these organisms resistance to the oxidative products of the respiratory burst. The recently characterized *Salmonella slyA* gene encodes a transcriptional regulator of oxidative stress defense systems that plays an important role in this adaptation (7).

The microaerophilic nature of *C. jejuni* and *C. coli* species implies an inherent sensitivity to oxygen and its reduction products, particularly the superoxide anion. It is likely, therefore, that cellular defenses against the damaging effects of oxidative stress play an important role in the survival of these bacteria during exposure to air. In this respect a number of enzymes, i.e., SOD, alkyl hydroperoxide reductases (AhpC and AhpF), catalase (KatA), glutathione synthetase, and glutathione reductase, are thought to provide the primary protection against oxygen toxicity in bacteria. To date, the products of three genes have been implicated in the oxidative defense of campylobacters. The deleterious effects of exposure to superoxide radicals are counteracted by the activity of SOD. Both *C. jejuni* and *C. coli* possesses a single iron–cofactored SOD (43, 45). Inactivation of the *sodB* gene, by allelic exchange, has demonstrated a clear role for SOD in the defense against oxida-

tive stress and aerotolerance (47). In addition, both catalase and alkylhydroperoxide reductase are involved in aspects of the oxidative defense of campylobacters (2, 17).

Insight into the mechanisms of regulation of gene expression in response to oxidative stress in campylobacters was first gained from analysis of the promoter regions of the genes encoding AhpC, KatA, and SodB. The promoter regions of all three genes possess sequences which closely resemble the *E. coli* Fur box consensus, implying Fur-mediated iron-responsive genetic regulation (2, 17, 43, 45). Furthermore, the expression of both AhpC and KatA is induced by iron limitation (2, 39). However, the finding that the expression of both AhpC and KatA is not derepressed in a *C. jejuni* Fur-deficient mutant implicates an alternative regulator in the expression of antioxidant enzymes in campylobacters (65). Analysis of the genome sequence, however, indicates that the key regulators of oxidative stress defense enzymes in *E. coli* and *S. typhimurium*, namely, SoxRS, OxyR, and SlyA, are not present in *C. jejuni*. Additional factors must therefore be involved in the regulation of the oxidative stress response. In this context, it is now apparent that a number of bacteria possess Fur-like homologues (42). For example, analysis of the complete genome sequence of *B. subtilis* reveals the presence of three open reading frames encoding proteins with significant homology to Fur (5, 30). While one of these is clearly equivalent to the iron uptake regulator Fur, a second Fur homologue, termed PerR, mediates the response to oxidative stress, including the induction of AhpC and catalase expression in *B. subtilis* (5). Consequently, the identification of a second Fur homologue in the *C. jejuni* genome sequence implies a role for this protein as a global regulator of the *Campylobacter* response to oxidative stress, which includes the regulation of AhpC and KatA expression (65).

THERMOREGULATION OF GENE EXPRESSION

C. coli and *C. jejuni* are able to grow at temperatures above 30°C and below 47°C, while an incubation temperature of 42 to 45°C is considered optimal. Since the temperature of the avian gastrointestinal tract is 42°C, this optimum growth requirement is probably related to the fact that these organisms colonize the gastrointestinal tract of birds. However, campylobacters are likely to be exposed to widely fluctuating temperatures, and their ability to regulate gene expression in response to temperature is therefore fundamental to their continuing survival.

Cold Shock

Since campylobacters can be isolated from a wide variety of aqueous environmental sources and refrigerated foods (49), they must be able to survive exposure to low temperatures for considerable periods. Although the survival of campylobacters at low temperatures is likely to play an important role in maintaining the contamination cycle of this pathogen, little is known about their metabolism and adaptation during exposure to this stress.

Many bacteria produce cold shock proteins when they are exposed to temperatures at or below their minimal growth temperature. In *E. coli,* for example, the major cold shock protein, CspA, is induced at low temperatures and is believed to act as an RNA chaperone to block the formation of secondary structures in mRNA (74). From analysis of the *C. jejuni* genome sequence, it is apparent that this bacterium does not contain genes encoding any previously characterized cold shock proteins. However, the organism is still motile and is able to consume oxygen, generate ATP, and synthesize proteins at 4°C, all of which are indicators that vital cellular processes are still functioning (22). Consequently, the mechanism of adaptation and regulation of gene expression during cold shock must be different from the paradigms established for other bacteria.

Heat Shock Response

The heat shock response is an important homeostatic mechanism that enables bacterial cells to survive a variety of environmental stresses and is characterized by the transiently increased synthesis of a number of proteins called heat shock proteins. Moreover, heat shock proteins are involved not only in the initial "shock" response but also in the steady-state adaptation to higher temperatures, since they remain at elevated levels if incubation is continued at the higher temperature. These proteins are known to play important roles in vivo and may act either as chaperones or as ATP-dependent proteases involved in the degradation of abnormal proteins.

At least 24 proteins are preferentially synthesized by *C. jejuni* immediately following heat shock (27). Some of these, such as GroELS, DnaJ, and Lon protease, have been characterized previously (27, 62, 63, 73). Furthermore, the importance of the heat shock response has been emphasized by the recent finding that *dnaJ* mutants are severely retarded in growth at 46°C and are unable to colonize chickens. This suggests that the heat shock response plays an important role in both thermotolerance and colonization (27).

Clp ATP-Dependent Proteases

The ability of bacteria to respond to environmental signals is dependent not only upon their ability to synthesize new proteins but also upon the rapid reversal of this process. One of the ways this is accomplished is by the targeted hydrolysis of regulatory proteins. The Clp ATP-dependent proteases are involved in the regulation of proteolysis in a number of bacteria during heat shock and adaptation to other stresses. These consist of the proteolytic subunit, ClpP, to which substrate specificity is conferred through association with either ClpC, ClpB, or ClpX ATPase subunits (67). In a number of bacteria, these protease components are implicated in the resistance of the cells to a variety of environmental stresses. For example, a *clpC* mutant of *Listeria monocytogenes* is hypersensitive to a number of stresses including heat shock (51). Homologues of ClpP (Cj0192C) and the ATPase subunits ClpB (Cj0509C), ClpA (Cj1108), and ClpX (Cj0275) were all found to be present in *C. jejuni* following analysis of the genome sequence, and it is therefore likely that they perform a similar role in campylobacters, i.e., the regulation of proteolysis in response to environmental stress.

Regulation of the Heat Shock Response

The heat shock response is characterized by the transiently increased synthesis of a number of heat shock proteins. In *E. coli,* the heat shock response is positively regulated and depends primarily upon the increased synthesis and stabilization of the otherwise scarce alternative σ factor σ^{32}. In contrast, *B. subtilis* contains three classes of heat shock genes. Class I heat shock genes are negatively regulated by HrcA, which interacts with a *cis*-active inverted repeat termed CIRCE (76). The expression of class II heat shock genes is positively regulated by σ^B (55), while class III heat shock genes are expressed from vegetative promoters and controlled by the negative regulator CtsR (29).

While it is clear that *C. jejuni* has a substantial repertoire of heat shock proteins and is thus likely to exhibit a heat shock response characteristic of that of most other bacteria, the mechanisms of regulation of the heat shock response have not been characterized experimentally and are still largely unknown. However, a number of recent studies and analysis of the *C. jejuni* genome sequence have provided some insight into the likely mechanisms regulating the heat shock response of campylobacters. For example, it is apparent from the genome sequence that *C. jejuni* does not possess a homologue of σ^{32}, the heat shock-specific σ factor (a detailed discussion of the σ factors present in *C. jejuni* appears below), suggesting that the mechanism of regulation of the heat shock response is markedly different from that seen in *E. coli.* Furthermore, analysis of the *C. jejuni* genome sequence reveals the presence of a number of heat shock proteins, some of which, by analogy to other bacterial heat shock regulatory mechanisms, may be expressed as components of heat shock-regulated operons. In *B. subtilis,* DnaK, an analogue of Hsp70 and a putative chaperonin, is expressed as part of the

dnaK heat shock operon. HrcA, encoded by the first gene acts as a negative regulator of other heat shock genes within the operon, namely, *grpE, dnaK,* and *dnaJ* (55). A similar operon, encoding homologues of HrcA (Cj0757) (this and the following designations correspond to a database of preliminary predicted proteins produced by the Pathogen Sequence Group at the Sanger Centre and can be obtained from ftp://ftp.sanger.ac.uk/pub/pathogens/cj/CJ.pep), GrpE (Cj0758), and DnaK (0759), is present in the genome of *C. jejuni,* and it is likely that it represents a heat shock operon wherein the HcrA homologue serves as negative regulator. However, *dnaJ* is absent from this operon but appears elsewhere on the *C. jejuni* chromosome (Cj1260C). The *dnaK* operon in *Streptomyces albus,* by way of comparison, comprises *dnaK, grpE, dnaJ,* and *hspR* in that order. In this instance, HspR a protein belonging to the MerR family of transcriptional regulators, is responsible for the negative control of the heat shock operon (6). Intriguingly, analysis of the *C. jejuni* genome sequence reveals the presence of another operon, encoding a CbpA homologue (Cj1229), a heat shock protein member of the DnaJ family, and a HspR homologue (Cj1230). If HspR performs the same function in *C. jejuni,* it is likely that it, too, regulates expression of the operon, which includes the heat shock protein CbpA, in response to heat shock.

There are potentially three regulatory systems controlling the induction of the heat shock response in *C. jejuni.* The RacRS regulon, previously characterized as a two-component regulatory system, is required for the differential expression of proteins at 37 and 42°C and is therefore likely to play a role in the regulation of the heat shock response (4). Since there are also homologues of HrcA and HspR, negative regulators of the heat shock response in *B. subtilis* and *S. albus,* respectively, and since they are linked to the expression of the known heat shock genes, *dnaJ* and *cbpA,* they are also likely to regulate some aspects of the heat shock response in *C. jejuni.* The identification of

CIRCE-like consensus sequences upstream of the *groESL* and *dnaK* operons of *C. jejuni* (61, 62) provides further support that the expression of these and maybe other heat shock genes is regulated by the HrcA homologue. However, it is also apparent from an analysis of the genome sequence that σ^{32}, the *E. coli* heat shock regulatory σ factor, σ_B, the regulator of *B. subtilis* class II heat shock genes, and CtsR, the regulator of *B. subtilis* class III heat shock genes, are all absent from *C. jejuni*. If the expression of components of the heat shock response is regulated by HrcA and/or HspR, *C. jejuni* would intriguingly have representatives of the heat shock regulatory systems from two different bacterial systems, namely, the class I heat shock regulon of *B. subtilis* and that from *S. albus*.

Thermoregulation and Virulence Gene Expression

The high energy cost of unnecessary virulence factor production requires that the expression of these specialized functions be strictly regulated and confined to periods during invasion and colonization of the host organism. In this context, transfer from the environment into the host offers a number of cues that bacteria can recognize as the requirement for the expression of virulence functions. One such signal is an increase in temperature.

The activity of some bacterial promoters which respond to changes in temperature, including those controlling the expression of invasion functions and other virulence loci (23), is correlated with the degree of DNA supercoiling. Thus, supercoiling has emerged as a central mediator of many temperature-regulated virulence regulons. Prokaryotic cells contain a number of proteins involved in the organization of the chromosomal DNA, and these are normally small, abundant, and basic. Among these, HU, IHF, FIS, and H-NS have been characterized in detail (21). In particular, one of the main nucleoid-associated proteins, H-NS, controls the temperature-dependent expression of a number of virulence genes. Most of these target genes are also regulated by

other environmental parameters such as pH and osmolarity. At present there is no information about the mechanisms controlling DNA supercoiling and the relationship between DNA conformation and temperature-regulated gene expression for campylobacters. Although a homologue of HU, a heterodimer capable of wrapping DNA into nucleosome-like particles, has been shown to be present in *C. jejuni* (28), a preliminary analysis of the genome sequence demonstrates that homologues of H-NS, FIS, and IHF are absent. This suggests either that the capacity of *C. jejuni* to modulate the level of DNA supercoiling in response to environmental parameters is restricted or that it occurs through as yet uncharacterized mechanisms.

ENVIRONMENTAL REGULATION OF GENE EXPRESSION THROUGH THE ACTION OF σ FACTORS

The DNA-dependent RNA polymerase is the key enzyme in transcription in eubacteria and, as such, controls an important step in gene regulation, that of transcriptional initiation. Transcription in prokaryotes is mediated by the RNA polymerase holoenzyme, which comprises two components: the core RNA polymerase and a σ factor. The frequency with which the holoenzyme initiates transcription is influenced by the promoter sequence and the conformation of the DNA in this region. Since the σ factor recognizes conserved nucleotides within the promoter consensus sequence, its presence will also govern the rate of transcriptional initiation by the holoenzyme at a particular sequence. In effect, therefore, the σ factor can confer specificity to the RNA polymerase. Consequently, the availability of a specific σ factor can lead to differential gene expression; many bacteria therefore possess a number of alternative σ factors which allow for coordinated changes in gene expression in response to different environmental stimuli.

The Primary σ factor, σ^{70}

At least one primary σ factor, generally termed σ^{70}, is present in a given bacterial species, is responsible for the transcription of most genes expressed in exponentially growing cells, and is essential for cell survival. The lack of typical *E. coli* σ^{70} consensus sequences in front of many *Campylobacter* genes raised the possibility that a different sequence forms the *Campylobacter* σ^{70} recognition sequence (71). Indeed, it is now known that the *C. jejuni* promoter region for many housekeeping genes is unlike the equivalent sequences encountered in other bacteria. Accordingly, it consists of three conserved regions centered 10, 16, and 35 bp upstream of the transcriptional start site. While the -10 site closely matches the typical σ^{70} *E. coli* promoter site, the -16 region is more often observed in the promoters of gram-positive bacteria and the -35 site is very different from the corresponding regions of both *B. subtilis* and *E. coli* (71). Characterization of the *rpoD* gene, encoding the primary σ factor of *C. jejuni,* has revealed some interesting features which may be correlated with the recognition of this unique canonical promoter sequence. For example, all known σ^{70} proteins contain a conserved region of 10 amino acids in subregion 4.2 except those in *C. jejuni* and *Helicobacter pylori* (72).

Analysis of the recently completed genome sequence for *C. jejuni* reveals the presence of only three σ factors, which parallels the situation in *H. pylori* (64). These are the major sigma factor RpoD or σ^{70}; σ^{54} or RpoN, which in enterobacteria and other organisms controls the expression of a wide variety of genes including those for nitrogen metabolism, and, finally, σ^{28} (RpoF or FliA), which generally controls the expression of genes required for flagellum formation and chemotaxis.

The Alternative σ factor σ^{54}

The alternative σ factor σ^{54} was first identified in enteric bacteria through its involvement in nitrogen fixation and assimilation. However, it is now apparent that the role of σ^{54} is much broader and that it is required by a variety of genes for transcriptional activation. For example, genes encoding proteins involved in dicarboxylate synthesis in *Pseudomonas putida,* the

formation of fimbriae in *Neisseria meningitidis,* and flagellar synthesis in *Caulobacter crescentus* all require RpoN for transcriptional activation (31). Further evidence for the diversity of σ^{54} mediated regulatory gene expression has recently been obtained in experiments with the pathogen *Vibrio cholerae* (26). A σ^{54} null mutant of this bacterium lacks a functional flagellum and is also defective for colonization in an infant-mouse model of cholera. However, the colonization defect is distinct from the nonmotile phenotype of the σ^{54} mutant, suggesting multiple and distinct roles for σ^{54} during the *V. cholera* pathogenic cycle.

The role that σ^{54} plays in the environmental regulation of gene expression in *C. jejuni* is poorly defined. However, the presence of a σ^{54} recognition sequence in the promoter sequence of the *flaB* gene, encoding a subunit of the *Campylobacter* flagellin, suggests that expression of *flaB* is regulated by σ^{54} (1, 37). Indeed, inactivation of the *C. jejuni rpoN* gene results in the abolition of FlaB expression (70). While this confirms the dependency of *flaB* expression on σ^{54}, other factors necessary for flagellum formation are also thought to be dependent on σ^{54} (25). By analogy to other bacteria, σ^{54} is also likely to play an important role in the environmental regulation of other genes. However, further characterization of σ^{54}-dependent genes is needed before a more complete understanding of the role of this protein in *Campylobacter* physiology can be gained.

The Alternative σ factor σ^{28}

The third sigma factor identified by analysis of the *C. jejuni* genome shows the greatest homology to σ^{28}. In *E. coli,* at least 50 genes are involved in the formation of a functional flagellum and σ^{28} is necessary for the expression of most of these (33). Similarly, SigD of *B. subtilis* is a member of this family and plays a similar role in the control of flagellin gene expression. While the exact function of σ^{28} in *C. jejuni* remains to be elucidated, it is likely that it too, plays a role in the regulation of flagellin gene expression and motility. In this context, the promoter of the *flaA* gene, encoding the major structural component of the flagellin, contains a consensus σ^{28} recognition sequence (37). It is probable, therefore, that expression of FlaA and other proteins involved in flagellum formation is dependent upon σ^{28}, although as yet there is no biochemical evidence to support this assumption.

Role of σ^{28} and σ^{54} in Regulation of Flagellar Gene Expression

The *Campylobacter* flagella are known to play an important role in pathogenicity. The existence of two tandemly arranged flagellin genes, namely, *flaA* and *flaB,* which are transcribed from σ^{28} and σ^{54}-dependent promoters respectively (1, 37), suggests that differential expression of the two genes may lead to the production of different types of flagella. Such a mechanism may provide the cell with a means of responding to changes in environmental parameters such as pH, viscosity, or the presence of neutralizing antibodies. In this context, expression of the *Campylobacter flaB* gene is influenced by environmental parameters (1, 39), and it is likely that σ^{54} plays some role.

Role of Three σ factors

It is possible that genome size and/or the ability of bacteria to adapt to a wide range of environmental conditions is related to the number of σ factors that they possess. Certainly, organisms which are able to adapt to and grow in the widest range of environments possess a correspondingly large number of σ factors. For example, *E. coli* and *B. subtilis,* which are both capable of growth and survival in a diverse range of environments, have 7 and 18 σ factors, respectively (3, 30). In contrast, *H. pylori,* which is not known to reside extensively in the external environment and, accordingly, is exposed to only a limited range of environments, possesses only three σ factors (64). Given its frequent isolation from a wide variety of environmental sources, it is apparent that *C. jejuni* is exposed to and can tolerate a much greater diversity of environments than *H. pylori*. It is intriguing, therefore, that like *H. pylori,* the genome of *C. jejuni* encodes only three

σ factors and that these are of the same type. The lack of specific σ factors, such as RpoS, which regulates the expression of genes involved in the resistance to inimical stress, and σ^{32}, which regulates the classical heat shock response, suggests that alternative regulatory mechanisms must exist in campylobacters. It also possible that although the number of σ factors types is limited in *C. jejuni,* the two alternative factors that are present play wider regulatory roles than those that have been characterized previously for *E. coli* and other bacteria.

REGULATION OF GENE EXPRESSION DURING STARVATION AND STATIONARY PHASE
Absence of RpoS

In other bacterial species, entry into the stationary phase or exposure to starvation conditions is accompanied by profound structural and physiological changes which result in increased resistance to heat shock and to oxidative, osmotic, and acidic stress. In *E. coli,* the expression of 30 or more genes is induced in response to entry into stationary phase or to starvation (32). The central regulator for many of these stationary-phase-induced changes in a number of gram-negative bacteria is the σ factor RpoS, which, accordingly, is critical for the survival of the bacterial cell in stationary phase and following exposure to many suboptimal conditions. A reflection of the importance of RpoS, in regulating the response of bacteria to a variety of inimical stresses is its widespread occurrence in a diverse range of bacterial species. To date, RpoS homologues have been found in most members of the *Enterobacteriaceae, Pseudomonas* species, *Vibrio* species, *Borrelia burgdoferi,* and *Aquifex aeolicus.* Despite its ability to survive in many oligotrophic environments, such as surface waters, it is apparent from analysis of the genome sequence that *C. jejuni* does not possess an RpoS homologue. Although we know little about the response of campylobacters to stationary phase and starvation, if they do exhibit adaptive responses to these environmental parameters, they will not be regulated by RpoS and must therefore rely on alternative and perhaps novel regulatory mechanisms instead.

Stringent Response

In many other bacteria, the cellular response to amino acid starvation is manifested when the ability to aminoacylate tRNA fails to keep up with the demands of protein synthesis in the growing cell and entails the coordinated regulation of numerous cellular activities known as the stringent response (16). The gaunosine nucleotide (p)ppGpp, synthesis of which is dependent upon Re1A, is considered to be central to this response. The enzymes of (p)ppGpp metabolism are now well characterized in a number of bacteria and are ppGpp synthase I (Re1A), (p)ppGpp 3′-pyrophosphohydrolase (SpoT), pppGpp 5′-phosphohydrolase (Gpp), and nucleoside 5′-diphosphate kinase (Ndk). However, while the *C. jejuni* genome contains genes encoding clear homologues of Ndk (Cj0332C), Gpp (0353C), and SpoT (1272C) and thus appears to have some of the apparatus necessary for (p)ppGpp metabolism, this cannot be taken as evidence that *C. jejuni* exhibits a true stringent response. Recently, it has been has shown that in *H. pylori*, guanosine polyphosphate levels do not rise as a result of amino acid starvation, and, as such, this organism constitutes the first example of a wild-type eubacterium showing a relaxed phenotype (56). In comparison, like *C. jejuni, H. pylori* has the enzymatic machinery for (p)ppGpp metabolism.

CsrA

Two homologues, CsrA (for "carbon storage regulator"), and RsmA (for "repressor of stationary-phase metabolites"), have been recently identified as part of a global regulatory system that controls bacterial gene expression posttranscriptionally (50). CsrA is thought to repress the expression of genes by binding to and destabilizing specific mRNA molecules. The second component of the Csr system CsrB, is a noncoding RNA molecule that forms a large globular ribonucleoprotein complex with CsrA and antagonizes its action. Numerous genes whose expression occurs in the stationary phase of growth are repressed by CsrA/RsmA, and, furthermore, CsrA may even activate certain exponential-phase metabolic pathways. In *E. coli,* glycogen catabolism, gluconeogenesis, glycolysis, motility, and adherence are modulated by CsrA, while in *Erwinia carotovora,* the production of several secreted virulence factors and, potentially, other secondary metabolites are regulated by RsmA. Given the lack of other key starvation and stationary-phase regulators, the identification of the CsrA homologue (Cj1103) from analysis of the genome sequence suggests that this novel kind of regulatory system is likely to play a key role in modulating gene expression in *C. jejuni* in response to starvation and stationary-phase conditions.

cAMP-CRP System

The cyclic AMP (cAMP)-cAMP receptor protein (CRP) system allows the use of alternative carbon sources and plays a role as an activator of approximately two-thirds of the carbon starvation-responsive genes in *E. coli* (34). However, glucose-linked catabolite repression, as it functions in *E. coli,* probably does not operate in *C. jejuni,* since glucose is not utilized as a carbon source and therefore may not be transported into the cell for this purpose. However, an analysis of the genome sequence does indicate the presence of a peptide with homology to the CRP/FNR (Cj0466) family of regulatory proteins, although the exact function of this protein is unknown. It is tempting to speculate, though, that since FNR is a positive regulator of genes encoding proteins involved in a variety of anaerobic electron transport systems in *E. coli* (57), this protein may be relevant to the response of campylobacters to reduced oxygen levels.

REGULATION OF GENE EXPRESSION BY TRANSCRIPTION REGULATORY PROTEINS

As mentioned above, certain global regulatory proteins such as OxyR and SoxS are absent from *C. jejuni*. Both proteins are examples of helix–turn–helix proteins, which form a large family of transcriptional regulatory proteins in prokaryotes. Other members of this family of proteins include Lrp, a global regulator of metabolism (8); the LysR family of transcriptional regulators (53); and the AraC/XylS family of positive transcriptional regulators (15). A preliminary analysis of the *C. jejuni* genome sequence demonstrates that while there are putative single representatives from both the LysR family (CJ1000) and the AraC family (CJ1042C), there does not appear to be a homologue of Lrp. In comparison with *B. subtilis,* which contains 19 members of the LysR family, 11 members of the AraC family, and 7 members of the Lrp family (30), the numbers of these classes of transcriptional regulators is very limited. Again, this is consistent with the general deficiency of global regulatory proteins in campylobacters.

REGULATION OF GENE EXPRESSION BY TWO-COMPONENT REGULATORY SYSTEMS

Prokaryotes have evolved highly sophisticated signal transduction systems, which, in response to environmental stress, control the coordinated regulation of cellular defense mechanisms. Although many different types of regulatory systems are involved in the adaptive responses of bacteria, these systems can be grouped into families depending on their mechanism of action. The family of two-component regulatory systems is made up of an important group of regulators, which direct the response of bacteria to a wide range of external and environmental stimuli (59). These usually comprise a cytoplasmic membrane-associated histidine protein kinase sensor (HK) and a cytoplasmic response regulator (RR). The sensor component is able to monitor changes in the environment and, in response to a specific environmental parameter, initiates the first step of phosphotransfer pathway, involving the autophosphorylation of a histidine residue within its C-terminal domain. The signal is then transduced via the transfer of the phosphate residue to an aspartic acid residue in the N-terminal domain of the RR, which subsequently modulates gene expression or protein-protein interaction.

Two-component regulatory systems are widespread in bacteria, and there appears to be a correlation between the number of these systems and the ability of bacteria to adapt to environmental conditions. For example, in *B. subtilis,* which can exist in and tolerate a wide range of environments, there are 34 genes encoding RRs, most of which have adjacent genes encoding HKs (30). In contrast, *H. pylori,* which occupies only a limited number of environmental niches, contains just four sensor proteins and seven RRs, which is approximately one-third of the number found in *E. coli* (64).

A preliminary analysis of the *C. jejuni* genome sequence reveals the presence of a number of genes encoding putative HKs and RRs. One such gene encodes a large (85-kDa) protein (Cj0284C) with an amino terminus that is homologous to the sensor protein CheA and a carboxyl terminus that is homologous to the RR CheY. It is likely, therefore, that this represents a bifunctional protein containing both HK and RR domains and is equivalent to CheF of *H. pylori* and CheAY of *Rhodospirillum centenum* (24). In addition, there are genes encoding 7 putative HK sensor proteins and 10 putative RR proteins in *C. jejuni*. In five cases, the genes encoding the RRs are adjacent to those encoding the HKs, while two HKs and five RRs are unpaired. In comparison to *H. pylori, C. jejuni* contains three additional HKs and three additional RRs, and it is likely that this reflects the greater adaptive potential of the latter.

The presence of a number of two-component regulatory systems suggests that these form a major regulatory family in *C. jejuni*. Although the function of many of these regulators is unknown, it is likely that they play a central role in the physiological response of campylobacters to the environment. The roles of some of the *C. jejuni* two-component regulatory systems have already been partially characterized. Chemotaxis, particularly towards the constituents of mucin, is considered to be an important factor controlling the colonization of the intestinal tract by campylobacters. One uncoupled RR (Cj1118C) is similar in both structure and sequence to CheY and is therefore likely to play a role in the regulation of chemotaxis. However, overexpression of this protein leads to the attenuation of adherence and invasion in cell culture assays, and it may therefore play some as yet uncharacterized role in modulating virulence gene expression (75). In addition, one of the coupled HK-RR systems, designated RacRS, plays a role in the regulation of temperature-induced changes in gene expression (4). Insight into the function of other two-component regulatory systems may be gained by analysis of their similarity to previously characterized systems and the location of the corresponding genes within the genome. Thus, given its striking homology to KdpD from *E. coli* and its location downstream of genes encoding structural components of a putative high-affinity transporter, KdpABC (Cj0671 to Cj0679), it is tempting to speculate that the uncoupled HK (Cj0679) has a similar function to KdpD. In *E. coli*, expression of the KdpABC transporter is regulated at the transcriptional level by turgor pressure and the osmolarity of the environment, via KdpD and KdpE, which form a paired HK and RR. If peptide Cj0679 is a KdpD homologue, it is likely to play a role in osmosensing and in the regulation of potassium uptake in campylobacters.

MUTATION-BASED REGULATION OF GENE EXPRESSION

To survive in a diverse range of environments, all bacterial species must be able to adapt in order to optimize their survival under a particular set of conditions. The classical mechanism for phenotypic adaptation requires that the bacterium be able to sense its surroundings and, in response, change its pattern of gene expression to bring about the increased synthesis of proteins necessary to counter the detrimental effects induced by the environment. However, it is now evident that at least some pathogens have evolved another solution to ensure their survival and that this comprises the operation

of mutational systems to diversify the phenotypes of individual cells within propagating populations (36, 52). This adaptive strategy, which acts via high-frequency genetic variation, can create repertoires of different strain types within a given population and has increasingly been documented in a number of bacterial species.

The presence of homonucleotide tracts and multiple short tandem repeats within open reading frames is often associated with a mutation-based strategy for gene regulation. These regions are hypermutable because of slippage within the DNA repeats. This results in the frequent shifting into and out of frame, which in turn generates on-off switching in the expression of the corresponding gene product and thereby generate antigenic or phase variation. Consequently, these types of repetitive element can be used as markers to indicate the presence of genes in which this process is likely to operate, and the availability of whole genome sequences now allows this kind of analysis to be carried out in silico (52). For example, the availability of the *H. pylori* genome sequence facilitated the initial identification of 17 putative phase-variable genes (64), while a more detailed in silico analysis identified a further 10 putative phase-variable genes (52).

Long before the availability of the *C. jejuni* genome sequence, it was apparent that the expression of at least some genes in campylobacters was governed by mechanisms which generated high levels of genetic variation. In particular, some strains of *Campylobacter* have long been known to undergo both antigenic variation (19) and phase variation of flagellar expression, with the latter involving a bidirectional transition between flagellate and aflagellate phenotypes (12). Events which lead to the loss of the flagellum and/or its antigenic variation may provide campylobacters with a mechanism to escape the host immune response. Furthermore, such an event would also allow the cell to save energy under circumstances where motility is not necessary. Interestingly, thermophilic campylobacters, which have the highest transition rate for flagellar phase variation in both directions, have the broadest host range in nature (12).

Evidence of the molecular mechanisms that operate to generate genetic variation and that are part of a mutation–based adaptive strategy has come to light recently. High-frequency reversible phase variation of flagellin gene expression in *C. coli* UA585, at least, can be correlated with insertion–deletion mutations in a poly(T) tract of seven or eight bases in the *flhA* gene (40). FlhA is a member of the LcrD/FlbF family, which are all integral cytoplasmic membrane proteins involved in the regulation or secretion of surface or extracellular proteins including flagellin (35). Whether or not *flhA* is a direct regulator of flagellin gene expression is unclear, but nevertheless the effect of slippage within the poly(T) tract is to prevent the expression of *flaA* and *flaB* and probably other flagellum–associated genes in a subpopulation of cells. The abrogation of *flhA* expression in this manner would therefore result in a significant reduction in macromolecular synthesis within such cells and would conserve their biosynthetic capacity under circumstances when motility is not necessary. Furthermore, flagellar phase variation may provide *C. coli* with the possibility of escaping the host immune response to the flagellum.

Given the high AT content of *Campylobacter* species, the genome will contain numerous poly(A/T) tracts. It is likely, therefore, that slippage within such DNA repeats operates at a number of other sites within the *Campylobacter* genome and consequently may give rise in part to the high degree of phenotypic variability that is seen with this organism (66). A preliminary analysis of the *C. jejuni* genome sequence reveals the presence of at least 25 polymorphic regions that correspond to repeat sequences. Most of the peptides encoded by the open reading frames containing repeat elements do not show significant homology to previously characterized proteins. There are, however, a number of exceptions. Repeat elements are present in genes encoding a type IIS restriction modification system (peptides Cj0031 and Cj0032); *recC*, encoding part of an exodeoxyri-

bonuclease V (peptide 0685C) and two open reading frames encoding proteins (Cj1139 and Cj1320) that may be involved in lipopolysaccharide biosynthesis. Peptide Cj1139C probably represents LgtD, a glycosyltransferase, and peptide Cj1320 represents an aminotransferase involved in lipopolysaccharide biosynthesis. In addition, there is a polymorphic region within an rRNA operon encoding rRNA. Intriguingly, there is also at least one family, containing five proteins with a high degree of identity, which are all encoded by genes containing a repeat region of nine G residues (Cj1305C, Cj1306C, Cj1310C, Cj1342C, and Cj0617/0618). These proteins do not show any significant homology to any previously characterized proteins, and so their function remains unclear. Another peptide, Cj1335, encoded by a gene containing a repeat region of nine G residues appears to be cotranscribed with PtmB (Cj1331) and PtmA (Cj1332), and, given that these two proteins are involved in posttranslational flagellin modification (19), it is tempting to speculate that the on–off switching of expression of this protein plays some role in the antigenic variation of the flagellin.

CONCLUSION

The ability to respond rapidly to changes in the environment is fundamental to the continuing survival of many bacteria and requires that the organism be able to sense its surroundings and modify its physiology accordingly. Although change in a specific environmental parameter might induce a particular regulon, many regulatory networks show some degree of cross-regulation, and generally a given environmental condition will induce more than one regulon. However, for the sake of simplicity, the responses of bacteria to changes in environmental conditions are often characterized in terms of oxidative stress, anaerobic stress, osmotic stress, DNA damage, heat stress, starvation and stationary-phase stress, nutrient limitation, and pH stress.

While *C. jejuni* and *C. coli* are acknowledged to be the most prevalent food-borne bacterial enteric pathogens in the developed world, our understanding of the ability of these bacteria to recognize and adapt to environmental conditions is only beginning; however, it will be greatly enhanced by the determination of the genome sequence. Already, this information has provided important data about a number of key regulatory systems. Thus, it is clear that a Fur homologue plays an important role in controlling gene expression in campylobacters in response to iron limitation and in a manner that is analogous to that in other bacteria. Consequently, when iron is limiting, the expression of a number of systems for transporting iron, in the form of siderophores and iron-containing host-derived compounds, is induced, this is mediated by Fur at the transcriptional level. In addition, it is likely that a second Fur homologue, termed PerR (65), is responsible for the regulation of expression of genes, including those encoding catalase and alkyl hyderoperoxide reductases, involved in the resistance to oxidative stress.

While campylobacters do not have any established cold shock proteins, it is clear from the analysis of the genome sequence that they do have a substantial repertoire of heat shock proteins and are thus likely to exhibit a heat shock response characteristic of that of most other bacteria. However, the absence of a σ^{32} homologue in *C. jejuni* suggests that the mechanism of regulation of the heat shock response is markedly different from that *E. coli*. There are, however, potentially three regulatory systems controlling the induction of the heat shock response in *C. jejuni*, namely, the RacRS regulon, HrcA, and HspR.

Despite the ability of *C. jejuni* to survive in a diverse range of environments, including the gastrointestinal tracts of animals and humans, food, and oligotrophic environments such as surface waters, its capacity for regulating gene expression in response to changes in environmental parameters appears to be limited in comparison to that of other bacteria, including *E. coli* and *B. subtilis*. For example, a number of key global regulatory proteins, such as OxyR, SoxRS, and Lrp, are absent. Furthermore, the capacity to modulate gene expression through

the use of alternative sigma factors also appears to be very limited, since only two alternative σ factors, σ^{54} and σ^{28}, are present. Compared to *E. coli* and *B. subtilis*, which possess 6 and 17 alternative σ factors, respectively, this number is minimal. Notably, the σ factor RpoS, which is a key regulator of stationary-phase and stress responses in other gram-negative bacteria, is absent. It is possible, however, that the two alternative σ factors present in *C. jejuni* play wider regulatory roles than those observed in other bacteria and that this may compensate to some extent for the numerical shortfall. The presence of a number of two-component regulatory systems suggests that these are a major regulatory family in this organism, and it is therefore likely that they play a central role in the physiological response of campylobacters to the environment. Again, in comparison to certain other bacteria, *C. jejuni* contains far fewer of these systems.

The related pathogen *H. pylori*, like *C. jejuni*, contains only a limited number of global regulatory proteins (64). It, too, has few two-component regulatory systems and no OxyR, SoxRS, RpoH, or RpoS homologues. The lack of such regulatory systems in *H. pylori*, however, can be rationalized by the fact that this organism is not known to reside extensively in the external environment between hosts and is therefore not exposed to a diverse range of environmental stresses. This is clearly not the case with *C. jejuni*, since this organism can be isolated from and encounters widely different environments, including the gastrointestinal tracts of animals, food, and water. The lack of established regulatory mechanisms in *C. jejuni* is therefore intriguing. However, the historical focus of bacterial physiology research has concentrated on a limited number of bacteria, notably *E. coli* and *B. subtilis*, and this has generated a legacy of assumptions which do not necessarily apply to all bacteria. Thus, in the absence of established adaptive mechanisms, other novel systems may account for the ability of campylobacters to survive in diverse environments. Also, since analysis of the genome sequence reveals an unusually large number of distinct frameshift mutator elements, a general solution for *Campylobacter* survival may lie in the operation of mutational systems to diversify the antigenic and phenotypic properties of individual cells within propagating populations.

REFERENCES

1. **Alm, R. A., P. Guerry, and T. J. Trust.** 1993. The *Campylobacter* σ⁵⁴ promoter is subject to environmental regulation. *J. Bacteriol.* **175:** 4448–4455.

2. **Baillon, M.-L., A. H. M. van Vliet, C. Constantinidou, J. M. Ketley, and C. W. Penn.** 1998. Cloning and sequencing of an iron-regulated AhpC homologue from *Campylobacter jejuni,* p. 523. *In* A. J. Lastovica, D. G. Newell, and E. E. Lastovica (ed.), *Campylobacter, Helicobacter and Related Organisms.* Institute of Child Health, Cape Town, South Africa.

3. **Blattner, F. R., G. Plunkett III, C. A. Bloch, N. T. Perna, V. Burland, M. Riley, J. Collado-Vides, J. D. Glasner, C. K. Rode, G. F. Mayhew, J. Gregor, N. W. Davis, H. A. Kirkpatrick, M. A. Goeden, D. J. Rose, B. Mau, Y. Shao, et al.** 1997. The complete genome sequence of *Escherichia coli* K-12. *Science* **277:**1453–1474.

4. **Bras, A., J. Henderson, B. W. Wren, and J. M. Ketley.** 1996. Identification of a response regulator gene in *Campylobacter jejuni,* p. 619–623. *In* D. G. Newell, J. M. Ketley, and R. Feldman (ed.), *Campylobacters, Helicobacters and Related Organisms.* Plenum Press, New York, N.Y.

5. **Bsat, N., A. Herbig, L. Casillas-Martinez, P. Setlow, and J. D. Helmann.** 1998. *Bacillus subtilis* contains multiple Fur homologues: identification of the iron uptake (Fur) and peroxide regulon (PerR) repressors. *Mol. Microbiol.* **29:**189–198.

6. **Bucca, G., Z. Hindle, and C. P. Smith.** 1997. Regulation of the *dnaK* operon of *Streptomyces coelicolor* A3(2) is governed by HspR, an autoregulatory repressor protein. *J. Bacteriol.* **179:** 5999–6004.

7. **Buchmeier, N., S. Bossie, C. Y. Chen, F. C. Fang, D. G. Guiney, and S. J. Libby.** 1997. SlyA, a transcriptional regulator of *Salmonella typhimurium,* is required for resistance to oxidative stress and is expressed in the intracellular environment of macrophages. *Infect. Immun.* **65:** 3725–3730.

8. **Calvo, J. M., and R. G. Matthews.** 1994. The leucine-responsive regulatory protein, a global regulator of metabolism in *Escherichia coli. Microbiol. Rev.* **58:**466–490.

9. **Chan, V. L., H. Louie, and H. L. Bingham.** 1995. Cloning and transcription regulation of the ferric uptake regulatory gene of *Campylobacter jejuni* TGH9011. *Gene* **164:**25–31.

10. **Demple, B.** 1996. Redox signalling and gene control in the *Escherichia coli* soxRS oxidative stress regulon. *Gene* **179:**53–57.

11. **Dickinson, J. H., K. A. Grant, and S. F. Park.** 1995. Targeted and random mutagenesis of the *Campylobacter coli* chromosome using integrational plasmid vectors. *Curr. Microbiol.* **31:**92–96.

12. **Diker, K. S., G. Hascelik, and M. Akan.** 1992. Reversible expression of flagella in *Campylobacter* spp. *FEMS Microbiol. Lett.* **78:**261–264.

13. **Doig, P., R. Yao, D. H. Burr, P. Guerry, and T. J. Trust.** 1996. An environmentally regulated pilus-like appendage involved in *Campylobacter* pathogenesis. *Mol. Microbiol.* **20:**885–894.

14. **Field, L. H., V. L. Headley, S. M. Payne, and L. J. Berry.** 1986. Influence of iron on growth, morphology, outer membrane protein composition, and synthesis of siderophores in *Campylobacter jejuni. Infect. Immun.* **54:**126–132.

15. **Gallegos, M. T., R. Schleif, A. Bairoch, K. Hofmann, and J. L. Ramos.** 1997. Arac/XylS family of transcriptional regulators. *Microbiol. Mol. Biol. Rev.* **61:**393–410.

16. **Goldman, E., and H. Jakubowski.** 1990. Uncharged tRNA, protein synthesis, and the bacterial stringent response. *Mol. Microbiol.* **4:**2035–2040.

17. **Grant, K. A., and S. F. Park.** 1995. Molecular characterization of *katA* from *Campylobacter jejuni* and generation of a catalase-deficient mutant of *Campylobacter coli* by intraspecific allelic exchange. *Microbiology* **141:**1369–1376.

18. **Guerry, P., J. Perez-Casal, R. Yao, A. McVeigh, and T. J. Trust.** 1997. A genetic locus involved in iron utilization unique to some *Campylobacter* strains. *J. Bacteriol.* **179:**3997–4002.

19. **Guerry, P., P. Doig, R. A. Alm, D. H. Burr, N. Kinsella, and T. J. Trust.** 1996. Identification and characterisation of genes required for post-translational modification of *Campylobacter coli* VC167 flagellin. *Mol. Microbiol.* **19:**369–378.

20. **Hani, E. C., and V. L. Chan.** 1995. Expression and characterization of *Campylobacter jejuni* benzoylglycine amidohydrolase (hippuricase) gene in *Escherichia coli. J. Bacteriol.* **177:**2396–2402.

21. **Hayat, M. A., and D. A. Mancarella.** 1995. Nucleoid proteins. *Micron* **26:**461–480.

22. **Hazeleger, W. C., J. A. Wouters, F. M. Rombouts, and T. Abee.** 1998. Physiological activity of *Campylobacter jejuni* far below the minimal growth temperature. *Appl. Environ. Microbiol.* **164:** 3917–3922.

23. **Hurme, R., and M. Rhen.** 1998. Temperature sensing in bacterial gene regulation—what it all boils down to. *Mol. Microbiol.* **30:**1–6.

24. **Jiang, Z. Y., and C. E. Bauer.** 1997. Analysis of a chemotaxis operon from *Rhodospirillum centenum. J. Bacteriol.* **179:**5712–5719.

25. **Kinsella, N., P. Guerry, J. Cooney, and T. J. Trust.** 1997. The *flgE* gene of *Campylobacter coli* is under the control of the alternative sigma factor σ^{54}. *J. Bacteriol.* **179:**4647–4653.

26. **Klose, K. E., and J. J. Mekalanos.** 1998. Distinct roles of an alternative sigma factor during both free-swimming and colonizing phases of the *Vibrio cholerae* pathogenic cycle. *Mol. Microbiol.* **28:** 501–520.

27. **Konkel, M. E., B. J. Kim, J. D. Klena, C. R. Young, and R. Ziprin.** 1998. Characterization of the thermal stress response of *Campylobacter jejuni. Infect. Immun.* **66:**3666–3672.

28. **Konkel, M. E., R. T. Marconi, D. J. Mead, and W. Cieplak, Jr.** 1994. Cloning and expression of the *hup* gene encoding a histone-like protein of *Campylobacter jejuni. Gene* **146:**83–86.

29. **Kruger, E., and M. Hecker.** 1998. The first gene of the *Bacillus subtilis clpC* operon, *ctsR,* encodes a negative regulator of its own operon and other class III heat shock genes. *J. Bacteriol.* **180:** 6681–6688.

30. **Kunst, F., N. Ogasawara, I. Moszer, A. M. Albertini, G. Alloni, V. Azevedo, M. G. Bertero, P. Bessieres, A. Bolotin, S. Borchert, R. Borriss, L. Boursier, A. Brans, M. Braun, S. C. Brignell, S. Bron, S. Brouillet, C. V. Bruschi, B. Caldwell, V. Capuano, N. M. Carter, S. K. Choi, J. J. Codani, I. F. Connerton, A. Danchin, et al.** 1997. The complete genome sequence of the gram-positive bacterium *Bacillus subtilis. Nature* **390:**249–256.

31. **Kustu, S., E. Santero, J. Keener, D. Popham, and D. Weiss.** 1989. Expression of σ^{54} (NtrA)-dependent genes is probably united by a common mechanism. *Microbiol. Rev.* **53:**367–376.

32. **Loewen, P. C., and R. Hengge-Aronis.** 1994. The role of the sigma factor σ^s (KatF) in bacterial global regulation. *Annu. Rev. Microbiol.* **48:**53–80.

33. **Macnab, R. M.** 1992. Genetics and biogenesis of bacterial flagella. *Annu. Rev. Genet.* **26:**131–158.

34. **Marschall, C., and R. Hengge-Aronis.** 1995. Regulatory characteristics and promoter analysis of *csiE,* a stationary phase-inducible gene under the control of σ^s and the cAMP-CRP complex in *Escherichia coli. Mol. Microbiol.* **18:**175–184.

35. **Miller, S., E. C. Pesci, and C. L. Pickett.** 1993. A *Campylobacter jejuni* homologue of the LcrD/FlbF family of proteins is necessary for flagellar biogenesis. *Infect. Immun.* **61:**2930–2936.

36. **Moxon, E. R., P. B. Rainey, M. A. Nowak, and R. E. Lenski.** 1994. Adaptive evolution of highly mutable loci in pathogenic bacteria. *Curr. Biol.* **4:**24–33.

37. **Nuijten, P. J., F. J. van Asten, W. Gaastra, and B. A. van der Zeijst.** 1990. Structural and functional analysis of two *Campylobacter jejuni* flagellin genes. *J. Biol. Chem.* **265:**17798–17804.

38. **Ochsner, U. A., and M. L. Vasil.** 1996. Gene repression by the ferric uptake regulator in *Pseudomonas aeruginosa:* cycle selection of iron-regulated genes. *Proc. Natl. Acad. Sci. USA* **93:** 4409–4414.

39. **Park, S. F.** 1999. The use of *hipO,* encoding benzoylglycine amidohydrolase (hippuricase), as a reporter of gene expression in *Campylobacter coli. Lett. Appl. Microbiol.* **28:**285–290.

40. **Park, S. F., D. Purdy, and S. Leach.** 2000. Localized reversible frame shift mutation in the *flhA* gene confers phase variability to flagellin gene expression in *Campylobacter coli. J. Bacteriol.* **182:** 207–210.

41. **Park, S. F., and P. T. Richardson.** 1995. Molecular characterization of a *Campylobacter jejuni* lipoprotein with homology to periplasmic siderophore-binding proteins. *J. Bacteriol.* **177:** 2259–2264.

42. **Patzer, S. I., and K. Hantke.** 1998. The ZnuABC high-affinity zinc uptake system and its regulator Zur in *Escherichia coli. Mol. Microbiol.* **28:** 1199–1210.

43. **Pesci, E. C., D. L. Cottle, and C. L. Pickett.** 1994. Genetic, enzymatic, and pathogenic studies of the iron superoxide dismutase of *Campylobacter jejuni. Infect. Immun.* **62:**2687–2695.

44. **Pickett, C. L., T. Auffenberg, E. C. Pesci, V. L. Sheen, and S. S. Jusuf.** 1992. Iron acquisition and hemolysin production by *Campylobacter jejuni. Infect. Immun.* **60:**3872–3877.

45. **Purdy, D., and S. F. Park.** 1994. Cloning, nucleotide sequence, and characterisation of a gene encoding superoxide dismutase from *Campylobacter jejuni* and *Campylobacter coli. Microbiology* **140:** 1203–1208.

46. **Purdy, D., and S. F. Park.** 1993. Heterologous gene expression in *Campylobacter coli:* the use of bacterial luciferase in a promoter probe vector. *FEMS Microbiol. Lett.* **111:**233–238.

47. **Purdy, D., S. Cawthraw, J. H. Dickinson, D. G. Newell, and S. F. Park.** 1999. Generation of a superoxide dismutase (SOD)-deficient mutant of *Campylobacter coli:* evidence for the significance of SOD in campylobacter survival and colonization. *Appl. Environ. Microbiol.* **65:**2540–2546.

48. **Richardson, P. T., and S. F. Park.** 1995. Enterochelin uptake in *Campylobacter coli:* characterisation of components of a binding protein-dependent transport system. *Microbiology* **141:** 3181–3191.

49. **Rollins, D. M., and R. R. Colwell.** 1986. Viable but nonculturable stage of *Campylobacter jejuni* and its role in survival in the natural aquatic environment. *Appl. Environ. Microbiol.* **52:**531–538.

50. **Romeo, T.** 1998. Global regulation by the small RNA-binding protein CsrA and the non-coding RNA molecule CsrB. *Mol. Microbiol.* **29:** 1321–1330.

51. **Rouquette, C., C. de Chastellier, S. Nair, and P. Berche.** 1998. The ClpC ATPase of *Listeria monocytogenes* is a general stress protein required for virulence and promoting early bacterial escape from the phagosome of macrophages. *Mol. Microbiol.* **27:**1235–1245.

52. **Saunders, N. J., J. F. Peden, D. W. Hood, and E. R. Moxon.** 1998. Simple sequence repeats in the *Helicobacter pylori* genome. *Mol. Microbiol.* **27:** 1091–1098.

53. **Schell, M. A.** 1993. Molecular biology of the LysR family of transcriptional regulators. *Annu. Rev. Microbiol.* **47:**597–626.

54. **Schena, M., D. Shalon, R. W. Davis, and P. O. Brown.** 1995. Quantitative monitoring of gene expression patterns with a complementary DNA microarray. *Science* **270:**467–470.

55. **Schulz, A., and W. Schumann.** 1996. *hrcA*, the first gene of the *Bacillus subtilis dnaK* operon, encodes a negative regulator of class I heat shock genes. *J. Bacteriol.* **178:**1088–1093.

56. **Scoarughi, G. L., C. Cimmino, and P. Donini.** 1999. *Helicobacter pylori*: a eubacterium lacking the stringer response. *J. Bacteriol.* **181:**552–555.

57. **Spiro, S., and J. R. Guest.** 1990. FNR and its role in oxygen-regulated gene expression in *Escherichia coli*. *FEMS Microbiol. Rev.* **6:**399–428.

58. **Stewart, G. S. A. B., and P. J. Williams.** 1992. *lux* genes and the applications of bacterial bioluminescence. *J. Gen. Microbiol.* **138:**1289–1300.

59. **Stock, J. B., A. J. Ninfa, and A. M. Stock.** 1989. Protein phosphorylation and regulation of adaptive responses in bacteria. *Microbiol. Rev.* **53:** 450–490.

60. **Storz, G., L. A. Tartaglia, and B. N. Ames.** 1990. The OxyR regulon. *Antonie Leeuwenhoek* **58:**157–161.

61. **Thies, F. L., H. Karch, H. P. Hartung, and G. Giegerich.** 1999. Cloning and expression of the *dnaK* gene of *Campylobacter jejuni* and antigenicity of heat shock protein 70. *Infect. Immun.* **67:** 1194–1200.

62. **Thies, F. L., A. Weishaupt, H. Karch, H. P. Hartung, and G. Giegerich.** 1999. Cloning, sequencing and molecular analysis of the *Campylobacter jejuni groESL* bicistronic operon. *Microbiology* **145:**89–98.

63. **Thies, F. L., H.-P. Hartung, and G. Giegerich.** 1998. Cloning and expression of the *Campylobacter jejuni lon* gene. *FEMS Microbiol. Lett.* **165:** 329–334.

64. **Tomb, J. F., O. White, A. R. Kerlavage, R. A. Clayton, G. G. Sutton, R. D. Fleisch-** mann, K. A. Ketchum, H. P. Klenk, S. Gill, B. A. Dougherty, K. Nelson, J. Quackenbush, L. Zhou, E. F. Kirkness, S. Peterson, B. Loftus, D. Richardson, R. Dodson, H. G. Khalak, A. Glodek, K. McKenney, L. M. Fitzegerald, N. Lee, M. D. Adams, J. C. Venter, et al. 1997. The complete genome sequence of the gastric pathogen *Helicobacter pylori*. *Nature* **388:**539–547.

65. **van Vliet, A. H. M., K. G. Wooldridge, and J. M. Ketley.** 1998. Iron-responsive gene regulation in a *Campylobacter jejuni fur* mutant. *J. Bacteriol.* **180:**5291–5298.

66. **Wassenaar, T. M., B. Geilhausen, and D. G. Newell.** 1998. Evidence of genomic instability in *Campylobacter jejuni* isolated from poultry. *Appl. Environ. Microbiol.* **64:**1816–1821.

67. **Wawrzynow, A., B. Banecki, and M. Zylicz.** 1996. The Clp ATPases define a novel class of molecular chaperones. *Mol. Microbiol.* **21:** 895–899.

68. **Wooldridge, K. G., and P. H. Williams.** 1993. Iron uptake mechanisms of pathogenic bacteria. *FEMS Microbiol. Rev.* **12:**325–348.

69. **Wooldridge, K. G., P. H. Williams, and J. M. Ketley.** 1994. Iron-responsive genetic regulation in *Campylobacter jejuni*: cloning and characterization of a *fur* homologue. *J. Bacteriol.* **176:** 5852–5856.

70. **Wosten, M. S. N.** 1998. Initiation of transcription and gene organization in *Campylobacter jejuni*. Ph.D. thesis. University of Utrecht, Utrecht, The Netherlands.

71. **Wosten, M. S. M., M. Boeve, M. G. A. Koot, A. A. van Nuenen, and B. A. M. van der Zeijst.** 1998. Identification of *Campylobacter jejuni* promoter sequences. *J. Bacteriol.* **180:**594–599.

72. **Wosten, M. S. M., M. Boeve, W. Gaastra, and B. A. M. van der Zeijst.** 1998. Cloning and characterisation of the gene encoding the primary sigma-factor of *Campylobacter jejuni*. *FEMS Microbiol. Lett.* **162:**97–103.

73. **Wu, Y. L., L. H. Lee, D. M. Rollins, and W. M. Ching.** 1994. Heat shock- and alkaline pH–induced proteins of *Campylobacter jejuni*: characterization and immunological properties. *Infect. Immun.* **62:**4256–4260.

74. **Yamanaka, K., L. Fang, and M. Inouye.** 1998. The CspA family in *Escherichia coli*: multiple gene duplication for stress adaptation. *Mol. Microbiol.* **27:**247–255.

75. **Yao, R., D. H. Burr, and P. Guerry.** 1997. CheY-mediated modulation of *Campylobacter jejuni* virulence. *Mol. Microbiol.* **23:**1021–1031.

76. **Zuber, U., and W. Schumann.** 1994. CIRCE, a novel heat shock element involved in regulation of heat shock operon *dnaK* of *Bacillus subtilis*. *J. Bacteriol.* **176:**1359–1363.

MECHANISMS OF ANTIBIOTIC RESISTANCE IN *CAMPYLOBACTER*

Catharine A. Trieber and Diane E. Taylor

22

The incidence of antibiotic resistance in most pathogenic bacteria has continually risen over the last few decades and has become a major medical challenge. In this chapter, we summarize the mode of actions for several antibiotics and the known determinants of antibiotic resistance found in *Campylobacter* species. The prevalence of antibiotic resistance in *Campylobacter* is reviewed in chapters 3 and 25.

TETRACYCLINE RESISTANCE

Mode of Action

Tetracyclines are broad-spectrum antibiotics, active against many gram-negative and gram-positive bacteria as well as chlamydiae, mycoplasmas, rickettsiae, and protozoan parasites (13, 47). Owing to their broad activity, relative safety, and low cost, tetracyclines have been widely used throughout the world for treatment of microbial infections. The emergence of bacterial resistance to tetracyclines has led to a decrease in their therapeutic use (48).

The typical tetracycline acts on the ribosome as a protein synthesis inhibitor, and its effects are bacteriostatic and reversible. The antibiotic is actively taken up and concentrated inside the cell, where it binds to the 30S subunit of the ribosome at a single high-affinity site and also to several low-affinity sites on both subunits (13, 53). The high-affinity site, which may be composed of both ribosomal proteins and the 16S rRNA, is most probably responsible for tetracycline inhibition (7, 36). Tetracycline binding prevents the binding of aminoacyl-tRNA (aa-tRNA) to the ribosomal A site, either directly or through a conformational change that may weaken the affinity of the aa-tRNA for the A site (12, 19). As a result, the elongation cycle is halted and nascent polypeptide synthesis stalls.

Genetics

The incidence of tetracycline resistance (Tc^r) in *Campylobacter* has been steadily increasing. In one Canadian report, it increased from 19% in 1985 to 1986 to 56% in 1995 to 1997 (20). High-level Tc^r is usually associated with self-transmissible plasmids in both *C. jejuni* and *C. coli* (63). These plasmids have a very narrow host range and transfer only between *Campylobacter* species (60). In one strain of *C. coli*, however, the resistance determinant was located on the chromosome, implying that a transposon may be involved in its dissemination (37). This

Catherine A. Trieber, Department of Medical Microbiology & Immunology, 128 Medical Sciences Building, University of Alberta, Edmonton, Alberta T6G 2H7, Canada. *Diane E. Taylor,* Departments of Medical Microbiology & Immunology and Biological Sciences, 128 Medical Sciences Building, University of Alberta, Edmonton, Alberta T6G 2H7, Canada.

Campylobacter, 2nd Ed., Edited by I. Nachamkin and M. J. Blaser
© 2000 American Society for Microbiology, Washington, D.C.

determinant was able to be transferred into a Tc^s *C. coli* strain by natural transformation and was shown to be inserted into the same site of the chromosome in each of four transformants. This suggests that the host cell recombination machinery, not a transposon, may be responsible for chromosomal insertion of the Tc^r determinant (59). The exact mechanism for insertion of the Tc^r determinant into the chromosome has not been resolved.

The plasmid-encoded Tc^r determinants from *C. jejuni* and *C. coli* were cloned and sequenced (35, 55). They are virtually identical, forming the basis for a new class of Tc^r determinants, Tet O (33a). This determinant consists of one gene, *tetO*, which encodes a polypeptide of 639 amino acid residues (approximately 72 kDa). Expression of this determinant in *Escherichia coli* produced a protein of approximately 70 kDa that was shown to be responsible for Tc^r by transposon and deletion analysis (35, 72). This expression was not tetracycline inducible but was constitutive at very low levels (62). The expressed TetO protein is not visible without radiolabling or immunoblotting. An element located upstream of the *tetO* gene was shown to be important for full expression of Tc^r, but it is not clear how this region exerts its effect (80).

The Tet O determinant has been identified not only in *Campylobacter* but also in a number of gram-positive organisms (47). Plasmids bearing the *tetO* gene were isolated from *Enterococcus faecalis* and *Streptococus* spp. and shown to have a similar size and restriction pattern to those isolated from *C. jejuni* and *C. coli* (84). The nucleotide sequence of the *Campylobacter tetO* genes has a G + C content of 40 mol%, while the genome G + C content is about 33 mol% (63). These findings have led to the suggestion that campylobacters aquired *tetO* from gram-positive sources (55, 63, 84).

Mechanism

Bacterial resistance to tetracycline commonly arises through one of four identified mechanisms: efflux of tetracycline, modification of tetracycline, ribosomal protection, or mutation

of the 16S rRNA (8, 50, 53). In *Campylobacter* spp., the soluble protein, TetO, mediates the resistance through ribosomal protection (67). There are several related classes of Tc^r determinants encoding ribosomal protection proteins (RPP), TetM, TetO, TetP, TetQ, TetS, TetT, TetW, and OtrA (14, 54, 67). These determinants have a high degree of sequence identity and appear to function in a similar manner. The OtrA determinant is particularly interesting since it is found in the chromosome of the oxytetracycline producer, *Streptomyces rimosus,* and may be the progenitor RPP (17). The most common determinants, Tet M and Tet O, encoding the TetM and TetO proteins, respectively, are also the best characterized.

TetO shows significant amino acid sequence similarity to the ribosomal elongation factors EF-Tu and EF-G (67). EF-Tu forms a ternary complex with aa-tRNA and GTP and catalyzes the binding of aa-tRNA to the A site. EF-G also binds GTP and is involved in the translocation step of protein synthesis, moving the tRNAs from the A and P sites to the P and E sites (15, 38). Figure 1 shows the domain structure of these proteins. The sequence identity to EF-Tu is mainly in the amino-terminal GTPase region, the G domain, which contains the five highly conserved sequence motifs G1 to G5. These five motifs are also present in EF-G. Like the elongation factors, TetO is a ribosome-stimulated GTPase (66). Mutation of a highly conserved residue in the putative GTP binding domain of TetO led to a decrease in Tc^r, indicating that the GTP binding function is important for Tc^r (24). The sequence similarity between EF-G and TetO stretches throughout the entire length of the protein, suggesting that TetO has a similar structure to that of EF-G and that they may undergo similar changes in conformation upon binding GTP and GDP. The structure of EF-G consists of five domains, the first two of which (domains I and II) form a structure similar to that of EF-Tu with an insertion of 90 amino acids, termed the G′ subdomain (2, 15). The G′ subdomain, believed to be responsible for GDP-GTP nucleotide exchange, is partially conserved in

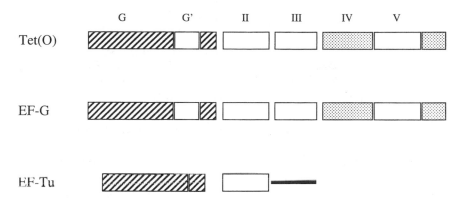

FIGURE 1 Domain structure of TetO and the elongation factors. TetO and EF-G can be divided into five domains (2). The first domain, G, is the GTPase domain and contains the G' subdomain, which is thought to be responsible for nucleotide exchange. The function of domain II is not known. Domain IV mimics the tRNA of the EF-Tu–GTP–aa-tRNA complex. Domains III and V may bind RNA and interact with the G domain. EF-Tu has only the G domain and domain II in common with TetO and EF-G.

TetO, indicating that it may also have this function. Domains III to V mimic the tRNA component in the ternary complex structure and are also conserved. Overall, it appears that the RPP have similar structural and presumably functional characteristics to EF-G, but the RPP TetM was not able to substitute for EF-G or EF-Tu (8, 10).

It has been demonstrated that mutations in the *miaA* gene of *Salmonella typhimurium* and *E. coli* can reduce TetM- and TetO-mediated Tc^r (9, 70). The *miaA* gene product is involved in the modification of most tRNAs that read codons staring with uridine (6). One characteristic of *miaA* mutants is an increase in translation accuracy, possibly due to alteration of the tRNA affinity for the A site (6). Mutations in ribosomal protein S12 (*rpsL* mutants) that alter translational accuracy were also shown to affect RPP-mediated Tc^r (70). In general, mutations which increase fidelity reduced TetO- and TetM-mediated Tc^r but mutations that decrease accuracy had no effect. Increased accuracy may be due to a lower affinity of the A site for common tRNA elements, thus increasing the requirement of specific codon interactions in binding. Conversely, an increase in affinity for the common tRNA elements would

decrease accuracy (30). The reduced affinity of the ribosomal A site for tRNA in *miaA* and *rpsL* mutants may hinder the ability of the EF-Tu–GTP–aa-tRNA complex to effectively compete with tetracycline, even in the presence of the RPP (70). An additional effect of the *rpsL* mutations may come from interference in the interactions between RPP and the ribosome. EF-Tu and EF-G are believed to bind to the same site on the ribosome (at or near S12), and some S12 mutants are abnormal in their ability to stimulate the EF-Tu GTPase activity (5, 15).

The molecular mechanism of RPP-mediated Tc^r is not yet clear, but valuable clues have been obtained from studies of the interaction of RPPs with *E. coli* ribosomes by using in vitro protein synthesis assays. Tetracycline was shown to bind to the ribosome and inhibit the ribosomal elongation rate, producing short chains (74). TetO restored the rate and processivity in the presence of tetracycline and GTP. TetM was shown to chase tetracycline from the ribosome in the presence of GTP (10). TetO also decreased tetracycline binding in the presence of GTP and nonhydrolyzable GTP analogs (74). The observation that the nonhydrolyzable analogs have a greater effect indicated that the hydrolysis of GTP is not necessary for TetO activity. The use of the nonhydrolyzable analogs converted the TetO activity from catalytic to stoichiometric. Binding assays demonstrated that TetO was bound to the ribosome with high affinity only in the presence of the nonhydrolyzable GTP analog GTPγS (74). This complex was stable enough to be isolated by gel filtration. TetO did not bind in the presence of GDP, indicating that it is only the GTP conformation of TetO that interacts with the ribosome.

Overall, the mechanism of TetO action resembles that of EF-G. EF-G–GTP binds to the pretranslocational state of the ribosome (tRNAs in the A and P sites) and catalyzes translocation to the posttranslocational state (tRNAs in the P and E sites) (15, 38). The GTPase activity of EF-G is stimulated by the posttranslocational ribosome. After hydrolysis of GTP, EF-G–GDP dissociates from the ribosome. The GTPase activities of both EF-G and TetO are greatly stimulated by the ribosome. Like EF-G, TetO binds GDP and GTP but interacts with the ribosome only in the GTP-bound form. The similarity between EF-G and TetO implies that both proteins may bind to the same ribosomal site. This is supported by the fact that EF-G has been cross-linked to the S12 protein and that S12 mutations were shown to interfere with TetO activity (15, 70). We propose that TetO-GTP binds to the pretranslocational ribosome, causing tetracycline to be displaced. TetO then hydrolyzes the GTP and dissociates from the ribosome.

To understand the workings of TetO, it is necessary to understand how tetracycline inhibits protein synthesis. In the model proposed in Fig. 2, tetracycline inhibits aa-tRNA binding to the A site of ribosomes in the posttranslocational state (74). The α-ε model of the elongation cycle proposes that there are two tRNA binding sites (α and ε) in a movable domain that shuffles α and ε between the A and P and the P and E sites (39). Tetracycline binds to the α domain at the A site and may induce a conformational shift of the ribosome toward the pretranslocation state (74). The ternary complex, aa-tRNA–EF-Tu–GTP, interacts with the posttranslocational ribosome, and the tRNA would be blocked from binding. TetO-GTP, like EF-G–GTP, would have a higher affinity for the pretranslocational state and could bind to the ribosome and displace tetracycline, inducing a conformational shift back to the posttranslocational state, which allows ternary complex to bind. We will test this hypothesis in future studies by addressing the interaction of TetO with the ribosome in both translocational states.

β-LACTAM RESISTANCE

Mode of Action

The β-lactam class of antibiotics includes four different groups, penicillins, cephalosporins, carbapenems, and monobactams, that contain the four-membered β-lactam ring. These antibiotics are bactericidal, and each has a wide spectrum of activity in gram-negative and gram-positive bacteria that varies with the antibiotic and class (45). β-Lactams are known to bind to a set of periplasmic proteins, the penicillin binding proteins, carboxypeptidases, and transpeptidases, which are involved in the synthesis and maintenance of the murein sacculus (16, 57). β-Lactams mimic a component of peptidoglycan, the D-Ala-D-Ala moiety, and are substrates for the transpeptidases that catalyze the synthesis of cross-links. The antibiotic irreversibly acylates and thus inactivates these enzymes. Cell wall synthesis is halted, and the murein hydrolases, responsible for nicking the peptidoglycan to allow growth, are unchecked. Bacterial lysis may then result from osmotic pressure.

Genetics

β-Lactam resistance is common in *Campylobacter* spp., but the number of resistant strains varies depending on the β-lactam agent in question. Many *C. jejuni* strains are resistant to penicillin G, piperacillin, cephalothin, cefazolin, and the other narrow-spectrum cephalosporins (31, 33, 58). Fewer organisms are resistant to ampicillin (15 to 40%) or amoxicillin

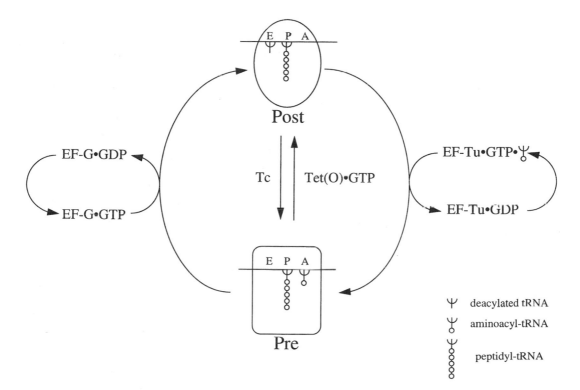

FIGURE 2 Model of tetracycline and TetO action. The elongation cycle is depicted with the ribosome in two distinct conformations, the posttranslocational state (Post) and the pretranslocational state (Pre). The EF-Tu–GTP–aa-tRNA ternary complex interacts with the Post ribosome, and the aa-tRNA binds to the A site, GTP is hydrolyzed, and EF-Tu–GDP is released. The Pre ribosome is acted upon by EF-G–GTP which catalyzes translocation. In the model, tetracycline (Tc) binds to the A site of the Post ribosome and causes a shift to the Pre ribosome, TetO-GTP then interacts with the tetracycline-bound Pre ribosome and displaces the tetracycline. The ribosome returns to the Post state, GTP is hydrolyzed, and TetO-GDP dissociates.

(10 to 14%), and none are resistant to imipenem. *C. coli* appears to be more susceptible to β-lactam antibiotics than *C. jejuni* does. *C. coli* strains are still resistant to penicillin G, piperacillin, and the narrow-spectrum cephalosporins, but 96% of the organisms are susceptible to ampicillin and amoxicillin and all are susceptible to imipenem (32). In many tetracycline- and ampicillin-resistant *C. jejuni* and *C. coli* isolates, the transfer of ampicillin resistance was not linked to a plasmid carrying Tc^r indicating that the resistance determinant may be chromosomally encoded (63). Inducible β-lactamase genes are present on the chromosomes of many other bacteria (42), and completion of the *C. jejuni* genome sequence by the Sanger

Centre could allow the identification of potentially related genes or enzymes. Small plasmids from *C. jejuni* which expressed both tetracycline resistance and ampicillin resistance in *E. coli* have been recently reported but are as yet uncharacterized (22).

Mechanisms

As many as 83 to 92% of *C. jejuni* and 68% of *C. coli* isolates produce a β-lactamase (31–33, 58), but it has not been demonstrated directly that this is the mechanism of resistance against most of the β-lactams. Resistance to β-lactams can occur through three methods: decreased uptake through modification of a porin, alteration of a penicillin binding protein so that the agent is no longer able to bind and inhibit, or production of a β-lactamase (42). The β-lactamase hydrolyzes the β-lactam rings of these antibiotics, rendering them inactive (16). Studies on the susceptibility of β-lactamase-producing *C. jejuni* to β-lactam agents demonstrate that penicillin G, piperacillin, and the narrow-spectrum cephalosporins are ineffective against these organisms regardless of β-lactamase production (31, 58). The presence of the β-lactamase correlated with higher resistance levels only for ampicillin and amoxicillin. Crude cell extracts were tested for activity against penicillins and cephalosporins, and only penicillin G, amoxicillin, and ampicillin (piperacillin was not tested) were substrates (31). The addition of the β-lactamase inhibitor clavulanate, a weak antibacterial agent in its own right, to the susceptibility test media greatly increased the activities of amoxicillin and ampicillin but not those of penicillin G and pipericillin (31). Other β-lactamase inhibitors, sulbactam and tazobactam, were only slightly effective at improving the efficacy of these agents. The β-lactamase appears to contribute to the resistance of *C. jejuni* to ampicillin and amoxicillin but not to penicillin G or piperacillin. Lucain et al. (34) have suggested that as many as four distinct β-lactamases may be produced by *C. jejuni* strains, based on slight differences in substrate specificity, isoelectric points, and molecular weight determinations. None of these enzymes have been purified, and further characterization is awaited.

Several factors must be considered in determining the efficacy of an antimicrobial agent. The permeability of the compound across the outer membrane is the first step. The porins of *C. jejuni* and *C. coli* have been demonstrated to be cation selective with molecular mass cutoffs of approximately 360 to 340 Da (40). β-Lactam antibiotics with a molecular mass of 360 Da or less and with an overall neutral charge, such as imipenem, ampicillin, and amoxicillin, would have a selective advantage over negatively charged agents such as penicillin G. Failure to penetrate may be the reason why antibiotics such as penicillin G, piperacil-

lin, and the narrow spectrum cephalosporins are not active against *C. jejuni*. The β-lactamase comes into action only on β-lactams that do pass the outer membrane and only against agents that fit the substrate specificity of the enzyme.

In general, β-lactams are not used to treat *Campylobacter* spp. due to widespread resistance. However, imipenem and combinations of β-lactams and β-lactamase inhibitors, such as amoxicillin-clavulanate, do give 100% susceptibility in vitro, even in high β-lactamase producers (31, 58), indicating a possible role for these compounds in treatment.

CHLORAMPHENICOL RESISTANCE

Mode of Action
Chloramphenicol is a broad-spectrum antibiotic with bacteriostatic activity against many gram-negative and gram-positive bacteria as well as rickettsiae, chlamydiae, and mycoplasmas (45). It binds to the ribosome in competition with the aa-tRNA for the A site. The peptidyltransferase activity is inhibited by chloramphenicol, leading to freezing of the protein translocation apparatus (56).

Genetics and Mechanism
Chloramphenicol resistance in *Campylobacter* spp. appears to be rare, and reported rates of resistance are low, 0.6 to 10% (33, 59). In general, Cm^r arises either through mutation of the 23S rRNA or, more commonly, through modification of chloramphenicol by an acetyltransferase (16, 56). The Cm^r determinant from a *C. coli* plasmid was cloned and sequenced (52, 78). It was found to consist of a single gene which is 67% identical to the chloramphenicol acetyltransferase (*cat*) genes of *Clostridium difficile* and *Clostridium perfringens* (78). In *C. coli*, as in the majority of Cm^r organisms, resistance is mediated by chloramphenicol acetyltransferase. The acetylation of chloramphenicol prevents it from binding to the ribosome and inhibiting protein synthesis. The enzyme has a molecular mass of 23.5 kDa and is produced constitutively in large amounts in both *C. coli*

and *E. coli* (78). No other Cm^r in *Campylobacter,* to our knowledge, has been characterized.

TRIMETHOPRIM RESISTANCE

Mode of Action

Trimethoprim is active against many gram-positive cocci and most gram-negative bacteria (45). It acts by selectively inhibiting dihydrofolate reductase, an essential enzyme which catalyzes the regeneration of the one-carbon carrier, tetrahydrofolate, from dihydrofolate (16). Tetrahydrofolate is required for amino acid and nucleotide biosynthesis. Campylobacters are considered to be intrinsically resistant to trimethoprim, and this compound is often used in selective media (33, 59).

Genetics and Mechanism

To identify the mechanism of resistance to trimethoprim in *C. jejuni,* several strains with high-level trimethoprim resistance (resistant to 500 to 1,000 μg/ml) were analyzed (22). The chromosomally located determinants were cloned, and six of them were found to mediate high-level trimethoprim resistance in *E. coli.* These determinants were sequenced and shown to be either the *dfr1* gene or the *dfr9* gene, both encoding trimethoprim-resistant dihydrofolate reductase. Screening of *C. jejuni* isolates for *dfr1* and *dfr9* demonstrated that the majority of strains had at least one of the two genes and 10% had both. The *dfr1* gene is the most common determinant in *C. jejuni,* and several integron-like features were noted flanking this gene. An additional imperfect, inverted repeat was located at the 3′ end of the gene which was identical to the 59-base element of the Tn7 *dfr1* gene, although an intact Tn7 was not present. The *dfr9* gene was also located in the remnants of a transposon, Tn*5393.* The *dfr9* gene has previously been found only in *E. coli* isolates from swine and one human pathogen but was present in the same configuration as with Tn*5393* (27). It has been suggested that the acquisition of the *dfr* genes by *C. jejuni* resulted from exposure of domestic animals to high levels of antibiotics (22). The G + C content of the *dfr* genes is higher than that of the *C. jejuni* chromosome, and *Campylobacter* spp. are naturally transformable (22, 79). This increase the likelihood of the genes being transferred from a resistant organism.

AMINOGLYCOSIDE RESISTANCE

Mode of Action

The aminoglycosides are chemically similar but vary with regard to antimicrobial spectrum, potency, and clinical usefulness (45). They are usually bactericidal. They penetrate the cell wall and bind irreversibly to the ribosome, but it is not clear how they actually kill the cell. Streptomycin, kanamycin, streptothricins, and spectinomycin belong to this group and are all protein synthesis inhibitors (56). Streptomycin, streptothricins, and kanamycin have pleiotropic effects on protein synthesis but are primarily A-site inhibitors. They interfere with A-site binding of the ternary complex and cause misreading, increasing translation errors. Spectinomycin interferes with a later step in the elongation cycle. It inhibits translocation by blocking EF-G–GTP from binding to the ribosome (56).

Genetics

Aminoglycoside resistance has been reported in *C. jejuni* and *C. coli* but is less common in *C. jejuni* than in *C. coli.* Studies of kanamycin resistance found that 5 of 225 and 3 of 92 *C. jejuni* strains and 6 of 54 and 2 of 10 *C. coli* strains were resistant (73, 75). The majority of resistance determinants are plasmid borne, but a few have been reported which seem to be chromosomally encoded (64, 73).

Mechanisms

Aminoglycoside resistance is fairly well characterized in *Campylobacter* spp. Resistance arises through modification of the antibiotic, which is then unable to interact with the ribosome. Three families of enzymes are responsible for aminoglycoside resistance in bacteria: the aminoglycoside phosphotransferases (APH), the aminoglycoside adenylyltransferases (AAD), and the acetyltransferases. Each family is divided into various subgroups depending on the site at which the antibiotic is modified and its characteristic substrate profile. A number of different enzymes have been identified in *Campylobacter* spp.

Kanamycin resistance in both *C. jejuni* and *C. coli* is mediated by APH(3′) type III and type IV and APH(3″) (46, 64, 73). The majority of these enzymes have broad substrate specificity; the most common aminoglycoside resistance determinant found in *Campylobacter* spp., APH(3′) type III, phosphorylates kanamycin, butyrosine, lividomycin, and amikacin but not tobramycin (64, 73). The ability to phosphorylate streptomycin but not spectinomycin is characteristic of an APH(3″) (46).

Also present in *C. jejuni* and *C. coli* are the adenylyltransferases. An investigation of streptomycin and spectinomycin resistance in *Campylobacter* spp. revealed two AAD enzymes, one active against only streptomycin and the other active against both streptomycin and spectinomycin (44). The *aadA* gene encodes an AAD(3″)(9), and the *aadE* gene encodes an AAD(6). The majority of streptomycin-resistant strains contain the *aadE* base on DNA hybridization. The AAD(6) enzyme is known to confer streptomycin resistance (44). The presence of the *aadA* gene in one *Campylobacter*-like strain confers resistance to both streptomycin and spectinomycin. The determinants for spectinomycin resistance in two strains and streptomycin resistance in one strain were unidentified and may be a 3″- or 6-streptomycin phosphotransferase or an as yet undescribed spectinomycin phosphotransferase (44).

Streptothricins are actually a combination of streptothricin antibiotics and have been used as additives to animal feeds in Germany. Resistance to these aminoglycosides occurs through modification by a streptothricin acetyltransferase. The *sat4* gene encoding this enzyme in *C. coli* has been identified, cloned, and sequenced (26). Southern hybridization with a *sat4* probe demonstrated that this gene is present in seven other streptothricin-resistant *Campylobacter* isolates from animal and clinical sources.

In addition to the modifying enzymes, chromosomal mutations of ribosomal proteins and rRNA may provide aminoglycoside resistance. These antibiotics all bind to specific sites on the ribosome, and modification of the binding site could greatly reduce the affinity of these compounds for the ribosome. In *E. coli* and other organisms, mutations in the 16S rRNA lead to resistance to streptomycin, spectinomycin, and neomycin while methylation of specific bases in the 16S rRNA causes gentamicin and kanamycin resistance (56). Mutations of ribosomal proteins S12, S4, and S5 lead to streptomycin dependence and resistance, while mutations in S5 also give spectinomycin resistance (56). Spontaneous chromosomal streptomycin resistance mutants of *C. coli* were generated by plating cells on streptomycin-containing media (79). The resistance determinant could be transferred by natural transformation to a second *C. coli*. Mapping and Southern hybridization indicated that the mutation was not present in S12 (59), but it may be present in the S4 or S5 proteins or in the 16S rRNA. This type of aminoglycoside resistance has not been further investigated in *Campylobacter*.

MACROLIDE RESISTANCE

Mode of Action

The macrolides, including erythromycin, azithromycin, and clarithromycin, have similar structures and are bacteriostatic agents active against gram-positive and some gram-negative bacteria, mycoplasmas, chlamydiae, treponemas, and rickettsiae (45). Erythromycin is considered to be one of the safest antibiotics and is the drug of choice against *C. jejuni* infections. Like tetracycline erythromycin is a protein synthesis inhibitor that binds reversibly to a site on the ribosome, which may include the 23S rRNA and proteins L2, L4, L15, L16, and L22 (56). Erythromycin binds to the ribosome and appears to cause dissociation of the peptidyl-tRNA rather than to block the peptidyltransferase activity, as is thought to occur with larger macrolides (56).

Genetics

Typically, the erythromycin resistance rates of *Campylobacter* spp. are fairly low, <1% in Canada and <3% in the United States, but they have been reported to be as high as 7 to 10% in Europe (20, 43, 76, 77). Erythromycin resistance also causes cross-resistance to clarithromycin and azithromycin and to lincosamide and streptogramin antibiotics (63, 65). In *C. jejuni* and *C. coli,* the erythromycin resistance is not associated with the presence of plasmid DNA and is thought to be chromosomally mediated (59). Recently, mobile erythromycin resistance determinants have been found in the presumptive periodontal pathogen *Campylobacter* (*Wolinella*) *rectus,* but no plasmids were identifiable in transconjugats and the determinants were located on the chromosome (49).

Mechanisms

In general, resistance to erythromycin is through modification of the target site, the ribosome, or through alteration of the antibiotic, e.g., esterification of erythromycin (3). Erythromycin resistance reported so far in *Campylobacter* is due to alteration of the ribosome. In *C. rectus,* the erythromycin resistance determinants ErmB, GrmC, GrmQ, and GrmFS have been identified (49). These determinants encode rRNA methylases, which methylate an adenine in the 23S rRNA and prevent the binding of the antibiotic.

In *C. jejuni* and *C. coli,* the resistance mechanism is not consistent with the presence of an rRNA methylase, with modification of the antibiotic, or with efflux (83). Whole ribosomes or 50S subunits were purified from erythromycin-resistant strains and shown to bind much less erythromycin than did ribosomes from sensitive strains, indicating that an alteration of the binding site had occurred. A mutation in either of the proteins mentioned above or the 23S rRNA is probably responsible for resistance (83). Resistance to clarithromycin in the closely related bacterium *Helicobacter pylori* (for-

merly *C. pylori*) was shown to be due to an alteration of one of two adenine residues in the 23S rRNA at the erythromycin binding site (69). Sequencing of the 23S rRNA genes from erythromycin-resistant *Campylobacter* spp. identified mutations at these sites which are most probably responsible for resistance (74a).

FLUOROQUINOLONE RESISTANCE

Mode of Action

The quinolones are bactericidal agents and exhibit a broad spectrum of activity against most gram-negative and some gram-positive bacteria (45). Fluoroquinolones, such as ciprofloxacin, ofloxacin, and norfloxacin, are a subgroup of quinolones derived from nalidixic acid and have a fluorine at the C-6 position of the quinolone structure. The targets of these agents are the type II topoisomerases DNA gyrase and topoisomerase IV (18). These enzymes are essential for DNA replication, recombination, and transcription. Both topoisomerases are tetramers composed of two subunits arranged into A_2B_2 holoenzymes; gyrase is $GyrA_2GyrB_2$, while topoisomerase IV is $ParC_2ParE_2$ (18). The quinolones do not bind directly to gyrase or to the DNA but, rather, form a ternary complex with the gyrase and the DNA (82). This complex is much more stable than the topoisomerase-DNA complex, and cleavage of the DNA follows complex formation (29). The quinolone-inhibited gyrase-DNA complex inhibits DNA replication and transcription, halting cell growth. It is the release of the double-stranded DNA breaks, highly toxic even in small numbers, which is thought to be responsible for the lethality of fluoroquinolones (18).

Genetics

Ciprofloxacin is one of the most widely used antibiotics in the world and is the second choice for treating gastroenteritis caused by *Campylobacter* spp. (1, 45). *C. jejuni* is highly susceptible to ciprofloxacin, which has an MIC of 0.5 μg/ml. Levofloxacin and ofloxacin exhibit similar potencies against *C. jejuni,* while other fluoroquinolones, such as trovafloxacin, clinafloxacin, and gatifloxacin, have even greater activities (4, 25). In addition to their use in human medicine, fluoroquinolones are used heavily in animal husbandry for medical reasons and as growth promoters (1). Resistance to one fluoroquinolone or to nalidixic acid usually gives cross-resistance to other fluoroquinolones, but there are exceptions. Only 86 and 53% of ofloxacin-resistant *Streptococcus pneumoniae* mutants were considered resistant, using established breakpoints, to levofloxacin and trovafloxacin respectively (28). Differences in the intrinsic resistance of a species to the quinolones also are common.

In *C. jejuni* and *C. coli,* the incidence of fluoroquinolone resistance has steadily risen, with reported rates in Spain being as high as 88% (1, 20, 41, 43, 51, 75). Resistance is usually chromosomally mediated, arising through mutation. Nalidixic acid-resistant mutants of *C. jejuni* and *C. coli* were shown to arise at a frequency of 10^{-8} and to be cross-resistant to fluoroquinolones (23, 61). In contrast, *C. fetus* subsp *fetus* isolates are intrinsically resistant to high levels of nalidixic acid but do not show cross-resistance to fluoroquinolones (61).

Mechanisms

Three basic mechanisms of bacterial resistance to quinolones have been described: modification of DNA gyrase or topoisomerase IV, reduced permeability, and efflux (1). The efflux of quinolones in *C. jejuni* is discussed in the context of multidrug resistance (see below). Fluoroquinolone resistance in *C. jejuni* appears to be due to mutations in the genes encoding subunits of DNA gyrase (*gyrA*) and topoisomerase IV (*parC*). DNA gyrase purified from quinolone-resistant mutants of *C. jejuni* was 100-fold less sensitive to inhibition by quinolones than was the wild-type gyrase (23). Cloning and sequencing of the *C. jejuni gyrA* gene demonstrated that mutations in *gyrA* at Thr-86, Asp-90, and Ala-70 were responsible for resistance (81). Mutations at Thr-86 are associated with a higher-level resistance to nalidixic acid (64 to 128 µg/ml) and ciprofloxacin (16 to 64 g/ml) than are mutations at Asp-90 or

Ala-70. The *gyrA* Thr-86 mutations were also found in a second study of quinolone-resistant *C. jejuni,* indicating that mutation of *gyrA* is a frequent cause of high-level resistance in clinical isolates (51). *C. jejuni* isolates resistant to even higher levels of quinolones (ciprofloxacin MIC of 125 µg/ml) were shown to carry two mutations, one in gyrA-encoded Thr-86 and the other in the *parC*-encoded topoisomerase IV subunit at Arg-139 (21). These two mutations appear to have a synergistic effect on resistance to ciprofloxacin, similar to that seen in fluoroquinolone-resistant *S. pneumoniae* mutants (28). The preponderance of fluoroquinolone-resistant mutants with mutations in either gyrase or topoisomerase IV appears to be characteristic of the bacterial species. The main target of quinolones in *E. coli* appears to be the gyrase, with topoisomerase IV being only a minor target, while the reverse is true in *Staphylococcus aureus* (18). The main target in *C. jejuni* is probably the gyrase.

The *gyrA* gene from the intrinsically nalidixic acid-resistant *C. fetus* was cloned and sequenced (68). The deduced protein sequence was found to be 78% identical to the *C. jejuni* GyrA protein sequence. All of the amino acids at positions important for fluoroquinolone resistance were conserved in the *C. fetus* GyrA, but variations at seven other proximal positions were noted. The *gyrA* genes from two ciprofloxacin-resistant *C. fetus* strains were sequenced and found to contain mutations at Asp-90, as was found in *C. jejuni*. Therefore, nalidixic acid resistance in *C. fetus* does not appear to be due to mutations in *gyrA*. The possibility that alterations in the *gyrB, parC,* or *parE* genes are responsible for resistance requires further clarification (68).

MULTIDRUG RESISTANCE

Multidrug resistance is rare in *C. jejuni* but has been reported, especially in isolates from immunosuppressed patients. One study documented the sequential emergence of resistance to fluoroquinolones, erythromycin, and tetracycline after treatment of patients with these agents (71). In addition to *C. jejuni,* a number of other microorganisms were isolated from these patients. The mechanism of acquisition of the resistance is unclear, and resistance could have arisen by mutation of chromosomal genes, as with fluoroquinolone resistance, or by transfer of a mobile element from other organisms present. Ribotyping was used to demonstrate that patients were infected with a single strain of *C. jejuni* and that this strain progressively acquired resistance to the antibiotics used in the treatment.

A different picture of multidrug resistance emerges from an in vitro study of *C. jejuni*. Passage of the bacteria on pefloxacin-containing agar led to the isolation of a fluoroquinolone-resistant strain (11). This strain was also resistant to tetracycline, erythromycin, chloramphenicol, and several β-lactams. Similar results were obtained by selecting with cefotaxime, with the exception of fluoroquinolone resistance. The pefloxacin-resistant strain carried a mutation at Thr-86 of the *gyrA*, product, which is probably responsible in part for the fluoroquinolone resistance. Uptake studies with this mutant showed a reduced accumulation of pefloxacin, ciprofloxacin, and minocycline that was energy dependent, suggesting an active efflux of the drugs. Two outer membrane proteins were overexpressed in the mutant strain that were absent in the parent. In addition to the resistance mechanisms mentioned in previous sections, resistance to fluoroquinolones, erythromycin, tetracycline, β-lactams, and chloramphenicol may be linked to a broad-specificity efflux pump in *C. jejuni* (11).

CONCLUSIONS

Much information has been acquired on Tc^r from studies with *C. jejuni* and *C. coli,* although determination of the exact mode of action of TetO requires further work. Chloramphenicol, aminoglycoside, and trimethoprim resistance are also fairly well understood. Additional research on resistance to fluoroquinolone, macrolide, and β-lactam antibiotics in *Campylobacter* is under way. Although *C. jejuni* and *C. coli* infections are usually self-limiting and antibiotics are not required, severe cases in children, immunosuppressed individuals, and the elderly often require treatment. In addition,

systemic infections by *C. fetus* are usually treated with antibiotics. Information on the prevalence of resistance and the poorly understood mechanisms of resistance will assist in designing more effective forms of therapy for eradicating *Campylobacter* spp.

ACKNOWLEDGMENTS

Support for this work was provided by the Natural Sciences and Engineering Research Council of Canada (to D.E.T.). D.E.T. is an Alberta Heritage Foundation for Medical Research Scientist, and C.A.T. is an AHFMR Fellow.

We thank Ge Wang for helpful discussion.

REFERENCES

1. **Acar, J. F., and F. W. Goldstein.** 1997. Trends in bacterial resistance to fluoroquinolones. *Clin. Infect. Dis.* **24**(Suppl. 1):S67–73.
2. **Ævarsson, A., E. Brazhnikov, M. Garber, J. Zheltonosova, Y. Chirgadze, S. Al-Karadaghi, L. A. Svensson, and A. Liljas.** 1994. Three-dimensional structure of the ribosomal translocase: elongation factor G from *Thermus thermophilus. EMBO J.* **13**:3669–3677.
3. **Arthur, M., A. Brisson-Noël, and P. Courvalin.** 1987. Origin and evolution of genes specifying resistance to macrolide, lincosamide and streptogramin antibiotics: data and hypotheses. *J. Antimicrob. Chemother.* **20**:783–802.
4. **Bauernfeind, A.** 1997. Comparison of the antibacterial activities of the quinolones BAY 12-8039, gatifloxacin (AM 1155), trovafloxacin, clinafloxacin, levofloxacin, and ciprofloxacin. *J. Antimicrob. Chemother.* **40**:639–651.
5. **Bilgin, N., F. Claesens, H. Pahverk, and M. Ehrenberg.** 1992. Kinetic properties of *Escherichia coli* ribosomes with altered forms of S12. *J. Mol. Biol.* **224**:1011–1027.
6. **Björk, G. R.** 1995. Genetic dissection of synthesis and function of modified nucleosides in bacterial transfer RNA. *Prog. Nucleic Acid Res.* **50**:263–338.
7. **Buck, M. A., and B. S. Cooperman.** 1990. Single protein omission reconstitution studies of tetracycline binding to the 30S subunit of *Escherichia coli* ribosomes. *Biochemistry* **29**:5374–5379.
8. **Burdett, V.** 1991. Purification and characterization of Tet(M), a protein that renders ribosomes resistance to tetracycline. *J. Biol. Chem.* **266**:2872–2877.
9. **Burdett, V.** 1993. tRNA modification activity is necessary for Tet(M)-mediated tetracycline resistance. *J. Bacteriol.* **175**:7209–7215.
10. **Burdett, V.** 1996. Tet(M)-promoted release of tetracycline from ribosomes is GTP dependent. *J. Bacteriol.* **178**:3246–3251.

11. **Charvalos, E., Y. Tselentis, M. M. Hamzeh-pour, Y. Köhler, and J.-C. Pechere.** 1995. Evidence for an efflux pump in multidrug-resistant *Campylobacter jejuni. Antimicrob. Agents Chemother.* **39:**2019–2022.

12. **Chopra, I.** 1985. Mode of action of the tetracyclines and the nature of bacterial resistance to them, p. 317–392. *In* J. J. Hlavka and J. H. Boothe (ed.), *The Tetracyclines.* Springer-Verlag KG, Berlin, Germany.

13. **Chopra, I., P. M. Hawkey, and M. Hinton.** 1992. Tetracyclines, molecular and clinical aspects. *J. Antimicrob. Chemother.* **29:**245–277.

14. **Clermont, D., O. Chesneau, G. De Cespedes, and T. Horaud.** 1997. New tetracycline-resistance determinants coding for ribosomal protection in streptococci and nucleotide sequence of *tet(T)* isolated from *Streptococcus pyogenes* A498. *Antimicrob. Agents Chemother.* **41:**112–116.

15. **Czworkowski, J., and P. B. Moore.** 1996. The elongation phase of protein synthesis. *Prog. Nucleic Acid Res.* **54:**293–332.

16. **Dever, L. A., and T. S. Dermody.** 1991. Mechanisms of bacterial resistance to antibiotics. *Arch. Intern. Med.* **151:**886–895.

17. **Doyle, K., K. J. McDowell, M. J. Butler, and I. S. Hunter.** 1991. Characterization of an oxytetracycline-resistance gene, *otrA,* of *Streptomyces rimosus. Mol. Microbiol.* **5:**2923–2933.

18. **Drlica, K., and X. Zhao.** 1997. DNA gyrase, topoisomerase IV, and the 4-quinolones. *Microbiol. Mol. Biol. Rev.* **61:**377–392.

19. **Epe, B., P. Woolley, and H. Hornig.** 1987. Competition between tetracycline and the tRNA at both P and A sites of the ribosome of *Escherichia coli. FEBS Lett.* **213:**443–447.

20. **Gaudreau, C., and H. Gilbert.** 1998. Antimicrobial resistance of clinical strains of *Campylobacter jejuni* subsp. *jejuni* isolated from 1985 to 1997 in Quebec, Canada. *Antimicrob. Agents Chemother.* **42:**2106–2108.

21. **Gibreel, A., E. Sjögren, B. Kaijser, B. Wretlind, and O. Sköld.** 1998. Rapid emergence of high-level resistance to quinolones in *Campylobacter jejuni* associated with mutational changes in *gyrA* and *parC. Antimicrob. Agents Chemother.* **42:**3276–3278.

22. **Gibreel, A., and O. Sköld.** 1998. High-level resistance to trimethoprim in clinical isolates of *Campylobacter jejuni* by acquisition of foreign genes (*dfr1* and *dfr9*) expressing drug-insensitive dihydrofolate reductases. *Antimicrob. Agents Chemother.* **42:**3059–3064.

23. **Gootz, T. D., and B. A. Martin.** 1991. Characterization of high-level quinolone resistance in *Campylobacter jejuni. Antimicrob. Agents Chemother.* **35:**840–845.

24. **Grewal, J., E. K. Manavathu, and D. E. Taylor.** 1993. Effect of mutational alteration of Asn-128 in the putative GTP-binding domain of tetracycline resistance determinant Tet(O) from *Campylobacter jejuni. Antimicrob. Agents Chemother.* **37:**2645–2649.

25. **Hosaka, M., T. Yasue, H. Fukuda, H. Tomizawa, H. Aoyama, and K. Hirai.** 1992. In vitro and in vivo antibacterial activities of AM 1155, a new 6-fluoro-8-methoxy quinolone. *Antimicrob. Agents Chemother.* **36:**2108–2117.

26. **Jacob, J., S. Evers, K. Bischoff, C. Carlier, and P. Courvalin.** 1994. Characterization of the *sat4* gene encoding a streptothricin acetyltransferase in *Campylobacter coli* BE/G4. *FEMS Microbiol. Lett.* **120:**13–18.

27. **Jansson, C., A. Franklin, and O. Sköld.** 1992. Spread of a newly found trimethoprim resistance gene, *dfrIX,* among porcine isolates and human pathogens. *Antimicrob. Agents Chemother.* **36:**2704–2708.

28. **Jorgensen, J. H., L. M. Weigel, M. J. Ferraro, J. M. Senson, and F. C. Tenover.** 1999. Activities of newer fluoroquinolones against *Streptococcus pneumoniae* clinical isolates including those with mutations in the *gyrA, parC,* and *parE* loci. *Antimicrob. Agents Chemother.* **43:**329–334.

29. **Kampranis, S. C., and A. Maxwell.** 1998. The DNA gyrase-quinolone complex. *J. Biol. Chem.* **273:**22615–22626.

30. **Karimi, R., and M. Ehrenberg.** 1994. Dissociation rate of cognate peptidyl-tRNA from the A-site of hyper-accurate and error-prone ribosomes. *Eur. J. Biochem.* **226:**355–360.

31. **Lachance, N., C. Gaudreau, F. Lamothe, and L. A. Larivière.** 1991. Role of the β-lactamase of *Campylobacter jejuni* in resistance to β-lactam agents. *Antimicrob. Agents Chemother.* **35:**813–818.

32. **Lachance, N., C. Gaudreau, F. Lamothe, and F. Turgeon.** 1993. Susceptibilities of β-lactamase-positive and -negative strains of *Campylobacter coli* to β-lactam agents. *Antimicrob. Agents Chemother.* **37:**1174–1176.

33. **Larivière, L. A., C. Gaudreau, and F. Turgeon.** 1986. Susceptibilities of clinical isolates of *Campylobacter coli* to twenty-five antimicrobial agents. *J. Antimicrob. Chemother.* **18:**681–685.

33a.**Levy, S. B., L. M. McMurry, T. M. Barbosa, V. Burdett, P. Courvalin, W. Hillen, M. C. Roberts, J. I. Rood, and D. E. Taylor.** 1999. Nomenclature for new tetracycline resistance determinants. *Antimicrob. Agents Chemother.* **43:**1523–1524.

34. **Lucain, C., H. Goosens, and J.-C. Pechère.** 1985. Beta-lactamases in *Campylobacter jejuni* p. 36 (abstract). *In* A. D. Pearson, M. B. Skirrow, H. Lior, and B. Rowe (ed.), *Campylobacter III.* Public Health Laboratory Service, London, United Kingdom.

35. **Manavathu, E. K., K. Hiratsuka, and D. E. Taylor.** 1988. Nucleotide sequence analysis and

expression of a tetracycline-resistance gene from *Campylobacter jejuni. Gene* **62**:17–26.

36. **Moazed, D., and H. F. Noller.** 1987. Interaction of antibiotics with functional sites in 16S ribosomal RNA. *Nature* **327**:389–394.

37. **Ng, L.-K., Stiles, M. E., and D. E. Taylor.** 1987. DNA probes for identification of tetracycline resistance genes in *Campylobacter* species isolated from swine and cattle. *Antimicrob. Agents Chemother.* **31**:1669–1674.

38. **Nierhaus, K. H.** 1996. The tricks of ribosomal elongation factors. *Angew. Chem. Int. Ed. Engl.* **35**:2198–2201.

39. **Nierhaus, K. H., D. Beyer, M. Dabrowski, M. Schäfer, C. M. T. Spahn, J. Wadzack, J. U. Bittner, N. Burkhardt, G. Diedrich, R. Jünemann, D. Kamp, H. Voss, and H. B. Stuhrmann.** 1995. The elongating ribosome: structural and function aspects. *Biochem. Cell Biol.* **73**:1011–1021.

40. **Page, W. J., G. Huyer, M. Huyer, and E. A. Worobec.** 1989. Characterization of the porins of *Campylobacter jejuni* and *Campylobacter coli* and implications for antibiotic susceptibility. *Antimicrob. Agents Chemother.* **33**:297–303.

41. **Piddock, L. J. V.** 1995. Quinolone resistance and *Campylobacter* spp. *J. Antimicrob. Chemother.* **36**:891–898.

42. **Piddock, L. J. V., R. N. Walters, Y.-F. Jin, H. L. Turner, D. M. Gascoyne-Binzi, and P. M. Hawkey.** 1997. Prevalence and mechanism of resistance to "third-generation" cephalosporins in clinically relevant isolates of *Enterobacteriaceae* from 43 hospitals in the UK, 1990–1991. *J. Antimicrob. Chemother.* **39**:177–187.

43. **Pigrau, C., R. Bartolome, B. Almirante, A.-M. Planes, J. Gavalda, and A. Pahissa.** 1997. Bacteremia due to *Campylobacter* species: clinical findings and antimicrobial susceptibility patterns. *Clin. Infect. Dis.* **25**:1414–1420.

44. **Pinto-Alphandary, H., C. Mabilat, and P. Courvalin.** 1990. Emergence of aminoglycoside resistance genes *aadA* and *aadE* in the genus *Campylobacter. Antimicrob. Agents Chemother.* **34**:1294–1296.

45. **Reese, R. E., and R. F. Betts.** 1993. *Handbook of Antibiotics.* Little, Brown & Co., Boston, Mass.

46. **Rivera, M. J., J. Castillo, C. Martin, M. Navarro, and R. Gomez-Lus.** 1986. Aminoglycoside-phosphotransferases APH(3′)-IV and APH(3″) synthesized by a strain of *Campylobacter coli. J. Antimicrob. Chemother.* **18**:153–158.

47. **Roberts, M. C.** 1994. Epidemiology of tetracycline-resistance determinants. *Trends Microbiol.* **2**:353–357.

48. **Roberts, M. C.** 1996. Tetracycline resistance determinants: mechanisms of action, regulation of expression, genetic mobility, and distribution. *FEMS Microbiol. Rev.* **19**:1–24.

49. **Roe, D. E., A. Weinberg, and M. C. Roberts.** 1995. Characterization of erythromycin resistance in *Campylobacter (Wolinella) rectus. Clin. Infect. Dis.* **20**(Suppl. 2):S370–S371.

50. **Ross, J. I., E. A. Eady, J. H. Cove, and W. J. Cunliffe.** 1998. 16S rRNA mutation associated with tetracycline resistance in a gram-positive bacterium. *Antimicrob. Agents Chemother.* **42**:1702–1705.

51. **Ruiz, J., F. Goñi, F. Gallardo, B. Mirelis, T. Jimenez De Anta, and J. Vila.** 1998. Increased resistance to quinolones in *Campylobacter jejuni*: a genetic analysis of *gyrA* gene mutations in quinolone-resistant clinical isolates. *Microbiol. Immunol.* **42**:223–226.

52. **Sagara, H., A. Mochizuki, N. Okamura, and R. Nakaya.** 1987. Antimicrobial resistance of *Campylobacter jejuni* and *Campylobacter coli* with special reference to plasmid-coded proteins of Japanese clinical isolates. *Antimicrob. Agents Chemother.* **31**:713–719.

53. **Schnappinger, D., and W. Hillen.** 1996. Tetracyclines: antibiotic action, uptake, and resistance mechanisms. *Arch. Microbiol.* **165**:350–369.

54. **Scott, K. P., R. M. Barbosa, K. J. Forbes, and H. J. Flint.** 1997. High-frequency transfer of a naturally occurring chromosomal tetracycline resistance element in the ruminal anaerobe *Butyrivibrio fibrisolvens. Appl. Environ. Microbiol.* **63**:3405–3411.

55. **Sougakoff, W., B. Papadopoulou, P. Nordmann, and P. Courvalin.** 1987. Nucleotide sequence and distribution of gene *tetO* encoding tetracycline resistance in *Campylobacter coli. FEMS Microbiol. Lett.* **44**:153–159.

56. **Spahn, C. M. T., and C. D. Prescott.** 1996. Throwing a spanner in the works: antibiotics and the translation apparatus. *J. Mol. Med.* **74**:423–439.

57. **Spratt, B. G.** 1989. Resistance to β-lactam antibiotics mediated by alterations of penicillin-binding proteins, p. 77–100. *In* L. E. Bryan (ed.), *Microbial Resistance to Drugs.* Springer-Verlag KG, Berlin, Germany.

58. **Tajada, P., J.-L. Gomez-Garces, J.-I. Alós, D. Balas, and R. Cogollos.** 1996. Antimicrobial susceptibilities of *Campylobacter jejuni* and *Campylobacter coli* to 12 β-lactams and combinations with β-lactamase inhibitors. *Antimicrob. Agents Chemother.* **40**:1924–1925.

59. **Taylor, D. E.** 1992. Antimicrobial resistance of *Campylobacter jejuni* and *Campylobacter coli* to tetracycline, chloramphenicol and erythromycin, p. 74–86. *In* I. Nachamkin, M. J. Blaser, and L. S. Tompkins (ed.), *Campylobacter jejuni: Current Status and Future Trends.* American Society for Microbiology, Washington, D.C.

60. **Taylor, D. E., S. A. DeGrandis, M. A. Kar-**

mali, and P. C. Fleming. 1981. Transmissible plasmids from *Campylobacter jejuni*. *Antimicrob. Agents Chemother.* **19**:831–835.

61. Taylor, D. E., L.-K. Ng, and H. Lior. 1985. Susceptibility of *Campylobacter* species to nalidixic acid, enoxacin, and other DNA gyrase inhibitors. *Antimicrob. Agents Chemother.* **28**:708–710.

62. Taylor, D. E., K. Hiratsuka, H. Ray, and E. K. Manavathu. 1987. Characterization of a cloned tetracycline resistance determinant from *Campylobacter jejuni* plasmid pUA466. *J. Bacteriol.* **169**:2984–2989.

63. Taylor, D. E., and P. Courvalin. 1988. Mechanism of antibiotic resistance in *Campylobacter* species. *Antimicrob. Agents Chemother.* **32**:1107–1112.

64. Taylor, D. E., W. Yan, L.-K. Ng, E. K. Manavathu, and P. Courvalin. 1988. Genetic characterization of kanamycin resistance in *Campylobacter coli*. *Ann. Inst. Pasteur Microbiol.* **139**:665–676.

65. Taylor, D. E., and N. Chang. 1991. In vitro susceptibilities of *Campylobacter jejuni* and *Campylobacter coli* to azithromycin and erythromycin. *Antimicrob. Agents Chemother.* **35**:1917–1918.

66. Taylor, D. E., L. J. Jerome, J. Grewal, and N. Chang. 1995. Tet(O), a protein that mediates ribosomal protection to tetracycline, binds and hydrolyses GTP. *Can. J. Microbiol.* **41**:965–979.

67. Taylor, D. E., and A. Chau. 1996. Tetracycline resistance mediated by ribosomal protection. *Antimicrob. Agents Chemother.* **40**:1–5.

68. Taylor, D. E., and A. Chau. 1997. Cloning and nucleotide sequence of the *gyrA* gene from *Campylobacter fetus* subsp. *fetus* ATCC27374 and characterization of ciprofloxacin resistant laboratory and clinical isolates. *Antimicrob. Agents Chemother.* **41**:665–671.

69. Taylor, D. E., Z. Ge, D. Purych, T. Lo, and K. Hiratsuka. 1997. Cloning and sequence analysis of two copies of a 23S rRNA gene from *Helicobacter pylori* and association of clarithromycin resistance with 23S rRNA mutations. *Antimicrob. Agents Chemother.* **41**:2621–2628.

70. Taylor, D. E., C. A. Trieber, G. Trescher, and M. Bekkering. 1998. Host mutations (*miaA* and *rpsL*) reduce tetracycline resistance mediated by Tet(O) and Tet(M). *Antimicrob. Agents Chemother.* **42**:59–64.

71. Tee, W., A. Mijch, E. Wright, and A. Yung. 1995. Emergence of multidrug resistance in *Campylobacter jejuni* isolates from three patients infected with human immunodeficiency virus. *Clin. Infect. Dis.* **21**:634–638.

72. Tenover, F. C., D. J. LeBlanc, and P. M. Elvrum. 1987. Cloning and expression of a tetracycline resistance determinant from *Campylobacter jejuni* in *Escherichia coli*. *Antimicrob. Agents Chemother.* **31**:1301–1306.

73. Tenover, F. C., and P. M. Elvrum. 1988. Detection of two different kanamycin resistance genes in naturally occurring isolates of *Campylobacter jejuni* and *Campylobacter coli*. *Antimicrob. Agents Chemother.* **32**:1170–1173.

74. Trieber, C. A., N. Burkhardt, K. H. Nierhaus, and D. E. Taylor. 1998. Ribosomal protection from tetracycline mediated by Tet(O): Tet(O) interaction with ribosomes is GTP-dependent. *Biol. Chem.* **379**:847–855.

74a. Trieber, C. A., and D. E. Taylor. 1999. Erythromycin resistance in *Campylobacter*, p. 3. *In* H. L. T. Mobley, I. Nachamkin, and D. McGee (ed.), *Proceedings of the 10th International Workshop on Campylobacter, Helicobacter and Related Organisms*. Baltimore, Md.

75. Velázquez, J. B., A. Jiménez, B. Chomón, and T. G. Villa. 1995. Incidence and transmission of antibiotic resistance in *Campylobacter jejuni* and *Campylobacter coli*. *J. Antimicrob. Chemother.* **35**:173–178.

76. Walder, M., and A. Forgren. 1978. Erythromycin-resistance campylobacters. *Lancet* **ii**:1201.

77. Wang, W.-L. L., L. B. Reller, and M. J. Blaser. 1984. Comparison of antimicrobial susceptibility patterns of *Campylobacter jejuni* and *Campylobacter coli*. *Antimicrob. Agents Chemother.* **26**:351–353.

78. Wang, Y., and D. E. Taylor. 1990. Chloramphenicol resistance in *Campylobacter coli*: nucleotide sequence, expression, and cloning vector construction. *Gene* **94**:23–28.

79. Wang, Y., and D. E. Taylor. 1990. Natural transformation in *Campylobacter* species. *J. Bacteriol.* **172**:949–955.

80. Wang, Y., and D. E. Taylor. 1991. A DNA sequence upstream of the *tet(O)* gene is required for full expression of tetracycline resistance. *Antimicrob. Agents Chemother.* **35**:2020–2025.

81. Wang, Y., W. M. Huang, and D. E. Taylor. 1993. Cloning and nucleotide sequence of the *Campylobacter jejuni gyrA* gene and characterization of quinolone resistance mutations. *Antimicrob. Agents Chemother.* **37**:457–463.

82. Willmott, C. J. R., and A. Maxwell. 1993. A single point mutation in the DNA gyrase A protein greatly reduces binding of fluoroquinolones to the gyrase-DNA complex. *Antimicrob. Agents Chemother.* **37**:126–127.

83. Yan, W., and D. E. Taylor. 1991. Characterization of erythromycin resistance in *Campylobacter jejuni* and *Campylobacter coli*. *Antimicrob. Agents Chemother.* **35**:1989–1996.

84. Zilhao, R., Papadopoulou, B., and P. Courvalin. 1988. Occurrence of the *Campylobacter* resistance gene *tetO* in *Enterococcus* and *Streptococcus* spp. *Antimicrob. Agents Chemother.* **32**:1793–1796.

THE HIPPURATE HYDROLASE GENE AND OTHER UNIQUE GENES OF CAMPYLOBACTER JEJUNI

Voon L. Chan, Eric Kurt Hani, Angela Joe, Jennifer Lynett, David Ng, and Marina Steele

23

Campylobacter jejuni is one of the 15 known species in the genus Campylobacter. The presence of hippurate hydrolase (N-benzoylglycine amidohydrolase [EC 3.5.1.32]) activity in C. jejuni is the critical biochemical reaction that distinguishes C. jejuni from other Campylobacter species. Hippurate hydrolase catalyzes the hydrolysis, at the peptide linkage, of hippuric acid to liberate benzoic acid and glycine.

C. jejuni is responsible for 80 to 90% of the Campylobacter infections in humans in developed countries (25); C. coli infections account for about 7%, and C. lari and C. upsaliensis represent about 1%. The main route of Campylobacter infection in humans is through consumption of undercooked poultry and pork and contaminated water. The distribution of C. jejuni and C. coli in pigs was observed to be about equal (27); raw poultry harbors 27% C. coli and 73% C. jejuni (11). Compared to the ratio of C. coli and C. jejuni in pork and poultry, the human host appears to be preferentially infected with C. jejuni rather than C. coli. This suggests that C. jejuni is more efficient in colonizing and causing enteritis in humans than the other Campylobacter species. Presumably, the genes that are unique to C. jejuni are at least partly responsible for the higher efficiency of this species in causing disease in humans. Species-specific sequences could be caused by accumulated point mutations over an evolutionary period. The majority of these sequences, however, are probably derived from acquired DNA fragments via interspecies horizontal gene transfer processes (18). Acquired DNA sequences would include lysogenic phages, plasmids, insertion elements, transposons, and pathogenicity islands. Therefore, an important first step is to identify the genes on the C. jejuni genome that are unique to the species and relate the function of the encoded products to the virulence of the bacterial organism. In this chapter, we review some of the genes that have been reported to be unique to C. jejuni. Their

Voon L. Chan, Department of Medical Genetics and Microbiology and Department of Laboratory Medicine and Pathobiology, Medical Sciences Building, University of Toronto, Toronto, Ontario M5S 1A8, Canada. Eric Kurt Hani, Department of Microbiology, University of Guelph, Guelph, Ontario N1G 2W1, Canada. Angela Joe, Department of Microbiology and Immunology, University of Melbourne, Parkville, Victoria 3052, Australia. Jennifer Lynett, Department of Laboratory Medicine and Pathobiology, University of Toronto, Toronto, Ontario M5S 1A8, Canada. David Ng, Department of Medical Genetics and Microbiology, University of Toronto, Toronto, Ontario M5S 3E2, Canada. Marina Steele, Department of Pathobiology, University of Guelph, Guelph, Ontario, Canada.

Campylobacter, 2nd Ed., Edited by I. Nachamkin and M. J. Blaser
© 2000 American Society for Microbiology, Washington, D.C.

positions on the genome and possible functions in pathogenesis are discussed.

THE *hipO* LOCUS

We theorized that the inability of the other *Campylobacter* species to hydrolyze hippurate was due to the lack of the hippurate hydrolase gene and hence of the corresponding enzyme. Cloning of the hippurate hydrolase gene should lead to the isolation of a gene unique to *C. jejuni*. Using the hippurate hydrolysis assay to screen pools of independent pBR322 recombinants, we were successful in isolating a recombinant, designated pHIP-O, that encodes hippurate hydrolase (10). The 4,447-bp insert in pHIP-O was completely sequenced on both strands (accession no. Z36940). Eight potential open reading frames (QRFs) were identified, and one, ORFU4, was found to encode hippurate hydrolase. The hippurate hydrolase gene, *hipO,* was used as a probe in DNA hybridization with DNA isolated from various species of *Campylobacter*. All the *C. jejuni* isolates tested hybridized and none of the isolates from the other species (*C. coli, C. lari, C. fetus, C. sputorum,* and *C. upsaliensis*) tested were positive (10).

Organization

The 4,447-bp insert of pHIP-O consists of eight potential ORFs (Fig. 1), four on each strand of the insert. The ORFs are designated ORFU1, ORFU2, ORFU3, and ORFU4 for those on the upper strand and ORFL1, ORFL2, ORFL3, and ORFL4 for those on the lower strand (9, 10). The ORF at the 3′ end of the pHIP-O insert, ORFL4, encodes a protein designated JlpA. Sequence analysis, using the pSORT algorithm, identified JlpA (374 amino acids [aa] 42.6 kDa) as a strong candidate for a lipoprotein located at either the outer membrane or the inner membrane. The amino acid sequence of ORFL4 was compared to the current database sequences by using BLAST, and no good sequence homology was identified. The protein product of *jlpA* was demonstrated by using a T7 expression system, and the presence of a lipid moiety on the JlpA

molecule was shown by incorporation of radioactive palmitic acid (12). It is notable that four of the ORFs (ORFU3, ORFU4 [HipO], ORFL1, and ORFU2) encoded by the pHIP-O fragment are putative cytoplasmic membrane proteins. This region, encoding cytoplasmic membrane proteins, hippurate hydrolase, and the lipoprotein, has been designated the MHL site. The G + C content of this 4,447-bp HIP-O fragment is 27.5%, compared to 31.9% for the total 43 protein-encoding genes of *C. jejuni* in the database, suggesting that it has been recently acquired from another genome. The codon usage of ORFL2, ORFL4, ORFU2, and ORFU3 is quite different from that of other *C. jejuni* genes.

Size of the MHL *C. jejuni*-Unique Region

A restriction enzyme map of the MHL region, which was obtained by mapping two overlapping lambda GEM11 recombinant clones (1A and 5A) of a genomic library of *C. jejuni* TGH9011, is shown in Fig. 2. Different restriction fragments isolated from inserts of recombinant phage 1A or 5A were used as probes in a Southern hybridization analysis of genomic digests of *C. jejuni* and *C. coli*. Probes B, C, and D hybridized only *C. jejuni* DNA, and not *C. coli* DNA. Probe A hybridized *C. jejuni* DNA strongly and *C. coli* DNA much more weakly, suggesting that the boundary of the *C. jejuni*-specific sequences is located within the *Eco*RI-*Xba*I fragment. To determine if the complete *jlpA* gene was conserved within *C. jejuni* strains, *jlpA*-specific primers P4 (GAGAAACATATGAAAAAAGGTATTTTT-CTC) and PR7 (AACTGCCGCCCATTAA-CATAGAAAAC) were used to amplify the gene from various genomic DNA samples. The 5′ end of P4 is located at the Shine-Dalgarno sequence of *jlpA,* and the 5′ end of PR7 is located at 10 nucleotides (nt) upstream from the stop codon of *jlpA*. A single PCR product of the expected size (1.1 kb) was observed in all 10 of the *C. jejuni* strains analyzed (12). Chromosomal DNA preparations from several *Campylobacter* species related to *C.*

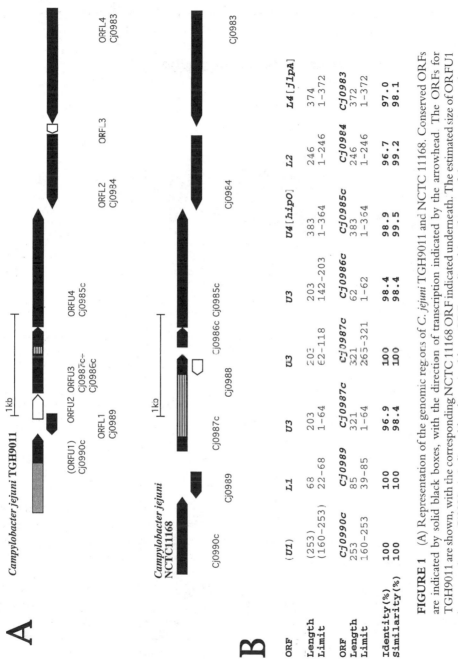

FIGURE 1   (A) Representation of the genomic regions of *C. jejuni* TGH9011 and NCTC 11168. Conserved ORFs are indicated by solid black boxes, with the direction of transcription indicated by the arrowhead. The ORFs for TGH9011 are shown, with the corresponding NCTC 11168 ORF indicated underneath. The estimated size of ORFU1 in comparison to Cj0990c is indicated by the striped box. ORFs predicted in only one of the two strains are shown by white boxes. The 200-aa coding sequence unique to Cj0987c and the 24-aa coding sequence unique to ORFU3 are indicated by striped boxes. (B) Comparison of the sequence identity of corresponding ORFs from strains TGH9011 and NCTC 11168. The partial sequences of ORFU1 are indicated by parentheses. The numbering for ORFU1 is idealized to facilitate comparison with Cj0990c. Lengths (in amino acid residues) are given for each ORF in TGH9011 and deduced polypeptide from NCTC 11168 genes.

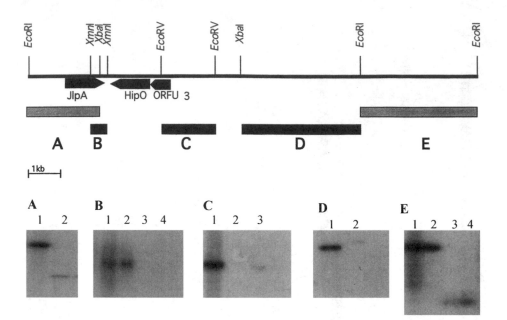

FIGURE 2 (Top) Restriction map for the approximately 13-kb region of the *C. jejuni* TGH9011 genome which includes the 4,447-nt region for which the sequence was previously determined (10). The ORFs *jlpA, hipO,* and ORFU3 and their direction of transcription are indicated (10). The bars labeled A to E represent fragments used as probes in Southern hybridizations of *C. jejuni* and *C. coli* genomic DNA. Bars A and E are shaded in gray and represent probes which hybridized to both *C. jejuni* TGH9011 and *C. coli* genomic DNA. Bars B, C, and D are shaded in black and represent probes which hybridized to *C. jejuni* TGH9011 genomic DNA only. These fragments were isolated by restriction enzyme digestion of pHIP-O or lambda GEM 1A and 5A (recombinant phages constructed from *C. jejuni* TGH9011 genomic DNA and lambda GEM 11). (Bottom) Results of Southern hybridization with fragments A to E as probes. Hybridization and washing conditions were performed under high stringency. Panels are as follows: (A) lane 1, *C. jejuni* TGH9011; lane 2, *C. coli* type strain; (B) lanes 1 and 2, *C. jejuni* TGH9011; lanes 3 and 4, *C. coli* type strain; (C) lane 1, *C. jejuni* TGH9011; lane 2, *C. lari* type strain; lane 3, *C. coli* type strain; (D) lane 1, *C. jejuni* TGH9011; lane 2, *C. coli* type strain; (E) lanes 1 and 2; *C. jejuni* TGH9011; lanes 3 and 4, *C. coli* type strain.

jejuni (*C. coli, C. lari, C. sputorum,* and *C. upsaliensis*) were also subjected to PCR analysis with the *jlpA*-specific primers. No detectable amplicons were generated from these samples (result not shown). To confirm that sequences homologous to the lipoprotein gene were absent in these *Campylobacter* strains, genomic DNAs were examined by Southern hybridization analysis. A digoxigenin-labeled 1.1-kb *jlpA*-specific DNA fragment was used to probe a blot of *Cla*I-digested chromosomal DNA. Under conditions of high stringency, a 2.2-kb hybridizing band was observed for *C. jejuni* TGH9011. The DNA probe did not hybridize to the genomic DNA samples from the other

species of *Campylobacter* (12). When Southern analysis was performed at lower stringency, identical results were obtained (data not shown), indicating that the *jlpA* gene is specific to *C. jejuni*. Probe E hybridized with both *C. jejuni* and *C. coli* DNA, suggesting that the 3′ boundary of the *C. jejuni*-unique sequence is located within the 5.5-kb *Eco*RI fragment (Fig. 2). The MHL *C. jejuni*-unique sequence is between 10 and 15 kb in length.

Comparison of the MHL Loci of TGH9011 and NCTC 11168

The organization of the ORFs in the 4447-bp fragment of TGH9011 is shown in Fig. 1; it is quite similar to that of the corresponding region in NCTC 11168. At the nucleotide level, the identity is about 97 to 98%. The deduced amino acid sequences encoded by *C. jejuni* TGH9011 ORFU1 (partial) and ORFL1 are completely identical to the corresponding predicted polypeptide products of the *C. jejuni* NCTC 11168 genes Cj0990c and Cj0989. ORFU2 has no corresponding predicted ORF in NCTC 11168. In strain TGH9011, the ORFU3 product is 203 aa and shows homology to the products of both NCTC 11168 genes Cj0987c (321 aa) and Cj0986c (62 aa). The N-terminal 64-aa stretch of the protein encoded by ORFU3 is 96.9% identical with the first 64 aa of the Cj0987c product. The Cj0987c product possesses an additional 200 aa not present in the ORFU3 product. The carboxy-terminal 56-aa stretch of the Cj0987c product is 100% identical to a 56-aa stretch of the ORFU3 product (residues 62 to 118 of 203). The ORFU3 product continues with a 24-aa stretch not predicted from the nucleotide sequence of NCTC 11168. However, a 70-bp intergenic region separates Cj0987c from Cj0986c, at which point the protein sequences realign, presumably due to a frameshift mutation. The 62 aa of the Cj0986c product are 98.4% identical to the last 62 aa of the ORFU3 product. Both ORFU3 and Cj0986c are immediately followed by *hipO*, whose product has 98.9% amino acid sequence identity between the two strains. The TGH9011 ORFs L2 and L4 have corresponding ORFs in strain NCTC 11168 (Cj0984 and Cj0983 respectively), whose products have 97% identity each. ORFL3 (with a 27-aa product) was not predicted in strain NCTC 11168.

Carboxypeptidase Activity

Purified recombinant hippurate hydrolase of *C. jejuni* TGH9011 was prepared to assay its protease activity by using a variety of commercially available synthetic protease substrates. No detectable enzyme activity was observed against Lys-*p*-nitroanilide, Leu-*p*-nitroanilide, and *N*-benzoyl (Bz)-Arg-*p*-nitroanilide, which are common aminopeptidase and endopeptidase substrates. Bz amino acids are common carboxypeptidase substrates. Bz-Gly, Bz-Met, Bz-Ala, Bz-Val, and Bz-Phe were readily hydrolyzed by the purified hippurate hydrolase, suggesting that the enzyme is a carboxypeptidase. Bz amino acids with small aliphatic amino acids such as glycine, alanine, or valine or the sulfur-containing amino acid methionine in the P1' position were hydrolyzed preferentially (26).

Possible Function of Hippurate Hydrolase (Hippuricase)

Some ideas on the possible function of hippurate hydrolase can be gained by examining the proteins which have high homology. These enzymes have a wide distribution in plants, animals, and microorganisms, and the substrate specificity among the amidohydrolases can vary from very broad to rather restricted enzymatic activity. These enzymes are involved in the cleavage of N-substituted amino acids from larger substrates, and they also participate in the biosynthesis of a number of amino acids. Hippurate hydrolase (EC 3.5.1.32) specifically cleaves Bz-Gly into benzoic acid and glycine. They also appear to play an important role in signaling events that control development steps in the division and elongation of cells of the dicot *Arabidopsis thaliana*. Amidohydrolases have found important applications in biotechnology. The chiral specificity of many amidohydrolases allows their use in the industrial production of stereoisomers from racemic mixtures. They have been used for the synthesis of amino acids from acetylated racemates for a long time. These interesting features of amidohydrolases have provided the incentive to search for such enzymes in a number of microorganisms and to clone their structural genes.

The Bz-Gly amidohydrolase (hippurate hydrolase) test is still of great importance in the biochemical differentiation of *C. jejuni* from all the other known campylobacters (22). Elucidation of the physiological role of hippurate hydrolase is likely to be helped by the examination of closely related proteins from other bacterial species. A comparison of hippurate hydrolase (HipO) with similar proteins from other microorganisms affords only a few instances of sequenced genetic elements whose polypeptide products have an experimentally determined concomitant function. In many cases, the isolated genes are categorized as "*hipO*-like." In this category, homology exists between the predicted polypeptide products of *C. jejuni hipO* and the *hipO*-like genes in the following organisms: a second copy in the genome of *C. jejuni* NCTC 11168 (http://www.sanger.ac.uk/Projects/C__jejuni), two unlinked copies in the genome of *Pyrococcus horikoshii* (14), and single copies in *Bacillus subtilis* (17), *Haemophilus influenzae* (5), and *Lactobacillus lactis* subsp. *cremoris* (23). A HipO homolog is located on an extrachromosomal element in *Rhizobium* sp. strain NGR234 (6).

The *C. jejuni* HipO protein does have several homologs whose functions have been experimentally determined to some degree. The archaebacterium *Sulfolobus solfataricus* possesses a carboxypeptidase gene (*cspA*) with strong homology to *hipO* from *C. jejuni* (3). The product of *S. solfataricus* gene has a substrate activity toward benzyloxycarbonyl-glycineglycinephenylalanine, carbobenzyloxy (Cbz)-arginine, and Cbz-aspartic acid and slight activity toward Cbz–phenylalanine.

Bacillus stearothermophilus aminoacylase (encoded by *amaA*) is also a strong homolog of HipO (24). The *amaA* gene was isolated by complementation of an *Escherichia coli argE* mutant, and the protein contains four subunits of identical size (molecular weight 42,000). Enzymatic activity was observed toward the substrates *N*-chloroacetyl-L-phenylalanine, *N*-acetyl-L-tyrosine, *N*-acetyl-L-alanine, *N*-acetyl-L-phenylalanine, *N*-acetyl-L-valine, *N*-acetyl-glycine, *N*-acetyl-L-leucine, *N*-acetyl-L-histidine, and *N*-acetyl-L-methionine. The reactivity of this enzyme with Bz-Gly was not determined.

Bacillus subtilis, in addition to containing a strong *hipO* homolog (17), contains an additional gene, *amhX* with homology to *hipO* (15). The amidohydrolase product of this gene has a predicted molecular mass of 41.5 kDa. Substrate studies were not performed on the overproduced protein, and so comparison to HipO is limited. Unlike the amidohydrolase gene from *B. stearothermophilus*, *amhX* from *B. subtilis* was not able to complement an *E. coli argE* mutant.

Enterobacter agglomerans possesses a HipO homolog, encoded by the gene for indole-3-acetyl-L-aspartic acid hydrolase (IAA-Asp hydrolase) (*iaaspH*) (2). IAA-Asp is a naturally occurring IAA amide conjugate present in soybean seeds and probably in several other plant species. In plants, the regulation of IAA-Asp synthesis and hydrolysis plays a key role in IAA metabolism. IAA is the major plant auxin, a signaling molecule that regulates developmental processes in plants. Not coincidentally, the *Arabidopsis thaliana* IAA-Leu hydrolase (encoded by *ilr1*) and its homologs (encoded by *ill1* and *ill2*) are highly homologous to HipO (1).

Several proteins have been described which exhibit Bz–amino acid amidohydrolase activity or a closely related activity but whose amino acid sequences have not been determined and encoding genes have not been isolated. This information would establish more concrete comparisons between these enzymes and HipO. The differences in the hippurate hydrolase activities of these enzymes could then be related to the primary sequence and predicted secondary and tertiary structures of these proteins. In particular, *Pseudomonas putida* possesses Bz-amidohydrolase activity (19). The enzyme contains four subunits with identical molecular weight (42,000). The enzyme hydrolyzes Bz-Gly, Bz-Ala, and Bz-L-aminobutyric acid but not other Bz amino acids, nor *N*-acetyl amino acids and *N*-carbobenzoxy amino acids. The p-NO_2-substituted substrates are hydrolyzed most rapidly.

Another pseudomonad species (strain KT801) possesses Bz-amino acid amidohyrolase activity (13). Substrate specificity was broad, with reactivity toward Bz-Ala, Bz-Met, Bz-Leu, Bz-Gly, and Bz-Val and slight reactions with other Bz–amino acids.

Streptococcus faecalis contains an *N*-benzoyloxycarbonyl amino acid urethanehydrolase that hydrolyzes Bz-Gly and Cbz-Gly at almost the same rate, and the reaction is accompanied by decarboxylation (21). A group B strepto-coccal isolate (strain GT-7909) from a urine isolate possesses Bz-Gly amidohydrolase activity (4). Enzyme activity is localized to the cytoplasmic fraction and displays trypsin sensitivity, heat lability, and a pH range of 7.1 to 9.0 for optimum activity.

Corynebacterium equi possesses a Bz-Ala amidohydrolase composed of six units with identical molecular weight (40,000) (20). The substrate specificity also includes Bz-Gly and Bz-aminobutyric acid. Substitution with p-NO$_2$ increases the rate of hydrolysis for Bz-Ala and Bz-Gly.

OTHER UNIQUE GENES

Korolik et al. (16) reported the first attempt to isolate a DNA probe that is specific for *C. jejuni*. A 6.1-kb *C. jejuni* DNA fragment was isolated from a *C. jejuni* genomic library constructed with the pBR322 plasmid. With this fragment as a probe in Southern hybridization, all the *C. jejuni* strains tested hybridized strongly. Under high stringency, no hybridization was observed to other species of *Campylobacter* except *C. coli*, which gave a distinct weak hybridization band. The 6.1-kb fragment was not sequenced, and therefore there is no information about the gene products that the fragment encodes.

Giesendorf et al. (7) reported the isolation of an 800-bp fragment from *C. jejuni* NCTC 11351 by a random amplified polymorphic DNA element generated by PCR with primers REP1R-I and REP2-I based on the prokaryotic repetitive extragenic palindrome (REP) motifs REP1R-I and REP2-I1 (30). By Southern hybridization analysis with the 800-bp unique element as probe, all 33 reference strains of *C. jejuni* tested were positive. No hybridization was observed with 30 reference strains of *C. coli*, 8 reference strains of *C. lari*, 37 strains from a broad range of other microorganisms including *Yersinia*, *Mycobacterium*, *Escherichia coli*, *Bacillus*, *Clostridium*, *Klebsiella*, *Listeria*, *Proteus*, *Pseudomonas*, *Salmonella*, *Shigella*, *Streptococcus*, *Staphylococcus*, and *Helicobacter*.

The fragment was not cloned, and the nucleotide sequence was not determined.

To develop a serological test to discriminate between *C. jejuni* and *C. coli*, Stucki et al. (28) were interested in identifying unique antigenic surface structures of *C. jejuni*. A library of genomic DNA of *C. jejuni* 81116 screened with hyperimmune serum against *C. jejuni* ATCC 29428 identified several recombinant clones expressing immunoreactive *C. jejuni* proteins. Of these, one clone expressed a protein designated MapA, which appeared to be unique to *C. jejuni*. Anti-MapA antibodies reacted with *C. jejuni* MapA in Western immunoblots but did not react with any *C. coli* proteins; thus, MapA appeared to be a species-specific antigen. The *mapA* gene encodes a membrane-associated protein of 214 aa with a molecular mass of 24 kDa, named MapA. The N-terminal 18 aa constitute a signal sequence characteristic of prokaryotic membrane lipoproteins. The lipoprotein nature of MapA was not confirmed experimentally by tritiated palmitic acid labeling. After posttranslational processing, the predicted molecular mass of the mature protein is 22 kDa. Mature MapA appears to be localized to the inner membrane of *C. jejuni*. A BLAST search with the amino acid sequence of protein MapA revealed no homology to known proteins. With the *mapA* gene fragment as a probe in colony blot hybridization assay, all 120 *C. jejuni* isolates tested, including 6 *C. jejuni* reference strains (ATCC 29428, NCTC 11351, CCUG 12085, CCUG 15114, CCUG 12082, and CCUG 12072), gave positive hybridization results. A total of 126 other *Campylobacter*, *Arcobacter*, and *Helicobacter* species (these include 34 *C. coli*, 63 *C. upsaliensis*, 8 *C. helveticus*, 3 *C. concisus*, 3 *A. butzleri*, 4 *H. canis*, 7 *H. cinaedi*-like, and 4 *H. pullorum* strains) were tested negative in the assay.

The MapA protein of *C. jejuni* 81116 has 100% amino acid sequence identity to the predicted sequence of the Cj1029c product of *C. jejuni* NCTC 11168, the *C. jejuni* strain sequenced by the Sanger Centre. The Cj1029c product is encoded by nt 960743 to 961655 of the genome.

CONCLUDING REMARKS

The *hipO* gene is located in the 10 to 15 kb MHL species-specific region of the genome and encodes a protein with hippurate hydrolase and carboxypeptidase activities. The in vivo substrates and function(s) of HipO remain to be established and are current interests of our laboratory. Two *C. jejuni*-specific loci have been identified, the *mapA* and the *hipO* (MHL) loci. It is interesting that these two loci are both found in a 40-kb region of the *C. jejuni* NCTC 11168 genome: *mapA* is at nt 960743 to 961655, and the MHL region is at nt 915570 to 922157. Sequences that are found in the genome of *Neisseria meningitidis* but not in that of *N. gonorrhoeae* are clustered in three distinct regions (29). Species-specific sequences are generally believed to be acquired by horizontal gene transfer followed by integration or recombination. New DNA sequences could be acquired through integration of a transducing phage, IS element, plasmid, transposon, or mobile pathogenicity island. The gene encoding Arg tRNA$_{GCG}$ is located at nt 943534 to 943610 (http://www.sanger.ac.uk/Projects/C_jejuni), which is between the *mapA* and MHL loci. Genes for tRNA are often sites for integration of bacteriophages and often flank pathogenicity islands (8). The *mapA-hipO* region may represent a favored region for integration by these genetic elements. It should be easier to identify other *C. jejuni*-specific sequences now that the complete genomic sequence of NCTC 11168 is available (http://www.sanger.ac.uk/Projects/C_jejuni). These sequences would encode proteins that are not homologous or have very little homology to any proteins in the database. Some of these proteins are probably *Campylobacter* genus specific, and some are *C. jejuni* specific. Characterization of *C. jejuni*-specific sequences should identify some genes that are important for colonization and infection of humans and also give some valuable information on the evolution and speciation of *Campylobacter* species.

ACKNOWLEDGMENTS

This work was supported by the Natural Sciences and Engineering Research Council of Canada. J.L. was supported by a research grant from the Crohn's and Colitis Foundation of Canada, and M.S. was partially supported by a contract grant from Vita-Tech Canada Inc.

REFERENCES

1. **Bartel, B., and G. R. Fink.** 1995. ILR1, an amidohydrolase that releases active indole-3-acetic acid from conjugates. *Science* **268:**1745–1748.

2. **Chou, J. C., W. W. Mulbry, and J. D. Cohen.** 1998. The gene for indole-3-acetyl-L-aspartic acid hydrolase from *Enterobacter agglomerans:* molecular cloning, nucleotide sequence, and expression in *Escherichia coli. Mol. Gen. Genet.* **259:**172–178.

3. **Colombo, S., G. Toietta, L. Zecca, M. Vanoni, and P. Tortora.** 1995. Molecular cloning, nucleotide sequence, and expression of a carboxypeptidase-encoding gene from the archaebacterium *Sulfolobus solfataricus. J. Bacteriol.* **177:**5561–5566.

4. **Ferrieri, P., L. W. Wannamaker, and J. A. Nelson.** 1973. Localization and characterization of hippuricase activity of group B streptococci. *Infect. Immun.* **7:**747.

5. **Fleischmann, R. D., M. D. Adams, O. White, R. A. Clayton, E. F. Kirkness, A. R. Kerlavage, C. J. Bult, J.-F. Tomb, B. A. Dougherty, J. M. Merrick, K. McKenney, G. Sutton, W. Fitzhugh, C. A. Fields, J. D. Gocayne, J. D. Scott, R. Shirley, L.-I. Liu, A. Glodek, J. M. Kelley, J. F. Weidman, C. A. Phillips, T. Spriggs, E. Hedblom, M. D. Cotton, T. R. Utterback, M. C. Hanna, D. T. Nguyen, D. M. Saudek, R. C. Brandon, L. D. Fine, J. L. Fritchman, J. L. Fuhrmann, N. S. M. Geohagen, C. L. Gnehm, L. A. McDonald, K. V. Small, C. M. Fraser, H. O. Smith, and J. C. Venter.** 1995. Whole-genome random sequencing and assembly of Haemophilus influenzae Rd. *Science* **269:**496–512.

6. **Freiberg, C., R. Fellay, A. Bairoch, W. J. Broughton, A. Rosenthal, and X. Perret.** 1997. Molecular basis of symbiosis between *Rhizobium* and legumes. *Nature* **387:**394–401.

7. **Giesendorf, B. A. J., A. van Belkum, A. Koeken, H. Stegeman, M. H. C. Henkens, J. van der Plas, H. Goossens, H. G. M. Biesters, and W. G. V. Quint.** 1993. Development of species-specific DNA probes for *Campylobacter jejuni, Campylobacter coli,* and *Cambylobacter lari* by polymerase chain reaction fingerprinting. *J. Clin. Microbiol.* **31:**1541–1546.

8. **Groisman, E. A., and H. Ochman.** 1996. Pathogenicity islands: Bacterial evolution in quantum leaps. *Cell* **87:**791–794.

9. **Hani, E. K.** 1997. Hippurate hydrolase gene of

Campylobacter jejuni. Ph.D. thesis. University of Toronto, Toronto, Ontario, Canada.

10. **Hani, E. K., and Chan, V. L.** 1995. Expression and characterization of *Campylobacter jejuni* benzoylglycine amidohydrolase (hippuricase) gene in *Escherichia coli. J. Bacteriol.* **177:**2396–2402.

11. **Harmon, K. M., G. M. Ransom, and I. V. Wesley.** 1997. Differentiation of *Campylobacter jejuni* and *Campylobacter coli* by polymerase chain reaction. *Mol. Cell. Probes* **11:**195–200.

12. **Joe, A., E. K. Hani, P. Sherman, and V. L. Chan.** 1999. Unpublished data.

13. **Kameda, Y., T. Kuramoto, K. Matsui, and T. Ebara.** 1968. Studies on acylase activity and microorganisms. XXV. Purification and properties of benzoylamino-acid amidohydrolase in KT 801 (*Pseudomonas* sp.). *Chem. Pharm. Bull.* **16:**1023–1029.

14. **Kawarabayasi, Y., M. Sawada, H. Horikawa, Y. Haikawa, Y. Hino, S. Yamamoto, M. Sekine, S. Baba, H. Kosugi, A. Hosoyama, Y. Nagai, M. Sakai, K. Ogura, R. Otuka, H. Nakazawa, M. Takamiya, Y. Ohfuku, T. Funahashi, T. Tanaka, Y. Kudoh, J. Yamazaki, N. Kushida, A. Oguchi, K. Aoki, Y. Nakamura, T. F. Robb, K. Horikoshi, Y. Masuchi, H. Shizuya, and H. Kikuchi.** 1998. Complete sequence and gene organization of the genome of a hyper-thermophilic Archaebacterium, *Pyrococcus horikoshii* OT3. *DNA Res.* **5:**55–76.

15. **Kempf, B., and E. Bremer.** 1996. A novel amidohydrolase gene from *Bacillus subtilis* cloning: DNA-sequence analysis and map position of *amhX. FEMS Microbiol. Lett.* **141:**129–137.

16. **Korolik V., P. J. Coloe, and V. Krishnapillai.** 1988. A specific DNA probe for the identification of *Campylobacter jejuni. J. Gen. Microbiol.* **134:**521–529.

17. **Lapidus, A., N. Galleron, A. Sorokin, and S. D. Ehrlich.** 1997. Sequencing and functional annotation of the *Bacillus subtilis* genes in the 200 kb *rrnB-dnaB* region. *Microbiology* **143:**3431–3441.

18. **Lawrence, J. G., and H. Ochman.** 1998. Molecular archaeology of the *Escherichia coli* genome. *Proc. Natl. Acad. Sci. USA* **95:**9413–9417.

19. **Miyagawa, E., J. Yano, T. Hamakado, Y. Kido, K. Nishimoto, and Y. Motoki.** 1985. Crystallization and properties of *N*-benzoylglycine amidohydrolase from *Pseudomonas putida. Agric. Biol. Chem.* **49:**2881–2886.

20. **Miyagawa, E., T. Harada, and Y. Motoki.** 1986. Purification and properties of *N*-benzoyl-L-alanine amidohydrolase from *Corynebacterium equi. Agric. Biol. Chem.* **50:**1527–1531.

21. **Murao, S., E. Matsumura, T. Shin, and T. Kawano.** 1984. A new enzyme, *N*-alpha-benzoylcarbonyl moiety hydrolytic enzyme, from *Streptococcus faecalis* R. *Agric. Biol. Chem.* **48:**1673.

22. **Penner, J. L.** 1988. The genus *Campylobacter:* a decade of progress. *Clin. Microbiol. Rev.* **1:**157–172.

23. **Raffeisbauer, D., A. Bubert, F. Engelbrecht, J. Scheinpflug, A. Simm, J. Hess, S. H. E. Kaufmann and W. Goebel.** 1998. The gene cluster *inlC2DE* of *Listeria monocytogenes* contains additional new internalin genes and is important for virulence in mice. *Mol. Gen. Genet.* **260:**144–158.

24. **Sakanyan, V., L. Desmarez, C. Legrain, D. Charlier, I. Mett, A. Kochikyan, A. Savchenko, A. Boyen, P. Falmagne, A. Pierard, and N. Glansdorff.** 1993. Gene cloning, sequence analysis, purification, and characterization of a thermostable aminoacylase from *Bacillus stearothermophilus. Appl. Environ. Microbiol.* **59:**3878–3888.

25. **Skirrow, M. B.** 1994. Diseases due to *Campylobacter, Helicobacter* and related bacteria. *J. Comp. Pathol.* **111:**113–149.

26. **Steele, M., J. Odumeru, C. Gyles, and V. L. Chan.** 1999. Unpublished data.

27. **Steinhauserova, I., J. Smola, and H. Stegnerova.** 1997. Serotyping and PCR detection of *Campylobacter jejuni* strains isolated in the Czech Republic, abstr. B11. *In 9th International Workshop on Campylobacter, Helicobacter and Related Organisms.* Abstract B11.

28. **Stucki, U., J. Frey, J. Nicolet, and A. P. Burnens.** 1995. Identification of *Campylobacter jejuni* on the basis of a species-specific gene that encodes a membrane protein. *J. Clin. Microbiol.* **33:**855–859.

29. **Tinsley, C. R., and X. Nassif.** 1996. Analysis of the genetic differences between *Neisseria meningitidis* and *Neisseria gonorrhoeae:* two closely related bacteria expressing two different pathogenicities. *Proc. Natl. Acad. Sci. USA* **93:**11109–11114.

30. **Versalovic, J., T. Koeuth, J. R. Lupski.** 1991. Distribution of repetitive DNA sequences in eubacteria and application to fingerprinting of bacterial genomes. *Nucleic Acids Res.* **19:**6823–6831.

CAMPYLOBACTER AND FOOD SAFETY

CAMPYLOBACTER IN THE FOOD SUPPLY

Wilma Jacobs-Reitsma

24

Campylobacter infections in humans are considered to be mainly food-borne diseases, in which foods of animal origin play an important role. Beside the food-related cases, close contact with pet animals and activities in relation with recreational waters, as well as unknown factors, do contribute to the large number of human illnesses due to *Campylobacter* each year.

Large community outbreaks are relatively rare in *Campylobacter* epidemiology, but the implicated sources are both epidemiologically and microbiologically identified to be raw milk and untreated surface water. The majority of *Campylobacter* infections are sporadic (single) cases or small family outbreaks, and the actual source of these types of infection is rarely microbiologically identified. Finding microbiological proof by culturing (the same types of) campylobacters from suspected sources as well as from the patients is not easy. Often, the original suspected food item was consumed as a whole, or leftovers are no longer available by the time of the illness. Moreover, after prolonged storage, it may be difficult to recover any campylobacters from the possibly implicated food items.

Epidemiological (case-control) studies have revealed a significant association between *Campylobacter* infection in humans and handling and eating raw or undercooked poultry. However, the extent to which poultry consumption is responsible for human campylobacteriosis is not exactly known. Nonetheless, poultry and poultry products have the doubtful honor of being considered the major cause of human *Campylobacter* infections, and therefore a lot of *Campylobacter* research has been poultry related. Indeed, large percentages of fresh and even frozen poultry products can be found to be contaminated with *Campylobacter*. Levels of contamination may vary between $\log_{10} 2$ and $\log_{10} 5$ CFU per carcass. In combination with the relatively low infectious dose of 500 CFU reported for *Campylobacter*, poultry products may pose a serious risk for consumers if unhygienically handled during preparation or insufficiently cooked. Besides poultry, other foods (mainly of animal origin) must be considered as potential sources of infection, because *Campylobacter* also has been isolated from food items such as raw milk, pork, beef, lamb, and seafood.

This chapter describes the detection and prevalence of *Campylobacter* in a wide range of different types of food. Possible strategies for minimizing the risks for human disease due to

Wilma Jacobs-Reitsma, ID-Lelystad Institute for Animal Science and Health, P.O. Box 65, 8200 AB Lelystad, The Netherlands.

Campylobacter, 2nd Ed., Edited by I. Nachamkin and M. J. Blaser
© 2000 American Society for Microbiology, Washington, D.C.

this pathogen will be discussed. Because food-borne campylobacteriosis is due mainly to the thermotolerant *Campylobacter* species (*C. jejuni, C. coli,* and, to a lesser extent, *C. lari*), this chapter focuses on these species.

DETECTION OF *CAMPYLOBACTER* IN FOODS

An extensive and detailed description of the developments in *Campylobacter* detection and the variety of existing media is given by Corry et al. (11). The media that are used for isolation of *Campylobacter* from food or water are derived from the media originally designed for detection of campylobacters from human stool samples. Fecal samples often contain large numbers of viable campylobacters, and detection is possible by direct plating on selective media. Food products, however, may harbor only small numbers of campylobacters, and the bacterial cells may be seriously injured by processing procedures such as freezing, cooling, heating, and salting. Therefore, liquid enrichment media have been developed to detect small numbers of *Campylobacter* cells and to promote the recovery of sublethally damaged cells. *Campylobacter* cells from the enrichment media are isolated on solid selective agars, often with comparable ingredients to the liquid medium. A variety of selective agents in different combinations as well as concentrations are incorporated into the various media for *Campylobacter,* with cefoperazone, cycloheximide, trimethoprim, and vancomycin often used. Several enrichment procedures delay the exposure to (some) selective agents until cell repair has occurred, in combination with the use of lower incubation temperatures during the first stages of enrichment. Incubation generally is carried out at 42°C, a temperature at which the thermotolerant campylobacters are able to grow well and which provides an enhanced selectivity. Sterile sheep or horse blood or charcoal is added to the media to neutralize the toxic effects of oxygen and light. Due to the microaerophilic nature of *Campylobacter,* it is necessary to incubate the samples in an oxygen-reduced atmosphere, most commonly in jars or in adapted CO_2 incubators. Several methods are available to achieve the optimal gas mixture of 5 to 7% oxygen, 10% carbon dioxide, and 80% nitrogen and/or hydrogen in the isolation of *Campylobacter;* these include replacement of the entire atmosphere by the appropriate bottled gas mixture, replacement of two-thirds of the atmosphere with a mixture of either nitrogen or hydrogen plus 5 to 15% carbon dioxide, and use of an appropriate gas-generating envelope or even candle jars (11, 69).

The 8th edition of the *FDA Bacteriological Analytical Manual* (35) gives a detailed description of the isolation of *Campylobacter* from food and water. In general, 25 g of food is combined with 100 ml of enrichment broth, but different sample preparations are described for various types of food. Whole chicken carcasses are rinsed with peptone water, the liquid is centrifuged, and the resuspended pellet is placed in enrichment broth. Water samples of preferably 2 to 4 liters are filtered, and the 0.45-μ-m-pore-size filters are enriched. For raw milk, immediately after sampling, the milk is adjusted to a pH of >7.6 with sterile NaOH to inactivate the lactoperoxidase system, which is toxic to *Campylobacter.* Preenrichment is carried out just for 3 h at 30°C followed by 2 h at 37°C (frozen samples, water, and shellfish) or just for 4 h at 37°C (all other cases). Finally, for both enrichment procedures, incubation is continued at 42°C for 20 to 42 h. The combination of Hunt enrichment broth base with lysed horse blood, FBP (ferrous sulfate, sodium metabisulfite, sodium pyruvate) growth supplement, and the selective agents vancomycin, trimethoprim lactate, cycloheximide, and cefoperazone is used for (selective) enrichment. For dairy products, rifampin is also added. The final cefoperazone concentration is reached when a second dose is added after the 3- or 4-h preenrichment step. Plating, either of direct counts or after enrichment, is done on both mCCDA (modified charcoal cefoperazone desoxycholate agar with additional yeast extract) and Abeyta-Hunt agar for 24 to 48 h at 42°C. Abeyta-Hunt agar contains sterile horse blood, whereas mCCDA is charcoal based. All incubations are carried out under microaerobic conditions, and details are given for the recommended shaking of enrichment in combination with a bubbler system for continuous gas flow. Identification is performed by microscopy and a number of biochemical tests, including a latex agglutination (35). The International Organization of Standardization prepared an International Standard describing a horizontal method for detection of thermotolerant *Campylobacter* in food and animal feed stuffs (37). This method also uses enrichment, either in Preston broth at 42°C for 18 h or in Park and Sanders broth. The latter is recommended for frozen samples or samples that otherwise may contain suble thally damaged cells, and the method includes a preenrichment incubation for 4 h at 32°C followed by 2 h at 37°C and finally 40 to 42 h at 42°C. Antibiotics are added at the start of the 37°C step. The sample is plated on the charcoal-based Karmali agar and on a second solid selective medium, which can be either modified Butzler (Virion) agar, Skirrow agar, CCDA, or Preston agar. All incubations are performed in a static microaerobic atmosphere. Sampling specifications are not part of this standard, but a 1 : 10 ratio for test portion to enrichment broth is given as a general rule (37). All the above mentioned methods are intended for isolation of thermotolerant campylobacters. However, some of these "thermotolerant" organisms are reported to be missed occasionally due to the antibiotics used in the selective media in combination with the elevated incubation temperature of 42°C. Membrane filtration followed by plating on nonselective (blood) media at 37°C is required to detect these and the other more sensitive members of the *Campylobacter* "family" (11).

FOODS CONTAMINATED BY *CAMPYLOBACTER*
Poultry Meat and Eggs

Live poultry, including broilers, laying hens, turkeys, and ducks, are often found to be colonized by large numbers of *Campylobacter* organisms without showing any signs of clinical illness. Colonization levels in the small intestine and especially the ceca range from 10^5 to $>10^9$ CFU/g (5, 51). Colonized birds enter the slaughterhouse with large numbers of *Campylobacter* organisms on their feathers and skin and, predominantly, in their intestinal tracts; consequently, campylobacters can be found throughout the slaughtering process. This also leads to contamination of equipment, working surfaces, process water, and air. The large amounts of water used during poultry processing contribute to the spread and survival of *Campylobacter* and complicate the in-plant control. (5, 54). Scalding of the birds, necessary to facilitate defeathering, is usually performed at a water temperature between 50 to 60°C for several minutes. At higher temperatures, a greater thermal reduction of *Campylobacter* numbers may occur, but the higher scalding temperature also affects the skin surface in a way that contaminating bacteria attach more firmly to the skin. During defeathering and evisceration, leakage of intestinal contents almost inevitably contributes to the contamination of carcasses. The next steps of washing and chilling tend to reduce the counts again but do not eliminate the contamination completely. Air chilling has been suggested to be more effective than water chilling because of the drying effects, but the structure of poultry skin, unlike pig skin, makes it much more difficult to dry completely, even after prolonged chilling (12, 56).

Overall, the slaughtering process may reduce the level of contamination about 1,000-fold. Mead et al. (51) found that during processing of broiler flocks colonized with $\log_{10}$ 6.8 CFU *Campylobacter* per g of cecal content, there was a reduction in the numbers of *Campylobacter* organisms on neck skin samples from $\log_{10}$ 3.7 after exsanguination to $\log_{10}$ 1.8 after packaging. The distribution and numbers of *Campylobacter* in 100 freshly slaughtered chickens originating from six different *Campylobacter*-positive flocks, was studied by Berndtson et al. (5). The cecal contents of the birds harbored $\log_{10}$ 5.8 to $>\log_{10}$ 9 CFU *Campylobacter* organisms per g. During processing, *Campylobacter* was isolated from 89% of neck skin samples, 93% of peritoneal cavity swab samples, and 75% of subcutaneous samples. The incidence in 340 muscle samples was very low, at 3%. *Campylobacter* numbers in neck skin and peritoneal cavities ranged from $\log_{10}$ 2.4 to $\log_{10}$ 3.4 CFU/g or CFU/4 cm^2, whereas numbers in the subcutaneous layer were only $\log_{10}$ 1.1 to $\log_{10}$ 1.8 CFU/4 cm^2 (5).

The reported levels of *Campylobacter* organisms in fresh poultry products vary between $\log_{10}$ 2 and $\log_{10}$ 5 CFU per carcass or $\log_{10}$ 1 to $\log_{10}$ 6 CFU/100 g of meat, depending on the different studies and the method used (5, 12). Freezing of the products diminishes the level of contamination, but survival at $-20°C$ for at least 3 months, although at a very low level, has been demonstrated (53). Campylobacters are also frequently found on edible offal, such as hearts and livers; this is more likely

to be caused by cross-contamination during processing rather than by infection of the tissue itself (9).

Table 1 summarizes the prevalence of *Campylobacter* in poultry products as reported in various studies over the past 10 years. Earlier studies (1977 to 1986) are summarized by Aho and Hirn (2) and Bryan and Doyle (9). A direct correlation of the various studies may be difficult because of the wide variety of methods that are used. Also, the differences in sampling procedures may account for the difference in isolation percentages. Examination of poultry may include 25 g of meat without skin, an area of skin (either the skin itself or swabs of the skin surface), thaw or drip water, or whole carcass rinses with shaking or massage. All studies summarized in Table 1 included some kind of enrichment procedure in their detection meth-

TABLE 1 Presence of thermotolerant *Campylobacter* in poultry products

Product	Stage of process	Sample type	No.[a]	% of positive samples	Country	Yr	Reference
Chicken carcasses	Before chilling	Swabs	203	80	USA	1990	45
Chicken carcasses	After chilling	Carcass rinse	50	52	USA	1991	40
Chicken carcasses	After chilling	Carcass rinse	80	86	USA	1995	71
Chicken breasts	After processing	Meat (10 g)	156	68	Japan	1991	73
Chicken breasts	At retail	Meat (25 g)	32	38	Italy	1996	78
Chicken breasts	At retail	Swabs	630	19	Germany	1996	27
Chicken breasts	At retail	Swabs	616	58	France	1996	27
Chicken breasts	At retail	Swabs	607	23	The Netherlands	1996	27
Chicken breasts	At retail	Meat (25 g)	2,016	28	Germany	1998	3
Chicken meat	At retail	Not specified	676	33	Denmark	1997	30
Chicken wings	At retail	Whole wings	153	65	N. Ireland	1994	25
Chicken carcasses	At retail	Carcass rinse	98	32	USA	1991	40
Chicken carcasses	At retail	Carcass rinse	50	98	USA	1992	70
Chicken carcasses	At retail	Carcass rinse	330	69	USA	1997	76
Chicken products	At retail	Meat (25 g)	279	61	The Netherlands	1990	14
Chicken products	At retail	Meat (25 g)	1,165	37	The Netherlands	1997	15
Chicken products	At retail	Meat (10 g)	120	38	N. Ireland	1998	48
Chicken carcasses	At retail, frozen	Carcass rinse	199	14	Finland	1989	2
Chicken livers	At retail, frozen	Exuded liquid	126	93	Chile	1996	23
Chicken carcasses	After storage[b]	Carcass rinse	80	28	USA	1995	71
Turkey carcasses	Before chilling	Swabs	236	3	USA	1990	45
Turkey breasts	At retail	Meat (25 g)	30	20	Italy	1996	78
Turkey meat	At retail	Not specified	311	25	Denmark	1997	30
Duck carcasses	Before chilling	Swabs	200	48	USA	1990	45
Goose carcasses	Before chilling	Swabs	200	38	USA	1990	45
Poultry	At retail	Meat (25 g)	758	56	UK	1989	26
Poultry[c] meat	At retail	Not specified	285	26	Denmark	1997	30

[a] Total number of samples examined.
[b] Storage at 4°C for 10 days.
[c] Ducks, pigeons, quails, and ostriches.

ods. Other avian species, such as gulls and pigeons (10, 42) as well as cockatiels, emus, ostriches, and parrots (58), harbor *Campylobacter* as a commensal. This may have implications when they are used for human consumption, but the risk of contracting a *Campylobacter* infection from these potential sources is probably higher via direct contact, since they are not eaten very often.

In general, commercial table eggs are not very likely to be associated with *Campylobacter* infections. Only one suggested case was reported by Finch and Blake (24); in this case, 26 of 81 individuals developed campylobacteriosis after consumption of undercooked eggs. Eggs presumed to be the cause of that outbreak were not available for examination. However, hens on the farm which supplied the eggs yielded a number of *Campylobacter* serotypes, one of which was identical to the isolate derived from a single patient. Like broilers, laying hens often excrete *Campylobacter* in large numbers, which may lead to externally contaminated eggs. Doyle (18) found that 2 of 226 eggshells from a flock of *Campylobacter*-excreting laying hens were contaminated with *Campylobacter*. One of the two eggs had a dirty shell. Jacobs–Reitsma (39) isolated *Campylobacter* from 3 of 179 shells of fecally contaminated eggs (not consumer quality). Survival of *Campylobacter* on eggshells, however, is considered to be poor because of the sensitivity of the organism to drying. Studies of artificially contaminated eggshells showed that *Campylobacter* could not be detected after storage at room temperature for 48 h (18, 64). Egg penetration studies revealed that *Campylobacter* organisms did not penetrate into the contents of eggs held at either 25, 37, or 4°C after artificial contamination. They were occasionally isolated for a short time from the inner shell and membranes of the refrigerated eggs (18). At room temperature, *Campylobacter* was recovered from 3 of 70 shell membranes and 1 of 70 egg contents but only for a short time (2 h) after artificial contamination (64). No *Campylobacter* organisms were isolated from 219 egg yolks (39) or 216 egg contents examined within 12 h of being laid (18). Izat

and Gardner (38) conducted five trials in two commercial egg-processing plants and detected no *Campylobacter* in the raw eggs or in any of the various processed egg products. So far, the case described by Finch and Blake (25) is the only egg-associated *Campylobacter* case, and commercial table eggs remain an uncommon source of infection.

Milk and Dairy Products

Unpasteurized milk is a well-documented cause of a number of outbreaks of campylobacteriosis (7, 24). The first documented milkborne outbreak associated with a *Campylobacter*-like organism occurred back in 1938 (7). A very large outbreak took place in 1979 in the United Kingdom, where over 2,500 children became infected by school milk (41).

Campylobacter can be isolated from the feces of healthy dairy cows, as well as from raw milk. Doyle and Roman (17) found that 50 (64%) of 78 milk-producing cows on nine farms excreted *Campylobacter* in their feces but isolated the organism from only 1 (0.9%) of 108 bulk tank milk samples from these farms. Beumer et al. (6) isolated *Campylobacter* from 22% of 904 fecal samples and 4.5% of the individual milk samples from 904 healthy dairy cows on 13 Dutch farms. Of 12 English dairy herds (examined by collection of a total of 668 rectal swab samples, 10 were *Campylobacter* positive, with a herd incidence of 10 to 72% of cows tested. No *Campylobacter* was detected in 30 bulk milk tanks of the two negative herds, but the organism was isolated from 9 (8%) of 111 samples from five farms with cows positive for *C. jejuni*. The mean level of contamination was a most-probable number (MPN) of 16 ± 30 organisms per 100 ml of milk (range, 1 to 100 CFU/100 ml) (33). Raw milk was considered to have become contaminated from feces. However, direct contamination of the milk as a consequence of udder infection by *Campylobacter* has also been described (36, 57). As well as raw cows' milk, unpasteurized goats' milk may transmit *Campylobacter* infection from the animals to humans (31).

TABLE 2 Presence of thermotolerant *Campylobacter* in raw milk

Product	Description	No.[a]	% of positive samples	Country	Yr	Reference
Raw cows' milk	Bulk tanks at 15 sites	237	0.4	USA	1987	50
Raw cows' milk	292 farm bulk tanks	292	12.3	USA	1992	63
Raw cows' milk	48 farm bulk tanks	48	0	Poland	1996	28
Raw cows' milk	27 farm bulk tanks	69	1.4	France	1997	16
Raw cows' milk	1,720 farm bulk tanks	1,720	0.5	Canada	1997	68
Raw cows' milk	12 farm bulk tanks	153	5.9	UK	1988	34
Raw cows' milk	Dairy bulk tank	130	1.5	Poland	1996	28
Raw cows' milk	Dairy milk supply	71	0	New Zealand	1987	72
Raw cows' milk	At retail	985	5.9	UK	1988	34
Raw goats' milk	Various sources	2,477	0.04	UK	1985	61
Raw goats' milk	Individual samples	1,078	0	Germany	1992	29
Raw goats' milk	Bulk tank samples	69	0	Germany	1992	29
Raw ewes' milk	Individual samples	1,391	0	Germany	1992	29
Raw ewes' milk	Bulk tank samples	56	0	Germany	1992	29

[a] Total number of samples examined.

Table 2 summarizes some larger studies on the presence of *Campylobacter* in raw milk. Differences in isolation percentages can be attributed to some extent to the different sampling procedures and the variety of isolation methods used. Fresh raw milk benefits from the availability of the lactoperoxidase system, which is toxic to *Campylobacter* (6). This system can be neutralized by addition of NaOH to the milk directly after sampling, and this leads to a higher percentage of isolation of *Campylobacter* from the milk (6, 35). It was not always specified whether such a neutralization procedure was used during the studies summarized in Table 2. Although *Campylobacter* can be detected in a low percentage of raw-milk samples, the actual numbers of campylobacters present are generally small (but are sufficient to cause disease). The common pasteurization process is sufficient to eliminate this risk. Several milk-related outbreaks in which the pasteurization process was inadequate have been described (7, 22). From the United Kingdom, outbreaks due to properly heat-treated milk, which became recontaminated presumably because of birds pecking at the foil tops of bottles delivered at the doorsteps of homes, were reported (32). The sensitivity of *Campylobacter* to low water activity suggests that the organism should not cause problems in foods with high solute concentrations such as cheese. In combination with its sensitivity to acid, *Campylobacter* is not very likely to survive in cheese or during production and ripening. Bachmann and Spahr (4) examined the ability of potentially pathogenic bacteria to grow and to survive during the manufacture and ripening of Swiss hard and semihard cheeses made from raw milk, inoculated with $\log_{10} 4$ to $\log_{10} 6$ CFU/ml. At the age of commercial ripeness (90 days), both the hard and the semihard cheeses were free of *Campylobacter* (4). Fermented milk products such as yogurt are not suspected sources of infection, also because of the low pH and the sensitivity of the organisms to organic acids like lactic acid (12).

In general, milk-borne infection can be adequately controlled by proper pasteurization and prevention of recontamination after the heat treatment.

Red Meat

Like dairy cows, meat-producing cattle may excrete *C. jejuni* in their feces, and this occurs with a higher incidence in summer than in winter (7). A carriage rate as high as 89% in samples of 360 cattle during 1 year was reported by Stanley et al. (67). Numbers of thermotolerant *Campylobacter* organisms were about $\log_{10}$ 2 MPN per g of fresh feces (67) and this is much lower than the $\log_{10}$ 6 to 9 commonly found in poultry feces (5). Also, swine are frequently found to harbor campylobacters, but in this animal reservoir, *C. coli* is isolated significantly more often than *C. jejuni* (26, 49). The number of organisms in the intestines are more comparable to the numbers in cattle than to the numbers in poultry (56).

Lambs at slaughter were found to carry thermotolerant *Campylobacter* in 91.7% of 360 samples of the small intestine, which appears to be the most important area colonized in these animals. The numbers average $\log_{10}$ 4.0 MPN per g of fresh intestinal content (66). The level of *Campylobacter* carriage in sheep and the presence of the bacterium on sheep meat at slaughter, however, are reported to be low (66). The slaughtering processes of cattle, swine, and sheep can lead to contamination of the meat with intestinal flora during manual evisceration, but this may occur less frequently than during poultry slaughtering, where the evisceration process often is mechanical and proceeds at a very high turnover rate. Lammerding et al. (46) isolated high percentages of *Campylobacter* from cattle, sheep, and pigs just after slaughter and before chilling. Overnight forced-air chilling of the carcasses is supposed to cause a significant reduction in the numbers of *Campylobacter* organisms on the carcasses (56, 69).

Table 3 summarizes the results of several large and recent studies on the presence of *Campylobacter* in various types of meat, excluding poultry. Early studies are summarized by Blaser (7). As stated for the results on poultry products (Table 1), these data should be interpreted with care due to the variety of method used. Numbers of *Campylobacter* on both pork and beef are reported to be small. These contamination levels, at about the detection limit of the method used, may contribute significantly to the differences in isolation rates in the various studies. It was mentioned that uncooked sausages may be contaminated with *Campylobacter* as a result of using fresh, unsalted swine intestine for sausage casing (54). Suffi-

cient heating of red-meat products, relatively infrequently contaminated with small numbers of *Campylobacter,* will eliminate this risk of human infection. Cooked-meat products (Table 3) are infrequently contaminated with *Campylobacter,* and the incidental cases were suspected of being caused by cross-contamination from raw-meat products.

Water and Seafood

Contaminated surface water is recognized as a source of *Campylobacter* outbreaks in humans and may also play a role in contamination of farm animals. The organism could also be isolated from various other water environments such as streams, seawater, and other recreational waters. These waters are not intended for human consumption, but accidental ingestion of a significant amount of water from these sources may pose a risk. Community water systems, sometimes chlorinated, are regarded as being free of *Campylobacter,* as long as safety procedures are maintained and mixing with potentially contaminated water sources is avoided. *Campylobacter* contamination of surface water is likely to originate from fecal contamination by wild birds or domestic animals or from sewage effluent (7, 43, 53).

As a consequence of the transient existence of *Campylobacter* in the marine environment, shellfish may become contaminated by the organism. Consumption of raw clams as well as raw Pacific oysters has been described as a cause of human *Campylobacter* infections (1). Several investigations on the detection of *Campylobacter* in different types of seafood have been carried out. The relatively high isolation percentages of *C. lari* in these products implicate gulls, which are often colonized with this *Campylobacter* species, as the primary source of contamination. In a Dutch study (21), *Campylobacter* was isolated from 41 (69%) of 59 batches of mussels and from 11 (27%) of 41 batches of oysters. High percentages of mussels from Germany, Denmark, and England and oysters from Northern Ireland were also culture positive for *Campylobacter* (65 and 25%, respectively). Further identification of 39 strains isolated from

TABLE 3 Presence of thermotolerant *Campylobacter* in meat products, excluding poultry

Product	Stage of process	No.[a]	% of positive samples	Country	Yr	Reference
Beef carcasses	Before chilling	114	0.9	USA	1990	45
Beef carcasses	After chilling	62	10	Belgium	1998	44
Beef carcasses	After overnight chilling	657	0.3	Australia	1998	74
Beef	After processing	52	0	Japan	1990	73
Beef	After processing	100	0	N. Ireland	1998	48
Beef meat	At retail	127	23.6	UK	1989	26
Beef meat	At retail	516	0.7	Denmark	1997	30
Beef meat	At retail	50	0	N. Ireland	1998	48
Pork diaphragm muscles	Before chilling	200	23.5	Canada	1989	49
Pork carcasses	Before chilling	105	2.9	USA	1990	45
Pork carcasses	After chilling	49[b]	2	Belgium	1998	44
Pork	After processing	94	2	Japan	1990	73
Pork	At retail	158	18.4	UK	1989	26
Pork loins	At retail	27	3.7	Italy	1996	78
Pork meat	At retail	433	1	Denmark	1997	30
Pork meat	At retail	50	0	N. Ireland	1998	48
Pig livers	At slaughter	400	6	N. Ireland	1998	52
Pork sausages	At retail	42	2.4	Italy	1996	78
Minced pork	At retail	104	1	The Netherlands	1990	14
Lamb	After processing	100	0	N. Ireland	1998	48
Lamb	After processing	30	0	Spain	1995	65
Lamb	At retail	103	15.5	UK	1989	26
Sheep	After chilling	465	3	Australia	1999	75
Offal[c]	At retail	689	47	UK	1989	26
Raw meat products[d]	At retail	2,330	0.6	UK	1998	47
Cooked meats	At retail	86	2.3	UK	1989	26
Cooked meats[e]	At retail	2,192	0	UK	1998	47

[a] Total number of samples examined.
[b] Each sample was a composite of gauze swab samplings of 5 half carcasses
[c] Liver, kidney, and heart from pigs, cows, or sheep.
[d] Sausages, hamburgers.
[e] Pies, sliced cooked meat, etc.

24 Dutch mussels batches revealed that all but 2 isolates were *C. lari* (21). A Danish survey of *Campylobacter* in foods from retail outlets (30) did not detect *Campylobacter* (<1 CFU/25 g) in any of 146 shellfish samples. In a British study in 1994 (77), 47% of 331 cockles, mussels, and scallops examined shortly after harvesting were found to contain *Campylobacter*. Of 49 samples of depurated and ready-to-eat oysters, 3 (6%) contained *Campylobacter*. Most isolations were during the cooler months of the year (November to March). The greatest percentage of strains (57%) were urease-positive thermophilic campylobacters, atypical strains which were described as not closely as-sociated with domestic or farm animals or humans. *C. lari* accounted for 24% of the isolated strains (77).

Campylobacter was also isolated from 50 (21%) of 240 samples of fresh hand-picked crab meat from 12 different blue-crab processing facilities in the United States (60). Quantitative levels in all cases were below the detection limit of 0.30 MPN/g. Based on the ability of *C. jejuni* to hydrolyze hippurate and on the failure of *C. coli* to produce H_2S on triple-sugar iron agar, the isolates were determined to be composed of 36 *C. jejuni* and 14 *C. coli* strains (60). Shellfish beds located near potential contamination sources such as sewage effluents, farmland runoffs, and waterfowl reservoirs were reported to present a particular health risk to persons consuming raw oysters (1). Moreover, depuration of oysters was shown to be not fully effective in eliminating potential bacterial pathogens such as *Campylobacter*. This indicates that some thermal processing of shellfish is generally advisable (77).

Other Foods

Relatively few studies are carried out on the presence or absence of *Campylobacter* in vegetable food types, although theoretically these products occasionally become contaminated by the application of natural fertilizers, by wild birds and animals, or by contaminated surface water.

In a large survey in Canada (59), a total of 1,564 fresh samples of 10 vegetable types from farmers' outdoor markets and supermarkets were examined for the presence of thermotolerant campylobacters. No *Campylobacter* was detected in the 1,031 samples from supermarkets. The detection rates in samples from the outdoor markets as follows: spinach, 3.3%; lettuce, 3.1%; radish, 2.7%; green onion, 2.5%; parsley, 2.4%; and potato, 1.6%. No *Campylobacter* was detected in celery, carrot, cabbage, or cucumber. *Campylobacter* was also detected in 14 (2.9%) of another 482 outdoor-market samples, but all these samples became negative for *Campylobacter* after being thoroughly washed with chlorinated water (59). Another Canadian study (55) detected no *Campylobacter* in any of 65 unprocessed or 296 fresh-cut and packaged ready-to-use vegetables such as lettuce, carrot, cauliflower, celery, broccoli, or sliced green peppers. During a nationwide survey on *Campylobacter* in food from retail outlets in Denmark in 1997 (30), no *Campylobacter* was detected in 123 vegetable or 103 fruit samples. *Campylobacter* could not be isolated from 106 samples of prepared salads at the retail level in the British study by Fricker and Park (26).

A study by the Seattle-King County Health Department revealed an elevated relative risk of developing campylobacteriosis in individuals who consume mushrooms (reported in refer-

ence 20). This study provided the impetus for Doyle and Schoeni (20) to examine retail mushrooms for the presence of *Campylobacter*. *C. jejuni* was isolated from 3 (1.5%) of 200 25-g samples from wrapped packages of fresh mushrooms obtained from local grocery stores. The 3 positive samples were packaged by the same mushroom producer, but it is unknown how the mushrooms became contaminated. The composted manure, used as the growth substrate for these mushrooms, had been heated to 60°C for 2 h and therefore was not considered a likely source of contamination (20). Several reported outbreaks of campylobacteriosis attributed to rare sources such as lettuce or tuna salad (62) are suggested to be in fact a result of cross-contamination during preparation, so that the food serves as a vehicle rather than being the original source of infection.

Besides the described reservoir of *Campylobacter* in animals for food production, wild animals, some of which may be consumed by humans, are frequent sources of *Campylobacter*. These include waterfowl, hares, wild boars, pheasants, guinea fowl, mallards, quails, and pigeons (13, 30).

SURVIVAL OF *CAMPYLOBACTER* ON FOODS

The optimum growth temperature of the thermotolerant campylobacters lies between 37 and 42°C, very close to the body temperature of the chicken (about 41°C). The thermotolerant campylobacters are not able to grow below 30°C, and so actual multiplication during handling or storage at room temperature in the kitchen will not readily occur in moderate climates. Especially during storage at room temperature, campylobacters are very sensitive to drying. In general, survival of *Campylobacter* is better at cooling temperatures than at room temperature. Nevertheless, refrigerated storage reduces the level of contamination. In a study by Stern, levels of *Campylobacter* on fresh broiler carcasses as high as $\log_{10} 5.8$ were in some cases reduced to nondetectable levels after storage for 10 days at 4°C (71).

Although freezing substantially reduces the numbers of *Campylobacter* cells, survival at -20°C is possible and *Campylobacter* could still be recovered at very low levels from frozen chicken drumsticks after 3 months of storage. Isolation rates for *Campylobacter* from frozen meat and poultry products were reported to be five fold lower than from the corresponding fresh products (53, 69). Fernandez and Pison (23) isolated *Campylobacter* from a large number of frozen chicken liver samples and identified 22% of the isolates as *C. jejuni* and 78% as *C. coli*. They suggested that *C. coli* survives better under frozen storage (and possibly also under other environmental circumstances) than *C. jejuni* (23).

Campylobacters are sensitive to heat and are inactivated by the pasteurization treatments used in practice. D-values (decimal reduction values) reported for the organism in skim milk at 48°C ranged from 7.2 to 12.8 min and at 55°C from 0.74 to 1.0 min. High-temperature short-time pasteurization for 80 s at 60°C also rapidly killed levels of $\log_{10}$ 6 CFU/ml inoculated in raw milk. D-values in meat ranged from 5.9 to 6.3 min for heating at 50°C and less than 1 min for heating at 60°C. D-values for *C. jejuni* in ground chicken heated at 49 or 57°C were about 20 min and 45 s, respectively. Meatballs of ground beef, inoculated with more than $\log_{10}$ 6 *Campylobacter* organisms per g, were cooked to an internal temperature of 60°C, and *Campylobacter* numbers were reduced to nondetectable levels within 10 min (53, 69).

The optimal concentration for growth of *Campylobacter* is 0.5%, but the organism is sensitive to higher concentrations of NaCl. The extent of sensitivity depends on both the temperature and the (food) medium. Certain spices, such as oregano, sage, and cloves, were reported to inhibit the growth of *Campylobacter* at 42°C in a 0.5% broth (69).

Properly chlorinated drinking water can be regarded as free of *Campylobacter*. Chlorination of the scalding or chilling water during processing of poultry carcasses is allowed in several countries, but the effects are reported to be minimal, most probably due to neutralization by organic matter in the chilling tank, and the campylobacters being protected by attachment to the skin. In an attempt to reduce the contamination of carcasses with *Campylobacter* during processing, Mead et al. (51) used chlorinated-water sprays on equipment and working surfaces, increased the chlorine concentrations in processing water, and removed any unnecessary carcass contact surface. These changes significantly reduced the levels of carcass contamination, but in practice the reduction was considered to be have little impact on consumer exposure to *Campylobacter* infection (51). Ascorbic acid at 0.05% inhibits the growth of *Campylobacter*, and a concentration of 0.09% is bactericidal (53). Lactic acid and acetic acid sprays or dips were evaluated for application during the slaughtering process, and *Campylobacter* contamination levels were found to be reduced (8, 69). Modified atmospheres or vacuum packaging have little effect on the survival of the microaerophilic campylobacters. When stored at 4°C, campylobacters survived just as well on beef or chicken packaged with oxygen-permeable wrap as under various modified atmospheres or vacuum (53, 69).

Campylobacter is quite sensitive to gamma irradiation, with a D-value of 32 kilorads. It was reported that *C. jejuni* in culture medium and in chicken paste survived an irradiation dose of 0.2 kG but not a dose of 1 kG. *Campylobacter* is also more sensitive to UV irradiation at 254 nm than is, e.g., *Escherichia coli* (53). Various disinfecting agents effectively inactivate *Campylobacter*. Phenolic compounds, iodophors, quaternary ammonium compounds, 70% ethyl alcohol, and glutaraldehyde in commonly applied concentrations were able to inactivate about $\log_{10}$ 7 CFU of *Campylobacter*/ml within 1 minute. Sodium hypochlorite at 1.25 ppm destroyed $\log_{10}$ 4 CFU/ml within 1 min, and 5 ppm killed $\log_{10}$ 7 CFU/ml within 15 min (69). The majority of studies on the growth characteristics and survival of *Campylobacter* were carried out during the early 1980s, and reviews can be found in papers by Doyle (19) and Stern and Kazmi (69). The overall results indicate that, depending on the *Campylobacter* strain, the initial number of cells, the type of food, and other environmental conditions, in particular the storage temperature, campylobacters may survive in food products for long periods (19).

PREVENTION OF FOOD-BORNE TRANSMISSION OF HUMAN CAMPYLOBACTERIOSIS

Since poultry products are believed to account for the majority of *Campylobacter* infections in humans, reduction of the *Campylobacter* contamination of these products is considered to have the greatest impact on this human health problem. Reduction of the potential risk of contaminated poultry products must be achieved by application of Good Hygienic Practices (GHP) by both the producers and the consumers of poultry meat products. The consumers need professional education programs, starting at elementary school levels, in combination with adequate information on proper handling of foods at risk. Product labeling sometimes is used to provide consumers with useful handling and preparation instructions. The National Advisory Committee on Microbiological Criteria for Foods (53) provides a fact sheet with essential basic information about *Campylobacter* for retail food, food service, and regulatory agency personnel, as well as a fact sheet for consumers about food-borne illness caused by *Campylobacter* bacteria.

The production of poultry meat products requires the application of Hazard Analysis Critical Control Points (HACCP) principles during all steps of production, processing, and distribution (53, 54). As described by the National Advisory Committee on Microbiological Criteria for Foods (54), the overall objective of the HACCP program is to ensure that production and processing is conducted to enhance the microbiological safety of the product. This is achieved through effective management of key operations that realistically prevent or control the introduction or growth of pathogens.

Total prevention of *Campylobacter* colonization of live broiler flocks at the farm level and hence delivery of *Campylobacter*-free material to the slaughterhouse would be the most certain way to reduce the level of contaminated poultry products. However, it appears to be complicated to achieve this in practice. The (im)possibilities of intervention strategies at the farm level are discussed in more detail by Newell and Wagenaar in chapter 26.

Improvements of processing procedures at the slaughterhouse level and decontamination treatment of end products might also be considered. Several procedures are suggested to minimize *Campylobacter* contamination during poultry processing. These include counterflow water systems during scalding and chilling, rinsing and washing of equipment to minimize or reduce cross-contamination, and disinfection of carcasses and related contact surfaces with chlorine or other bacterial control treatments such as trisodium phosphate or lactic acid (8, 53, 54). In addition, "logistical" slaughter of known *Campylobacter*-free flocks in the morning, followed by the positive flocks at the end of the day, may further reduce the risk of cross-contaminated end products. To be applicable in practice logistical slaughter requires a very accurate and punctual surveillance system for all broiler flocks and a relatively low percentage of *Campylobacter*-infected flocks. In the United States and several other countries, irradiation of the packaged fresh or frozen poultry products at 1.5 to 3.0 kGray may be applied as an effective treatment to eliminate *Campylobacter* from the end product (8, 53).

Other recognized food-related sources of human campylobacteriosis, in particular raw milk and contaminated water, can be avoided relatively easily by refraining from drinking any raw milk, by consuming only properly heat-treated milk, and by drinking water only from approved sources. These suggestions are made under the realistic assumption that treatment procedures in milk and drinking-water production are properly controlled and that re-contamination is avoided.

CONCLUSIONS

Campylobacter bacteria are widespread in warm-blooded animals used for food production, and the food products may easily become contaminated during processing. Also, different types of seafood can be contaminated with this human pathogen. Campylobacters may survive in food products for long periods, depending on the initial number and type of cells, the specific food product, and environmental conditions such as the storage temperature. Only a small number of campylobacters ingested via (cross-) contaminated food may lead to infection and disease in humans.

The risk of consuming raw foods of animal origin in relation to human campylobacteriosis is evident. This risk can be avoided by only consuming pasteurized milk; thoroughly heated red meat, poultry, and seafood; and water from approved sources. In addition, good food handling practices in the home and in food services will reduce the risk of illness.

REFERENCES

1. **Abeyta, C., F. G. Deeter, C. A. Kaysner, R. F. Stott, and M. M. Wekell.** 1993. *Campylobacter jejuni* in a Washington State shellfish growing bed associated with illness. *J. Food Prot.* **56:** 323–325.
2. **Aho, M., and J. Hirn.** 1988. Prevalence of campylobacteria in the Finnish broiler chicken chain from the producer to the consumer. *Acta Vet. Scand.* **29:**451–462.
3. **Atanassova, V., J. Alterneier, K. P. Kruse, and B. Dolzinski.** 1998. The detection of *Salmonella* and *Campylobacter* in fresh poultry. *Fleischwirtschaft* **78:**364–366.
4. **Bachmann, H. P., and U. Spahr.** 1995. The fate of potentially pathogenic bacteria in Swiss hard and semihard cheeses made from raw milk. *J. Dairy Sci.* **78:**476–483.
5. **Berndtson, E., M. Tivemo, and A. Engvall.** 1992. Distribution and numbers of *Campylobacter* in newly slaughtered broiler chickens and hens. *Int. J. Food Microbiol.* **15:**45–50.
6. **Beumer, R. R., J. J. Cruysen, and I. R. Birtantie.** 1988. The occurrence of *Campylobacter je-*juni in raw cows' milk. *J. Appl. Bacteriol.* **65:** 93–96.
7. **Blaser, M. J., D. N. Taylor, and R. A. Feldman.** 1983. Epidemiology of *Campylobacter jejuni* infections. *Epidemiol. Rev.* **5:**157–176.
8. **Bolder, N. M.** 1997. Decontamination of meat and poultry carcasses. *Trends Food Sci. Technol.* **8:** 221–227.
9. **Bryan, F. L., and M. P. Doyle.** 1995. Health risks and consequences of *Salmonella* and *Campylobacter jejuni* in raw poultry. *J. Food Prot.* **58:** 326–344.
10. **Casanovas, L., M. de Simon, M. D. Ferrer, J. Arques, and G. Monzon.** 1995. Intestinal carriage of campylobacters, salmonellas, yersinias and listerias in pigeons in the city of Barcelona. *J. Appl. Bacteriol.* **78:**11–13.
11. **Corry, J. E. L., D. E. Post, P. Colin, and M. J. Laisney.** 1995. Culture media for the isolation of campylobacters. *Int. J. Food Microbiol.* **26:** 43–76.
12. **Cuk, Z., A. Annan-Prah, M. Janc, and J. Zajc Satler.** 1987. Yoghurt: an unlikely source of *Campylobacter jejuni/coli*. *J. Appl. Bacteriol.* **63:** 201–205.
13. **de Boer, E., W. M. Seldam, and H. H. Stigter.** 1983. *Campylobacter jejuni*, *Yersinia enterocolitica* and *Salmonella* in game and poultry. *Tijdschr. Diergeneesk.* **108:**831–836.
14. **de Boer, E., and M. Hahné.** 1990. Cross-contamination with *Campylobacter jejuni* and *Salmonella* spp. from raw chicken products during food preparation. *J. Food Prot.* **53:**1067–1068.
15. **de Boer, E., P. van Beek, and K. Pelgrom.** 1997. Comparison of culture media for the isolation of campylobacters from chicken meat, p. 370–371. *In* A. J. Lastovica, D. G. Newell, and E. E. Lastovica (ed.), *Campylobacter, Helicobacter, and Related Organisms.* Institute of Child Health, Cape Town, South Africa.
16. **Desmasures, N., F. Bazin, and M. Gueguen.** 1997. Microbiological composition of raw milk from selected farms in the Camembert region of Normandy. *J. Appl. Microbiol.* **83:**53–58.
17. **Doyle, M. P., and D. J. Roman.** 1982. Prevalence and survival of *Campylobacter jejuni* in unpasteurized milk. *Appl. Environ. Microbiol.* **44:** 1154–1158.
18. **Doyle, M. P.** 1984. Association of *Campylobacter* with laying hens and eggs. *Appl. Environ. Microbiol.* **47:**533–536.
19. **Doyle, M. P.** 1984. *Campylobacter* in foods, p. 163–180. *In* J. P. Butzler (ed.), *Campylobacter Infection in Man and Animals.* CRC Press, Inc., Boca Raton, Fla.
20. **Doyle, M. P., and J. L. Schoeni.** 1986. Isolation

of *Campylobacter jejuni* from retail mushrooms. *Appl. Environ. Microbiol.* **51**:449–450.

21. **Endtz, H. P., J. S. Vliegenthart, P. Vandamme, H. W. Weverink, N. P. van den Braak, H. A. Verbrugh, and A. van Belkum.** 1997. Genotypic diversity of *Campylobacter lari* isolated from mussels and oysters in The Netherlands. *Int. J. Food Microbiol.* **34**:79–88.

22. **Fahey, T., D. Mongan, C. Gunneburg, G. K. Adak, F. Majid, and E. Kaczmarski.** 1995. An outbreak of *Campylobacter jejuni* enteritis associated with failed milk pasteurisation. *J. Infect.* **31**:137–143.

23. **Fernandez, H., and V. Pison.** 1996. Isolation of thermotolerant species of *Campylobacter* from commercial chicken livers. *Int. J. Food Microbiol.* **29**:75–80.

24. **Finch, M. J., and P. A. Blake.** 1985. Foodborne outbreaks of campylobacteriosis: the United States experience, 1980–1982. *Am. J. Epidemiol.* **122**:262–268.

25. **Flynn, O. M. J., I. S. Blair, and D. A. McDowell.** 1994. Prevalence of *Campylobacter* species on fresh retail chicken wings in Northern Ireland. *J. Food Prot.* **57**:334–336.

26. **Fricker, C. R., and R. W. A. Park.** 1989. A two-year study of the distribution of 'thermophilic' campylobacters in human, environmental and food samples from the Reading area with particular reference to toxin production and heat-stable serotype. *J. Appl. Bacteriol.* **66**:477–490.

27. **Geilhausen, B., H. Schutt Gerowitt, S. Aleksic, R. Koenen, G. Mauff, and G. Pulverer.** 1996. *Campylobacter* and *Salmonella* contaminating fresh chicken meat. *Zentl. Bakteriol.* **284**:241–245.

28. **Gomolka, M., and J. Uradzinski.** 1996. Occurrence of *Campylobacter* species in raw milk in North Eastern Poland. *Milchwissenschaft* **51**:366–368.

29. **Hahn, G., H. Kirchhoff, P. Hammer, E. H. Ubben, and W. H. Heeschen.** 1992. Bacteriological findings and their evaluation for milk and dairy products. *Arch. Lebensmittelhyg.* **43**:89–93.

30. **Hald, T., H. C. Wegener, and B. Beck Joergensen (ed.).** 1998. *Danish Ministry of Food, Agriculture and Fisheries. Annual Report on Zoonoses in Denmark 1998.* Danish Zoonosis Centre, Copenhangen, Denmark.

31. **Harris, N. V., T. J. Kimball, P. Bennett, Y. Johnson, D. Wakeley, and C. M. Nolan.** 1987. *Campylobacter jejuni* enteritis associated with raw goat's milk. *Am. J. Epidemiol.* **126**:179–186.

32. **Hudson, S. J., N. F. Lightfoot, J. C. Coulson, K. Russell, P. R. Sisson, and A. O. Sobo.** 1991. Jackdaws and magpies as vectors of milk-borne human *Campylobacter* infection. *Epidemiol. Infect.* **107**:363–372.

33. **Humphrey, T. J., and P. Beckett.** 1987. *Campylobacter jejuni* in dairy cows and raw milk. *Epidemiol. Infect.* **98**:263–269.

34. **Humphrey, T. J., and R. J. Hart.** 1988. *Campylobacter* and *Salmonella* contamination of unpasteurized cows' milk on sale to the public. *J. Appl. Bacteriol.* **65**:463–467.

35. **Hunt, J. M., and C. Abeyta.** 1995. *Campylobacter*, p. 7.01–7.27. *In* Food and Drug Administration (ed.), *FDA Bacteriological Analytical Manual*, 8th ed. AOAC International, Gaithersburg, Md.

36. **Hutchinson, D. N., F. J. Bolton, P. M. Hinchliffe, H. C. Dawkins, S. D. Horsley, E. G. Jessop, P. A. Robertshaw, and D. E. Counter.** 1985. Evidence of udder excretion of *Campylobacter jejuni* as the cause of milk borne *Campylobacter* outbreak. *J. Hyg.* **94**:205–215.

37. **International Organization for Standardization.** 1995. *Microbiology of Food and Animal Feeding Stuffs. Horizontal Method for Detection of Thermotolerant Campylobacter.* ISO 10727:1995(E). International Organization for Standardization, Geneva, Switzerland.

38. **Izat, A. L., and F. A. Gardner.** 1988. Incidence of *Campylobacter jejuni* in processed egg products. *Poult. Sci.* **67**:1431–1435.

39. **Jacobs-Reitsma, W. F.** 1994. Epidemiology of *Campylobacter* in poultry. Ph.D. Thesis. Wageningen Agricultural University, Wageningen, The Netherlands.

40. **Jones, F. T., R. C. Axtell, D. V. Rives, S. E. Scheideler, F. R. Tarver Jr., R. L. Walker, and M. J. Wineland.** 1991. A survey of *Campylobacter jejuni* contamination in modern broiler production and processing systems. *J. Food Prot.* **54**:259–262, 266.

41. **Jones, P. H., A. T. Willis, D. A. Robinson, M. B. Skirrow, and D. S. Josephs.** 1981. *Campylobacter* enteritis associated with the consumption of free school milk. *J. Hyg.* **87**:155–162.

42. **Kapperud, G., and O. Rosef.** 1983. Avian wildlife reservoir of *Campylobacter fetus* subsp. *jejuni*, *Yersinia* spp., and *Salmonlla* spp. in Norway. *Appl. Environ. Microbiol.* **45**:375–380.

43. **Koenraad, P. M. F. J., F. M. Rombouts, and S. H. W. Notermans.** 1997. Epidemiological aspects of thermophilic *Campylobacter* in water related environments: a review. *Water Environ. Res.* **69**:52–63.

44. **Korsak, N., G. Daube, Y. Ghafir, A. Chahed, S. Jolly, and H. Vindevogel.** 1998. An efficient sampling technique used to detect four foodborne pathogens on pork and beef carcasses in nine Belgian abattoirs. *J. Food Prot.* **61**:535–541.

45. **Kwiatek, K., B. Wojton, and N. J. Stern.** 1990. Prevalence and distribution of *Campylobacter*

spp. on poultry and selected red meat carcasses in Poland. *J. Food Prot.* **53:**127–130.

46. **Lammerding, A. M., M. M. Garcia, E. D. Mann, Y. Robinson, W. J. Dorward, R. B. Truscott, and F. Tittiger.** 1988. Prevalence of *Salmonella* and thermophilic *Campylobacter* in fresh pork, beef, veal and poultry in Canada. *J. Food Prot.* **51:**47–52.

47. **Little, C. L., and J. de Louvois.** 1998. The microbiological examination of butchery products and butchers' premises in the United Kingdom. *J. Appl. Microbiol.* **85:**177–186.

48. **Madden, R. H., L. Moran, and P. Scates.** 1998. Frequency of occurrence of *Campylobacter* spp. in red meats and poultry in Northern Ireland and their subsequent subtyping using polymerase chain reaction restriction fragment length polymorphism and the random amplified polymorphic DNA method. *J. Appl. Microbiol.* **84:**703–708.

49. **Mafu, A. A., R. Higgins, M. Nadeau, and G. Cousineau.** 1989. The incidence of *Salmonella, Campylobacter,* and *Yersinia enterocolitica* in swine carcasses and the slaughterhouse environment. *J. Food Prot.* **52:**642–645.

50. **McManus, C., and J. M. Lanier.** 1987. *Salmonella, Campylobacter jejuni,* and *Yersinia enterocolitica* in raw milk. *J. Food Prot.* **50:**51–55.

51. **Mead, G. C., W. R. Hudson, and M. H. Hinton.** 1995. Effect of changes in processing to improve hygiene control on contamination of poultry carcasses with *Campylobacter. Epidemiol. Infect.* **115:**495–500.

52. **Moore, J. E., and R. H. Madden.** 1998. Occurrence of thermophilic *Campylobacter* spp. in porcine liver in Northern Ireland. *J. Food Prot.* **61:** 409–413.

53. **National Advisory Committee on Microbiological Criteria for Foods.** 1994. *Campylobacter jejuni/coli. J. Food Prot.* **57:**1101–1121.

54. **National Advisory Committee on Microbiological Criteria for Foods.** 1997. Generic HACCP application in broiler slaughter and processing. *J. Food Prot.* **60:**579–604.

55. **Odumeru, J. A., S. J. Mitchell, D. M. Alves, J. A. Lynch, A. J. Yee, S. L. Wang, S. Styliadis, and J. M. Farber.** 1997. Assessment of the microbiological quality of ready to use vegetables for health care food services. *J. Food Prot.* **60:** 954–960.

56. **Oosterom, J., G. J. A. de Wilde, E. de Boer, L. H. de Blaauw, and H. Karman.** 1983. Survival of *Campylobacter jejuni* during poultry processing and pig slaughtering. *J. Food Prot.* **46:** 702–706, 709.

57. **Orr, K. E., N. F. Lightfoot, P. R. Sisson, B. A. Harkis, J. L. Tweddle, P. Boyd, A. Carroll, C. J. Jackson, D. R. A. Wareing, and R.**

Freeman. 1995. Direct milk excretion of *Campylobacter jejuni* in a dairy cow causing cases of human enteritis. *Epidemiol. Infect.* **114:**15–24.

58. **Oyarzabal, O. A., D. E. Conner, and F. J. Hoerr.** 1995. Incidence of campylobacters in the intestine of avian species in Alabama. *Avian Dis.* **39:**147–151.

59. **Park, C. E., and G. W. Sanders.** 1992. Occurrence of thermotolerant campylobacters in fresh vegetables sold at farmers' outdoor markets and supermarkets. *Can. J. Microbiol.* **38:**313–316.

60. **Reinhard, R. G., T. J. McAdam, G. J. Flick, R. E. Croonenberghs, R. F. Wittman, A. A. Diallo, and C. Fernandes.** 1996. Analysis of *Campylobacter jejuni, Campylobacter coli, Salmonella, Klebsiella pneumoniae,* and *Escherichia coli* O157:H7 in fresh hand picked blue crab (*Callinectes sapidus*) meat. *J. Food Prot.* **59:**803–807.

61. **Roberts, D.** 1985. Microbiological aspects of goats' milk—a public health laboratory service survey. *Goat Vet. Soc. J.* **6:**10–13.

62. **Roels, T. H., B. Wickus, H. H. Bostrom, J. J. Kazmierczak, M. A. Nicholson, T. A. Kurzynski, and J. P. Davis.** 1998. A foodborne outbreak of *Campylobacter jejuni* (O:33) infection associated with tuna salad: a rare strain in an unusual vehicle. *Epidemiol. Infect.* **121:**281–287.

63. **Rohrbach, B. W., F. A. Draughon, P. M. Davidson, and S. P. Oliver.** 1992. Prevalence of *Listeria monocytogenes, Campylobacter jejuni, Yersinia enterocolitica,* and *Salmonella* in bulk tank milk: risk factors and risk of human exposure. *J. Food Prot.* **55:**93–97.

64. **Shane, S. M., D. H. Gifford, and K. Yogasundram.** 1986. *Campylobacter jejuni* contamination of eggs. *Vet. Res. Commun.* **10:**487–492.

65. **Sierra, M. L., E. Gonzalez Fandos, M. L. Garcia Lopez, M. C. Garcia Fernandez, and M. Prieto.** 1995. Prevalence of *Salmonella, Yersinia, Aeromonas, Campylobacter,* and cold growing *Escherichia coli* on freshly dressed lamb carcasses. *J. Food Prot.* **58:**1183–1185.

66. **Stanley, K. N., J. S. Wallace, J. E. Currie, P. J. Diggle, and K. Jones.** 1998. Seasonal variation of thermophilic campylobacters in lambs at slaughter. *J. Appl. Microbiol.* **84:**1111–1116.

67. **Stanley, K. N., J. S. Wallace, J. E. Currie, P. J. Diggle, and K. Jones.** 1998. The seasonal variation of thermophilic campylobacters in beef cattle, dairy cattle, and calves. *J. Appl. Microbiol.* **85:**472–480.

68. **Steele, M. L., W. B. McNab, C. Poppe, M. W. Griffiths, C. Shu, S. A. Degrandis, L. C. Fruhner, C. A. Larkin, J. A. Lynch, and J. A. Odumeru.** 1997. Survey of Ontario bulk tank raw milk for food borne pathogens. *J. Food Prot.* **60:**1341–1346.

69. **Stern, N. J., and S. U. Kazmi.** 1989. *Campylobacter jejuni*, p. 71–110. *In* M. P. Doyle (ed.), *Food-Borne Bacterial Pathogens,* Marcel Dekker Inc., New York, N.Y.

70. **Stern, N. J., and J. E. Line.** 1992. Comparison of three methods for recovery of *Campylobacter* spp. from broiler carcasses. *J. Food Prot.* **55:** 663–666.

71. **Stern, N. J.** 1995. Influence of season and refrigerated storage on *Campylobacter* spp. contamination of broiler carcasses. *J. Appl. Poultry Res.* **4:** 235–238.

72. **Stone, D. L.** 1987. A survey of raw whole milk for *Campylobacter jejuni, Listeria monocytogenes* and *Yersinia enterocolitica. N. Z. J. Dairy Sci. Technol.* **22:**257–264.

73. **Tokumaru, M., H. Konuma, M. Umesako, S. Konno, and K. Shinagawa.** 1991. Rates of detection of *Salmonella* and *Campylobacter* in meats in response to the sample size and the infection level of each species. *Int. J. Food Microbiol.* **13:** 41–46.

74. **Vanderlinde, P. B., B. Shay, and J. Murray.** 1998. Microbiological quality of Australian beef carcass meat and frozen bulk packed beef. *J. Food Prot.* **61:**437–443.

75. **Vanderlinde, P. B., B. Shay, and J. Murray.** 1999. Microbiological status of Australian sheep meat. *J. Food Prot.* **62:**380–385.

76. **Willis, W. L., and C. Murray.** 1997. *Campylobacter jejuni* seasonal recovery observations of retail market broilers. *Poultry Sci.* **76:**314–317.

77. **Wilson, I. G., and J. E. Moore.** 1996. Presence of *Salmonella* spp. and *Campylobacter* spp. in shellfish. *Epidemiol. Infect.* **116:**147–153.

78. **Zanetti, F., O. Varoli, S. Stampi, and G. De Luca.** 1996. Prevalence of thermophilic *Campylobacter* and *Arcobacter butzleri* in food of animal origin. *Int. J. Food Microbiol.* **33:**315–321.

ANTIMICROBIAL RESISTANCE IN ANIMALS AND RELEVANCE TO HUMAN INFECTIONS

Kirk E. Smith, Jeffrey B. Bender, and Michael T. Osterholm

25

The human health relevance of antimicrobial-resistant bacteria from food production animals has long been, and continues to be, a point of contention between the public health and animal health communities. Most public health officials recognize the primary role of antimicrobial use in food animals in the increasing resistance in food-borne bacterial pathogens, but many representatives of the animal health community deny this relationship, citing a perceived lack of scientific evidence. It has been established that administration of antimicrobials to food animals can select for resistance among bacteria which are subsequently transmitted to humans through food or animal contact. However, the exact magnitude of the resulting human health problems has been difficult to quantify. That there is a risk to human health from antimicrobial-resistant food-borne bacteria as a result of the selective pressure applied by antimicrobial use in food animals is logical. However, because the chain of events from antimicrobial use in animals to clinically significant resistant bacterial infections in humans is complex, documenting comprehensive evidence of cause and effect is

very difficult. When evaluating the public health consequences of antimicrobial use in animals, it is important to consider each pathogen-antimicrobial situation individually. With *Campylobacter jejuni,* most of the work in this regard has concerned resistance to the fluoroquinolones.

C. jejuni is the most commonly recognized cause of bacterial gastroenteritis in the United States (3, 26) and is a frequently diagnosed cause of traveler's diarrhea. When antibiotics are indicated for treatment of campylobacter gastroenteritis, erythromycin or a fluoroquinolone is cited as the drug of choice (29). Fluoroquinolones are also cited as the drugs of choice for the prevention or treatment of traveler's diarrhea (30) and are used empirically for the treatment of bacterial gastroenteritis because of their effectiveness against a range of bacterial enteric pathogens (8, 9, 29).

FLUOROQUINOLONE RESISTANCE WORLDWIDE

Increasing resistance to fluoroquinolones among human *Campylobacter* isolates was first documented in the late 1980s and continues to be a problem (19). Emerging resistance to fluoroquinolones has been documented in numerous countries (19); in some countries the rise in resistance has been remarkably rapid (15,

Kirk E. Smith, Jeffrey B. Bender, and Michael T. Osterholm, Acute Disease Epidemiology Section, Minnesota Department of Health, 717 Delaware Street SE, Minneapolis, MN 55414.

Campylobacter, 2nd Ed., Edited by I. Nachamkin and M. J. Blaser
© 2000 American Society for Microbiology, Washington, D.C.

21). Investigators from numerous countries have provided evidence suggesting that fluoroquinolone use in veterinary medicine, especially poultry, largely explains the increasing fluoroquinolone resistance among human *Campylobacter* isolates. Country-specific data supporting this association are presented here.

The Netherlands

The initial study providing evidence of a link between fluoroquinolone use in veterinary medicine and increasing fluoroquinolone resistance in human isolates of *Campylobacter* was done in the Netherlands (4). Enrofloxacin was introduced for use in veterinary medicine in the Netherlands in 1987 and is used extensively there for the treatment of *Escherichia coli* and *Mycoplasma* infections in poultry and to a lesser extent in pigs. Sales of enrofloxacin for animal use in the Netherlands in 1989 amounted to about half of sales of all quinolones for human use. Endtz et al. documented the prevalence of ciprofloxacin resistance among human and poultry product isolates of *Campylobacter* during the years bracketing the introduction of enrofloxacin into veterinary medicine (4). In this study, *C. jejuni* comprised 92% of human isolates and 72% of poultry product isolates; the remainder were *C. coli*. Among human *Campylobacter* isolates, no ciprofloxacin resistance was found during 1982 to 1983 or 1985. The percentage of resistant isolates increased to 8% during 1987 to 1988 and to 11% during 1989. Ciprofloxacin resistance among *Campylobacter* isolates from poultry products closely paralleled that found among human isolates. No resistance was found in poultry isolates from 1982 to 1983; the percentage of resistant isolates increased to 8.4% during 1987 to 1988 and to 14% during 1989. Among human and poultry isolates from all years combined, resistance was more common in *C. coli* (14%) than *C. jejuni* (6%). As in other countries, poultry is the primary source of *Campylobacter* for human infections in the Netherlands. The authors of this study attributed the emergence of quinolone resistance in *Campylobacter* in the Netherlands

primarily to the extensive use of enrofloxacin in poultry.

Since the initial study, additional work on this topic has been done in the Netherlands. During 1992 to 1993, 181 (29%) of 617 *Campylobacter* isolates from broiler chickens were resistant to nalidixic acid, ciprofloxacin, flumequine, and enrofloxacin; resistant isolates were identified from 57 (38%) of 150 broiler flocks (11). Of 268 isolates tested, 177 (66%) were *C. jejuni* and 91 (34%) were hippurate negative and thus most likely to be *C. coli* (11). Of the 177 *C. jejuni* isolates, 70 (39.5%) were resistant to all four quinolones, as were 17 (18.7%) of the hippurate-negative isolates. The latest information on human isolates of *Campylobacter* from the Netherlands indicated that by 1997 the proportion resistant to fluoroquinolones had increased to 29% (25).

Spain

In Spain, a number of studies have documented a marked and rapid increase in rates of quinolone resistance among human isolates of *Campylobacter* following the introduction of enrofloxacin for veterinary use into that country in 1990 (17, 18, 21–23). Figure 1 illustrates combined data from these studies demonstrating this pattern. Resistance in this figure generally refers to ciprofloxacin resistance, except for one study in which resistance to nalidixic acid was used for 1989 to 1992 (18). Before 1990, fewer than 3% of isolates from humans were resistant to quinolones. During 1990, 9% of isolates from humans were resistant. A marked jump occurred from 1990 to 1991, when 39% of isolates were resistant. Since that time, the percentage of resistant isolates has risen steadily, reaching 83% in 1996. The highest annual percentage of resistant isolates in a single study was reported by Ruiz et al., who documented ciprofloxacin resistance in 88% of *C. jejuni* isolates (22). In a study of patients with campylobacter bacteremia, 12 (67%) of 18 *C. jejuni* isolates from blood during 1989 to 1996 were resistant to ciprofloxacin; of these, all resistant isolates were from 1991 or later (20).

Investigators in Spain have stated that the

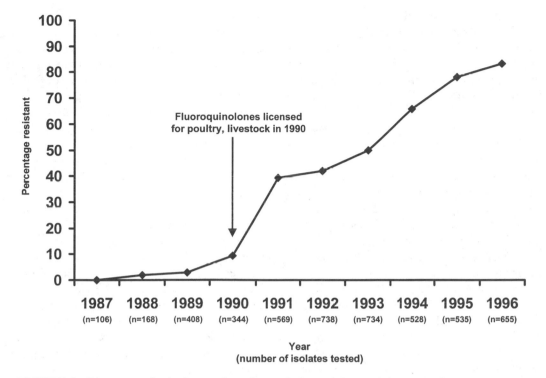

FIGURE 1 Percentage of quinolone-resistant human isolates of *C. jejuni/coli* in Spain from 1987 to 1996. This represents combined data from five studies (17, 18, 21–23). Quinolone resistance was defined as resistance to ciprofloxacin, except for one study (18), in which resistance to nalidixic acid was used for 1989 to 1992.

use of fluoroquinolones in veterinary medicine is most likely to be the driving force behind the dramatic increase in quinolone resistance in human isolates of *Campylobacter* (18, 22, 32). In some of the above-mentioned studies, most (23) or all (21) patients with quinolone-resistant *Campylobacter* infections were pediatric, an age group in which fluoroquinolone use is not recommended. Therefore, the resistant *Campylobacter* infections cannot be attributed directly to quinolone use among humans. Enrofloxacin was first licensed for veterinary use in Spain in 1990 for oral administration and in 1991 as injectable solutions. Enrofloxacin and other quinolones are used widely in Spain to prevent respiratory and enteric disease in broilers, reproductive chickens, laying hens, and pigs (32). Perez-Trallero et al. found that 20 (50%) of 40 *Campylobacter* isolates from retail poultry products obtained in 1993 were resis-

tant to ciprofloxacin and enrofloxacin, compared to 81 (49%) of 165 human isolates obtained during the first 6 months of 1993 (18).

United Kingdom
In the United Kingdom, fluoroquinolone resistance among human *Campylobacter* isolates was first demonstrated in 1991, when the percentage of resistant isolates ranged from 1.9 to 4.1% in three different studies (2, 7, 13). In 1992, 4.9% of isolates were resistant to fluoroquinolones (13). During 1991 to 1992, 33 to 55% of patients with quinolone-resistant cases had a recent history of foreign travel (2, 7, 13). In the largest study, 61 (67%) of 91 quinolone-resistant *Campylobacter* isolates were domestically acquired, and none of the patients had taken a quinolone prior to detection of the isolate (7). In this study, 1 (3%) of 37 *Campylobacter* isolates from 64 retail chicken products from

chickens bred in the United Kingdom was resistant to ciprofloxacin whereas 7 (27%) of 26 *Campylobacter* isolates from 50 imported (from Denmark and France) chicken products were resistant to ciprofloxacin (7). Enrofloxacin was first licensed for use in food animals in the United Kingdom in November, 1993; thus, the rarity of quinolone resistance in *Campylobacter* strains recovered from domestic chicken products in 1991 is not surprising. In a simple model put forth by Gaunt and Piddock (7), estimates of the amount of imported chicken consumed in the United Kingdom resulted in a predicted percentage of ciprofloxacin-resistant human *Campylobacter* isolates (2.4%) that was very close to the observed percentage among domestically acquired cases (2.7%).

After the approval of enrofloxacin for use in food animals in the United Kingdom in 1993, Piddock (19) stated that the United Kingdom could serve as a "control" to determine the effect of fluoroquinolone use in veterinary medicine on the emergence of fluoroquinolone-resistant food-borne pathogens. Testing of 5,800 isolates of *Campylobacter* isolated from humans in 1996 and 1997 revealed that 12% were resistant to ciprofloxacin (at a level of >8 μg/ml) (31), providing strong support for a link between veterinary use of fluoroquinolones and increasing fluoroquinolone resistance among human *Campylobacter* isolates.

Taiwan

In Taiwan, 52% of 73 *C. jejuni* and 75% of 20 *C. coli* isolates from pediatric patients in 1994 to 1996 were resistant to ciprofloxacin whereas 92% of 12 *C. jejuni* and 91% of 23 *C. coli* isolates from retail chicken products were resistant to ciprofloxacin (12). The authors suggested that the large amount of quinolones used in poultry may play an important role in the emergence of ciprofloxacin-resistant *Campylobacter* strains in Taiwan.

United States

In the United States, two surveys encompassing 474 human *Campylobacter* isolates from 1982 to 1992 yielded only one ciprofloxacin-resistant isolate (16, 28). The one resistant isolate was subsequently identified as *C. lari,* which is intrinsically resistant to quinolones (3a). Therefore, no fluoroquinolone-resistant *C. jejuni* or *C. coli* isolates were identified in either study.

In Minnesota, we studied quinolone resistance rates among *C. jejuni* isolates from Minnesota residents submitted to the Minnesota Department of Health from 1992 to 1998 (24). The Minnesota Department of Health Public Health Laboratory serves as a statewide reference laboratory for *Campylobacter* confirmation and identification. Beginning in 1995, disease-reporting rules were changed to require the submission of all *Campylobacter* isolates as part of the reporting process. All isolates were screened for resistance to nalidixic acid, which proved to be an excellent marker for resistance to ciprofloxacin. In this manner we were able to obtain sound population-based data on rates of quinolone resistance among human *Campylobacter* isolates.

The annual percentage of *C. jejuni* isolates that were resistant to nalidixic acid increased from 1.3% in 1992 to 10.2% in 1998 (χ^2 for linear trend, 75.3; $P < 0.001$) (Fig. 2). By quarter, the percentage of resistant isolates exhibited a marked seasonality characterized by peaks during the first quarter and valleys during the third quarter of each calendar year. To understand the seasonality observed in Fig. 2, we undertook a case comparison study during 1996 to 1997. Each case with a ciprofloxacin-resistant *C. jejuni* isolate was matched to two cases with nalidixic acid- and ciprofloxacin-sensitive isolates; cases were matched by age of patient, location of patients residence, and date of specimen collection. Patients with resistant isolates in 1998 were interviewed but were not compared to those with sensitive isolates.

Foreign travel was the most prominent risk factor for acquiring quinolone-resistant *C. jejuni* infection; 75% of such patients had a history of foreign travel within the 7 days preceding the onset of illness. Travel to the specific geographic locations of Mexico, South or Central America other than Mexico, Asia, and

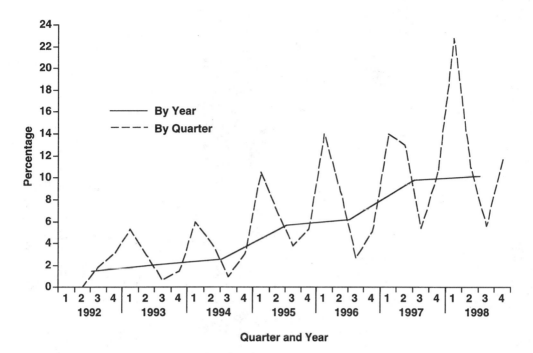

FIGURE 2 Percentage of *C. jejuni* specimens isolated from Minnesota residents and submitted to the Minnesota Department of Health that were resistant to nalidixic acid, by year and quarter, 1992 to 1998. For outbreaks, only the isolate from the index patient is included in calculations. Adapted from reference 24 with permission of the publisher.

Spain were all significantly associated with quinolone-resistant *C. jejuni* infection, with Mexico being the most frequent destination. Use of a quinolone during the month before specimen collection was also a significant risk factor but accounted for a maximum of 20% of quinolone-resistant cases from 1996 to 1997. Prior quinolone use did not differ significantly between foreign travel-associated and domestically acquired cases or from 1996 to 1997. In 1998, 94% of patients with quinolone-resistant isolates did not use a quinolone before culture; combined with the 1996 to 1997 data, 179 (85%) of 210 patients with quinolone-resistant isolates did not use a quinolone during the month before culture. For patients from 1997 who were treated with a fluoroquinolone after the collection of stool specimens, the duration of diarrhea was longer in the patients with quinolone-resistant *C. jejuni* infections (median, 10 days) than in the patients with quino-lone-sensitive *C. jejuni* infections (median, 7 days; $P = 0.03$).

Figure 3 illustrates the epidemic curve of infections with quinolone-resistant *C. jejuni* from 1996 through 1998, by month and foreign travel history. To negate the influence of prior quinolone use, data for patients who used quinolones during the month before culture are excluded. Outbreak-associated cases are also excluded; with regard to clusters, only the index is included. By using these criteria, the percentage of all confirmed *C. jejuni* cases among Minnesota residents that were domestically acquired and caused by quinolone-resistant isolates increased from 0.8% in 1996 to 3.0% in 1998 (χ^2 for linear trend, 9.8; $P = 0.002$). Of note, the seasonality of domestically acquired infections closely tracks the summer/fall seasonality for all *C. jejuni* infections in the United States.

Fluoroquinolones were first licensed in the

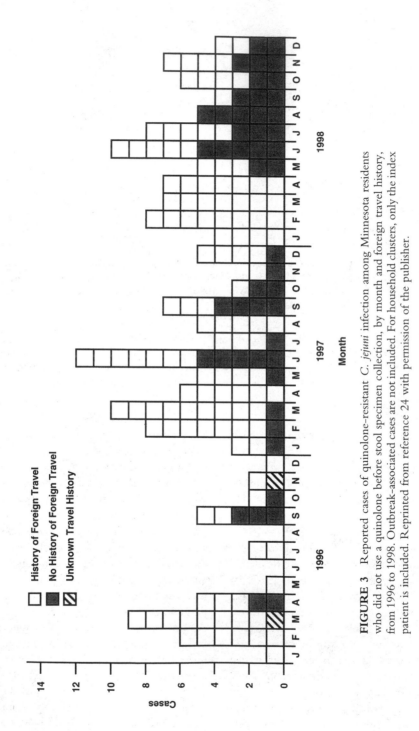

FIGURE 3 Reported cases of quinolone-resistant *C. jejuni* infection among Minnesota residents who did not use a quinolone before stool specimen collection, by month and foreign travel history, from 1996 to 1998. Outbreak-associated cases are not included. For household clusters, only the index patient is included. Reprinted from reference 24 with permission of the publisher.

United States for use in poultry in 1995. Sarafloxacin was licensed in August 1995, followed by enrofloxacin in 1996. These quinolones, both of which are available in formulations to be applied in drinking water, are licensed for use in young chickens and turkeys for the treatment of bacterial respiratory infections. To determine whether chickens could be a source of domestically acquired human cases of quinolone-resistant *C. jejuni* infections in humans in the United States, we cultured 91 chicken products obtained from 16 retail markets in the Minneapolis-St. Paul metropolitan area during September to November 1997. These products were composed of a variety of fresh or thawed items with and without the skin. The products originated in 15 poultry-processing plants in nine states. Multiple colonies were picked from all positive products, but 15 products were tested quantitatively to systematically capture diversity.

Campylobacter spp. were isolated from 80 (88%) of the 91 chicken products, including *C. jejuni* from 67 (74%) and *C. coli* from 19 (21%). Both species were isolated from six products. Ciprofloxacin-resistant *Campylobacter* was isolated from 18 (20%) of the products, including resistant *C. jejuni* from 13 (14%) and resistant *C. coli* from 5 (6%). Products that yielded resistant isolates were purchased at 11 retail markets representing eight franchises; they originated in seven poultry-processing plants in five states. Eight (73%) of 11 *Campylobacter*-positive chicken products tested quantitatively yielded a combination of species and/or ciprofloxacin resistance types; for example, one product yielded sensitive *C. jejuni,* sensitive *C. coli,* and resistant *C. coli.*

Molecular subtypes of *C. jejuni* isolates from human and chicken product isolates were determined by PCR with restriction length polymorphism flagellin gene typing (PCR-FLA). Forty-five PCR-FLA subtypes were identified among 269 typeable *C. jejuni* isolates from 1996 to 1997 case-comparison study patients. Among the human isolates from 1997, 5 subtypes were detected among quinolone-resistant isolates only, 24 were detected among quinolone-sensitive isolates only, and 12 were detected among both resistant and sensitive isolates.

Twelve PCR-FLA subtypes were identified among *C. jejuni* isolates from 13 positive chicken products: three subtypes were detected among quinolone-resistant isolates only, five were detected among quinolone-sensitive isolates only, and four were detected among both resistant and sensitive isolates. Up to three subtypes were identified per product. Six of seven subtypes of quinolone-resistant *C. jejuni* identified among isolates from retail chicken products were also identified among quinolone-resistant *C. jejuni* isolates from humans. For human cases with onset during 1997 and excluding patients who had used quinolones before culture, patients with domestically acquired quinolone-resistant *C. jejuni* infection were more likely to have a *C. jejuni* subtype also found among quinolone-resistant *C. jejuni* from chicken products than were patients with domestically acquired quinolone-sensitive *C. jejuni* infection (12 of 13 and 40 of 90, respectively; odds ratio, 15.0; 95% confidence interval, 1.9 to 321.8) or patients with foreign travel-associated resistant *C. jejuni* infection (12 of 13 and 14 of 40, respectively; odds ratio, 22.3; 95% confidence interval, 2.5 to 507.8).

For 96% of the ciprofloxacin-resistant *C. jejuni* strains isolates from humans during 1992 to 1998, the ciprofloxacin MIC was ≥ 32 μg/ml, as was the MIC for all ciprofloxacin-resistant chicken product isolates. Ciprofloxacin-resistant isolates from human cases ($n = 20$) and chicken products ($n = 8$) in 1997 were also resistant to enrofloxacin, sarafloxacin, and the newer human fluoroquinolones grepafloxacin, levofloxacin, and trovafloxacin.

In summary, we documented an overall increase in quinolone-resistant *C. jejuni* infections in Minnesota residents from 1992 to 1998. Domestically acquired resistant infections increased from 1996 to 1998. Ciprofloxacin-resistant *C. jejuni* was isolated from 14% of retail chicken products collected during 1997. By molecular subtyping, we showed that strains of domestically acquired ciprofloxacin-resistant *C. jejuni* from infected humans closely corresponded to ciprofloxacin-resistant strains isolated from retail chicken products. We attributed the increase in domestically acquired quinolone-resistant infections in humans largely to the use of fluoroquinolones in poultry in the United States. Since fluoroquinolone use in poultry in the United States has been implemented recently (late 1995), we probably documented the early emergence of quinolone-resistant *Campylobacter* in this country.

In a 1997 study of *Campylobacter* isolates from humans in California, Connecticut, Georgia, and Oregon, 20 (12%) of 164 isolates were resistant to ciprofloxacin; resistance was documented in isolates from all four states (6). Of 16 patients who were interviewed, only 1 (6%) used a quinolone before culture and 9 (56%) had domestically acquired cases; 5 (31%) of the 16 patients were hospitalized overnight, compared to only 1 (3%) of 31 patients with fluoroquinolone-sensitive *Campylobacter* infections (matched odds ratio, ∞; lower-limit 95% confidence interval, 3.0) (6).

In 1998, 13.4% of 330 *C. jejuni* isolates submitted to the Centers for Disease Control and Prevention as part of the National Antimicrobial Resistance Monitoring System were resistant to ciprofloxacin (3a).

Mexico

Our 1996 to 1997 case comparison study of quinolone-resistant *C. jejuni* cases in Minnesota residents provided indirect evidence of a link between fluoroquinolone use in poultry in Mexico and human infections with quinolone-resistant *C. jejuni* (24). A substantial proportion (36%) of quinolone-resistant *C. jejuni* infections in Minnesota residents in 1996 to 1997 were probably acquired in Mexico. Of *C. jejuni* isolates from 77 patients with a history of travel to Mexico during the week before the onset of illness, 47 (61%) were resistant to ciprofloxacin. Few of the returning travelers infected with quinolone-resistant *C. jejuni* patients had taken a quinolone before culture; therefore, most *C. jejuni* strains were resistant to fluoroquinolones when they were acquired. Mexico does produce a substantial amount of poultry meat; production increased from 1.7×10^9 lb in 1990 to 3.2×10^9 lb in 1997 (5). Sales of quinolones for use in poultry in Mexico, including the fluoroquinolones ciprofloxacin, enrofloxacin, and danofloxacin, increased dramatically from 86×10^6 medicated liters in 1993 to 326×10^6 medicated liters in 1997 (14). These data led us to consider that fluoroquinolone use in poultry in Mexico may be an important contributor to infections with resistant *C. jejuni* in travelers to that country.

SYNOPSIS OF THE LINK BETWEEN FLUOROQUINOLONE USE IN POULTRY AND QUINOLONE-RESISTANT *CAMPYLOBACTER* INFECTIONS IN HUMANS

The cumulative evidence strongly suggests that fluoroquinolone use in veterinary medicine, especially for poultry, is a major contributor to the increase in human infections with quinolone-resistant *Campylobacter*. This evidence can be summarized as follows.

(i) Poultry repeatedly has been documented as a major food reservoir of *Campylobacter* for human infections (26). Person-to-person transmission occurs relatively uncommonly and is not epidemiologically important (26).

(ii) It has been shown experimentally that enrofloxacin treatment of chickens infected with quinolone-sensitive *C. jejuni* does not eradicate the organism; rather, fluoroquinolone resistance in *C. jejuni* can consistently be selected (10).

(iii) Fluoroquinolone use in poultry and livestock for treatment of disease is widespread in many regions of the world, including Europe, the United States, Asia, Latin America, and South Africa (35). In some regions, fluoroquinolones are also used for disease prevention. Generic or counterfeit quinolone products are known to be used substantially in many countries; the use of these nonproprietary products is believed to exceed that of proprietary products in many countries (35).

(iv) A temporal relationship between the licensure of fluoroquinolones for use in food animals, particularly poultry, and a subsequent increase in quinolone resistance among *Campy-*

lobacter isolates from humans has been demonstrated in the Netherlands, Spain, the United Kingdom, and the United States. This effect has been most dramatic in Spain, where fluoroquinolones are reportedly used widely in all facets of poultry production.

(v) Fluoroquinolone-resistant *Campylobacter* has been isolated from retail chicken products in the Netherlands, Spain, Taiwan, the United Kingdom, and the United States. The percentage of *Campylobacter* isolates from chicken products from any given country that are quinolone resistant generally corresponds well to the percentage of human isolates that are resistant in that country; i.e., countries with a high percentage of resistance among chicken isolates have a high percentage of resistance among human isolates.

(vi) In the United States, molecular subtyping by PCR-FLA identified indistinguishable strains of quinolone-resistant *C. jejuni* among isolates from domestically acquired human cases and locally available retail chicken products. In fact, a statistically significant association was made between molecular subtypes of quinolone-resistant *C. jejuni* isolated from patients with domestically acquired cases and from retail poultry products. This association is not surprising, since many studies using a variety of laboratory characterization techniques have demonstrated similarities among *Campylobacter* isolates from humans and retail poultry products (26).

EVIDENCE FOR A LIMITED LINK BETWEEN FLUOROQUINOLONE USE IN HUMANS AND QUINOLONE-RESISTANT *CAMPYLOBACTER* INFECTIONS IN HUMANS

Despite the evidence above implicating fluoroquinolone use in poultry, some may suggest that the increased use of quinolones among humans may be driving the increasing quinolone resistance among human *Campylobacter* isolates. However, fluoroquinolones have been widely used in humans in the United States since 1986. Fluoroquinolone resistance in human isolates of *Campylobacter* was not documented until 1992, and the low level of resistance observed in Minnesota in the early 1990s was probably due largely to foreign travel (24). In Minnesota, higher levels of resistance, including a significant increase in the number of domestically acquired infections with resistant strains, have occurred only since the approval of fluoroquinolones for use in poultry in 1995 (24).

It has been recognized that treatment of *Campylobacter* infections can lead to the selection of quinolone-resistant *Campylobacter* isolates (19). In Minnesota, we found that quinolone use prior to culture was shown to be a significant risk factor for infection with quinolone-resistant *C. jejuni* (24). However, during 1996 to 1998, this phenomenon could account for a maximum of 15% of resistant isolates. In reality, many of these isolates were from patients who had a history of foreign travel as well as quinolone use prior to culture; therefore, a proportion of these patients were likely to already have had an infection with resistant *C. jejuni* prior to treatment. In many of the other studies previously mentioned in this chapter, quinolones had not been used by infected patients or the subjects were pediatric patients, in whom quinolone use is not recommended. Because person-to-person transmission of *Campylobacter* is uncommon (26), patients infected with resistant *Campylobacter* are not important as a source of resistant *Campylobacter* for other humans. Thus, while human quinolone use has undoubtedly contributed to the increase in resistance among *Campylobacter* isolates, the relative contribution compared to quinolone use in veterinary medicine appears to be small.

HUMAN HEALTH RELEVANCE OF RESISTANCE TO NONQUINOLONE ANTIMICROBIALS IN ANIMALS

Published information specifically addressing the human health relevance of resistance of animal *C. jejuni* isolates to nonquinolone antimicrobials is relatively sparse. There are some animal data on resistance to macrolide antibiotics such as erythromycin, a treatment of choice for campylobacter gastroenteritis. In general, rates of resistance to erythromycin among human isolates of *C. jejuni* have been low and quite stable, usually less than 5%. However resistance to erythromycin among isolates of *C. coli*, which is much less frequently recovered from humans, is documented more commonly. Rates of resistance to erythromycin of up to 79% have been reported for *C. coli* isolates from pigs, a primary reservoir for this species (1, 27, 33). Among *Campylobacter* isolates from chicken products in Taiwan, 2 (17%) of 12 *C. jejuni* and 19 (83%) of 23 *C. coli* isolates were resistant to erythromycin (12). Among human isolates of *Campylobacter* in Taiwan, 7 (10%) of 73 *C. jejuni* and 10 (50%) of 20 *C. coli* isolates were resistant to erythromycin (12). In Denmark, the percentage of erythromycin-resistant *C. jejuni* isolates from cattle, broilers, and pigs was 3, 6, and 33%, respectively, but no erythromycin resistance was observed among human isolates (1). In the same study, the percentage of erythromycin-resistant *C. coli* isolates from broilers, pigs, and humans was 18, 74, and 14%, respectively. (1). In the Netherlands, 26 (4.2%) of 617 *Campylobacter* isolates from broiler flocks were resistant to erythromycin; 1.7% of *C. jejuni* isolates and 12.1% of hippurate-negative isolates (likely to be *C. coli*) were resistant (11). Macrolides, especially tylosin, are used therapeutically and subtherapeutically as feed additives for livestock and poultry, and some investigators (21) have attributed macrolide resistance in *Campylobacter* isolates from animals and humans to use of macrolides in food animals, especially pigs; however, this relationship has not been explored in detail.

Tetracyclines have been listed as an alternative treatment for campylobacter gastroenteritis in the past, but recent studies in some countries have revealed high rates of resistance to tetracyclines among human isolates of *Campylobacter* (12, 16, 22, 24). For example, in our studies in Minnesota, 61% of *C. jejuni* isolates from humans in 1992 to 1997 were resistant to tetracycline, with rates remaining stable over this period (24). In Taiwan, 95% of *C. jejuni* and 85% of *C. coli* isolates from humans were resistant to tetracyclines, as were 83% of *C. jejuni*

and 96% of *C. coli* isolates from chicken products (12). In the Netherlands, 99 (16%) of 617 *Campylobacter* isolates from broiler flocks were resistant to tetracycline and 11.9% of *C. jejuni* isolates and 18.7% of hippurate-negative isolates (likely to be *C. coli*) were resistant (11). As with macrolides, tetracyclines are used widely both therapeutically and subtherapeutically as feed additives for livestock and poultry, but any potential relationship between tetracycline use in veterinary medicine and resistance among human isolates of *Campylobacter* has not been adequately evaluated.

Clindamycin is also cited as an alternative treatment for campylobacter gastroenteritis, but there are few data on resistance rates in *Campylobacter* from animal sources. In Taiwan, 10% of *C. jejuni* and 50% of *C. coli* isolates from humans were resistant to clindamycin, as were 8% of *C. jejuni* and 83% of *C. coli* isolates from chicken products (12). Lincomycin, a close relative of clindamycin, is used as a feed additive in livestock and poultry, but the significance of this has not been determined.

FUTURE DIRECTIONS

The World Health Organization (WHO) reported on research and monitoring needs to further evaluate the relationship between fluoroquinolone use in animals and human infections with food-borne quinolone-resistant bacteria and to address identified problems (35). Much of the discussion from the WHO meeting is equally applicable to the use of other antimicrobials in animals. It is clear that monitoring quinolone usage in animals is critical in evaluating its effect on human health. However, usage data are known to be grossly incomplete, and there are a number of obstacles to acquiring the needed data. Because pharmaceutical companies may view usage data as proprietary information, regulatory and public health agencies often have limited access to these data. In some countries, attempts are being made to overcome this problem by processing these data in a manner that protects confidentiality. Even this, however, would not address the quantification of generic or counterfeit quinolones used in animals. The usage of nonproprietary quinolones is substantial in some countries and overall is believed to exceed the use of veterinary proprietary products worldwide.

The WHO also recommended consideration of a number of public health safeguards that should be considered as part of developing prudent use of antimicrobials in livestock guidelines (35). Among these recommendations were that quinolones should be registered for therapeutic use only and not for performance enhancement. In addition, extra-label use of quinolones in food animals should be discouraged. On a broader scale, the WHO recommended that any antimicrobial agent should not be used for growth promotion in animals if it is used in human therapeutics or is known to select for cross-resistance to antimicrobials used in human medicine (34).

In November 1998, the U.S. Food and Drug Administration proposed a Framework for Evaluating and Assuring the Human Safety of the Microbial Effects of Antimicrobial New Animal Drugs Intended for Use in Food-Producing Animals. This framework will establish a series of thresholds for antimicrobial resistance, with required mitigating actions when each threshold is met. This process will ultimately result in the withdrawal of the antimicrobial if the mitigating actions do not succeed in preventing continued increasing resistance. The public health effects of fluoroquinolone use in poultry should be a top priority for evaluation by the Food and Drug Administration. However, it is not clear what mitigating options are available for the use of fluoroquinolones in poultry, since the widespread selection of fluoroquinolone-resistant Campylobacter may be impossible to avoid when fluoroquinolones are administered in the drinking water on a flock-wide basis.

To optimally detect or assess potential or existing human health problems related to antimicrobial use in animals, a well-coordinated international surveillance and monitoring program is key. This pertains to bacterial isolates from cases of human illness as well as from food or animal sources. Because of increasing foreign travel and the increasing international food trade, it is clear that control measures implemented only in individual countries will not be sufficient to curtail the development of resistance in food-borne bacterial pathogens. For example, efforts to slow or stop the development of quinolone-resistant Campylobacter in poultry in the United States would largely interrupt the increasing problem of domestically acquired quinolone-resistant C. jejuni infections in Minnesota residents but would not address the problem of resistant infections acquired in foreign countries. Interventions must be applied both domestically and internationally to achieve a comprehensive solution.

REFERENCES

1. **Aarestrup, F. M., E. M. Nielson, M. Madsen, and J. Engberg.** 1997. Antimicrobial susceptibility patterns of thermophilic Campylobacter spp. from humans, pigs, cattle, and broilers in Denmark. *Antimicrob. Agents Chemother.* **41:** 2244–2250.

2. **Bowler, I., and D. Day.** 1992. Emerging quinolone resistance in campylobacters. *Lancet* **340:**245.

3. **Centers for Disease Control and Prevention.** 1999. Incidence of foodborne illnesses: preliminary data from the foodborne diseases active surveillance network (Foodnet)—United States, 1998. *Morbid. Mortal. Weekly Rep.* **48:**189–194.

3a. **Centers for Disease Control and Prevention.** Unpublished data.

4. **Endtz, H. P., G. J. Ruijs, B. van Klingeren, W. H. Jansen, T. van der Reyden, and R. P. Mouton.** 1991. Quinolone resistance in Campylobacter isolated from man and poultry following the introduction of fluoroquinolones in veterinary medicine. *J. Antimicrob. Chemother.* **27:**199–208.

5. **Food and Agriculture Organization of the United Nations.** 1993–1998. *FAO Production Yearbook,* vol. 46–51. FAO Statistics Series. Food and Agriculture Organization of the United Nations, Rome, Italy.

6. **Friedman, C. R., S. Yang, J. Rocourt, K. Stamey, D. Vugia, R. Marcus, S. Segler, B. Shiferaw, and F. J. Angulo.** 1998. Fluoroquinolone-resistant Campylobacter infections in the United States: a pilot case-control study in Food-Net sites, abstr. no. 545, p. 179. *In Abstracts of the 36th Annual Meeting of the Infectious Diseases Society of America.*

7. **Gaunt, P. N., and L. V. J. Piddock.** 1996. Ciprofloxacin resistant Campylobacter spp. in humans:

an epidemiological and laboratory study. *J. Antimicrob. Chemother.* **37:**747–757.

8. **Guerrant, R. L.** 1995. Inflammatory enteritides, p. 987–998. *In* G. L. Mandell, J. E. Bennett, and R. Dolin (ed.), *Principles and Practice of Infectious Diseases,* 4th ed. Churchill Livingstone Inc., New York, N.Y.

9. **Hooper, D. C., and J. S. Wolfson.** 1991. Fluoroquinolone antimicrobial agents. *N. Engl. J. Med.* **324:**384–394.

10. **Jacobs-Reitsma, W. F., C. A. Kan, and N. M. Bolder.** 1994. The induction of quinolone resistance in *Campylobacter* bacteria in broilers by quinolone treatment. *Lett. Appl. Microbiol.* **19:**228–231.

11. **Jacobs-Reitsma, W. F., P. M. F. J. Koenread, N. M. Bolder, and R. W. A. W. Mulder.** 1994. In vitro susceptibility of *Campylobacter* and *Salmonella* isolates from broilers to quinolones, ampicillin, tetracycline, and erythromycin. *Vet. Q.* **16:**206–208.

12. **Li, C. C., C. H. Chiu, J. L. Wu, Y. C. Huang, and T. Y. Lin.** 1993. Antimicrobial susceptibilities of *Campylobacter jejuni* and *coli* by using E-test in Taiwan. *Scand. J. Infect. Dis.* **30:**39–42.

13. **McIntyre, M., and M. Lyons.** 1993. Resistance to ciprofloxacin in *Campylobacter* spp. Lancet **341:**188.

14. **Mercadeo Estadistico.** 1994–1998. (Software.) Mercadeo Estadistico, Colonia. Minerva, Mexico, D.F.

15. **Murphy, G. S., Jr., P. Echeverria, L. R. Jackson, M. K. Arness, C. LeBron, and C. Pitarangsi.** 1996. Ciprofloxacin- and azithromycin-resistant *Campylobacter* causing traveler's diarrhea in U.S. troops deployed to Thailand in 1994. *Clin. Infect. Dis.* **22:**868–869.

16. **Nachamkin, I.** 1994. Antimicrobial susceptibility of *Campylobacter jejuni* and *Campylobacter coli* to ciprofloxacin, erythromycin and tetracycline from 1982 to 1992. *Med. Microbiol. Lett.* **3:**300–305.

17. **Perez-Trallero, E., F. Otero, C. Lopez-Lopategui, M. Montes, J. M. Garcia-Arenzana, and M. Gomariz.** 1997. High prevalence of ciprofloxacin resistant *Campylobacter jejuni/coli* in Spain, abstr. C-21, p. 49. *In Program and Abstracts of the 37th Interscience Conference on Antimicrobial Agents and Chemotherapy.* American Society for Microbiology, Washington, D.C.

18. **Perez-Trallero, E., M. Urbieta, C. L. Lopategui, C. Zigorraga, and I. Ayestaran.** 1993. Antibiotics in veterinary medicine and public health. *Lancet* **342:**1371–1372.

19. **Piddock, L. V. J.** 1995. Quinolone resistance and *Campylobacter* spp. *J. Antimicrob. Chemother.* **36:**891–898.

20. **Pigrau, C., R. Bartolome, B. Almirante, A. M. Planes, J. Gavalda, and A. Pahissa.** 1997. Bacteremia due to *Campylobacter* species: clinical findings and antimicrobial susceptibility patterns. *Clin. Infect. Dis.* **25:**1414–1420.

21. **Reina, J., M. J. Ros, and A. Serra.** 1994. Susceptibilities to 10 antimicrobial agents of 1,220 *Campylobacter* strains isolated from 1987–1993 from feces of pediatric patients. *Antimicrob. Agents Chemother.* **38:**2917–2920.

22. **Ruiz, J., P. Goni, F. Marco, F. Gallardo, B. Mirelis, T. J. De Anta, and J. Vila.** 1998. Increased resistance to quinolones in *Campylobacter jejuni*: a genetic analysis of *gyrA* gene mutations in quinolone-resistant clinical isolates. *Microbiol. Immunol.* **42:**223–226.

23. **Sanchez, R., V. Fernandez-Baca, M. D. Diaz, P. Munoz, M. Rodriguez-Creixems, and E. Bouza.** 1994. Evolution of susceptibilities of *Campylobacter* spp. to quinolones and macrolides. *Antimicrob. Agents Chemother.* **38:**1879–1882.

24. **Smith, K. E., J. M. Besser, C. W. Hedberg, F. T. Leano, J. B. Bender, J. H. Wicklund, B. P. Johnson, K. A. Moore, and M. T. Osterholm.** 1999. The epidemiology of quinolone-resistant *Campylobacter jejuni* infections in Minnesota, 1992–1998. *N. Engl. J. Med.* **340:**1525–1532.

25. **Talsma, E., W. G. Goettsch, H. Niest, and M. J. W. Sprenger.** 1998. Increasing fluoroquinolone resistance in *Campylobacter* spp. in the Netherlands, abstr. C-78, p. 91. *In Program and Abstracts of the 38th Annual Interscience Conference on Antimicrobial Agents and Chemotherapy.* American Society for Microbiology, Washington, D.C.

26. **Tauxe, R. T.** 1992. Epidemiology of *Campylobacter jejuni* infections in the United States and other industrialized nations, p. 9–19. *In* I. Nachamkin, M. J. Blaser, and L. S. Tompkins (ed.), *Campylobacter jejuni: Current Status and Future Trends.* American Society for Microbiology, Washington, D.C.

27. **Taylor, D. N., M. J. Blaser, P. Echeverria, C. Pitarangsi, L. Bodhidatta, and W. L. Wang.** 1987. Erythromycin-resistant *Campylobacter* infections in Thailand. *Antimicrob. Agents Chemother.* **31:**438–442.

28. **Tenover, F. C., C. N. Baker, C. L. Fennell, and C. A. Ryan.** 1992. Antimicrobial resistance in *Campylobacter* species, p. 66–73. *In* I. Nachamkin, M. J. Blaser, and L. S. Tompkins (ed.), *Campylobacter jejuni: Current Status and Future Trends.* American Society for Microbiology, Washington, D.C.

29. **The Medical Letter, Inc.** 1998. The choice of antibacterial drugs. *Med. Lett. Drugs Ther.* **40:**33–42.

30. **The Medical Letter, Inc.** 1998. Advice for travelers. *Med. Lett. Drugs Ther.* **40:**47–50.

31. **Threlfall, E. J., J. A. Frost, and B. Rowe.** 1999. Fluoroquinolone resistance in salmonellas and campylobacters from humans. *Br. Med. J.* **318:** 943–944.

32. **Velazquez, J. B., A. Jiminez, B. Chomon, and T. G. Villa.** 1995. Incidence and transmission of antibiotic resistance in *Campylobacter jejuni* and *Campylobacter coli. J. Antimicrob. Chemother.* **35:**173–178.

33. **Wang, W. L., L. B. Reller, and M. J. Blaser.** 1984. Comparison of antimicrobial susceptibility patterns of *Campylobacter jejuni* and *Campylobacter coli. Antimicrob. Agents Chemother.* **26:**351–353.

34. **World Health Organization.** 1997. The medical impact of the use of antimicrobials in food animals health. Report of a WHO Meeting.

35. **World Health Organization.** 1998. Use of quinolones in food animals and potential impact on human health. Report of a WHO Meeting.

POULTRY INFECTIONS AND THEIR CONTROL AT THE FARM LEVEL

Diane G. Newell and Jaap A. Wagenaar

26

Much of the world's poultry production is contaminated with campylobacters and this has been implicated as a major source of human infections. Removal of these organisms from the poultry food chain or at least reduction in their frequency, has now become a significant objective of campylobacter research. There are three practical levels at which infection control could be targeted and implemented: at the poultry farm, during poultry meat processing, and during meat handling and cooking by the end consumer. The development of control strategies during meat processing, especially at the abattoir, is reviewed elsewhere (see chapter 24). With the exception of decontamination of the end product, the most effective impact will be achieved by intervention measures directed at poultry production at the farm level. Because *Campylobacter jejuni* appears to be adapted to optimally colonize the avian gut, this task will not be an easy one. In 1992, Stern (61) comprehensively reviewed the state of knowledge regarding *C. jejuni* in poultry. In this chapter we aim to extend that knowledge base and to speculate on current strategies attempting to deal with this problem.

ROLE OF POULTRY CAMPYLOBACTERS IN HUMAN CAMPYLOBACTERIOSIS

The evidence that poultry is a major source of human campylobacteriosis is largely circumstantial. Early data based on some case-control studies indicate that at least half of all sporadic cases of campylobacter infection are attributable to the handling or consumption of chicken meat (5, 17, 25, 30). However, the degree of risk appears to vary between studies. For example, de Boer and Hahne (16) considered that only 15% of infections were traceable to poultry meat. Moreover, in one recent study, contact with whole raw chicken in the home was significantly associated with a decrease in the risk of becoming ill with campylobacter (2). Certainly a significant proportion of chicken meat is contaminated with campylobacters at retail, and at least some of the serotypes of these poultry strains are identical to those found in humans (30, 47, 48). However, the pathogenicity of all poultry campylobacters is debatable. The distribution of serotypes in *C. jejuni* strains from poultry and humans are not necessarily the same (46a), and recent data obtained by using genotypic techniques support some

Diane G. Newell, Veterinary Laboratories Agency (Weybridge), New Haw, Addlestone KT15 3NB, United Kingdom. *Jaap A. Wagenaar,* Institute for Animal Science and Health (ID-Lelystad), P.O. Box 65, 8200 AB Lelystad, The Netherlands.

Campylobacter, 2nd Ed., Edited by I. Nachamkin and M. J. Blaser
© 2000 American Society for Microbiology, Washington, D.C.

host specificity among clones of campylobacter. For example, genotypes, based on *fla* typing (see chapter 2), frequently present in poultry strains are not always detectable in strains isolated from human waste effluent (34) or human fecal samples (15) with apparent geographical and temporal relationships. Conversely, there are *fla* types frequently present in human isolates which are not observed in poultry. Similarly Korolik et al. (36, 37), investigating campylobacters from Australia and the United States by using a hybridization probe technique, found that certain hybridization patterns were more common in poultry strains than in human strains.

The importance of poultry campylobacters in human disease may be further disputed as efforts to control infections become more effective. For example, significant reductions in poultry flock colonization in some countries, such as Sweden, have not been reflected in parallel reductions in human infections (18a).

EPIDEMIOLOGY OF POULTRY FLOCK COLONIZATION

Data on the prevalence of campylobacter-positive poultry flocks worldwide is limited. Some early surveys have been previously reviewed (56). There have been few national surveillance studies, and such studies are fraught with difficulties. This is because in most countries the poultry industry is fragmented, geographically dispersed, and poorly organized, so that random sampling and sample collection at the farm level is difficult. Such problems make it difficult

to survey even for statutory diseases like salmonellosis. In addition, although fresh cecal droppings are as sensitive for screening purposes as cloacal swabs (19), campylobacters are very sensitive to dehydration and atmospheric conditions, and so swabs are preferable; this requires catching and handling of birds. Finally, flock positivity is clearly age related. Because of these problems, flock sampling may be best undertaken at slaughter, and because most birds in a flock will be infected, flock sampling can be reduced to very few birds (19).

In Europe the most accurate information is available from the northern countries (Table 1). In all studies birds are found to be colonized primarily with *C. jejuni,* less often with *C. coli* and rarely with other species. The relative distribution of *C. jejuni* and *C. coli* strains recovered varies between countries. For example in Denmark, the United Kingdom, and the Netherlands, the proportion of *C. jejuni* is 85, 95, and 65% respectively (19, 48, 71a).

Comparison of data on flock colonization between countries is difficult because of the different isolation methods used. Nevertheless, in Europe there appears to be a consistently lower prevalence of positive flocks in Europe compared to the United Kingdom and The Netherlands (56). The reason for this is unknown. Zootechnical parameters (number of animals per farm, climatic conditions, and distance between farms) may all influence the infection rate. It is also possible that the poultry industries in these Northern European coun-

TABLE 1 Flock colonization on farms in northern Europe

Country	% of positive flocks	Total no. of flocks	Survey type	Reference
The Netherlands	57	112	Longitudinal	69
	82	187	Longitudinal	28
United Kingdom	27	251	Longitudinal	53
	45	151	Cross-sectional	19
	95	200	Longitudinal	19
Denmark	47 (average)		National survey 1996–1998	24
Norway	18	176	Longitudinal	31
Sweden	27	287	Longitudinal	9
	10–16	622	Longitudinal	8

tries are less mature and more closely regulated than elsewhere in Europe. No recent data on flock positivity is available from the United States and Canada except for the contamination levels on poultry carcasses at retail. Given the opportunity for cross-contamination within the abattoir, this is not a good measure of flock colonization.

Several surveys have indicated a seasonal variation in the prevalence of poultry flock colonization. This seasonality generally demonstrates a higher rate of infection in summer than in winter (9, 24, 28). Some studies failed to demonstrate a seasonality in the prevalence of poultry campylobacters (26), but this may reflect of the sample size and flock selection. The reason for this seasonal variation is unknown but probably reflects levels of environmental contamination. Certainly poultry houses have more ventilation in the summer, increasing the contact of the birds with the outside environment. Interestingly, no accurate comparisons with the seasonality in human infections have been published. The recent Danish report (24) suggests that the seasonal variation in humans coincides with or even precedes, rather than following, that in poultry. Similar observations have been made by Swedish researchers (18a). Such data appear to be inconsistent with a close association between the consumption of contaminated poultry meat and human disease.

Given the high levels of colonization in chickens and the optimal growth temperature of these organisms, it is assumed that the thermophilic campylobacters have evolved to optimally grow in the avian gut microenvironment. Significant levels of infection occur in poultry other than chickens, including ducks, pigeon, quails, ostriches, and turkeys (24, 72, 78). There are a few studies of infection rates in wild birds and noncommercial birds held in capture. Without exception, campylobacters have been found in all these avian hosts, albeit with some differences in prevalence (3, 22, 51). Usually such colonization does not cause clinical disease in the birds. However, in ostriches, campylobacter infection can be associated with hepatitis (59) or acute, sometimes fatal, enteritis (71).

NATURE AND MECHANISM OF COLONIZATION

The sites and extent of naturally occurring colonization in poultry remain largely uninvestigated. Experimentally, colonization is found largely in the ceca and is confined primarily to the intestinal mucus layer in the crypts of the intestinal epithelium (7). There is no close association with intestinal epithelial cells. However, campylobacters have been recovered from extraintestinal sites (7), including the liver and spleen, even in asymptomatic birds (14a), suggesting that some translocation across the intestinal epithelium is a normal part of the colonization process. This may be the reason for the strong systemic specific immune response despite the apparent commensal nature of the infection in chickens (12).

It is clear from longitudinal studies in commercial broiler houses that there is an age-related increase in prevalence. In most flocks investigated, there is no detectable colonization until at least 10 days of age. In preliminary studies in the Netherlands, only about 10% of flocks are detectably colonized by 2 weeks of age (71a). The reason for this lag phase is unknown but is unlikely to be due to lack of exposure to this ubiquitous organism. Experimentally, birds are susceptible to infection with even very low doses of organisms during this early phase of life (14), but under field conditions, the birds undergo several changes in management during this period, including feed composition, and the effect of these on susceptibility has not been investigated. Nevertheless, the mechanisms of this lag phase may be exploitable to provide a method of infection control. Putative mechanisms of resistance to colonization during this lag phase include the presence of maternal antibodies, antibiotic feed additives, and competitive members of the gut flora. Considerably more research is required to establish the nature and mechanism of this effect.

The duration of colonization and shedding in poultry is not fully determined. It is generally

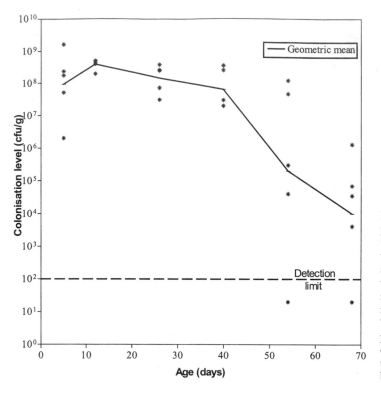

FIGURE 1 Colonization of experimentally infected chickens. One-day-old chickens were dosed with 10^4 CFU of *C. jejuni* 81116, and the cecal contents were harvested over time. The dosing and recovery of organisms were performed as previously described (75). The limit of detection was 10^2 CFU per g of cecal contents; therefore, data below this limit indicate negative birds. Figure kindly provided by S. Cawthraw.

accepted that chickens, once colonized with campylobacters, remain chronically infected for many weeks. For broiler chickens, this condition continues until slaughter. However, in experimentally infected birds, colonization may gradually reduce in terms of both the level of organisms recoverable from the cecal contents and the number of infected birds (Fig. 1). In one study (1) the prevalence of infection in birds housed individually was less than 40%, a major decline from the rate of more than 80% in birds housed communally. Self-limitation of infection has been reported in other naturally infected birds. For example, gulls can become negative for *Campylobacter* within a period of 4 weeks (23).

In several studies in which campylobacter colonization of broilers has been investigated in detail, mixed infections are frequently described (8, 29, 68). Strains may differ in their capacity to colonize chickens (35, 42) and strains with a high colonization potential are able to replace others (35). Such facts may be

important when subtyping methods are used for strain tracing, since minor bacterial populations may not be detected.

MODELS OF AVIAN COLONIZATION

Many targeted intervention measures developed, especially those affecting susceptibility to colonization, will require the establishment of appropriate models for experimentally testing the efficacy of the control strategy. Suitable models should be quantitative and, if possible, dose related to ensure that minor differences in the colonization potential of strains and mutants are detected (46). They should also mimic the natural infection as closely as possible, and birds of known infection and immune status should be used. Several models have been described, and these vary substantially in the method and level of dose, the age, immune status, and housing of the birds, and the method of measurement of colonization. One major difference is in the method of infection, i.e., either by the oral administration of bacteria by gavage of all birds at one time or by the introduction of birds with an established infection (seeder birds) to uninfected birds. These two methods model quite separate phases of flock infection. The latter mimics the transmission of the organisms through the flock. Under natural conditions, the route of transmission is probably fecal-oral aided by the fact that birds in the confined conditions of the broiler house are extremely coprophagic. In vivo passage through chickens increases the colonization potential of some strains, particularly those which are laboratory attenuated. This increase can be as much as 10,000-fold (14). Thus, the seeder bird model can provide a measure of the infectiveness of the bacteria. Nevertheless, oral administration more closely mimics the primary events leading to initial infection of the flock. Because the campylobacters, transmitted from an environmental source, are likely to be at low dose levels and stressed by hostile conditions such as temperature, nutrient depletion, osmotic shock, or disinfectants, these bacteria may have a reduced colonization potential in chickens (20). This could be important in the assessment of the efficacy of protection measures like vaccination and competitive exclusion. The levels of protection required to control this initial infection may be far less demanding at this initial phase of an outbreak than during subsequent phases, where transmission occurs more readily.

The biological background of the birds used in such studies is also inherently important to the outcome of colonization studies. Age, genetic lineage, and immune status (passive or active immunity) may all be relevant to their susceptibility to colonization. The campylobacter infection status of the parent flocks is rarely stated, and insufficient work has been done in comparing the susceptibility of chickens from commercial breeds with that of specific-pathogen-free chickens bred for experimental purposes. There is an urgent need for comparative studies between laboratories to test the range of models available.

Despite these difficulties, the models which have been developed have already proved useful for identifying bacterial factors involved in avian-gut colonization. Several such factors have been investigated by using a series of defined mutants with mutations in the genes for putative colonization factors for the animal models described below. It is clear that some bacterial factors are essential for optimal chicken colonization; these include products of the *flaA*, *flaB*, *sod*, *htrA*, and *racR* genes but not those of the *cat* or *peb1A* genes (10, 41, 45, 46, 54, 75). Definition of essential colonization factors is likely to become an important component of any targeted intervention strategy in the future.

INTERVENTION STRATEGIES

In principle, intervention to control *C. jejuni* contamination of poultry meat could occur at any stage from farm to fork. However, it is generally considered that, excluding meat decontamination methods such as irradiation (see chapter 24), control strategies should be applied primarily at the farm level. This is largely because abattoir contamination from the gut contents of the first colonized flock which enters the poultry line affects all subsequent flocks regardless of their campylobacter status. Although significant proportions of campylobacters can survive in the abattoir environment, it is unlikely that they can grow under these conditions, and so the numbers decline during processing (see chapter 24). Several intervention strategies at the poultry production level are currently being developed. The most effective approach will probably be a stratified one with initial measures to minimize exposure of the flock to the organism and subsequent measures to prevent any such exposure from leading to maximal colonization.

BIOSECURITY

The sources of infection of poultry flocks are still debatable. Vertical transmission via contaminated eggs although reported (53), is highly controversial (63). Certainly, isolation of campylobacters from eggs is very infrequent and results mainly from fecal contamination of the shells (29, 68). Moreover, surveys indicate that there is no direct relationship between flock positivity and hatchery source, suggesting that vertical transmission is unlikely.

All the evidence suggests that the primary transmission route is horizontal, from organisms contaminating the environment around and within the broiler house. The roles of many of the potential sources are reviewed elsewhere (56, 61). Several more recent epidemiological studies have been undertaken to identify management and other factors associated with flock infection (19, 26, 27, 31, 52, 68). There are some differences in the risk factors identified between studies, but poor broiler house maintenance (as indicated by large rodent populations and poor building repair), inadequate staff training (including the use of boot dips and changing of outer clothing), insufficient cleansing and disinfection between flocks (including reuse of old litter), close location to other poultry sites or farm animals, and contaminated water supplies (poorly cleaned water pipes or polluted stored water) are all implicated. Rapid dissemination of organisms throughout the flock is then facilitated by communal drinkers and feed lines.

The role of viable-but-nonculturable campylobacters (VNC) as a source of poultry infection has also been controversial. Epidemiological studies (52) implicated such forms as waterborne sources. However, results of in vivo studies with chickens and experimentally induced VNC to demonstrate the colonization potential of such forms have been contradictory (21, 40, 64). Given the differences in models, strains, VNC induction, and doses administered, it is difficult to compare the data, but although extremely large numbers of VNC administered to chickens may induce some colonization, the colonization potential of VNC forms is at best severely reduced and is most likely to be negligible. Moreover, the types of environmental stresses, such as nutrient depletion, which induce VNC formation rapidly negate the colonization potential even of culturable campylobacters (20).

The primary intervention strategy adopted to date has been to enhance biosecurity in an attempt to prevent the entrance of the organism into the broiler house from the environment. This approach has been relatively empirical, focusing on simple intervention measures such as use of closed houses, provision of clean feed and water, elimination of rodents and wild birds, restrictions on the staff and equipment entering the house, and improved hygiene procedures by poultry house workers, concentrating on changing of outer clothes and efficient dipping of boots. Significant reduction in campylobacter infection in broilers after the application of strict hygienic measures has been reported (70). However, the maintenance of such measures on the farm is extremely difficult, and during a follow-up inspection shortly after this study finished, infection returned to the original level (68a). It also is claimed that such measures have been successful in some countries (Sweden, Norway, and Finland), but data supporting this information is not yet publicly available. Similar measures in other countries, such as the United Kingdom, although generally effective in reducing *Salmonella* infections of flocks, only appear to delay the onset of colonization by campylobacters (Fig. 2) and do not predictably prevent positive flocks at slaughter. These results suggest that intervention will have to be more targeted in the future to be effective.

Targeted biosecurity requires the identification of specific sources and accurate tracing of transmission routes. Such information demands appropriate strain-subtyping techniques. Serotyping has been used for this purpose but is largely ineffective due to the occurrence of a large proportion of nontypeable strains among poultry isolates. The recent introduction of molecular typing techniques, like *fla* typing, pulsed-field gel electrophoresis, randomly amplified polymorphic DNA, riboprinting, and amplification fragment length polymorphism (see chapter 2) is proving successful. One major problem appears to be that the environment surrounding broiler houses containing positive flocks becomes so heavily contaminated that determining the routes of strain transmission—for example, puddles to chickens or

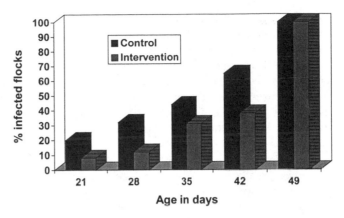

FIGURE 2 Effect of improved biosecurity, including boot dipping and changing of outer clothing, on flock positivity. Data kindly provided by J. Gibbens.

chickens to puddles—is very difficult without performing longitudinal studies prior to flock colonization. However, preliminary studies with such molecular epidemiological tools in the United Kingdom and the Netherlands confirm the roles of wild birds, surface standing water, boots of personnel and other animals in the immediate locality as sources of infection and, in addition, have highlighted the role of unauthorized entrance points into the poultry houses (46b, 70).

Biosecurity can provide only a preliminary barrier. The organisms are too ubiquitous in the environment to be totally excluded. Moreover, the measures recommended have proved difficult to enforce and monitor and are generally too draconian for the industry in most countries to maintain. Supplementary measures, to prevent poultry colonization by any campylobacters penetrating the primary barriers, will almost certainly be required.

COMPETITIVE EXCLUSION AND USE OF PROBIOTICS

Competitive exclusion has been a relatively successful approach for the control of some bacterial infections, particularly salmonellosis, in poultry. The principle was developed from original observations by Nurmi and Rantala (50) and exploits the competition between microbiological agents for similar ecological niches. The concept seems most appropriate for microorganisms colonizing the gut, where

nutrients are generally limited and competitors are numerous. Early experiments indicated that some undefined members of the avian intestinal flora can partly protect birds from campylobacter colonization, particularly when applied under field conditions (44). However, this effect is unpredictable, and to be practically feasible, competitive exclusion agents should be isolated and maintained by in vitro culture. Isolates derived under various conditions from chicken feces, intestinal contents, or members of the mucosa-associated flora have been tried. Their efficacy against campylobacter colonization appears variable at best. Some preparations can reduce the level of colonization (39, 60), and apparently even commercially available competitive exclusion agents can achieve substantial reductions in both the level and prevalence of campylobacter colonization in some experiments (23a, 77). However, in other experiments, similar agents had no effect despite showing efficacy against salmonellosis (4). Such inconsistencies may reflect the variable content of the competitive agents, which is, of course, significantly influenced by the status of the donor birds, the site from which the starter material is collected, and the culture conditions used (39, 57). Because the nature of such agents is complex and generally undefined, maintenance of material active against campylobacters during bulk production may be particularly difficult, especially if obligate anaerobes are involved (39). In vitro assays suggest that effective agents may produce anticampylobacter metabolites (39, 58), which may enable more effective screening of potential agents.

Obviously, a defined flora, which would provide predictable efficacy against *C. jejuni*, would be optimal. Preliminary studies (57) have identified some of the bacteria located in the mucus layer of the cecum which appear to have anticampylobacter activity. Up to nine of these bacteria, when administered orally as a mixture, partially protect chickens against experimental colonization by *C. jejuni*. Further work is obviously needed on this approach.

Although the ability of other microorganisms to protect chickens from campylobacter colonization may be limited, they may have therapeutic potential. The oral administration of the yeast *Saccharomyces boulardii* to campylobacter-infected broilers reduces the level, although not the prevalence, of cecal colonization (38). Similar results have been obtained with a mixture of *Lactobacillus acidophilus* and *Streptococcus faecium* (43). Such activity would be extremely useful to reduce the effects of stress induced by transportation from the farm to the abattoir (62), especially when coupled with management practices such as feed withdrawal (11), which enhance the excretion of campylobacters by poultry. However, the effect of administration of such probiotics on the overall contamination levels on the retail product has yet to be assessed.

The difficulties in the development of a competitive exclusion agent for campylobacter is surprising, given the success of this approach for salmonellosis, but they probably reflect the unique ecological niche occupied by campylobacters. A possible alternative approach (74) is to use campylobacter strains, which have a high colonizing potential but are nonpathogenic, as competitive excluders of potentially pathogenic environmental strains (homologous competitive exclusion). The success of such an approach is dependent on (i) the identification of highly colonizing strains which will exclude or replace other strains, (ii) the identification and elimination of virulence factors from these strains, and (iii) the stability of this nonpathogenic phenotype. By using oral models of

chicken colonization, highly colonizing strains have been identified (14, 35). Such strains can replace existing colonizing strains (35) and outcompete others during multiple-strain challenge experiments (15a). Further experiments have shown that the mutation of at least some potential virulence genes, for example the *fla* genes (75), *peb1A* (41), and *cat* (4), have little or no effect on colonization potential in the avian gut. Finally, by using mutants marked with antibiotic cassettes, there is evidence that natural transformation does not occur in the avian gut (73), so that an avirulent phenotype should remain stable during in vivo passage. Obviously, considerable further work is needed to confirm and expand these results so that such homologous competitive excluders can be effectively designed.

VACCINATION

Chickens colonized with *C. jejuni* induce both systemic and mucosal humoral responses (12, 76) of immunoglobulin G (IgG), IgA, and IgM isotypes. Strong systemic antibody induction, generally unexpected in commensal gut bacteria, may be a consequence of bacterial translocation across the intestinal epithelium. These antibodies are directed against a variety of *C. jejuni* antigens, including flagellin. Interestingly, this specificity may be compartmentalized, such that a narrower spectrum of antigens is detected by mucosal than by circulating antibodies (12).

The potentially protective nature of these anticampylobacter antibodies is debatable. Colonization in broilers appears to be chronic, at least to the point of slaughter, once established, but the levels of colonization decline by at least 8 weeks of age in experimentally infected birds (Fig. 1), which is consistent with the kinetics of the antibody responses. Such antibody responses appear to protect the birds at least partly from rechallenge with the homologous strain (13) following clearance of the primary infection with antibiotics.

Effective vaccine strategies directed against campylobacters in broiler chickens have yet to be developed. Such strategies must either provide protection from exposure, presumably from the first day of age to the point of slaughter, or must eliminate colonization by the time of slaughter. Given that the average life span of broiler chickens is only 6 weeks, this is a very short period in which to induce effective antibody responses, especially in an immunologically immature animal. An alternative, or complementary, strategy is passive immunization. Orally administered anticampylobacter antibodies have both therapeutic and prophylactic properties in chickens (66, 67). Therefore, one approach may be to immunize parent flocks to produce passively protected chickens. Detectable circulating IgG antibodies are present in young chickens (12) and are presumably maternally derived. It is not unlikely that these antibodies contribute to the lag phase in infection. The improvement and extension of the protective capacity of any such maternally derived immune protection requires further investigation.

The choice of the vaccine candidates and delivery systems will dictate the outcome of any immunization. Killed vaccines and subunit vaccines, such as flagellin, administered parenterally may provide partial protection (76). However, parenteral immunization, although feasible for breeder flocks, would be too costly for broilers. Oral delivery systems would be less expensive and easier to administer. Orally delivered killed vaccines have little if any protective capacity, even when delivered with mucosal adjuvants (13, 55) unless they are coupled (33). Nevertheless, in ovo vaccination may overcome some of these problems and can certainly induce immune responses, although the protective capacity of such responses has yet to be determined (49).

Oral live vaccines currently appear to be the candidates of choice. Two possible approaches are being considered: (i) live campylobacters which would colonize chickens but be nonpathogenic to humans and (ii) live vectors, such as attenuated *Salmonella,* genetically engineered to express campylobacter antigens. Live vaccines may also act as competitive exclusion agents, giving additional protection (6). The choice of antigens is critical. Antigens inducing protective immune responses are unidentified. However, preliminary experimental studies of passive immunity initiated by mouse monoclonal antibodies suggest that such antibodies directed against flagella may induce partial protection in chickens (59a). The *flaA* gene has been expressed in *Salmonella* vectors like *S. enteritidis* (18) or *S. typhimurium* (32). The engineered product can confer partial protection. This protection is more significant against challenge with the homologous strain than against challenge with a heterologous strain (32). Whether the efficacy of this response can be enhanced by improving antigen presentation or expression has yet to be determined.

The results to date suggest that vaccination of chickens may be a feasible strategy for reducing, but is unlikely to prevent, colonization. However, under field conditions, the challenge dose is likely to be low and the bacteria are likely to be environmentally stressed, which may enhance vaccine efficacy.

OTHER POTENTIAL INTERVENTION MEASURES

Several other novel intervention strategies have been suggested for control of campylobacter colonization in chickens (6). By using inbred chicken lines, genetically linked resistance to some avian bacterial infections, such as salmonellosis, has been demonstrated. However, the basis for this resistance and its role in a commensal organism like *C. jejuni* have been relatively poorly investigated, although there is preliminary evidence that the host lineage can influence resistance to this infection (65). The administration of virulent bacteriophages has been successfully used in some serious bacterial infections. Campylobacters are susceptible to a range of bacteriophages. However, bacteriophage activity is campylobacter subtype dependent, and resistance can be induced, possibly as a consequence of genomic instability (see chapter 18). Thus, the frequent therapeutic application of such agents may result in amplification of bacteriophage-resistant campylobacters in the environment.

CONCLUSION

In conclusion, campylobacteriosis in humans is a serious and apparently increasing problem with huge social and economic consequences worldwide. The contamination of meat products, especially poultry, by campylobacters appears to be a significant risk factor. The problem of campylobacters in the food chain must be urgently addressed, but there seem to be no immediate solutions available. The strategies so successful for controlling salmonella infection in poultry are generally ineffective against campylobacters. To identify a practical and sustainable strategy, more information about the epidemiology, physiology, and ecology of this group of organisms in the avian host is required.

ACKNOWLEDGMENTS

We thank S. Cawthraw and J. Gibbens (Veterinary Laboratories Agency, Weybridge) for Fig. 1 and 2. We acknowledge the financial support of the Ministry of Agriculture, Fisheries and Foods, London, United Kingdom.

REFERENCES

1. **Achen, M., T. Y. Morishita, and E. C. Ley.** 1998. Shedding and colonization of *Campylobacter jejuni* in broilers from day-of-hatch to slaughter age. *Avian Dis.* **42**:732–737.

2. **Adak, G. K., J. M. Cowden, S. Nicholas, and H. S. Evans.** 1995. The Public Health Laboratory Service national case-control study of primary indigenous sporadic cases of campylobacter infection. *Epidemiol. Infect.* **115**:15–22.

3. **Adesiyun, A. A., K. Caesar, and L. Inder.** 1998. Prevalence of *Salmonella* and *Campylobacter* species in animals at the Emperor Valley Zoo. *Trinidad J. Zoo Wildl. Med.* **29**:237–239.

4. **Aho, M., L. Nuotio, E. Nurmi, and T. Kiiskinen.** 1992. Competitive exclusion of campylobacters from poultry with K-bacteria and Broilact. *Int. J. Food Microbiol.* **15**:265–275.

5. **Annan-Prah, A., and M. Janc.** 1988. The mode of spread of *Campylobacter jejuni/coli* to broiler flocks. *Zentralbl. Veterinarmed Reihe* B **35**:11–18.

6. **Barrow, P. A.** 1997. Novel approaches to control of bacterial infections in animals. *Acta Vet. Hung.* **45**:317–329.

7. **Beery, J. T., M. B. Hugdahl, and M. P. Doyle.** 1988. Colonization of gastrointestinal tracts of chicks by *Campylobacter jejuni*. *Appl. Environ. Microbiol.* **54**:2365–2370.

8. **Berndtson, E.** 1996. *Campylobacter in Broiler Chickens.* Ph.D. thesis. Swedish University of Agricultural Sciences, Uppsala, Sweden.

9. **Berndtson, E., M. L. Danielsson-Tham, and A. Engvall.** 1996. Campylobacter incidence on a chicken farm and the spread of *Campylobacter* during the slaughter process. *Int. J. Food Microbiol.* **32**:35–47.

10. **Bras, A. M., S. Chatterjee, B. W. Wren, D. G. Newell, and J. M. Ketley.** 1999. A novel *Campylobacter jejuni* two component regulatory system important for temperature-dependent growth and colonization. *J. Bacteriol.* **181**:3298–3302.

11. **Byrd, J. A., D. E. Corrier, M. E. Hume, R. H. Bailey, L. H. Stanker, and B. M. Hargis.** 1998. Effect of feed withdrawal on *Campylobacter* in the crops of market-age broiler chickens. *Avian Dis.* **42**:802–806.

12. **Cawthraw, S., R. Ayling, P. Nuijten, T. Wassenaar, and D. G. Newell.** 1994. Isotype, specificity, and kinetics of systemic and mucosal antibodies to *Campylobacter jejuni* antigens, including flagellin, during experimental oral infections of chickens. *Avian Dis.* **38**:341–349.

13. **Cawthraw, S. A., C. Gorringe, and D. G. Newell.** 1998. Prior infection, but not a killed vaccine, reduces colonization of chickens by *Campylobacter jejuni*, p. 364–367. *In* A. J. Lastovica, D. G. Newell, and E. E. Lastovica (ed.), *Campylobacter, Helicobacter and Related Organisms.* University of Cape Town, Cape Town, South Africa.

14. **Cawthraw, S. A., T. M. Wassenaar, R. Ayling, and D. G. Newell.** 1996. Increased colonization potential of *Campylobacter jejuni* strain 81116 after passage through chickens and its implication on the rate of transmission within flocks. *Epidemiol. Infect.* **117**:213–215.

14a. **Cawthraw, S. A.** Unpublished data.

15. **Clow, K., S. F. Park, P. R. Hawtin, V. Korolik, and D. G. Newell.** 1998. The genotypic comparison of *Campylobacter jejuni* strains from poultry and humans, p. 368–369. *In* A. J. Lastovica, D. G. Newell, and E. E. Lastovica (ed.), *Campylobacter, Helicobacter and Related Organisms.* University of Cape Town, Cape Town, South Africa.

15a. **Clow, K.** Personal communication.

16. **de Boer, E., and M. Hahné.** 1990. Cross-contamination with *Campylobacter jejuni* and *Salmonella* spp. from raw chicken products during food preparation. *J. Food Prot.* **53**:1067–1068.

17. **Deming, M. S., R. V. Tauxe, P. A. Blake, S. E. Dixon, B. S. Fowler, T. S. Jones, E. A. Lockamy, C. M. Patton, and R. O. Sikes.** 1987. *Campylobacter* enteritis at a university: trans-

mission from eating chicken and from cats. *Am. J. Epidemiol.* **126:**526–534. (Erratum, **126:**1220.)

18. **Ellen-Vercoe, E., S. Cawthraw, D. G. Newell, and M. J. Woodward.** 1996. Expression of *Campylobacter jejuni flaA* epitopes within a modified salmonella flagellin in *Salmonella enteritidis*, p. 667–672. *In* D. G. Newell, J. M. Ketley, and R. A. Feldman (ed.), *Campylobacters, Helicobacters and Related Organisms*. Plenum Press, New York, NY.

18a. **Engvall, A.** Personal communication.

19. **Evans, S. A.** 1997. *Epidemiological studies of Salmonella and Campylobacter in poultry.* Ph.D. thesis. University of London, London, United Kingdom.

20. **Fearnley, C., S. Cawthraw, and D. G. Newell.** 1998. Sub-lethal injury to, and colonization potential of, *Campylobacter jejuni* strain 81116, p. 181–183. *In* A. J. Lastovica, D. G. Newell, and E. E. Lastovica (ed.), *Campylobacter, Helicobacter and Related Organisms*. University of Cape Town, Cape Town, South Africa.

21. **Fearnley, C., R. Ayling, S. Cawthraw, and D. G. Newell.** 1996. The formation of viable but non-culturable *C. jejuni* and their failure to colonize one-day-old chicks, p. 101–104. *In* D. G. Newell, J. M. Ketley, and R. A. Feldman (ed.), *Helicobacters, Campylobacters, and Related Organisms*. Plenum Press, New York, N.Y.

22. **Fernandez, H., K. Kahler, R. Salazar, and M. A. Rios.** 1994. Prevalence of thermotolerant species of *Campylobacter* and their biotypes in children and domestic birds and dogs in southern Chile. *Rev. Inst. Med. Trop. Sao Paulo* **36:**433–436.

23. **Glunder, G., U. Neumann, and S. Braune.** 1992. Occurrence of *Campylobacter* spp. in young gulls, duration of *Campylobacter* infection and reinfection by contact. *J. Vet. Med. Soc. B* **39:**119–122.

23a. **Hakkinen, M., and C. Schneitz.** Personal communication.

24. **Hald, T., H. C. Wegener, and B. B. Jorgensen.** 1999. *Annual Report on Zoonoses in Denmark 1998.* Ministry of Food, Agriculture and Fisheries, Copenhagen, Denmark.

25. **Harris, N. V., D. Thompson, D. C. Martin, and C. M. Nolan.** 1986. A survey of Campylobacter and other bacterial contaminants of premarket chicken and retail poultry and meats, King County, Washington. *Am. J. Public Health* **76:**401–406.

26. **Humphrey, T. J., A. Henley, and D. G. Lanning.** 1993. The colonization of broiler chickens with *Campylobacter jejuni:* some epidemiological investigations. *Epidemiol. Infect.* **110:**601–607.

27. **Jacobs-Reitsma, W. F.** 1997. Aspects of epidemiology of *Campylobacter* in poultry. *Vet Q.* **19:**113–117.

28. **Jacobs-Reitsma, W. F., N. M. Bolder, and R. W. Mulder.** 1994. Cecal carriage of Campylobacter and Salmonella in Dutch broiler flocks at slaughter: a one-year study. *Poult. Sci.* **73:**1260–1266.

29. **Jacobs-Reitsma, W. F., A. W. van de Giessen, N. M. Bolder, and R. W. Mulder.** 1995. Epidemiology of *Campylobacter* spp. at two Dutch broiler farms. *Epidemiol. Infect.* **114:**413–421.

30. **Juven, F. T., and M. Rogol.** 1984. Incidence of *Campylobacter jejuni* and *Campylobacter coli* serogroups in a chicken processing factory. *J. Food Prot.* **49:**290–292.

31. **Kapperud, G., E. Skjerve, L. Vik, K. Hauge, A. Lysaker, I. Aalmen, S. M. Ostroff, and M. Potter.** 1993. Epidemiological investigation of risk factors for campylobacter colonization in Norwegian broiler flocks. *Epidemiol. Infect.* **111:**245–255.

32. **Kauc, L., and I. Nachamkin.** 1998. A recombinant *Salmonella typhimurium* strain expressing *Campylobacter jejuni* flagellin confers partial colonization protection in chicks, p. 166–170. *In* A. J. Lastovica, D. G. Newell, and E. E. Lastovica (ed.), *Campylobacter, Helicobacter and Related Organisms*. University of Cape Town, Cape Town, South Africa.

33. **Khoury, C. A., and R. J. Meinersmann.** 1995. A genetic hybrid of the *Campylobacter jejuni flaA* gene with LT-B of *Escherichia coli* and assessment of the efficacy of the hybrid protein as an oral chicken vaccine. *Avian Dis.* **39:**812–820.

34. **Koenraad, P. M., R. Ayling, W. C. Hazeleger, F. M. Rombouts, and D. G. Newell.** 1995. The speciation and subtyping of campylobacter isolates from sewage plants and waste water from a connected poultry abattoir using molecular techniques. *Epidemiol. Infect.* **115:**485–494.

35. **Korolik, V., M. R. Alderton, S. C. Smith, J. Chang, and P. J. Coloe.** 1998. Isolation and molecular analysis of colonising and non-colonising strains of *Campylobacter jejuni* and *Campylobacter coli* following experimental infection of young chickens. *Vet. Microbiol.* **60:**239–249.

36. **Korolik, V., J. Chang, N. Stern, and P. J. Coloe.** 1996. Differentiation of *Campylobacter* strains from chickens in the USA using a DNA probe, p. 203–207. *In* D. G. Newell, J. M. Ketley, and R. A. Feldman (ed.), *Campylobacters, Helicobacters and Related Organisms*. Plenum Press, New York, NY.

37. **Korolik, V., L. Moorthy, and P. J. Coloe.** 1995. Differentiation of *Campylobacter jejuni* and *Campylobacter coli* strains by using restriction endonuclease DNA profiles and DNA fragment polymorphisms. *J. Clin. Microbiol.* **33:**1136–1140.

38. **Line, J. E., J. S. Bailey, N. A. Cox, and N. J.**

Stern. 1997. Yeast treatment to reduce *Salmonella* and *Campylobacter* populations associated with broiler chickens subjected to transport stress. *Poult. Sci.* **76:**1227–1231.

39. **Mead, G. C., M. J. Scott, T. J. Humphrey, and McAlpine.** 1996. Observations on the control of *Campylobacter jejuni* infection of poultry by 'competitive exclusion'. *Avian Pathol.* **25:**69–79.

40. **Medema, G. J., F. M. Schets, A. W. van de Giessen, and A. H. Havelaar.** 1992. Lack of colonization of 1 day old chicks by viable, nonculturable *Campylobacter jejuni. J. Appl. Bacteriol.* **72:**512–516.

41. **Meinersmann, R. J., Z. Pei, and M. J. Blaser.** 1996. Capacity of a *peb1A* mutant of *Campylobacter jejuni* to colonize chickens, p. 597–598. *In* D. G. Newell, J. M. Ketley, and R. A. Feldman (ed.), *Campylobacters, Helicobacters, and Related Organisms.* Plenum Press, New York, NY.

42. **Meinersmann, R. J., W. E. Rigsby, N. J. Stern, L. C. Kelley, J. E. Hill, and M. P. Doyle.** 1991. Comparative study of colonizing and noncolonizing *Campylobacter jejuni. Am. J. Vet. Res.* **52:**1518–1522.

43. **Morishita, T. Y., P. P. Aye, B. S. Harr, C. W. Cobb, and J. R. Clifford.** 1997. Evaluation of an avian-specific probiotic to reduce the colonization and shedding of *Campylobacter jejuni* in broilers. *Avian Dis.* **41:**850–855.

44. **Mulder, R. W. A. W., and N. M. Bolder.** 1991. Experience with competitive exclusion in the Netherlands, p. 77–89. *In* L. C. Blankenship (ed.), *Colonization Control of Human Bacterial Enteropathogens in Poultry.* Academic Press, Inc., San Diego, Calif.

45. **Nachamkin, I., X. H. Yang, and N. J. Stern.** 1993. Role of *Campylobacter jejuni* flagella as colonization factors for three-day-old chicks: analysis with flagellar mutants. *Appl. Environ. Microbiol.* **59:**1269–1273.

46. **Newell, D. G., S. Cawthraw, C. Fearnley, T. Wassenaar, and R. A. Ayling.** 1996. Bacterial factors involved in the colonisation of poultry by *Campylobacter jejuni/coli* and strategies for control, p. 51–55. *In* B. Nagy, E. Nurmi, and R. W. A. W. Mulder (ed.), *COST Action 97. Pathogenic Microorganisms in Poultry and Eggs. Protection of Poultry from Foodborne Pathogens.* European Commission, Brussels, Belgium.

46a. **Newell, D. G., and J. A. Frost.** Unpublished data.

46b. **Newell, D. G., and W. F. Jacobs-Reitsma.** Unpublished data.

47. **Nielsen, E. M., J. Engberg, and M. Madsen.** 1997. Distribution of serotypes of *Campylobacter jejuni* and *C. coli* from Danish patients, poultry, cattle and swine. *FEMS Immunol. Med. Microbiol.* **19:**47–56.

48. **Nielsen, E. M., and N. L. Nielsen.** 1999. Serotypes and typability of *Campylobacter jejuni* and *Campylobacter coli* isolated from poultry products. *Int. J. Food Microbiol.* **46:**199–205.

49. **Noor, S. M., A. J. Husband, and P. R. Widders.** 1995. *In ovo* oral vaccination with *Campylobacter jejuni* establishes early development of intestinal immunity in chickens. *Br. Poult. Sci.* **36:**563–573.

50. **Nurmi, E., and M. Rantala.** 1973. New aspects of *Salmonella* infection in broiler production. *Nature* **241:**210–211.

51. **Oyarzabal, O. A., D. E. Conner, and F. J. Hoerr.** 1995. Incidence of campylobacters in the intestine of avian species in Alabama. *Avian Dis.* **39:**147–151.

52. **Pearson, A. D., M. Greenwood, T. D. Healing, D. Rollins, M. Shahamat, J. Donaldson, and R. R. Colwell.** 1993. Colonization of broiler chickens by waterborne *Campylobacter jejuni. Appl. Environ. Microbiol.* **59:**987–996.

53. **Pearson, A. D., M. H. Greenwood, R. K. Feltham, T. D. Healing, J. Donaldson, D. M. Jones, and R. R. Colwell.** 1996. Microbial ecology of *Campylobacter jejuni* in a United Kingdom chicken supply chain: intermittent common source, vertical transmission, and amplification by flock propagation. *Appl. Environ. Microbiol.* **62:**4614–4620.

54. **Purdy, D., S. Cawthraw, J. H. Dickinson, D. G. Newell, and S. F. Park.** 1999. Generation of a superoxide dismutase (SOD)-deficient mutant of *Campylobacter coli:* evidence for the significance of SOD in *Campylobacter* survival and colonization *Appl. Environ. Microbiol.* **65:**2540–2546.

55. **Rice, B. E., D. M. Rollins, E. T. Mallinson, L. Carr, and S. W. Joseph.** 1997. *Campylobacter jejuni* in broiler chickens: colonization and humoral immunity following oral vaccination and experimental infection. *Vaccine* **15:**1922–1932.

56. **Saleha, A. A., G. C. Mead, and A. L. Ibrahim.** 1998. *Campylobacter jejuni* in poultry production and processing in relation to public health. *World's Poult. Sci. J.* **54:**49–57.

57. **Schoeni, J. L., and M. P. Doyle.** 1992. Reduction of *Campylobacter jejuni* colonization of chicks by cecum-colonizing bacteria producing anti-*C. jejuni* metabolites. *Appl. Environ. Microbiol.* **58:**664–670.

58. **Schoeni, J. L., and A. C. Wong.** 1994. Inhibition of *Campylobacter jejuni* colonization in chicks by defined competitive exclusion bacteria. *Appl. Environ. Microbiol.* **60:**1191–1197.

59. **Stephens, C. P., S. L. W. On, and J. A. Gibson.** 1998. An outbreak of infectious hepatitis in

commercially reared ostriches associated with *Campylobacter coli* and *Campylobacter jejuni*. *Vet. Microbiol.* **61**:183–190.

59a. Stern, N. Personal communication.

60. Stern, N. J. 1994. Mucosal competitive exclusion to diminish colonization of chickens by *Campylobacter jejuni*. *Poult. Sci.* **73**:402–407.

61. Stern, N. J. 1992. Reservoirs for *Campylobacter jejuni* and approaches for intervention in poultry, p. 49–60. *In* I. Nachamkin, M. J. Blaser, and L. S. Tompkins (ed.), *Campylobacter jejuni: Current Topics and Future Trends.* ASM Press, Washington, DC.

62. Stern, N. J., M. R. Clavero, J. S. Bailey, N. A. Cox, and M. C. Robach. 1995. *Campylobacter* spp. in broilers on the farm and after transport. *Poult. Sci.* **74**:937–941.

63. Stern, N. J., and W. F. Jacobs-Reitsma. 1998. Poultry infections and their control, p. 353–356. *In* A. L. Lastovica, D. G. Newell, and E. E. Lastovica (ed.), *Campylobacter, Helicobacter and Related Organisms.* University of Cape Town, Cape Town, South Africa.

64. Stern, N. J., D. M. Jones, I. V. Wesley, and D. M. Rollins. 1994. Colonization of chicks by non-culturable *Campylobacter* spp. *Lett. Appl. Microbiol.* **18**:333–336.

65. Stern, N. J., R. J. Meinersmann, N. A. Cox, J. S. Bailey, and L. C. Blankenship. 1990. Influence of host lineage on cecal colonization by *Campylobacter jejuni* in chickens. *Avian Dis.* **34**:602–606.

66. Stern, N. J., R. J. Meinersmann, and H. W. Dickerson. 1990. Influence of antibody treatment of *Campylobacter jejuni* on the dose required to colonize chicks. *Avian Dis.* **34**:595–601.

67. Tsubokura, K., E. Berndtson, A. Bogstedt, B. Kaijser, M. Kim, M. Ozeki, and L. Hammarstrom. 1997. Oral administration of antibodies as prophylaxis and therapy in *Campylobacter jejuni*-infected chickens. *Clin. Exp. Immunol.* **108**:451–455.

68. van de Giessen, A., S. I. Mazurier, W. Jacobs-Reitsma, W. Jansen, P. Berkers, W. Ritmeester, and K. Wernars. 1992. Study on the epidemiology and control of *Campylobacter jejuni* in poultry broiler flocks. *Appl. Environ. Microbiol.* **58**:1913–1917.

68a. van de Giessen, A. Personal communication.

69. van de Giessen, A. W., B. P. Bloemberg, W. S. Ritmeester, and J. J. Tilburg. 1996. Epide-miological study on risk factors and risk reducing measures for campylobacter infections in Dutch broiler flocks. *Epidemiol. Infect.* **117**:245–250.

70. van de Giessen, A. W., J. J. Tilburg, W. S. Ritmeester, and J. van der Plas. 1998. Reduction of campylobacter infections in broiler flocks by application of hygiene measures. *Epidemiol. Infect.* **121**:57–66.

71. van der Walt, M. L., D. J. Verwood, J. Cloete, A. Olivier, and M. M. Henton. 1998. The association of *Campylobacter jejuni* with outbreaks of enteritis in ostrich chicks, p. 415–417. *In* A. J. Lastovica, D. G. Newell, and F. E. Lastovica (ed.), *Campylobacter, Helicobacter and Related Organisms.* University of Cape Town, Cape Town, South Africa.

71a. Wagenaar, J. Unpublished data.

72. Wallace, J. S., K. N. Stanley, and K. Jones. 1998. The colonization of turkeys by thermophilic campylobacters. *J. Appl. Microbiol.* **85**:224–230.

73. Wassenaar, T. M., B. Geilhausen, and D. G. Newell. 1998. Evidence of genomic instability in *Campylobacter jejuni* isolated from poultry. *Appl. Environ. Microbiol.* **64**:1816–1821.

74. Wassenaar, T. M., D. G. Newell, and B. A. M. van der Zeijst. 1994. Towards the use of attenuated campylobacter mutants as a probioticum in poultry, p. 85–90. *In* J. F. Jensen, M. M. Hinton, and R. W. A. W. Mulder (ed.), FLAIR no 6. *Prevention and Control of Potentially Pathogenic Microorganisms in Poultry and Poultry Meat Processing* vol. 12. *Probiotics and Pathogenicity.* COVP-DLO Het Spelderholt, The Netherlands.

75. Wassenaar, T. M., B. A. van der Zeijst, R. Ayling, and D. G. Newell. 1993. Colonization of chicks by motility mutants of *Campylobacter jejuni* demonstrates the importance of flagellin A expression. *J. Gen. Microbiol.* **139**:1171–1175.

76. Widders, P. R., R. Perry, W. I. Muir, A. J. Husband, and K. A. Long. 1996. Immunisation of chickens to reduce intestinal colonisation with *Campylobacter jejuni*. *Br. Poult. Sci.* **37**:765–778.

77. Wieliczko, A. 1995. The role of *Campylobacter* spp. in the pathology of poultry. III. Effects of selected feed supplements on the colonization of the alimentary tract of chickens by *C. jejuni*. *Med. Weten.* **51**:693–696.

78. Yogasundram, K., S. M. Shane, and K. S. Harrington. 1989. Prevalence of *Campylobacter jejuni* in selected domestic and wild birds in Louisiana. *Avian Dis.* **33**:664–667.

CAMPYLOBACTER PREVENTION AND CONTROL: THE USDA-FOOD SAFETY AND INSPECTION SERVICE ROLE AND NEW FOOD SAFETY APPROACHES

Gerri M. Ransom, Bruce Kaplan, Ann Marie McNamara, and I. Kaye Wachsmuth

27

The U.S. Department of Agriculture (USDA) was established in 1862 by a Congressional act signed by President Abraham Lincoln. During the development of this major department of government, the present Food Safety and Inspection Service (FSIS) has evolved into the public health agency within USDA (46). FSIS regulates and inspects meat, poultry, and egg products for use as human food. The purpose is to protect consumers from food-borne illness with the defined mission to ensure that meat, poultry, and egg products are safe, wholesome, and properly marked, labeled, and packaged. Legal authority is granted under the Federal Meat Inspection Act, the Poultry Products Inspection Act, and the Egg Products Inspection Act. The remaining food products in the marketplace fall under the regulatory authority of the Food and Drug Administration (FDA), an agency of the U.S. Department of Health and Human Services (HHS).

To better meet FSIS goals to protect consumer health, the Office of Public Health and Science (OPHS) was created in 1997. The OPHS provides expert scientific support to USDA and FSIS based on the collection and analysis of data. Evaluations of the microbiological, physical, and chemical contamination of meat, poultry, and egg products are conducted by a unique complementary mix of scientists, including microbiologists, epidemiologists, veterinarians, physicians, nurses, parasitologists, pathologists, and chemists. OPHS interacts and coordinates with other public health and government agencies including the Centers for Disease Control and Prevention (CDC), FDA, state and local health and agriculture departments, the Agricultural Research Service (ARS), the Animal and Plant Health Inspection Service (APHIS), the Environmental Protection Agency (EPA), and various law enforcement agencies.

OPHS and FSIS play a leading role in the nation's efforts in improving the safety of meat, poultry, and egg products. Involvement is broad in scope and spans the farm-to-table continuum. One OPHS focus is on human health end points such as those determined through participation in FoodNet and PulseNet Surveillance projects (discussed below). A major goal is to be responsive to

Gerri M. Ransom, Emerging Microbial Issues Branch, Microbiology Division, Office of Public Health and Sciences (OPHS), Food Safety and Inspection Service (FSIS), USDA, 1400 Independence Ave. S.W., Washington, DC 20250-3700. *Bruce Kaplan,* USDA, FSIS, OPHS (Washington, D.C.), 4748 Hamlets Grove Drive, Sarasota, FL 34235. *Ann Marie McNamara,* Sara Lee Foods, Cordova, TN 38018, *formerly* Microbiology Division, OPHS, FSIS, USDA, 1400 Independence Ave. S.W., Washington, DC 20250-3700. *I. Kaye Wachsmuth,* OPHS, FSIS, USDA, 1400 Independence Ave. S.W., Washington, DC 20250-3700.

Campylobacter, 2nd Ed., Edited by I. Nachamkin and M. J. Blaser
© 2000 American Society for Microbiology, Washington, D.C.

food-borne pathogens as they emerge, as has been the case with *Escherichia coli* O157:H7 and *Campylobacter jejuni/coli*. FSIS food safety approaches are exemplified by programs supporting food safety research, nationwide microbial testing, participation in national initiatives, establishment of innovative science-based (risk-based) regulations, promotion of pathogen control techniques, management of food-borne disease incidents, and communication about consumer risk. Summarized below are some FSIS food safety activities, including those focused on *Campylobacter* food-borne disease.

FSIS *CAMPYLOBACTER* WORK

In the 1970s, with the advent and subsequent use of improved culturing techniques, campylobacters were gaining recognition as a common cause of human diarrheal illness (12, 22, 69). During the early 1980s, the FSIS Microbiology Division (presently part of OPHS) began extensive evaluation of available *Campylobacter* testing methods for analysis of meat and poultry products (60). In 1984, FSIS laboratories, in conjunction with the ARS Meat Science Research Laboratory, published the results of a survey of *C. jejuni/coli* in raw meat and poultry products (75). A goal of this work was to determine the prevalence of this pathogen at the point of slaughter from samples collected nationwide to reveal potential sources of the organism in human disease. Campylobacters were isolated from avian, bovine, porcine, and ovine meat species, and no *Campylobacter* prevalence for any meat species was detected above 21.3%. The low prevalences reported, particularly in poultry products, can probably be attributed to the suboptimal recovery methods available at the time. As evidence pointing to *Campylobacter*, particularly *C. jejuni*, as a major food-borne disease threat mounted (11, 68, 77, 79), FSIS continued to recognize *Campylobacter* as a significant food-borne pathogen (48, 54, 59) and conducted studies to improve methodology. In 1992, the *FSIS Method for the Isolation, Identification, and Enumeration of C. jejuni/coli from Meat and Poultry Products* was issued (63).

An updated version of this method was published in the 1998 *FSIS Microbiology Laboratory Guidebook* (MLG) (64). The FSIS MLG *Campylobacter* method is considered a "gold standard" method and is accepted internationally by food microbiologists. However, the method is labor-intensive, especially if quantitative results are desired, and so FSIS continues to work to establish improved protocols.

Today, campylobacters, particularly *C. jejuni*, are known to be a leading cause of human gastroenteritis worldwide (15, 17, 33, 77, 78, 80), and data from the 1996 FoodNet surveillance program established *Campylobacter* as the most commonly diagnosed cause of sporadic food-borne illness in the United States (33). Infections with this organism, as well as those with *Salmonella*, produce effects by tissue invasion (43). Signs include fever, abdominal cramps, and diarrhea. Guillain-Barré syndrome, a central nervous system disorder, and other serious sequelae have been associated epidemiologically with *Campylobacter* infections (1–3, 56). Like *Salmonella* gastroenteritis, formerly identified as the most frequent food-borne enteric infection in the United States, *Campylobacter* infection has been strongly associated with consumption of contaminated poultry (3, 59, 77). *Campylobacter* antimicrobial resistance issues are a recent public health concern, especially relating to fluoroquinolones and the possible links to approval of this drug for use in poultry (3, 70). Campylobacters are ubiquitous in the animal environment, since they are commensal inhabitants of the gastrointestinal tracts of wild and domestic cattle, sheep, swine, goats, dogs, cats, rodents, poultry, and other birds (42, 47). Most human *Campylobacter* infections probably originate as a result of some form of fecal contamination by an animal through food or by direct contact. However, the source of infecting organisms in sporadic cases is frequently obscure (6).

The above information, along with other established food safety frameworks and milestones mentioned below, have helped to strengthen the FSIS commitment to reduce food-borne disease and provide the impetus for accelerated efforts to improve food safety, including those that specifically target *Campylobacter.*

ARS/FSIS COOPERATIVE RESEARCH

In 1988, FSIS and ARS Administrators put into force a Memorandum of Understanding that strengthened and established an official interrelationship between the two agencies to cooperate indefinitely on food safety research efforts. This agreement provides for a continuous exchange of technical information through reports, workshops, seminars, and appointment of FSIS scientific liaisons for the purpose of overseeing ARS research being performed on behalf of FSIS. This arrangement allows FSIS scientific managers knowledgeable about FSIS food safety research priorities related to meat, poultry, and egg products (34) to steer and expand ARS research projects toward the goal of reducing food-borne illnesses associated with meat and poultry. Some recent examples of collaborative efforts include PCR identification of campylobacters (45), predictive modeling work on clostridia (49, 50), competitive exclusion work with poultry (10), and evaluation of the chicken crop as a source of *Salmonella* contamination in broilers (44). Two notable joint projects in progress include methods development for an improved quantitative direct-plating method for detection of *Campylobacter* in poultry (52) and a rapid and sensitive electrochemiluminescence method for detection of *E. coli* O157:H7 in ground beef (19).

A valuable outcome of the ARS/FSIS working relationship has been annual USDA-FSIS/ARS/APHIS Food Safety Research Planning Meetings. During these meetings, ARS scientists present research and FSIS and APHIS scientific liaisons evaluate projects and provide feedback on future directions. ARS food safety research is designed to cover the farm-to-table continuum and has recently been categorized as follows: (i) control of food-borne pathogens in live animals, (ii) pathogen control during slaughter and processing, (iii) post-slaughter pathogen modeling and control, (iv) residue detection and chemical analysis; and (v) new

areas of research (covering fruits and vegetables, animal manure safety, and viruses in shellfish) (4).

Prompted by a 1997 *Campylobacter* research meeting at CDC (see "*Campylobacter* research needs meeting" below) and the importance of and expanded interests in *Campylobacter*, separate *Campylobacter* research meeting sessions were established at the annual food safety research planning meetings, beginning in 1997. *Campylobacter* work presented at the December 1998 USDA-FSIS/ARS/APHIS Food Safety Research Planning Meeting included a new quantitative method for *Campylobacter* spp. in poultry (52) and method developments based on immunochemistry (71), monoclonal antibodies (53), and matrix-assisted laser desorption mass spectroscopy (53). Also noteworthy was preliminary work with a commercial herbal extract, Protecta, which demonstrated significant reductions in the numbers of *Campylobacter, E. coli,* coliforms, and total aerobes in poultry carcasses when added during a simulated processing chill step (14). Work on the USDA/CDC/FDA National Antimicrobial Resistance Monitoring System was presented (23). Antimicrobial testing of *Campylobacter* spp. was added to this program in 1998. FSIS has been submitting *Salmonella* isolates to this program since early 1998 and has recently committed to provide *C. jejuni/coli* isolates. Details of a joint ARS/industry nationwide epidemiological survey of *Campylobacter* and *Salmonella* levels in broiler production facilities were also presented (74). Goals of this in-progress study are (i) the identification of significant sources of these pathogens in the broiler production environment that may result in poultry contamination at the processing plant and (ii) the development of effective on-farm interventions. Optimal molecular and other subtyping systems for *Campylobacter* and *Salmonella* are also being studied.

FSIS BASELINE STUDIES

Beginning in 1992, FSIS conducted a series of Nationwide Microbiological Baseline Data Collection Programs and Surveys. These stud-

TABLE 1 Raw product pathogen prevalence from FSIS national baseline and survey data

Pathogen	Prevalence (% positive) of pathogen on raw product[a]							
	Steer or heifer (24, 2,060)	Cow or bull (26, 2,112)	Ground beef (28, 560)	Market hog (32, 2,112)	Broiler chicken (29, 1297)	Ground chicken (30, 285)	Ground turkey (31, 296)	Young turkey (37, 1221)
Salmonella	1.0	2.7	7.5	8.7	20.0	44.6	49.9	18.6
C. jejuni/coli	4.0	1.1	0.002	31.5	88.2	59.8	25.4	90.3
E. coli O157:H7	0.2	0.0	0.0	0.0	0.0	0.0	0.0	0.0
L. monocytogenes	4.1	11.3	11.7	7.4	15.0	41.1	30.5	5.9
S. aureus	4.2	8.4	30.0	16.0	64.0	90.0	57.3	66.7
C. perfringens	2.6	8.3	53.3	10.4	42.9	50.6	28.1	22.9

[a] Numbers in parentheses are reference number followed by the approximate number of samples analyzed.

ies were designed to estimate the prevalence and levels of bacteria, especially those of public health concern, in raw meat and poultry from establishments operating under federal inspection. Organisms were chosen for study based on involvement in human illness and their value as indicators of general hygiene or process control. Baseline studies or surveys and data analysis have been completed on the following raw products: broiler chickens, ground chicken, turkeys, ground turkey, ground beef, cows and bulls, steers and heifers, and market hogs. In these studies, the prevalence and levels of the following were determined: *Salmonella, E. coli* O157:H7, *C. jejuni/coli, Listeria monocytogenes, Staphylococcus aureus, Clostridium perfringens,* total coliforms, *E. coli* biotype I, and aerobic plate counts. These programs generated microbial profiles of a variety of raw products in the food supply. A summary of FSIS baseline and survey pathogen prevalence data (Table 1) for raw products is available. Baseline and survey data have been essential to the Pathogen Reduction/Hazard Analysis and Critical Control Points (PR/HACCP) regulation (see below) in assisting with hazard identification and assessment of microbial contamination at slaughter, as well as allowing the development of raw-product performance standards and criteria. The data also support pathogen risk assessments and allow for comparisons after pre- and postharvest interventions have been instituted. Furthermore, the data have proven valuable for setting lethality and stabilization performance standards for ready-to-eat products, since they allowed an estimation of worst-case pathogen levels on incoming raw products (39). FSIS is committed to continue to conduct new baseline studies for pathogens to update existing data, support risk assessments, develop new performance standards, and provide information for additional products as warranted.

NATIONAL ADVISORY COMMITTEE ON MICROBIOLOGICAL CRITERIA FOR FOODS

The 1993 National Advisory Committee on Microbiological Criteria for Foods (NACMCF) project, jointly sponsored by USDA, HHS, the Department of Defense, and the Department of Commerce, addressed the issue of food-borne campylobacteriosis. At the request of sponsors, the NACMCF produced a comprehensive review, entitled *Campylobacter jejuni/coli* (57). This publication covered the ecology, epidemiology, and pathogenesis of *C. jejuni/coli,* recommended control strategies, and identified pertinent research needs. Control strategies included pre- and postharvest considerations for poultry, with an emphasis on biosecurity and sanitation/antibacterial treatments, respectively. HACCP was espoused as being important to food production and processing, as well as distribution. The list of research needs outlined in the publication encompassed efforts on the farm, processing-plant controls, and education strategies, as well as epidemiologic and clinical research in humans. This document was useful to FSIS in designing its food safety research agenda (34).

FOOD-BORNE DISEASES ACTIVE SURVEILLANCE NETWORK (FOODNET)

An important public health initiative is the CDC/FDA/FSIS Foodborne Diseases Active Surveillance Network, known as FoodNet (15, 17, 33). This unique collaboration began in July 1995. In 1996, FoodNet included population-based active surveillance for select food-borne pathogens in Minnesota and Oregon, and several counties in California, Connecticut, and Georgia (total population, 15.9 million). In 1998, selected counties in Maryland and New York State were added, and Connecticut went statewide to include a catchment area of 20.5 million persons (based on 1997 estimates). In 1999, data collection expanded to include more counties in New York State, the entire state of Georgia, and selected counties in Tennessee to include approximately 30 million persons (by 1997 estimates).

The components of FoodNet include active laboratory-based surveillance, clinical laboratory surveys, physician surveys, population surveys, and case-control studies. An objective is to actively, rather than passively, gather data in order to identify the incidence of sporadic food-borne illness in the United States and determine the proportion of cases attributable to specific food commodities, e.g., from consumption of meat, poultry, and egg products. In 1997, case-control studies of *E. coli* O157:H7 and *Salmonella* serogroups B and D were started, and these were followed by the addition of a *Campylobacter*-targeted study in 1998.

Data from 1997 showed that reported laboratory-confirmed human bacterial gastroenteritis cases were made up as follows: 46% were campylobacteriosis, 26% were salmonellosis, 15% were shigellosis, 4.0% were *E. coli* O157:H7 infections, 1.6% were yersiniosis, and approximately 1% each were listeriosis and vibrio infections (15). Historically, the FoodNet project represents the first active-surveillance study of sporadic food-borne diseases, compiling data to make national estimates. Moreover, national epidemiological trends are expected to be established more accurately as data accumulate over a number of years, especially as new sites are added. FoodNet data will be used to evaluate the effectiveness of public health control strategies such as the PR/HACCP regulation.

A preliminary assessment of 1998 data shows that the overall incidence rates of laboratory-confirmed infections under surveillance have decreased from 1996 to 1998 (17). Specifically, declines in the numbers of cases of *Salmonella* and *Campylobacter* infections are evident. FSIS-mandated changes in U.S. meat and poultry plants through the PR/HACCP regulations may have contributed to this decrease in food-borne disease.

Data provided by the 1996 FoodNet surveillance program established *Campylobacter* as the most commonly isolated sporadic food-borne pathogen in the United States (33), and this trend continued in 1997 and 1998 (15, 17). Food-borne *Campylobacter* infection results in substantial health care costs and lost productivity for consumers in the United States (13). FoodNet and other influences helped FSIS in its 1997 development of a refocused food safety research agenda to specifically target significant pathogens, including *Campylobacter* (34). Important *Campylobacter*-related topics identified for investigation included broad aspects of incidence attributed to cross-contamination such as food preparation in the kitchen; human sequelae of acute infection, as well as serotypes associated with Guillain-Barré syndrome; the way the organism colonizes animals and humans; intervention techniques and their impact in the food chain, particularly on farms and how this would affect human infections; the best method of subtyping for epidemiological purposes; and the most economical detection methods for foods and clinical testing.

PATHOGEN REDUCTION/HAZARD ANALYSIS AND CRITICAL CONTROL POINTS (PR/HACCP)

A significant food safety advancement was instituted with FSIS development of the

PR/HACCP Systems for federally inspected meat and poultry plants. The new regulation for this program was announced and published in the *Federal Register* in July 1996 (25). HACCP represents the beginnings of the modernization of the USDA meat and poultry inspection system and is a "preventative system" for improved food safety.

HACCP incorporates science-based standards to improve the delivery of safer meat and poultry products to American consumers. All federally inspected slaughter and processing plants will be required to develop and operate under HACCP plans based on the principles articulated by the NACMCF (58). The principles are (i) hazard analysis, (ii) critical control point identification, (iii) establishment of critical limits, (iv) monitoring procedures, (v) corrective actions, (vi) record keeping, and (vii) verification procedures.

HACCP COMPONENTS

In addition to the system of process controls accomplished through a HACCP plan, establishments producing raw meat and poultry products will be required to develop and follow sanitation standard operating procedures (SSOPs), required to perform generic *E. coli* testing and meet performance criteria for *E. coli* levels on carcasses, and required to meet *Salmonella* performance standards.

SSOP requirements will ensure that a comprehensive written plan for plant sanitation exists and that records are being kept to verify that it is consistently being carried out. FSIS designed the PR/HACCP regulations to better address hazards within slaughter and processing plants but recognizes that these measures are only part of a comprehensive food safety strategy that also addresses other points in the farm-to-table continuum. FSIS continues to evaluate and plan for an expanded broad-based approach by also concentrating efforts on hazards arising during transportation and distribution and at the retail level.

Generic *E. coli* testing by slaughter plants is required to verify process controls for fecal contamination on carcasses. Performance criteria for generic *E. coli* were based on data from FSIS national baselines and surveys. Quantitative levels of generic *E. coli* are considered in an assessment of a "moving window" of data. Generic *E. coli* performance criteria have been set so that more than 3 marginal results in the last 13 consecutive results constitute a process control deviation. Repeated failures in meeting acceptable levels of generic *E. coli* or inability to meet *Salmonella* performance standards would necessitate reevaluation of a plant's HACCP plan and corrective actions.

Salmonella performance standards must be below the prevalence of contamination of raw products as determined based on FSIS nationwide baseline and survey data. Separate performance standards apply to each meat species and class of product. The *Salmonella* performance standards are expressed in terms of the maximum number of positive samples permitted in a defined sample set. The sample set sizes are statistically determined and range from 51 samples for broilers to an 82-sample requirement for steers and heifers. The *Salmonella* performance standards that processors must meet under PR/HACCP are shown in Table 2. FSIS raw-product testing verifies compliance with *Salmonella* performance standards.

The *Salmonella* pathogen reduction performance standards complement the process control performance criteria for fecal contamination and generic *E. coli* testing. The FSIS rationale for selecting salmonellae included the fact that they are enteric pathogens and that as a group they cause a large portion of the preventable illnesses associated with meat and poultry (25). Furthermore, the following factors are pertinent: (i) at the time decisions were made, *Salmonella* was considered the most common bacterial cause of food-borne illness (*Campylobacter* has recently been shown to be the most commonly isolated sporadic food-borne pathogen in the United States [15, 17, 33]); (ii) FSIS baseline data show that salmonellae can be found on raw food animal products and occur at frequencies which permit changes to be detected and monitored; (iii) current methods can recover salmonellae from a variety

TABLE 2 PR/HACCP raw-product *Salmonella* performance standards[a]

Class of product	Performance standard (% positive for *Salmonella*)[b]	No. of samples tested	Maximum no. of positives to achieve standard
Steer or heifer carcasses	1.0	82	1
Cow or bull carcasses	2.7	58	2
Ground beef	7.5	53	5
Hog carcasses	8.7	55	6
Fresh pork sausages	NA[c]	NA	NA
Broilers	20.0	51	12
Ground chicken	44.6	53	26
Ground turkey	49.9	53	29
Turkeys	NA	NA	NA

[a] Data from reference 25.

[b] Performance standards are the FSIS calculation of the national prevalence of *Salmonella* on the indicated raw products based on data developed by FSIS in its nationwide microbiological baseline data collection programs and surveys.

[c] NA, not available. Baseline targets for fresh pork sausages and turkeys will be added upon completion of the data analysis for these products.

of meat and poultry products; and (iv) interventions aimed at reducing fecal contamination and other sources of *Salmonella* on raw products should be effective against other pathogens.

FSIS is committed to working with other agencies and the scientific community to improve the scientific basis for establishing food safety performance standards. FSIS intends to revise *Salmonella* performance standards periodically, as new data become available. The Agency anticipates making downward adjustments to performance standards in keeping with progress in pathogen reduction. Other plans include assessing the public health benefits of setting additional pathogen performance standards. A *Campylobacter* performance standard for raw chicken carcasses is currently under consideration (see "Potential HACCP *Campylobacter* performance standard for chickens" below).

PR/HACCP PROGRESS REPORT
The PR/HACCP regulations are being instituted through a phased-in implementation. The requirements for generic *E. coli* testing and SSOPs became effective for all plants on 27 January 1997. Requirements for operation under HACCP and compliance with *Salmonella* performance standards are being phased in based according to plant size as follows: large

plants with 500 employees or more, January 1998; small plants with 10 to 499 employees, January 1999; and very small plants with fewer than 10 employees (or annual sales of less than $2.5 million), January 2000. HACCP plan process controls, in conjunction with microbial testing and SSOPs, have already shown evidence of reduced *Salmonella* contamination of raw meat and poultry in federally inspected plants. Data should be interpreted cautiously, because first-year *Salmonella* HACCP test results for large plants overall are from a subset of the establishments used to calculate the nationally representative *Salmonella* performance standard. However, for poultry, the majority of U.S. production is from large plants, and these have been under HACCP for over 1 year. The currently available data for large plants are presented (Table 3). It is not known how *Salmonella* and *Campylobacter* data correlate, but new studies may provide useful information.

PRESIDENT'S FOOD SAFETY INITIATIVE
On 25 January 1997, President William Jefferson Clinton announced a new public-private initiative for improving the safety of the nation's food supply. As a result, USDA, HHS, and EPA food safety experts joined forces with consumers, industry, and academia to identify

TABLE 3 Prevalence of *Salmonella* in meat and poultry products[a]

Class of product	*Salmonella* performance standard (%)	Post-HACCP implementation *Salmonella* prevalence (%)[b]
Broilers	20.0	10.9 (n^b = 5,697)
Swine carcasses	8.7	6.5 (n = 1,532)
Ground beef	7.5	4.8 (n = 1,184)
Ground turkey	49.9	36.4 (n = 748)

[a] Post-PR/HACCP implementation results from large plants, 1 February 1998 through 25 January 1999 (21). The results reflect testing from products with 10 or more completed sample sets.
[b] n is the number of samples.

critical elements of an effective food safety initiative and to develop strategies for prevention of food-borne disease. The resultant plan from this partnership has evolved into a logical and sound science-based strategy that targets weaknesses in existing systems and emphasizes filling in data gaps related to food-borne illness. Some specific focuses include developing an effective nationwide surveillance and outbreak response capability, increased food safety inspections, expanded food safety research, the use of microbial risk assessment, and expanded food safety training and education. This initiative has proven valuable in steering the allied agencies to concentrate food safety efforts on priority areas. The initiative specifically directs attention to *Campylobacter* as well as other predominant food-borne pathogens, promotes the expansion of FoodNet, and promotes the use of HACCP-based systems of preventative controls in the food industry (81, 83).

CAMPYLOBACTER RESEARCH NEEDS MEETING

In recognition of the need to establish research priorities for *Campylobacter,* OPHS organized an interdisciplinary meeting held at the CDC, Atlanta, Ga., in January 1997 (35). Participants included key *Campylobacter* researchers from the United States (FSIS, ARS, CDC, and FDA) and Canada. This meeting served to reinforce the significance of food-borne *Campylobacter* disease, to identify data gaps, and

to formulate strategies to best address this major public health concern. FSIS management communicated HACCP-related needs to evaluate the effects of process control and interventions on *Campylobacter* prevalence, particularly in poultry (82). It was also recommended that to fully understand the impact and occurrence of *Campylobacter* throughout the farm-to-table continuum, FSIS would have to conduct quantitative risk assessments and evaluate intervention strategies to determine the most cost-effective control and prevention approaches. Immediate FSIS needs expressed were for reliable quantitative methods for detection of *Campylobacter* in meat and poultry, nondestructive sampling methods, and efficacious sample transport protocols.

Technologies suggested as useful to *Campylobacter* detection, enumeration, and characterization included direct-plating techniques, magnetic-bead and/or antibody-based technology, PCR-based screening, flow cytometry, and optimal subtyping systems. Areas identified as essential to *Campylobacter* control included research in poultry preharvest and postharvest interventions, *Campylobacter* biology, and expanding human case-control studies through FoodNet by using broad-based sampling. Risk assessment data gaps were highlighted to include (i) growth modeling, (ii) inactivation modeling to include viable but not yet culturable campylobacters, and (iii) quantitative *Campylobacter* data for poultry from processing to the consumer.

NEW QUANTITATIVE *CAMPYLOBACTER* METHOD

As an outcome of the January 1997 *Campylobacter* Research Needs meeting, the ARS-Poultry Microbiological Safety Research Unit and the FSIS-OPHS, Microbiology Division, Special Projects and Outbreak Support Laboratory, committed to collaborate on an ARS project to develop an improved quantitative direct-plating method for detection and enumeration of *Campylobacter* on poultry carcasses. The protocol has evolved into a direct-plating procedure with a backup enrichment to ensure the detection of campylobacters below the direct-plating detection threshold (52). This procedure uses a blood-free Bolton enrichment broth in vented tissue culture flasks and a new ARS-developed Campy-Line agar in conjunction with use of charged tri-gas (5% O_2, 10% CO_2, 85% N_2) incubators. The agar contains highly selective antibiotics and a triphenyltetrazolium chloride indicator. FSIS collaborative is conducting a trial of this method on poultry carcasses in consideration for its adoption as a standard method and for use in FSIS *Campylobacter* testing programs.

FSIS *CAMPYLOBACTER* TESTING PROGRAMS FOR POULTRY

Responding to *Campylobacter* as a significant public health threat, a heightened awareness of food-borne *Campylobacter* disease, and frameworks such as the President's Food Safety Initiative and the USDA Pathogen Reduction Program, FSIS-OPHS and the FSIS-Office of Policy, Program Development, and Evaluation recently initiated two focused and targeted nationwide *Campylobacter* testing programs for poultry. These nonregulatory programs were set up to collect current information on *C. jejuni/coli* quantitative levels and prevalence in poultry. Data will be informative for future development of policies and regulations within FSIS.

These programs include nondestructive rinse sampling of post-chiller chicken carcasses and overnight shipment of refrigerated rinse samples to one of the three FSIS Technical Service Laboratories (Athens, Ga., St. Louis, Mo., or Alameda, Calif.). Collaborative work with the ARS-Poultry Microbiological Safety Research Unit (73) established that the current FSIS poultry rinse sampling technique for *Salmonella,* using buffered peptone water (36), is acceptable for *Campylobacter* work. A most-probable-number (MPN) method based on the current FSIS MLG *C. jejuni/coli* testing protocol, relying on a Hunt broth enrichment and subsequent plating onto modified *Campylobacter* charcoal differential agar (MCCDA) (64)

is being used as the analytical method in these programs.

CAMPYLOBACTER MONITORING PROGRAM FOR CHICKENS

The FSIS Chicken Monitoring Program for *Campylobacter* began in October 1998. This program will run indefinitely to monitor the presence and levels of *C. jejuni/coli* in all classes of raw whole poultry carcasses processed in plants operating under federal inspection. Poultry plants are sampled randomly; initially, 120 monthly samples are being taken, and future increases are planned.

NEW NATIONWIDE YOUNG CHICKEN *CAMPYLOBACTER* BASELINE DATA COLLECTION PROGRAM

The FSIS Nationwide Young Chicken *Campylobacter* Baseline Data Collection Program began in late January 1999 and is expected to continue for at least 1 year. This program is modeled after the 1994 to 1995 Nationwide Broiler Chicken Microbiological Baseline Data Collection Program (29) and includes all establishments that slaughter young chickens (approximately 205 establishments). Random sampling by establishment and bird will be undertaken. Establishments are selected with probabilities in proportion to the total number of birds slaughtered. It was determined that a sample size of 1,200 would ensure reasonable levels of precision for yearly estimates based on expected *Campylobacter* prevalence. This program was initiated to update the *Campylobacter* prevalence (88.2% [Table 1]) and quantitative data for young chickens that was generated from the July 1994 to June 1995 Nationwide Broiler Chicken Microbiological Baseline Data Collection Program (Table 4).

POTENTIAL HACCP *CAMPYLOBACTER* PERFORMANCE STANDARD FOR CHICKENS

Data generated from the the above-described FSIS Nationwide Young Chicken *Campylobacter* Baseline Data Collection Program may be used to support the development of a

TABLE 4 FSIS nationwide broiler chicken data showing the *C. jejuni/coli* distribution in enumerated positive broiler carcass rinse fluids[a]

Range (MPN/ml)[b]	No. of samples	% of total	Cumulative %
<0.03[c]	153	11.8	11.8
0.03–0.30	75	5.8	17.6
0.301–3.0	145	11.2	28.8
3.01–30.0	422	32.5	61.3
>30.0[d]	502	38.7	100.0
Total	1,297	100.0	

[a] Data from reference 29.
[b] Value multiplied by 400 equals the number of campylobacters detected per 400 ml of carcass rinse sample or per carcass.
[c] Negative by quantitative MPN method.
[d] Maximum level detected = 230,000 MPN/ml.

HACCP performance standard for *C. jejuni/coli* in young chickens. FSIS management is committed to evaluating the concept of a *Campylobacter* performance standard for young chickens, in light of the high incidence of food-borne *Campylobacter* disease and the significant physiological differences between *Salmonella* and *Campylobacter*. FSIS has emphasized the need to address this pathogen and to specifically consider the setting of a *Campylobacter* performance standard (9, 83). Prevalence and quantitative data from the baseline study of young chickens will be used by FSIS scientific and risk managers in determining the feasibility of a *Campylobacter* performance standard for young chickens. Data will address issues such as the usefulness of a standard based on a prevalence figure, like the HACCP *Salmonella* performance standard, or one based on a threshold quantitative level. There is some concern that the seasonality of *Campylobacter* infection in poultry will present difficulties is setting a performance standard based on prevalence. On the other hand, with the limitations in our current knowledge, it would be difficult to make the justification for an "acceptable or safe quantitative level" for raw poultry, making a quantitative risk assessment important. A risk assessment might provide a prediction of the level of reduction of food-borne *Campylobacter* disease that could be afforded by allowing a particular level of the organism to be present on raw poultry. A *Campylobacter* performance standard should encourage specific and effective control measures and thus would have a positive public health effect.

OTHER FOOD SAFETY MEASURES FROM FARM TO TABLE

Pathogen Reduction Tools

Food-borne pathogens exist at multiple entry points throughout the continuum from the farm environment until food reaches the consumer's table. Thus, a multifaceted intervention approach is essential to adequately control contamination. For example, in poultry, the period during which day-old chickens are raised to 6- to 8-week-old broiler chickens must include proper sanitation, biosecurity, vaccinations for contagious diseases, appropriate drug therapy, and biological control procedures aimed at preventing colonization by pathogenic microorganisms (76, 85). New FSIS PR/HACCP and performance standards-based regulations were designed to encourage industry innovations in process controls and in-tervention and control strategies. A combination of pre- and postharvest treatments may be necessary before effective control of pathogens on raw meats and poultry is achieved. Such pathogen reduction tools might include preharvest efforts such as vaccinations, competitive exclusion, and feed and litter treatments. Postharvest activities available today, such as incorporating antimicrobial treatments into processing by use of chlorine, trisodium phosphate, lactic or acetic acid or steam-pasteurizing or vacuuming techniques may become essential to meeting microbiological standards (67).

FSIS continues to evaluate and plan for an expanded, broad-based approach to improving food safety during transportation and storage, through a joint FSIS/FDA effort. In the past the FDA good manufacturing practice regulations have addressed requirements for food handling during transportation and storage. FSIS formerly played a limited regulatory role in handling meat and poultry products outside official establishments.

The basis of many state and local laws is the FDA Food Code. This is a set of model ordinances, developed by FDA (revised in 1997), that include recommendations from the Conference for Food Protection and the Association of Food and Drug Officials. These also address food health inspection of various food service facilities such as grocery stores and restaurants. FSIS collaborates with FDA and encourages implementation of the Food Code nationwide in all jurisdictions. The Department of Transportation has regulations affecting the conditions under which edible products are transported in commerce.

Regulatory Reform Initiatives

FSIS is in the process of a comprehensive reevaluation of meat, poultry, and egg product regulations in an attempt to incorporate science-based preventative measures to enhance safety and reinforce the responsibilities of the processors under the inspection laws (27). The emphasis is to depart from the Agency's traditional "command and control" approach and shift to performance standards-based regulations. The preventative system of process controls created in the PR/HACCP regulations is among the first of these initiatives. In the performance standards concept, the objective level of performance to produce a safe product is provided. It is then the responsibility of the processor to meet the conditions of the performance standard. Built into this is flexibility for the processor in the methods of processing procedures, as long as the performance standard is met. It is the intent of the FSIS that performance standards based regulations will provide an incentive for development of improved processes, provide flexibility for innovation, and allow the industry to more efficiently meet food safety responsibilities. In this regulatory transition, FSIS is transforming and improving food safety regulations to ensure that they are based on performance standards and are consistent with HACCP. Additional goals include the elimination of obsolete and redundant regulations which may have outlived their effectiveness. These efforts are part of the "Rein-vention of Government" initiative, and they are in keeping with national food safety improvement.

FSIS Risk Analysis

OPHS has created the Epidemiology and Risk Assessment Division (ERAD), which is specifically designed to study food-borne illnesses linked to meat, poultry, and egg products. Public health experts rely on risk analysis principles to help guide and enhance the overall decision-making process to support the farm-to-table continuum in safeguarding the public health. This Division complements and works with the USDA Office of Risk Assessment and Cost-Benefit Analysis (ORACBA), which was established by the Federal Crop Insurance Reform and Department of Agriculture Act of 1994.

ERAD scientists participated in a comprehensive risk assessment of *Salmonella enteritidis* that was initiated in December of 1996. This project was developed in response to the increasing reports of human *S. enteritidis* illnesses associated with the consumption of shell eggs. The product of this work was a risk assessment model for *S. enteritidis* in shell eggs (5). A computerized version of this model can be downloaded from the FSIS website on the World Wide Web at http://www.fsis.usda.gov. The model allows simulation of the occurrence of *S. enteritidis* in shell eggs from production through consumption and the effects of possible mitigations.

An in-progress farm-to-table risk assessment for *E. coli* O157:H7 in beef, with a focus on ground beef, was initiated in June 1998 (38). ERAD and other OPHS members serve on the multidisciplinary core risk assessment team. Major goals of this work include a mathematical modeling of human illness caused by *E. coli* O157:H7 in beef in the United States, identification of the occurrence and levels of the organism at points along the farm-to-table continuum and their contribution to human illness, and quantification of the effects of evolving mitigation strategies on decreasing cases of human illness. A final report of this work is anticipated by the end of 1999.

An FSIS risk assessment for food-borne *Campylobacter* disease is being considered. This project is in the planning and formulation stages; the appropriate scope is being determined. Assembly of an expert panel and data collection will further the process. Poultry slaughter and production will be carefully analyzed for this project. Collection of new nationwide baseline quantitative and prevalence data on *Campylobacter* in young chickens is under way (See "FSIS *Campylobacter* testing programs for poultry" above). FSIS recognizes raw pork as a source of *Campylobacter* spp. (Table 1), but the limited association between pork products and human food-borne disease (20, 77, 84) may not warrant inclusion of pork in this first-generation risk assessment. However, pigs may be colonized up to 100% with campylobacters, primarily *C. coli,* and they may serve as a reservoir for other livestock, particularly poultry (84). It is anticipated that risk factors and potential mitigations for *Campylobacter* will be elucidated through a risk assessment. Compiling of the FoodNet *Campylobacter* case-control study data in 1999 will support this work. The *Campylobacter* risk assessment project is considered critical for FSIS to identify the most effective means of controlling this important food-borne disease organism.

FSIS recognizes risk assessment as an integral feature in determining the public health hazards of food-borne pathogens, since this technique was prominent in the framework of its research agenda (34). The interdisciplinary risk reduction approach to devise barriers to introduction and multiplication of pathogens in meat, poultry, and eggs is recognized as essential to the development of cost-effective pathogen control and intervention strategies, which should have positive public health impacts. The technique is also proving critical to food safety, since it identifies research needs and serves to communicate risks to interested parties.

Irradiation

A highly effective and safe pathogen reduction tool available today is the use of irradiation (cold pasteurization) technology (62, 66, 72). The FDA has approved and confirmed the safe use of this technology in poultry and red meats. FSIS determines and proposes regulatory rules for how irradiation can be carried out effectively in FSIS-regulated plants. FSIS subsequently enforces final rules for accurate product labeling and for the way in which this technology is to be applied by federally inspected slaughter and processing facilities. Under the Federal Food, Drug, and Cosmetic Act, sources of radiation are considered "food additives." For this reason, the FDA must first approve irradiation and FSIS must then undertake rule making. FDA does have regulations specific to the National Aeronautics Space Administration space flight program, allowing packaged meat to be irradiated at high doses to sterilize the product (i.e., to destroy all enteric viruses and spores). Currently FSIS recognizes irradiation as an approved additive in the processing of carcasses and fresh or previously frozen cuts of pork for *Trichinella spiralis* control. FSIS also allows the technology to reduce the numbers of pathogenic microorganisms in fresh or frozen uncooked packaged poultry products and mechanically separated poultry. A new FSIS proposed rule expands the use of ionizing radiation for controlling food-borne pathogens in meat and meat by-products of cattle, sheep, swine, goats, and horses (40, 41). It also makes irradiation regulations compatible with HACCP and modifies poultry requirements to be as consistent as allowable by FDA regulations with those for red meat.

Low-dose irradiation (absorbed doses of ionizing energy typically used for reducing but not eliminating all pathogens) is capable of achieving significant reductions in the numbers of many food-borne pathogens of concern including *Campylobacter, Salmonella, E. coli* O157: H7, *L. monocytogenes,* and *S. aureus* (18, 41). Control of parasites such as *Trichinella spiralis* and *Toxoplasma gondii,* as well as of tapeworms, can be achieved. However, enteric viruses and spores of the genera *Clostridium* and *Bacillus* are highly resistant to low levels of ionizing radiation (41, 55, 61).

In addition to USDA-FSIS recognition, endorsements for the use of this powerful food safety technology have come from the World Health Organization, the American Medical Association, the American Veterinary Medical Association, the NACMCF, the Institute of Food Technologists, the American Council on Science, and the Council on Agricultural Science and Technology. Public health officials need to encourage the meat and poultry industry to institute low-dose irradiation technology in order to achieve attributable human health results.

Emergency and Laboratory Response

The Emergency Response Division was created within OPHS to lead and coordinate investigation and tracebacks related to meat and poultry associated with food-borne illnesses and product recall activities. A multidisciplinary team of scientists and technical experts mobilize to form a recall committee in response to reports of food contamination or illness linked to products in commerce. The recall committee evaluates each potential recall situation and recommends Agency action. While recalls are voluntary for industry, FSIS plays a significant role in evaluating and recommending the need for establishments to recall product. FSIS has no regulatory authority to enforce a recall, but it does have the authority to detain or seize adulterated product in commerce. Also, FSIS may withhold or withdraw federal inspection at a plant where products are suspected to pose a public health risk; this would have the effect of shutting down a plant.

Press releases and postings on the World Wide Web at http://www.fsis.usda.gov are used to alert the public about recalls by describing the product, packaging, nature of the potential contamination or illness, or other adulteration or misbranding. The FSIS compliance program performs effectiveness checks to verify that the identified product is removed from wholesale and retail outlets. The program may also detain and prevent further distribution of the suspect product in the unlikely event that a plant should refuse to carry out a recommended voluntary recall. FSIS also performs follow-up testing of in-plant or retail-collected product as appropriate. The CDC has estimated that recalls have a significant effect on the prevention of subsequent additional illnesses and deaths from consumption of adulterated meat, poultry, and egg products that have entered or been distributed in commercial channels (7). Since *Campylobacter* illness is generally sporadic, especially when related to meat and poultry, and is not linked to food vehicles proactively, there have been no FSIS-prompted product recalls due to *Campylobacter* contamination.

In response to food-borne disease incidents, the OPHS Special Projects and Outbreak Support Laboratory performs sample analyses for pathogens and participates in the CDC PulseNet Program. The PulseNet program began in 1995 and is a national network of public health laboratories that maintain an electronic exchange of pulsed-field gel electrophoresis (PFGE) patterns of *E. coli* O157:H7 isolates. The sharing of PFGE patterns through this national database allows timely surveillance and investigation of food-borne illness and provides an early warning of possible multistate outbreaks as DNA fingerprint pattern matches are made. All FSIS laboratories will soon be submitting *Salmonella* PFGE patterns to CDC in an effort to share data. The Special Projects and Outbreak Support Laboratory recently played an important role in performing PFGE on *L. monocytogenes* isolates suspected to be involved in the large multistate outbreak linked to hot dogs and deli meats in late 1998 and early 1999. As of 2 March 1999, CDC reported 97 illnesses and 20 deaths associated with this largest-ever *L. monocytogenes* outbreak linked to ready-to-eat products. CDC reported that the number of illnesses caused by this outbreak decreased after the recall was in place (16).

FSIS Consumer Education

A vital aspect of prevention of food-borne illness is the availability and distribution of food safety risk information to consumers. These communications focus primarily on how to properly handle, prepare, and thoroughly cook meat and poultry products without causing cross-contamination. A recent study suggested that *C. jejuni* organisms can withstand repeated freeze-thawing similar to domestic household handling of poultry products (51) and reinforced the need for updated consumer education. While *C. jejuni* infections are most frequently associated with improper preparation or consumption of mishandled poultry, outbreaks and sporadic cases are also associated with consumption of raw (unpasteurized) milk or unchlorinated water (2, 8). Another vital concern of all public health agencies is educating and encouraging consumers about the significant benefits of frequent hand-washing (65).

FSIS established a Food Safety Education and Communications Staff to most effectively disseminate important food safety information to consumers. FSIS, CDC, and FDA continually produce and update educational pamphlets and brochures for public distribution. Among other initiatives, FSIS participates in the public-private partnership Fight BAC food safety campaign. FSIS also operates a widely publicized Meat and Poultry Hotline, which encourages consumer inquiries nationwide (1-800-535-4555). FSIS continually offers consumer advice through newspapers, television, radio, magazines, and various trade publications. Additionally, updated food safety information for consumers is available on the World Wide Web at http://www.fsis.usda.gov.

CONCLUSION

The nationwide public response to increased reports of epidemics and sporadic cases of foodborne illness has resulted in demands for more efficacious governmental prevention and control measures. As a result, food safety maintains a high profile with our current Administration. The public health agencies responsible for food safety measures include FSIS, HHS (CDC and FDA), and EPA. Significant pathogens such as *Campylobacter* and others present an immense challenge. FSIS and the other public health agencies have individually and jointly accepted

this challenge, and a food safety revolution has been taking place. The Agency is no longer willing to consider any level of pathogen contamination on raw meat and poultry products an unavoidable defect or outcome of processing. This became evident in 1994, when FSIS declared *E. coli* O157:H7 an adulterant in raw ground beef, and with the 1996 landmark PR/HACCP Rule. The current understanding of the epidemiology and control and prevention of *Campylobacter* infections and other foodborne illnesses has been enhanced by (i) management of slaughterhouse operations to minimize contamination of meat and poultry, especially with ingesta and feces; (ii) adoption of the Pathogen Reduction/HACCP system; (iii) increased use and encouragement of available pathogen reduction technology tools in federal meat and poultry plants; (iv) appropriate prompt recall actions for contaminated products; (v) ever-improving active surveillance for food-borne diseases (FoodNet); (vi) ongoing scientific risk analyses and applications; and (vii) repetitive, effective consumer risk communications.

Collaborative, cooperative government efforts (FSIS/CDC/FDA/EPA/ARS/APHIS, etc.), along with prompt recognition and implementation of innovative approaches to food safety by industry, offer the best hope for future advancement of food safety protection on the eve of and during the new millennium.

REFERENCES

1. **Allos, B. M.** 1997. Association between *Campylobacter* infection and Guillain-Barré syndrome. *J. Infect. Dis.* **176:**125–128.
2. **Altekruse, S. F., M. L. Cohen, and D. L. Swerdlow.** 1997. Emerging foodborne diseases. *Emerg. Infect. Dis.* **3:**285–293.
3. **Altekruse, S. F., N. J. Stern, P. I. Fields, and D. L. Swerdlow.** 1999. *Campylobacter jejuni*—an emerging foodborne pathogen. *Emerg. Infect. Dis.* **5:**28–35.
4. **Arnold, J. W., J. F. Robens, and J. A. Lindsay (ed.).** 1998. *1998 Progress Report on Food Safety Research Conducted by ARS.* Agricultural Research Service, U.S. Department of Agriculture, Beltsville, Md.
5. **Baker, A. R., E. D. Ebel, A. T. Hogue, R. M. McDowell, R. A. Morales, W. D. Schlos-**

ser, and R. D. Whiting. 1998. *Salmonella Enteritidis Risk Assessment: Shell Eggs and Egg Products, Final Report.* Food Safety and Inspection Service, U.S. Department of Agriculture, Washington, D.C.

6. **Beers, M. H., and R. Berkow (ed.).** 1999. *The Merck Manual, 17ᵗʰ ed.,* p. 1174–1175. Merck Research Laboratories, Whitehouse Station, N.J.

7. **Bell, B. P., M. Goldoft, P. M. Griffin, M. A. Davis, D. C. Gordon, P. I. Tarr, C. A. Bartleson, J. H. Barrett, J. G. Wells, R. Baron, and J. Kobayashi.** 1994. A multistate outbreak of *Escherichia coli* O157:H7-associated bloody diarrhea and hemolytic uremic syndrome from hamburgers: the Washington experience. *JAMA* **272:**1349–1353.

8. **Benenson, A. S., and J. Chin (ed.).** 1995. *Control of Communicable Diseases Manual, 16ᵗʰ ed.,* p. 74–76. American Public Health Association, Washington, D.C.

9. **Billy, T. J.** 1998. Food Safety and inspection Service, U.S. Department of Agriculture. *The USDA Food Safety Strategy—Improving the Focus on Public Health.* Association of State and Territorial Public Health Laboratory Directors, Breckenridge, Colo.

10. **Blankenship, L. C., J. S. Bailey, N. A. Cox, N. J. Stern, R. Brewer, and O. Williams.** 1993. Two step mucosal competitive exclusion flora treatment to diminish salmonellae in commercial broilers. *Poult. Sci.* **72:**1667–1672.

11. **Blaser, M. J., J. G. Wells, R. A. Feldman, R. A. Pollard, J. R. Allen, and the Collaborative Diarrheal Disease Study Group.** 1983. *Campylobacter* enteritis in the United States: a multicenter study. *Ann. Intern. Med.* **98:**360–365.

12. **Butzler, J.-P., P. Dekeyser, M. Detrain, and F. Dehaen.** 1973. Related vibrio in stools. *J. Pediatr.* **82:**493–495.

13. **Buzby, J. C., and T. Roberts.** 1997. Guillain-Barré syndrome increases foodborne disease costs. *Food Rev.* **20:**36–42.

14. **Cason, J. A.** 1998. Scalding/picking, "Protecta" herbal extracts for chiller water. *In Nineteenth Annual USDA Food Safety Research Planning Meeting.*

15. **Centers for Disease Control and Prevention.** 1998. *1997 Final FoodNet Surveillance Report.* Foodborne Diseases Active Surveillance Network. Centers for Disease Control and Prevention, Atlanta, Ga.

16. **Centers for Disease Control and Prevention.** 1999. *Update: Multistate Outbreak of Listeriosis.* CDC Media Relations Release, 2 March 1999. Centers for Disease Control and Prevention, Atlanta, Ga.

17. **Centers for Disease Control and Prevention.** 1999. Incidence of foodborne illnesses: preliminary data from the Foodborne Diseases Active Surveillance Network (FoodNet)—United States, 1998. *Morbid. Mortal. Weekly Rep.* **48:**189–194.

18. **Charbonneau, D. P. and C. Thibault.** 1994. Effect of ionizing dose rate on the radioresistance of some food pathogenic bacteria. *Can. J. Microbiol.* **40:**369–374.

19. **Crawford, C. G.** 1998. Personal communication. Rapid method for *Escherichia coli* O157:H7 in ground beef. *In Nineteenth Annual USDA Food Safety Research Planning Meeting.*

20. **Davies, P.** 1999. Foodborne pathogens and pork production: what is our Achilles' heel? *Am. Assoc. Swine Pract.* **1:**275–285.

21. **Davis, H.** Unpublished data.

22. **Dekeyser, P., M. Gossuin-Detrain, J. P. Butzler, and J. Sternon.** 1972. Acute enteritis due to related vibrio: first positive stool cultures. *J. Infect. Dis.* **125:**390–392.

23. **Fedorka-Cray, P. J., D. A. Dargatz, N. E. Wineland, M. A. Miller, L. Tollefson, and K. E. Petersen.** 1998, Antimicrobial resistance monitoring program. *In Nineteenth Annual USDA Food Safety Research Planning Meeting.*

24. **Food Safety and Inspection Service, U.S. Department of Agriculture.** 1994. *Nationwide Beef Microbiological Baseline Data Collection Program: Steers and Heifers* (October 1992–September 1993). Food Safety and Inspection Service, U.S. Department of Agriculture, Washington, D.C.

25. **Food Safety and Inspection Service, U.S. Department of Agriculture.** 1996. Pathogen reduction; hazard analysis and critical control point (HACCP) systems; Final Rule. *Fed. Regist.* **61:** 38806–38989.

26. **Food Safety and Inspection Service, U.S. Department of Agriculture.** 1996. *Nationwide Beef Microbiological Baseline Data Collection Program: Cows and Bulls (December 1993–November 1994).* Food Safety and Inspection Service, U.S. Department of Agriculture, Washington, D.C.

27. **Food Safety and Inspection Service, U.S. Department of Agriculture.** 1996. *Reforming the Meat and Poultry Inspection System To Improve Food Safety.* FSIS Backgrounder, March 1996. Food Safety and Inspection Service, U.S. Department of Agriculture, Washington, D.C.

28. **Food Safety and Inspection Service, U.S. Department of Agriculture.** 1996. *Nationwide Federal Plant Raw Ground Beef Microbiological Survey (August 1993–March 1994).* Food Safety and Inspection Service, U.S. Department of Agriculture, Washington, D.C.

29. **Food Safety and Inspection Service, U.S. Department of Agriculture.** 1996. *Nationwide Broiler Chicken Microbiological Baseline Data Collection Program (July 1994–June 1995).* Food Safety

and Inspection Service, U.S. Department of Agriculture, Washington, D.C.

30. **Food Safety and Inspection Service, U.S. Department of Agriculture.** 1996. *Nationwide Raw Ground Chicken Microbiological Survey.* Food Safety and Inspection Service, U.S. Department of Agriculture, Washington, D.C.

31. **Food Safety and Inspection Service, U.S. Department of Agriculture.** 1996. *Nationwide Raw Ground Turkey Microbiological Survey.* Food Safety and Inspection Service, U.S. Department of Agriculture, Washington, D.C.

32. **Food Safety and Inspection Service, U.S. Department of Agriculture.** 1996. *Nationwide Pork Microbiological Baseline Data Collection Program: Market Hogs (April 1995–March 1996).* Food Safety and Inspection Service, U.S. Department of Agriculture, Washington, D.C.

33. **Food Safety and Inspection Service, U.S. Department of Agriculture.** 1997. *FSIS/CDC/ FDA Sentinel Study: the Establishment and Implementation of an Active Surveillance System for Bacterial Foodborne Diseases in the United States.* Report to Congress. Food Safety and Inspection Service, U.S. Department of Agriculture, Washington, D.C.

34. **Food Safety and Inspection Service, U.S. Department of Agriculture.** 1997. *Food Safety Research Agenda, Directions for the Future.* Food Safety and Inspection Service, U.S. Department of Agriculture, Washington, D.C.

35. **Food Safety and Inspection Service, U.S. Department of Agriculture, Office of Public Health and Science, Scientific Research Oversight Staff.** 1997. Summary notes. *Interdisciplinary Meeting on Campylobacter Methods and Research Needs.*

36. **Food Safety and Inspection Service, U.S. Department of Agriculture.** 1997. *Salmonella Analysis, Collecting Raw Meat and Poultry Product Samples.* Food Safety and Inspection Service, U.S. Department of Agriculture, Washington, D.C.

37. **Food Safety and Inspection Service, U.S. Department of Agriculture.** 1998. *Nationwide Young Turkey Microbiological Baseline Data Collection Program (August 1996–July 1997).* Food Safety and Inspection Service, U.S. Department of Agriculture, Washington, D.C.

38. **Food Safety and Inspection Service, U.S. Department of Agriculture.** 1998. *Risk Assessment of E. coli O157:H7 in Beef. Quarterly Progress Report—November 1998.* Food Safety and Inspection Service, U.S. Department of Agriculture, Washington, D.C.

39. **Food Safety and Inspection Service, U.S. Department of Agriculture.** 1999. Performance standards for the production of certain meat and poultry products. Final Rule. *Fed. Regist.* **64:** 732–749.

40. **Food Safety and Inspection Service, U.S. Department of Agriculture.** 1999. USDA issues meat and poultry irradiation proposal. *FSIS Backgrounder. February 1999.* Food Safety and Inspection Service, U.S. Department of Agriculture, Washington, D.C.

41. **Food Safety and Inspection Service, U.S. Department of Agriculture.** 1999. Irradiation of meat and poultry products. Proposed Rule. *Fed. Regist.* **64:**9089–9105.

42. **Franco, D. A.** 1988. *Campylobacter* species: considerations for controlling a foodborne pathogen. *J. Food Prot.* **51:**145–153.

43. **Greenberg, R. N.** 1999. Food-borne illness, p. 77–82. *In* R. E. Rakel (ed.), *Conn's Current Therapy,* The W. B. Saunders Co., Philadelphia, Pa.

44. **Hargis, B. M., D. J. Caldwell, R. L. Brewer, D. E. Corrier, and J. R. Deloach.** 1995. Evaluation of the chicken crop as a source of *Salmonella* contamination for broiler carcasses. *Poult. Sci.* **74:** 1548–1552.

45. **Harmon, K. M., G. M. Ransom, I. V. Wesley.** 1996. Differentiation of *Campylobacter jejuni* and *Campylobacter coli* by multiplex polymerase chain reaction. *Mol. Cell. Probes* **11:**195–200.

46. **Hollingsworth, J. and B. Kaplan.** 1998. Food safety in the United States, p. 109–118. *In* J. B. Kaper and A. D. O'Brien (ed.), *Escherichia coli O157:H7 and other Shiga Toxin-Producing E. coli Strains.* American Society for Microbiology, Washington, D.C.

47. **James, W., and B. Kaplan.** 1998. Poultry farm study probes sources of *Campylobacter. J. Am. Vet. Med. Assoc.* **212:**164.

48. **Johnston, R. W.** *Campylobacter and the Safety of Meat and Poultry.* Personal communication. Memorandum of screening and surveillance, vol. III part 4, p. 5–8. Food Safety and Inspection Service, U.S. Department of Agriculture, Washington, D.C.

49. **Juneja, V. K., and H. M. Marks.** Proteolytic *Clostridium botulinum* growth at 12 to 48°C simulating the cooling of cooked meat: development of a predictive model. *J. Food Microbiol.* in press.

50. **Juneja, V. K., R. C. Whiting, H. M. Marks, and O. P. Snyder.** Predictive model for the growth of *Clostridium perfringens* at temperatures applicable to the cooling of cooked meat. *J. Food Microbiol.,* in press.

51. **Lee, A., S. C. Smith, and P. J. Coloe.** 1998. Survival and growth of *Campylobacter jejuni* after artificial inoculation onto chicken skin as a function of temperature and packaging condition. *J. Food Prot.* **66:**1609–1614.

52. **Line, J. E.** 1998. Cultural detection and quantification of *Campylobacter*. *In Nineteenth Annual USDA Food Safety Research Planning Meeting*.

53. **Mandrell, R.** 1998. Mab and mass spectroscopy. *In Nineteenth Annual USDA Food Safety Research Planning Meeting*.

54. **McNamara, A. M.** 1994. The Microbiology Division's perspective on *Listeria monocytogenes, Escherichia coli* O157:H7, and *Campylobacter jejuni/coli. Dairy Food Environ. Sanit.* **14:**259–261.

55. **Monk, J. D., L. R. Reuchat, and M. P. Doyle.** 1995. Irradiation inactivation of food-borne microorganisms. *J. Food Prot.* **58:**197–208.

56. **Nachamkin, I., B. M. Allos, and T. Ho.** 1998. *Campylobacter* species and Guillain-Barré syndrome. *Clin. Microbiol. Rev.* **11:**555–567.

57. **National Advisory Committee on Microbiological Criteria for Foods.** 1994. *Campylobacter jejuni/coli. J. Food Prot.* **57:**1101–1121.

58. **National Advisory Committee on Microbiological Criteria for Foods.** 1997. Generic HACCP application in broiler slaughter and processing. *J. Food Prot.* **60:**579–604.

59. **Norcross, M. A., R. W. Johnston, and J. L. Brown.** 1992. Importance of *Campylobacter* spp. to the food industry, p. 61–65. *In* I. Nachamkin, M. J. Blaser, and L. S. Tompkins (ed.), *Campylobacter jejuni: Current Status and Future Trends*. American Society for Microbiology, Washington, D.C.

60. **Okrend, A. J.** 1999. Personal communication.

61. **Osterholm, M. T. and M. E. Potter.** 1997. Irradiation pasteurization of solid foods: taking food safety to the next level. *Emerg. Infect. Dis.* **3:**1–4.

62. **Patterson, M. F.** 1995. Sensitivity of *Campylobacter* spp. to irradiation in poultry meat. *Lett. Appl. Microbiol.* **20:**338–340.

63. **Ransom, G. M., and B. E. Rose.** 1992. *FSIS Method for the Isolation, Identification, and Enumeration of Campylobacter jejuni/coli from Meat and Poultry Products*. Laboratory communication 69. U. S. Department of Agriculture, Food Safety Inspection Service, Microbiology Division, Washington, D.C.

64. **Ransom, G. M. and B. E. Rose.** 1998. FSIS method for the isolation, identification, and enumeration of *Campylobacter jejuni/coli* from meat and poultry products, p. 6.1–6.10. *In* B. P. Dey and C. P. Lattuada (ed.), *U.S. Department of Agriculture, Food Safety Inspection Service, Microbiology Division, Microbiology Laboratory Guidebook, 3rd ed.* Government Printing Office, Pittsburgh, Pa.

65. **Reed, C. R., and B. Kaplan.** 1996. Neglected but commonsense steps to prevent foodborne illness. *J. Am. Vet. Med. Assoc.* **209:**1053.

66. **Reed, C. R., and B. Kaplan.** 1996. A useful food safety tool: irradiation technology. *J. Am. Vet. Med. Assoc.* **209:**1785.

67. **Reed, C. R., and B. Kaplan.** 1997. Prevention is best against foodborne illness. *J. Am. Vet. Med. Assoc.* **210:**316.

68. **Riley, L. W., and M. J. Finch.** 1985. Results of the first year of national surveillance of *Campylobacter* infections in the United States. *J. Infect. Dis.* **151:**956–959.

69. **Skirrow, M. B.** 1977. *Campylobacter* enteritis: a "new" disease. *Br. Med. J.* **2:**9–11.

70. **Smith, K. E., J. M. Besser, C. W. Hedberg, F. T. Leano, J. B. Bender, J. H. Wicklund, B. P. Johnson, K. A. Moore, M. T. Osterholm, and the Investigation Team.** 1999. Quinolone-resistant *Campylobacter jejuni* infections in Minnesota, 1992–1998. *N. Engl. J. Med.* **20:**1525–1532.

71. **Stanker, L.** 1998. Immunochemical methods for bacterial detection. *In Nineteenth Annual USDA Food Safety Research Planning Meeting*.

72. **Steel, J. H. and R. E. Engel.** 1992. Radiation processing of foods. *J. Am. Vet. Med. Assoc.* **201:**1522–1529.

73. **Stern, N. J.** Unpublished data.

74. **Stern, N. J., J. S. Bailey, N. A. Cox, S. E. Craven, P. F. Cray, and R. J. Meinersmann.** 1998. Flow of *Campylobacter* and *Salmonella* through poultry operations to the processed carcass: overview and status. *In Nineteenth Annual USDA Food Safety Research Planning Meeting*.

75. **Stern, N. J., S. S. Green, N. Thaker, D. J. Krout, and J. Chiu.** 1984. Recovery of *Campylobacter jejuni* from fresh and frozen meat and poultry collected at slaughter. *J. Food Prot.* **47:**372–374.

76. **Stern, N. J., and R. B. Russel.** 1994. Control of *Campylobacter jejuni* in poultry. *WHO/CDS/VPH* **135:**121–131.

77. **Tauxe, R. V.** 1992. Epidemiology of *Campylobacter jejuni* infections in the United States and other industrialized nations, p. 9–19. *In* I. Nachamkin, M. J. Blaser, and L. S. Tompkins (ed.), *Campylobacter jejuni: Current Status and Future Trends*. American Society for Microbiology, Washington, D.C.

78. **Tauxe, R. V.** 1997. Personal communication. *In Interdisciplinary Meeting on Campylobacter Methods and Research Needs*.

79. **Tauxe, R. V., N. Hargrett-Bean, C. M. Patton, and I. K. Wachsmuth.** 1988. *Campylobacter* isolates in the United States, 1982–1986. CDC Surveillance Summaries, June 1988. *Morbid. Mortal Weekly Rep.* **37**(SS-2):1–13.

80. **Taylor, D. N.** 1992. *Campylobacter* infections in developing countries, p. 20–30. *In* I. Nachamkin, M. J. Blaser, and L. S. Tompkins (ed.), *Campylobacter jejuni: Current Status and Future Trends*.

American Society for Microbiology, Washington, D.C.

81. **U. S. Department of Agriculture, Department of Health and Human Services, and U. S. Environmental Protection Agency.** 1997. *Food Safety from Farm to Table: a New Strategy for the 21st Century.* Discussion draft and current thinking on a national food safety initiative. USDA and U. S. EPA, Washington, D.C.

82. **Wachsmuth, I. K.** 1997. Personal communication. *In Interdisciplinary Meeting on Campylobacter Methods and Research Needs.*

83. **Wachsmuth, I. K.** 1998. The relevance and role of microbial data in implementing the national food safety initiative. *In The National Food Safety Initiative Conference: Implications for Microbial Data Collection, Analysis, and Application, International Life Sciences Institute.*

84. **Wesley, I.** 1998. Overview. Public health significance of *Campylobacter* in livestock and poultry, p. 216–234. *In Proceedings of the One Hundred and Second Annual Meeting of the United States Animal Health Association.*

85. **White, P. L., A. R. Baker, and W. O. James.** 1997. Strategies to control *Salmonella* and *Campylobacter* in raw poultry products. *Rev. Sci. Tech. O.I.E.* **16:**525–541.

A NATIONAL MOLECULAR SUBTYPING NETWORK FOR FOOD-BORNE BACTERIAL DISEASE SURVEILLANCE IN THE UNITED STATES

*Bala Swaminathan, Timothy J. Barrett, and the CDC PulseNet Task Force**

28

Molecular subtyping (typing of bacterial isolates by characterization of proteins or nucleic acids) has been successfully applied to aid epidemiologic investigations of food-borne disease outbreaks since the initial use of plasmid fingerprinting nearly 20 years ago (6, 7). Since that time, several methods for identifying restriction fragment length polymorphisms on chromosomal DNA have been developed and molecular subtyping has become an essential component of epidemiologic investigations of infectious diseases (1, 10, 11, 19, 20).

Because molecular subtyping does not require specialized reagents or high levels of specialized training, many more laboratories have become involved in this method of typing bacterial isolates (18). Unfortunately, this widespread use of molecular typing has resulted in a plethora of techniques and protocols for subtyping even the same species of bacteria. Further, because each laboratory uses its own protocols for molecular typing and customized designations of patterns, the results cannot be compared with those of another laboratory, even if both laboratories have used essentially the same methods. This has greatly diminished the power of molecular subtyping methods.

In 1993, during the investigation of an *Escherichia coli* O157:H7 outbreak caused by contaminated hamburgers served in a regional fast-food restaurant in the western United States, Barrett et al. (3) used pulsed-field gel electrophoresis (PFGE) to characterize clinical and food isolates of *E. coli* O157:H7 and demonstrated its utility in outbreak investigations. When a paper describing this application of PFGE was published, our laboratory started receiving numerous requests from state health departments for subtyping *E. coli* O157:H7. Although we attempted to comply with these requests as rapidly as possible, it often took several weeks for completion of subtyping of isolates. Therefore, the results were mostly useful only for providing laboratory confirmation of the conclusions deduced from epidemiologic investigations several weeks after the investigations were complete and the outbreaks were over.

We reasoned that decentralization of subtyping activities and transfer of standardized molecular subtyping methodology to public

*Bala Swaminathan, Timothy J. Barrett, and the CDC PulseNet Task Force, Foodborne and Diarrheal Diseases Branch, Division of Bacterial and Mycotic Diseases, National Center for Infectious Diseases, Centers for Disease Control and Prevention, Atlanta, GA 30333.
*In addition to the authors, the CDC PulseNet Task Force includes Daniel Cameron, Wallis DeWitt, Mary Ann Lambert-Fair, Lewis Graves, Peggy Hayes, Susan Hunter, Susan Maslanka, Loretta McCroskey, Jeremy Miller, Efrain Ribot, and Susan Van Duyne.

Campylobacter, 2nd Ed., Edited by I. Nachamkin and M. J. Blaser
© 2000 American Society for Microbiology, Washington, D.C.

health laboratories should enable more timely subtyping of clinical and food isolates and that the information would be more useful to epidemiologists while they were investigating outbreaks. Also, we thought that routine subtyping of isolates of food-borne pathogenic bacteria received by public health laboratories would lead to identification of outbreaks not readily recognizable by other means. Use of standardized subtyping methods would allow the comparison of isolates from different parts of the country, thus enabling the recognition of nationwide outbreaks attributable to a common source of infection, particularly those in which cases are geographically separated.

In 1995, the Centers for Disease Control and Prevention (CDC), with the assistance of the Association of Public Health Laboratories, an organization that represents public health laboratories in the United States, selected the state public health laboratories in Massachusetts, Minnesota, Washington, and Texas as Area Laboratories for PulseNet. Standardized PFGE typing and pattern analysis technology would be transferred to the Area Laboratories, which would assume responsibility for subtyping food-borne pathogenic bacteria from their states and for providing the subtyping service to neighboring states that requested assistance. At about the same time, CDC, as part of its response to emerging infectious–disease threats (2), began implementing a food-borne disease active-surveillance program called FoodNet. The objectives of FoodNet were to accurately estimate the burden of food-borne disease in the United States, investigate the sources of infection in outbreaks and sporadic cases, and build public health infrastructure for dealing with issues involving emerging food-borne disease. Participants in FoodNet immediately recognized the advantages offered by participation in PulseNet, and several obtained funding to participate in PulseNet. The first 5-day workshop on standardized methods for PFGE for food-borne pathogenic bacteria was held at CDC in January 1996 and was attended by laboratory personnel from the PulseNet Area Laboratories, the USDA-FSIS Laboratory, and three state public health laboratories that were participating in FoodNet. Later, with funds from the CDCs epidemiology and laboratory capacity (building) initiative under the emerging-infections program (2) and with funds from states and other nonfederal sources, several additional state and local public health laboratories were able to join PulseNet. At present, PulseNet includes 32 state public health laboratories and the public health laboratories in New York City, N.Y., and Los Angeles County, Calif. (Fig. 1).

We spent much of 1996 in evaluating the standard protocol for *E. coli* O157:H7. A set of 50 *E. coli* O157:H7 strains was assembled to evaluate how well the standardized methodology worked. This set of strains (the reproducibility evaluation set) was sent to the laboratories that had completed the CDC training. The laboratories were asked to type the strains by the standardized methods and return the raw electronic images of the PFGE patterns to CDC for analysis. Analysis of the data from the reproducibility study showed that when a highly standardized protocol is followed by participating laboratories, the results are highly reproducible and that it is possible to compare DNA patterns generated at different laboratories.

STANDARDIZED EQUIPMENT FOR LABORATORIES PARTICIPATING IN PULSENET

PulseNet laboratories use CHEF-DRII, CHEF-DRIII, or CHEF-Mapper (Bio-Rad Laboratories, Hercules, Calif.) for PFGE of restricted bacterial DNA. Although any of the three instruments will be able to run current PulseNet protocols, CHEF-Mapper allows greater flexibility in the development of electrophoretic separation conditions and nonlinear ramping. After electrophoresis, the gels are stained with ethidium bromide and the PFGE patterns are digitized in a TIFF format (uncompressed .tif file) by using a GelDoc 1000 or other image acquisition equipment capable of 768 by 640 or higher pixel resolution and creating an uncompressed TIFF file. Molecular Analyst Fingerprinting Plus with Data Sharing

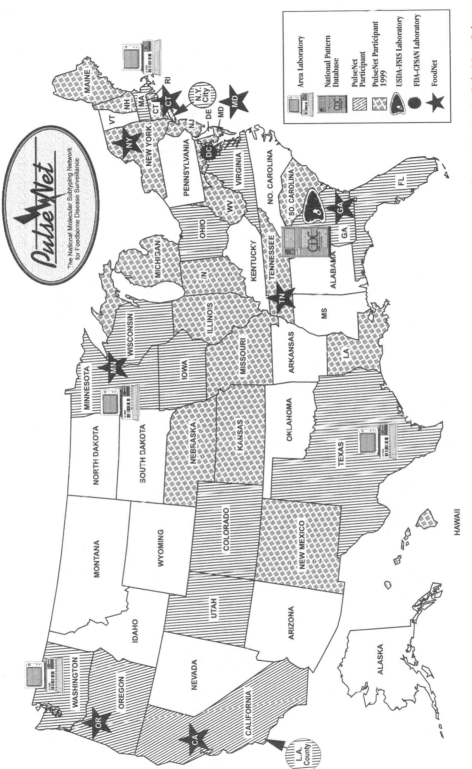
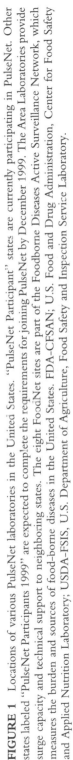

FIGURE 1 Locations of various PulseNet laboratories in the United States. "PulseNet Participant" states are currently participating in PulseNet. Other states labeled "PulseNet Participants 1999" are expected to complete the requirements for joining PulseNet by December 1999. The Area Laboratories provide surge capacity and technical support to neighboring states. The eight FoodNet sites are part of the Foodborne Diseases Active Surveillance Network, which measures the burden and sources of food-borne diseases in the United States. FDA-CFSAN; U.S. Food and Drug Administration, Center for Food Safety and Applied Nutrition Laboratory; USDA-FSIS, U.S. Department of Agriculture, Food Safety and Inspection Service Laboratory.

Tools (DST version; Bio-Rad Laboratories [sold as GelCompar in Europe]) is the software used by PulseNet laboratories for analysis of PFGE patterns. Each PulseNet laboratory has all of the above equipment and has the capability to normalize the patterns, compare them to other patterns, and maintain local databases of PFGE patterns for each bacterial pathogen of interest.

NATIONAL DATABASE OF PFGE PATTERNS AND ASSOCIATED EPIDEMIOLOGIC INFORMATION

At CDC, we are building national databases of PFGE patterns for each food-borne bacterial pathogen beginning with *E. coli* O157:H7. These databases reside on a PulseNet server at CDC. For each bacterial pathogen, there is a normalized PFGE pattern database and a separate database of epidemiologic and clinical information for isolates that are associated with each normalized PFGE pattern. One isolate may be associated with more than one PFGE pattern in the database because PulseNet protocols may call for the use of more than one restriction enzyme to achieve appropriate discrimination between epidemiologically unrelated isolates. The *E. coli* O157:H7 database is currently functional; databases for nontyphoidal *Salmonella* serotypes and *Listeria monocytogenes* are under construction.

At present, seven PulseNet laboratories (the four Area Laboratories, FDA-CFSAN, USDA-FSIS, and CDC) have direct access to the PulseNet database server. These laboratories are able to directly access the CDC PulseNet server through the Internet and submit normalized PFGE patterns (the DST version of the Molecular Analyst software creates special "bundle" files for comparison with the national database) and associated epidemiologic information. These laboratories are able to query the national database for identical matches or closely related patterns (>95% related under specified conditions) to the submitted patterns. If identical or close matches to the submitted patterns are found, the submitter is able to access epidemiologic information asso-

ciated with that patterns from the text database. The PulseNet server will be programmed to automatically issue e-mail alerts of possible multisite food-borne disease outbreaks to all PulseNet laboratories if two or more PulseNet laboratories submit identical or closely related patterns within a prespecified time period.

PulseNet laboratories that do not presently have direct access to the PulseNet server may electronically submit normalized PFGE patterns (bundle files) or raw TIFF images to the CDC PulseNet Database Administration Team by e-mail or through file transfer protocols (ftp). The PulseNet Database Administration Team will compare the submitted patterns to the national database and send the results by e-mail to the submitter as quickly as possible. We expect to provide direct access to the CDC PulseNet server to 23 more laboratories by the end of 1999.

STEPS IN DEVELOPING A STANDARDIZED PROTOCOL

Currently, PulseNet standardized PFGE protocols have been developed for *E. coli* O157:H7, *Salmonella typhimurium* (the same protocol is applicable to most other nontyphoidal *Salmonella* serotypes, and *Listeria monocytogenes*. Standard PFGE protocols for *Shigella* spp. and *Clostridium perfringens* are under development and validation. All PulseNet protocols are 1-day protocols and are based on the 1-day PFGE protocol developed by the Washington State Public Health Laboratory (a PulseNet Area Laboratory) in response to the identification of a need for such an accelerated method at the first PulseNet update meeting held at CDC in 1997 (4). All protocols undergo initial evaluation at the developing laboratory, a second evaluation at CDC, α-testing at one or two PulseNet laboratories, and β-testing at several PulseNet laboratories before they are adopted as official PulseNet protocols. Evaluation criteria include reproducibility of patterns, appropriateness of the strain used as the reference standard for normalization of DNA fragment patterns of unknowns, and robustness of the procedure. Once a protocol is officially adopted as the standard PulseNet protocol, no changes can be made to it except by a petition to the PulseNet Task Force, discussion of the proposed changes, and adoption of the proposal by PulseNet laboratories.

QUALITY ASSURANCE/QUALITY CONTROL PROGRAM FOR PULSENET LABORATORIES

A quality assurance/quality control (QA/QC) program has been instituted for the PulseNet Project to ensure the quality and integrity of the results obtained by the standardized PFGE techniques used to subtype food-borne bacterial pathogens by the PulseNet-affiliated laboratories. This program consists of (i) training standards, (ii) a set of standardized protocols, (iii) an initial certification set for each organism, and (iv) an ongoing proficiency-testing program. Two documents have been prepared that describe the QA/QC Program, a QA/QC manual and a Proficiency Testing manual. As laboratories join PulseNet, they are sent the standardized protocols and certification sets appropriate to the organism(s) being tested. Appropriate training is scheduled, and follow-up is provided via the certification sets and a regularly scheduled proficiency-testing program.

PRIORITY ORDER FOR DEVELOPING PULSENET SUBTYPING PROTOCOLS AND NATIONAL DATABASE OF SUBTYPE PATTERNS FOR FOOD-BORNE PATHOGENIC BACTERIA

A priority order has been developed for inclusion of food-borne bacterial pathogens in PulseNet (Table 1). The prioritization takes into account the availability of an acceptable molecular subtyping method for a pathogen, the severity of the disease caused by that pathogen, the propensity for the pathogen to cause outbreaks, and the potential for recognizing outbreaks by routine subtyping and taking corrective action. *Campylobacter jejuni* and *C. coli* are scheduled to be added to PulseNet in 2000.

UTILITY OF ROUTINE SUBTYPING OF *CAMPYLOBACTER*

Perhaps due to the high diversity of *C. jejuni/coli* subtypes, routine subtyping of these

TABLE 1 Priority order for inclusion of food-borne bacterial pathogens in PulseNet

Pathogen	Expected yr of inclusion in PulseNet
Escherichia coli O157:H7	1997
Nontyphoidal *Salmonella* serotypes[a]	1998
Listeria monocytogenes	1999
Shigella sonnei	1999
Clostridium perfringens	2000
Campylobacter jejuni/coli	2000
Vibrio cholerae	2000
Vibrio parahaemolyticus	2000
Other pathogenic *E. coli*	2001
Salmonella enteritidis	2001

[a] Excluding *Salmonella enteritidis*. At this time, no satisfactory molecular subtyping method is available for this highly clonal serotype.

species has not proven useful in detecting outbreaks or in associating particular subtypes with likely animal origins. Subtypes of *C. jejuni* from apparently sporadic cases are highly diverse (13). Although *C. jejuni* has been the most commonly isolated enteric pathogen in England and Wales since 1981, outbreaks of *C. jejuni* infection have rarely been detected (15). Outbreaks have also been infrequently reported to CDC (unpublished data). The reasons for this paradox are uncertain. While it is likely that most diarrheal disease caused by *C. jejuni* is truly sporadic, it may also be true that clusters of infection are not being recognized due to the diversity of subtypes contaminating a food product. Multiple subtypes have been reported in broiler flocks (14), in red meats and poultry (9), and variety of environmental sources in broiler production facilities (17). There are also reports indicating a lack of stability in *C. jejuni* subtypes (12, 21). It thus seems likely that persons whose infections actually came from the same source could have different subtypes identified in their stools. Considering the sporadic nature of *C. jejuni* infections and the potential diversity of subtypes, *Campylobacter* was not considered a high priority for development of a national database of subtype patterns and is not among the organisms currently covered by PulseNet.

OUTBREAK INVESTIGATIONS

Although it may not be useful to routinely sub-type clinical isolates of *C. jejuni* and *C. coli*, epidemiologic investigations of *Campylobacter* outbreaks can be greatly facilitated by subtyping, since sporadic *Campylobacter* infections are typically occurring at the same time as the outbreaks and it is helpful to know which infections are likely to be related. Serotyping can be useful if the outbreak strain is not one of the common serotypes (16), but often a more discriminating method is needed. We have found both PFGE and *flaA* gene typing to be useful in outbreak investigations (unpublished data), and others have reported the use of RAPD (random amplified polymorphic DNA) (5) and restriction endonuclease analysis (8). Given the high level of diversity of *Campylobacter* subtypes, the choice of a subtyping method for outbreak investigations does not appear to be critical.

REFERENCES

1. **Ackers, M. L., B. E. Mahon, E. Leahy, B. Goode, T. Damrow, P. S. Hayes, W. F. Bibb, D. H. Rice, T. J. Barrett, L. Hutwagner, P. M. Griffin, and L. Slutsker.** 1998. An outbreak of *Escherichia coli* O157:H7 infections associated with leaf lettuce consumption. *J. Infect. Dis.* **177:**1588–1593.

2. **Anonymous.** *Preventing Emerging Infectious Diseases: a Strategy for the 21st Century. Overview of the Updated CDC Plan.*

3. **Barrett, T. J., H. Lior, J. H. Green, R. Khakhria, J. G. Wells, P. Bell, K. D. Greene, J. Lewis, and P. M. Griffin.** 1994. Laboratory investigation of a multi-state food-borne outbreak of *Escherichia coli* O157:H7 by using pulsed-field gel electrophoresis and phage typing. *J. Clin. Microbiol.* **32:**3013–3017.

4. **Gautom, R. K.** 1997. Rapid pulsed-field gel electrophoresis protocol for *E. coli* O157:H7 and other gram-negative organisms in one day. *J. Clin. Microbiol.* **35:**2977–2890.

5. **Hilton, A. C., D. Mortiboy, J. G. Banks, and C. W. Penn.** 1997. RAPD analysis of environmental, food, and clinical isolates of *Campylobacter* spp. *FEMS Immunol. Med. Microbiol.* **18:**119–124.

6. **Holmberg, S. D., I. K. Wachsmuth, F. W. Hickman-Brenner, and M. L. Cohen.** 1984. Comparison of plasmid profile analysis, phage typing, and antimicrobial susceptibility testing in characterizing *Salmonella typhimurium* isolates from outbreaks. *J. Clin. Microbiol.* **19:**100–104.

7. **Holmberg, S. D., and K. Wachsmuth.** 1989. Plasmid and chromosomal DNA analyses in the epidemiology of bacterial diseases, p. 105–129. *In* B. Swaminathan and G. Prakash (ed.), *Nucleic Acid and Monoclonal Antibody Probes: Applications in Diagnostic Microbiology*. Marcel Dekker, Inc., New York, N.Y.

8. **Jimenez, A., J. Barros-Velazquez, J. Rodriguez, and T. G. Villa.** 1997. Restriction endonuclease analysis, DNA relatedness and phenotypic characterization of *Campylobacter jejuni* and *Campylobacter coli* isolates involved in food-borne disease. *J. Appl. Microbiol.* **82:**713–721.

9. **Madden, R. H., L. Moran, and P. Scates.** 1998. Frequency of occurrence of *Campylobacter* ssp. in red meats and poultry in Northern Ireland and their subsequent subtyping using polymerase chain reaction-restriction fragment length polymorphism and the random amplified polymorphic DNA method. *J. Appl. Microbiol.* **84:**703–708.

10. **Muramatsu, K.** 1999. Comparison of epidemiological markers for *Vibrio parahaemolyticus* isolated from food poisoning. *Kansenshogaku Zasshi* **73:**179–186. (In Japanese.)

11. **Nakama, A., M. Matsuda, T. Itoh, and C. Kaneuchi.** 1998. Molecular typing of Listeria monocytogenes isolated in Japan by pulsed-field gel electrophoresis. *J. Vet. Med. Sci.* **60:**749–752.

12. **On, S. L.** 1998. In vitro genotypic variation of *Campylobacter coli* documented by pulsed-field gel electrophoretic DNA profiling: implications for epidemiological studies. *FEMS Microbiol. Lett.* **165:**341–346.

13. **Owen, R. J., E. Slater, D. Telford, T. Donovan, and M. Barnham.** 1997. Subtypes of *Campylobacter jejuni* from sporadic cases of diarrhoeal disease at different locations in England are highly diverse. *Eur. J. Epidemiol.* **13:**837–840.

14. **Payne, R. E., M. D. Lee, D. W. Dreesen, and H. M. Barnhart.** 1999. Molecular epidemiology of *Campylobacter jejuni* in broiler flocks using random amplified polymorphic DNA-PCR and 23S rRNA-PCR and role of litter in its transmission. *Appl. Environ. Microbiol.* **65:**260–263.

15. **Pebody, R. G., M. J. Ryan, and P. G. Wall.** 1997. Outbreaks of *Campylobacter* infection: rare events for a common pathogen. *Commun. Dis. Rep.* CDR *Rev.* **7:**R33–R37.

16. **Roels, T. H., B. Wickus, H. H. Bostrom, J. J. Kazmierczak, M. A. Nicholson, T. A. Kurzynski, and J. P. Davis.** 1998. A foodborne outbreak of *Campylobacter jejuni* (O:33) infection associated with tuna salad: a rare strain in an unusual vehicle. *Epidemiol. Infect.* **121:**281–287.

17. **Stern, N. J., M. A. Myszewski, H. M. Barn-**

hart, and D. W. Dreesen. 1997. Flagellin A gene restriction fragment length polymorphism patterns of *Campylobacter* spp. isolates from broiler production series. *Avian Dis.* **41:**899–905.

18. **Swaminathan, B., and G. M. Matar.** 1993. Molecular typing methods, p. 26–50. *In* D. H. Persing, T. F. Smith, F. C. Tenover, and T. J. White (ed.), *Diagnostic Molecular Microbiology: Principles and Applications.* American Society for Microbiology, Washington, D.C.

19. **Threlfall, E. J., L. R. Ward, M. D. Hampton, A. M. Ridley, B. Rowe, D. Roberts, R. J. Gilbert, P. Van Someren, P. G. Wall, and P.**

Grimont. 1998. Molecular fingerprinting defines a strain of *Salmonella enterica* serotype Anatum responsible for an international outbreak associated with formula-dried milk. *Epidemiol. Infect.* **121:** 289–293.

20. **Wachsmuth, K.** 1986. Molecular epidemiology of bacterial infections: examples of methodology and of investigations of outbreaks. *Rev. Infect. Dis.* **8:**682–692.

21. **Wassenaar, T. M., B. Geilhausen, and D. G. Newell.** 1998. Evidence of genetic instability in *Campylobacter jejuni* isolated from poultry. *Appl. Environ. Microbiol.* **64:**1816–1821.

INDEX